UVEITIS

SECOND EDITION

DEDICATION

To my patients past and present, and their families for their courage and dedication.

UVEITIS

SECOND EDITION

NICHOLAS JONES FRCOphth
Director, Uveitis Service
Consultant Ophthalmic Surgeon
Manchester Royal Eye Hospital, UK
Honorary Senior Lecturer in Ophthalmology
University of Manchester, Manchester, UK

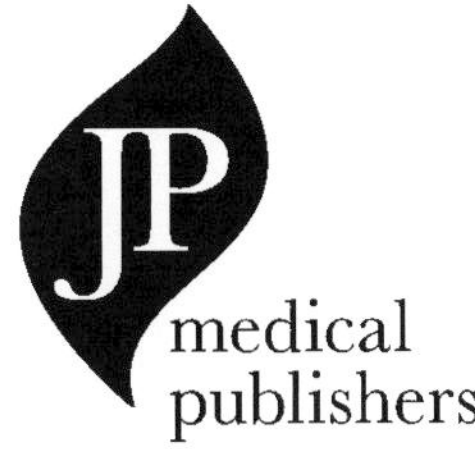

London • Panama City • New Delhi

Published by JP Medical Ltd, 83 Victoria Street, London, SW1H 0HW, UK
Tel: +44 (0)20 3170 8910 Fax: +44 (0)20 3008 6180
Email: info@jpmedpub.com Web: www.jpmedpub.com

ISBN: 978-1-907816-18-5

British Library Cataloguing in Publication Data
A catalogue record for this book is available from the British Library

Library of Congress Cataloging in Publication Data
A catalog record for this book is available from the Library of Congress

JP Medical Ltd is a subsidiary of Jaypee Brothers Medical Publishers (P) Ltd, New Delhi, India.

Publisher:	Richard Furn
Senior Editorial Assistant	Katrina Rimmer
Design:	Designers Collective Ltd

Typeset, printed and bound in India.

Foreword

The field of uveitis research and treatment has grown immensely, in part due to recent advances in molecular and immunological investigation and imaging techniques and to the introduction of novel biological agents for the management of uveitis and related intraocular inflammations. A book that succinctly incorporates these developments is highly desirable for clinicians interested in treating and managing patients with uveitis. That goal is accomplished in this, the second edition of *Uveitis*, by the internationally recognized uveitis expert from Manchester, England, Nicholas Jones. Dr Jones should be congratulated for this accomplishment, and even more so for providing a highly illustrated book that covers the gamut of uveitis entities and related intraocular inflammations, as well as their complications and their management.

This book is unique in presenting a well-synthesized, state-of-the-art, etiologic approach. Its ultimate goal is to provide a practical method for establishing the diagnosis of uveitis and for proceeding with treatment. The author introduces the topics in an orderly fashion, allowing readers to grasp the clinically relevant details by providing a global approach to the management of uveitis. This approach incorporates clinical history taking, examination, and imaging methods, along with their indications and their use in diagnosis and treatment. Such details are followed by chapters on the various uveitis entities, classified on the basis of their etiology and pathogenesis. The book includes images vividly displaying bacterial, viral, fungal, and parasitic diseases that present with clinical features of uveitis. The chapters on the treatment of uveitis with anti-inflammatory, immunomodulatory, and biological agents present a practical approach to the management of recalcitrant uveitis. The chapters on sarcoidosis and other systemic disorders with ocular changes are superbly illustrated, supporting the clinical features of both systemic manifestations and ocular findings.

This second edition of *Uveitis* by Dr Jones will be useful in the clinical setting for ophthalmologists, internists, and ophthalmology residents and fellows; all should find the book very helpful in their patient care.

Narsing A Rao, MD
Steiger Professor of Vision Research and Director of Uveitis Service, Doheny Eye Institute
Professor of Ophthalmology and Pathology, University of Southern California, LA, USA
President,
International Ocular Inflammation Society
2012

Foreword to first edition

It is a pleasure and an honour to write the Foreword for this book. Uveitis is a fascinating condition with many diverse causes and clinical manifestations. Certain type of uveitis are extremely serious and unless appropriately managed may result in severe ocular morbidity. Uveitis is frequently a source of frustration to ophthalmologists and is often misdiagnosed and mismanaged.

Our knowledge of uveitis has increased enormously since the days when the most common causes were thought to be either syphilis or tuberculosis. It is now apparent that the array of diseases that can affect the uveal tract is enormous. Added to this is the rapidly advancing field of immunology and the discovery of new, or the re-definition of old, uveitis entities. The clinician managing patients with uveitis therefore requires a broad and up-to-date knowledge not only of ophthalmology but also of immunology and general medicine. Nicholas Jones has all of these credentials in abundance. Seven years ago, he created the Uveitis Clinic at the Royal Eye Hospital in Manchester; the clinic serves the Northwest of England and has dealt with over a thousand patients with uveitis. His work on Fuchs' heterochromic uveitis has been acknowledged worldwide. He is also one of the founder members of the British Uveitis Group. He is a superb clinician and an inspiring teacher.

Uveitis: An Illustrated Manual presents a complex subject in a logical, systematic and, digestible manner. I have learned much from reading it myself and some of my rather hazy ideas on the subject have been crystallized. Above all, the book contains a lot of common sense. It is an excellent resume of current knowledge which, I am sure, will be extremely useful to consultants, ophthalmologists in training, physicians and all who deal with uveitis.

Jack J. Kanski MD, MS, FRCS, FRCOphth

Preface

In 1998 my book *Uveitis: An Illustrated Manual* was published. Although never intended to be a *vade-mecum* (handbook), the primary intention was to provide a book of direct clinical usefulness to the ophthalmologist managing intraocular inflammation. The book was well received but the passage of time has seen remarkable developments in uveitis diagnosis and management. The time is opportune to reflect these developments with a new book, based on the structure and essentials of the first but with an enlarged format, a more detailed text, and a plethora of new or replacement illustrations based on a further 14 years of experience in a busy uveitis clinic, which has now treated over 3000 patients. Added to this is a series of illustrative case reports, each chosen to demonstrate a diagnostic or management dilemma. They are structured to be interactive and will hopefully be found useful to the reader. My current and recent fellows and trainees have enthusiastically contributed to these case reports, and I am indebted to them. They are: Romi Chhabra, Tim de Klerk, Assad Jalil, Karl Mercieca, Laura Steeples and Robyn Troutbeck.

This book is intended to serve both the practicing ophthalmologist who deals with uveitis, and those in ophthalmological training. Specialist nurses and optometrists will also find it of practical use. Many physicians who deal with multisystem inflammatory disease will encounter uveitis, and it is hoped that the book may prove useful and interesting to these, and to all involved in the care of patients with this fascinating but debilitating group of diseases. Our experience has led to the development of a substantial number of written management protocols and patient information pamphlets that we have found enhance our practice considerably. For the first time these are now available, in fully editable format, for readers to use and adapt if they wish, for their own clinical practice (see management protocols and patient information pamphlets on attached disk).

The great majority of illustrations in this book are taken from patients attending the Uveitis Clinic at the Manchester Royal Eye Hospital, and I am indebted to Jane Gray and her staff in the Ophthalmic Imaging Department for their excellent photography. Where gaps have existed I am immensely grateful to colleagues and friends worldwide who have so kindly contributed images. I would like to record the enthusiasm and support of Richard Furn and his team at JP Medical, who have made this project possible. In particular I would like to thank Katrina Rimmer for her indefatigable hard work. I must express my thanks to colleagues in the north of England and beyond who continue to refer patients to the Manchester Uveitis Clinic. I thank, again, my wife, who has borne my long periods in the study with a familiar resignation. Finally I must thank my patients, who have educated me, rebuked me, shared with me their most personal trials, made me laugh and made me cry. They bear their sometimes appalling problems with such forbearance.

Nicholas Jones
2012

Preface to first edition

The diagnosis and management of intraocular inflammatory disease can at times be the most frustrating, and at others the most rewarding of medical tasks. Uveitis can present substantial challenges to the ophthalmologist; most do not encounter cases frequently, and are justifiably concerned when encountering young patients with severe inflammation; understanding of the immunology of inflammatory disease proceeds apace, so that it is difficult for the practicing ophthalmologist to maintain an up-to-date knowledge; approaches to treatment develop and evolve constantly, sometimes using methods which require particular care. Many ophthalmologists find the field somewhat daunting.

The purpose of this book is to provide a basis of up-to-date immunological knowledge which is adequate for the practicing clinician; to lay out firm guidelines on the general principles of diagnosis and treatment; and to provide a structured approach to individual uveitis diagnoses, with a practical and well-illustrated strategy for the management of each. The book is primarily intended both for the practicing ophthalmologist who deals with uveitis, and for those in ophthalmological training. However, many physicians who deal with multisystem inflammatory disease will encounter uveitis, and it is hoped that the book will also prove useful and interesting to these, and to all involved in the care of patients with this fascinating but debilitating group of diseases.

The great majority of illustrations in this book are taken from patients attending the Uveitis Clinic at the Manchester Royal Eye Hospital, and I am indebted to the staff of the Ophthalmic Imaging Department for their excellent photography. However, where gaps have existed I am immensely grateful to colleagues in Manchester and elsewhere who have so kindly contributed illustrations. I am also grateful to those who have advised me on sections of the text, in particular to my colleague Andrew Tullo. I would like to record the enthusiasm and support of Caroline Makepeace and her team at Butterworth Heinemann, who have made this project possible. I must thank my wife for her immense support and for tolerating my prolonged absences in my study, and my sons who despite being frequently denied access to our computer to play games, have been constantly supportive and enthusiastic.

Finally I must express my heartfelt thanks to colleagues in the north of England and beyond who continue to refer patients to the Uveitis Clinic, and also to my patients, who bear their sometimes appalling problems with such patience and forbearance.

Nicholas P Jones
1998

Contents

On the accompanying CD-ROM

All the protocols and pamphlets listed below are included as Microsoft Word files on the CD-ROM attached to the inside front cover. The files are provided in fully editable format for adaptation and use in clinical practice.

Management protocols
Acute anterior uveitis – unilateral
Aqueous sampling
Azathioprine
Bevacizumab – intraocular
Cardiovascular disease in the uveitis clinic
Cataract surgery
Ciclosporin
Ganciclovir – intraocular
Health review form – instructions
Health review form
Methotrexate
Methylprednisolone – intravenous
Mycophenolate mofetil
Prednisolone
Sarcoidosis – diagnosis
Tacrolimus
Toxoplasmosis
Triamcinolone – intraocular
Varicella-zoster virus
Viral retinitis

Patient information pamphlets
Anti-TNF alpha
Azathioprine
Behçet's disease
Birdshot retinopathy
Cataract
Ciclosporin
Fuchs' heterochromic uveitis
Glaucoma
HLA-B27
Immunosuppression, vaccination and travel abroad
Intermediate uveitis
Juvenile idiopathic arthritis screening
Macular oedema
Methotrexate
Mycophenolate mofetil
New patient questionnaire
Prednisolone
Sarcoidosis
Tacrolimus
Toxoplasmosis
Triamcinolone – intraocular
Uveitis
Viral retinitis
Vitrectomy

CD-ROM system requirement: Windows XP or later.

Note on introductory boxes

This text is intended primarily to be clinically useful and instructive in a readable and well-illustrated form. For those forms of inflammation of greatest importance, the relevant section is prefaced by a chart containing summary information.

Included in this is a histogram of the age distribution at commencement of the disease. This information is distilled from a combination of the available literature and our own experience in the Manchester Uveitis Clinic. Some data smoothing has been applied for convenience, and the graphs are intended only as an approximate guide. The y-axis is not scaled, so graphs cannot be compared for disease frequency.

Also included is a world map giving an approximate guide to disease prevalence. Such data are unavailable from many countries and figures emanating from different regions may not be directly comparable. It is therefore reasonable only to express prevalence in three ways: first, areas where the disease is known to be very common or important (colored in red); second where the disease is well recognized (yellow); and last where it is very uncommon or unreported (gray). The reader should understand that a degree of artistic license and over-interpretation of available data has been used, and the maps should be interpreted with this in mind. Nevertheless, it is hoped that stark regional differences will be well represented and that at a glance the reader can form a picture of the approximate distribution of a disease.

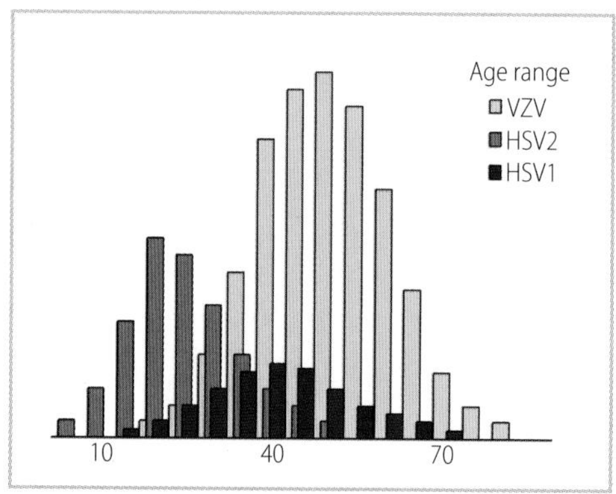

Example histogram: acute retinal necrosis.

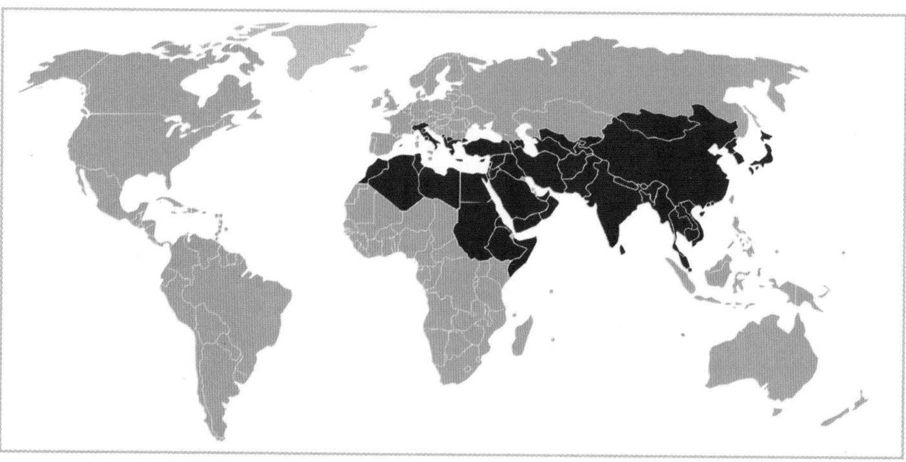

Example map: Behçet's disease.

List of abbreviations

Some medical and ophthalmological abbreviations are used commonly within this text and are in virtually universal usage. They may not be defined repeatedly within the text, but are listed below. Other abbreviations are defined within each chapter subsection in which they are used. SI units are used throughout.

Ab antibody
AC anterior chamber
ACE angiotensin-converting enzyme
Ag antigen
AIDS acquired immune deficiency syndrome
ANA antinuclear antibody
ANCA antineutrophil cytoplasmic antibody
APC antigen-presenting cell
APMPPE acute posterior multifocal placoid pigment epitheliopathy
ARN acute retinal necrosis
ATP adenosine triphosphate
AZOOR acute zonal occult outer retinopathy
BCG bacille Calmette–Guérin
BP blood pressure
C complement constituents (e.g. C3)
CD cluster differentiation (for cell labeling, e.g. CD4+)
CF visual acuity – counting fingers
CMV cytomegalovirus
CNS central nervous system
COX cyclooxygenase
CSF cerebrospinal fluid
CT computed tomography
Da dalton (unit of molecule size)
DMARD disease-modifying anti-rheumatic drug
DNA deoxyribose nucleic acid
DUSN diffuse unilateral subacute neuroretinitis
EAU experimental autoimmune uveitis
ELISA enzyme-linked immunosorbent assay
EOG electro-oculogram
ERG electroretinogram
ESR erythrocyte sedimentation rate
FEV1 forced expiratory volume in 1 second
FVC forced vital capacity
HAART highly active antiretroviral therapy
HHV human herpesvirus
HIV human immunodeficiency virus
HLA human leukocyte antigen
HM visual acuity – hand movements
HSV herpes simplex virus
ICAM intercellular adhesion molecule
ICG indocyanine green
IFN interferon
Ig immunoglobulin (e.g. IgG)
IL interleukin
IOL intraocular lens
IOP intraocular pressure
IRIS immune recovery inflammation syndrome
JIA juvenile idiopathic arthritis
KP keratic precipitate
LFT liver function test
MAb monoclonal antibody
MEWDS multiple evanescent white dot syndrome
MHC major histocompatibility complex
MRI magnetic resonance imaging
MUC Manchester Uveitis Clinic
Nd:YAG neodymium:yttrium–aluminium–garnet laser
NPL visual acuity – no perception of light
NSAID non-steroidal anti-inflammatory drug
OCT ocular coherence tomography
PAS peripheral anterior synechia
PCR polymerase chain reaction
PDT photodynamic therapy
PIC punctate inner choroidopathy
PL visual acuity – perception of light
POHS presumed ocular histoplasmosis syndrome
PS posterior synechia
PVR proliferative vitreoretinopathy
RBC red blood cell
RNA ribonucleic acid
RPE retinal pigment epithelium
SEM scanning electron micrograph
SLE systemic lupus erythematosus
TB tuberculosis
TEM transmission electron micrograph
TGF transforming growth factor
TNF tumor necrosis factor
TORCH *Toxoplasma*, other, rubella, cytomegalovirus, herpes
U&Es urea and electrolytes
VEGF vascular endothelial growth factor
VEP visual evoked potential
VKH Vogt–Koyanagi–Harada syndrome
VZV varicella-zoster virus
WBC white blood cell
WCC white cell count

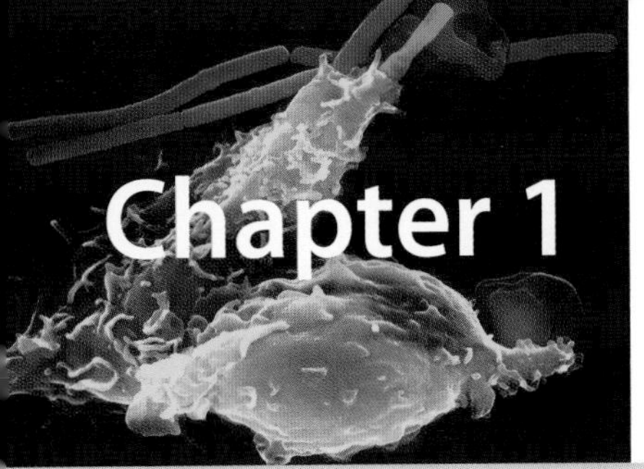

Chapter 1 The anatomy and immunology of uveitis

A sound knowledge of the microscopic anatomy and histology of the uvea, and of the mechanisms of inflammation that are relevant to it, is essential for the optimal management of the patient with uveitis. Although the clinician treating uveitis need not be overburdened with the minutiae of immunology and inflammation, an understanding of the basics is essential to permit logical treatment selection. For those interested to pursue more detailed knowledge in this confusing and constantly developing field, there are excellent sources elsewhere. However, this chapter seeks to provide a basic understanding of the mechanisms currently thought to play a part in the pathogenesis of uveitis, so that strategies for treatment, both present and future, can be understood.

ANATOMY

The uveal tract (**Fig. 1.1**) is a highly vascular, heavily pigmented layer comprising three regions each with a distinct appearance and function: the iris, ciliary body and choroid. The uvea is derived from both neuroectoderm and mesoderm; the neuroectodermal optic cup forms the epithelial layers of the ciliary body and iris and the sphincter and dilator pupillae muscles. The mesoderm forms the uveal vasculature, stroma and ciliary muscle.

The iris

The iris (**Fig. 1.2**) is covered posteriorly by the deeply pigmented epithelium which ensures its opaqueness and therefore its effectiveness as a light-excluding diaphragm. The anterior border of the pigmented epithelium (the only part visible on slit-lamp biomicroscopy) is the pupil ruff, which forms a darkly pigmented corrugated border to the pupil. Atrophy of this ruff is a feature of some forms of anterior uveitis. The fibers of dilator pupillae are in close contact with the anterior aspect of the pigmented epithelium, and pass radially towards the iris periphery. Atrophy of the pigmented epithelium is frequently associated with damage to dilator fibers and poor mydriasis. The iris sphincter is separated from the epithelium and lies anterior to it.

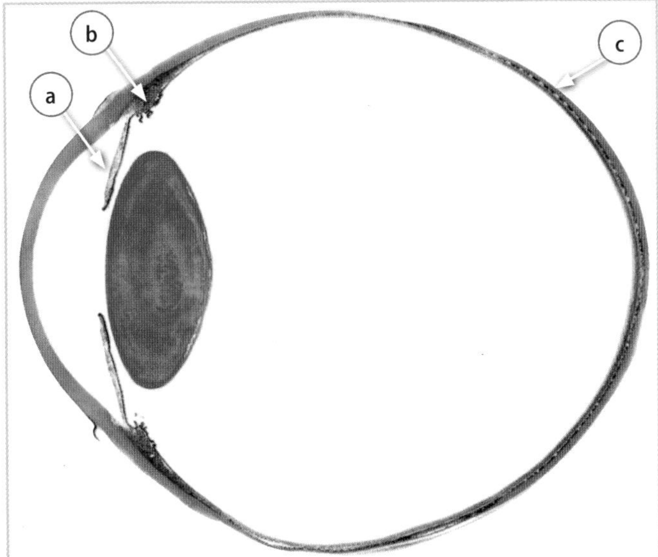

Figure 1.1 A human eyeball in horizontal section demonstrating the three regions of the uvea with their characteristic pigment deposition. The iris (a) is anterior to the lens, the base of which is contiguous with the ciliary body (b). The choroid (c) lies internal to the sclera throughout the posterior segment. (Courtesy of Dr R Bonshek.)

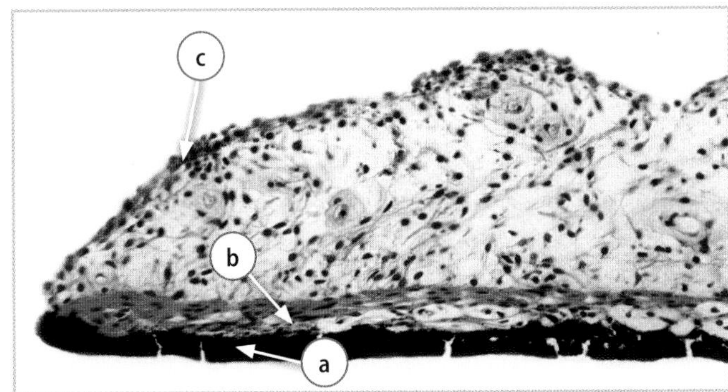

Figure 1.2 A cross-section of the pupillary region of the human iris. The pigmented epithelium (a) is opaque. Anterior to this lie the fibers of dilator pupillae (b), and then a loose fibrillary stroma containing blood vessels. The anterior border layer (c) is a condensation of this, not an epithelium. (Courtesy of Dr R Bonshek.)

The iris stroma is a loose collagenous meshwork with a broadly radial pattern, with condensations around its radial blood vessels and nerves, and an annular pattern near the pupil. Anteriorly the collagen becomes much more dense to form the anterior border layer, which is of variable depth and pattern. It is usually thickest at the collarette, the embryological remnant of the pupillary membrane, and may have radial spokes with intervening crypts, within which the less dense stroma and its blood vessel plexus remain visible. In some eyes the stroma is sufficiently diaphanous to allow visualization of the pigmented epithelium from its anterior aspect. The iris blood vessels have tight junctions and are non-permeable, in contrast to those of the ciliary body and choroid. Importantly, there is no anterior epithelium to the iris.

The degree of pigmentation of the iris is very variable. The normal iris always has a deeply pigmented posterior epithelium and there is little racial variation in this. However, although both stroma and anterior border layer contain melanocytes, pigmentation in white people may vary enormously; in some, pigmentation of both stroma and anterior border layer is negligible and the iris appears blue or gray (**Fig. 1.3**). Commonly there is a concentration of pigment in the anterior border layer, with little in the underlying stroma (**Fig. 1.4**) and it is this circumstance that leads to the perceived wide variety of iris 'color' in light-skinned races. In some white people and in all dark-skinned races, both stroma and anterior border layer melanocytes are packed with pigment so that not only is the iris dark brown (**Fig. 1.5**) but it appears much smoother and its radial fibrillary structure is obliterated by pigment-filled cells. These differences in iris appearance and structure are relevant in inflamed eyes: dark brown eyes will respond to mydriatics less well

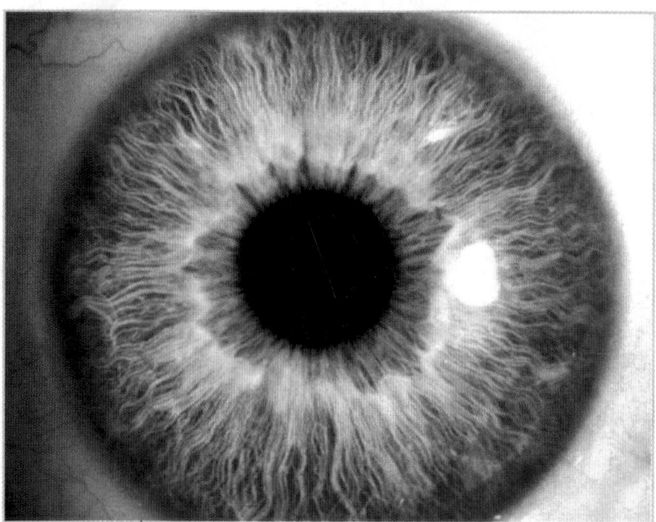

Figure 1.3 A poorly pigmented iris in a white patient is seen as blue, the anterior border layer being creamy, especially at the region of the collaret.

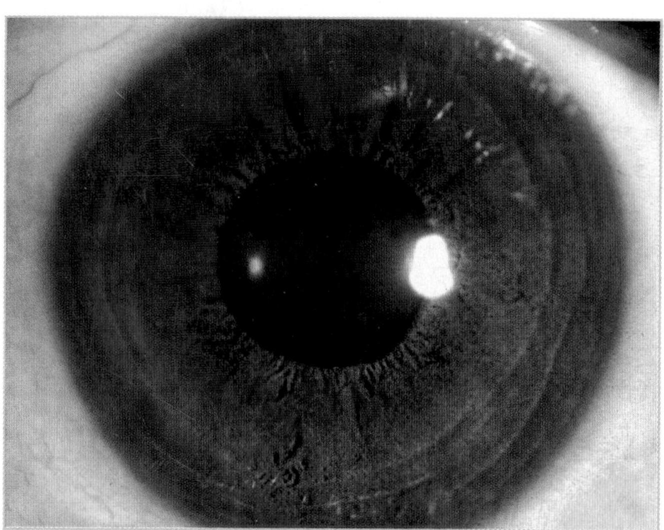

Figure 1.5 A deep brown iris in an eye of a Middle Eastern patient is packed with pigment-containing stromal cells which blur the radial fibrillary structure.

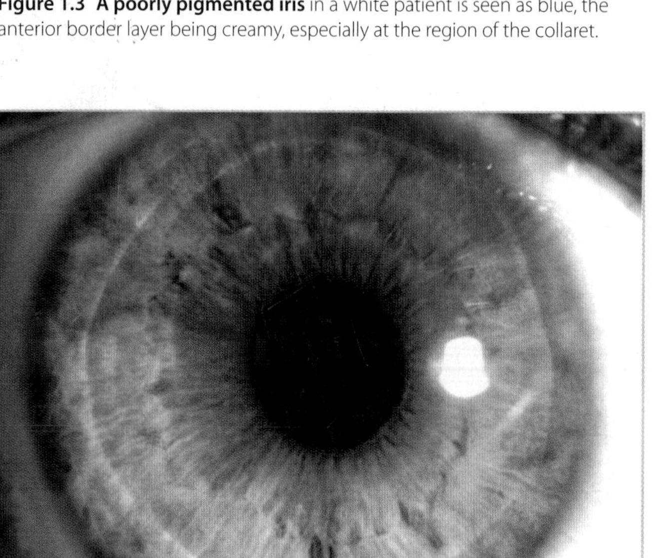

Figure 1.4 A more heavily pigmented iris in a white patient has a brown-colored anterior border layer overlying a poorly pigmented stroma.

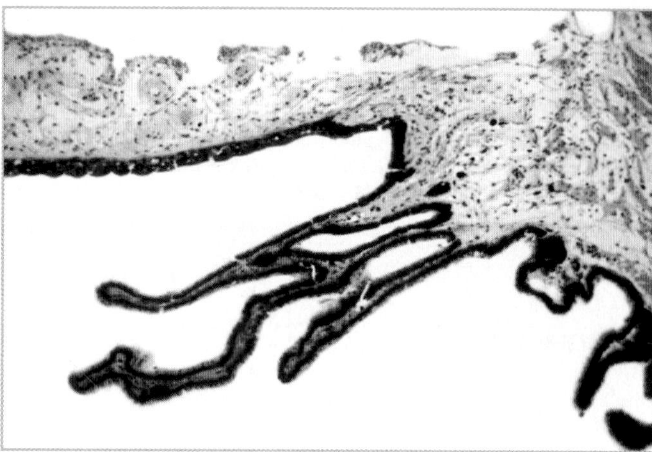

Figure 1.6 A cross-section of iris root above contiguous with pars plicata of the ciliary body showing ciliary processes. The non-pigmented secretory epithelium overlies the pigmented cell layer. Beneath this are vascular stroma and muscle fibers. (Courtesy of Dr R Bonshek.)

than others; the visibility of inflammatory deposits and nodules on the anterior surface of dark brown irides is greater; and iris swelling in acute inflammation or iris atrophy as a result of chronic inflammation will lead to widely varying appearances dependent on the pre-existing iris structure, which may otherwise be overlooked.

The ciliary body

The ciliary body (**Fig. 1.6**) is bordered anteriorly by the iris root and posteriorly by the ora serrata. The (more anterior) pars plicata, about 1.5 mm wide, is corrugated by 70–80 prominent secretory ciliary processes; the (more posterior) pars plana, about 3.5 mm wide, is flat and limited behind by the ora serrata of the retina.

The ciliary body is lined by two layers of epithelium: superficially a non-pigmented epithelium which, over the pars plicata, is responsible for the formation of aqueous humor and, over the pars plana, may be responsible for the formation of vitreous glycosaminoglycans. It is continuous anteriorly with the pigmented posterior epithelium of the iris and posteriorly with the neurosensory retina; underneath this is the deeply pigmented epithelium which is the anterior continuation of the retinal pigment epithelium (RPE) and diffuses anteriorly into the dilator pupillae. The ciliary body is very deeply pigmented, almost black, and very vascular. In the ciliary processes capillaries are fenestrated. The circular ciliary muscle fibers lie within the pars plicata. Inflammation leading to ciliary body swelling affects both accommodative function and resting lens position. Severe cyclitis will disrupt the epithelia and release pigment.

The choroid

The choroid extends from the optic nerve head to ora serrata. It is usually quite heavily pigmented (less so internally) but most of its bulk is composed of blood vessels with loose connective tissue support (**Fig. 1.7**). It is particularly rich in mast cells, especially near

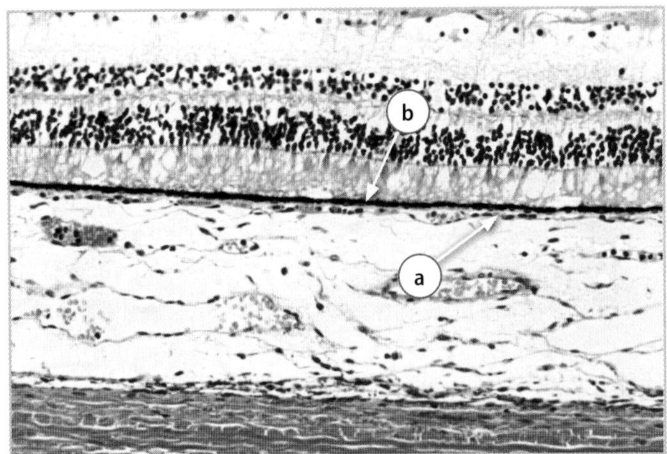

Figure 1.7 A cross-section of the posterior ocular coats. At the bottom is the dense sclera. Above this is the pigmented vascular choroid with its choriocapillaris plexus (a) lying superiorly. Directly above is the retinal pigment epithelium (b), most of the layers of neurosensory retina also being seen. (Courtesy of Dr R Bonshek.)

the posterior pole. Its thickness varies from some 0.2 mm under the macula to 0.1 mm at the ora, reflecting the metabolic needs of the overlying retina. The choroid is firmly attached to the sclera at the optic disk margin, and has some attachments where vessels (including the vortex veins) and nerves penetrate; these are strongest and most numerous behind the equator. Thus in some circumstances fluid can accumulate in the suprachoroidal space over a wide area, and may extend forwards as far as the scleral spur, also detaching the ciliary body.

The choroid has a very high blood flow. Its external large vessels become progressively smaller in caliber, reaching the choriocapillaris internally. These very wide-bore capillaries (up to 50 μm) are saccular and fenestrated, and form a meshwork underlying Bruch's membrane. The choriocapillaris has a lobular structure, each lobule being supplied by a single central precapillary arteriole and drained by peripheral postcapillary venules. This supply structure probably explains the clinical appearances of some forms of multifocal chorioretinitis. The distinct hexagonal lobular architecture of the posterior pole becomes gradually more attenuated in the anterior choroid, and has disappeared by the ora serrata. The vascular caliber of the choriocapillaris is thought to explain the propensity for choroid to entrap fungal emboli.

The retina

The retina (see Fig. 1.7) is inescapably involved in many forms of uveitis, of which a large subset seem to affect specifically the chorioretinal junction, and primary retinitis or retinal vasculitis is managed within clinics dealing with uveitis. Pragmatically, therefore, the retina is awarded 'honorary membership' of the uvea. There is no need to reiterate here the detailed anatomy of this complex layer which is well related elsewhere, but an appreciation of those characteristics that affect its behavior during inflammation is important. This includes particularly: the formation and maintenance of the inner limiting lamina and vitreoretinal interface; the different laminar relationships and metabolism at the macula; the normal structure and disruption of retinal blood vessels; and the retinal pigment epithelium, its function, metabolism and reaction to postinflammatory damage.

The variable pigmentation within both RPE and choroid combine to change profoundly the appearance of the normal fundus between individuals. This is partly a racial characteristic, partly genetic and, in the uveitis clinic, it is important because the visibility of chorioretinal abnormalities against a variable background and the variable propensity to pigmentation within scar tissue can make interpretation difficult. The range is infinite, but examples of four broad categories are shown in **Fig. 1.8**, including pale/albinoid (low level pigment in both RPE and choroid with clear visibility of choroidal vessels), typical features in white people (moderate pigment in both RPE and choroid, choroidal vessels not visible), tesselated/tigroid (low pigment level in RPE, deep pigment in choroid so that visible choroidal vessels are separated by deeply pigmented zones) and lastly the typical fundus of the dark-skinned individual (high pigment levels in both RPE and choroid giving a deep brown or green color with invisible choroidal vessels). The pigment level in RPE will also affect the behavior of angiography sequences so that for instance, in a deeply pigmented fundus in a non-white person, fluorescein passage will not show as an early choroidal blush.

The vitreous humor

Filling 80% of ocular volume as it does, the vitreous and its behavior during inflammation cannot be ignored. During the last 15 years huge advances into the structure and physiology of vitreous have been made, crucially into the molecular structure of the vitreoretinal interface.

The vitreous is a composite, its gel structure being maintained by a complex collagen matrix of fibrils, the interfaces being filled with a further glycosaminoglycan network (predominantly of hyaluronan). This polymeric molecular matrix generates its gel structure and behavior despite occupying only 0.1% of vitreous space. The ageing human vitreous undergoes progressive remodeling with formation of thicker collagen fibrils and, elsewhere, collagen degeneration to form fluid-filled lacunae. Especially in basal and cortical vitreous, the glycoprotein opticin, secreted by the ciliary body, forms part of the vitreoretinal interface. Increasing knowledge of these molecular structures has facilitated the development of enzymatic interventions either to liquefy vitreous or to disrupt abnormal vitreoretinal adhesions in disease, and this is discussed in Chapter 7. Modern imaging techniques have for the first time permitted in vivo examination of human vitreous (Mojana et al. 2010).

The blood–ocular barrier

The blood–ocular barrier is an effective cellular barrier to the movement of macromolecules between the intravascular space and the intraocular compartment. It exists in different forms depending on location. In the iris, the thick-walled capillaries comprise vascular endothelium with (in humans but not in some laboratory animals) effective zonulae occludentes. In the ciliary body and choroid the capillaries are extensively fenestrated, allowing free flow of some macromolecules into the extracellular compartment; in the ciliary body the barrier is therefore the bilayered epithelium and, in the choroid, the Bruch's membrane/RPE complex, especially the tight junctions of the latter. The RPE forms the outer part of the blood–retinal barrier, the inner being formed by the impermeable vascular endothelium of the intraretinal blood vessels. The retina itself is therefore protected by the blood–ocular barrier, but the posterior uvea is not.

Breakdown of the blood–ocular barrier is a common accompaniment to uveitis. Damage to vascular endothelium or uveal/retinal epithelium may then allow macromolecules to pass into the intraocular

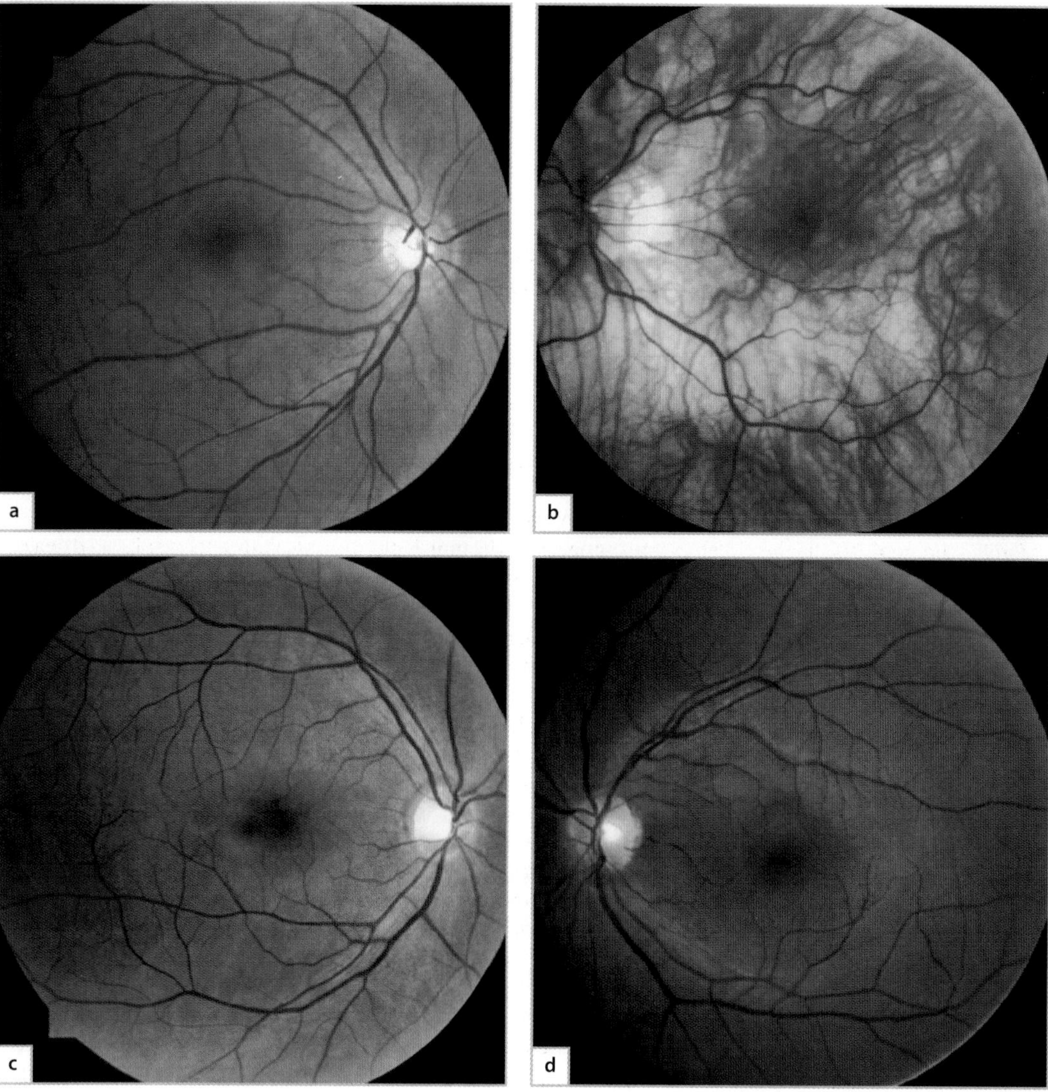

Figure 1.8 Four variants of normal fundal pigmentation: (a) in a white patient; (b) albinotic; (c) tesselated; (d) in a African–Caribbean patient.

compartment, which is normally virtually protein free. In the anterior segment, extravasation from iris vessels is a universal accompaniment to iritis. Fibrinogen (the longest plasma protein molecule, so released in quantity only if breakdown is severe) is troublesome, leading to intraocular coagulation and synechia formation. α_2-Macroglobulin will also extravasate; this globulin both carries interleukin-1 (IL-1) and neutralizes transforming growth factor-β (TGF-β), giving a dual proinflammatory effect. After most episodes of acute inflammation with focal breakdown of the blood–ocular barrier, restoration takes place. However, when severe and/or very chronic, inflammation can lead to structural changes in the blood–aqueous barrier, which becomes permanently ineffective. Chronic anterior chamber (AC) flare, representing an abnormally high aqueous protein concentration, is the result, and is particularly common in the chronic uveitis associated with juvenile chronic arthritis. Retinal vasculitis is usually accompanied by multifocal breakdown of the blood–retinal barrier, as shown by perivascular exudation and abnormal leakage of fluorescein.

IMMUNOLOGY

The development of knowledge about the immune system continues apace, the result being increasing complexity rather than clarification; the practicing clinician encounters constantly changing mechanisms for the immune system compared with those studied as a medical student. The changing nomenclature and ever-developing knowledge within this field are daunting to one who merely wishes to understand something of the basis of the diseases that he or she treats. There are many excellent sources for detailed information on modern immunological knowledge. This section intends to serve only as a basic introduction to those aspects of immunology that are pertinent to the ophthalmologist dealing with uveitis.

The immune system began to develop phylogenetically as soon as unicellular organisms began to bump into each other within the primordial soup. Such mundane interactions soon became competitive, each combatant requiring either the ability to lyse and phagocytose, or the mechanisms to deter or defend against such an attack. As simple multicellular organisms came into being, the need to recognize and dispose of harmful foreign 'non-self' material, mainly microorganisms, became the *raison d'être* of the immune system. The natural, or **innate** immune system, developed first and uses non-specific, scattergun methods to destroy foreign material. These, both cellular and humoral, include, for example, the secretion of lysozyme by macrophages, histamine and prostaglandins by mast cells, and interferons by many tissue cells, the complement system and leukocyte phagocytosis, with its associated effects, including the release of cytotoxic free radicals.

The **adaptive** immune system is phylogenetically much more modern, thought to have begun development only after vertebrates appeared. On exposure to a specific antigen, an adaptive immune response can develop or augment defense mechanisms. The key to adaptation is the creation of specific memory of the event, leading to future acquired resistance to the particular antigen. The system is dependent on the T and B lymphocytes, populations of which can selectively react to myriads of different antigens. The adaptive immune system can function in isolation, but normally exerts its destructive effects on antigens in interaction with elements of the natural immune system, especially via activation of the complement system, and using the phagocytic capabilities of granulocytes and macrophages.

In the race to eliminate dangerous microorganisms, normally all foreign material (including that which is harmless) induces an immune response. However, it is essential for a complex multicellular organism to differentiate between three types of antigen: first, components of self; second, harmless foreign material that can be either neutral (implying contact with but no need, such as pollen) or useful (such as food); and third, foreign material that is harmful, including pathogenic organisms. The organisms need to develop **tolerance** to the first two of these categories. **Central tolerance** is the process of tolerating self (or, rather, discouraging recognition of self). Controlled mainly by the thymus and bone marrow, and largely initiated during fetal development (but continuing throughout life) the process both encourages expansion of those lymphocyte clones showing tolerance to self-antigens (especially human leukocyte antigen or HLA antigens) and detects and destroys lymphocytes that recognize self. **Acquired tolerance** develops with exposure to each successive external antigen. One crucial component of this mechanism is oral tolerance, whereby lymphoid tissue in the gut lining permits the passage of harmless antigens without a reaction. This phenomenon can, up to a point, be used to generate tolerance as a form of therapy.

Central tolerance may break down in certain circumstances; the resulting **autoimmune** reaction may lead to severe damage to tissues bearing the target antigen. The phenomenon is important in some forms of uveitis. When acquired tolerance breaks down, the immune system over-reacts to an antigen that is otherwise harmless. The resulting **hypersensitivity** reaction leads to damage greater than that which would have been induced by the antigen itself.

The complement system

The complement system includes some 15 serum proteins which can be rapidly activated by several stimuli. These include immunoglobulin IgG/-A or IgM/-A complexes (via the classic pathway), IgA and some antigenic polysaccharides (via the alternate pathway). Activation of the system leads to three main effects, which are all short-lived and localized owing to the very short life of the complement constituents. First, anaphylatoxins (C3a and C5a) are created. These are peptides that act on polymorphs, mast cells and smooth muscle to promote an inflammatory response. Second, C3b is deposited on to adjacent cell membranes; this acts as a powerful **opsonin**, an attractant for macrophages and polymorphs; these cells carry C3b receptors and will phagocytose cells thus labeled (in general, any surface protein that induces phagocytosis is an opsonin; it is the immunological equivalent of ketchup). Last, the release of C5b stimulates the creation of a C5b/C6/C7/C8/C9 'membrane attack complex,' which forms many open rings within the target cell membrane. This prevents cellular control of ingress and egress and causes lysis of that cell (**Fig. 1.9**).

As a response to inflammation, neutrophils and macrophages release a combination of proinflammatory cytokines into the bloodstream. In response the liver produces and releases a selection of **acute phase proteins** (those proteins with serum concentrations that rise during acute inflammation). Complement factors account for several of these, as do coagulation factors including fibrinogen and prothrombin, amyloid A, plasminogen and C-reactive protein (a pentameric globulin that is capable of surface binding to many bacteria). This fixes complement and therefore (as another opsonin) promotes phagocytosis.

Cells of the immune system

The white 'blood' cells represent phylogenetically distinct cell lines, although all develop from a common precursor stem cell. In morphology, immune behavior and extravascular activity they have substantial differences. Differentiation began in invertebrates, originally creating phagocytes to combat bacterial and fungal infection, this function being preserved in granulocytes (particularly neutrophils) and macrophages. Subsequently, parasitic infestations led to the development of the eosinophil in amphibians and early fishes. Lymphocyte differentiation took place somewhat later but similar basic properties are seen in all vertebrates. The beginnings of adaptive immunity were therefore in the Ordovician and Silurian periods between 500 and 400 million years ago. Today in the Pleistocene, evolution has produced substantial interspecific variation even within mammals, reflecting their different environments and immunological requirements.

Granulocytes

The granulocytes (neutrophils, eosinophils and basophils) usually comprise some four-fifths of the circulating leukocytes, and neutrophils form the vast majority of these. Originally evolved to counter bacterial and fungal infection, they will phagocytose opsonized foreign material and release inflammatory mediators when appropriately stimulated. Eosinophils developed originally to defend against parasitic infestation and raised counts are still a marker for such diseases. However, they have also become the predominant inflammatory cell in allergic reactions. Basophils are also active in both parasitic diseases and allergy, with additional actions including vasodilation (via histamine) and anticoagulation (via heparin). The extravascular equivalent of the basophil is the mast cell, and both rapidly degranulate on stimulation, releasing their characteristic cytokine and lipid mixture.

Monocytes/macrophages

Monocytes do not have cytoplasmic granules, and after migration into the extravascular space become macrophages, which are powerful and multifunctional immune cells. They share some functions with neutrophils but have additional unique functions and are much longer lived. They are active phagocytes and release antibacterial enzymes such as lysozyme; they can destroy bacteria without interaction with other components of the immune system. They are general scavengers and remove necrotic cellular debris. The macrophage is capable of secreting a number of **cytokines** that contribute to the inflammatory reaction. They also act as antigen-presenting cells (APCs), and are therefore important in the recruitment and activation of other inflammatory cells. The macrophage is the characteristic cell of chronic inflammation, which in certain circumstances becomes epithelioid and forms granulomas, sometimes including multinucleate giant cells. The widespread and multifunctional nature of macrophages and their lineage is manifest in the varying names used for them in various locations, including Kupffer's cells, microglia, osteoclasts and histiocytes.

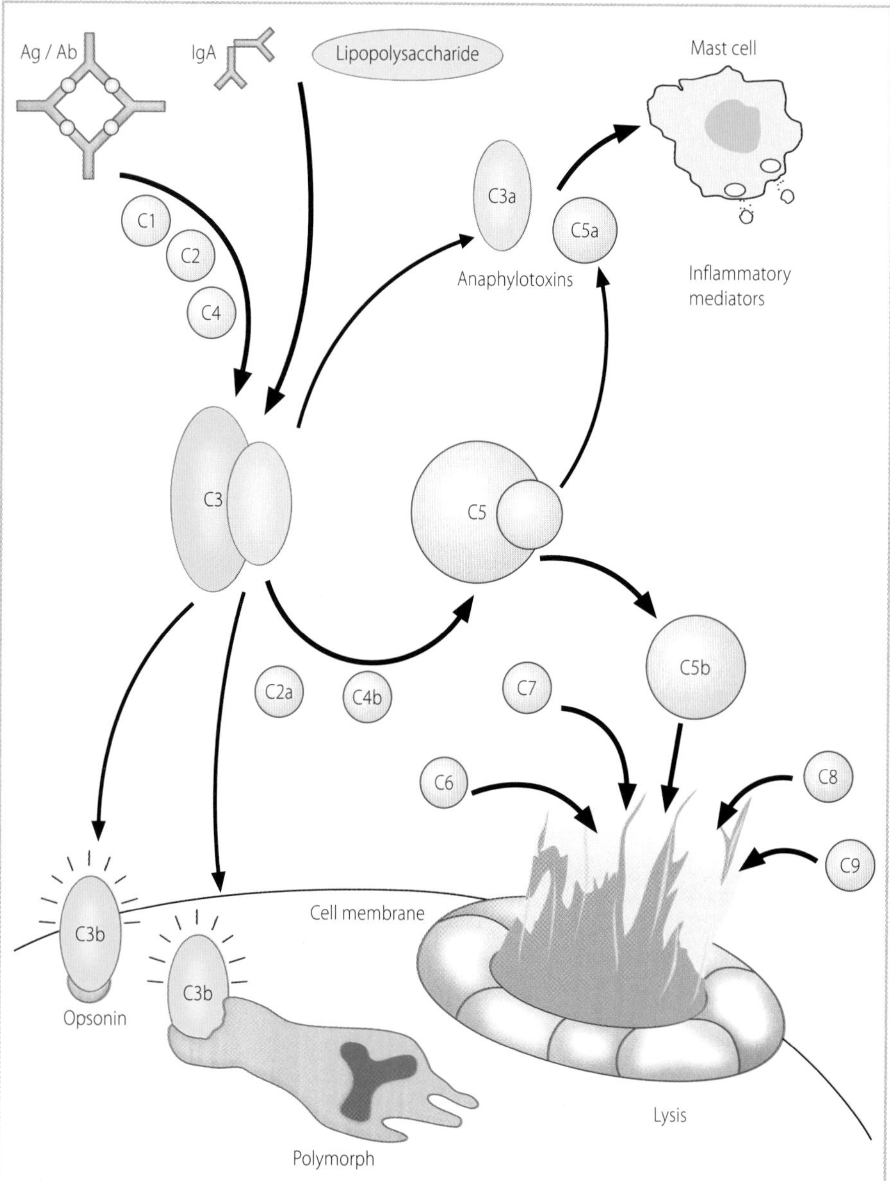

Figure 1.9 A schematic summarizing the most important steps in the complement cascade, which may be activated via classic or alternate pathways. The primary end-point is the C5–9 complex which disrupts cell membrane integrity by forming open pores.

Dendritic cells

These **antigen-presenting cells** do not necessarily belong here because they may derive from either hemopoietic or plasmacytoid lineage. However, it is appropriate to discuss them here before passing on to the most complex and important cells of the adaptive immune system, the lymphocytes.

Dendritic cells are the resident APCs mainly situated in those tissues directly contacting external stimuli, including skin (Langerhans' cells), mucosae, and gastrointestinal and respiratory tracts. Being permanently 'on watch' in such tissues they are sometimes referred to as 'professional' APCs. A foreign antigen activates the dendritic cell which then migrates to regional lymph nodes to prime lymphocytes and initiate clonal expansion. Only dendritic cells are capable of performing this initial priming process. Within the eye, dendritic cells reside mainly in mesenchyme-derived connective tissue, but within the retina there are virtually none (though there are microglia, which serve a similar function). In addition to APC functions, some dendritic cells may be involved in immune tolerance, probably either by inducing T-cell anergy or apoptosis.

Lymphocytes

The lymphocyte is a long-lived cell which repeatedly recirculates from tissues to blood, and has surface receptors that can respond only to a single antigen. The lymphoid cell precursor can differentiate into one of three types of lymphocyte. Morphologically lymphocytes are either small (comprising T and B cells) or large (large granular lymphocytes, including natural killer (NK) cells).

T cells

The T cell accounts for some two-thirds of the lymphocyte population at any one time, and is responsible for cell-mediated immune mechanisms and other functions. These cells carry a surface **T-cell receptor** (TCR). This is composed of α and β polypeptide chains, which can, in combination with HLA class II molecules (see below), recognize a foreign antigen. Following this interaction the lymphocyte can, by gene rearrangement, form a surface receptor unique to the antigen to which it has been exposed, thus limiting its future immune responsiveness to the same antigen. These **memory T cells** are very long lived, sometimes living for the lifetime of the animal, allowing the specific memory of antigen exposure to be retained for very long periods. A tiny subset of T cells has a different TCR comprising γδ, and these Tγδ cells currently seem confined to gut mucosa. They are probably involved in oral tolerance.

About two-thirds of T lymphocytes bear the CD4 surface antigen (see Table 1.1), and are known as **helper T cells** (Th), which are essential for cell-mediated immune reactions, to prime cytotoxic T cells, and for the regulation of B-cell responses. These cells respond to antigens complexed with major histocompatibility complex (MHC) class II molecules. They are also involved in some autoimmune disease processes. The rest of the T cells bear the CD8 surface antigen; these cells are either **regulatory T cells** (Tr, previously known as suppressor T cells) or **cytotoxic T cells** (Tc); CD8 cells may be either bifunctional (Ts/c) or of two distinct types, both bearing the CD8 antigen. These cells respond to antigens complexed with MHC class I molecules (see below). Tr cells are essential for immune tolerance and inhibit activated Th cells. Tc cells destroy virally infected and cancer cells and are involved in transplant rejection.

Th cells comprise at least two populations, named Th1 and Th2. Th1 cells produce the cytokines tumor necrosis factor β (TNF-β) and interferon-γ (IFN-γ), and are involved in the provocation of the type IV hypersensitivity response (and are almost certainly involved in both experimental and clinical uveitis). They specifically provoke macrophage and Tc activity, provoking target cell destruction. In contrast, Th2 cells produce the cytokines IL-4, IL-6 and IL-10, are involved in type I hypersensitivity, interact specifically with B cells to induce proliferation and antibody production, but may be suppressive for some forms of inflammation. Recent development show that the Th1 and Th2 subdivision is, alone, inadequate to describe all functions of Th cells. A variety of different Th markers have been described with as yet poorly defined functions. Each phase of research uncovers increased complexity within the adaptive immune system.

B cells

The B cell comprises less than a fifth of the total lymphocyte population. They are the only cell to carry a surface **immunoglobulin** marker which represents the Ig that the cell is capable of producing; after appropriate stimulation, they convert to **plasma cells** which develop extensive cytoplasm containing many ribosomes and rough endoplasmic reticulum, which is essentially an Ig-producing factory. The type of Ig expressed is decided only after specific activation, but, induced by certain cytokines, B cells are capable of changing the type of Ig that they express and manufacture. Usually B-cell proliferation and Ig manufacture require the presence of activated T cells, but certain molecules and viruses can cause non-specific (polyclonal) proliferation of B cells, stimulating Ig production.

There are five types of Ig: IgA, IgD, IgE, IgG and IgM. Most B cells/ plasma cells produce IgG and most reside in the spleen and lymph nodes. However, after first exposure to a new antigen, IgM is the first Ig to be manufactured, followed later by IgG. Serological identification of the levels of IgG and IgM helps to indicate a new from a previously acquired infection (**Fig. 1.10**). Both IgG and IgM can activate the complement pathway, and by interacting with foreign surface antigens, they attract phagocytes.

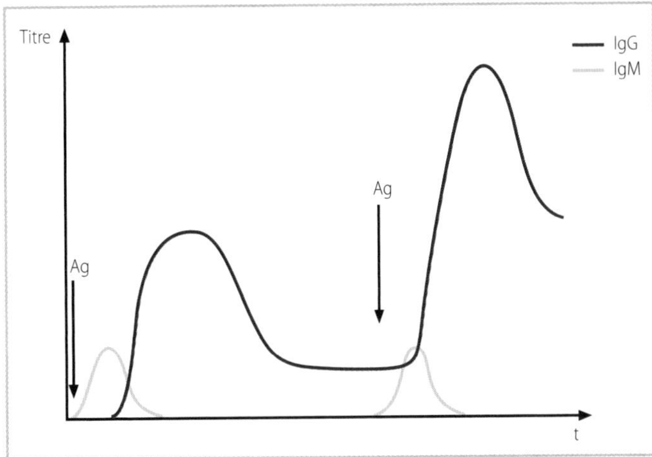

Figure 1.10 The antigens of a microorganism causing primary infection induce antibody formation: first IgM and then IgG. The IgM response is rapid but short-lived and again becoming undetectable. In contrast the IgG response is slightly delayed but greater and more sustained, falling slowly to a level that is sustained usually throughout life. Secondary exposure to the same antigen produces a similar response but the IgG peak may be greater.

Natural killer cells

The third type of lymphocyte is the NK cell, comprising about a fifth of the population. They are 'null' cells in that they have neither immunoglobulin nor T-cell receptors on their surface. They are part of the innate rather than the adaptive immune system, targeting cancer cells and virus-infected cells. They respond to interferon expression, releasing cytotoxic granules that destroy the target cell.

Antigen-presenting cells

Normally antigens must be modified and 'presented' to T and B lymphocytes before an appropriate immunological response can be generated. Several different forms of cell have the capability to act as APCs. The main 'professional' APCs are macrophages and dendritic cells.

In order to function as an APC a cell must bear MHC class II surface antigens. These cells bind foreign antigens and dismember them into peptides which, when associated with the HLA class II molecules expressed on the cell surface, are then recognized by T lymphocytes. Constant recirculation of lymphocytes, especially through the spleen and lymph nodes, enhances contact with APCs and therefore speeds the process of presentation. Presentation induces activation of the T cells, leading to B-cell activation and antibody production (**Fig. 1.11**).

Other cells can be induced to express HLA class II antigens, and therefore can act in some circumstances as APCs. Some resident ocular cells fall into this category, including RPE cells and vascular endothelium; the presence of IFNγ has been found to induce MHC class II expression by these cells, and they can then act in this way.

Cell surface markers

Proteinaceous, lipid or other molecules on or within the cell membrane create cell individuality. Such molecules may individually have a single function, or several functions; each cell may bear several types rendering it multifunctional and highly communicative. Such markers may also be found within cell cytoplasm, especially on endoplasmic reticulum or lysosomes, facilitating intracellular functions. A surface **receptor** is a protein molecule with an **epitope** that is specific to another of specific shape – a **ligand**. It may be on the surface

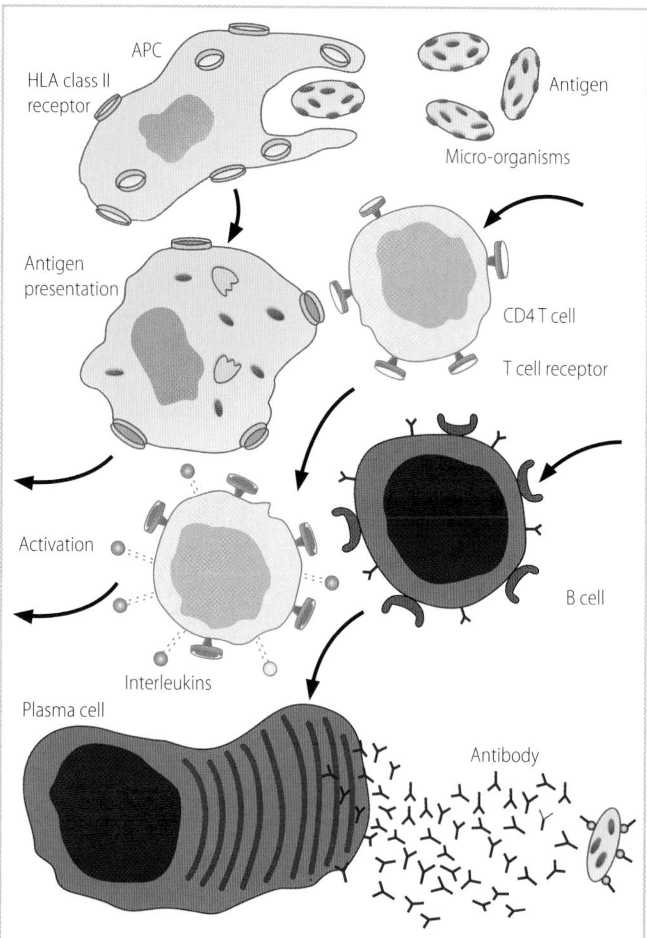

Figure 1.11 The cells involved in antibody response to an antigen: the antigen-presenting cell (APC) phagocytoses the antigen and then expresses this together with its HLA II surface receptor. A helper T cell interacts and therefore becomes activated, secreting proinflammatory cytokines. This activated T cell also interacts with a B cell which then, similar to the T cell, undergoes clonal proliferation, converting to plasma cells that produce specific antibody in large quantities.

or transmembrane. Each surface marker has designated function, whether it be interaction with a pre-identified antigen, a hormone, a neurotransmitter or a drug, and whether it leads to chemotaxis, degranulation, adhesion or ingress of calcium or γ-aminobenzoate.

Different leukocyte types often bear several surface markers, and the identification of these can elucidate the function of the cell. Such antigens can be recognized (and therefore labeled) by **monoclonal antibodies** (MAbs). To produce these, B cells and tumor cells are fused to form a **hybridoma,** which will then (in a monoclonal culture) continue to produce, in large quantities, the antibody of the specific B cell. Many different MAbs are now available and can be used to identify leukocyte types for either research or therapy. It was the widespread laboratory generation of MAbs that provoked the creation of a labeling system known as cluster of differentiation (CD). Several CD numbers are synonymous with cell surface markers named for functionality and this sometimes causes confusion. Some of the most important CD designations are shown in **Table 1.1**.

The ability of the adaptive immune system to recognize and respond uniquely to such a large variety of individual antigens is the product of three heterogeneous cell surface marker systems, all adapted from a common phylogenetic precursor. The immunoglobulin and T-cell receptor are two of these, and the third is the **human leukocyte antigen**.

Human leukocyte antigens

On the short arm of chromosome 6 is located the **major histocompatibility complex**, a region that contains the genes responsible for the production of the HLA antigens (**Fig. 1.12**). Class I HLA antigens are carried on the surface of almost all nucleated cells. Genes for these antigens are carried in loci A, B and C of the MHC. These surface antigens serve as recognition labels (tissue types) for each cell, and are the main provokers of allograft rejection (mediated by Tc cells).

Class II HLA antigens are coded in the HLA-D locus of the MHC (including HLA-DM, -DR, -DQ, -DP) and are carried only by some component cells of the immune system, including macrophages, B cells, activated T cells, Langerhans' cells and dendritic cells. It is necessary to express HLA class II antigens if a cell is to act as an APC. The antigens are responsible for ensuring immune specificity, so that cells that need to interact in an immune process will do so only if both carry the same HLA class II antigen. This process is known as MHC restriction.

Humans may carry two alleles at each HLA locus if heterozygous, or, if homozygous, only one. Epidemiological and disease-based studies have demonstrated that the racial and geographic distribution of HLA types is often strikingly different, and that certain antigens are particularly associated with some forms of inflammation, at least within a defined population. This is also true of some forms of uveitis, and these associations are discussed in Chapter 3.

Cell adhesion molecules

These cell surface glycoproteins, including the integrins and selectins, stimulate the attachment of leukocytes to vascular endothelium, provoking migration of the leukocytes through the endothelium into adjacent inflamed tissue. The expression of cell adhesion molecules (CAMs) seems to be controlled by cytokines. One such molecule, intercellular adhesion molecule-1 (ICAM-1) is also expressed on corneal endothelium (where it may stimulate the adhesion of keratic precipitates), on the vascular endothelium of iris and ciliary body, and on the ciliary epithelium. The importance of CAMs in experimental uveitis has been demonstrated, and the severity of inflammation can be reduced by the use of MAbs directed against these CAMs.

Fas ligand

Fas ligand (FasL) is a transmembrane protein, one of a group structurally similar to TNFs. This surface marker is expressed by activated T cells as a self-destructive mechanism that initially permits clonal expansion and the performance of its immune function, but then, by inducing apoptosis of the cells, terminating the acute episode and preventing the unnecessary damage that would result from a prolonged response. FasL is therefore an important regulator of T-cell activity. It is also expressed by some ocular tissues, such as keratocytes, which contribute to ocular immune privilege (see below) by inhibiting primed lymphocyte infiltration.

Cytokines

The cytokines are protein molecules that cells secrete to influence the activity of other cells, either locally or at a distance. They are essentially signaling molecules. The terminology of cytokines has been confusing, mainly being complicated by the monofunctional naming

Table 1.1 Cluster of differentiation labeling

CD number	Cell type	Function ± alternative name
CD2	T cells, NK cells	Signal transduction and cell adhesion
CD3	Mature T cells	Part of the T-cell receptor
CD4	Helper T cells, some macrophages	A co-receptor for MHC II
CD8	Suppressor/cytotoxic T cells	A co-receptor for MHC I
CD11 (a, b, c)	Myeloid and lymphoid series leukocytes	Integrins, interacting with ICAMs, complement, etc.
CD14	Monocytes	Binds to bacterial surface components
CD15	All granulocytes	Facilitates chemotaxis and phagocytosis
CD16	NK cells, macrophages, neutrophils	An Ig receptor
CD19	B cells	A B-cell surface antigen marker
CD20	B cells	Transmembrane protein permitting Ca^{2+} transport across cell membrane
CD25	Activated T cells, B cells, etc.	IL-2 receptor
CD45	All leukocytes	Transmembrane protein, facilitates cell activation
CD52	Mature lymphocytes, monocytes, APCs	Cell identity marker
CD54	Activated T cells, B cells, APCs	ICAM-1: adheres to vascular endothelium
CD62E	Vascular endothelium	E-selectin: when activated, adheres to passing leukocytes
CD95L	T cells, some ocular tissue cells	Fas ligand: immune regulator, induces T-cell apoptosis
CD120	Many cell types	A TNF receptor

APC, antigen-presenting cell; ICAM, intercellular adhesion molecule; IL, interleukin; NK, natural killer; TNF, tumor necrosis factor.

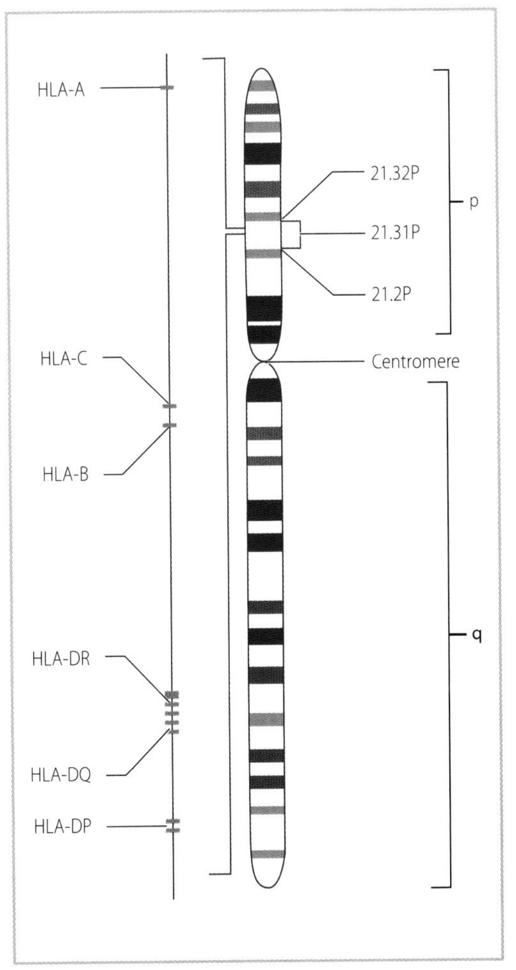

Figure 1.12 The MHC is located at 21.31p on chromosome 6. The relevant segment has been expanded left to show the comparative locations of the HLA alleles.

of cytokines that have later been discovered to be multifunctional. These functions may depend on the local environment, and cytokines frequently have overlapping or sometimes conflicting effects. Some are synergistic with others, some antagonistic. Examples of the most important cytokines, their source cells and their most important actions are shown in **Tables 1.2** and **1.3**. Some cells also secrete chemical mediators of the inflammatory response. Mast cells secrete histamine, heparin, leukotrienes and chemotactic factors; macrophages and others secrete prostaglandins and thromboxanes. The chemical 'traffic' from and between cells involved in inflammation and immune responses is extremely complex and incompletely understood. It is clear that cytokines play an active part in ocular inflammation, either as stimulants (e.g. IL-2, IL-6, TNF-α, IFN-γ) or as suppressants (e.g. IL-10, TGF-β). Various resident ocular cells are capable of producing cytokines, including ciliary body epithelium, RPE, retinal Müller cells and lens epithelium.

As cytokines are a fundamental part of the immune response, and are clearly implicated in uveitis, methods of antagonizing their action to alleviate inflammation have been studied (Heiligenhaus et al. 2010). This ever-expanding field has already led to the development of clinically useful anti-cytokine therapy and the drugs available are discussed in Chapter 6.

Hypersensitivity

This term is now used broadly to mean any immune mechanism that leads to uncontrolled host damage. Gell and Coombs described four types of hypersensitivity based on the mechanism that leads to such damage, and all four varieties may occur in the human uvea.

Type I (anaphylactic)

Typified by classic allergic reactions. A harmless foreign protein, e.g. grass pollen, stimulates IgE production which binds to and

Table 1.2 Cytokines: examples of interleukins (IL)

Designation	Cell type	Function ± alternative name
IL-1	Many cell types	Endogenous pyrogen, stimulates proliferation of T and B lymphocytes
IL-2	Activated T cells	Activates macrophages, T cells, B cells. Enhances specific immune responses
IL-3	Activated T cells, mast cells	Stimulates production of macrophages and granulocytes
IL-4	Possibly basophils, unconfirmed	Induces transformation of Th0 cells into Th2 cells; regulates inflammatory response
IL-5	Th2 cells	Eosinophil differentiation factor: regulates eosinophil maturation, stimulates B-cell maturation
IL-6	T cells and macrophages	IFN-β_2: B-cell stimulatory factor: converts B cells into plasma cells
IL-7	Marrow and thymus stromal cells	Hemopoietic growth factor: stimulates T- and B-cell maturation
IL-8	Macrophages, epithelial cells	Chemotaxis for neutrophils and others, induces phagocytosis, angiogenic
IL-9	Th1 cells	Stimulates T-cell proliferation and inhibits apoptosis
IL-10	Monocytes/macrophages, some lymphocytes	Human cytokine synthesis inhibitory factor: anti-inflammatory
IL-12	APCs and activated B-cells	T-cell-stimulating factor, chemotactic for NK cells, stimulates IFN-γ and TNF-α
IL-17	Activated T cells	Several subtypes; proinflammatory, synergistic with TNF-α, mediates delayed hypersensitivity
IL-27	APCs	A subset of IL-12. Regulates both T- and B-cell functions

APC, antigen-presenting cell; CD, cluster differentiation; Th, T-helper; NK, natural killer.

Table 1.3 Cytokines: examples of others

Designation	Cell type	Function ± alternative name
Interferon (IFN)		
IFN-α	Leukocytes, mainly macrophages	Fourteen subtypes; innate antiviral immunity
IFN-β	Fibroblasts	Two subtypes; innate antiviral immunity
IFN-γ	Th cells, NK cells and Tc cells	The Th-cell-defining marker, inducing clonal expansion; macrophage activating factor; innate immunity against intracellular microorganisms (viruses and bacteria), pyrogen. Induces HLA class II antigen expression on cell surfaces
Colony-stimulating factor (CSF)		
G-CSF	Macrophages, endothelium and others	Stimulates marrow to generate and release granulocytes into blood
Tumor necrosis factor (TNF)		
TNF-α	Macrophages and many others	Cachexin: multifunctional, including inflammatory mediation, pyrogen, weakly cytotoxic to vascular endothelium supplying tumors
Transforming growth factor (TGF)		
TGF-β	T cells, many others	Multifunctional: inhibits several cytokines and some T cells, downregulates IL-2-induced immune responses, inhibits TNF, induces fibroblast growth

IL, interleukin.

degranulates mast cells; the resulting release of inflammatory mediators causes tissue damage.

Type II (cytotoxic)

Mediated by IgG or IgM. The antibodies interact with surface antigen of target cells, thus activating complement and killer cells, inducing phagocytosis.

Type III (immune complex mediated)

The attachment of an antibody (Ab) to an antigen (Ag) to form an Ag/Ab (immune) complex normally brings about immediate phagocytosis, especially where complement is activated. Most complexes are large, with many separate Ab and Ag molecules aggregating together. This facilitates phagocytosis. However, where complexes are small, they may persist in the circulation or tissues, activate complement and cause tissue damage. This mechanism may be involved in some forms of uveitis including Behçet's disease.

Type IV (cell mediated)

T cells re-encounter an antigen and recruit macrophages, which phagocytose the antigen. Where the macrophage is incapable of destroying the antigen, the cells become epithelioid and form granulomas. This mechanism plays a part, for example, in sarcoidosis and inflammatory bowel disease, and is involved in several forms of uveitis, notably sympathetic uveitis and Vogt–Koyanagi–Harada (VKH) syndrome.

Autoimmunity

The components of 'self' are normally protected against the immune system by several mechanisms: self-antigens are not presented by APCs; potentially self-reactive lymphocyte clones are selectively eliminated; both T-cell and B-cell receptors may be blocked; and any self-reactive activity is suppressed by Tr cells. These mechanisms together lead to tolerance of self-antigens which protects against autoimmune reactions.

These protective mechanisms occasionally fail, for several possible reasons, any one or combination of which can lead to autoimmune disease (**Fig. 1.13**). The first and most well-known mechanism is that of **molecular mimicry**: an invading microorganism may share some antigenic features with the host, presumably a very similar epitope, such that generation of an immune response against the foreign antigen also causes damage to host cells bearing the similar surface antigen. This mechanism is thought to be important in the generation of some HLA-associated diseases, where infection by some Gram-negative bacilli can induce, via the HLA system, inflammatory effects against host tissue.

Second, self-antigens may be sequestered from the immune system, and presented to it later, then being automatically treated as foreign. The phenomenon is particularly important in the eye, and is portentous in sympathetic uveitis, retinal antigens normally being sequestered from the immune system until local damage exposes it. Indeed, this phenomenon may be used to induce **experimental autoimmune uveoretinitis** (EAU): the inoculation of retinal S-antigen and/or inter-photoreceptor binding protein, together with a stimulatory immunological 'soup' (such as Freund's adjuvant), into the footpad of an experimental animal, will lead to a severe and destructive form of uveitis.

Other mechanisms of autoreactivity exist: a self-cell may also display non-self antigens, e.g. a virus-infected cell during the 'budding' of viral particles, and will be destroyed by the immune process; antigens may be presented by non-professional APCs (possibly induced to bear MHC II 'accidentally' by IFN-γ) and lead to host cell damage; self-reactive B-cell clones that have not been eliminated may be stimulated by any polyclonal activator, inducing autoimmune activity from that clone; regulatory mechanisms, including the suppressor T-cell system, may break down.

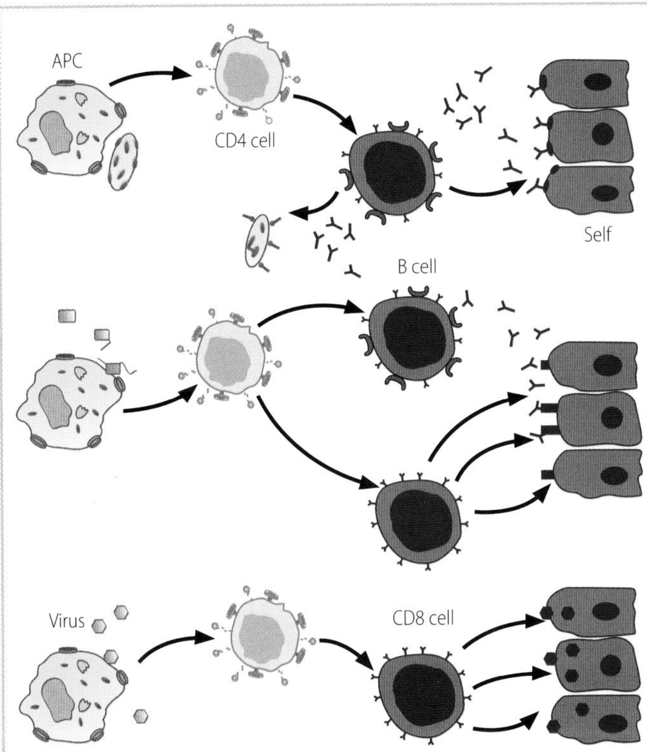

Figure 1.13 Three possible methods of autoimmunity. Top: foreign antigens expressed, e.g. by a bacterium, share characteristics with surface antigens on a self-cell. Via Th cells, B cells are activated to produce antibody which not only destroys foreign but also self-antigen. In the middle example, self-antigens previously sequestered from the immune system (e.g. within a privileged environment) become available and induce an immune reaction via both antibody and cytotoxic cells. Bottom, a virus infection induces infected cells to express viral antigen at the surface; these cells are then destroyed by the immune reaction, typically mediated by cytotoxic cells.

Some pathogenic bacteria can produce **superantigens**, which first cause non-specific T-cell activation and therefore a polyclonal response, and can even bypass the need for T-cell activation by directly inducing polyclonal B-cell proliferation. In this instance the autoimmune component is global rather than directed, but nevertheless potentially very damaging to tissue.

A breakdown of normal host immune regulation can in various ways induce self-directed inflammation: the normal cytokine regulation system can become dysregulated so that normal regulator effects break down; APCs may persist for inappropriate periods because apoptosis is suppressed, allowing decline in tolerance of self-antigens.

It can be seen that potential mechanisms for autoimmunity are legion and new modes of breakdown of tolerance systems continue to be discovered. It may be that several are in effect simultaneously in any one disease. The above examples include both 'true', directed autoimmunity involving a specific self-antigen, and 'collateral' autoimmunity in which polyclonal expansion produces general tissue damage. Perhaps the term 'autoimmunity' should more accurately apply only to the former type, which requires a specific process of monoclonal immune cell activation.

Immunosuppression

It is possible to damage or reduce the efficiency of the cell-mediated immune system in several different ways; the medical challenge is to do this selectively so that the unwanted immune mechanism (autoimmune disease or transplant rejection) is affected, but the essential remainder of the immune system is not. One example of an extremely potent but inadequately specific treatment is Campath-1H (anti-CD52 monoclonal antibody), which rapidly removes virtually all lymphocytes from the circulation with very potent anti-inflammatory effects but causes high mortality from intercurrent infection. The division of lymphocytes during their initial clonal expansion can be retarded (but not yet aborted), although such drugs also prevent other essential cells from dividing. Various elements of the effector pathway of inflammation can be depressed, again non-selectively. Ideally a treatment that acts against, or defends, against only those lymphocyte clones reacting to self-antigens is needed. Increasingly selective forms of immunosuppression, predominantly in the field of biologics (monoclonal antibodies) are becoming available, and the practicalities of current and future treatment modalities are discussed in Chapter 6.

Immunodeficiency

The normal immune system is extremely complex. Occasionally one or more components of it are deficient. These problems can be inherited (primary) or acquired (secondary). Of most importance in the field of uveitis is AIDS. The human immunodeficiency virus (HIV), an RNA retrovirus, selectively infects Th cells, gradually depleting their number and leading to secondary immunodeficiency via increasing malfunction of the T-cell-mediated components of the immune system. The disease itself, and the opportunistic infections encountered as a result, are discussed in the relevant chapters.

The field of primary immune deficiency (requiring no external precipitator such as HIV infection) is immensely complex and, because of the high mortality associated with so many subtypes, primarily a pediatric specialty. Most of the severe forms predispose to overwhelming bacterial infection, but some that permit survival into adulthood, including T-cell cytopenias, may be associated with uveitis. The pathogenesis in these cases is obscure, and decision-making on therapeutic immunosuppression can be difficult.

The ocular immune environment

It is proven that some body tissues are much less susceptible to immune-mediated injury; clearly such tissues have developed special protection, and the brain and eye are examples. Put simply, an uncontrolled intraocular inflammatory response first would obliterate the transparent media and tissues that are fundamental to image transmission, and second would rapidly and permanently destroy the complex retinal anatomy. Local damage to this small spoonful of tissue would place the person more at risk than perhaps any other of similar size within the body, with the exception of the brain stem. Evolution has therefore developed an immunological protection method that is multifactorial, permitting the intraocular compartment to have **immune privilege**.

With the possible exception of exogenous bacterial endophthalmitis, virtually no form of intraocular inflammation is permitted to develop unconstrained – all inflammations are regulated by immune privilege. Understanding of the underlying immunological basis for this has, however, changed substantially. The historical presumption was that this was mainly a passive anatomical phenomenon: first that the eye had no effective lymphatic drainage (which is now known to be partially incorrect), and second that because of a functioning blood–ocular barrier the intraocular compartment had no intrinsic leukocyte exposure. This led to the assumption that the intraocular environment was simply 'hidden' from the immune system. Such was the basis for early theories on the initiation of sympathetic uveitis, which 'for the first time' exposed intraocular antigens to the immune system. These hypotheses are now known to be untrue. Nevertheless there are indeed structural components of ocular immune privilege: it is true that the blood–ocular barrier exists and provides a genuine barrier up to a point, that ocular lymphatic drainage is *virtually* absent and, importantly, the aqueous humor drains not into the lymphatics but into the bloodstream so that primed lymphocytes do not migrate directly to regional lymph nodes.

It is now clear that, although the intraocular compartment is anything but hidden from the immune system, it has special immunological properties that may suppress or modify some inflammatory responses. It is also clear that both migrant and resident ocular cells actively participate in immunological processes. In addition to macrophages and dendritic cells, which are numerous within the uveal tract (McMenamin 1997), RPE cells, Müller cells and intraocular vascular endothelium may all play a part. Müller cells are able to downregulate intraretinal inflammatory responses. RPE cells, in contrast, can be potent mediators and initiators of inflammation; they can become mobile, can phagocytose, will release free radicals and can produce IL-6, a powerful inflammatory mediator. In the presence of IFN-γ and TNF-α, they can express MHC class II antigens and can act as APCs. They can secrete IL-8, a leukocyte chemotactic, and can also express ICAM-1. The demonstrated functions of RPE cells make it clear that, in the correct circumstances, they may play a pivotal role in both the pathogenesis and the perpetuation of posterior uveitis. Uveal dendritic cells lie closely apposed to the RPE and it seems likely that they are the primary site of granuloma formation in some forms of multifocal posterior uveitis and the VKH syndrome.

Several intraocular antigens, normally protected from immune reactivity, are capable of leading to autoimmune inflammation. Interphotoreceptor-binding protein (IRBP) is involved in chemical transfer between RPE and photoreceptors, and retinal S-antigen arises from the photoreceptors themselves, being a component of the photo-induced enzyme cascade. Both are potent antigens capable of generating EAU when inoculated elsewhere. Other intraretinal molecules capable of inducing similar responses are rhodopsin, phosducin and recoverin, and soluble lens proteins have similar properties.

The experimental model of EAU has close similarities to several forms of human uveitis, and immune responses to retinal S-antigen have been detected in some patients with sympathetic uveitis, the VKH syndrome and several other uveitides. It is known that activated T cells are necessary for the development of posterior uveitis, but the mechanism of the breakdown in tolerance necessary for the initiation of inflammation is unknown.

The intraocular compartment is capable of modifying systemic immune responses. In fact there is no better demonstration of the interaction between the intraocular environment (previously presumed to be 'hidden') and the systemic immune system than the cardinal work of the late J Wayne Streilein's group (Eichorn et al. 1993) which by a series of elegant experiments demonstrated **anterior chamber-associated immune deviation** (ACAID): the normal response to unmatched allografting (e.g. a mouse skin graft) is rejection of the transplant. However, placing the same tissue within the anterior chamber of the eye of the graft recipient causes a depression of cell-mediated immunity and leads to tolerance of that allograft from the same donor placed elsewhere in the host. This principle also applies to intraocular inflammation, e.g. the inoculation of retinal antigens into a mouse footpad will normally lead to the development of EAU. However, the prior injection of the same antigens into the host anterior chamber will prevent the uveitis from developing. The mechanism of ACAID is unknown, but cytokines are involved, and the presence in aqueous humor of TGF-β, which is capable of downregulating immune responses, appears to be important; Tr cells are also upregulated. Aqueous humor is also known to suppress complement activation (Streilein 1997) and macrophage activity by macrophage migration inhibitory factor. Normal aqueous humor is known to contain a mixture of immunosuppressive cytokines including TGF-β, vasoactive intestinal peptide and α-melanocyte-stimulating hormone. These presumably provide a powerful barrier to local immune responses, but in eyes acutely inflamed, the cytokine mix is profoundly changed; whether this is the cause or the result is as yet unproven. The relevance (if any) of ACAID to uveitis is the subject of speculation, but the ACAID ability may well serve to downregulate the intraocular cell-mediated immune response to antigens as a means of reducing the local inflammatory response in so delicate an organ.

It is now known that ocular immune privilege is anything but passive: a complex immunological protective mechanism has evolved to permit limited immune intervention and inflammation where necessary but to attempt to prevent extensive damage by curtailing over-enthusiastic immune responses. These regulatory changes to adaptive immunity are both humoral and cellular. A greater understanding may permit better-directed approaches to the management of uveitis (Taylor and Kaplan 2010), which is especially important because it has been persuasively argued that some forms of uveitis, especially retinal autoimmunity, are an unavoidable consequence of immune privilege (Caspi 2006).

The anterior chamber is not the only locality capable of inducing tolerance to foreign antigen. Certain sites, particularly the oropharyngeal and gastrointestinal mucosa, are exposed to enormous numbers of foreign antigens, most of which are harmless. Tolerance to antigens may be induced locally at these sites, which are adjacent to the mucosa-associated lymphoid tissues (MALT). Via ingestion or inhalation of antigen, this mechanism (which is not entirely local, requiring a functional spleen) has been found to suppress the development, or even the continuation, of EAU (Nussenblatt et al. 1990). The prospect of orally or inhalation-induced tolerance for human patients with uveitis was initially exciting, but unfortunately clinical studies have shown an unimpressive effect. However, studies are ongoing and the addition of adjuvant such as cholera toxin B subunit to the selected antigen has been found to induce superior effect (Sun et al. 2010); perhaps the technique may again become therapeutically interesting.

REFERENCES

Caspi RR. Ocular autoimmunity: the price of privilege? *Immunol Rev* 2006;**213**:23–5.

Eichorn M, Horneber M, Streilein JW, et al. Anterior chamber associated immune deviation elicited via primate eyes. *Invest Ophthalmol Vis Sci* 1993;**34**:2926–30.

HeiligenhausA, Thurau S, Hennig M, et al. Anti-inflammatory treatment of uveitis with biologicals: new treatment options that reflect pathogenetic knowledge of the disease. *Graefes Arch Clin Exp Ophthalmol* 2010;**248**:1531–51.

McMenamin PG. The distribution of immune cells in the uveal tract of the normal eye. *Eye* 1997;**11**:183–93.

Mojana F, Kojak I, Oster SF, et al. Observations by spectral-domain ocular coherence tomography combined with simultaneous scanning laser ophthalmoscopy: imaging of the vitreous. *Am J Ophthalmol* 2010;**149**: 641–50.

Nussenblatt RB, Caspi RR, Mahdi R, et al. Inhibition of S-antigen-induced experimental autoimmune uveoretinitis by oral induction of tolerance with S-antigen. *J Immunol* 1990;**144**:1689–95.

Streilein JW. Regulation of ocular immune responses. *Eye* 1997;**11**:171–5.

Sun JB, Czerkinsky C, Holmgren J. Mucosally-induced immunological tolerance, regulatory T-cells and the adjuvant effect by cholera toxin B subunit. *Scand J Immunol* 2010;**71**:1–11.

Taylor AW, Kaplan HJ. Ocular immune privilege in the year 2010: ocular immune privilege and uveitis. *Ocul Immunol Inflamm* 2010;**18**:488–92.

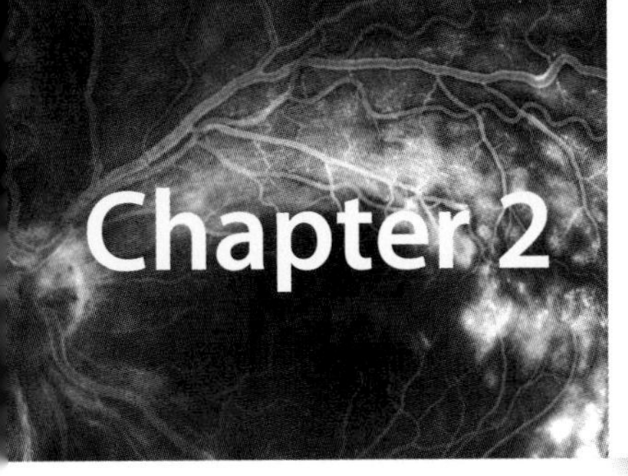

History, examination and ophthalmic imaging

HISTORY-TAKING

The busy practice of ophthalmology is such that most practitioners rarely use the skill, hard acquired at medical school, of constructing a comprehensive and structured history. Ophthalmological diagnosis is, more than in most specialties, a visual art, yet in the diagnosis of uveitis the patience to delve deeply into a medical history will reap frequent rewards. This process may be time-consuming. Many patients are diffident in reporting apparently irrelevant illnesses to an ophthalmologist, and yet these episodes, some forgotten, some never reported to a doctor, may be of great diagnostic importance. In some instances, only repeated and probing questions may prise out the important details of a history.

It is important to define clearly the presenting complaint; this in itself can be typical of a particular diagnosis. Except for those with acute presentations, patients often underestimate the duration of their symptoms, either because of an unsure memory or, in some cases, in the knowledge that they should really have come sooner. Some episodes may be recurrent, previous ones having been forgotten; perhaps the other eye was involved first. Some patients may admit to fluctuating symptoms that in retrospect may have started years earlier.

For every patient presenting with uveitis, it is important to enquire about general health. Some forms of uveitis are preceded or accompanied by specific systemic symptoms, perhaps a flu-like illness, a bowel upset or a skin rash with arthralgia. A systems review is important to identify any associated symptomatology, past or present, that could be associated with uveitis, but that many patients would not think to volunteer to an ophthalmologist. Some symptoms may have been misleadingly diagnosed and treated by another doctor, such as the occasional patient with sarcoidosis who has been treated for asthma. Previous diagnoses should therefore not be taken at face value; a clear picture of symptoms should be sought and previous medical records examined if necessary.

Other elements of the general history may be helpful in diagnosis; uveitis is not often a familial problem, but the inheritance of HLA-B27 is an exception, and familial cases of Behçet's disease, sarcoidosis, heterochromic uveitis, multiple sclerosis and acute posterior multifocal placoid pigment epitheliopathy (APMPPE) are well known. Some infections, particularly tuberculosis, show a history of family contact. Some racial groups are more prone to certain types of uveitis, e.g. sarcoidosis in black people and, in Japanese individuals, Behçet's disease and the Vogt–Koyanagi–Harada (VKH) syndrome. Some forms of uveitis are almost confined to certain populations, e.g. again in Japanese individuals, HTLV-I (human T-lymphotropic virus I)-associated uveitis.

There may, for a variety of reasons, be a sex bias to some forms of uveitis, including sarcoidosis, toxocariasis, tuberculosis and several multifocal retinochoroidopathies. Some forms of uveitis have well-defined age ranges: toxocariasis, juvenile chronic arthritis and APMPPE are examples. Recent foreign travel may expose the patient to new antigens (e.g. Gram-negative bacillary dysentery leading to reactive arthropathy and uveitis) and some forms of uveitis are seen within limited areas (such as the presumed ocular histoplasmosis syndrome) or in particular environments (e.g. Lyme borreliosis).

On occasion the sexual history of the patient must be explored. It may be necessary to ascertain the risk of HIV infection; although the great majority of HIV-positive patients presenting to an ophthalmologist are already aware of their diagnosis, the ophthalmologist will occasionally have to broach the subject anew. In some uveitides, the possibility of intravenous drug abuse should be explored, and sometimes an initial denial is reversed only after an examination of the scarred antecubital fossae.

The wide-ranging systemic associations of uveitis have engendered patient health questionnaires in various units including our own. For new patients, the opportunity to remember potentially relevant events and to present the information when attending for the first time may be helpful. The Manchester Uveitis Clinic New Patient Questionnaire is available as a supplement to this text (see patient information pamphlets on the attached disk).

OCULAR EXAMINATION

Some patients have uveitis for many years, and accurate and repeatable assessments of their status are of great importance in maintaining effective treatment with minimum risk. The diligent and structured recording of examination data is therefore crucial. The quantification of activity is one aspect of this. Several methods of quantification have been devised, and each is meritorious, but the selection of a particular method of quantification is perhaps of lesser importance than the repeatability of a method for a single patient from visit to visit, often involving several ophthalmologists. Accurate, labeled drawings of anterior segment and fundus are a great help in the follow-up of patients with uveitis, whereas hasty and careless sketches are at best an irritation, and at worst dangerously misleading. Photography, the images being either stored with patient records or otherwise readily available for comparison, is often helpful.

Visual acuity

The assessment of disease activity, and the observation of subtle macular edema, can be challenging in those with chronic uveitis. For this reason, the careful measurement of visual acuity is of great importance in the monitoring of progress. The assessment of best-corrected acuity is particularly significant in patients who may demonstrate several causes of visual loss, and therefore regular refraction is helpful, especially in those with chronic uveitis.

The Snellen chart is widely used to assess distance acuity, but suffers from the disadvantage of being an insensitive indicator of acuity change in the upper half of the chart (6/18–6/60) because of the small number of letters available (**Fig. 2.1**). In this clinic the LogMAR chart (**Fig. 2.2**) is used, which includes five letters at each acuity level and therefore allows more sensitive incremental recording of acuity. For such sensitive recording of acuity, particular attention must be paid to the reproducibility of ambient lighting levels. The measurement of near acuity is frequently omitted, but is a valuable indicator of macular function and seems to be a good marker of the progress of macular edema. It should be a routine part of acuity assessment in a uveitis clinic.

High-contrast acuity testing is repeatable and accepted as the monitoring method of choice. However, some argue that real-life vision

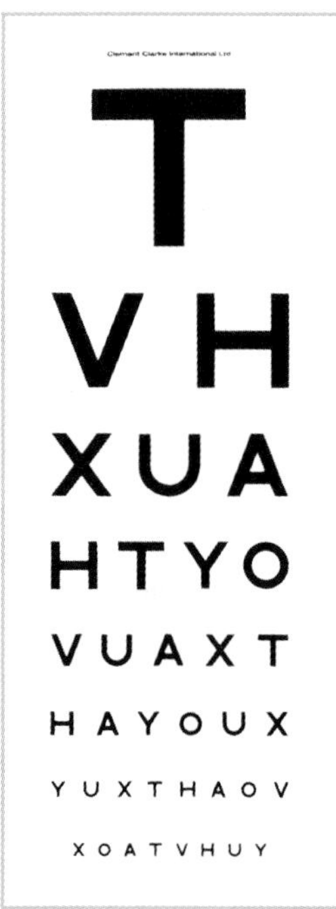

Figure 2.1 Standard illuminated 6-meter Snellen visual acuity chart.

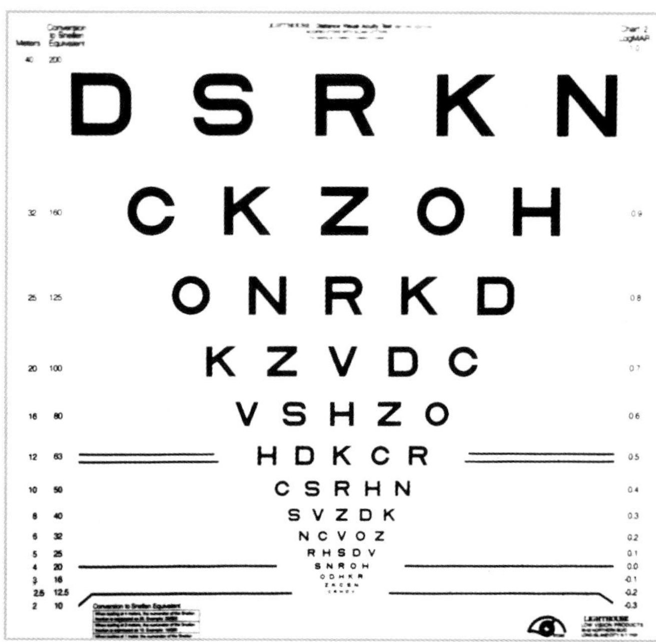

Figure 2.2 LogMAR 4-meter illuminated visual acuity chart.

can be reflected only by contrast acuity testing. In some assessments of visual function the Pelli–Robson chart may be helpful (Gardiner et al. 2002) but it is not routinely used in our clinic and is largely limited to research use.

Intraocular pressure

The measurement of intraocular pressure (IOP) is an essential component of ocular examination in every patient with uveitis. Sudden rises may occur, even in those with previously stable IOP over a long period. Applanation tonometry is preferable and most children can, with care and persistence, be taught to accept applanation as a normal part of ocular examination. However, sometimes this is not possible and non-applanation tonometry, although somewhat less accurate, is an acceptable alternative in this age group. We have found that rebound tonometers are better tolerated and easier to use than air-puff tonometry in children.

Topical fluorescein penetrates the anterior chamber quite rapidly, and the greenish tinge within the anterior chamber (AC) mimics protein flare. This should be borne in mind when assessing inflammation after instillation. If necessary it is entirely possible to perform applanation tonometry in white light without the use of fluorescein.

Slit-lamp biomicroscopy

The best quality slit-lamp biomicroscopes, used under ideal conditions, allow unsurpassed viewing capability. However, there is great variability in design and in performance. Most ophthalmologists are strong supporters of either parallel or converging eyepiece systems and the different depth perceptions that they can produce, the choice often being somewhat dependent on their own exophoria. All good slit-lamps have a wide variability in the brightness of illumination, which is particularly important for estimating aqueous and vitreous opacification; the worst slit-lamps do not. Convenient systems for rapid changes in magnification are useful, and the ability to tilt or decenter the viewing angle is occasionally important. The siting of the slit-lamp in a position that allows practical ambient illumination, with comfort for both patient and examiner, is essential.

Our own studies on slit-lamp illumination capability have shown a wide range in maximum luminance, between manufacturer types and in the same type between new and old bulbs. The task of recording AC inflammation accurately is rendered more challenging by these variations. When in doubt, the usefulness of switching off ambient illumination cannot be over-estimated.

Conjunctiva, episclera and sclera

The distribution of redness in an inflamed eye is best estimated with the naked eye and a pen-torch, but in some circumstances a critical examination using the slit-lamp is useful. Magnification and slit-beam illumination can clarify which plexus of vessels is inflamed, and can confirm episcleritis or scleritis (**Fig. 2.3**), which may be associated with uveitis. Conjunctival vessel shutdown (**Fig. 2.4**) or curlicue formation is a feature of some vasculitic or connective tissue diseases that may present with uveitis. Ciliary injection is of course a classic sign of iris or corneal inflammation although it may vary in severity or extent (**Fig. 2.5**).

Cornea

The cornea may be involved in several forms of uveitis: epithelial ulceration and/or stromal keratitis will accompany herpetic keratouveitis (**Fig. 2.6**); keratoneuritis may be seen in acanthamoeba keratouveitis; interstitial keratitis (**Fig. 2.7**) is now rare in syphilis but is a feature of Cogan's syndrome; and sclerokeratitis may accompany uveitis in the connective tissue diseases. Corneal endothelial changes, including guttata, may follow chronic uveitis. Localized corneal decompensation (**Fig. 2.8**) is an unusual manifestation of Fuchs' heterochromic uveitis, and also of the rare corneal endotheliitis, and in both conditions a peripheral whitish opacification of Descemet's membrane is visible. Generalized decompensation is fortunately very uncommon in uveitis but may require keratoplasty.

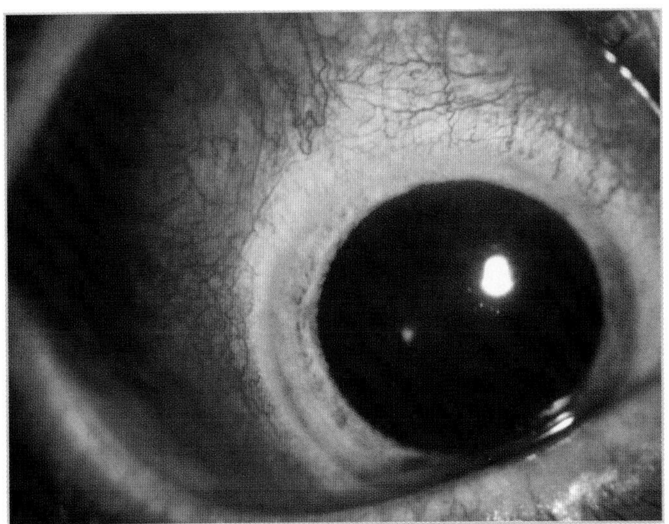

Figure 2.3 Diffuse scleritis and episcleritis associated with anterior uveitis.

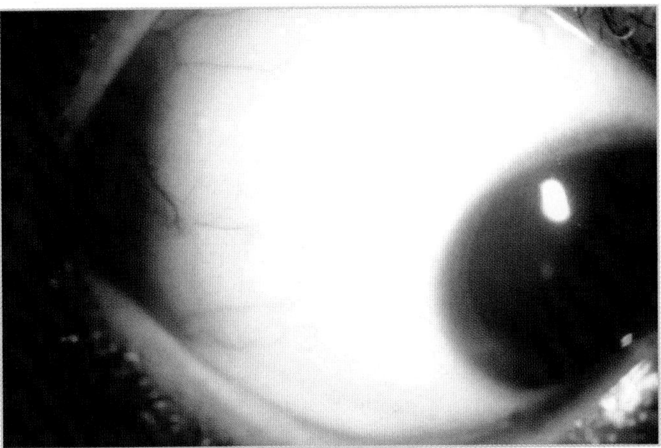

Figure 2.4 Widespread conjunctival vessel shutdown in a patient with systemic lupus erythematosus.

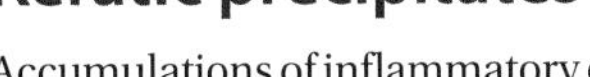

Keratic precipitates

Accumulations of inflammatory cells adherent to corneal endothelium are a feature of all forms of anterior uveitis, but their position, quantity, shape, size, color and activity can all contribute to the process of diagnosis.

Position

In the great majority of patients with acute uveitis, most or all keratic precipitates (KPs) are adherent to the inferior cornea, sometimes in a fine vertical spindle, or more often in a base-down pyramidal distribution (**Fig. 2.9**). It is assumed that this position is a result of aqueous convection currents, probably more pronounced when fuelled by a warmer iris containing engorged, inflamed blood vessels. Even in those with chronic uveitis with larger KPs, the great majority are invariably on the inferior endothelium (**Fig. 2.10**). The distribution of KPs in Fuchs' heterochromic uveitis (and, uncommonly, in some with intermediate uveitis) is therefore a stark contrast; although there is often a slight preponderance inferiorly, KPs are usually scattered over the whole endothelium (**Fig. 2.11**). This leads one to hypothesize that the deposition of KPs in Fuchs' heterochromic uveitis may be by an entirely different mechanism than that in other forms of uveitis.

Local inflammation leads to local KPs : disciform keratitis will accumulate precipitates underneath the affected area, as will localized endotheliopathy. The sentinel KPs in Posner–Schlossman syndrome may be located near the angle, reflecting the probable associated trabeculitis.

Quantity

In acute unilateral iridocyclitis, KPs may be myriad; in chronic 'granulomatous' uveitis or Fuchs' heterochromic uveitis they may be very numerous; in the Posner–Schlossman syndrome by contrast they are usually very few, but prominent (**Fig. 2.12**) and are often inferior and peripheral. The gradual disappearance of KPs follows successful treatment of uveitis, but their disappearance, as with their accumulation, follows some time after changes in AC inflammation.

Shape and size

KPs in acute iridocyclitis are usually tiny, resembling a superfine dust on the endothelium; those in 'granulomatous' uveitis may be very large

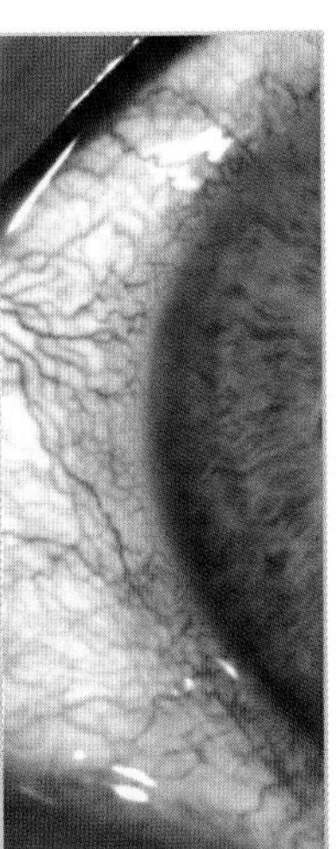

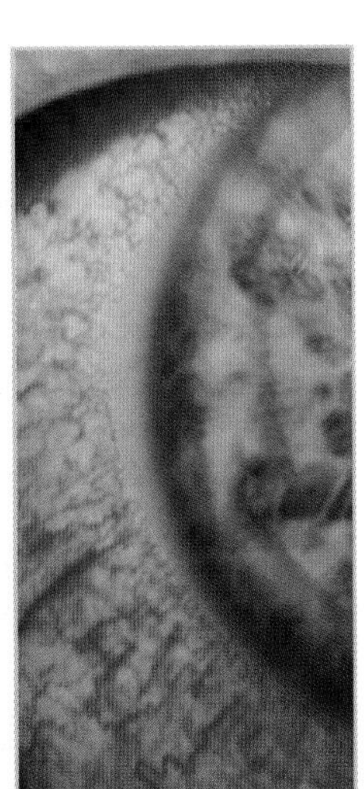

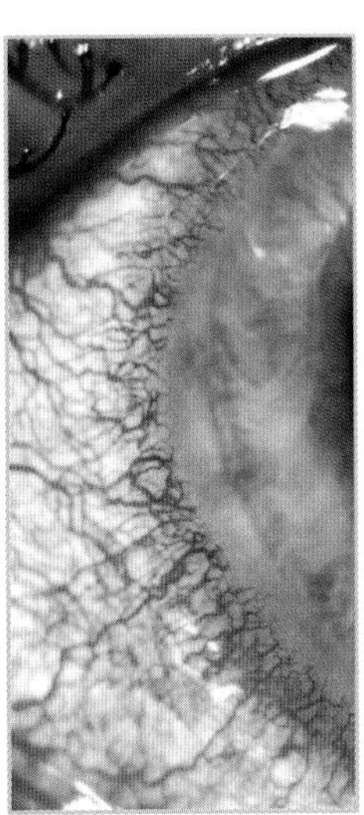

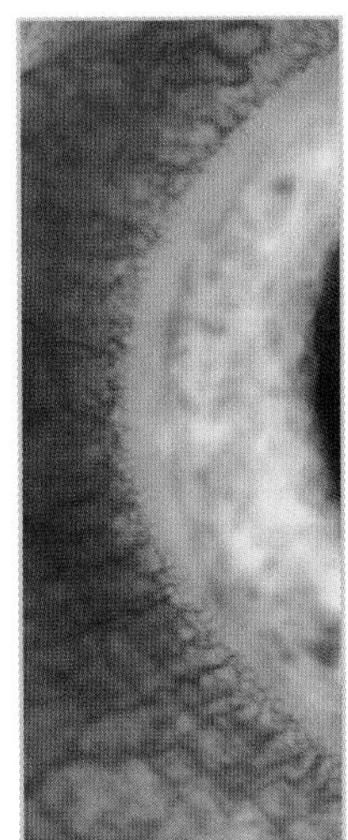

Figure 2.5 Four eyes with acute anterior uveitis showing varying degrees of ciliary injection.

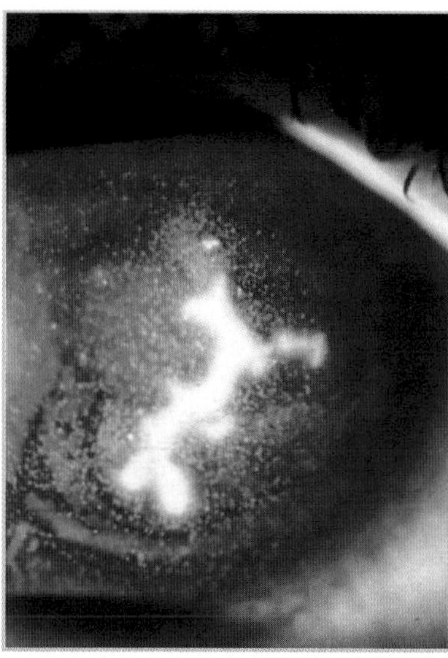

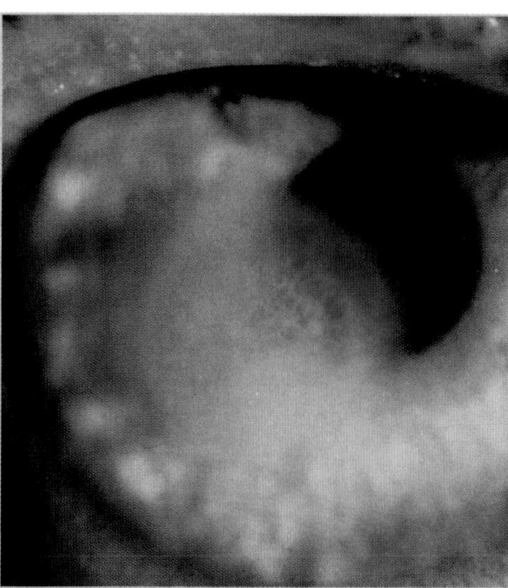

Figure 2.6 Signs of herpetic keratitis; dendritic epithelial ulceration and old disciform keratitis.

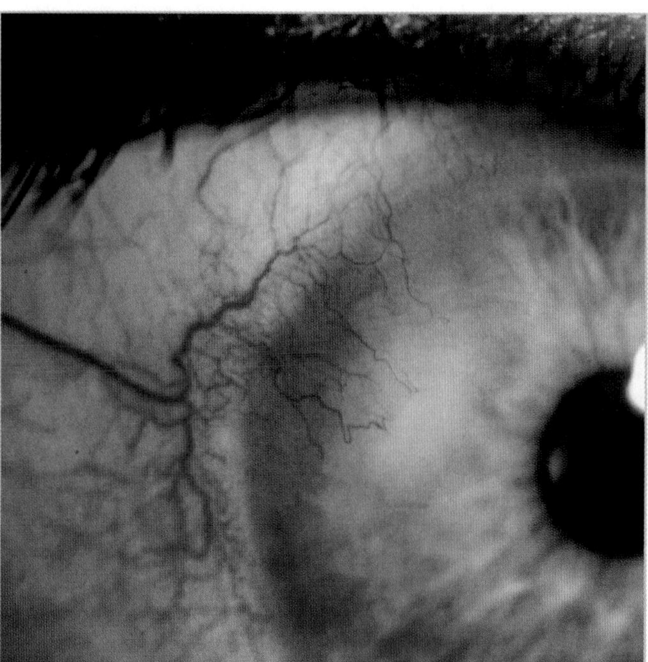

Figure 2.7 Active interstitial keratitis with both superficial and stromal corneal neovascularization.

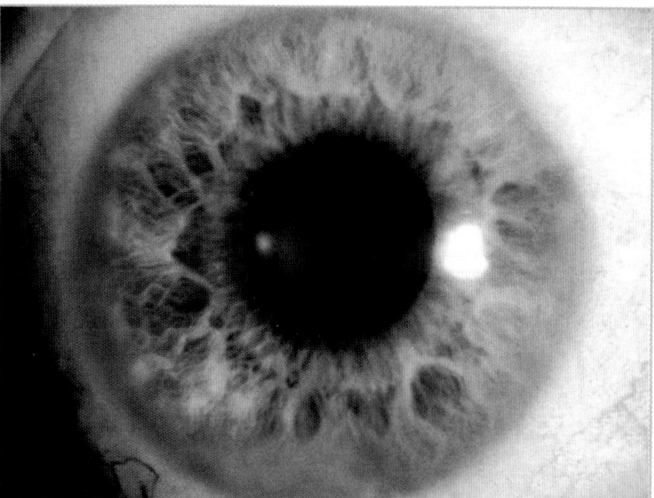

Figure 2.8 Inferior localized corneal decompensation in an eye affected by Fuchs' heterochromic uveitis.

(**Fig. 2.13**), roundish but often irregular in outline, and with a grayish or creamy translucency that has been likened to 'mutton fat'; when severe and chronic they may be virtually confluent. Smaller granular KPs may, however, also be seen in sarcoidosis (**Fig. 2.14**). The KPs in Fuchs' heterochromic uveitis are large enough to show individual shape and, although many are roundish and pearly translucent, some are strikingly 'stellate,' with projections that seem to extend for a considerable distance over the endothelium. Under very high magnification, tiny fibrillary structures may be seen running across the endothelium, although it is unclear whether these are a continuum with the KPs themselves (**Fig. 2.15**). Rarely a patient is seen with most peculiar large branching KPs. They should be treated with suspicion; we have anecdotally encountered intraocular lymphoma with this presentation (**Fig. 2.16**).

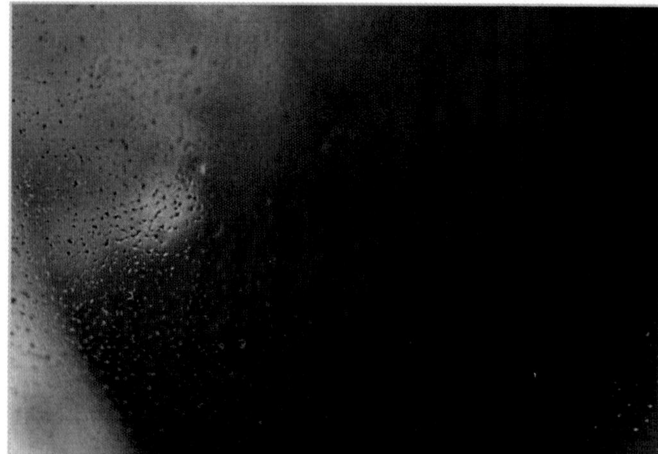

Figure 2.9 Fine keratic precipitates on inferior corneal endothelium in acute anterior uveitis.

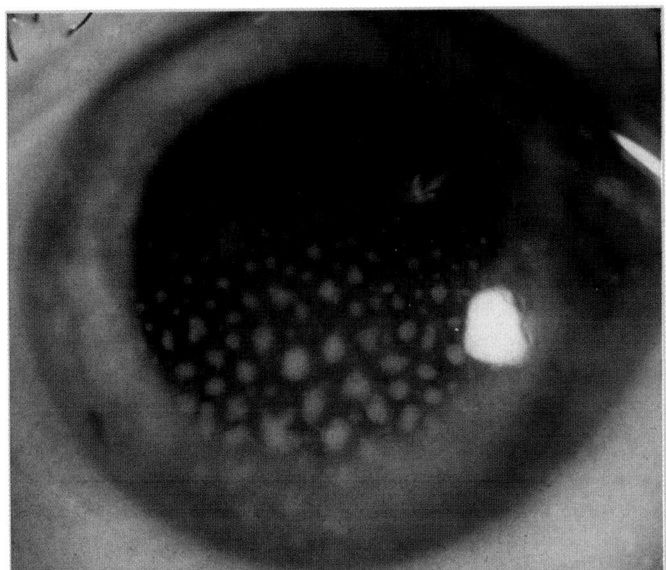

Figure 2.10 Mutton-fat type keratic precipitates in an eye with sarcoid-associated uveitis.

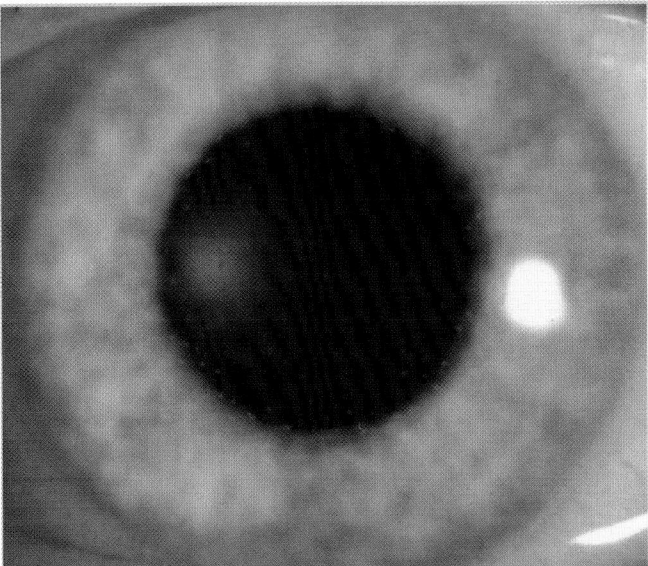

Figure 2.11 In Fuchs' heterochromic uveitis the keratic precipitates are usually spread over the whole endothelium.

Traditionally, large, 'mutton-fat'-type KPs have been described as 'granulomatous.' This is not a histological description of their structure, but describes their perceived association with granulomatous disease, emanating from a time when tuberculosis and syphilis were much more common. Following the decline in these diseases some have suggested that the term is now archaic and should be discarded. Nevertheless, in this clinic, KPs of this type are more frequently an indicator of sarcoidosis (a granulomatous disease) than of any other diagnosis and, in the absence of a better term, the current one is adequately understood and best retained.

Color and activity

All active KPs large enough to examine individually, have form and a variable degree of opacification. Most KPs disappear entirely, but some leave their 'imprint' permanently, either in the form of a blob of uveal pigment or a tiny granular structure, or as a flat, damaged area of Descemet's membrane (usually bare of endothelium when examined with the specular microscope) large enough to be visible on the slit-lamp. It is clearly important to distinguish such archaeological artifacts from active inflammation. Those forms of uveitis that include uveal depigmentation [including, for instance, heterochromic uveitis and VKH syndrome (**Fig. 2.17a**)] may create pigmented KPs, the residue of which may persist for life (**Fig. 2.17b**) and do not indicate current activity. However, cytomegalovirus (CMV)-associated anterior uveitis in contrast deposits a multitude of pigmented KPs early in its course (**Fig. 2.17c**), and the degree of associated AC activity will make it clear that the disease is most certainly active. Finally, the strange large corneal endothelial plaques that are seen in a few patients with Fuchs'

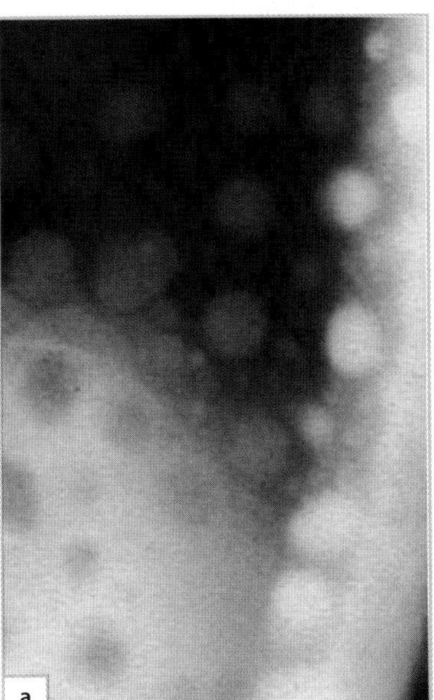

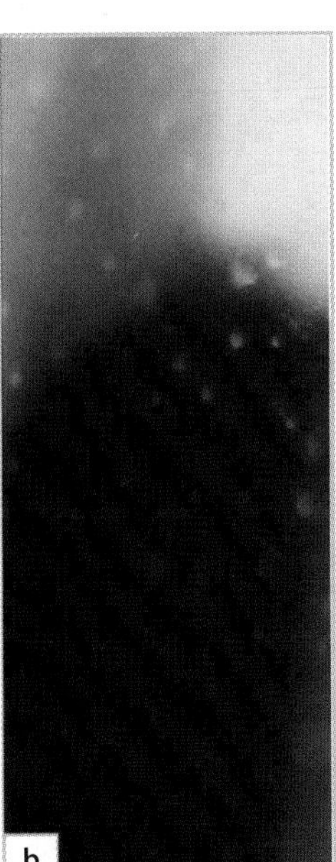

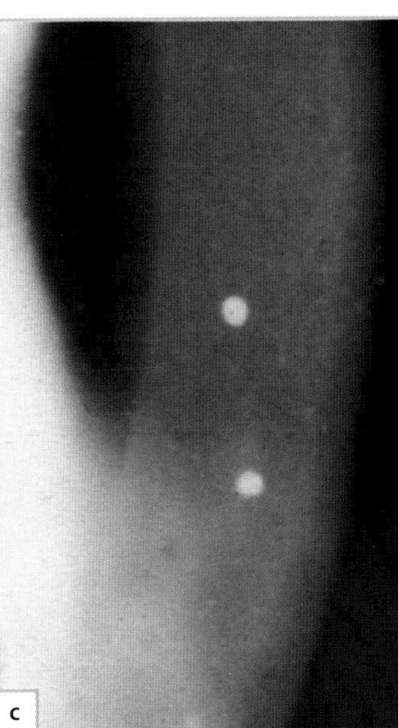

Figure 2.12 The typical keratic precipitates in (a) granulomatous uveitis, (b) heterochromic uveitis and (c) the Posner–Schlossman syndrome.

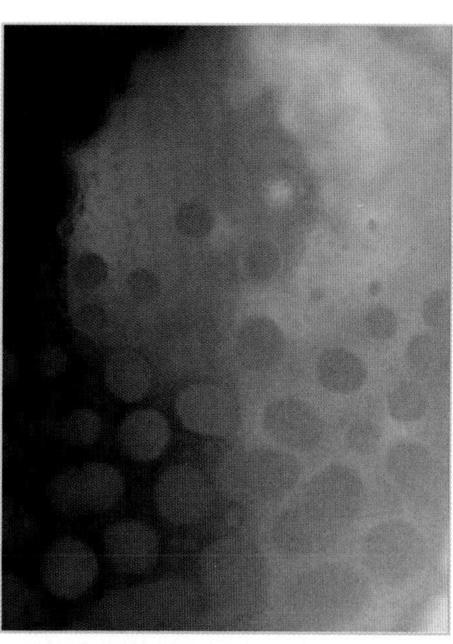

Figure 2.13 Large 'greasy' keratic precipitates in tuberculosis.

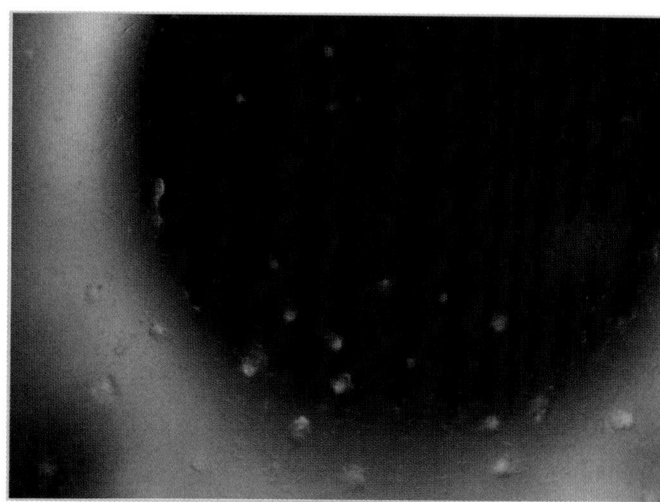

Figure 2.15 The typical morphology of keratic precipitates in heterochromic uveitis: irregular-shaped, sometimes stellate, pearly translucent with tiny fibrils on the intervening endothelium.

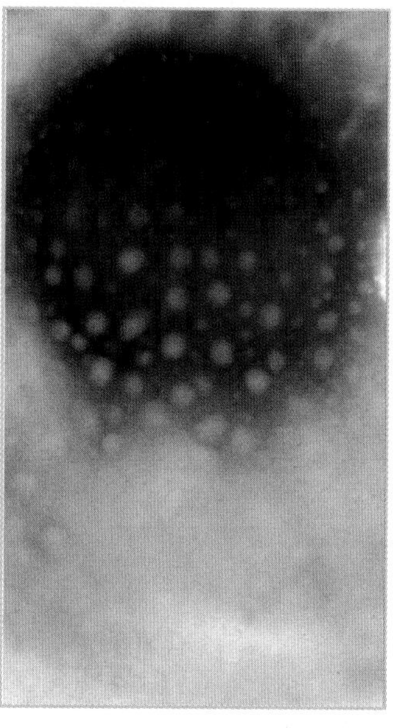

Figure 2.14 Two eyes with sarcoidosis: on the left, small granular keratic precipitates (KPs); on the right, more typical mutton-fat KPs.

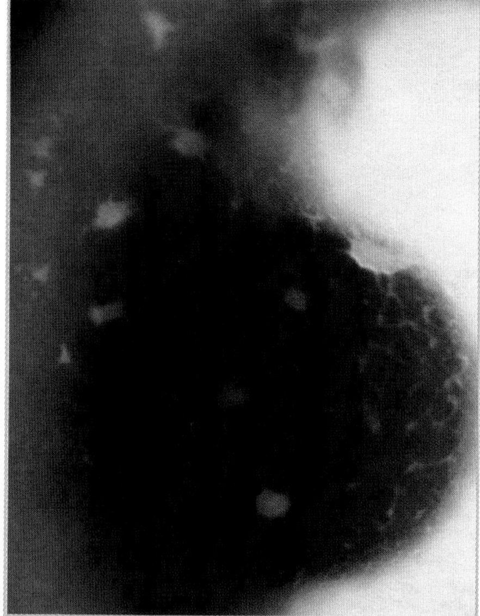

Figure 2.16 The bizarre keratic precipitates in a patient who subsequently died of primary central nervous system/ ocular lymphoma.

heterochromic uveitis (**Fig. 2.18**) should be mentioned; cell bare on specular microscopy, they are too large to correspond to areas previously covered by KPs and their origin is unknown.

Anterior chamber

Cells and flare

The anterior chamber, an extracellular fluid compartment, is normally free of cells, the barrier being the tight junctions of iris vessels. During inflammation of the iris and ciliary body, inflammatory cells migrate into that extracellular space and become visible by slit-lamp biomicroscopy. Cellular activity within the aqueous humor is therefore a sensitive, although indirect and slightly delayed, marker of anterior uveitis. Although occasionally a cell or two are seen in those without inflammation (especially after mydriasis) the presence of several cells is abnormal.

Aqueous humor contains very low levels of protein (10 mg/100 ml) in comparison to plasma (7 g/100 ml), and therefore aqueous is essentially transparent. A greater level of aqueous protein, leaked from inflamed and porous uveal blood vessels, gives aqueous humor a 'flare' of opacification. Except under the most stringent lighting conditions, aqueous flare is not seen in non-inflamed eyes. However, topical fluorescein may mimic flare, and therefore estimations of flare should be carried out before the measurement of intraocular pressure (IOP). Very low flare levels are detectable only after removing ambient lighting.

The assessment of AC activity is most easily performed by directing a bright (the brightest available setting) but narrow slit of light into the AC at 45° to the angle of view, to highlight suspended cells and protein flare (**Fig. 2.19**). A reduction in ambient lighting can substantially affect the ophthalmologist's estimation of activity; lowered lighting levels are therefore important for this component of the ocular examination. Estimation of cell count is facilitated by a darker background, and the pupil is better than the iris for this purpose. Eyes with chronic

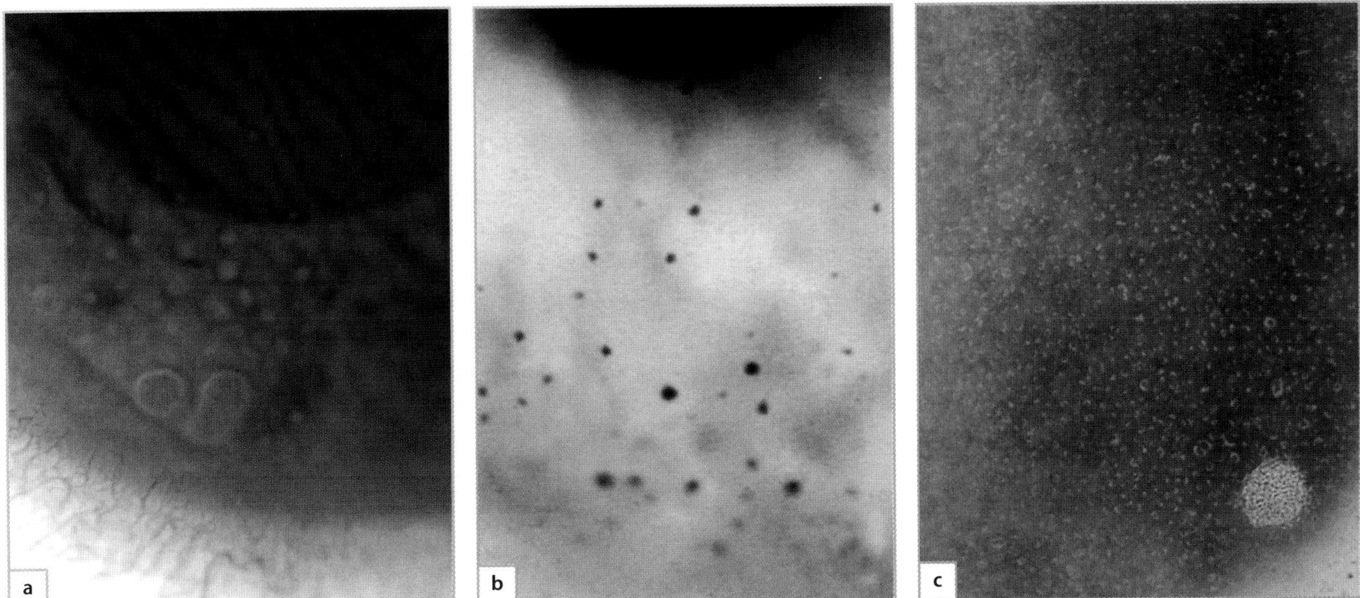

Figure 2.17 Pigmented keratic precipitates in three eyes: (a) in acute Vogt–Koyanagi–Harada syndrome, (b) in longstanding Fuchs' heterochromic uveitis and (c) in chronic cytomegalovirus anterior uveitis.

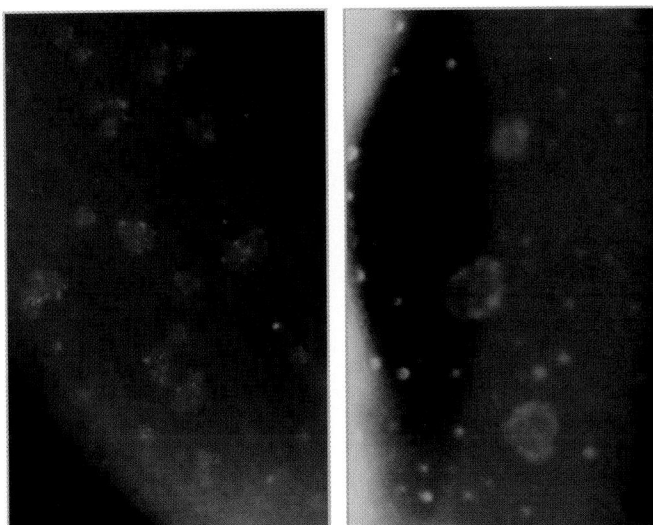

Figure 2.18 Corneal plaques in two eyes with heterochromic uveitis.

uveitis and pupillary membrane may not provide a dark background for activity estimation, which can therefore be difficult.

Estimates of AC activity can vary widely between observers, and methods of recording activity may be inconsistent. These measurements are important, and efforts should always be made to improve consistency. The individual observer should aim to use an identical method for each observation, including ambient lighting, beam angle, height, width and brightness, and method of recording, and ophthalmologists working within the same clinic should ensure interobserver consistency as far as is possible. To facilitate consistency, several methods of quantification have been devised and, although superficially similar, all rely on individual interpretation, including the most commonly used (BenEzra et al. 1991). Systems that rely on an actual cell count within a narrow stationary beam (usually 1 mm × 1 mm) are sensitive for lower levels of inflammation, but become less quantifiable at higher cell counts. To standardize measurements of inflammation and other parameters used in uveitis publications, a standardization of uveitis nomenclature (SUN) was published in 2005 (Jabs et al. 2005) The system continues in practice to estimate the number of AC cells at higher levels, but assumes (correctly or not) the

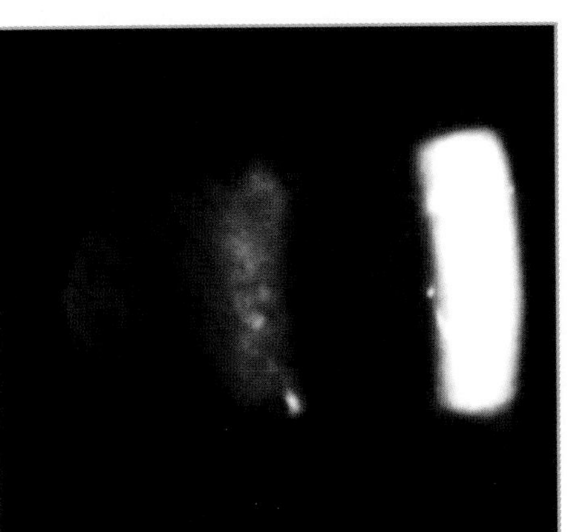

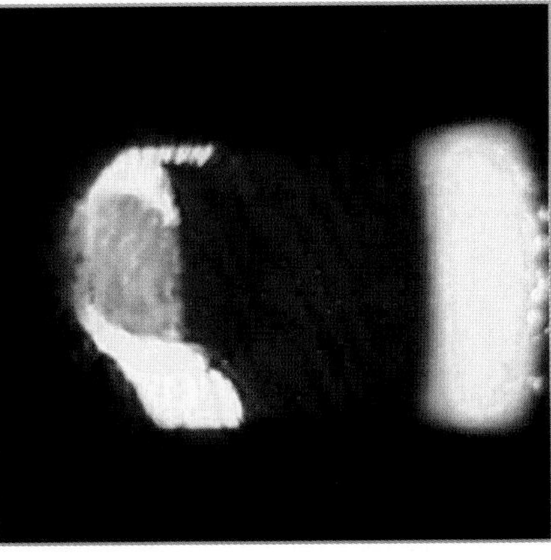

Figure 2.19 Two eyes under treatment for acute HLA-B27-associated uveitis: on the left, flare +, cells ±, on the right, flare ++, cells ++.

observer's ability to fit such estimates into numerical categories. This system is shown in **Table 2.1** alongside the system used clinically by the author's institution.

Flare is caused by the leakage of protein into aqueous humor, because of a breakdown of the blood–ocular barrier. Such an event is frequently part of the acute or chronic inflammatory process, but inflammation is not necessarily present. In some forms of chronic uveitis, particularly the uveitis seen in association with juvenile chronic arthritis, permanent breakdown of the blood–ocular barrier ensues, with aqueous flare that is unresponsive to topical steroids. In such circumstances, the presence of flare cannot be used as an indicator of activity. Nevertheless it is important; if substantial it will continue to predispose to adhesions and will substantially affect attempts at surgical intervention. The SUN system is based on subjective observation and is shown in **Table 2.2**. It is very similar to previous systems including our own.

Devices to measure AC flare and cells

Various devices are available to measure objectively the scatter of laser directed into aqueous humor. Such devices are more sensitive at low levels of flare, have high consistency, are of proven value in clinical research and have improved with development. Although more reliable than human observation at low levels of activity, such devices have yet to identify their place in the routine clinical appraisal of uveitis patients; put simply, despite the enthusiasm of some ophthalmologists (Wakefield et al. 2010), the expense and time required to undertake the process in busy uveitis services have not convinced the majority. Fluorophotometry is a non-invasive method of quantifying blood–ocular barrier breakdown, and measures fluorescein leakage from circulation into the anterior or posterior segment. It is useful as a research tool in the quantification of uveitis.

Fibrin deposition, hypopyon and hyphema

Some forms of uveitis, particularly acute recurrent iridocyclitis associated with HLA-B27, are characterized by severe breakdown of the blood–ocular barrier, with leakage of substantial quantities of plasma protein into aqueous humor. Such 'plasmoid' aqueous humor impedes the thermal circulation of AC cells which may appear almost to be suspended as though in a gel. Fibrinogen is the longest of the plasma protein molecules. If the inflamed iris blood vessels are sufficiently 'leaky,' the AC may contain enough fibrinogen to coagulate into a fibrin clot (**Fig. 2.20**). Fibrin formation in acute uveitis also causes widespread adhesions including both anterior and posterior synechiae (**Fig. 2.21**), and web-like strands may form within the AC.

In some cases of anterior uveitis the leakage of protein is not so prominent, but there are very substantial numbers of inflammatory cells, which, in the absence of a fibrin mass, sink to form an inferior white pool, a hypopyon (**Fig. 2.22**). Behçet's disease is characterized by explosive neutrophil and macrophage migration but without fibrinogen leakage, and in this disease the hypopyon may be entirely mobile because of the absence of clot. Sometimes small hypopyons are visible only on gonioscopy. In severe HLA-B27-related uveitis there may also be an inferior collection of white cells, but typically embedded in an amorphous mass of fibrin clot, with an irregular top. Again in HLA-B27-related uveitis, very severe blood–ocular barrier breakdown can cause

Table 2.1 Quantification of anterior chamber cellular activity

SUN system (cells counted in 1 mm x 1 mm beam)*		Manchester Royal Eye Hospital clinical system	
0	< 1		No cells seen on scanning the whole anterior chamber
Trace:	So few cells that all within the anterior chamber could easily be counted (alternative – state total cells seen in anterior chamber)		
0.5+	1–5	±	Very few cells within a narrow beam
1+	6–15	+	Cells numerous but countable within a narrow beam
2+	16–25	++	Cells very numerous – a severe uveitis
3+	26–50	+++	Cells very concentrated within a narrow beam – very severe uveitis
4+	> 50	++++	An exceptional number of cells, seen rarely in only the most severe anterior uveitis
Hypopyon	Record separately		Measure vertical central depth; if irregular, draw or photograph

[a]Adapted in part from Jabs et al. (2005).

Table 2.2 Quantification of anterior chamber flare and protein deposition

SUN system (cells counted in 1 mm x 1 mm beam)[a]		Manchester Royal Eye Hospital clinical system	
0	None		No flare visible under low ambient lighting
±	Flare only just visible under low ambient lighting	±	Flare only just visible under low ambient lighting
1+	Faint	+	Significant flare, visible with low room lighting
2+	Moderate (iris details clear)	++	Prominent flare, but not affecting the view of the iris
3+	Marked (iris details hazy)	+++	Substantial flare, enough to slightly blur the details of the iris; there may also be fibrin deposition
4+	Intense (often with fibrin or plastic aqueous	++++	An exceptional level of flare, usually only seen in association with very substantial plasmoid changes (the anterior chamber cells seem suspended and immobile)
Fibrin	If present, draw or photograph	Fibrin	If present, draw or photograph

[a]Adapted in part from Jabs et al. (2005).

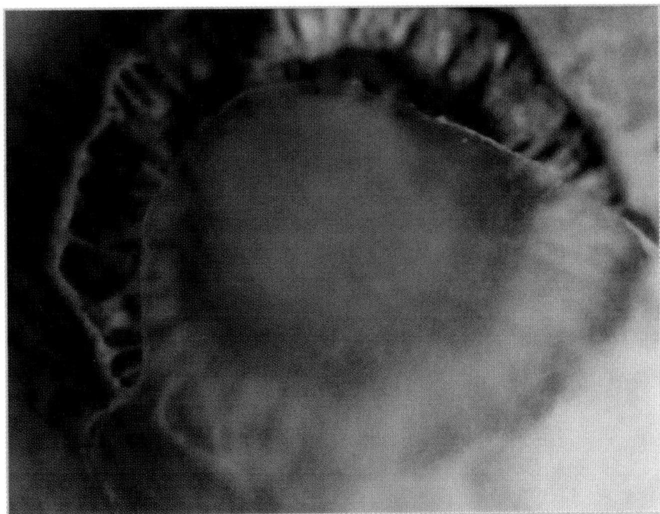

Figure 2.20 A large fibrin clot has formed during an acute recurrence of iridocyclitis in HLA-B27-associated uveitis. After several days of intensive topical steroid it is starting to reabsorb.

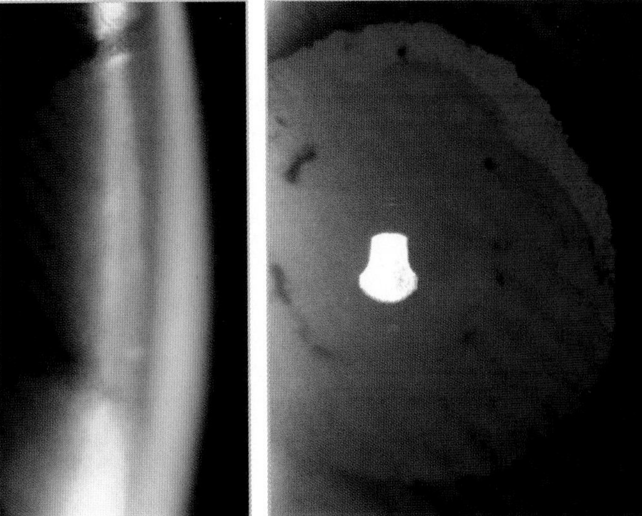

Figure 2.21 Fibrinous deposits during acute iridocyclitis have formed a pupil membrane that is being detached by intensive mydriasis and topical steroid.

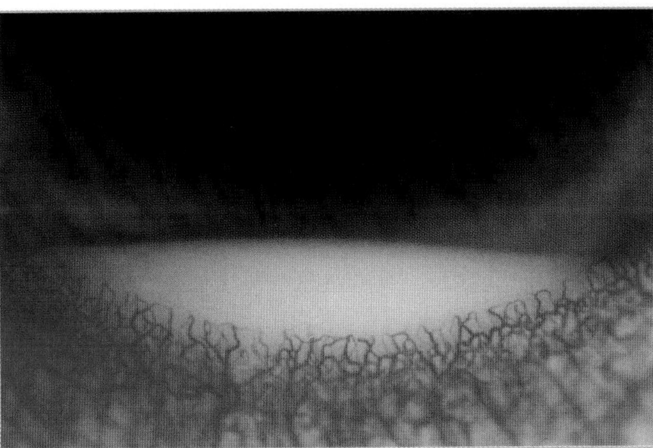

Figure 2.22 A large hypopyon during an acute flare-up of Behçet's disease. There is no fibrin, and it is 'clean' and white with a horizontal top.

erythrocytes to leak, and there will be blood within the fibrin clot and a bloody hyphema (**Fig. 2.23**). Unless the characteristics of HLA-B27-associated uveitis are clear, a bloody hypopyon should be treated with suspicion as a possible sign of infection or leukemia, and an AC tap will be necessary. Blood in a hypopyon is also considered a sign of possible herpetic uveitis.

Iris and pupil

Signs of acute inflammation

Identifiable structural iris changes during acute inflammation are unusual, but the extravasation of fluid and protein may sometimes cause a subtle swelling of iris stroma, which may blunt the fibrillary radial structure. Pupil reactions may become sluggish simply because of this mechanical effect. The AC reaction will be the prominent feature in such cases and this makes iris observation less clear. Uncommonly, a translucent sheet of inflammatory cells covers the anterior iris surface and this again may be missed. In very severe iridocyclitis, bleeding into the iris stroma (**Fig. 2.24**) may occur, for the same reason as the hyphema discussed above, and again most commonly in severe HLA-B27-associated iridocyclitis.

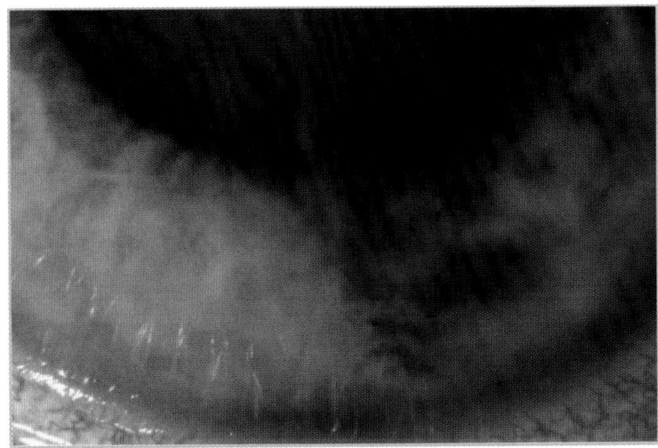

Figure 2.23 Blood and fibrinous exudate are mixed in this eye with severe HLA-B27-associated iridocyclitis.

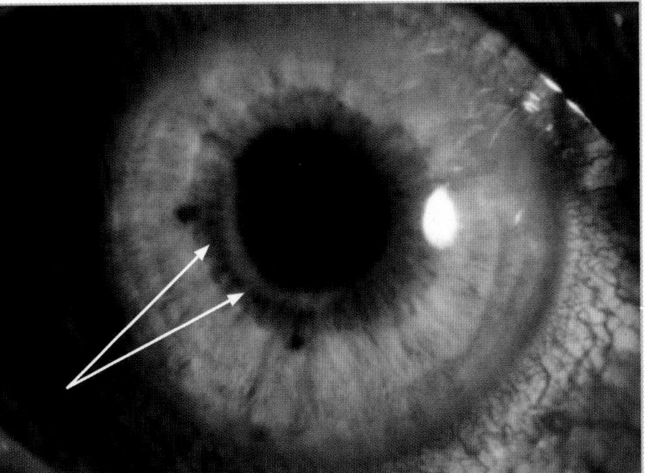

Figure 2.24 Bleeding into the iris stroma is an unusual feature of severe breakdown of blood–ocular barrier in acute anterior uveitis. A hypopyon is also seen.

Iris atrophy, transillumination and heterochromia

Any layer of the iris may become atrophic during anterior uveitis, and this atrophy may be patchy or generalized. Atrophy and depigmentation of the anterior border layer, that mesenchymal condensation of anterior stroma, is typical of Fuchs' heterochromic uveitis (**Fig. 2.25**) but may also occur, in a more subtle way, in the Posner–Schlossman syndrome and in intermediate uveitis. The visibility of such heterochromic atrophy is largely a function of the pre-existing iris color; irides that are blue–grey may become very atrophic without significant change in color; thickly pigmented brown irides require profound stromal atrophy before any color change is detectable; by contrast, the iris that has an orange–brown anterior border layer on top of a blue stroma may show striking heterochromia if affected by Fuchs' heterochromic uveitis; in this situation, one blue and one brown iris may be seen (**Fig. 2.26**).

Iris stromal atrophy is a late feature of Fuchs' heterochromic uveitis, but is less helpful in diagnostic terms, being seen in may eyes with chronic uveitis. Loss of parts of the posterior pigmented epithelium, leading to transillumination defects, may accompany any chronic anterior uveitis, and detached posterior synechiae often leave pigmented debris attached to the lens, with corresponding transillumination defects of adjacent iris, which are permanent. Iris adjacent to posterior synechiae is in any case often 'moth eaten' and atrophic (**Fig. 2.27**). In heterochromic uveitis of long standing, pigment epithelial atrophy also occurs, and the pattern is typical of this form of uveitis (although the pattern is also seen in pigment dispersion syndrome): loss of the pupillary ruff and transillumination of the thinnest parts of pigment epithelium – around the pupil and in the iris periphery (**Fig. 2.28**). Sectoral atrophy of all layers is characteristic of herpetic uveitis and may lead to sectoral depigmentation, denervation of the pupil sphincter giving irregular mydriasis, excavated stromal atrophy and sectoral transillumination (**Fig. 2.29**).

Iris nodules and crystals

Nodular lesions of the iris are an uncommon finding in uveitis which can be extremely useful in differential diagnosis. Much unnecessary attention normally centers on their correct historical nomenclature, the so-called 'mesodermal floccules' of Busacca on the iris surface being distinguished from the 'ectodermal nodules' of Koeppe, the assumption being that the latter are limited to the surface of the neuroectodermal iris, its visible anterior border being the pupillary ruff. There is, however, no evidence that these two eponymous lesions are pathogenetically different, and they may be morphologically indistinguishable and coexist in the same eye. The terms are anachronistic and, with respect to their eponymous authors, should be abandoned.

Iris nodules may be characterized by their size, position in relation to iris structure, number and regularity. The most common underlying diagnosis is Fuchs' heterochromic uveitis. Iris nodules occur in a significant minority with this disease (Rothova et al. 1994), and can remain for years. They are typically small, very numerous, translucent (and therefore quite easy to miss, especially on a blue iris), perched on the anterior iris surface, always on the pupillary side of the collarette (**Fig. 2.30**), and sometimes on the pupil margin itself. No other form of uveitis appears to be associated with this particular pattern of iris nodules and it is therefore virtually pathognomonic.

Other iris nodules are likely to be associated with granulomatous disease, and in most uveitis practices sarcoidosis is the most common association. However, other uveitides that may be associated with such signs include sympathetic uveitis, VKH syndrome, lens-induced uveitis, tuberculosis, syphilis, toxoplasmosis and multiple sclerosis. Collections of inflammatory cells may adhere to the iris surface to create quite large but irregular, creamy nodules (**Fig. 2.31**), or in some cases histological granulomas form within the iris stroma, which bulge forwards (**Fig. 2.32**), and these may even be vascularized (**Fig. 2.33**).

Rarely, in some forms of chronic anterior uveitis, iris crystals may be seen as tiny, glistening lesions on the anterior iris surface. Usually few in number (**Fig. 2.34**), they are thought to represent masses of crystalline immunoglobulin (Russell bodies) manufactured by activated plasma cells involved in the uveitis (Lam et al. 1993). The main differential diagnosis is the even rarer cystinosis, but in this disease the crystals are also in the cornea and conjunctiva. Iris pearls are rare but pathognomonic of leprosy. They are pearly white, small round and

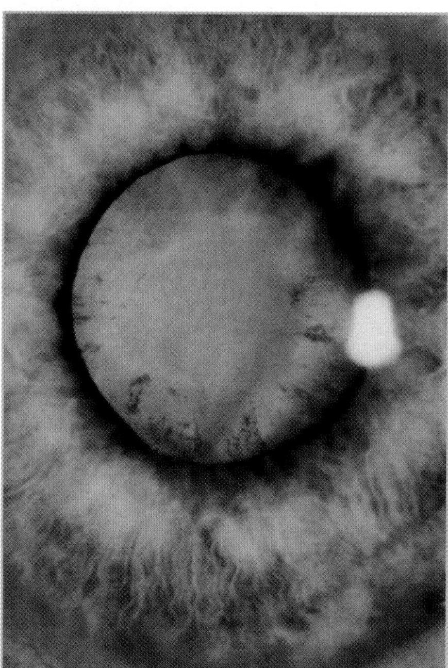

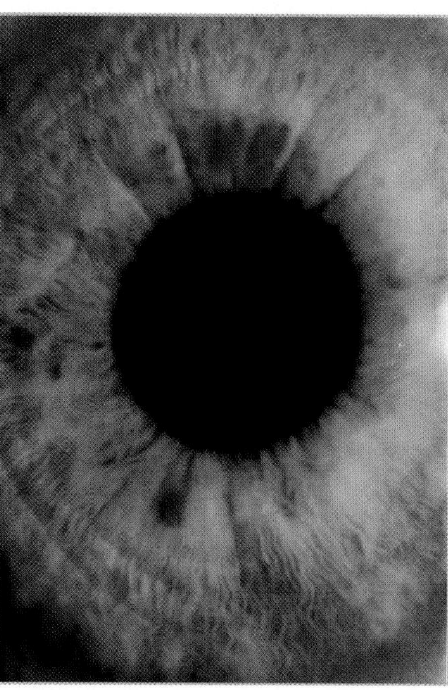

Figure 2.25 The right eye (with Fuchs' heterochromic uveitis) has lost its anterior border layer pigment, which appears white in comparison to the normal left eye. Also in the affected eye are radial lines of pigment on the lens surface, probably smeared on by active iris nodules on the posterior surface.

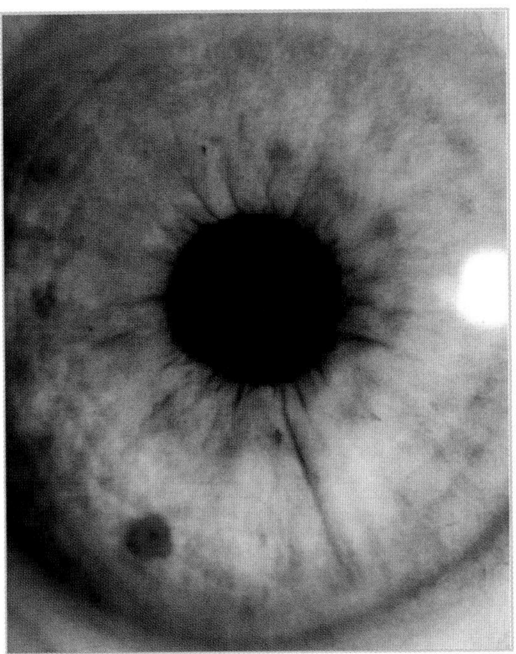

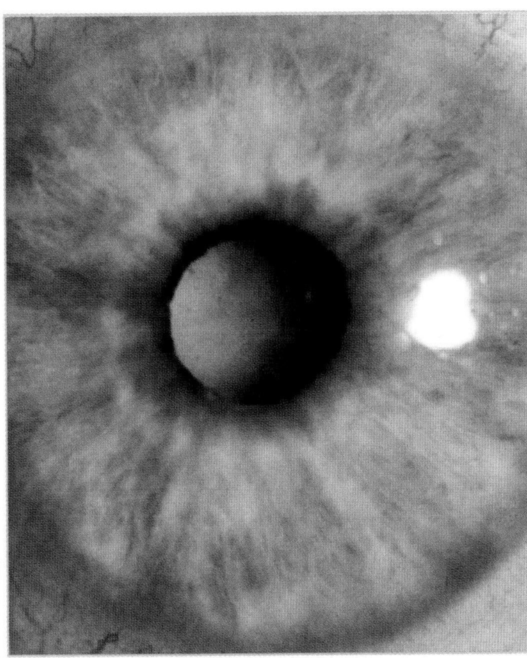

Figure 2.26 The classic appearance of heterochromic uveitis.

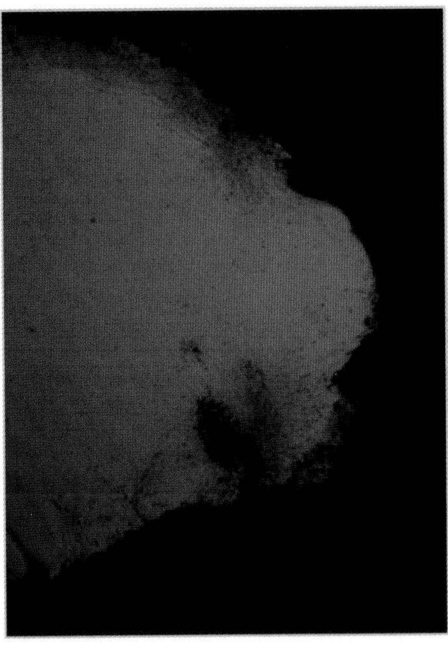

Figure 2.27 An irregular, atrophic pupil margin adherent to the lens after previous acute anterior uveitis.

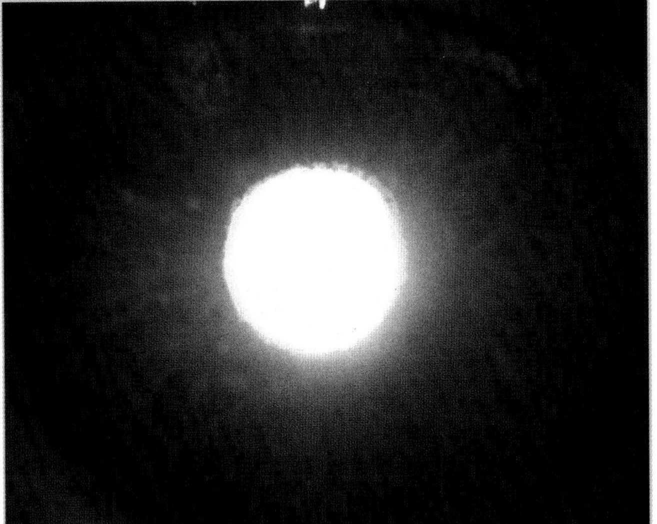

Figure 2.28 Iris pigment epithelial atrophy in chronic heterochromic uveitis causing transillumination.

well defined, not 'fluffy,' granulomatous nodules on the iris surface, sometimes pedunculated, sometimes detaching to fall to the bottom of the anterior chamber.

Iris vasculature

Vascular involvement in acute iridocyclitis may cause engorgement of normal iris vessels, which may be misinterpreted as rubeosis. Normal but engorged iris vessels, although distorted and sinuous, follow anatomical paths, unlike genuine rubeosis, which does also occur in chronic anterior uveitis, without any evidence of posterior segment ischaemia, and this is a recognized feature of heterochromic uveitis (**Fig. 2.35**). Rubeosis may be detectable only on gonioscopy, or may involve any part of the iris surface, if severe sometimes also passing onto the lens surface (**Fig. 2.36**). Anti-inflammatory treatment may lead to emptying of rubeotic vessels.

Posterior synechiae and pupil membranes

Adhesions between iris and anterior lens capsule are a frequent finding in acute or chronic anterior uveitis. When identified early enough and treated vigorously with mydriasis, adhesions can often be broken (**Fig. 2.37**). Nevertheless, permanent adhesions are frequent (**Fig. 2.38**) and these compromise both dilation, for examination purposes, and accommodative miosis. Recurrently or slowly extending posterior synechiae can lead to pupil block, iris bombé (**Fig. 2.39**) and acute glaucoma. In some situations a pupil is almost blocked but a remaining open 'chink' prevents acute glaucoma (**Fig. 2.40**); preventing this from closing with nocturnal mydriasis, and/or applying prophylactic laser or surgical iridectomy, is essential. Where posterior synechiae have been broken by treatment in acute anterior uveitis, pigment deposits may remain on the anterior lens surface. In Fuchs' heterochromic uveitis, although cicatricial posterior synechiae are not seen, occasional

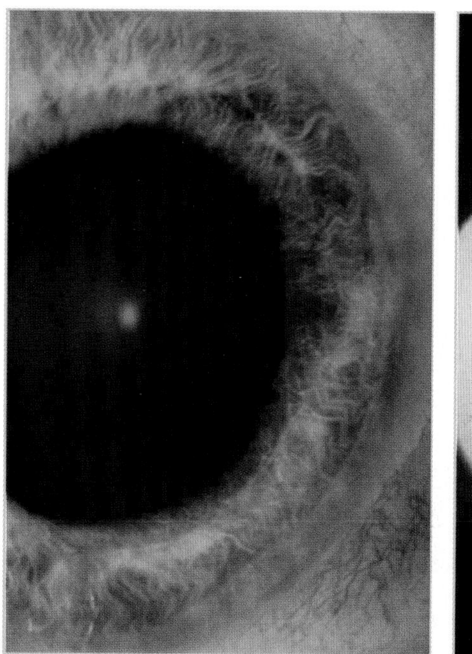
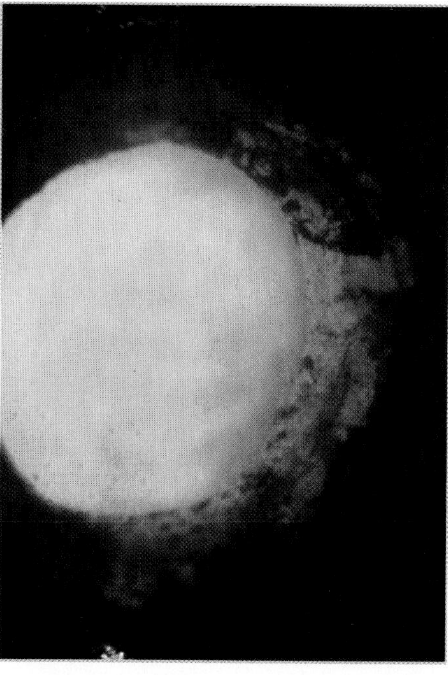

Figure 2.29 The typical appearance of herpetic anterior uveitis: the transilluminated iris corresponds to the area of atrophy and depigmentation visible by direct illumination.

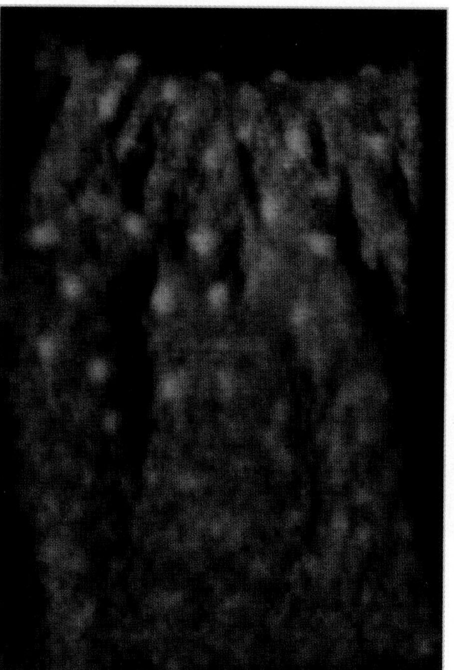
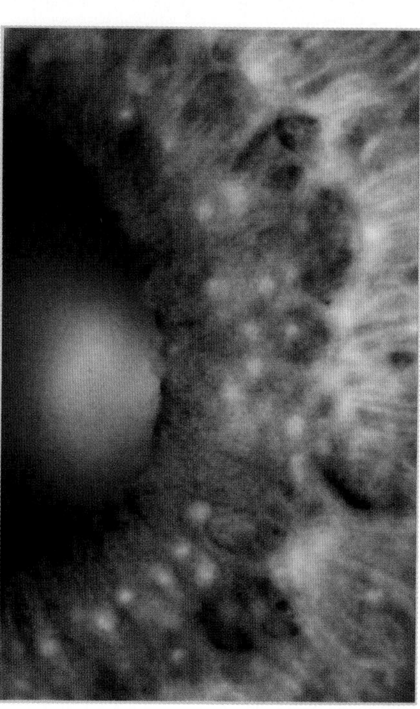

Figure 2.30 Small iris nodules – virtually pathognomonic of Fuchs' heterochromic uveitis.

temporary iris/lens adhesions do occur, resulting in smears of pigment in a radial pattern on the lens capsule (see Fig. 2.25).

Chronic or recurrent anterior uveitis not only leads to pupil block, but also to fibrotic membrane formation over the anterior lens surface. This is often pigmented, and may virtually obliterate the pupil (**Fig. 2.41**). Congenital epicapsular stars are occasionally confused with post-inflammatory debris, but the pupil anatomy will be normal in the former, clearly scarred in the latter (**Fig. 2.42**).

Pupil testing

Pupil testing is frequently compromised in uveitis patients, by posterior synechiae, atrophy of sphincter or dilator fibers, or the use of mydriatics. Where testing is possible, several forms of pupil defect may be of relevance. Optic nerve involvement occurs in a variety of uveitides, and the identification of an afferent defect is an important sign of either acute or chronic changes. Sectorial paralysis commonly follows herpetic uveitis, but occasionally a fixed dilated pupil results, and this is not unique to herpetic uveitis, occurring sometimes in toxocariasis and anecdotally in other situations. Horner's syndrome is in the differential diagnosis of inflammatory heterochromia.

Anterior chamber angle

The use of gonioscopy is important in establishing the cause of glaucoma secondary to uveitis. Peripheral anterior synechiae (**Fig. 2.43**)

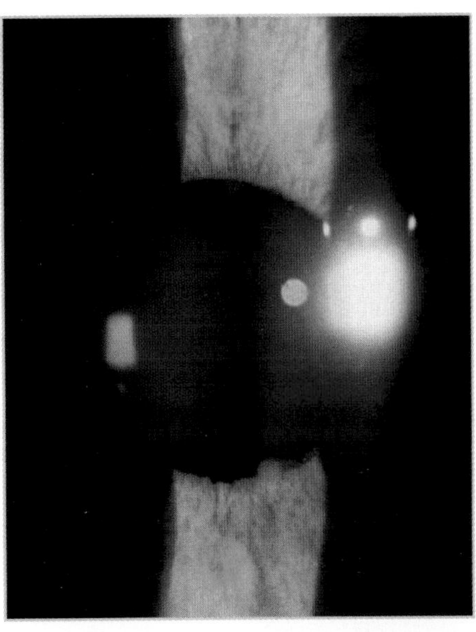

Figure 2.31 Two translucent nodules on the pupil margin in a patient with sarcoidosis.

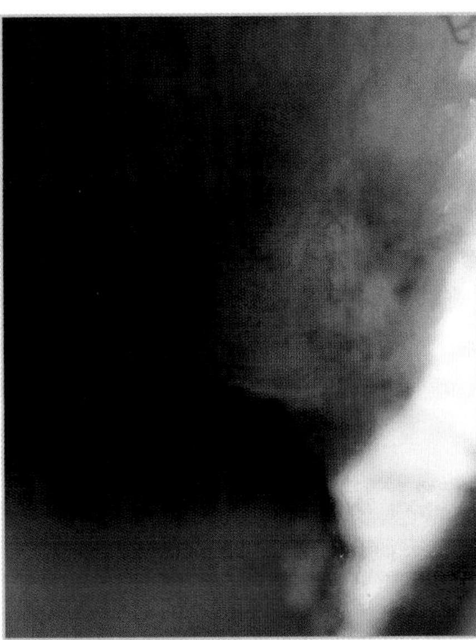

Figure 2.32 A large intrastromal granuloma, also in a patient with sarcoidosis.

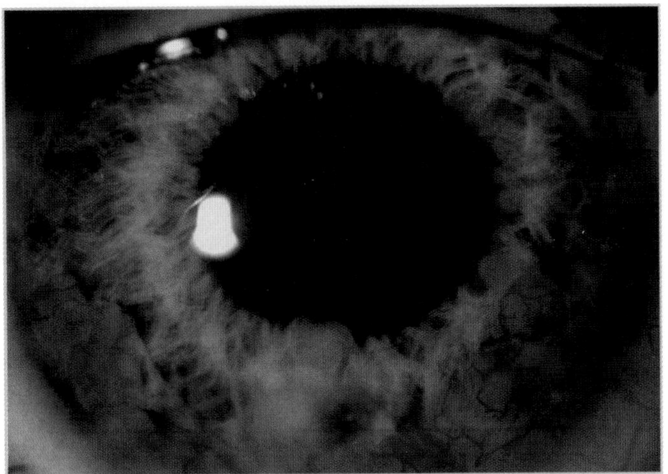

Figure 2.33 A collection of large, confluent vascularized iris granulomas in a patient with sarcoidosis.

Figure 2.34 Immunoglobulin crystals on the iris surface are an unusual finding in very chronic uveitis.

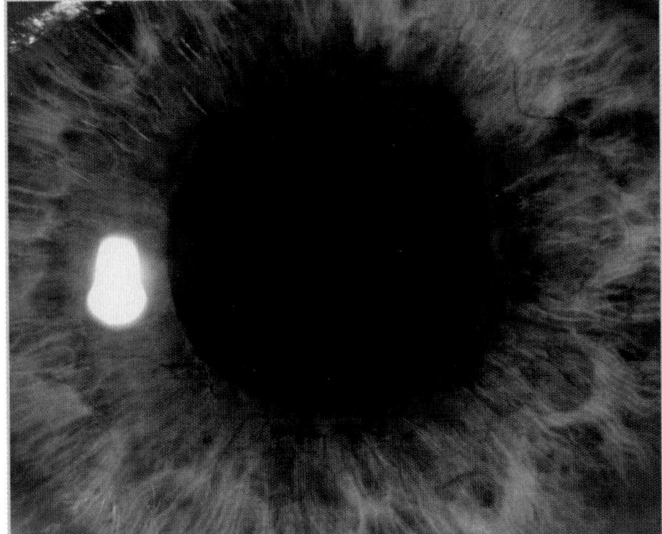

Figure 2.35 Iris rubeosis.

or rubeotic vessels may be visible only using this method. Similarly, some small hypopyons may not be visible by direct viewing. Some forms of inflammation may concentrate in the angle, and a trabeculitis, manifested as a fluffy white deposit covering the meshwork, may be detected by gonioscopy.

Lens

Cataract is common in uveitis, as a result of both inflammation and its treatment with steroids. Most cataracts begin in typical posterior subcapsular form and progression may be rapid. The management of cataract in uveitis, in the context of active inflammation, structural changes and possibly several causes of visual loss, may be complex and is discussed in Chapter 7. Those with mature or hypermature cataract may have an element of phakodonesis as a result of cumulative zonular damage and, rarely, hypermaturity itself can lead to lens-induced uveitis or glaucoma.

Vitreous humor

Inflammation of ciliary body, retina or choroid is often accompanied by the migration of inflammatory cells into vitreous humor. The structure of vitreous limits, to some extent, the spread of cells throughout the

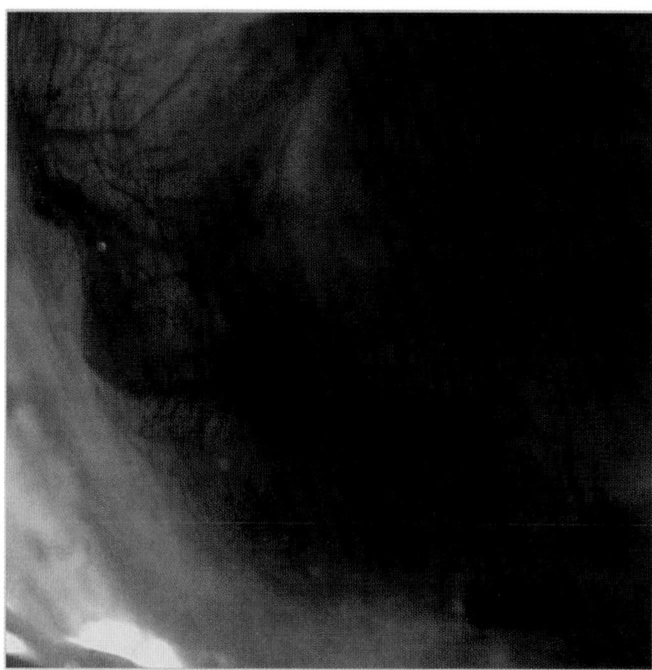

Figure 2.36 Severe rubeosis involving the lens surface in an eye with uncontrolled longstanding uveitis.

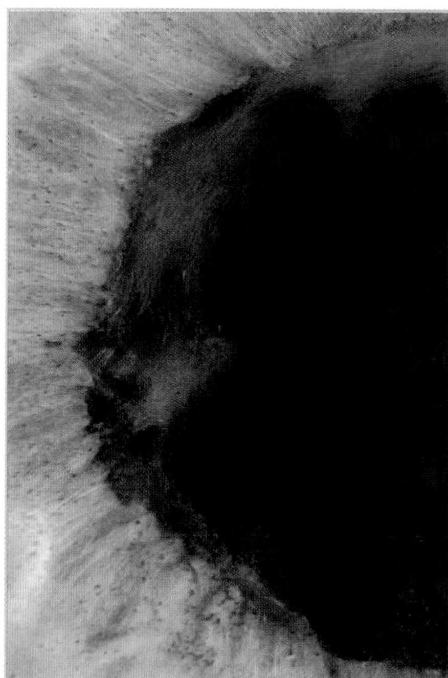

Figure 2.38 Permanent, firmly attached posterior synechiae are associated with partial pupillary fibrosis and pigment dispersion.

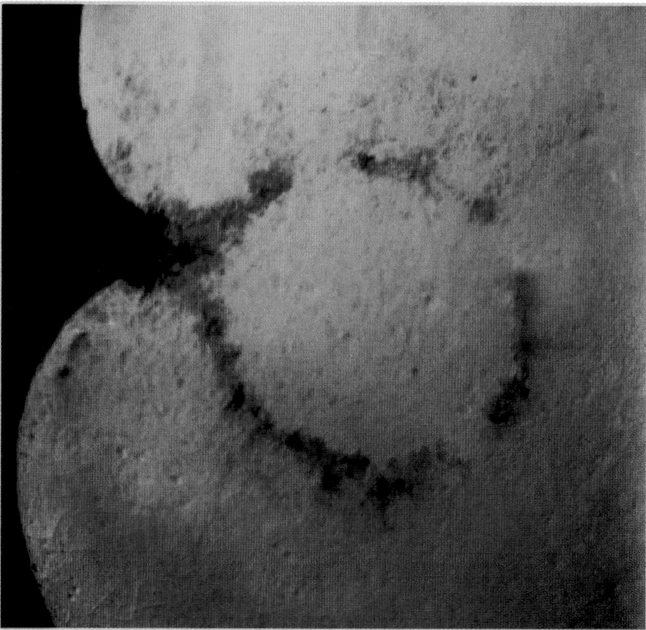

Figure 2.37 The attempt to break posterior synechiae has been almost successful, leaving one firm attachment and a ring of residual pigment.

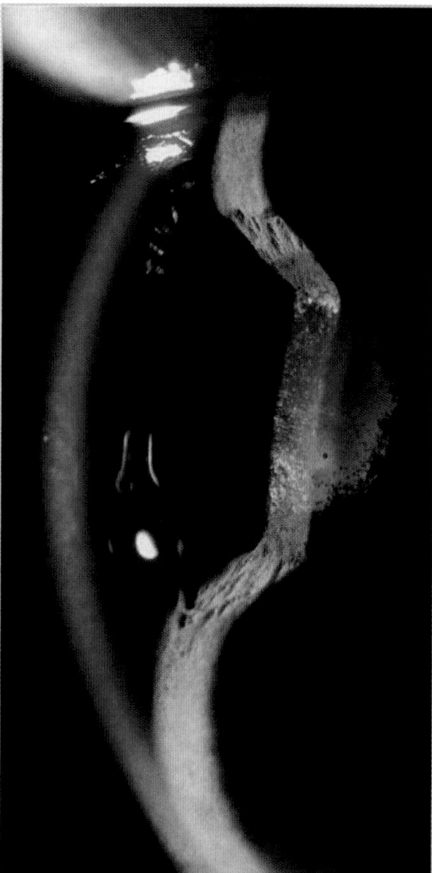

Figure 2.39 Iris bombé is the result of complete posterior synechiae.

posterior segment, and therefore the greatest concentration of cells will be seen near any focus of inflammation. Acute inflammation is typically accompanied by non-aggregated cells within liquid vitreous; in chronic inflammation such cells often aggregate around the vitreous structure (**Fig. 2.44**) to form clumps, snowballs or cylinders, which may be characteristic of some forms of inflammation. Large, stellate cell clumps in the anterior vitreous are frequent in Fuchs' heterochromic uveitis and sometimes seen in intermediate uveitis. The latter more commonly creates snowballs, large fluffy white globular opacities (**Fig. 2.45**), always most concentrated over the inferior pars plana, but sometimes compromising the visual axis, especially in juveniles. Multiple small preretinal opacities, smaller than the snowballs typical of intermediate uveitis, are seen most often in sarcoid uveitis. The particular collections of snowball-like opacities described as 'strings of pearls' are

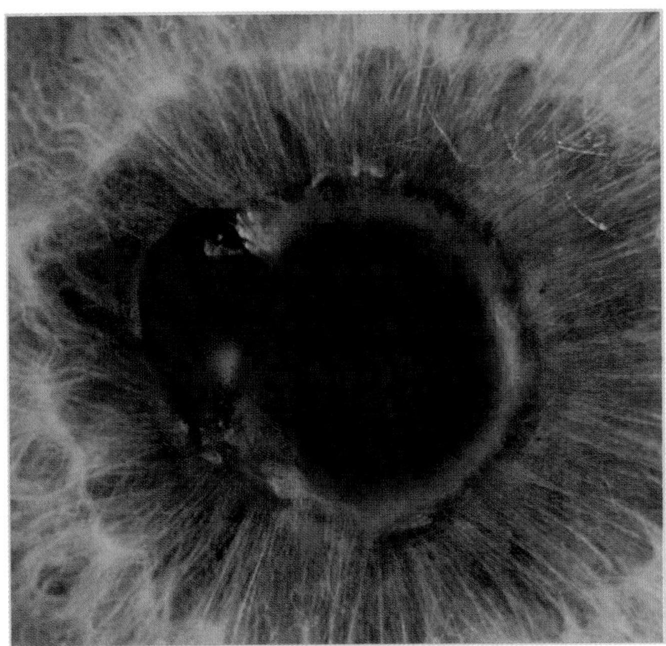

Figure 2.40 One passage for aqueous flow remains open and must be protected by treatment.

suggestive of fungal infection (**Fig. 2.46**), most commonly by *Candida* spp. Vitreous cylinders are striking accumulations of cells surrounding vitreous fibrils (**Fig. 2.47**), and are reported most frequently in association with toxoplasmosis. Pigmented debris may appear, especially in the anterior vitreous in some patients. This may represent shedding from an inflamed ciliary body, and is not necessarily indicative of a retinal break, although this too may occur in uveitis.

The vitreous, similar to aqueous humor, may show flare and this can be quantified in a similar way by slit-lamp transillumination. As for aqueous humor, this breakdown of blood-ocular barrier does not necessarily indicate active inflammation. Vitreous opacification may therefore be a combination of both active inflammation, and the accumulated debris of repeated or chronic inflammation. Vitreous opacification can be quantified by various methods, the most useful, a 0 (clear) to 5 (view of fundus entirely obscured) system, being based on indirect ophthalmoscopy, and devised and well illustrated by Nussenblatt and colleagues (1985). Any system needs to take into account other causes of media opacification, and does not easily distinguish active from passive changes. Such a distinction, and the main location of the cells, is probably best detected by a combination of slit-lamp transillumination (mainly for anterior to mid-vitreous) and fundus lens. The SUN workshop (Jabs et al. 2005) could not reach a consensus on the categorization of vitreous cellular activity, not least because of difficulties in the visualization and interpretation of vitreous opacities.

Posterior vitreous detachment is a common finding in many patients with intermediate or posterior uveitis, and the event may occur in young adults or even earlier. This condenses any opacification closer to the nodal point and usually precipitates new visual problems with floaters. It often leads to the patient's first presentation to the ophthalmologist for intermediate uveitis and Fuchs' heterochromic uveitis. For those already under supervision, it is often mistakenly interpreted by both patient and ophthalmologist as a worsening of the uveitis itself. In some forms of inflammation, posterior vitreous condensations may form, sometimes overlying retinal vessels if these have been inflamed, and these vitreous 'sails' and more dramatic condensations in some forms of uveitis (**Fig. 2.48**) may be a source of traction.

The vitreous in toxocariasis is a special case, one possibility being that migratory efforts by a larva before incarceration leave behind it a trail of antigen and resultant vigorous fibrotic reaction. However, the complexity of the vitreous latticework that sometimes results suggests

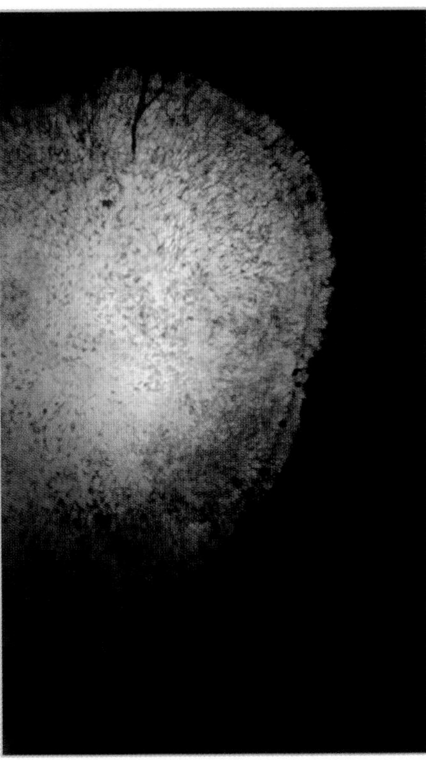

Figure 2.41 Pigmented fibrocytic proliferation across this pupil renders it almost opaque to direct illumination.

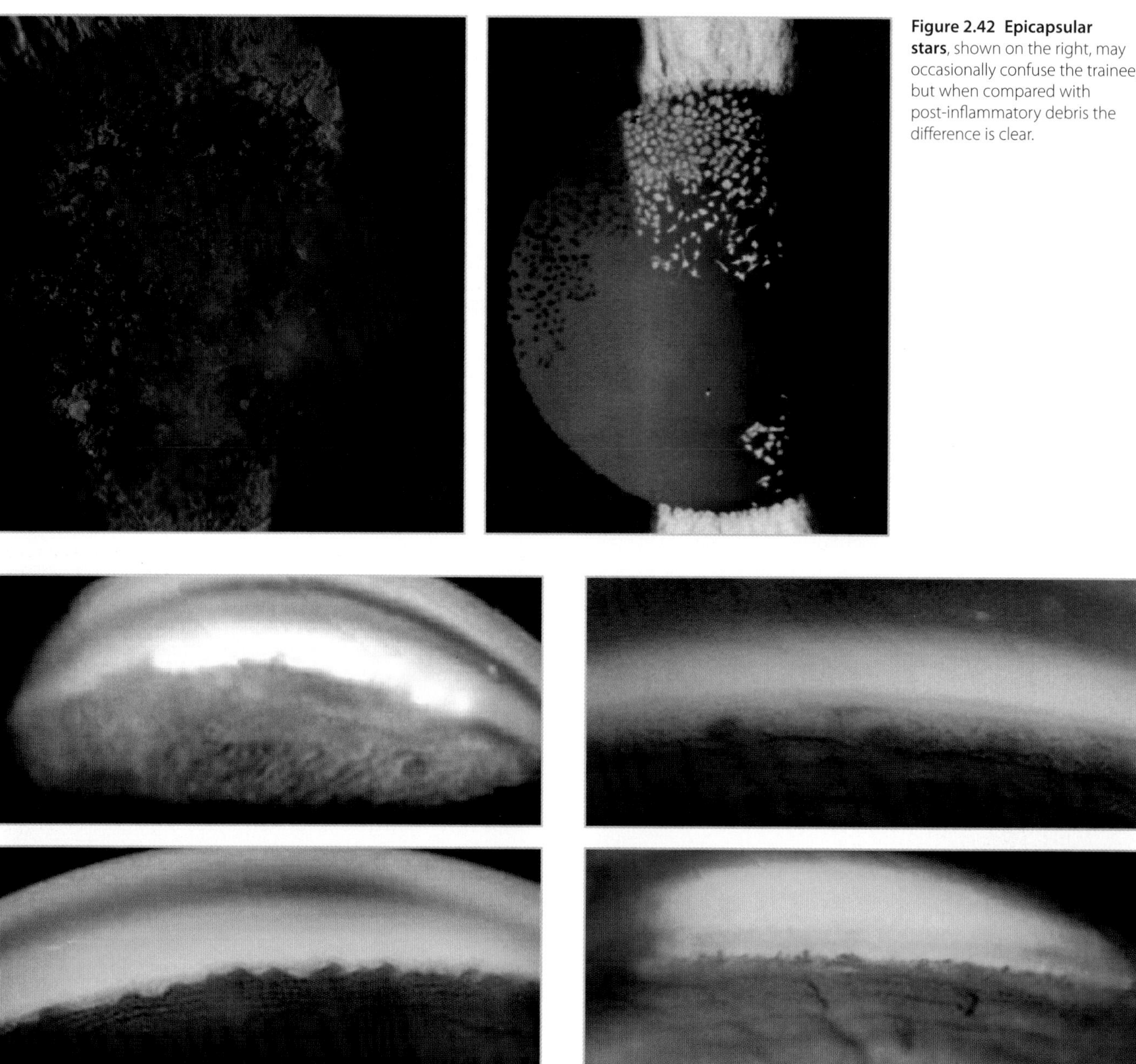

Figure 2.42 Epicapsular stars, shown on the right, may occasionally confuse the trainee, but when compared with post-inflammatory debris the difference is clear.

Figure 2.43 Peripheral anterior synechiae, seen in varying quantity and configuration in four patients with chronic anterior uveitis.

a more generalized mechanism. Single fibrotic strands may pass between periphery and disk, often inducing considerable traction, and there may be other fibers, any of which may induce dystopia (**Fig. 2.49**).

Retina and choroid

Viewing the retina and choroid can be a challenge in many patients with uveitis, and a piecemeal gathering of information using fundus lenses, indirect ophthalmoscopy and fluorescein angiography may be necessary. Most ophthalmologists have their preferred choice of fundus lens for use with the slit-lamp biomicroscope. The Goldmann contact lens has been virtually supplanted by the various hand-held lenses, for reasons of convenience, but the performance of the latter may be poorer in conditions where the view is difficult, and those ophthalmologists of a certain vintage appreciate the superior capability of the Goldmann contact lens in some circumstances.

Indirect ophthalmoscopy will penetrate vitreous opacities far better than a slit-lamp system and should supplement funduscopy in most circumstances where the view is difficult. It is imperative in intermediate uveitis, in order to identify the presence of active snowbanking, pars plana scarring, peripheral neovascularization or traction. Peripheral lesions in toxocariasis, granulomatous disease or, very occasionally, toxoplasmosis may be visible only with indentation. The use of a 28-diopter (28-D) lens often allows more effective viewing through pupils tied down by synechiae.

The macula

Macular edema is common in uveitis (**Fig. 2.50**), and if longstanding will cause permanent visual loss. The detection of mild macular edema behind hazy vitreous is difficult, but, in this situation, near and pinhole acuity act as effective surrogates. The introduction of ocular

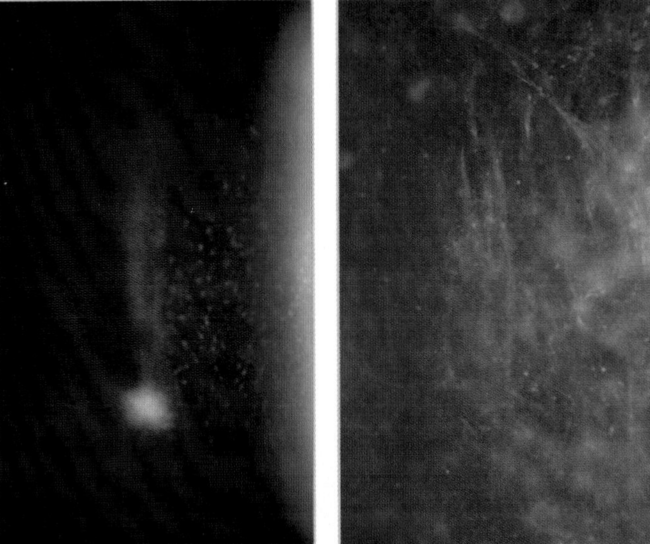

Figure 2.44 Two images of vitreous inflammatory infiltrate: acute vitritis on the left causes myriad distinct cells to be seen within the vitreous lacunae. On the right, more chronic inflammation sees cell aggregates attached largely to fibrillary vitreous opacities.

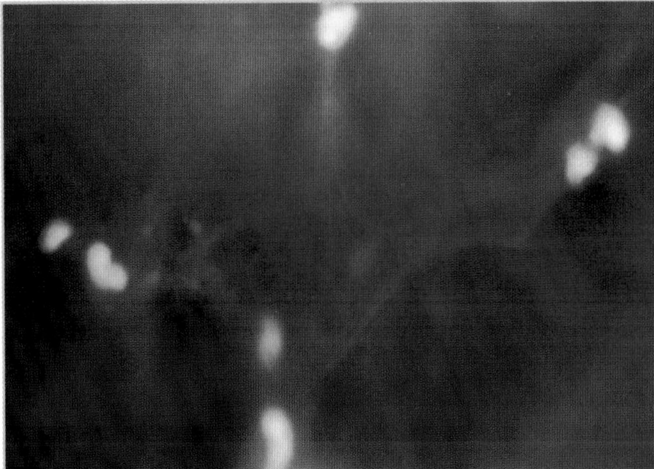

Figure 2.45 Vitreous snowballs in a child with intermediate uveitis.

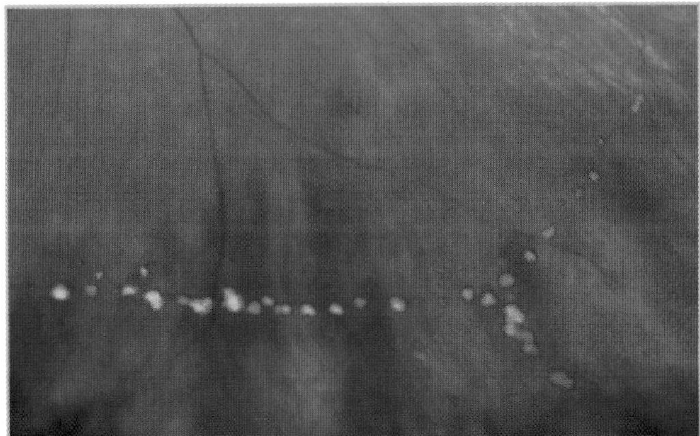

Figure 2.46 String-of-pearls appearance of opacities in candida endophthalmitis.

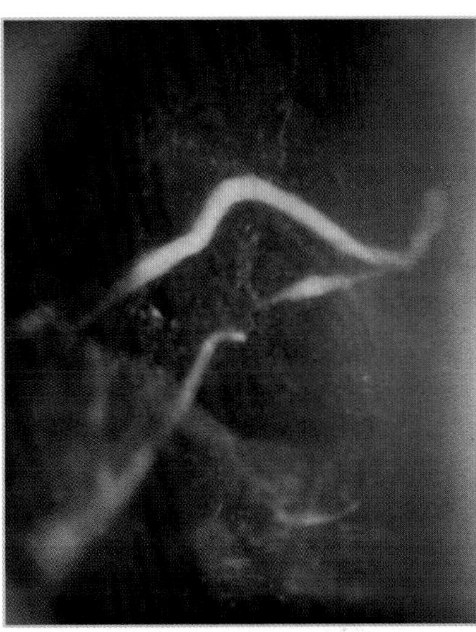

Figure 2.47 Vitreous cylinders in ocular toxoplasmosis.

coherence tomography (OCT) permits more effective assessment and is discussed below; for this function it has essentially replaced fluorescein angiography. Of course a constellation of macular problems accompanies many forms of uveitis (**Fig. 2.51**) and these are discussed in the relevant chapters.

Retinal vasculitis

Inflammation of retinal vessels, either veins or arterioles, is seen as a perivascular whitish cuff, usually affecting only segments of vessels. Any part of the fundus may be affected, but the temporal or nasal periphery is a particularly fruitful area for examination. Sheathing may be extremely subtle, or dramatic exudative changes may be seen (**Fig. 2.52**), especially in sarcoidosis. The 'fluffy,' poorly defined nature of this active vascular inflammation can be distinguished from the thinner, 'harder' outline of perivascular sheathing indicative of past, inactive vasculitis (**Fig. 2.53**).

Vascular inflammation may cause apparent (because of overlying exudate) or actual caliber changes in vessels, and obliteration of the lumen is an important indicator of severity that transforms the prognosis and the level of treatment required. In florid vasculitis, intraretinal hemorrhage may occur (**Fig. 2.54**). Acute vascular occlusion may occur secondary to adjacent retinitis (e.g. in toxoplasmosis) or because of vasculitis itself (**Fig. 2.55**). Ischaemic retinal edema or cotton-wool spots may be seen. Complete shutdown of major arterioles may be followed by silver wiring (**Fig. 2.56**). Macroaneurysm formation (**Fig. 2.57**) is a recognized feature of sarcoid-associated retinal vasculitis, and of the rare IRVAN (idiopathic retinal vasculitis, aneurysms, and neuroretinitis) syndrome. The complete evaluation of a patient with retinal vasculitis is not possible without the use of fluorescein angiography, which can indicate subclinical areas of vasculitis and vessel shutdown, the extent of ischemia (**Fig. 2.58**), and subtle neovascularization.

Focal or multifocal lesions

Some forms of uveitis cause focal or multifocal inflammation of the retina or choroid. The distinction between actively inflamed and inactive lesions is extremely important. Not all such lesions are associated with cells in vitreous humor when active. Features of activity include an impression of substance, poorly defined edges, associated retinal edema or vasculitis, and new symptoms and

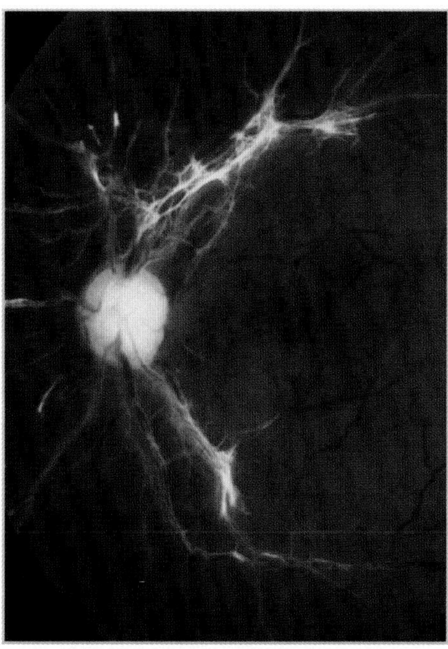
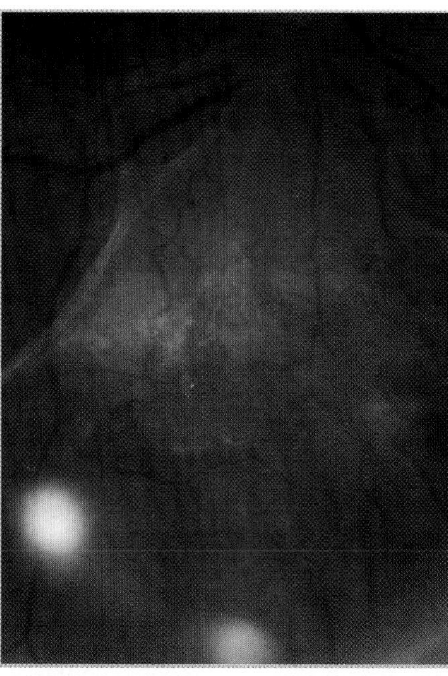

Figure 2.48 Fibroglial change accompanying intraocular inflammation: on the left, perivascular fibrosis in primary retinal vasculitis; on the right, posterior hyaloid condensation and retinal traction in intermediate uveitis.

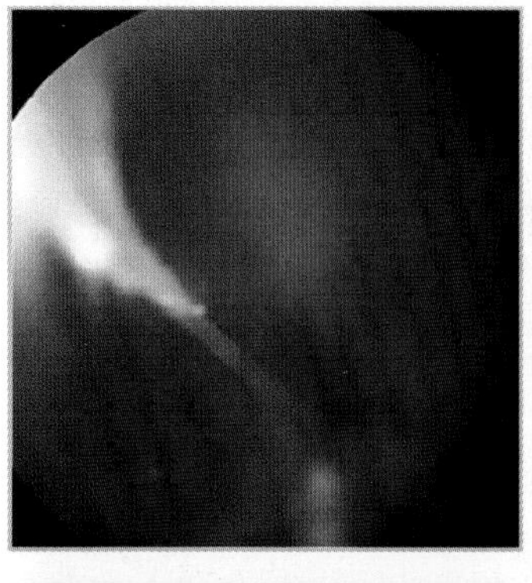
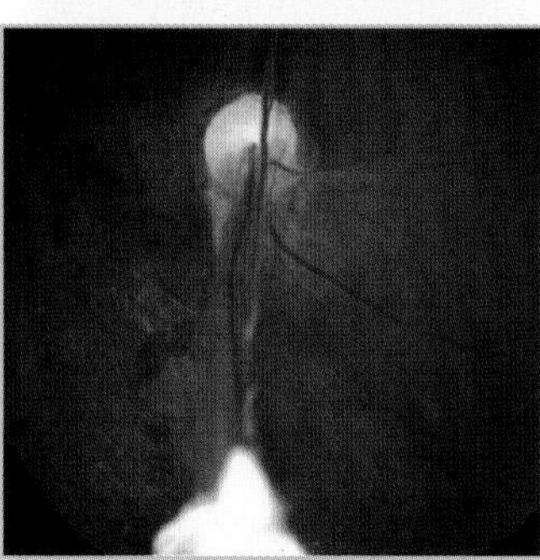
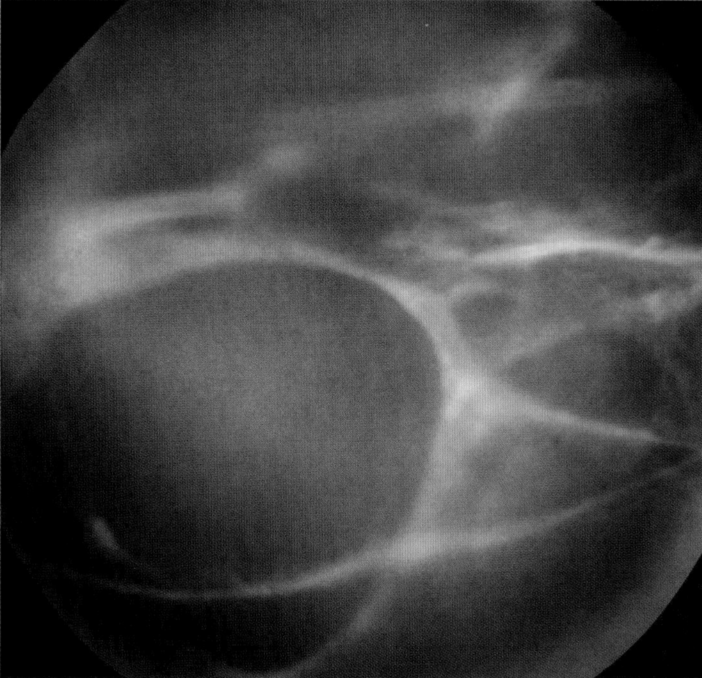

Figure 2.49 Three eyes with toxocariasis: all have tractional vitreous strands. (Images on left courtesy of Mr C Pavesio.)

signs of active inflammation within the vitreous or aqueous humor. Signs of quiescence include atrophic excavation, depigmentation or hyperpigmentation (**Fig. 2.59**), well-defined lesions and an absence of supporting signs.

Detecting the level at which inflammation is most prominent is of great importance in diagnosis, but can be difficult. Superficial retinal inflammations may be influenced by nerve fiber layer anatomy, as for cotton-wool spots and flame hemorrhage, and such lesions will cover underlying retinal vessels. Significant vitreous cellular activity may overlie retinal lesions. Many areas of multifocal inflammation appear predominantly to affect the retinal pigment epithelium (RPE) or choriocapillaris. Such lesions are typically subtly opaque, with little or no substance (but sometimes 'placoid') and little or no vitreous activity. Severe inflammations may be accompanied by overlying serous retinal elevation (**Fig. 2.60**). When suspecting lesions of the RPE, examination under red-free illumination can often substantially enhance the contrast of subtle lesions. Lesions of the RPE or choriocapillaris can be evanescent, leaving no scarring, tiny and punctate, or progressively atrophic, leading to depigmentation as in birdshot retinochoroidopathy; sometimes they can leave considerable pigment dispersion after acute posterior multifocal placoid pigment epitheliopathy (APMPPE). Some lesions of the choriocapillaris appear limited by the lobular architecture, and are thought to represent vasculitis of lobular supply arterioles.

Some inflammatory lesions involve a greater thickness of choroid and can exhibit more substance, raising the overlying retina (**Fig. 2.61**).

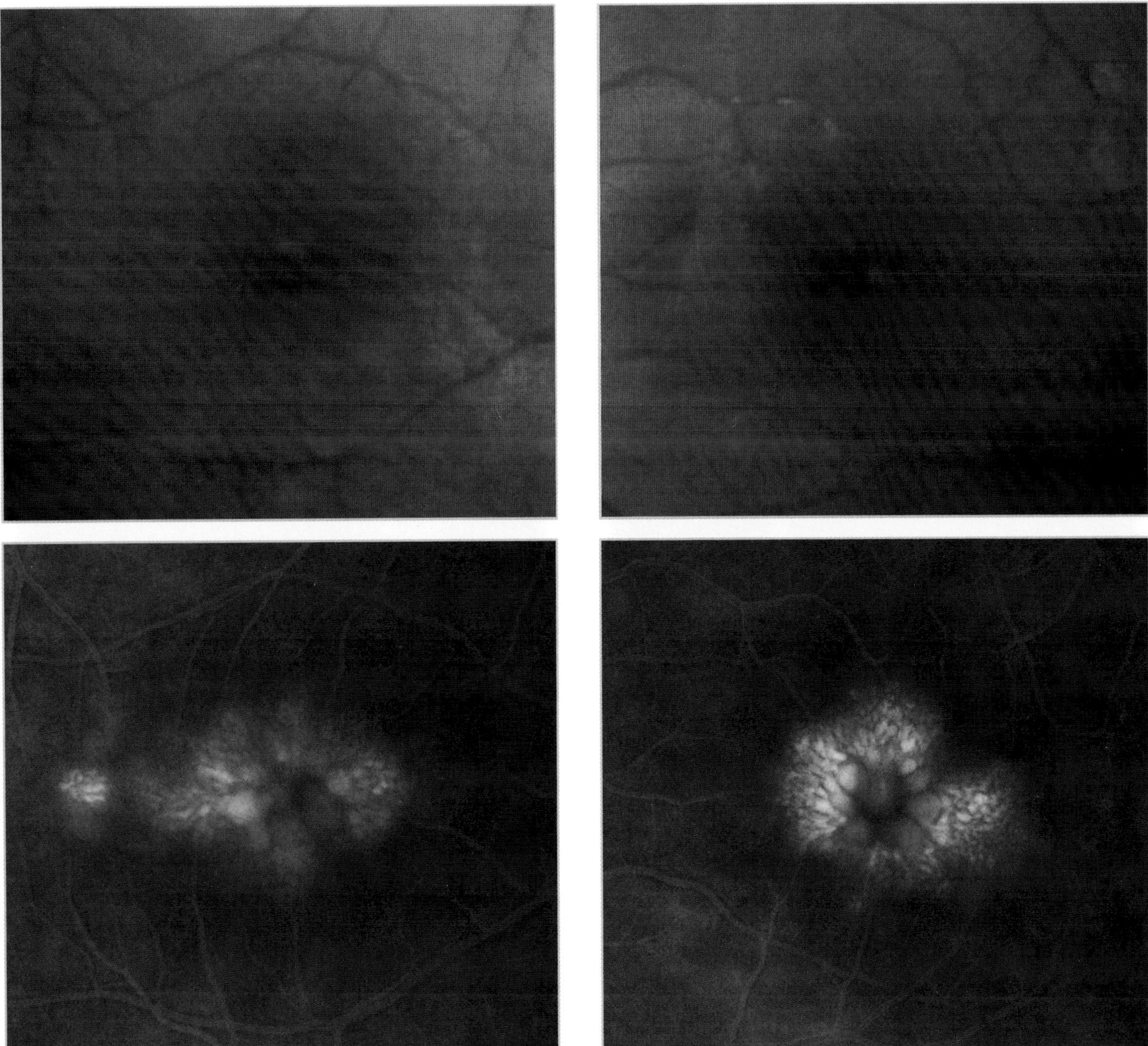

Figure 2.50 Bilateral cystoid macular edema in chronic uveitis: angiography shows both the extent and the severity more accurately than funduscopy.

Choroidal scarring tends to leave completely depigmented, sometimes excavated, scars, which characteristically have deeply pigmented edges with sclera visible centrally (**Fig. 2.62**). Such scars are typically seen after multifocal choroiditis. Occasionally, if the RPE is not too dense, perivascular exudation around larger choroidal vessels is observed, and presumably represents a choroidal vasculitis.

Any post-inflammatory or post-traumatic scar involving superficial choroid and RPE is at some risk for the future development of subretinal neovascularization and, although this risk is well known in the presumed ocular histoplasmosis syndrome and punctate inner choroidopathy, it may occur in other conditions, e.g. toxoplasmosis (**Fig. 2.63**) and Behçet's disease. New visual symptoms in the presence of what are apparently old scars should therefore be treated with some suspicion, and fluorescein angiography may detect subclinical subretinal changes.

Optic nerve head

The optic nerve head may be affected in several ways. Disk swelling may occur in panuveitis, intermediate uveitis or even accompanying anterior uveitis in juveniles. Granulomas or focal inflammation may directly involve the nerve head, and peripapillary edema and atrophy may occur. Disk neovascularization may occur due to an ischemic vasculitis or in intermediate uveitis. Glaucomatous disk damage may be seen. Papilledema may occur because of coexisting neurological disease, including neurosarcoid (**Fig. 2.64**). A specific form of inflammation, neuroretinitis, includes optic nerve head swelling and hypervascularity with or without peripapillary edema, with associated exudation into the macular area forming a star shape. Several infections or post-infective states can cause this manifestation but toxoplasmosis and bartonellosis should be specifically excluded.

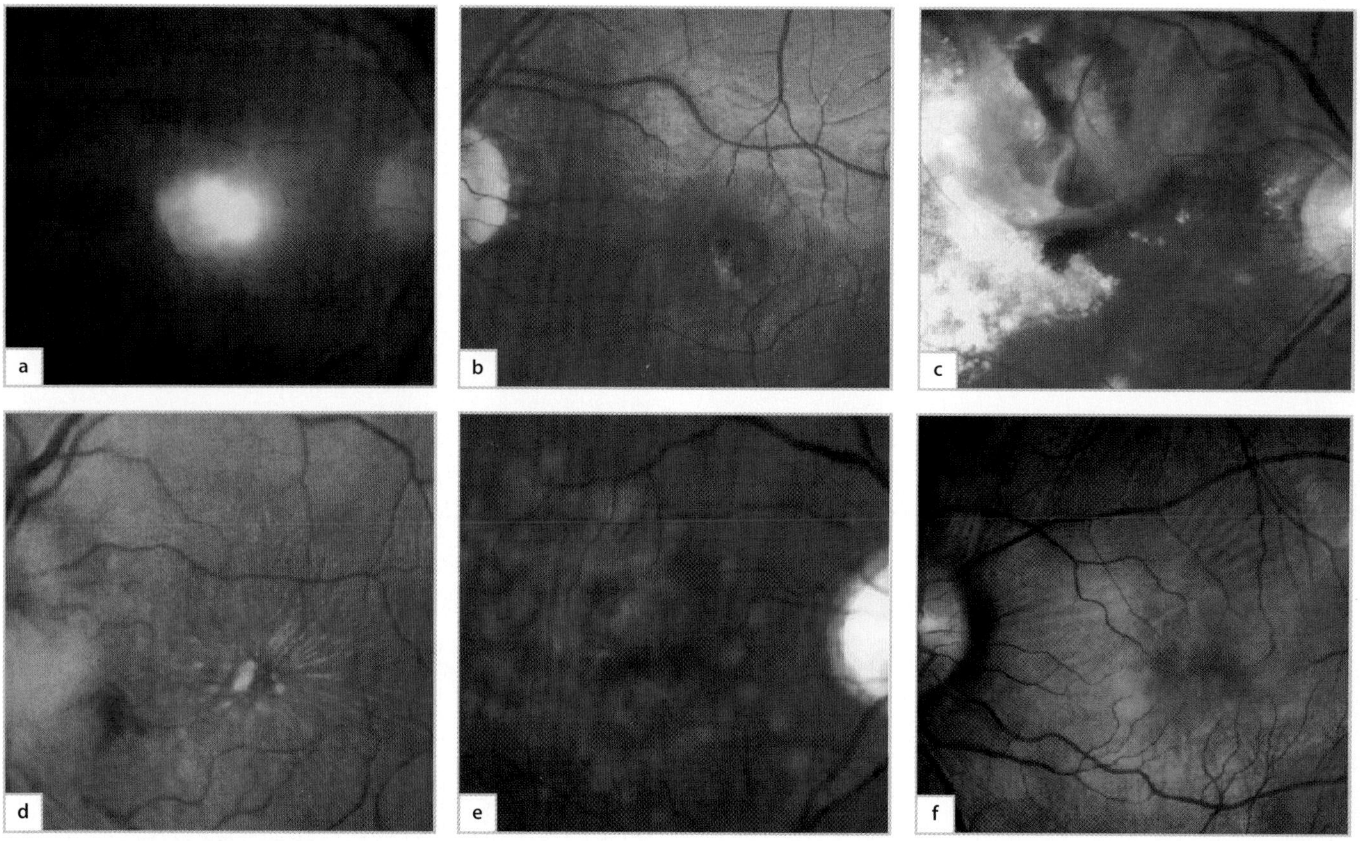

Figure 2.51 A selection of macular lesions in uveitis: (a) primary ocular toxoplasmosis; (b) retinal pigment epitheliitis; (c) choroidal neovascular membrane in punctate inner choroidopathy; (d) neuroretinitis in cat-scratch disease (courtesy of Dr A Curi); (e) persistent placoid maculopathy; (f) serous macular detachment in Vogt–Koyanagi–Harada syndrome.

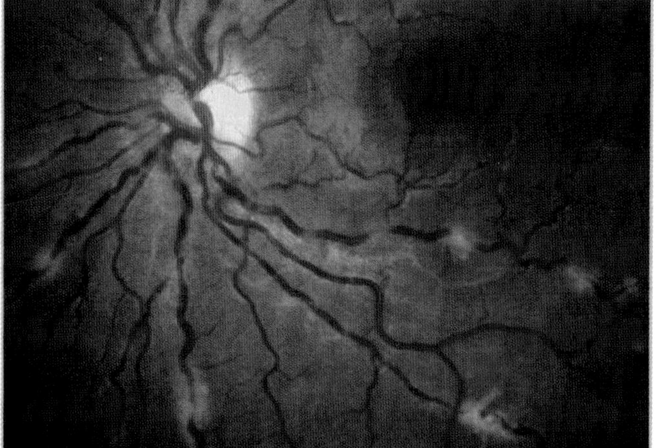

Figure 2.52 Active segmental vasculitis in sarcoidosis with fluffy perivenous sheathing.

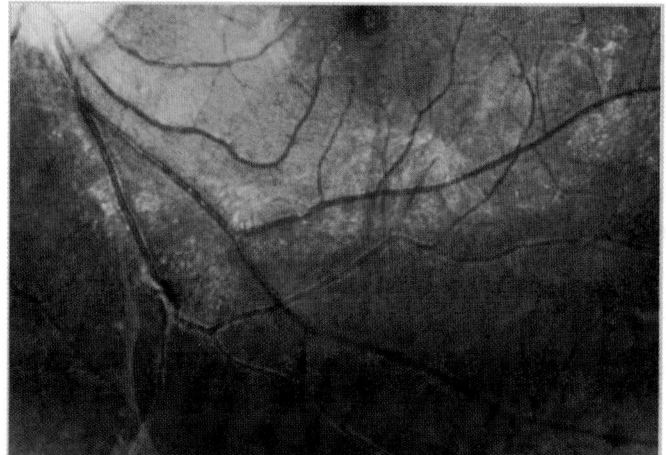

Figure 2.53 Old perivascular sheathing after previous active vasculitis.

GENERAL EXAMINATION

In some circumstances the ophthalmologist will call upon the services of doctor colleagues in order to aid diagnosis or treatment of multisystem disease. However, in many instances clear physical signs may be quite amenable to examination by the ophthalmologist. It is essential to have, within the ophthalmic clinic, an adequate facility for a general physical examination in patients with a suggestion of accompanying systemic disease. Many physical signs are readily available to the skills of the ophthalmologist, and the different perspective of the ophthalmologist may be of great value in multisystem disease where diagnosis has as yet eluded the physician. As an *aide-memoire,* **Table 2.3** is a summary of the more important physical findings that may be associated with uveitis or its treatment, and the most likely associated diagnosis. In particular the ophthalmologist should be aware of the differential diagnosis of various skin and mucocutaneous lesions,

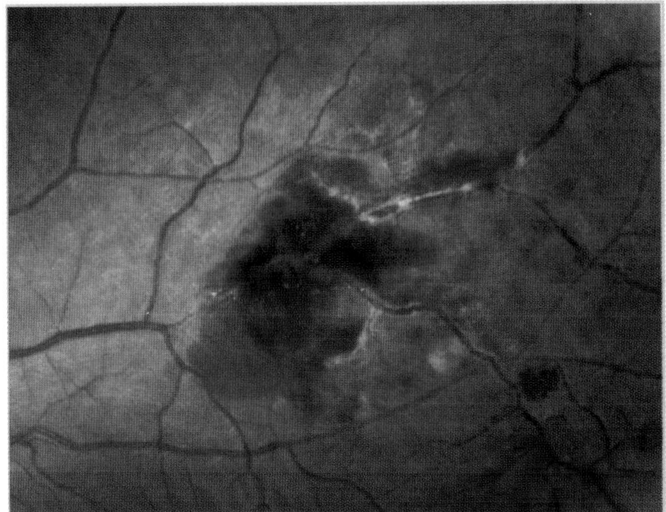

Figure 2.54 Perivascular hemorrhage accompanying acute vasculitis in Behçet's disease.

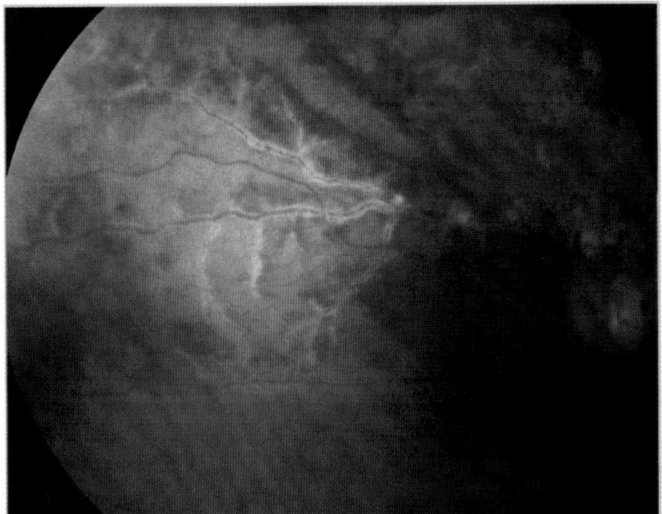

Figure 2.55 Acute hemisphere vein occlusion in Behçet's disease.

and able to diagnose (or formulate a logical differential diagnosis for) and understand the implications of psoriasis, erythema nodosum, lupus pernio, folliculitis, secondary syphilis, oral ulceration and lupus. A collection of relevant lesions is shown in **Fig. 2.65**. Some exposure to dermatology clinics is valuable for the ophthalmologist wishing to specialize in uveitis.

AUXILIARY OCULAR EXAMINATION

Direct examination of the eye alone may be an inadequate source of information in patients with uveitis. The pupil may be incapable of dilation, the ocular media may prevent an adequate fundal view, and optic nerve involvement may be suspected but unconfirmed. Even with a reasonable fundal view, subtle macular edema, vasculitis, and the level and behavior of fundal lesions may be difficult to ascertain. In these circumstances some auxiliary or indirect methods of ocular examination may add valuable information.

Figure 2.56 Silver wiring after progressive vascular occlusion. Shunting is also seen.

Visual field testing

Visual field testing may be used for a variety of purposes in the patient with uveitis. The estimation of glaucomatous visual field loss is frequently needed, but this may be compromised by media opacities. Some inflammation may be progressive and, particularly in those in whom retinal signs may be absent or subtle, visual field examination may give valuable evidence, e.g. in CMV retinitis or acute zonal occult outer retinopathy. Blind spot size may be enlarged in some circumstances, alone as acute idiopathic blind spot enlargement, in combination with multifocal retinochoroidopathies or because of direct optic nerve inflammation. Some uveitides may be associated with intracranial lesions, such as neurosarcoidosis, multiple sclerosis and toxoplasmosis (**Fig. 2.66**). The identification of visual pathway lesions may therefore be facilitated.

Microperimetry

The ability to test accurately and repeatedly the paracentral retinal sensitivity (up to either 5° or 10° from fixation) is met by microperimetry, which permits stimulation of known retinal foci using an on-screen macular image that identifies and tracks high-contrast components including disk margin and vessels to ensure accurate localization (**Fig. 2.67**). Testing requires a subjective response from the patient and therefore is subject to repeatability error. However, the technique adds potentially useful information to visual acuity testing and macular OCT, e.g. in birdshot retinochoroidopathy (Giuliari et al. 2010) in which widespread macular dysfunction may not be adequately reflected in visual acuity testing.

Fluorescein angiography

Fluorescein angiography (FA) is an essential method of examination for many patients with posterior uveitis. Sodium fluorescein is a hydrocarbon which, when injected, becomes about 60% plasma protein bound and has its spectral peaks of excitation and emission at about 480 nm and 530 nm, respectively. High-quality FA films provide additional information over funduscopy in several situations. Angiography should always if possible be combined with color fundus photographs for comparison. The red-free frames that precede

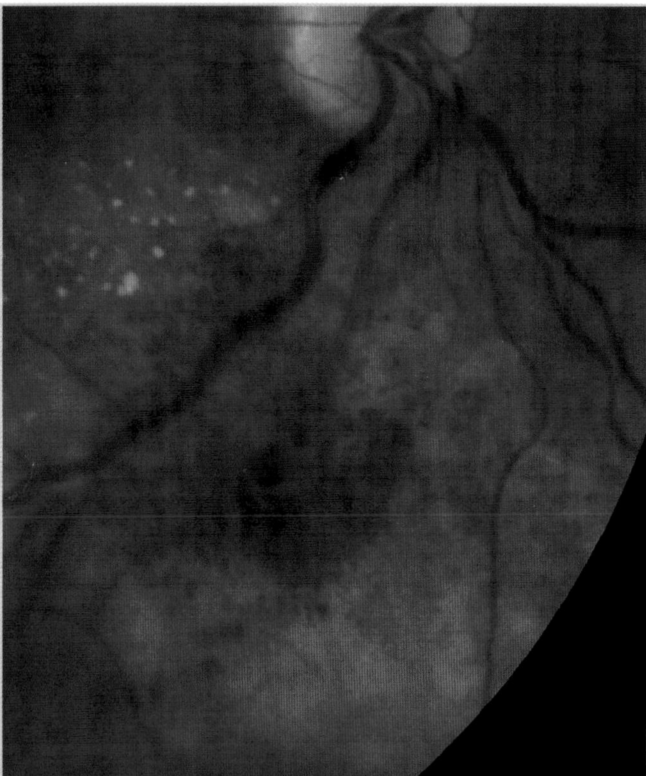

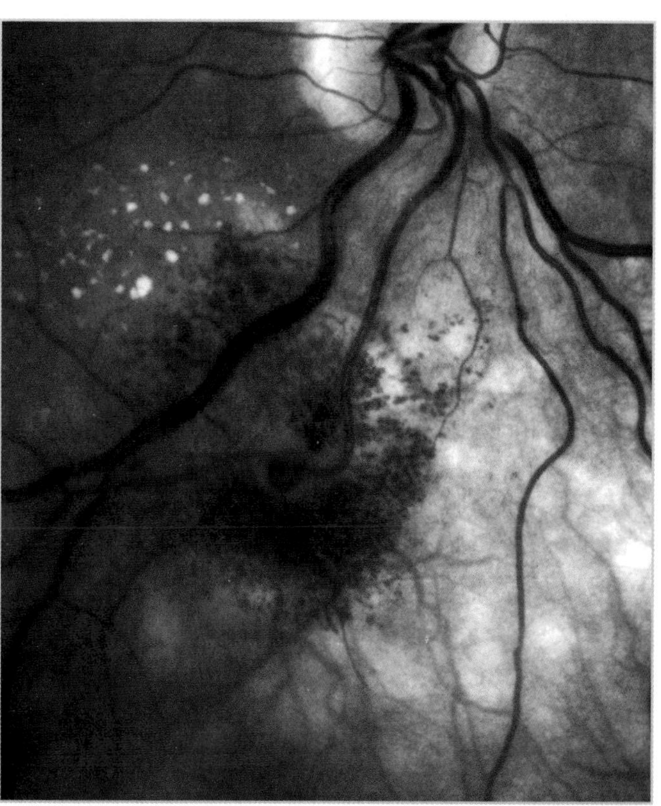

Figure 2.57 A single retinal macroaneurysm in a patient with sarcoidosis.

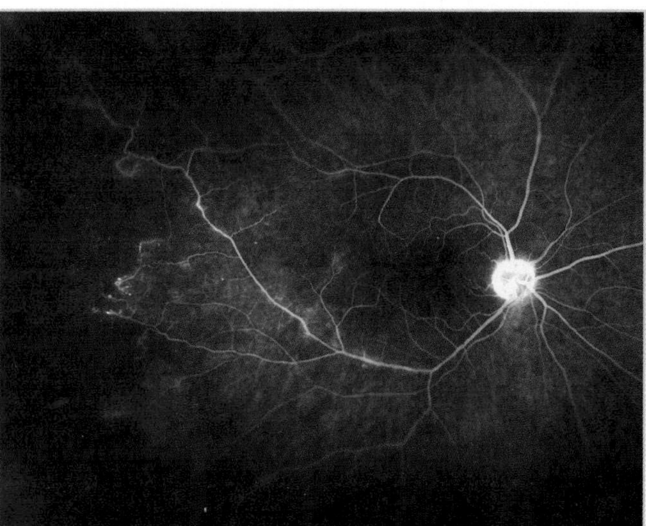

Figure 2.58 Wide-field fluorescein angiography showing substantial peripheral vascular closedown in a patient with primary retinal vasculitis.

the fluorescein run also often highlight fundal lesions at the level of the RPE (**Fig. 2.68**). This principle should also be remembered while examining an inflamed fundus on the slit-lamp; the red-free filter highlights RPE as well as nerve fiber layer. The FA run itself often shows characteristic changes in choriocapillaris/RPE-level inflammations such as APMPPE (**Fig. 2.69**) and the procedure is an essential identifier of choroidal neovascular membrane in punctate inner choroidopathy (PIC) and several other forms of chorioretinitis (**Fig. 2.70**).

Macular edema, which may be difficult to detect through opacified vitreous, and needs treatment if present, may be diagnosed using FA (**Fig. 2.71**). Areas of subclinical retinal edema or peripapillary edema, themselves important markers of inflammation in some circumstances, may also be detected. However, for perifoveal macular edema, OCT is non-invasive, quicker to perform and at least as accurate in diagnosis; it has therefore virtually replaced FA for this purpose. Retinal vasculitis may be present without clear funduscopic evidence of perivascular exudate and, in either active or prior vasculitis, FA will show cardinal signs (**Fig. 2.72**) that may not be obvious on direct examination. These include staining of vessel walls and perivascular leakage at either small vessel or capillary level, large or small vessel shutdown with resultant ischemia and subtle foci of retinal neovascularization.

FA cannot provide a complete picture of choroidal vasculature, particularly at the posterior pole, for two reasons: first because macular xanthophyll is an effective partial barrier to excitation and fluorescence, and second because fluorescein, being only 60% protein bound, is capable of early and profuse leakage from the fenestrated vessels in the choriocapillaris. This immediately stains choroidal interstitial tissue and obscures the development of any vascular choroidal pattern. For the purposes of choroidal examination, indocyanine green has clear advantages.

Iris FA has been used to identify changes in chronic uveitis, including neovascularization and fluorescein leakage from abnormal vessels, but the investigation has not proved valuable enough to find itself a routine place in clinical management.

Wide-field photography and fluorescein angiography

For macular diseases requiring successive angiograms to portray the temporal development of staining or leakage, standard FA is entirely

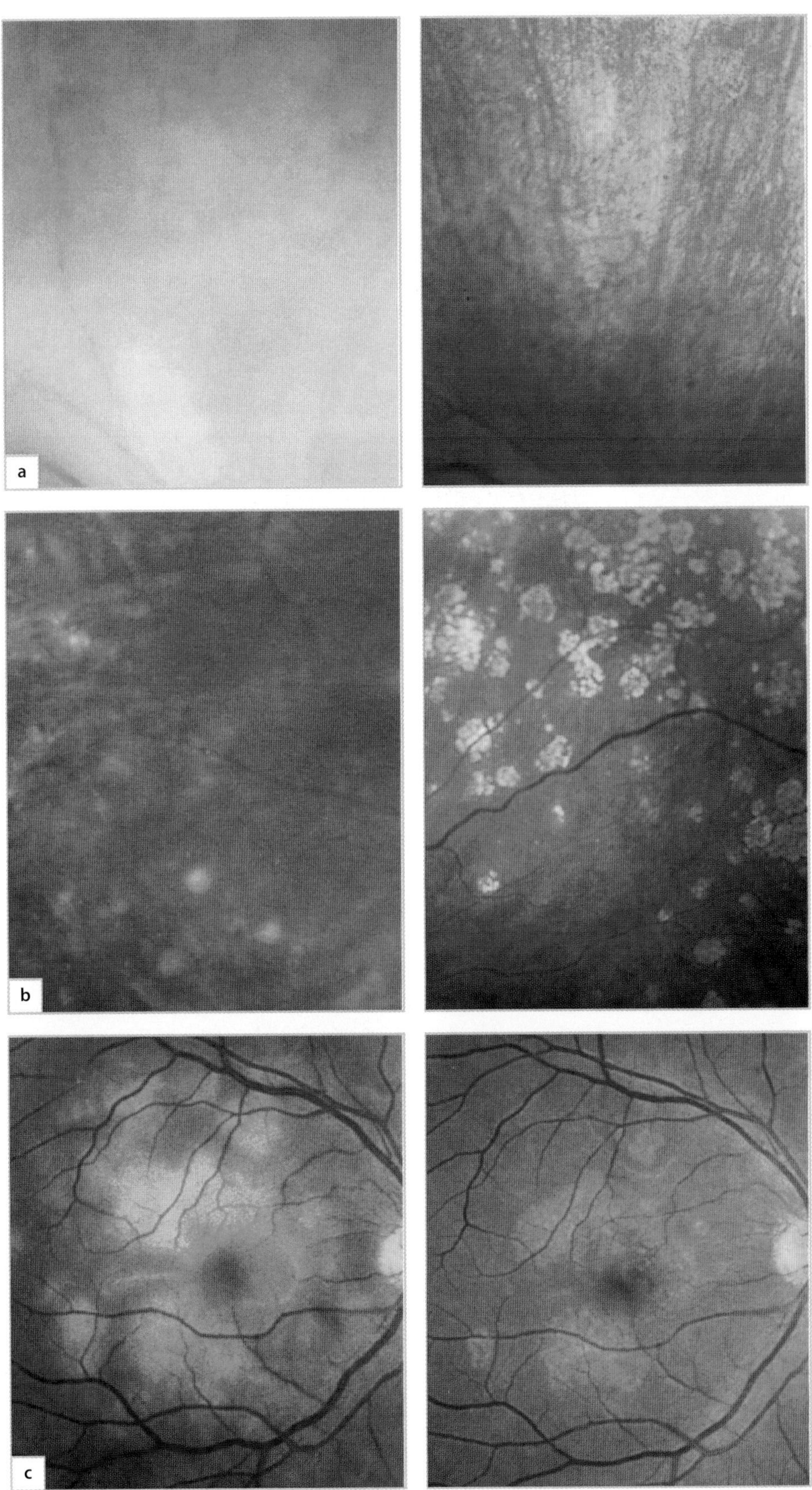

Figure 2.59 Acute retinal or retinal pigment epithelium inflammation (left) and after scarring (right) in (a) syphilis, (b) sympathetic uveitis and (c) acute posterior multifocal placoid pigment epitheliopathy.

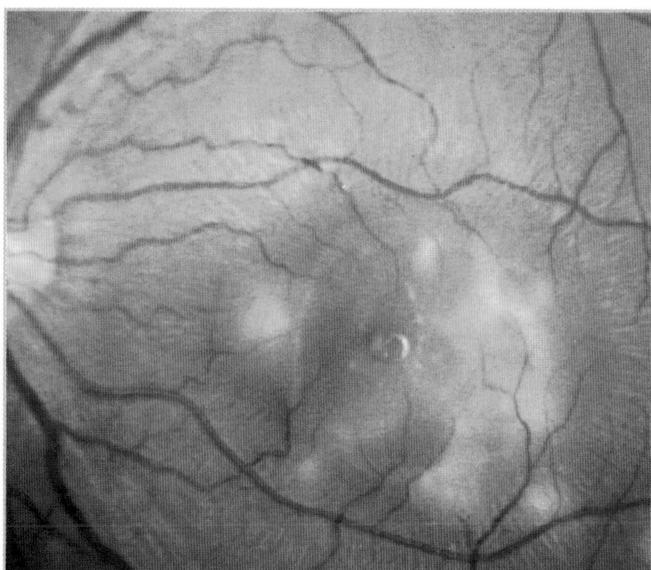

Figure 2.60 Loculated serous retinal elevation overlying acute posterior multifocal placoid pigment epitheliopathy.

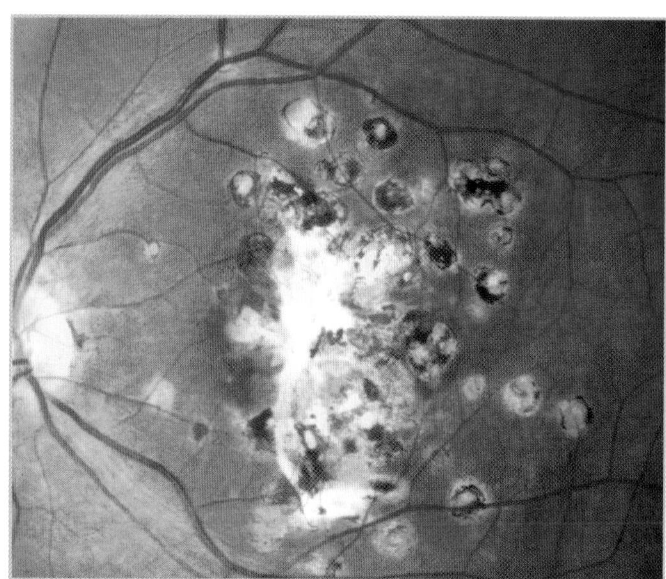

Figure 2.62 Typical deep choroidal scars with pigmented edges and pale centers after multifocal choroiditis.

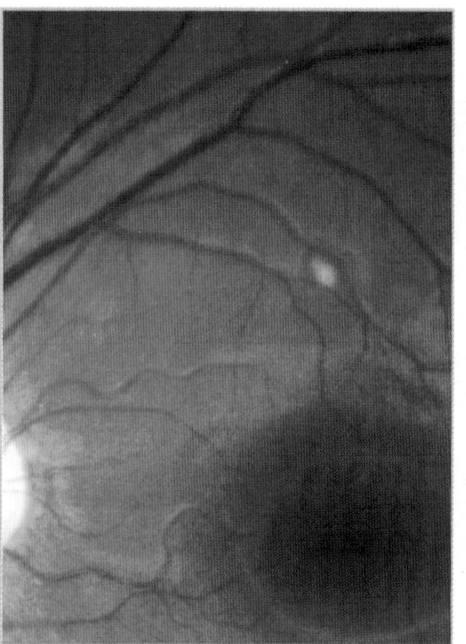

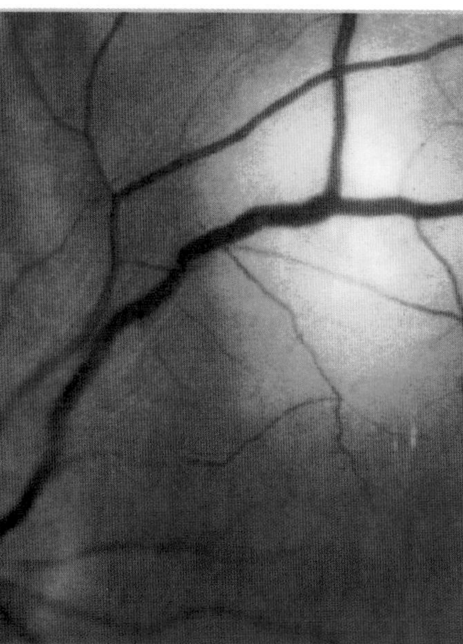

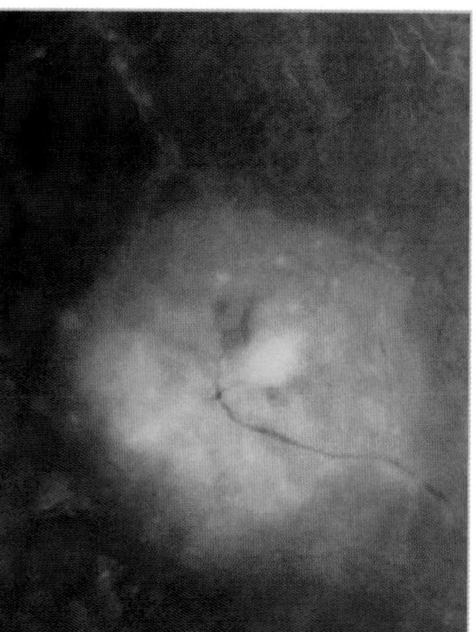

Figure 2.61 Three choroidal granulomas elevating the overlying retina.

appropriate and remains necessary in the management of choroidal neovascular membranes. However, in the management of widespread fundal disease or in occlusive vasculitis, the development of wide-field photography has been very beneficial. The technique uses an Optos confocal scanning laser that uses a moving pinhole system to optically conjugate incoming images. It performs both vertical and horizontal raster scans with red and green lasers to capture an almost panfunduscopic image in 0.25 s, the rapidly moving elliptical mirror system enabling a virtual focal point posterior to the pupil. This and its very good depth of focus create what, to the new initiate, are astounding images that for the first time place fundal lesions into direct anatomical perspective (**Fig. 2.73**). In contrast to standard fundal photography, which is merely blurred by vitreous opacification, such opacities are well delineated in wide-field images (**Fig. 2.74**). Until this invention the ophthalmologist has relied on a mental picture built up by the conjugation of images glimpsed via a fundus lens or indirect ophthalmoscope. Current disadvantages of the wide-field photography system include the unnatural red/green balance of the resultant image and the intrusion of eyelashes, both of which may be alleviated in development.

FA is also possible with the Optos (**Fig. 2.75**) and is excellent at mapping retinal ischemia in occlusive vasculitis (**Fig. 2.76**), but not as yet indocyanine green angiography. Wide-field FA cannot be excelled for quantifying and monitoring retinal vasculitis with peripheral occlusion (**Fig. 2.77**), and where available will render Goldmann visual field testing (our historical method of monitoring progressive occlusion until

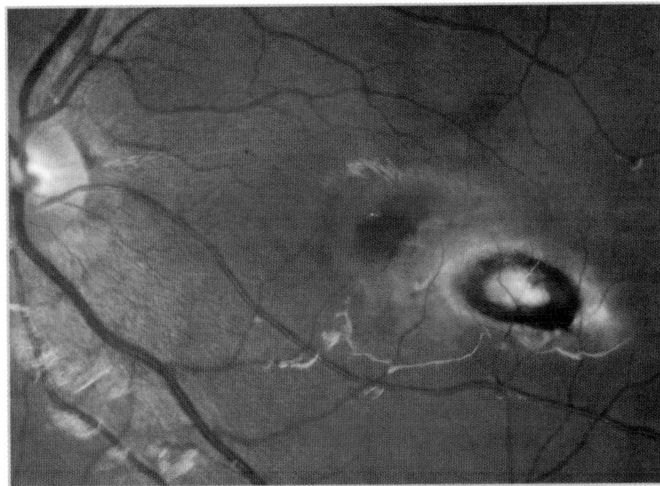

Figure 2.63 Choroidal neovascular membrane formation on the macular side of an old toxoplasma scar.

recently) redundant. The digital reconstruction of images means that resolution at high magnification currently remains inferior to standard photography, but a niche for this new technique has rapidly developed (Kaines et al. 2009) and doubtless images will continue to improve.

Indocyanine green angiography

Indocyanine green (ICG) is a small-molecule cyanine dye from a group initially developed for photographic development. ICG angiography complements fluorescein angiography in being superior at choroidal imaging. ICG has its peak excitation (805 nm) and fluorescence (835 nm) wavelengths in the near infrared, and at these wavelengths xanthophyll and melanin are relatively transparent, allowing better transretinal viewing of the choroid. The dye, when injected, becomes 98% plasma protein bound and therefore remains almost entirely intravascular even within fenestrated choriocapillaris vessels. These two parameters together allow more accurate and prolonged assessment of choroidal vasculature. Typically active lesions are hypofluorescent (**Fig. 2.78**) and often remain so for longer in the disease process than was realized before the technique became available (Herbort et al. 1998). The hypofluorescence represents either focal inflammation or ischemia, or both. It has been claimed that ICG findings more accurately reflect visual function than either funduscopy or FA, suggesting a clear role for ICG in the follow-up of sight-threatening inflammations affecting choroid, choriocapillaris and RPE. Modern ICG techniques have substantially improved resolution and further enhanced its potential. Allergy to iodine or shellfish is usually considered a contraindication to the technique, although in fact evidence of

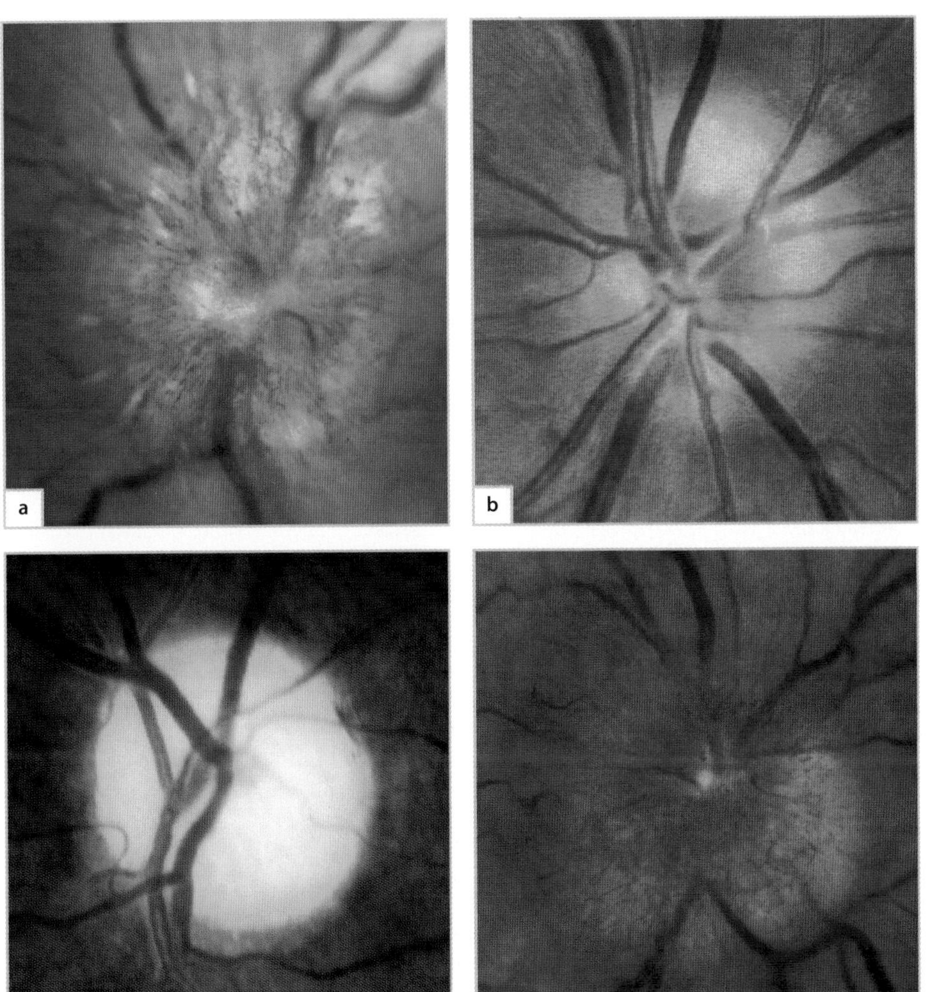

Figure 2.64 Four optic nerve head abnormalities associated with uveitis: (a) papillitis in syphilis; (b) optic nerve head drusen in a child with intermediate uveitis – a common mimic of optic nerve head swelling; (c) optic atrophy in multiple sclerosis with uveitis; and (d) papilledema in neurosarcoidosis.

Table 2.3 Systemic physical signs associated with uveitis

Signs	Possible diagnosis
Mouth and fauces	
Oral/faucal/pharyngeal ulceration	Behçet's disease
	Reactive arthropathy
	Herpes simplex
	Crohn's disease, ulcerative colitis
	Systemic lupus erythematosus (SLE)
	Primary or secondary syphilis
White plaques, erythema	Candidiasis
Integument	
Erythema nodosum	Sarcoidosis
	Behçet's disease
	Tuberculosis
	Streptococcal infection
	Inflammatory bowel disease
	Acute posterior multifocal placoid pigment epitheliopathy (AMPPE)
Maculopapular/scaly rash	Psoriasis
	Secondary syphilis
	Cutaneous candidiasis
	Drug induced (especially sulfonamides)
	Cutaneous larva migrans
Discoid/localized skin lesion (raised/flat)	Lupus pernio (sarcoidosis)
	Discoid/systemic lupus erythematosus
	Lupus vulgaris (tuberculosis)
	Erythema migrans (Lyme borreliosis)
Multifocal vasculitic rash	Systemic vasculitis, SLE
	Behçet's disease
	Sarcoidosis (unusual)
Follicular/pustular/acneiform rash	Behçet's disease
	Steroid-induced
	Pustular psoriasis
Vesicular dermatitis	Herpes simplex, herpes zoster
Lesions on palms/soles (in reactive arthritis)	Keratoderma blenorrhagicum
	Secondary syphilis
	Pustular psoriasis
Malar rash	SLE
	Lupus pernio
Leg ulcers	Cutaneous vasculitis
	Polyarteritis nodosa
	Syphilitic gumma
	Pyoderma gangrenosum (in inflammatory bowel or Behçet's disease)
	Leprosy, yaws
Kaposi's sarcoma	AIDS
Vitiligo	Vogt–Koyanagi–Harada (VKH) syndrome
	Sympathetic uveitis
	AMPPE
Hyperpigmentation	Whipple's disease
Alopecia	Vogt-Koyanagi-Harada syndrome
	Psoriasis, lupus, syphilis
	Cytotoxic treatment, steroid treatment

Table 2.3 *Continued.*

Signs	Possible diagnosis
Hirsutism	Treatment with ciclosporin, steroids
Subcutaneous nodules	Sarcoidosis
	Onchocerciasis
	Polyarteritis nodosa
Nail abnormalities	Pitting (psoriasis)
	Nail splinter hemorrhage (bacterial endocarditis, vasculitis)
Joints	
Axial arthropathy/spondylitis	Ankylosing spondylitis
	Reactive arthropathy,
	Inflammatory bowel disease (HLA-B27+)
	Psoriatic arthropathy (HLA-B27+)
Destructive hand arthropathy, rheumatoid type, sacroiliitis	Psoriatic arthropathy
Lower limb arthritis, spondylitis	Reactive arthritis
Monoarthritis, oligoarthritis	Juvenile chronic arthritis (especially knee)
	Endogenous sepsis, Lyme borreliosis
Polyarthritis	Reactive arthritis, SLE, drug reactions
	Whipple's disease
	Sarcoidosis
	Behçet's disease
	Juvenile chronic arthritis
Abdomen and genitals	
Genital ulceration	Behçet's disease
Perianal ulceration	Crohn's disease, Behçet's disease
Circinate balanitis	Reactive arthritis and uveitis
Epididymo-orchitis	Behçet's disease
Organomegaly	Sarcoidosis, malignancy
	Visceral larva migrans
	Cytomegalovirus (CMV) infection
Nervous system	
Central nervous system (CNS) abnormalities (various)	Sarcoidosis, herpes zoster, toxoplasmosis
	Multiple sclerosis
	Behçet's disease
	Systemic vasculitis, lupus
	Intraocular/CNS lymphoma
	AIDS, cryptococcosis, cysticercosis
	Ciclosporin/tacrolimus induced
	Tertiary syphilis, Lyme borreliosis
Peripheral neuropathy	Sarcoidosis, multiple sclerosis
	Leprosy, malignancy
	Ciclosporin/tacrolimus/isoniazid induced
Meningitis/meningoencephalitis	VKH syndrome, APMPPE
	Toxoplasmosis, herpes simplex, cryptococcosis
	Lyme borreliosis, brucellosis
Others	
Abnormal chest sounds	Sarcoidosis, tuberculosis
	Churg–Strauss syndrome, malignancy
Salivary gland enlargement	Sarcoidosis, malignancy, Behçet's disease
Lymphadenopathy	Sarcoidosis, tuberculosis
	AIDS, malignancy
	Bartonellosis

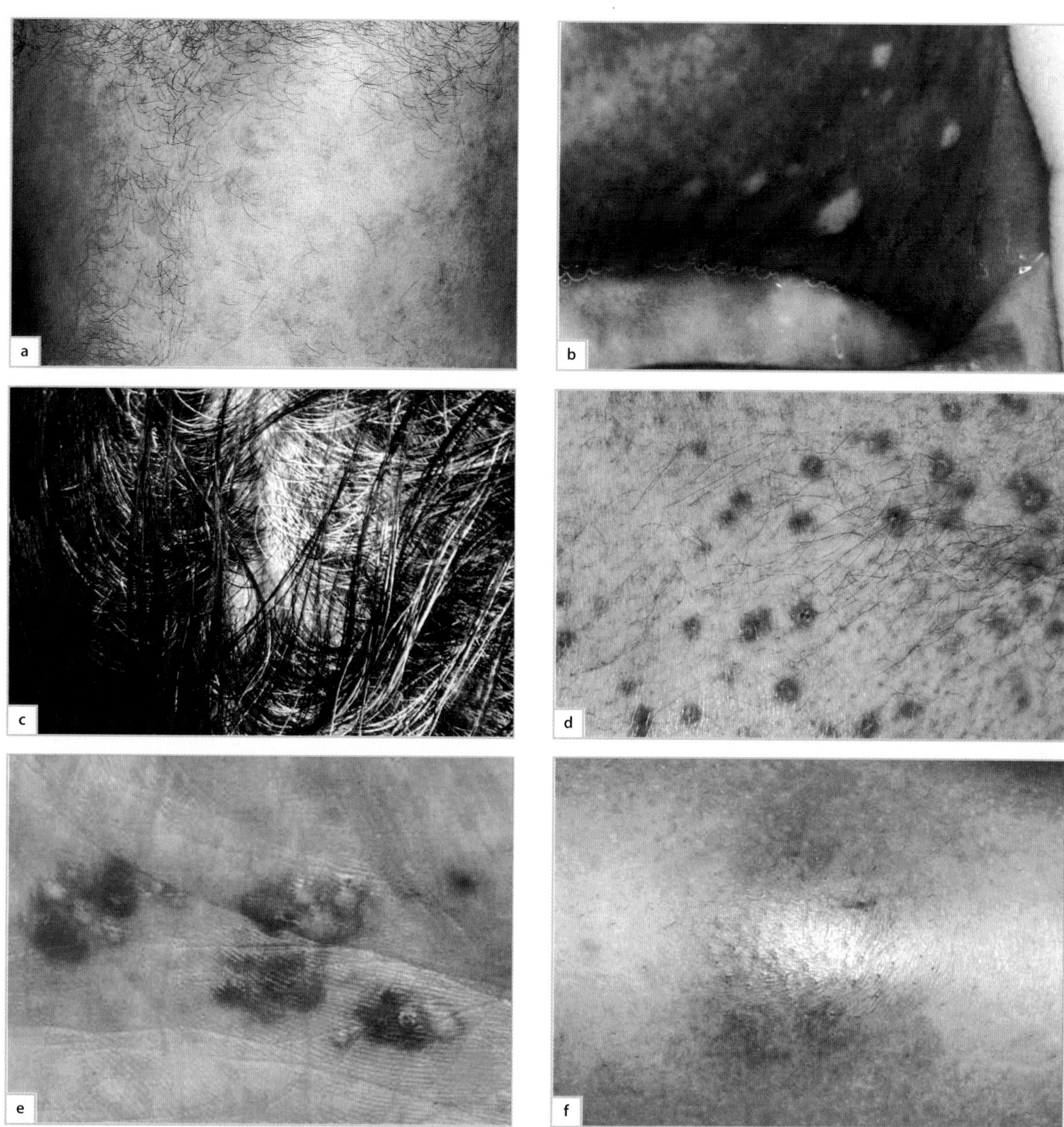

Figure 2.65 A collection of mucocutaneous and dermatological manifestations that the uveitis specialist will encounter: (a) maculopapular rash in secondary syphilis; (b) aphthous ulcers in Behçet's disease; (c) alopecia and poliosis in Vogt–Koyanagi–Harada syndrome; (d) cutaneous sarcoidosis; (e) keratoderma blenorrhagicum in reactive arthritis; and (f) erythema nodosum in sarcoidosis.

cross-reactivity with shellfish is not strong and requires reappraisal because about 2% of patients will claim such an allergy. Currently the view is that ICG is a better reflection of active choroidal disease than either FA or autofluorescence. However, new developments in OCT (see below) may enable better identification of choroidal structures, so that future of ICG angiography for inflammatory disease is unsure.

Fundus autofluorescence

Angiography is invasive and there is some associated risk. The prospect of a non-invasive imaging technique useful in posterior segment inflammation is attractive, and hence new attention has been drawn to the old technique of fundus autofluorescence (FAF). The substances capable of inducing FAF are fluorophores within lipofuscin, which

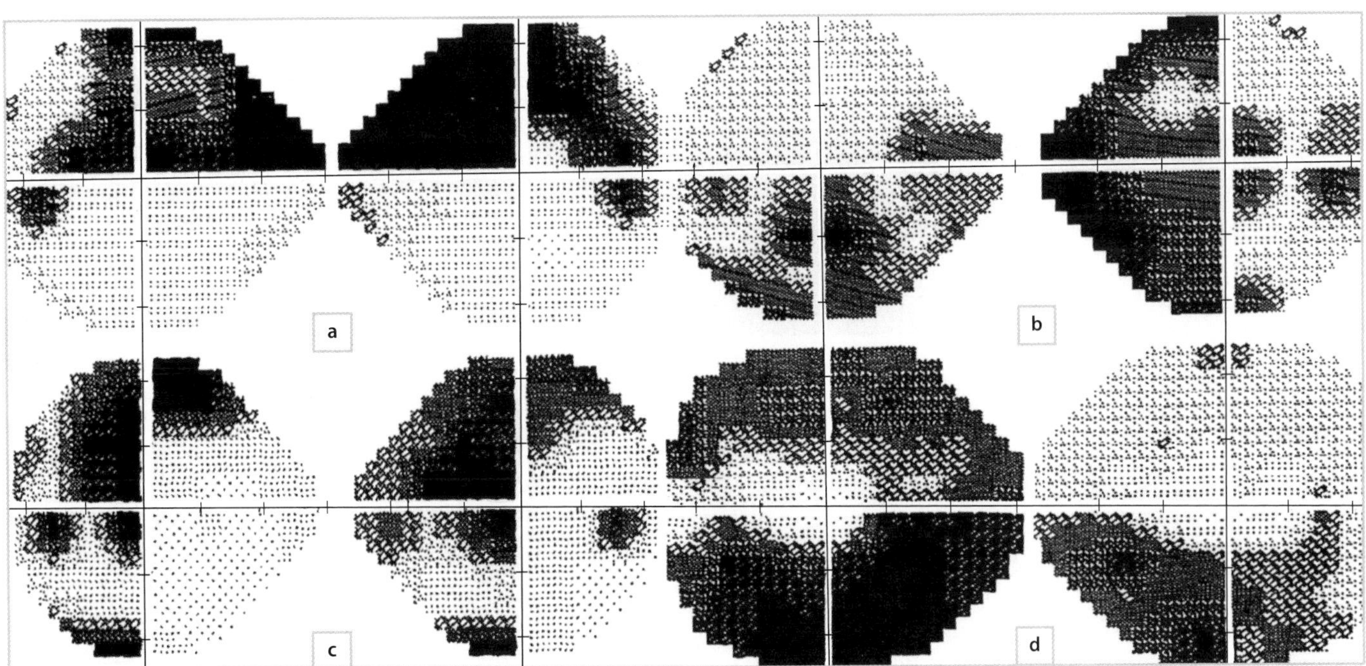

Figure 2.66 Visual field defects in patients with uveitis: (a) Advanced secondary glaucoma; (b) multifocal choroiditis with uveitis; (c) cerebrovascular disease and optic neuropathy in Behçet's disease; and (d) acute zonal occult outer retinopathy.

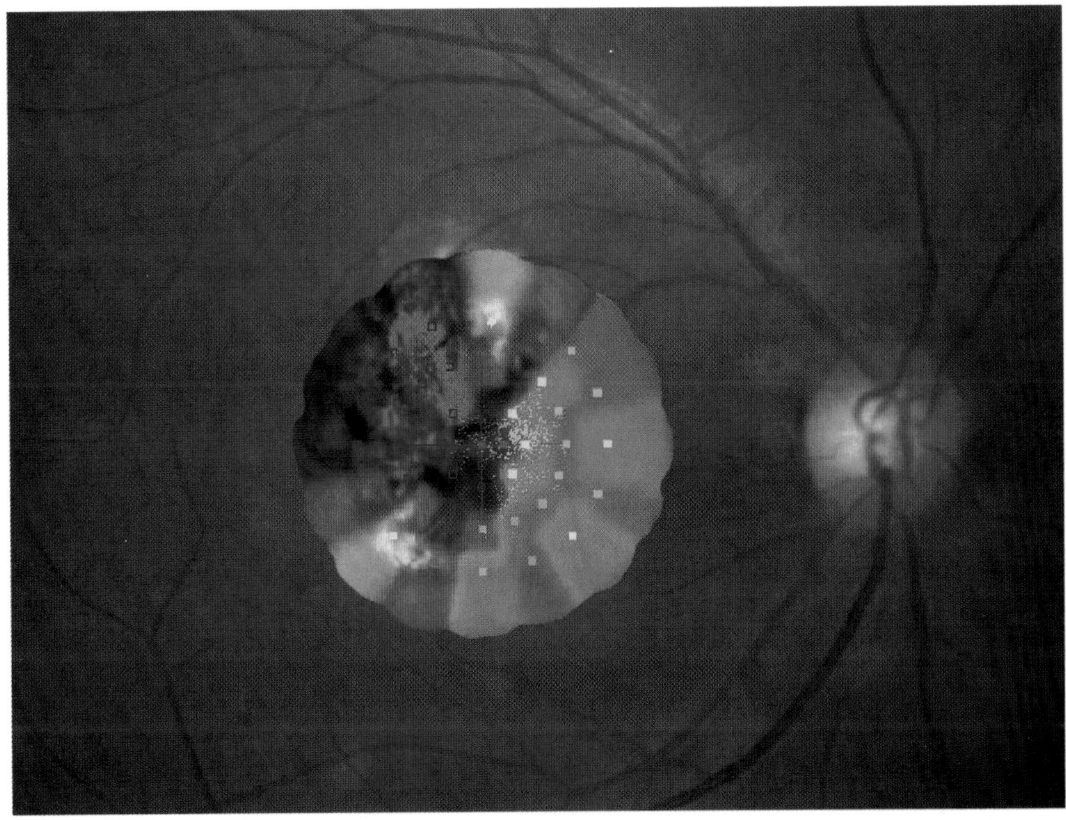

Figure 2.67 Microperimetry in a patient with severe macular involvement in punctate inner choroidopathy.

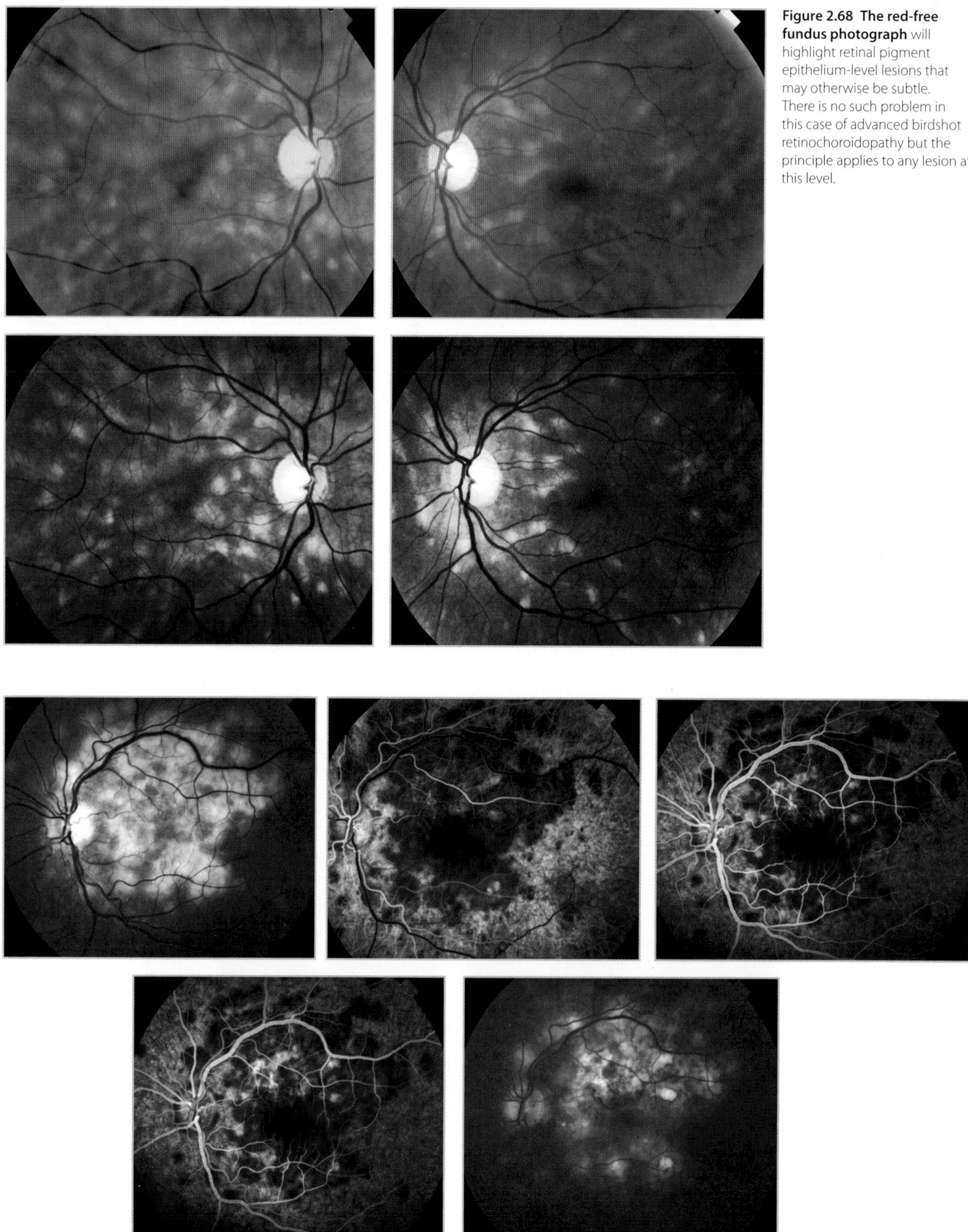

Figure 2.68 The red-free fundus photograph will highlight retinal pigment epithelium-level lesions that may otherwise be subtle. There is no such problem in this case of advanced birdshot retinochoroidopathy but the principle applies to any lesion at this level.

Figure 2.69 A typical fluorescein angiography sequence in acute posterior multifocal placoid pigment epitheliopathy, preceded by a red-free photograph. Early dark areas during the 'choroidal blush' phase indicate lobular ischemia, followed by patchy incomplete filling and then late lesion staining.

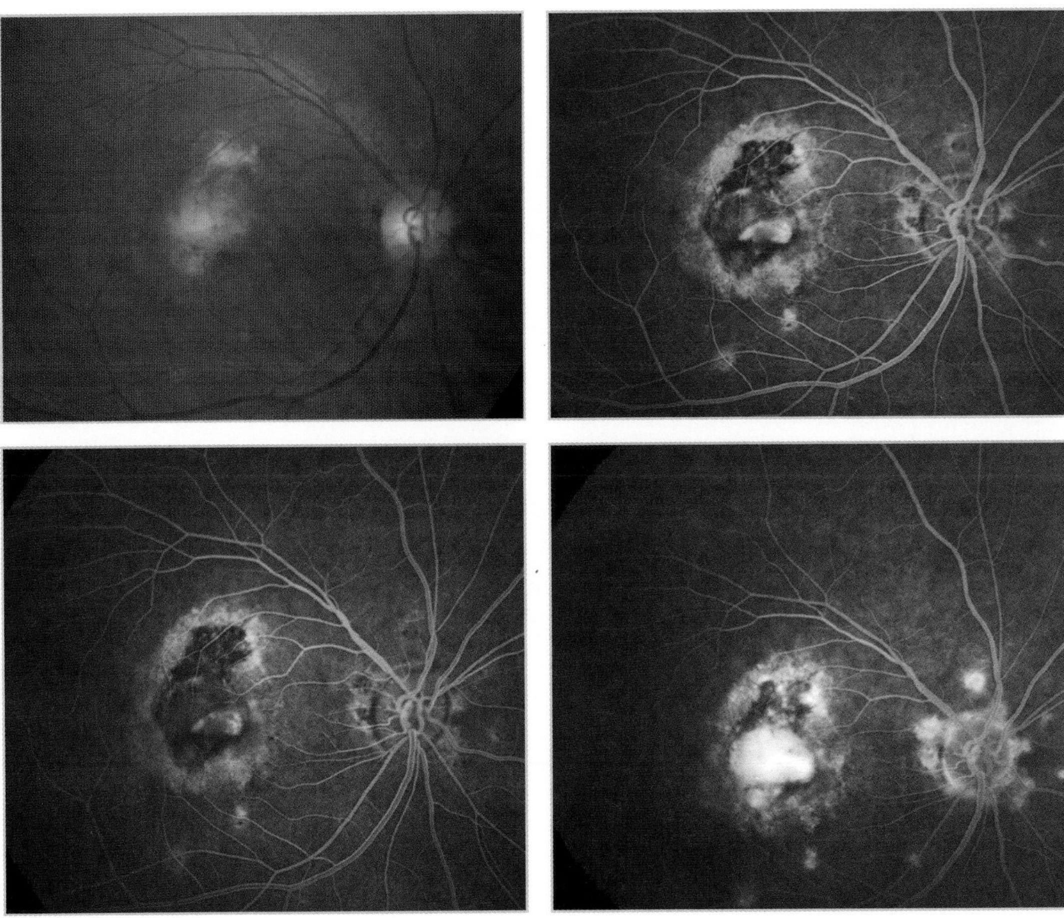

Figure 2.70 A fluorescein run showing a choroidal neovascular membrane in an eye with punctate inner choroidopathy scars.

accumulates metabolically within the RPE. Collagen and elastin are minor fluorophores normally not visible where the RPE is intact. Luteal pigments at the fovea mask normal RPE autofluorescence but damage to this area exposes FAF at the RPE level. There is a range of both excitation and emission wavelengths for FAF but generally excitation when using a scanning laser ophthalmoscope (SLO) is at 490 nm and the emission filter set at between 500 and 700 nm. Using a conventional fundus camera to detect FAF, excitation is normally about 550 nm and emission 650–700 nm. The quality and pattern detected will vary between these two systems but the SLO generally provides more discriminatory images. Atrophic RPE is dark on FAF and the edges of diseased areas are often hyperfluorescent, indicating high levels of metabolite accumulation (**Fig. 2.79**). The technique is particularly useful in the early diagnosis and monitoring of dystrophic or degenerative RPE maculopathies but its place in the management of inflammatory diseases is as yet unsure. Its capability of showing edge activity in multifocal lesions may be useful (Yeh et al. 2010) and it is clearly capable of showing activity invisible to FA (**Fig. 2.80**). There may be a place in the diagnosis of relatively occult inflammations such as acute zonal occult outer retinopathy (AZOOR) where conventional imaging is not useful (**Fig. 2.81**).

High-resolution ICG angiography is probably of greater current relevance in the field of posterior segment inflammation because of the primary location of disease in the choriocapillaris in so many entities. Three methods are compared in **Fig. 2.82**. There is a codicil to this: the increasing quality of SLO techniques now allows high-resolution near-infrared FAF where melanin may be the main fluorophore. Although the RPE will usually therefore remain the highest emitter, choroidal visibility may be enhanced by this technique and ICG may have a non-invasive competitor to image choroidal inflammations in the future.

Optical coherence tomography

Optical coherence tomography medical instruments share the property of using either visible or near-infrared light to create sectional images from translucent or nominally opaque tissue. They use low-coherence interferometry to effectively remove all non-coherent scattered light, so that only coherent reflected light is included in the resultant image. The intensity and reflection distance thus combine to give tomographic images (essentially optical coherence B-scans), and those produced by instruments for ocular use have evolved enormously since their first description 20 years ago. A false-color system differentiates high or low reflectivity, which is an expression of tissue junctions rather than anatomical layers. This is time-domain OCT. The RPE in particular has high reflectivity, as has choriocapillaris (normally the greatest penetrable depth by standard OCT), but less so the retinal nerve fiber layer. The outer retinal reflective layer is actually bilaminar, the inner (upper) layer probably representing the inner/outer photoreceptor junction and the lower probably corresponding to Bruch's membrane. Epiretinal membranes and posterior hyaloid are also distinguishable (**Fig. 2.83**). Cystoid accumulations of intraretinal edema are completely non-reflective. Retinal thickness measurements are reliably repeatable.

Those readers who have a higher qualification in physics will doubtless regard the above disdainfully as an absurd oversimplification of an exquisitely powerful and sensitive instrument, and they are correct. The subsequent introduction of spectral-domain (or Fourier-domain)

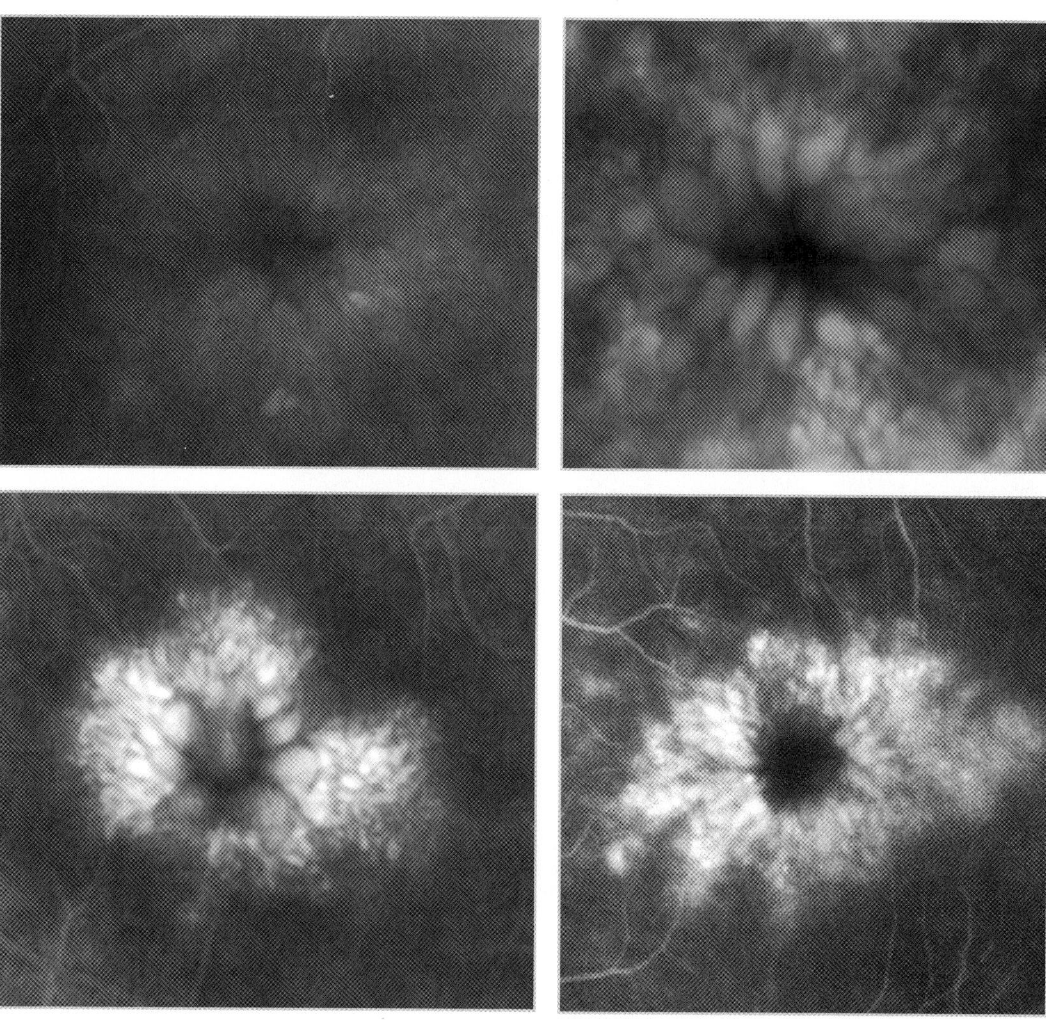

Figure 2.71 Grades of macular edema visible with fluorescein angiography.

software, however, stretches the demand on the reader (and most certainly the author) unfamiliar with Fourier analysis to a yet higher level. Broadly speaking, a Fourier transform is a process capable of fragmenting a complex mathematical function into constituent trigonometric parts, and complex multi-wavelength signals such as those generated by OCT are one variety of such a complex function that can be broken down into constituent frequencies. In the context of OCT, the simultaneous use of spectrometry and a high-speed charge-coupled device enables the use of oscillatory magnitude as a surrogate measure of the echo time delay (the normal OCT depth differentiator) using Fourier transform software. This enables the calculation of A-scan measurements without the need to move the reference mirror, which is both a time- and resolution-limiting feature of older machines. Thus spectral domain OCT instruments are much faster in image acquisition, produce images of better resolution and can be presented with simultaneous SLO ophthalmoscopy (**Fig. 2.84**).

The uveitis practitioner will use the OCT machine as a virtual replacement of FA in the monitoring of macular edema and to differentiate treatable from non-treatable chronic edema, and to detect both macular holes and pseudoholes, epiretinal membrane (ERM) and tractional change attributable to it, serous retinal elevation in acute or chronic inflammations and pigment epithelial detachment. Media opacities can substantially degrade OCT images so that occasionally FA is superior to OCT in detecting macular edema, but this is unusual. Broadly speaking, currently available OCT machines provide an understanding of the retinal and preretinal complications of inflammatory posterior segment disease in a way never previously available (**Fig. 2.85**).

The technique of OCT is not confined to retinal examination. Although most OCT instruments are capable of accurately imaging a depth of up to 2 mm and therefore cannot image choroid, new developments in image acquisition can enable images of increasing depth (**Fig. 2.86**); clearly, if this becomes clinically useful, this form of OCT will combat ICG angiography as the prime imager of choroidal disease. Anterior segment OCT is also capable of producing high-resolution images (**Fig. 2.87**) as far back as the anterior lens surface and resolution is good enough to map peripheral anterior synechiae (**Fig. 2.88**). For imaging of the ciliary body, ultrasound biomicroscopy is superior (Bianciotto et al. 2011) although both may have a role for uveitis imaging in the future.

Confocal scanning laser ophthalmoscopy

The principle of confocal microscopy is to permit recording of planar alterations in high detail compared with optical photography, enabling simultaneous recording of surfaces at variable depth. In addition to permitting intraretinal layer discrimination, modern instruments using confocal scanning laser ophthalmoscopy (cSLO) also allow FAF and angiography. The Spectralis instrument from Heidelberg Engineering now permits simultaneous cSLO and

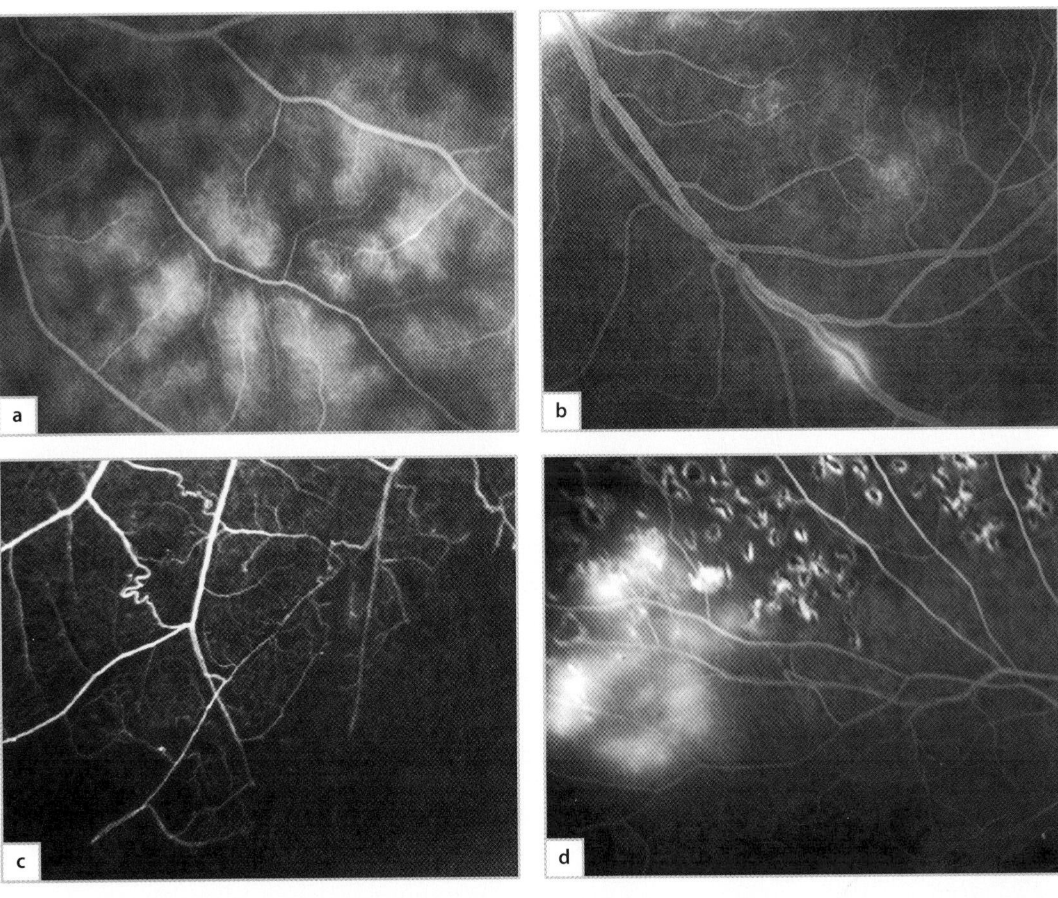

Figure 2.72 Manifestations of retinal vasculitis which aid diagnosis or management: (a) capillaritis in Behçet's disease; (b) focal retinal vasculitis in birdshot retinochoroidopathy; (c) peripheral ischemia and shunting in sarcoidosis; and (d) neovascularization in Eales' disease

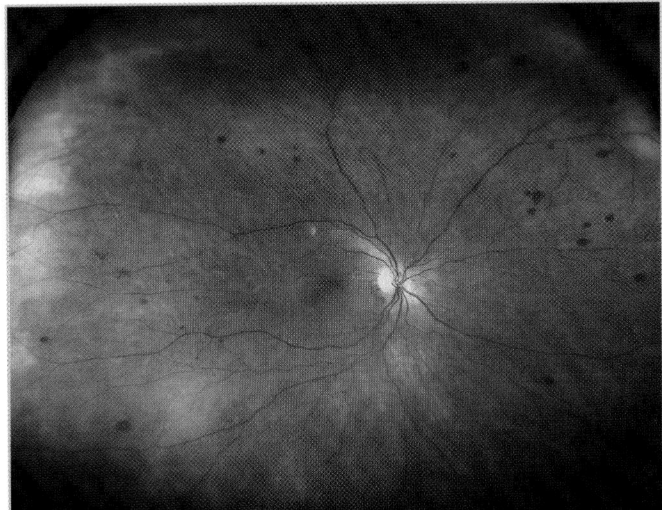

Figure 2.73 An Optos wide-field Optomap in a patient with retinal vasculitis.

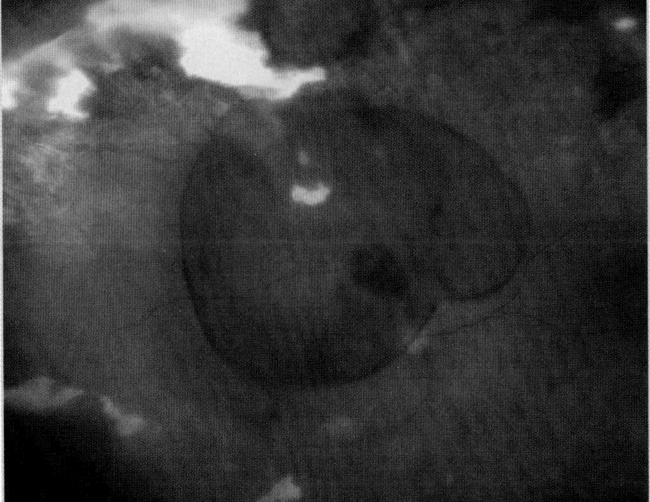

Figure 2.74 An Optos wide-field Optomap showing vitreous collapse following viral retinitis.

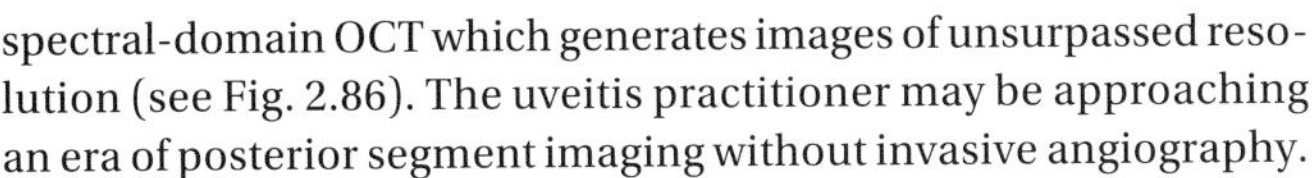

spectral-domain OCT which generates images of unsurpassed resolution (see Fig. 2.86). The uveitis practitioner may be approaching an era of posterior segment imaging without invasive angiography.

Ultrasonography

In some circumstances ultrasonography provides valuable additional information in patients with uveitis. It may be useful in assessing lesional density where neoplastic disease is part of the differential diagnosis, and may provide additional information on granulomas, e.g. in toxocariasis or sarcoidosis. It will identify posterior vitreous detachment and diagnose retinal detachment in those with opaque media. It will also identify the pattern of vitreous condensations, which may be of diagnostic significance. It is able to detect choroidal or scleral thickening and may be useful in the differential diagnosis of optic nerve head enlargement. Higher-frequency examination can

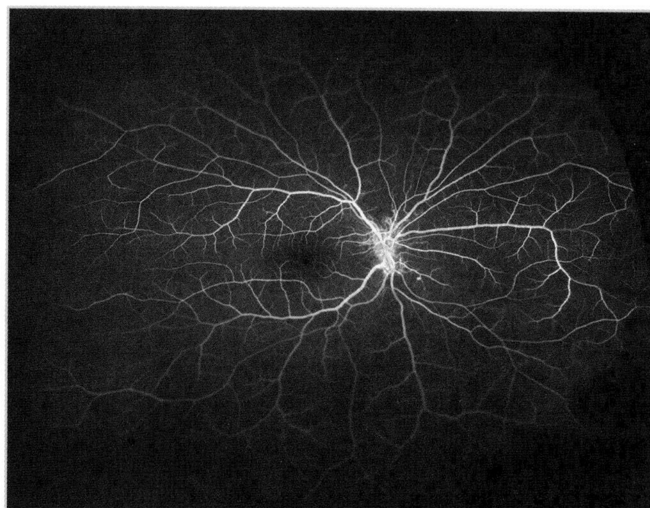

Figure 2.75 A normal fundus undergoing Optos wide-field fluorescein angiography. The eyelashes usually intrude inferiorly.

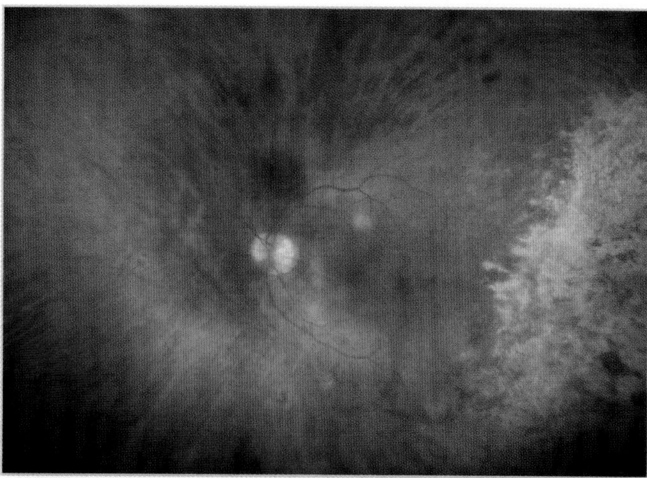

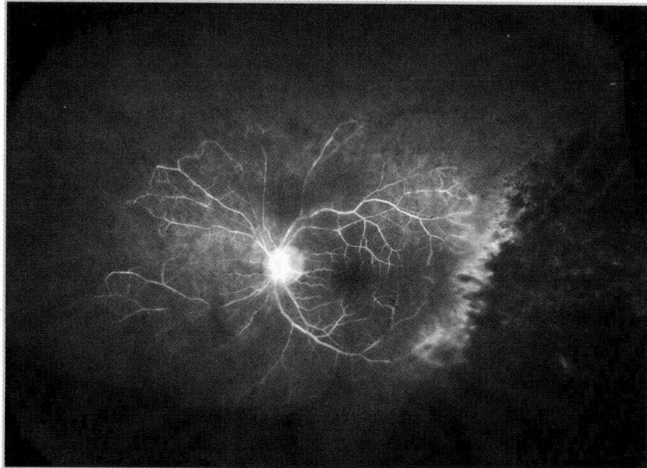

Figure 2.76 Cytomegalovirus retinitis with profound retinal ischaemia shown on Optos images.

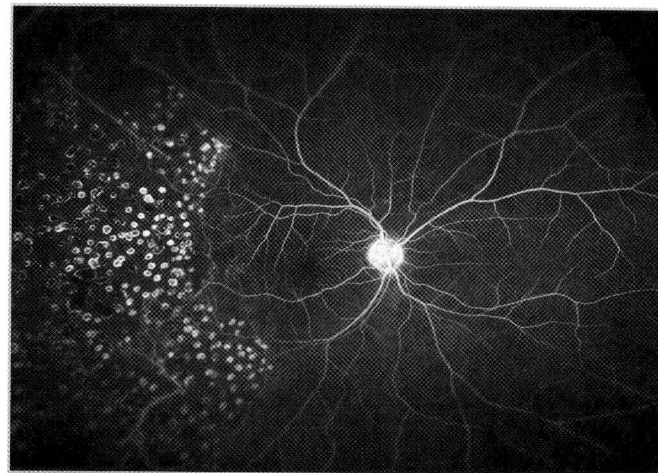

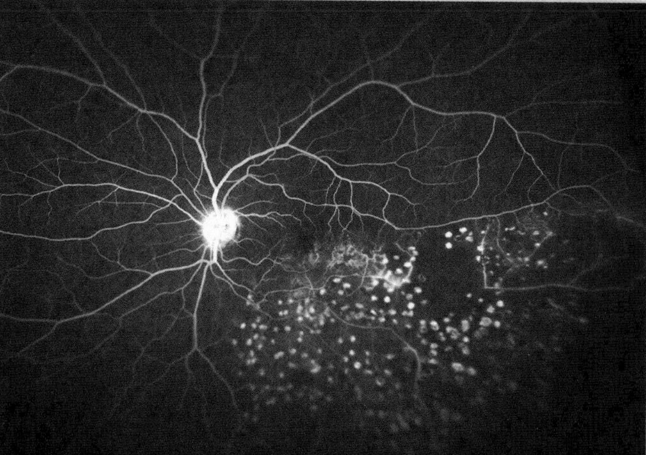

Figure 2.77 Optos wide-field angiograms of a patient with bilateral occlusive primary retinal vasculitis who has undergone sectoral laser ablation.

Figure 2.78 Multifocal dark areas on indocyanine green angiography in a patient with birdshot retinochoroidopathy.

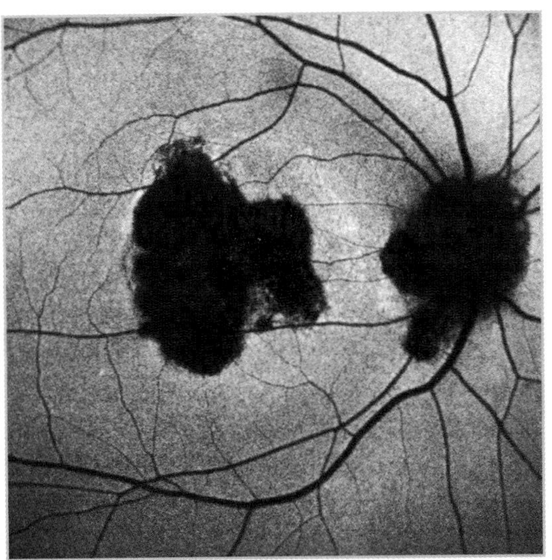

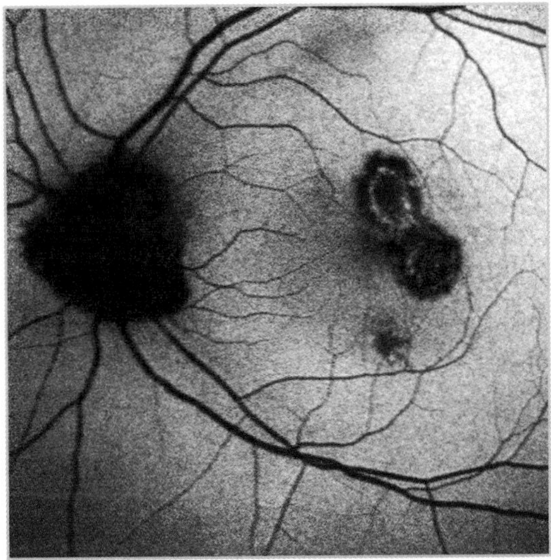

Figure 2.79 Autofluorescence of a lesion edge indicating residual activity in punctate inner choroidopathy. (Courtesy of Dr E Priel.)

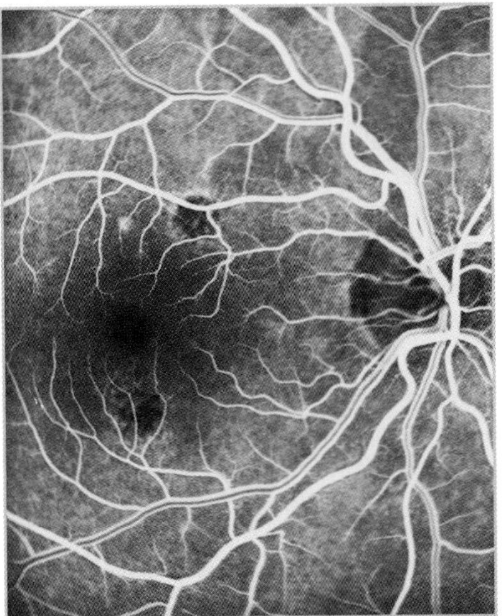

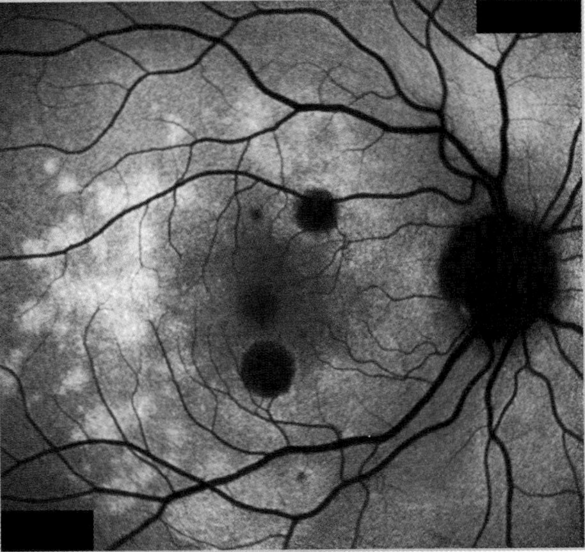

Figure 2.80 Multifocal autofluorescence indicating areas of damage not seen on fluorescein angiography in punctate inner choroidopathy. (Courtesy of Dr E Priel.)

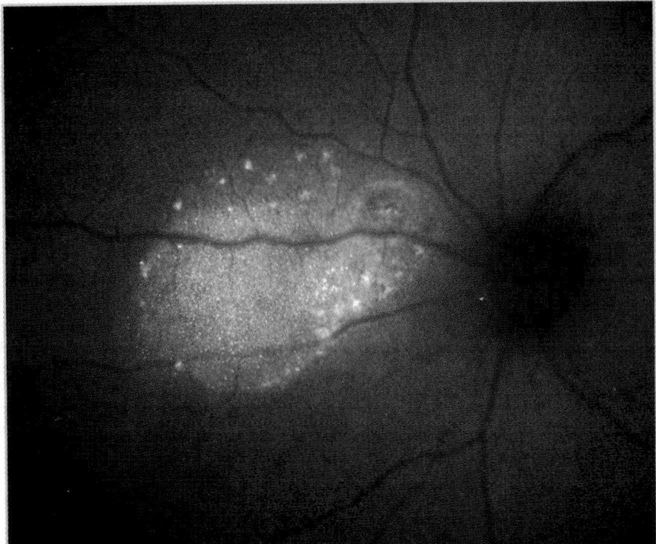

Figure 2.81 An area of punctate hyper-autofluorescence in a patient with symptoms indicative of acute zonal occult outer retinopathy. Funduscopy was entirely normal.

provide detailed assessment of pars plana where funduscopy is difficult (Doro et al. 2006).

Anterior and mid-segment ultrasound biomicroscopy permits imaging of peripheral anterior segment anatomy otherwise inaccessible to examination. Ciliary body abnormalities (**Fig. 2.89**), iris–lens diaphragm position, peripheral anterior synechiae, peripheral vitreoretinal traction and detachment are all identifiable. The technique has uses in planning surgical approaches in both cataract and glaucoma surgery, although recently the development of anterior segment OCT has led to comparisons of image quality and penetration. The superior definition of OCT is balanced by the greater penetration of ultrasonography, and there will be an ongoing use for both methods of imaging.

Electrophysiology

Electroretinal tests are frequently abnormal in widespread retinochoroiditis and reflect the degree of retinal involvement, but changes may be non-specific and therefore diagnostically unhelpful. However, visual field loss without clinical evidence of intraocular cause, such as acute idiopathic blind spot enlargement or acute zonal occult outer retinopathy, occurs in isolation or in combination with multifocal inflammation, and these conditions

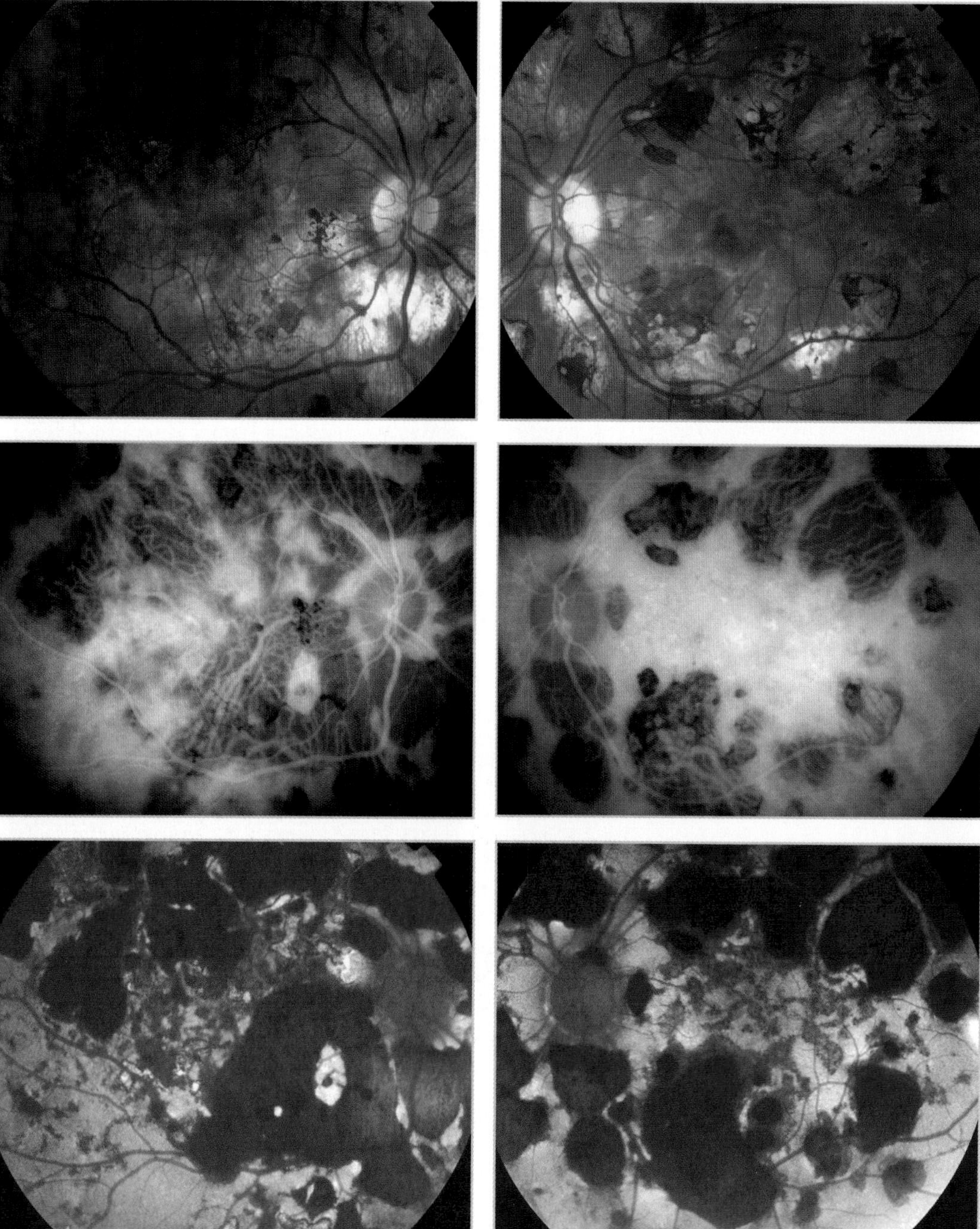

Figure 2.82 Imaging compared: a patient with atypical acute posterior multifocal placoid pigment epitheliopathy is examined with indocyanine green (ICG) angiography (center, showing large choroidal vessels and basically imaging these and choriocapillaris) and fundus autofluorescence (below, which shows large dead areas of retinal pigment epithelium including subtle areas not seen on ICG, but no choroidal details).

have been associated with abnormal electroretinal tests. The differentiation of such presumed retinal abnormalities from optic nerve or intracranial causes of visual field loss is important. Also, the use of visual evoked potentials in those with putative optic nerve damage is sometimes helpful.

Developments in ERG techniques have recently permitted a more specific assessment of inflammatory retinal dysfunction which is helpful both diagnostically and in treatment monitoring, e.g. in birdshot retinochoroidopathy (Holder et al. 2005). However, in general electrophysiological assessments mirror examination methods of retinal and visual function which are both quicker to perform and more accurate in assessment, and these latter are developing more rapidly; the future of electrophysiology in the uveitis clinic is not secure.

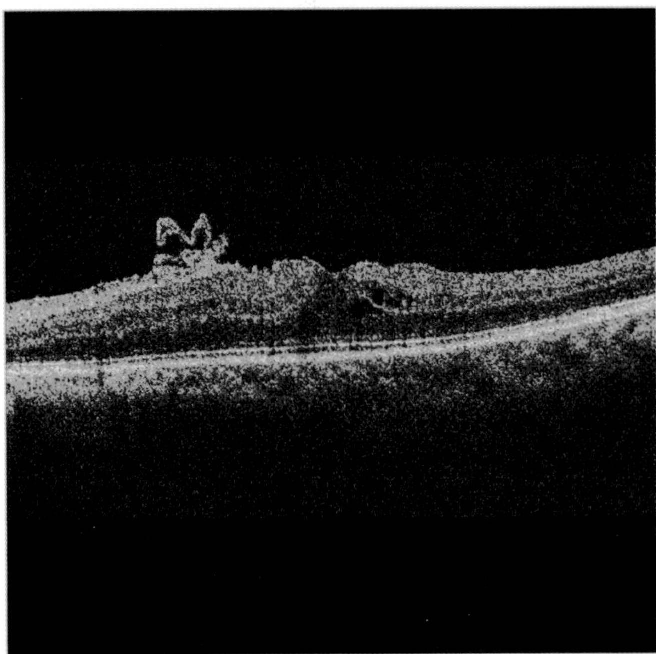

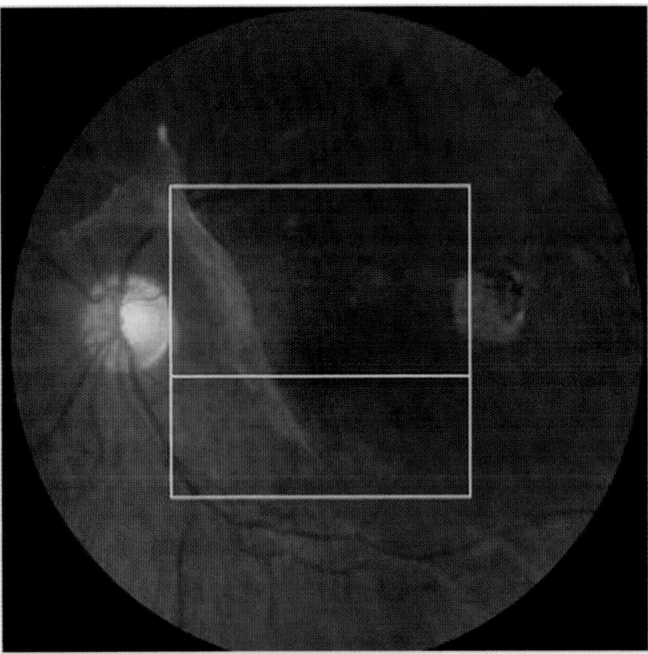

Figure 2.83 An optical coherence tomographic scan of a partially avulsed inflammatory epiretinal membrane showing the wrinkled detached cross-section with associated macular edema.

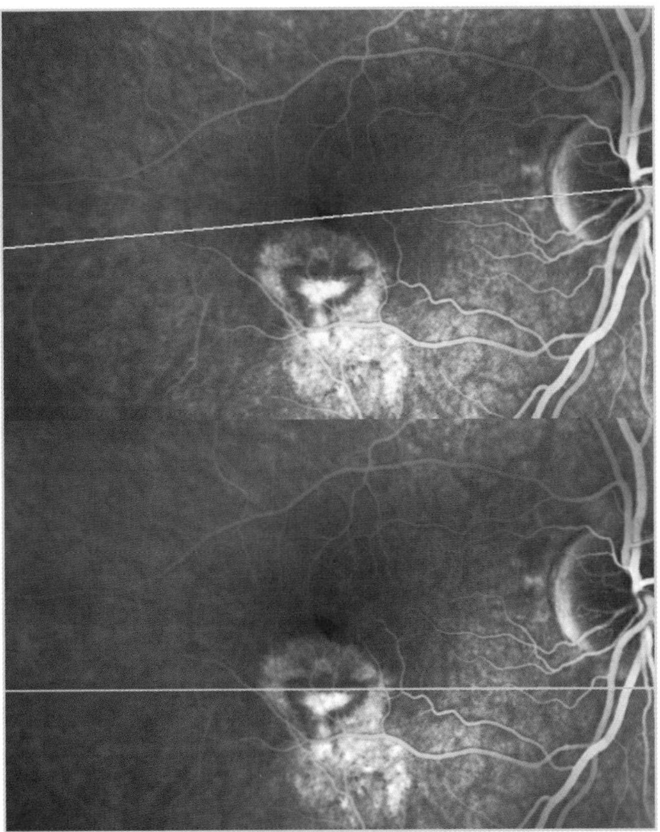

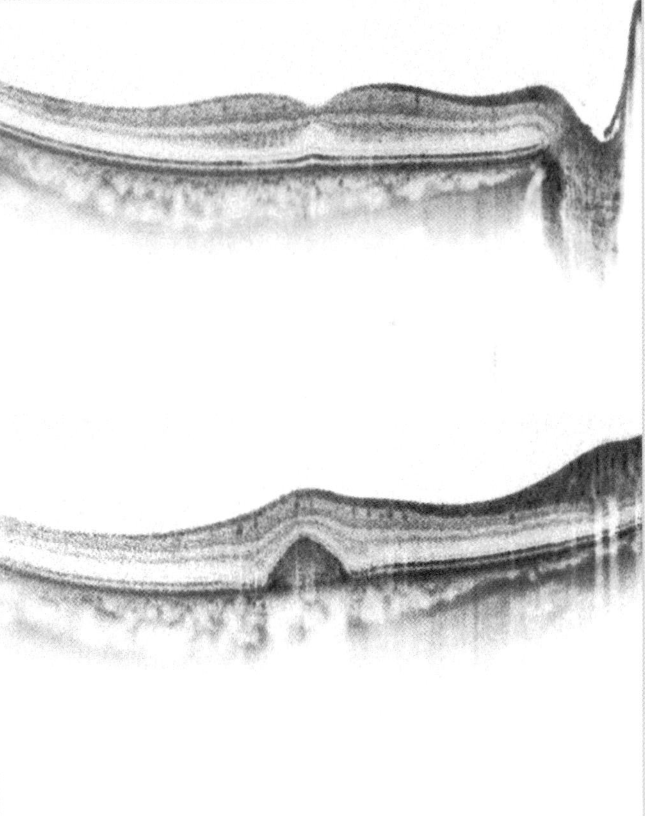

Figure 2.84 Simultaneous spectral-domain optical coherence tomography and scanning laser ophthalmoscopy show high-resolution imaging of retinal layers with excellent delineation of abnormal lesions, such as a neovascular membrane in punctate inner choroidopathy. (Courtesy of Dr E Priel.)

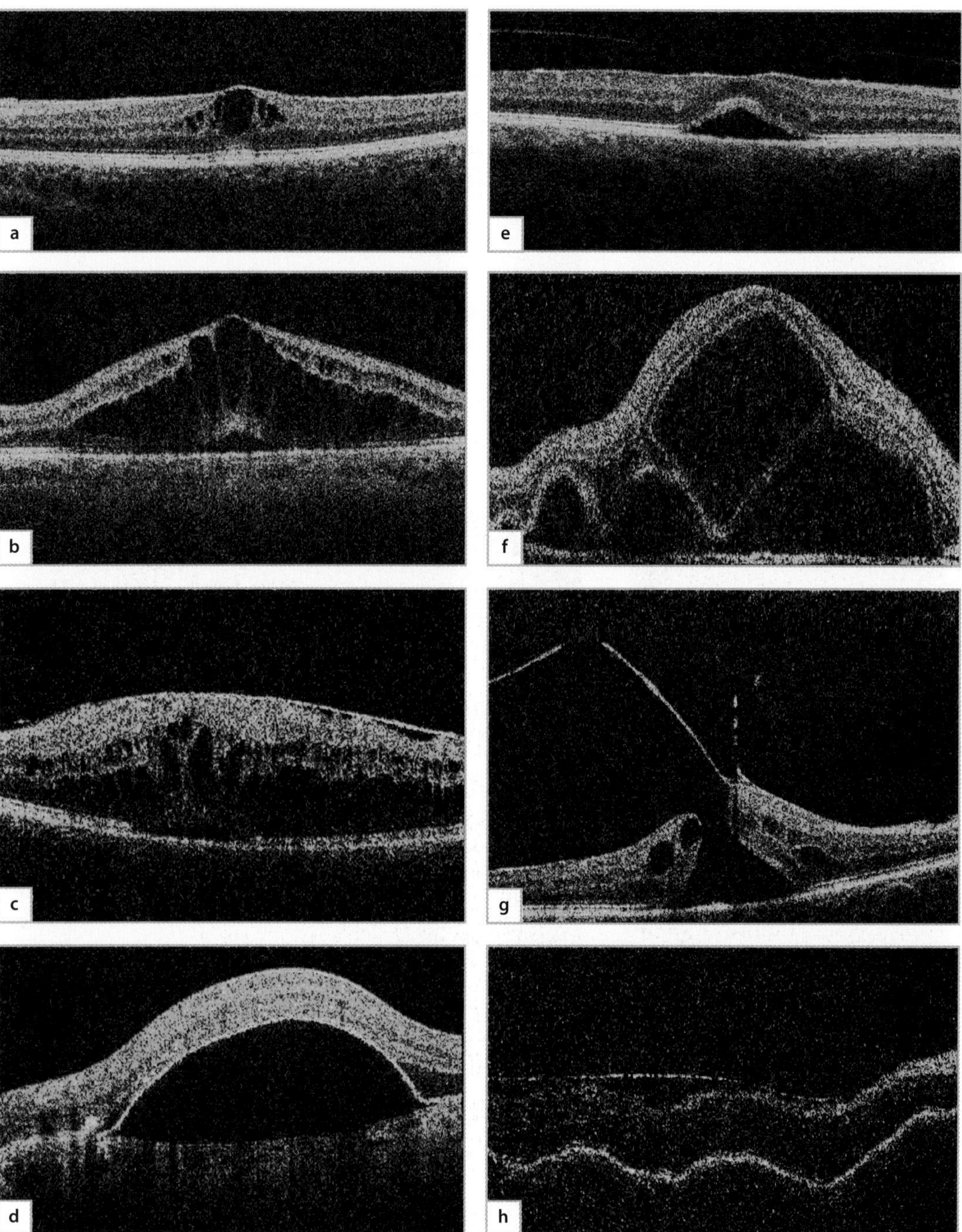

Figure 2.85 Optical coherence tomography in patients with uveitis: (a) moderate cystoid macular edema (CMO);(b) very severe CMO with associated PED; (c) very chronic CMO with disrupted retinal architecture; d) severe chronic pigment epithelial detachment (PED) after vitrectomy with removal of epiretinal membrane (ERM); (e) chronic unresponsive PED; (f) multiloculated serous retinal detachment in Vogt–Koyanagi–Harada syndrome; (g) severe tractional ERM with retinal hole; and (h) phthisis with retinal wrinkling and ERM.

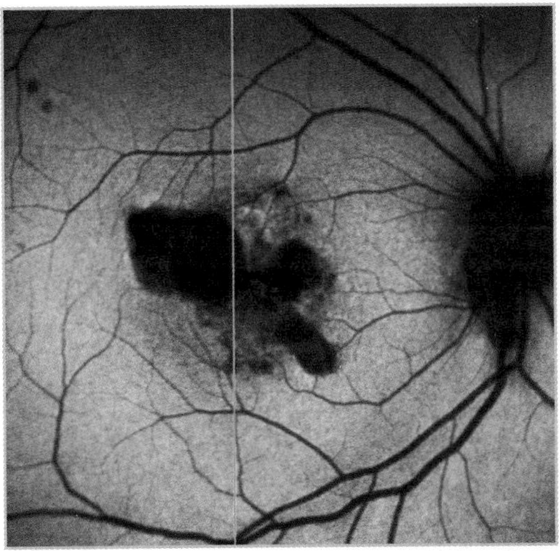

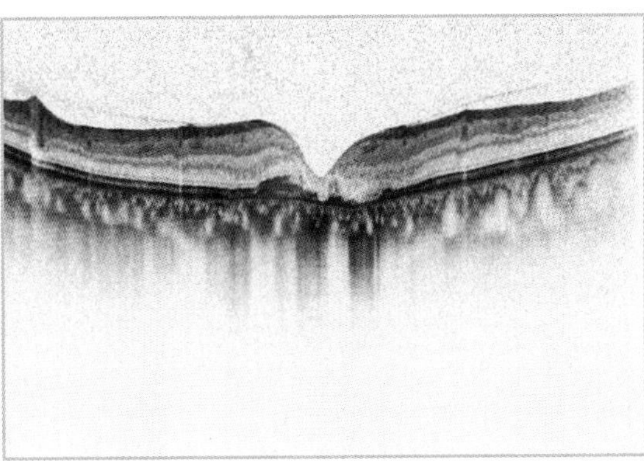

Figure 2.86 New developments in optical coherence tomography are allowing scans of increasing depth; the choriocapillaris structure is already visible. (Courtesy of Dr E Priel.)

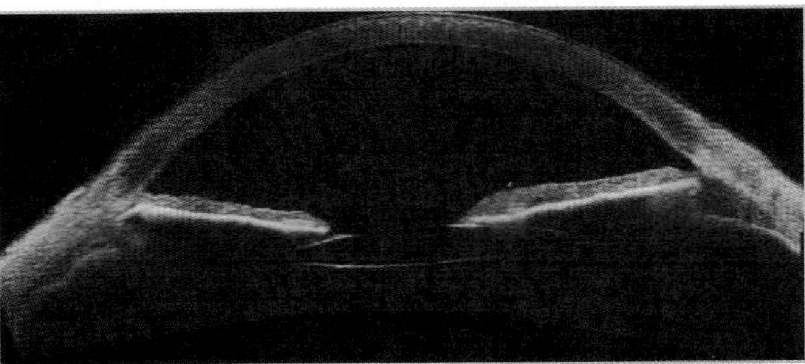

Figure 2.87 Anterior segment optical coherence tomography is capable of high-resolution images but only back to the anterior lens surface. The peripheral anterior synechiae on the left of the image are distinguishable. (Courtesy of Mr L Au.)

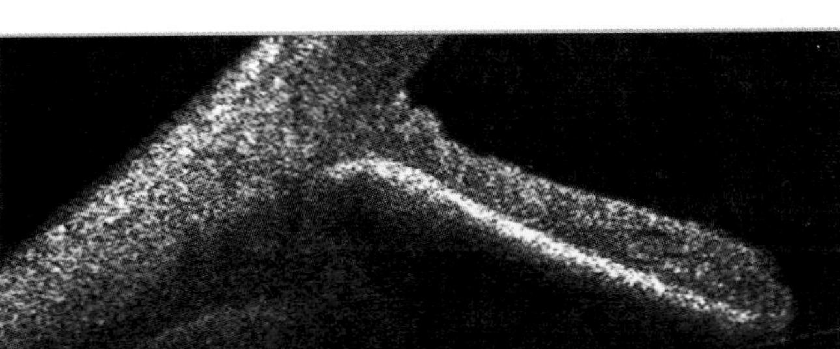

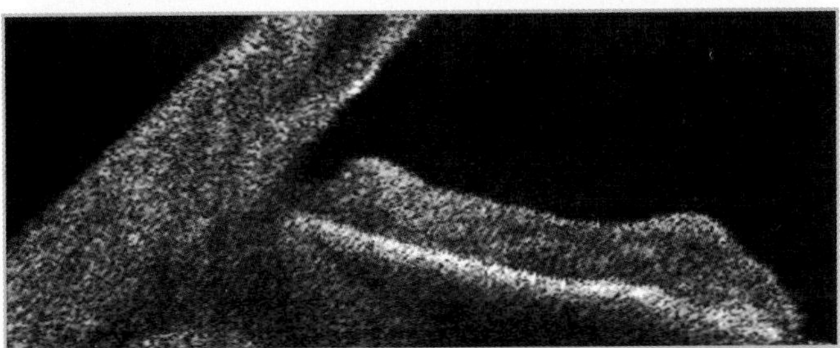

Figure 2.88 Magnified anterior segment optical coherence tomographic scans before (top) and after (bottom) goniosynechialysis clearly show the resolution of peripheral anterior synechiae. (Courtesy of Mr L Au.)

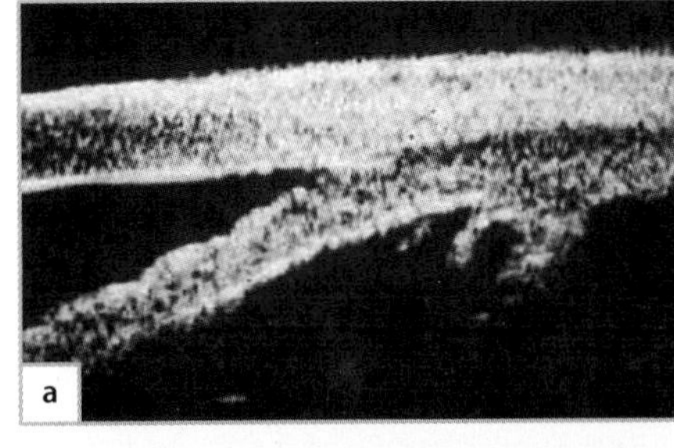

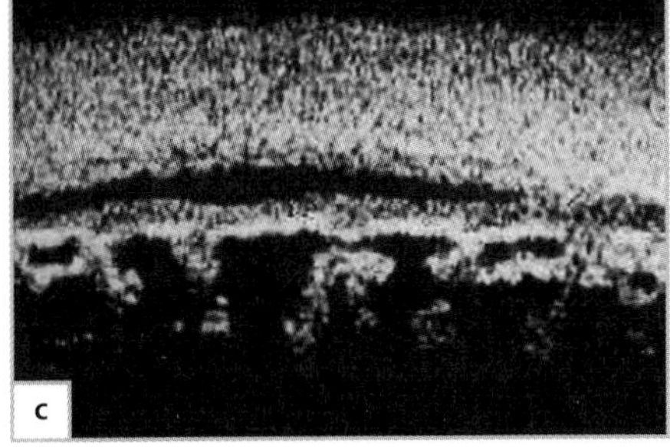

Figure 2.89 Three ultrasound biomicroscopy images of anterior segment: (a) normal configuration; (b) ciliary body cyst; and (c) transverse section showing ciliary cleft and processes. (Courtesy of Dr C Tromans.)

REFERENCES

BenEzra D, Forrester JV, Nussenblatt RB, et al. *Uveitis Scoring System*. Berlin: Springer-Verlag, 1991.

Bianciotto C, Shields CL, Guzman JM, et al. Assessment of anterior segment tumours with ultrasound biomicroscopy versus anterior segment optical coherence tomography in 200 cases. *Ophthalmology* 2011;**118**:1297–302.

Doro D, Manfre A, Deligianni V, Secchi A. Combined 50- and 20-MHz frequency ultrasound imaging in intermediate uveitis. *Am J Ophthalmol* 2006;**141**:953–55.

Gardiner AM, Armstrong RA, Dunne MC, Murray PI. Correlation between visual function and visual ability in patients with uveitis. *Br J Ophthalmol* 2002;**86**:993–6.

Giuliari GP, Pujari S, Shaikh M, et al. Microperimetry findings in patients with birdshot chorioretinopathy. *Can J Ophthalmol* 2010;**45**:399–403.

Herbort CP, LeHoang P, Guex-Crozier Y. Schematic interpretation of indocyanine green angiography in posterior uveitis using a standard angiographic protocol. *Ophthalmology* 1998;*105*:432–40.

Holder GE, Robson AG, Pavesio C, Graham EM. Electrophysiological characterisation and monitoring in t he management of birdshot chorioretinopathy. *Br J Ophthalmol* 2005;**89**:709–18.

Jabs DA, Nussenblatt RB, Rosenbaum JT, et al. Standardization of uveitis nomenclature for reporting clinical data. Results of the first international workshop. *Am J Ophthalmol* 2005;**140**:509–16.

Kaines A, Tsui I, Sarraf D, Schwartz S. The use of ultra wide field fluorescein angiography in evaluation and management of uveitis. *Semin Ophthalmol* 2009;**24**:19–24.

Lam S, Tessler HH, Winchester K, et al. Iris crystals in chronic iridocyclitis. *Br J Ophthalmol* 1993;**77**:181–2.

Nussenblatt RB, Palestine AG, Chan CC, et al. Standardisation of vitreal inflammatory activity in intermediate and posterior uveitis. *Ophthalmology* 1985;**92**:467–71.

Rothova A, La Hey E, Baarsma GS, et al. Iris nodules in Fuchs' heterochromic uveitis. *Am J Ophthalmol* 1994;**118**:338–42.

Wakefield D, Herbort CP, Tugal-Tutkun I, Zierhut M. Controversies in ocular inflammation and immunology: laser flare photometry. *Ocul Immunol Inflamm* 2010;**18**:334–40.

Yeh S, Forooghian F, Wong WT, et al. Fundus autofluorescence imaging of the white dot syndromes. *Arch Ophthalmol* 2010;**128**:46–56.

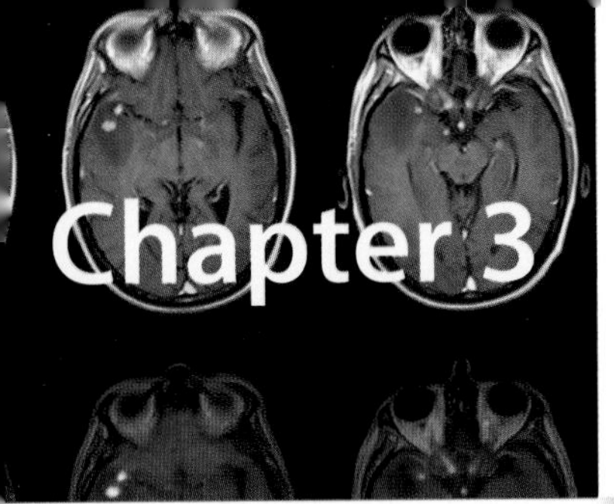

Chapter 3 Investigations in uveitis

The relevance and importance of investigations in the diagnosis and management of uveitis are a complex matter, and the issue is not one that readily lends itself to standard protocols. The performance of any investigation should require a proper understanding of the relevance of possible test results for an individual patient. The concept of a 'diagnostic' test with 100% sensitivity and specificity is known by all of us to be merely whimsical, yet there is a natural and widespread tendency to over-interpret test results, for a variety of reasons: the clinician's knowledge of the test itself may be suboptimal; new testing methods arrive regularly on the scene, and laboratories may fix local criteria for normality and abnormality. Sometimes laconic methods of laboratory reporting, and a lack of communication between laboratory experts and clinicians, can lead to a poor understanding of modern testing methods. The laboratory that includes explanatory notes with test results is thoroughly appreciated by the clinician.

The etiological diagnosis of uveitis is sometimes a frustrating business, and the perceived need to apply a 'label' to a particular uveitis is a pressure on the ophthalmologist: self-applied, from the patient and relatives, and sometimes from other doctors. The temptation to apply a label that, in the cold light of day, may not be justified is sometimes heightened by the result of a test performed and interpreted out of context. This problem applies particularly to ophthalmologists in training, who may allow their enthusiasm to express, in case notes, a differential diagnosis that is unrealistic. With the passage of time, such written statements, if left uncorrected, seem to acquire a validity of their own which in the future may misdirect diagnostic efforts. They should therefore be immediately edited.

CHOOSING AND INTERPRETING TESTS

It is assumed here that the ophthalmologist considering investigations for a patient is driven only by practical altruism, the desire to facilitate diagnosis and management. In making decisions about investigations in a particular patient, it is useful for the ophthalmologist to ask the following questions.

Are there more simple ways (for both patient and doctor) of reaching a diagnosis instead of performing this test?

Has a really thorough examination been performed, to search for physical signs that may influence the differential diagnosis? Is there another test that would be equally effective, but more straightforward? Are the ocular features so clear that the test is really only confirmatory?

For example: classic ocular toxoplasmosis exhibits an active focus of retinitis near to a pre-existing chorioretinal scar, with significant vitritis in a young adult. Toxoplasma seropositivity in different populations in this age group ranges from the fairly common to the virtually universal. As the inflammation is recurrent, not newly acquired, there will be no IgM response and the IgG response is variable and cannot be used to confirm the association. Serological testing is frequently reported positive by laboratories only if a certain titer is reached, and false negatives are quite possible. A positive test will not influence management because the diagnosis is clinically obvious and treatment has usually been started before the serology is reported. However, a negative test will cause concern to the ophthalmologist that the diagnosis is incorrect, and may provoke a raft of further unnecessary investigations. In this patient, was the toxoplasma serology really necessary?

Answer: no, it was not necessary other than as a reassurance to the prescribing doctor. However, if no chorioretinal scar was seen, or if the inflammation was multifocal or in any other way atypical, then not only toxoplasma serology, but also a panel of investigations addressing the differential diagnosis, should be performed.

Is the test invasive, painful or inconvenient, and might it do harm? If any of these are true, is the test therefore justified for this patient?

The presence of sight-threatening uveitis will substantially raise the tolerance threshold for such questions. However, each interventional test has a risk profile: radiological investigation carries a radiation dose, sometimes there are severe reactions to intravenous fluorescein or indocyanine green, and intraocular sampling may risk further visual loss. The risk–benefit balance for each test must be fair to the patient and the test performed with informed consent.

For example: a 12-year-old girl presents with acute right visual loss and is found to have a vitreous hemorrhage secondary to bilateral intermediate uveitis. Bilateral pink optic disk swelling is noted. The child is systemically well and neurological examination is normal. Should cerebrospinal fluid (CSF) analysis and/or brain imaging be performed?

Answer: reactive optic nerve head swelling is common in children with intermediate uveitis. In the absence of focal neurological signs there is no justification for either brain imaging or lumbar puncture, each being unpleasant for a child. Nevertheless, a frequent finding is that children with these characteristics have frequently undergone just such investigations before referral to a uveitis clinic.

Is this test, for an unusual or rare condition, really justified in this patient?

Diagnostic frustration (or thoughtless broad-based investigation) often produces results that are not useful, and sometimes actively misleading (and therefore harmful), for a particular patient, e.g. there is a commonly held misconception that searching for anti-neutrophil cytoplasmic antibodies (ANCAs) in patients with uveitis is a productive investigation. In fact the association between systemic small-vessel vasculitis and uveitis, in the absence of clear symptoms and signs, is negligible. The occasional positive p-ANCA (perinuclear ANCA) is therefore merely a diversion that could have been avoided.

For example: a young farmer in Bavaria presents with bilateral nongranulomatous anterior uveitis. He is fit and well with no history of recent illness, chest problems, skin rash or arthropathy. In a panel of investigations borrelia serology is performed. The enzyme-linked immunosorbent assay (ELISA) result shows positivity at a low titer, and this is the only positive result. How should the patient be treated?

Answer: the ocular presentation is not in any way suggestive of Lyme disease, and as a random test, Lyme serology has a predictive value (see below) of less than 10%. In parts of Germany (as in many rural and forested parts of northern Europe) seropositivity with no previous history of erythema chronicum migrans is not uncommon, but ocular Lyme disease is rare. There is no evidence to support the contention that this is *Borrelia* spp.-related uveitis. Antibiotic treatment is not justified.

In what way would a particular result from this test influence the management of this patient?
Information provided from testing may influence management in several ways. Most importantly (but uncommonly) an infection is proven, which leads to specific antimicrobial treatment. Some doctors (usually laboratory scientists who do not have the responsibility of direct patient care with face-to-face contact) would argue that, unless a test would influence treatment so directly, it is not justified. However, from the ophthalmologist's point of view, any information that enables a degree of explanation to the patient may be welcome. This may allow more confident prognostication, e.g. in discussing the risk of the second eye becoming involved, the likelihood of chronicity, of the development of ocular complications or systemic disease, or of a risk of familial transmission. It may also allow logical decisions to be taken on the best form of management with steroid or immunosuppressive therapy.

For example: a fit 30-year-old American black woman presents with bilateral granulomatous anterior uveitis. She has no significant systemic symptoms and signs and no risk factors (other than racial) for any disease. Sarcoidosis is high on the differential diagnosis list but in the absence of systemic involvement biopsy confirmation is unlikely. The chest radiograph is normal but the angiotensin-converting enzyme (ACE) level is 125 IU. Does the differential diagnosis need to remain open?

Answer: there is a significant list of diseases that can be associated with a raised serum ACE including lymphoma, tuberculosis and liver storage diseases. However, an ACE level raised above 100 IU has a very high predictive value for sarcoidosis and is strongly supportive of the diagnosis. If syphilis serology is negative and there is no evidence of a tuberculosis risk, the diagnosis of ocular sarcoidosis can be assumed.

If this test is not performed, would it be likely that an important diagnosis, perhaps requiring specific treatment, might be missed?
Such a question is almost always directed at uveitis with a potential infective etiology, and although in some instances (e.g. classic recurrent toxoplasma retinochoroiditis or cytomegalovirus [CMV] retinitis) investigation is usually not required, in those infections (such as syphilis) that can cause less specific forms of uveitis, but require specific treatment, a lower testing threshold is justified. Indeed, despite the rarity of syphilitic uveitis, some would argue that syphilis serology is one of the few tests that should be routinely considered in the testing regime.

For example: a 75-year-old woman presents with gradual blurring of vision in both eyes with floaters. She has no indicators of systemic illness. Bilateral vitritis with cell clumps and strands are seen, with no clear retinal abnormality. Could this be intraocular lymphoma?

Answer: intraocular large-cell lymphoma is lethal and early diagnosis can influence both visual retention and survival. Suggestive vitreous appearance in this age group mandates vigorous investigation, including diagnostic vitrectomy (repeated if necessary), computed tomography (CT) scan and lumbar puncture for CSF cytology.

Is the test expensive?
The expense of testing cannot be ignored and, for this and other reasons, an unyielding and widespread investigation protocol for uveitis is both unhelpful and wasteful; it may even influence the future availability of a test for those patients who really need it, e.g. the identification of HLA-B27, which is readily and cheaply performed, may have direct and important relevance to some forms of uveitis and associated disease. However, requests for expensive full HLA typing merely to identify haplotypes that have only tenuous associations with certain diseases is unjustified.

For example: in the UK a young adult male presents with acute unilateral non-granulomatous panuveitis with occlusive retinal phlebitis, orogenital ulceration and erythema nodosum. An HLA type is requested to seek HLA-B51 in support of a diagnosis of Behçet's disease, and he is B51 negative. Was this test helpful, and would it have been more so if he were HLA-B51 positive?

Answer: not helpful in either circumstance. In a UK-born white person the association with HLA-B51 is only weak to moderate. The physical signs are entirely typical of the diagnosis; the test is unnecessary and more likely than not to be negative and therefore misleading.

Do I understand the basics of the method of testing, and am I able to interpret the result as reported by the laboratory?
Which is a more reliable detector of IgG on the toxoplasma serology report form, the ELISA or the dye test? Why is the IgM ELISA for *Toxoplasma* spp. negative but the ISAGA (IgM immunosorbent agglutination assay) positive, and what does this mean? This retinal lesion looks absolutely typical of toxoplasmosis. What has been gained by performing this test?

This patient with uveitis and a nondescript rash has positive serology for *Borrelia* spp. Was syphilis serology performed at the same time (because this appearance is far more suggestive of syphilis and *Treponema* spp., another spirochete, can cause false positivity in borrelia serology)?

The significance of laboratory tests is almost always modified by the clinical context, and it is absolutely fundamental that the clinician should understand this. Laboratory staff have a tendency to benign paternalism which assumes (usually correctly) that the interpreting clinician has only a basic knowledge of the investigation and may over-interpret the result if provided with too much detail, e.g. the report may read 'No serological evidence of exposure to toxoplasmosis' whereas it might read 'Toxoplasma latex agglutination test negative at 1:64 dilution' or perhaps even 'Toxoplasma latex agglutination test positive at 1:4 dilution' (all three being compatible with each other and each saying something slightly different). In short, laboratory experts may choose criteria of 'positivity' or 'negativity' (sometimes set locally) in an entirely understandable and altruistic effort to protect physicians from the need to interpret. Ophthalmologists should be wary of this approach. Their task is to understand the test properly and to request more accurate information. They should also be aware that requests for laboratory testing may come frequently from certain groups of doctors (and usually for quite narrow diagnostic reasons) and less commonly from others, who may actually require different information. Testing may be both performed and reported in a way that is more useful for the frequent user.

For example: a 50-year-old man presents with bilateral subacute panuveitis with patchy diffuse retinitis and headache. He gives a history of treatment 3 years ago for an unknown sexually transmitted infection, and syphilis serology is performed. It shows ICE (in-cell ELISA) positive for syphilis and a rapid plasmin reagin (RPR) of 1:4. Does he have syphilitic uveitis?

ELISA testing for *Treponema* spp. is largely replacing old treponemal serology testing. Various commercially available ELISAs have both sensitivity and specificity above 97%, and in general a positive ELISA for syphilis can be taken as evidence of exposure to syphilis past and/or present (syphilis can be caught more than once). It remains positive for life but does not distinguish between old and new syphilis. The RPR test is not specific to syphilis (e.g. it may be positive in severe rheumatoid arthritis) and so must always be performed together with a *Treponema* spp.-specific test. However, in contrast to ELISAs it is quantifiable and a marker of current activity, so it is used both to diagnose newly acquired syphilis and to monitor treatment efficacy. A titer of 1:4 is low and does not indicate active disease. However, the clinical context is entirely in keeping with syphilitic uveitis. The correct course of action upon receipt of these results is for the ophthalmologist first to consider other causes of such a presentation (e.g. herpetic retinitis) and second to liaise with genitourinary medicine colleagues to explain the suspicion, which will probably lead to investigations for neurosyphilis including CSF analysis and CT (and naturally, repeated serology). Intraocular sampling for polymerase chain reaction (PCR) is also warranted.

How specific and sensitive is this test and how good at predicting disease likelihood?

It is timely here to insert a brief reminder about standard medical statistical terms. The reliability of a test to detect only that which is being looked for is its **specificity**. The ability to detect that which is actually present is its **sensitivity**. Increased sensitivity is usually gained at the expense of a drop in specificity, and a middle ground that is considered most useful for clinical purposes may be pre-set by the laboratory, both in the choice of test and in its interpretation and reporting. Sensitivity and specificity are defined in terms of true and false positivity and negativity as shown in **Fig. 3.1**.

	Disease present	Disease absent
Test +ve	A. True positive	B. False positive
Test −ve	C. False negative	D. True negative

Figure 3.1 The definitions of sensitivity, specificity and predictive value are functions of the above parameters and appear in the text.

The sensitivity is defined as A/(A + C) expressed as a percentage, and the specificity as D/(B + D)%. The results from Fig. 3.1 can also be used to calculate the **positive predictive value** (or precision rate), which is the proportion of those with positive tests who are true positives [A/(A + B)%]. In contrast the **negative predictive value** is the proportion of those with negative tests who are true negatives [D/(C + D)%]. The predictive values can be calculated only if the disease **prevalence** is known for the population studied. Prevalence is defined as the total number within the population who have the disease at any one time (usually expressed as cases per 100 000 population). This is different from the **incidence** which is the number of new cases within a defined population over a specified time period (in medicine, often shown as cases per 100 000 population per year).

Some people carry increased risk of certain diseases. This may be racial, genetic, occupational or linked to social behavior. The **relative risk** (RR) is the chance of developing a disease if exposed to the increased risk, compared with those who are not (RR = risk if exposed/risk if not exposed).

For example: about 5% of a population are HLA-B27 positive. However, about 80% of that same population who have ankylosing spondylitis (AS) are HLA-B27 positive. Only 1% of those who are HLA-B27 positive actually develop AS whereas a mere 0.011 % of those who are HLA-B27 negative develop AS:

RR = Risk of AS in those who are HLA-B27 +ve = 1% = **90**
Risk of AS in those who are HLA-B27 −ve = 0.011%

In this population the HLA-B27-+ve person is 90 times more likely to develop AS than one who is HLA-B27 −ve.

Is the relative risk for this patient different from the average, and does this affect interpretation of the test?

Understanding the RR of a patient having a particular condition is an essential part of interpreting a test for that condition. Such factors will be assimilated as a matter of course by the astute ophthalmologist. Geography, race, climate, travel and sexual history may all modify the diagnostic approach.

For example: a 50-year-old veterinary surgeon in a small animal practice develops neuroretinitis with posterior uveitis but no history of systemic upset. Bartonellosis is part of the differential diagnosis and serology is requested. The laboratory routinely reports serology for both *Bartonella henselae* and *B. quintana* and finds IgG positivity for both at titers of 1:50 and 1:4, respectively, but no IgM response. Is cat-scratch disease the cause of the neuroretinitis?

Several aspects of this case need to be set into context. First, the population seroprevalence for *Bartonella* spp. varies widely according to climate and country of origin. In the highest affected over a quarter may be seropositive. Some of course will have a substantially greater risk of exposure and seroprevalence in veterinarians may be over 40%. Most patients with cat-scratch disease and intraocular involvement have either recent lymphadenopathy and malaise or cat-scratch, or both. Most patients affected by cat-scratch disease have IgM positivity but this is not universal and the possibility of late-onset ocular involvement (with falling IgG titers) cannot be excluded. *B. henselae* can cross-react with *both B. quintana* and *Coxiella burnetii* (but in practice there is usually no clinical diagnostic confusion). The typical intraocular manifestations of cat-scratch disease include focal retinitis, neuroretinitis and retinal vasculitis with occlusion. Does this veterinarian have cat-scratch disease?

Answer: there is no sure answer but, on the balance of probabilities, no. However, the most common cause of neuroretinitis with uveitis in most countries is either toxoplasmosis or bartonellosis. In the absence of other pointers a course of co-trimoxazole with or without oral steroid will treat both conditions and is pragmatic.

How should the test be interpreted for this particular patient?
Knowledge of the sensitivity and specificity of the test is only part of a proper interpretation. The test is performed for a patient who has unique circumstances, and up to the point of testing the ophthalmologist will have gained an impression of how likely a particular diagnosis is. As the testing is therefore already selective, the pre-test probability of the disease being present is already substantially greater than the population prevalence. Features of the patient's age, sex, race, locality, uveitic features, and associated symptoms and signs may have raised that probability very markedly (indeed, so markedly that sometimes no testing is thought necessary for diagnosis). It is in this context that the test is performed and interpreted, in the light of its known specificity and sensitivity. If the pre-test diagnostic probability is actually known, then Bayes' theorem can be applied, but, as such a figure is usually speculative at best, the process is more usually an informal bayesian 'analysis' performed by the clinician, from a background of experience. In other words, diagnosis remains as much an art as a science.

For example: a young adult male who was born in Gujurat but came to the UK as a teenager presents to the uveitis clinic with bilateral, exudative, non-occlusive, retinal phlebitis and uveitis. He is fit and well. He is already on treatment with prednisolone 40 mg/day started by his local ophthalmologist. He has no history of tuberculosis or of known contact with TB. He has been back to visit family in India a few times. He is not sure whether he received BCG immunization but there is a poorly defined small scar over the right deltoid. His chest radiograph probably shows mild, unilateral, hilar adenopathy but no parenchymal lesion and his serum ACE is 75 IU. He is tested by the Mantoux test which gives 8 mm of induration. Could he have TB or is this likely to be sarcoidosis?

Answer: Gujurat and other western areas of India have a high endemic rate of TB. Most intraocular involvement with tuberculosis occurs in fit patients with no evidence of pulmonary disease. BCG immunization leads in most patients to permanent Mantoux positivity, but usually weak to moderate (< 12 mm), not severe. Oral steroid treatment adversely affects the Mantoux reaction so that an 8-mm reaction (not suggestive) in a patient on oral steroid might have been 15 mm (highly suggestive) without. Raised serum ACE can occur in both TB and sarcoidosis. These data are non-diagnostic. Perform an interferon-γ test if possible, which eliminates the confounding factor of previous BCG and should not be affected by moderate-dose steroid treatment. High-resolution chest CT may show characteristic peribronchial granulomas of sarcoidosis. If these tests are not possible, be pragmatic: in the UK newly identified latent TB in the under-35-year age group requires 3 months of two-drug anti-tuberculous treatment. In this age group treatment is usually well tolerated. A suggestive Mantoux test in a patient requiring moderate- to high-dose oral steroid treatment (carrying a small risk of reactivated TB), with a uveitis that is potentially sight threatening, makes a full 6-month course of anti-tuberculous chemotherapy entirely appropriate.

Does this test more properly lie within the field of expertise of another physician, and should I therefore refer the patient and allow that physician to request tests from that greater position of expertise?
There is sometimes a tendency for the ophthalmologist to over-investigate outside his or her field of expertise. In most circumstances the prior advice of an expert will reduce the need for investigation. The need to involve a physician in the diagnosis of uveitis will vary according to the skills and approach of the ophthalmologist, but clearly the latter must identify his or her own boundaries of expertise. Selectively used, such a diagnostic liaison can be extremely useful and many physicians are interested in the subject.

For example: a young adult male presents with a first episode of acute unilateral anterior uveitis. Systemic questioning reveals increasing morning stiffness and low backache. He may well have ankylosing spondylitis, but the ophthalmologist is not best placed to request a radiograph of the lumbar spine, which carries a significant radiation dose. The patient will require a rheumatological opinion in any case, and the decision to X-ray should be made by this expert.

SPECIFIC TESTS

The details of investigations appropriate to the diagnosis of a particular form of uveitis are included in the diagnostic sections of each chapter. Included below are the details of investigations that have more general application, or where certain laboratory methods are common to various tests. Chapter references are given for those investigations dealt with at greater length elsewhere.

Hematology

Myriad full (or complete) blood count (FBC or CBC) and differential white cell counts appear in the case notes of patients with uveitis, only to gather dust. There are, however, circumstances in which non-specific investigations into associated systemic disease are important. Any patient with a recent or current pyrexial illness, lymphadenopathy or symptoms or signs of infection should be so investigated, and very rarely a leukemia may masquerade as uveitis. Eosinophilia is a recognized feature of any systemic parasite infestation, and is seen in the rare Churg–Strauss syndrome. In any patient with suspected systemic inflammatory disease it is reasonable to examine the erythrocyte sedimentation rate (ESR) and acute-phase proteins.

Urea and electrolyte (U&E) balance is again non-specific and only occasionally rewarding. Calcium metabolism is detectably abnormal in a minority of patients with sarcoidosis, but this is best identified using full calcium metabolic studies including serum phosphate levels and 24-hour urinary calcium collection. Such abnormalities are usually found only where other, more straightforward, investigations have already shown the diagnosis. Those with biochemical renal dysfunction, e.g. those with renal vasculitis, sarcoidosis, tubulointerstitial nephritis or lupus, are likely to have physical features that should direct such investigations. ACE and lysozyme levels may be extremely useful in the diagnosis of sarcoidosis. Liver function in the well patient with uveitis is highly unlikely to provide useful data. However, all organ function tests provide a baseline before potential treatment with steroid or immunosuppressive, and of course, for some drugs, prior normality is essential.

Microbiology

Diagnosis in the patient with suspected intraocular infection is approached in different ways depending upon the likely organism. Some infections present a characteristic clinical picture, e.g. the diagnosis of toxoplasmosis or CMV retinitis is almost always presumptive and does not involve direct microbiological methods. Where direct identification of an organism needs to be pursued (in patients with severe, apparently infective, ocular disease where indirect tests have not been informative), microbiological sampling is necessary, the source being dependent on the clinical characteristics of the patient.

Endophthalmitis

The patient with endogenous endophthalmitis usually presents with a likely primary source for the infection, many have an organism already identified, and some are extremely ill, e.g. with septicemia. Others may have suffered a significant recent infection, e.g. involving the urinary tract. In the absence of a clear history, a particularly stringent general examination is essential, and urgent hospitalization to allow full investigation and treatment is necessary. A physician should be involved, and all likely possibilities should be vigorously pursued. Subacute bacterial endocarditis should be excluded, and any risk factors for fungal infection noted. Repeated blood cultures are important. In some circumstances intraocular sampling is necessary, either for microscopy, culture and antibiotic sensitivity, or for PCR tests. The surgical methods are discussed below.

The microbiologist should be fully involved in the investigation and appraised of the suspicions of the clinician, especially where fungal culture is required. Each unit may have developed its own protocol for sample reception and inoculation. The use of fluid rather than agar-based culture media for intraocular specimens is said to produce a substantially higher pick-up rate (Kratz et al. 2006).

Polymerase chain reaction

The principle and crude practice of DNA amplification were known in the 1960s, but the development and refinement of the PCR by Kary Mullis in 1983 transformed the method into one absolutely fundamental to medical molecular diagnostic technique and led to his Nobel prize. First used to make copies of genes for research, the main diagnostic interest in the context of uveitis is the ability of PCR to use DNA probes to locate DNA fragments specific to certain microorganisms (which may be undetectable by other methods) and to amplify the relevant DNA strands to a quantity that permits identification.

If microorganism X is suspected of being responsible for a case of uveitis, then a sample of intraocular fluid may be mixed with a DNA probe (or primer) known to complement a unique DNA sequence from microorganism X. The enzyme polymerase, and a quantity of nucleotides to fuel the polymerization, are added. The polymerization process is heat sensitive, and automated PCR is performed in thermal cycles of a few minutes, ranging from 55°C to 94°C. Over a few hours and some 30 cycles, the exponential polymerization will (if any DNA from microorganism X is present) have generated enough DNA to be detectable by electrophoresis.

By definition PCR is exquisitely sensitive. This allows the detection of minute DNA fragments but also allows the potential for false positivity. It is therefore imperative to avoid contamination at all stages of the process and, as the laboratory must run positive controls to validate each PCR procedure, particularly stringent methods are required to ensure complete separation of PCR investigations from potential sources of contaminating material. In addition, PCR is not capable of differentiating between DNA from active microorganisms responsible for a current infection and fragments remnant from a previous one. However, messenger RNA (mRNA) can be detected using reverse transcriptase-PCR (rtPCR), and this may become a useful tool in differentiating active from previous infection.

PCR is now well established as a crucial component of microbiological investigation in many fields of medicine. Primers for a large selection of species are now available and constant refinement leads to increasing sensitivity and specificity. In the context of intraocular infection, the developing use of PCR, in particular for the herpesviruses, fungi and mycobacteria, has improved diagnostic sensitivity. Other PCRs such as *Toxoplasma gondii* require some refinement but are still useful in atypical clinical cases.

As PCR techniques have evolved, greater diversity can be achieved by multiplex testing which enables the simultaneous application of several primers to investigate for their relevant organisms in a way that would otherwise require consecutive testing and larger samples (of great relevance to the ophthalmologist). The specificity of testing is greatly enhanced by nested PCR, in which two consecutive thermal cycles are performed on the same test specimen using two different primers with different binding sites. This technique minimizes the possibility of inadvertent amplification of spurious DNA fragments. Further refinement occurs in real-time quantitative PCR, in which the target DNA amplified is identified not at the end of the whole set of thermal cycles by electrophoresis, but as the PCR process proceeds, usually by indirect fluorescence methods. This technique provides perhaps the most accurate of PCR methods (Dworkin et al. 2002).

Human leukocyte antigen testing

Several human leukocyte antigens (HLAs) of the major histocompatibility complex (MHC) are known to be significantly associated with various forms of inflammatory disease, including some forms of uveitis. In addition, some HLA types (e.g. HLA-B27) appear capable of modifying the presentation of a disease process. Theories abound on the relevance of these associations, which may be because of a direct pathogenetic link, or may be merely a marker for disease, perhaps in linkage disequilibrium with the relevant gene. The former seems increasingly likely for some diseases and HLA types.

Except for specific testing for HLA-B27, conventional full HLA typing is time-consuming and expensive. However, newer molecular methods promise a greater accessibility to clinicians. In particular, PCR methods are in use and nested PCR for simultaneous allele testing is increasingly used.

The HLA associations most likely to be encountered in the patient with uveitis are listed in **Table 3.1**. In some cases the relative risk is very significant. In others a weaker association has been found in research, and this does not usually justify HLA testing for diagnostic purposes. The association between HLA-A29 (present in only about 5% of the indigenous UK population) and birdshot retinochoroidopathy is virtually constant, with the highest known relative risk for an HLA association.

Some HLA types have quite confined geographical distributions, and figures appropriate to the locality (or at least the country) should be consulted before judging the relevance of a particular test (Solberg et al. 2008), e.g. HLA-B51 (specifically B*5101) has a concentrated epicenter in Turkey, the Caucasus and western Silk Road (prevalence in 35% of population), which decreases with distance, through 20% in most Mediterranean countries, to only 5–10% in the UK (**Fig. 3.2**). The relative risk of HLA-B51 positivity for Behçet's disease is very different at

Table 3.1 HLA associations with uveitis, or diseases that may be associated with uveitis

Disease	Region	HLA type	Relative risk (if known)
Acute anterior uveitis	Europe	B27	8
Ankylosing spondylitis	Europe	B27	90
APMPPE	Europe	B7	3
		DR2	3
Behçet's disease	Turkey	B51	14
	UK	B51	2
JIA with uveitis	Europe	DRB1*13	–
Birdshot retinochoroidopathy	Europe	A29	224
Intermediate uveitis	USA	DR15	–
Multiple sclerosis (and uveitis with optic neuritis)	Europe	DR15	4
		DQ6	–
Reactive arthritis	Europe	B27	35
Sarcoid uveitis	Sweden	DRB1*04	–
Systemic lupus erythematosus	Europe	DR3	6
Sympathetic uveitis	USA	DR4	–
		Dw53	–
Tubulointerstitial nephritis and uveitis	USA	DRB*0102	4
Vogt–Koyanagi–Harada syndrome	China	DRB1*0405	46
	USA	DRB1*0404	–

HLA-DR2 may now be listed as DR15 or DR16.

AMPPE, acute posterior multifocal placoid pigment epitheliopathy; JIA, juvenile idiopathic arthritis.

these extremes, and for British white individuals the test is not usually felt to be helpful in diagnosis. Another example is HLA-B29 (specifically A*2902) which has a major epicenter in southern Africa, but the prevalence of birdshot retinochoroidopathy in no way reflects this (**Fig. 3.2**), supporting the notion of a two-hit or three-hit provocation.

For some diseases the claimed HLA associations are significantly different between populations and this heterogeneity increases as alleles are subtyped. For each disease association the precise link between the HLA genetics and the phenotype remains unknown but it is agreed that the genetic basis provides only a predisposition and at least one if not several immune 'hits' are also required to initiate disease. Broadly speaking, with the above few exceptions HLA associations are important research tools but with generally low predictive values, or limited diagnostic use (Zamecki et al. 2010).

Serological tests for antibody detection

The formation of IgM and IgG antibody to the antigens of an infective agent follow predictable temporal patterns (see Figure 1.10), but the different ways in which these antibodies can be detected may affect results; antigens themselves are structurally complex, and various antigenic determinant sites may be detectable in different ways by different serological tests. Some serological tests use an exponential dilution series, and the result is expressed as a titer, which is the most diluted solution to show a positive reaction. Changing titer levels are seen during the acute and convalescent phases of acquired infection, and serial testing may be used to confirm such cases.

There are various ways in which antigen/antibody (Ag/Ab) reactions can be detected. They vary in their complexity, sensitivity, expense and speed. Several serological methods are now automated.

Agglutination and flocculation tests

Insoluble particles such as sheep erythrocytes or latex can be coated with a specific Ag. The addition of patient serum, if containing the relevant Ab, will cause a visible clumping (agglutination) of these particles. The ability to agglutinate particles is a function of the number of binding sites on the Ab molecule. IgM is polyvalent and causes agglutination in smaller quantities than does IgG. Indirect, or passive, agglutination is used in the latex agglutination test for *Toxoplasma* spp., and to detect IgM rheumatoid factor. The Venereal Disease Research Laboratory (VDRL) test for syphilis is a flocculation test, which combines the features of agglutination and precipitation tests to give a visible foaming rather than clumping reaction. Agglutination tests remain useful for the diagnosis of several infections and autoimmune diseases but other methods (including ELISA) are gradually displacing them.

Fluorescent antibody tests

Test antigen is combined with patient serum and a fluorescent dye, usually fluorescein or rhodamine. A positive reaction is shown by fluorescence under the appropriate light. Indirect variants of this test are the fluorescent treponemal antibody (FTA) test used to detect syphilis and the indirect fluorescent antibody test for toxoplasmosis. Although new ELISAs continue to erode the usefulness of these tests, some are historically considered as 'gold standard' and have therefore not yet been displaced.

Enzyme-linked immunosorbent assay

During the past 20 years ELISA tests have become increasingly used for several reasons; first because of high sensitivity and second because of the availability of automated multiplex plates which speed the process and reduce the cost. Sensitivity is comparable to that of radioimmunoassay, which it has supplanted because it requires no radioactive

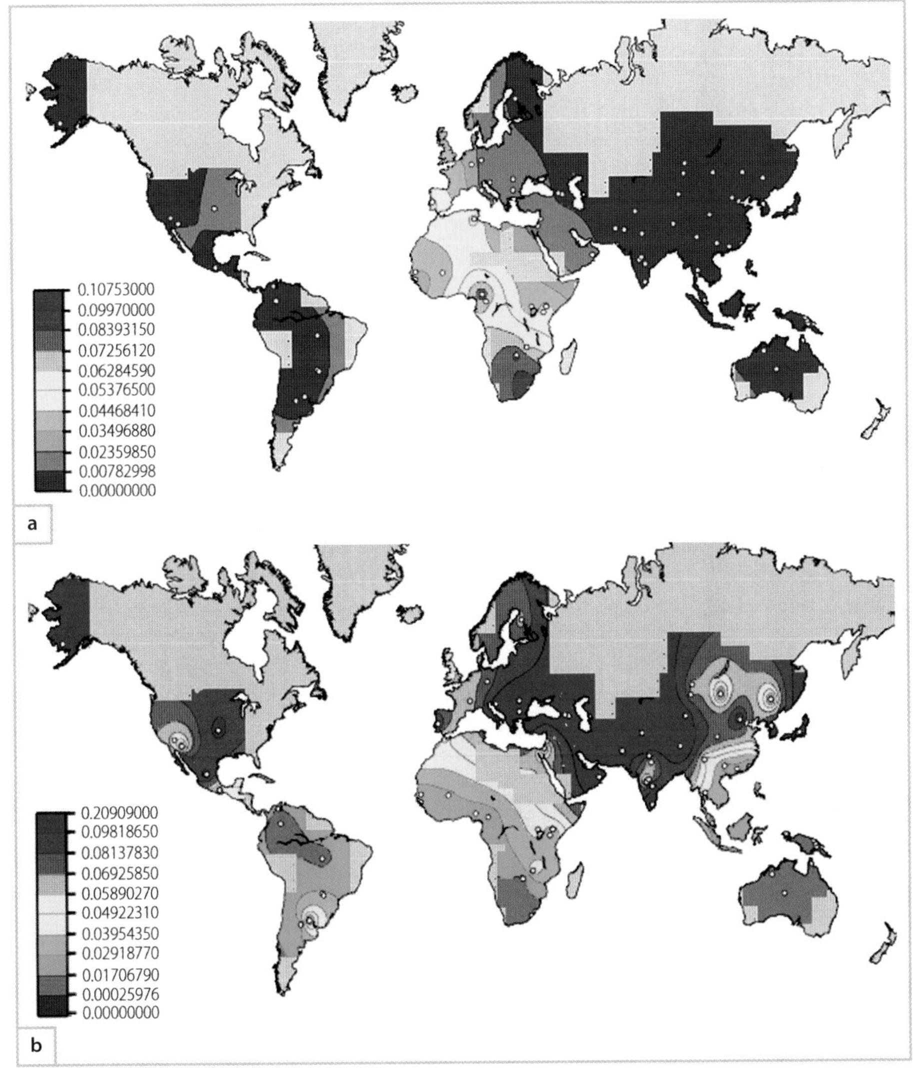

Figure 3.2 The known world distributions of two important HLA alleles, HLA-A*2902 (a) being associated with birdshot retinochoroidopathy and HLA-B*5101 (b) with Behçet's disease. (Modified from Solberg et al. [2008], with permission.)

isotopes. Usually a polystyrene microtiter plate is pre-coated with, for example, test Ag. Diluted patient serum is added, which bonds with the Ag only if Ab is present. An enzyme (historically, horseradish peroxidase) is covalently attached if bonding has occurred, and after washing the substrate the marker is then added, which will react if enzyme has remained. Detection is by visible or fluorescent color. Standard positive and negative wells are used as controls. Results are expressed only as positive or negative. Industry ELISA kits are available for many microorganisms and autoantigens, and newer forms can be reported quantitatively. A variety of ELISA known as enzyme-linked immunosorbent spot (ELISPOT) is exquisitely sensitive and in clinical medicine is used as an interferon-γ detector.

Immunoelectrophoresis

This is a special form of precipitation test. Serum is fractionated within a gel by electrophoresis, then Ag-containing reactant is placed alongside the fractionated components and allowed to diffuse towards it. Precipitation lines form where interaction has occurred. It is increasingly supplanted by gel electrophoresis and electroblotting because of time and expense.

Interferon-γ release assays

These tests are used to identify an immune reaction against *Mycobacterium tuberculosis* and the ELISPOT and QuantiFERON-TB methods use slightly different techniques. Both rely on the ability of patients' lymphocytes (if previously exposed to TB) to secrete interferon-γ when exposed to tubercular antigens (early secretory antigen target 6 [ESAT-6] and culture filtrate protein 10 [CFP-10]) which are species specific. Neither is quantifiable enough to differentiate latent from active disease but both have added accuracy to TB diagnosis.

Immunology

The study of immune mechanisms in disease is one of the most rapidly advancing fields in medicine. Frequent modifications and developments in immune theory make it challenging to maintain an up-to-date understanding of the relevance of immune mechanisms in uveitis. In basic terms, immunological tests are used diagnostically in uveitis for the following reasons:

- To search for a specific autoantibody which, if present, would indicate quite a narrow range of underlying possibilities. There are two obvious examples here. The ANCA is closely (but not uniquely) associated with some forms of systemic vasculitis, and the antinuclear antibody (ANA) is associated with both systemic lupus erythematosus and juvenile chronic arthritis. There is no value whatever in testing for their presence in fit adults with uveitis.

- To identify humoral or cellular immunodeficiency, to explain unusual manifestations of ocular infection. There are many forms of inherited deficiencies of immunoglobulins, complement, phagocytes and lymphocytes, or combinations of these. Some are associated with ocular problems, usually in childhood, and most cause a spectrum of recognizable systemic problems, but a search for such rare conditions in the patient with uveitis without accompanying features is fruitless.

Some apparently fit patients may show manifestations of ocular infection that are atypical, such as a recurrent multifocal toxoplasmosis. In such circumstances the possibility of HIV infection must be considered, but the procedure of investigation and diagnosis must be pursued with care and in consultation with expert physicians. In the absence of HIV infection, isolated investigations into cellular immunity by the ophthalmologist are not likely to be helpful and liaison with an immunologist is recommended.

Some patients with uveitis may have circulating antibodies to ocular components, e.g. antibodies to retinal S-antigen have been identified in patients with birdshot retinochoroidopathy and some other forms of posterior uveitis. However, the identification of such antibodies, although contributing significantly to an understanding of pathogenetic mechanisms, is a research tool, and not a clinical diagnostic test.

Antibodies to various non-ocular self-antigens have been described in association with some forms of uveitis, and have been investigated particularly in those with ocular vasculitis. Such autoantibodies include anticardiolipin antibodies and von Willebrand's factor, both of which are markers for vascular damage and possible mediators of vascular thrombosis. They are the subject of research, but requests for such testing are unlikely to be helpful in the individual patient with uveitis or vasculitis.

Radiology and nuclear medicine

Radiological and nuclear procedures are invasive, but mostly of very low risk. Directed investigations are sometimes very valuable in the diagnosis of uveitis. Arranging a chest radiograph as a standard investigation for uveitis is not justified, but it is an essential examination for any patient with a uveitis that could be caused by TB or sarcoidosis, particularly granulomatous uveitis. In some patients with possible ocular sarcoidosis, pulmonary involvement can be confirmed by high-resolution chest CT without the need for bronchoscopy or biopsy. Gallium-67 scintigraphy scan may show isotope uptake in certain specific areas in sarcoidosis, but the test results are usually most impressive in those in whom the diagnosis is already obvious by other, easier diagnostic methods. The test is now rarely justified in the patient with uveitis.

Intracranial radiology is sometimes important: calcification may be evident in those with congenital toxoplasmosis. CT or magnetic resonance imaging (MRI) may be imperative in patients with signs indicating intraocular lymphoma, or where associated neurological symptoms and signs suggest possible neuro-Behçet's disease, neurosarcoid or demyelination. Positron emission tomography (PET) can assist in lymphoma diagnosis and monitoring.

Some patients with anterior uveitis and symptoms of spondyloarthropathy undergo radiological investigation at the instigation of ophthalmologists. In our clinic, referral to a rheumatologist is thought appropriate, and it is that specialist who is better able to order appropriate radiographs if thought necessary.

Skin testing

The provocation of an inflammatory reaction by the intradermal inoculation of antigens is the in vivo equivalent of serological testing for previous exposure to that antigen, and is of importance in the diagnosis of TB. The provocation of a weal by intradermal trauma (the pathergy test) may be useful to help the diagnosis of Behçet's disease in some populations.

Tuberculin test

Tuberculin antigen (purified protein derivative or PPD) is inoculated intradermally either by raising an intradermal bleb with a cannula (Mantoux test) or by multiple punctures with primed points (Heaf test). The latter has been abandoned in the UK because the Mantoux test is regarded as more accurately quantifiable.

Kveim test

A small quantity of macerated spleen obtained from a sarcoidosis patient was injected intradermally and biopsied 6 weeks later; characteristic non-caseating granulomas were considered diagnostic. The test has been abandoned largely owing to the potential risk of transferring prions.

Histoplasmin test

A small quantity of antigen from killed *Histoplasma capsulatum* was injected intradermally and an inflammatory reaction, observed 24–48 hours later, was indicative of previous infection. Largely superseded by serology even in areas endemic for histoplasmosis, this test is largely historical and of no current value in patients with possible presumed ocular histoplasmosis.

Pathergy

A sterile pustule forms at the site of dermal puncture. The test is neither pathognomonic for nor particularly sensitive for Behçet's disease and is therefore not often practiced in the west. Occasionally a patient will report this phenomenon as a response to previous trauma.

Extraocular tissue biopsy

Multisystem diseases such as sarcoidosis may have protean manifestations and, as indirect methods of diagnosis may be frustratingly inadequate, any reasonable opportunity to obtain tissue samples should be taken. In patients with suspected sarcoidosis, blind conjunctival biopsy is not performed in our clinic, but biopsy would be performed on a visible conjunctival nodule. Lacrimal biopsy is a procedure associated with well-reported risks and any decision to undertake such a procedure should be taken with care, and with informed consent. We prefer to avoid this procedure unless absolutely necessary.

Skin biopsy

Cutaneous lesions in suspected sarcoidosis are often amenable to easy biopsy. Skin biopsy remains the standard diagnostic method for both onchocerciasis and leprosy.

Organ biopsy

Internal biopsy is sometimes performed in the diagnosis of multisystem inflammation, at the recommendation of a physician. Liver or renal biopsy is occasionally performed, mainly to diagnose sarcoidosis. Whipple's disease may be confirmed by peroral jejunal biopsy. Transbronchial biopsy under sedation is commonly used by respiratory physicians in the diagnosis of sarcoidosis, and sometimes in other lung inflammations. *Pneumocystis* pneumonia can if necessary be confirmed in this way. Brain biopsy may rarely be essential for some forms of uveitis with focal central nervous system (CNS) involvement, especially neurosarcoidosis.

Lumbar puncture for CSF analysis

Cytological examination of CSF is imperative in patients suspected of having CNS large-cell lymphoma. Non-specific pleocytosis is often seen in patients with the Vogt–Koyanagi–Harada syndrome and has also been found in those few patients with acute posterior multifocal placoid pigment epitheliopathy (AMPPE) who develop symptoms of meningeal irritation. However, the signs are non-diagnostic. Syphilis serology can be performed on CSF and lumbar puncture is an essential component of neurosyphilis diagnosis. Lumbar puncture is not necessary for patients with papillary swelling in association with uveitis, in the absence of focal neurological signs. This phenomenon is common in children and lumbar puncture is fruitless.

Intraocular sampling

Intraocular fluid or tissue can provide important diagnostic evidence in the patient with uveitis (Manku and McCluskey 2005, Rothova et al. 2008). Any procedure involving intraocular sampling carries surgical risks, and these must always be balanced against possible benefits.

There are several reasons for wishing to obtain an intraocular sample. It is imperative to have in place, before surgery, complete plans on the type of specimen to be obtained, its division into appropriate fractions, the correct containers, rapid and completely reliable transport arrangements, and laboratories (preferably an individual) that are primed to receive the specimen and have a full understanding of the investigations that have been requested by prior discussion. If these stringent preparations are not followed, our experience is that the capacity for error is limitless, and such precious samples must not be allowed to be wasted. Tests may include the following.

Microscopy and culture for microorganisms

The principles of direct microbiological investigation are discussed above, and for individual organisms, in Chapter 10. Vitreous humor is in general much more likely to be a fruitful source than aqueous humor even where a hypopyon is present.

PCR for microorganisms

For many organisms the reliability of PCR from intraocular fluid is now very high. Exceptions awaiting further refinement are mycobacterial and toxoplasmic PCRs. There is little evidence of superior sensitivity from vitreous sampling and aqueous tap is almost always adequate. Quite rightly PCR is frequently used especially in patients with suspected intraocular infection, or in those in whom clinical characteristics are atypical, or where immune deficiency renders serology unhelpful. This problem occurs with particular frequency in those with AIDS.

One problem compromising attempts at broad investigation is the limited volume of aqueous humor available for testing. A sample of 0.15 ml is usually all that can be obtained and this may not be adequate for multiple separate PCRs. The potential development of a multiplex panel for aqueous humor would be very beneficial and technically entirely achievable.

Serological tests

Sampling of intraocular fluid may be used to compare specific antibody levels against a particular microorganism, with levels in the serum. The ratio of these levels, each having been compared with the total immunoglobulin levels in each sample, is Desmont's coefficient (a specific form of the Goldmann–Witmer coefficient); this is based on the theory that, if the infective process is active within the eye, levels of specific antibody here will be significantly higher than in the serum. Aqueous humor sampling for serological reasons is most frequently used in mainland Europe where there is great enthusiasm for the technique, which is not shared elsewhere. The possibility of a polyclonal rather than a monoclonal response and the imposition of an arbitrary cut-off ratio for positivity are among the reasons for skepticism. Many claims for a microbiological basis for uveitis are based entirely on the results of comparative serology without PCR support. This author's perspective is that, although the technique provides interesting research results, these should not be used as the sole basis for patient management.

Cytological or histological examination in suspected masquerade syndromes

Some forms of malignancy may mimic uveitis, and these masquerade syndromes are discussed in Chapter 20. In particular, large-cell lymphoma is a dangerous malignancy that is notorious for its ability to evade early diagnosis. Vigorous diagnostic investigation should include vitrectomy for cytological examination. Careful extraction and handling must be followed by very expert cytological examination for optimal results, and in the best hands the investigation is crucial for some forms of inflammation (Wittenberg et al. 2008). In some patients, the more invasive technique of chorioretinal biopsy (see below) is justified.

Research

Increasing knowledge of the role of individual components of the immune system has led to intensive study in the field of uveitis. The investigation of intraocular fluids for immune components is a part of this process, and cytokine levels, inflammatory cell markers and evidence of local antibody production are examples of targets for research.

In order to perform the above investigations, there are essentially three methods of sampling:

Aqueous humor sampling

Extracting aqueous humor is, compared with the removal of vitreous humor, a straightforward procedure, and one that may be performed under local anesthesia. Several methods have been described, but all require the atraumatic entry of the anterior chamber under magnification, either by first penetrating most of the corneal thickness with a sharp blade, or by the gentle rotation of a narrow-gauge cannula. Usually a 27- or 30-gauge cannula is mounted on a 1-ml tuberculin syringe. However, one method uses a cannula mounted on an emptied, squeezed saline drop dispenser, which it is claimed is safe for use on the slit-lamp. In our clinic, aqueous sampling is performed in the operating theatre under sterile conditions. Up to 0.2 ml of aqueous humor may be withdrawn under favorable conditions, but less in those with shallower anterior chambers. With care, lens or iris touch is a theoretical rather than an actual risk.

Vitreous humor sampling

For microscopy and culture of vitreous in those with presumed bacterial endophthalmitis, a vitreous aspirate may be adequate. However, for all other circumstances in the investigation of uveitis (including cytology for malignancy and in the investigation of all other infections) a three-port pars plana total vitrectomy is required. Usually the surgery is performed for a combination of diagnostic and therapeutic reasons. For most diagnostic purposes, an aliquot of neat vitreous is desirable, and this is achieved by allowing controlled globe collapse with the infusion off. The neat sample is withdrawn from the aspiration tube, and then the infusion switched on allowing the next, diluted portion of vitreous to be similarly collected. The cassette fluid should also be kept because it may be spun down to provide some cells. The diagnostic vitreous sample should therefore ideally be sent as three components.

Chorioretinal biopsy

Open transscleral chorioretinal biopsy, which required hypotensive anesthesia and carried significant risk to the patient, has been largely abandoned in favor of closed biopsy via pars plana vitrectomy. Newer closed techniques (Cole et al. 2008) have improved ocular safety and enabled substantial specimens to be removed without the complications of hypotensive anesthesia. The investigation is usually reserved for those with severe bilateral uveitis, for which problems with diagnosis and management have been encountered, the surgery usually being performed on the less-useful eye.

AN INVESTIGATION GUIDELINE FOR UVEITIS

The word 'guideline' rather than 'protocol' has been chosen here because, even though our clinic has protocols, they are based on the known epidemiology of this particular hospital, i.e. a university hospital in a large western city at 53° north latitude within an unusually temperate large island. Sarcoidosis is not uncommon. The population is mostly indigenous white people derived from Anglo-Saxon or Celtic genetics, but there is a substantial and increasing minority of those particularly from the Indian subcontinent, but also from within the European Union, eastern Europe and Africa. There is a small but important number of immigrants with a high rate of TB infection. As with most European cities there is a significant gay community with its HIV and syphilis risk. The city has a large international airport, regularly importing those with new infections, but the UK climate does not permit any tropical viral diseases, and arthropod-borne infections are not endemic with the exception of borreliosis, which in Europe has a tendency to lead to erythema chronicum migrans but not Lyme disease. There is no histoplasmosis. There are no wild raccoons. The UK has a longstanding and largely effective childhood immunization policy, but recently the policy of universal BCG immunization has been abandoned. The UK healthcare service is free of charge at the point of delivery for qualifying residents and visitors, so disease tends to present early rather than late.

This combination of factors defines our patient population and their risk of disease, and has led to our approach to investigation. The reader's population may be entirely different, so the text below is intended as a guideline rather than a proscriptive recommendation. A knowledge of local needs is essential to pragmatic investigation and, in particular, to avoid over-investigation (Fooroghian et al. 2006). The following summarizes our approach to **initial investigation** in a patient presenting with a particular form of uveitis.

1. Unilateral acute, new or recurrent non-granulomatous anterior uveitis in a fit young adult

- No investigations required

In the UK this group of patient accounts for the majority of all cases of uveitis. The great majority of these patients will be HLA-B27 positive, but testing to confirm this is unnecessary. A brief history will exclude significant associated systemic disease; any suggestion of spondyloarthropathy should lead to referral to a rheumatologist, but a radiograph does not need to be performed by the ophthalmologist.

2. Bilateral simultaneous anterior uveitis of any type, or granulomatous anterior uveitis affecting either eye, in a fit patient

- FBC (CBC), U&Es, liver function tests (LFTs), ACE, ESR, C-reactive protein (CRP), syphilis serology, chest radiograph

Always exclude syphilis in any patient outside group 1. Exclude sarcoidosis and test organ function to exclude low-grade asymptomatic systemic inflammation. Always take a detailed systems review. Do not look for autoantibodies including ANA and ANCA – it is a waste of expense.

3. Anterior uveitis of any type in a child

- FBC, U&Es, LFTs, ACE, ANA (streptococcal serology)

Involve a pediatrician in investigation and diagnosis. Other tests are performed as directed by associated symptoms if any. Post-streptococcal uveitis is not uncommon. Any child presenting with uveitis after a recent fever, sore throat or lymphadenopathy should have serology performed.

4. Intermediate uveitis

- FBC, U&Es, LFTs, syphilis serology, ACE, chest radiograph
- CT of the brain if focal neurological symptoms

In the absence of defining features such as retinal vasculitis or peripheral granuloma, most intermediate uveitis is idiopathic. Multiple sclerosis eventually occurs in a substantial minority but it is our practice not to perform brain imaging unless a patient has a clear history of focal neurological symptoms. Sarcoidosis accounts for up to 10% of cases. Other causes are unusual and almost always have other defining features. Syphilis can cause any form of uveitis.

5. Acute unilateral panuveitis

- FBC, U&Es, LFTs, ESR, CRP, HLA-B27, urine microscopy and culture
- Blood culture if pyrexial
- Vitreous tap for microbiology
- Echocardiography if indicated

Exclude endogenous endophthalmitis. Identify risk factors including intravenous drug abuse or cannulation. If organisms grown but source unidentified, request cardiological investigation. Remember that very severe HLA-B27-associated uveitis can mimic infection.

6. Necrotizing retinitis

- Anterior chamber tap for herpesviruses, syphilis serology
- Consider lymphoma or *Toxoplasma* spp. if unresponsive to antiviral
- Consider immunodeficiency if atypical

Typical acute retinal necrosis in immunocompetent individuals does not necessarily require confirmation by PCR but it is always reassuring. Rarely other diagnoses can cause spreading necrotizing disease but these are usually in immunodeficient individuals.

7. Posterior uveitis and retinal vasculitis

- Pattern recognition with directed investigations
- TB testing if progressive

It is not possible to standardize a logical guideline for posterior uveitis in general. The great majority of diagnoses are presumed autoimmune and pattern recognition on examination is fundamental. In cases of occlusive retinal vasculitis or progressive chorioretinitis always consider TB.

REFERENCES

Cole CJ, Kwan AS, Laidlaw DA, Aylward GW. A new technique of combined retinal and choroidal biopsy. *Br J Ophthalmol* 2008;**92**:1357–60.

Dworkin LL, Gibler TM, Van Gelder RN. Real-time quantitative polymerase chain reaction diagnosis of infectious posterior uveitis. *Arch Ophthalmol* 2002;**120**:1534–9.

Fooroogian F, Gupta R, Wong DT, Derzko-Dzulynsky L. Anterior uveitis investigation by Canadian ophthalmologists: insights from the Canadian National Uveitis Survey. *Can J Ophthalmol* 2006;**41**:576–83.

Kratz A, Levy J, Belfair N, et al. Broth culture yield vs traditional approach in the work-up of endophthalmitis. *Am J Ophthalmol* 2006;**141**:1022.

Manku H, McCluskey P. Diagnostic vitreous biopsy in patients with uveitis: a useful investigation? *Clin Exp Ophthalmol* 2005;**33**:604–10.

Rothova A, de Boer JH, Ten-Dam van Loon NH, et al. Usefulness of aqueous humour analysis for the diagnosis of posterior uveitis. *Ophthalmology* 2008;**115**:306–11.

Solberg OD, Mack SJ, Lancaster AK, et al. Balancing selection and heterogeneity across the classical leukocyte loci: a meta-analytic review of 497 population studies. *Hum Immunol* 2008;**69**:443–64.

Wittenberg LA, Maberley DA, Ma PE, et al. Contribution of vitreous cytology to final clinical diagnosis: fifteen-year review of vitreous cytology specimens from one institution. *Ophthalmology* 2008;**115**:1944–50.

Zamecki KJ, Jabs DA. HLA typing in uveitis: use and misuse. *Am J Ophthalmol* 2010;**149**:189–93.

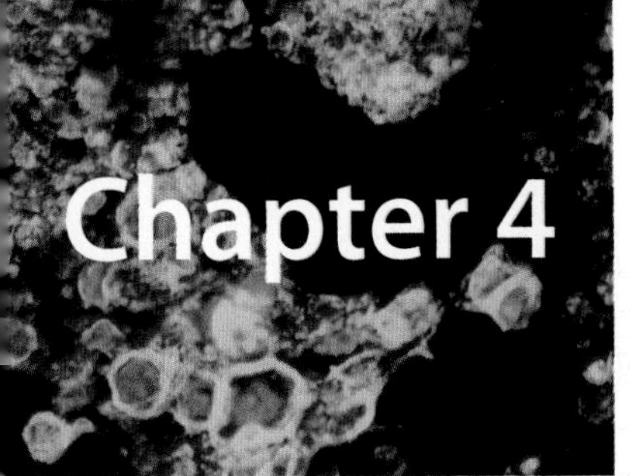

Chapter 4 Diagnosing uveitis

MAKING A DIAGNOSIS

The identification of a diagnosis is perceived by doctor and patient alike as a crucial step in the management of an illness. The former is taught that this stage of a structured process is imperative for the logical and scientific practice of medicine. The latter is concerned that the doctor should understand the illness and give appropriate treatment, and the application of a diagnostic label, no matter how uninformative, can serve to reassure.

Unfortunately the field of uveitis is a paradigm for the difficulties that can pervade the medical diagnostic process. Even after careful examination and well-selected investigation, in only a minority of cases are we able to uncover a proven etiological and pathogenetic diagnosis. Often despite intensive attempts at diagnosis, many cases of uveitis have no known cause. Nevertheless, almost always a level of knowledge may be accumulated about an individual uveitis, which is enough to aid management. It is important to have a logical approach to the acquisition of this knowledge, and to work within its limitations, resisting the ever-present temptation to venture speculatively outside those limits. In this context, the word 'diagnosis' might therefore be pragmatically defined: 'Reaching a level of knowledge about the uveitis which allows the development of confident, informed decisions on management.'

One of the most confusing aspects of uveitis diagnosis is the mixture of terms that have been progressively added to our lexicon. A variety of descriptive labels is in use, and many of these have overlapping or confused boundaries. Such terms include the anatomical (e.g. intermediate uveitis), the descriptive (e.g. birdshot retinochoroidopathy), the behavioral (e.g. chronic anterior uveitis), the eponymous (e.g. Posner–Schlossman syndrome), the systemic association (e.g. sarcoid uveitis), the pathogenetic or etiological (e.g. cytomegalovirus retinitis) and the purely speculative. Diagnosis is potentially a most confusing process, and therefore research and comparative study are difficult in this field. Such communicative difficulties have been likened to a 'tower of Babel' (Rosenbaum et al. 1996). In contrast to some areas of general medicine, there have been few collaborative efforts to identify strict diagnostic criteria for the various forms of uveitis.

There is pressure to compartmentalize an individual case of uveitis into a descriptive category, and this challenge has been increased by the progressive addition of apparently new uveitis entities, particularly over the last 20 years. although some cases may be characteristic of such a diagnosis, many are less easy, and some may have features that are shared between different diagnoses. Almost always it is the uveitic features themselves, and not the descriptive category into which the patient most neatly fits, that are more informative and that will be of most use in directing the management of the patient.

Uveitis is an uncommon disease, but, as with so many medical conditions, and especially for the trainee, rare forms are perceived to be less rare, first because of publication bias and second because surveys into uveitis incidence and prevalence usually emanate from specialist referral centers with a patient population that is already pre-selected by referral. This difficulty has been highlighted by a study comparing a population of unselected consecutive cases of uveitis with a population of uveitis patients in a referral centre (McCannel et al. 1996). There is a tendency, by no means unique to the field of uveitis, to over-diagnose rare forms, which is not helpful to patient management. In teaching on this subject to groups of ophthalmologists, my portrayal of a learner's diagnostic curve (**Fig. 4.1**) may cause much amusement but is rooted in real experience; the parallel with the phases of bereavement will not be lost on some readers. Those as yet ignorant of a diagnosis will clearly never reach it (the 'abyss of ignorance'). However, once learning of the possibility (the 'age of enlightenment') there is an irresistible tendency to reach the diagnosis at the slightest provocation, almost always wrongly ('the peak of enthusiasm'). Reality imposes its cold hand fairly quickly, however, and a 'vale of depression' often follows, with the inevitable irony that, on the first occasion when the disease is truly encountered, it will be missed. With the grey hairs of experience comes the green 'path of acceptance'; the ageing ophthalmologist will make the diagnosis at a rate approximating to its true incidence, but never quite reaching perfection. Keeping on this pathway while trudging towards a professional sunset is perhaps the most that mere mortals can achieve.

The effects of diagnostic over-enthusiasm are not merely temporarily diverting. The absolute beginner in the clinic will happily write down a suggested diagnosis which may on the day be peremptorily rejected by his or her supervisor, but which nevertheless will remain visible in the yellowing clinical records in perpetuity, acquiring an entirely undeserved validity with the passage of time. Future browsers will happen across it and raise the possibility again in the future, serving the patient not at all. A structured acquisition of diagnostic information and a responsible method of note keeping will lessen this tendency. Several efforts among the uveitis community have been made to standardize the classification of uveitis, and the terms used to describe it. In 2005 the first international workshop of the Standardization of Uveitis Nomenclature (SUN) Working Group met to form agreement about the basics of classification (SUN Working Group 2005), and the work is ongoing with the aim of ensuring properly comparable publications on the subject. A clear iteration of the

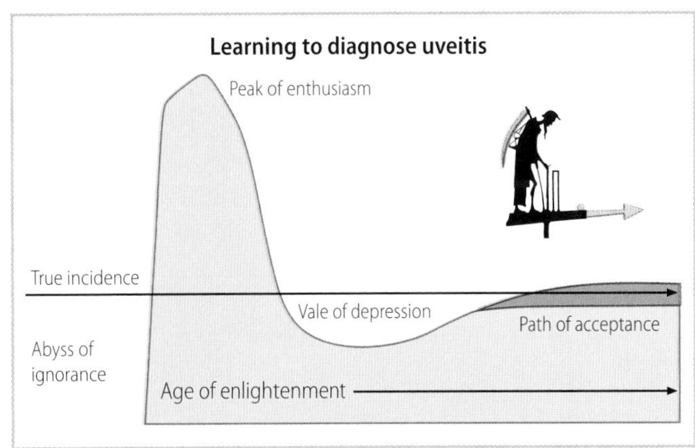

Figure 4.1 The diagnostic curve – a life of learning.

basic descriptive terms in uveitis was published, in some instances slightly amending the meaning of words as previously used by many authors. These terms are summarized in **Table 4.1**. The broad-brush results of these efforts are essential for comparable research but, wherever descriptive (or indeed any) boundaries are drawn, can be found the seeds of dispute (Khairallah 2010). It is clear that within a working clinic a more detailed approach is required and an adequate diagnostic label applied from several different directions. The variables to be considered include the following.

Anatomical location

Some forms of uveitis are typically confined to either the anterior or the posterior segment. Others may be more widespread, and either anterior or posterior segment inflammation may have 'spillover' effects. to clarify the anatomical description of uveitis, the International Uveitis Study Group (IUSG) recommended in 1987 a nomenclature that is now being increasingly adopted, with amendment from the SUN group, and shown in **Table 4.2**. It should be stressed that this classification refers to the primary site of inflammation and does not refer to the site of complications (e.g. macular edema). In the posterior segment, the primary location of inflammatory disease involving both retina and choroid may be difficult to determine, and for some types of inflammation is the subject of continued debate. Primary retinal inflammations may have widespread intraocular effects. The retina is therefore considered, in the field of 'uveitis', to be an honorary member of the uveal tract.

Laterality

Some forms of uveitis, such as Fuchs' heterochromic uveitis, are typically unilateral. Others, e.g. intermediate uveitis, while often asymmetrical, are almost always bilateral. Some forms of uveitis, e.g. that associated with HLA-B27, may be typically unilateral at each recurrence, but may involve either eye. Others presenting unilaterally have a significant risk of future contralateral involvement. The laterality of the disease process is therefore not only useful in diagnostic terms, but also important for prognostication.

Table 4.1 Descriptor terms in uveitis

Preferred SUN term	Synonyms or definition
Chronic	Inflammation relapsing less than 3 months after stopping treatment
Insidious onset	Slow onset
Persistent	A duration of an attack of inflammation lasting more than 3 months
Recurrent	Repeated episodes of inflammation separated by at least 3 months of inflammation-free period
Remission	Inflammation free despite being off all treatment for 3 months or more
Sudden onset	Acute onset
Adapted from SUN Working Group (2005).	

Table 4.2 Anatomical classification of uveitis

Anterior uveitis: Iritis Iridocyclitis Anterior cyclitis
Intermediate uveitis
Posterior uveitis: Focal, multifocal or diffuse choroiditis, chorioretinitis, retinochoroiditis, or neurouveitis
Panuveitis
Adapted from SUN Working Group (2005).

Pattern of onset

The thorough evaluation of a patient with uveitis at the onset of the disease process is of the greatest importance. The clinical characteristics of the eye and patient at this stage should be carefully documented. For those inflammations that become chronic (lasting more than 3 months) the clinical findings are often at their most distinctive at the onset of the disease, frequently becoming nondescript with the passage of time and the application of treatment. It is in these early stages where possible associations with recent systemic illness, or significant foreign travel, can most easily be uncovered, and the ability to perform any relevant acute and convalescent serological testing is confined to this period.

Behavior and course

Some forms of uveitis have courses that are typically acute (of sudden onset), acute recurrent, persistent (lasting more than 3 months), fluctuating (persistent but fluctuating in intensity) or chronic (relapsing less than 3 months after an attempt to discontinue medication). Acute unilateral anterior uveitis with fibrinous exudate (almost always associated with HLA-B27) is a self-limiting process that will require treatment for only weeks but has a relatively high risk of future recurrence. The teenager with floaters who is found to have intermediate uveitis may have a fluctuating disease course interspersed with episodes requiring treatment, but long-term inflammation at some level is to be expected. The patient with presumed Behçet's disease and ocular involvement is likely to develop future explosive recurrences of inflammation unless immunosuppressed.

There are some forms of uveitis in which characteristic features allowing a firmer diagnosis appear only after a period of time. The Asian patient with severe hypertensive anterior uveitis may only later develop alopecia and poliosis, suggesting the Vogt–Koyanagi–Harada syndrome. The middle-aged patient with chronic nondescript vitritis may only later develop the typical subtle depigmented retinal pigment epithelium (RPE) lesions characteristic of birdshot retinochoroidopathy. The diagnostic process is therefore not necessarily based on a single 'snapshot' of a patient with uveitis; the regular re-evaluation of a patient, with a healthy skepticism for an earlier diagnosis, is an important and often rewarding part of uveitis management.

Characteristic clinical descriptions

Certain findings on physical examination may serve to narrow the diagnostic spectrum considerably, e.g. large mutton-fat keratic precipitates (KPs) are suggestive of 'granulomatous' disease, and in most practices sarcoidosis heads the differential diagnosis list. Heterochromia is by no means unique to Fuchs' heterochromic uveitis, but strongly suggests that possibility. Inferior snowbanking and snowballs are almost pathognomonic of intermediate uveitis.

In the posterior segment, lesions can exhibit a variety of characteristics that will aid diagnosis: single or multiple; unilateral or bilateral; atrophic, placoid or raised; involving primarily choroid or retina; distributed only within the vascular arcades, or mainly peripherally, or perhaps in a 'birdshot' distribution. The forms of uveitis that exhibit multifocal posterior segment inflammation have perhaps the most confusing nomenclature, and several also seem to share some common features. Despite this, a careful observation of the characteristics of these lesions will help the diagnostic process.

Presence of complications

Although complicating phenomena are common in uveitis, the ability of some forms of uveitis to cause such complications may vary widely, and their presence may therefore serve to aid diagnosis, e.g. band keratopathy is particularly common in uveitis associated with juvenile chronic arthritis and cataract is almost universal in those with Fuchs' heterochromic uveitis. Macular edema is rare in the latter, but very common in intermediate uveitis, with which it is sometimes confused. Glaucoma is perceived to be particularly characteristic of some forms of uveitis, and these include the Posner–Schlossman syndrome, herpetic uveitis, Fuchs' heterochromic uveitis and the Vogt-Koyanagi–Harada syndrome.

Severity

The severity of an inflammation can be expressed in several different ways. More severe forms of uveitis have more acute and more extreme symptoms. Medial opacities may be more dense, the breakdown of the blood–ocular barrier may be more profound and a hypopyon may be observed. However, the single tiny foveal retinal focus, with minimal inflammatory signs, may be just as destructive to vision. The usefulness of the word 'severity' in diagnosis is therefore limited, and is best used to define the grade of intraocular inflammation, the quantification of which is dealt with in Chapter 2.

Age, sex, race, geography

Some forms of uveitis characteristically involve certain age groups. Each form of uveitis has its age spectrum, and for some this is relatively confined (and therefore potentially useful for diagnosis) whereas in others it is widespread. This book illustrates the age range for many different forms of uveitis in the relevant section, but examples of the diagnostically useful age disparities are illustrated (**Fig. 4.2**).

Although several forms of uveitis have unequal sex incidence ratios, in most this is not striking enough to be particularly helpful in diagnosis. There are some exceptions, e.g. most of the sexually transmitted infections are more common in men, and the incidence of AIDS-related uveitis and retinitis is much lower in women. Most of the multifocal white dot syndromes are somewhat more common in women, some strikingly so, e.g. multiple evanescent white dot syndrome (MEWDS) (**Fig. 4.2**).

The predilection of some forms of uveitis for certain racial groups is again sometimes useful in diagnosis, e.g. the high incidence of Behçet's disease in Asia and the Middle East is striking, and this increased incidence holds true for those emigrating from these areas to Europe or the USA. The predilection of sarcoidosis for African-Caribbean individuals, and of some multifocal posterior segment inflammations (particularly birdshot retinochoroidopathy) for white people, are other examples. Some diseases may closely follow archaic populations and migration routes, e.g. the Vogt-Koyanagi–Harada syndrome is at its most common in the Far East, particularly in Japan where the disease causes over 10% of all cases of uveitis. The significant migration of this population, during a previous ice age, over the Bering Straits, to form the first indigenous population of North America, carried with it the predisposition to the disease, and al though the Vogt-Koyanagi–Harada syndrome is only infrequently

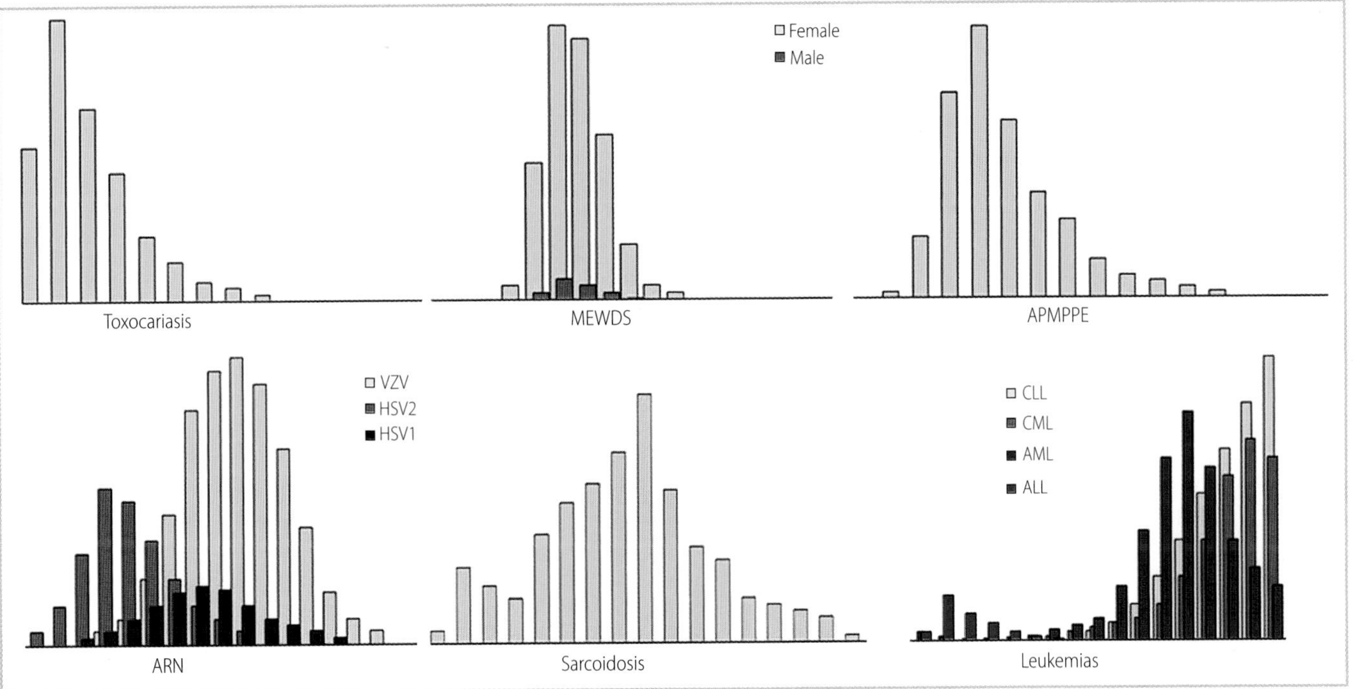

Figure 4.2 The disparity in age at presentation for some forms of uveitis.

seen in the USA, a record of indigenous North American ancestry has been found in most, and may be present in all affected patients in that country.

Differences in the incidence of infection may be international, regional or environmental. Travel to, or habitation within, endemic areas must therefore be taken into consideration. Examples of those forms of uveitis with a quite confined geographical distribution are the presumed ocular histoplasmosis syndrome, Lyme disease, human T-lymphotropic virus type I (HTLV-I)-associated uveitis and diffuse unilateral subacute neuroretinitis. Uveitis surveys emanating from different countries will show strikingly different patterns, and these have been neatly analyzed (Chams et al. 2009). Some examples of disparate geographical distributions are shown (**Fig. 4.3**).

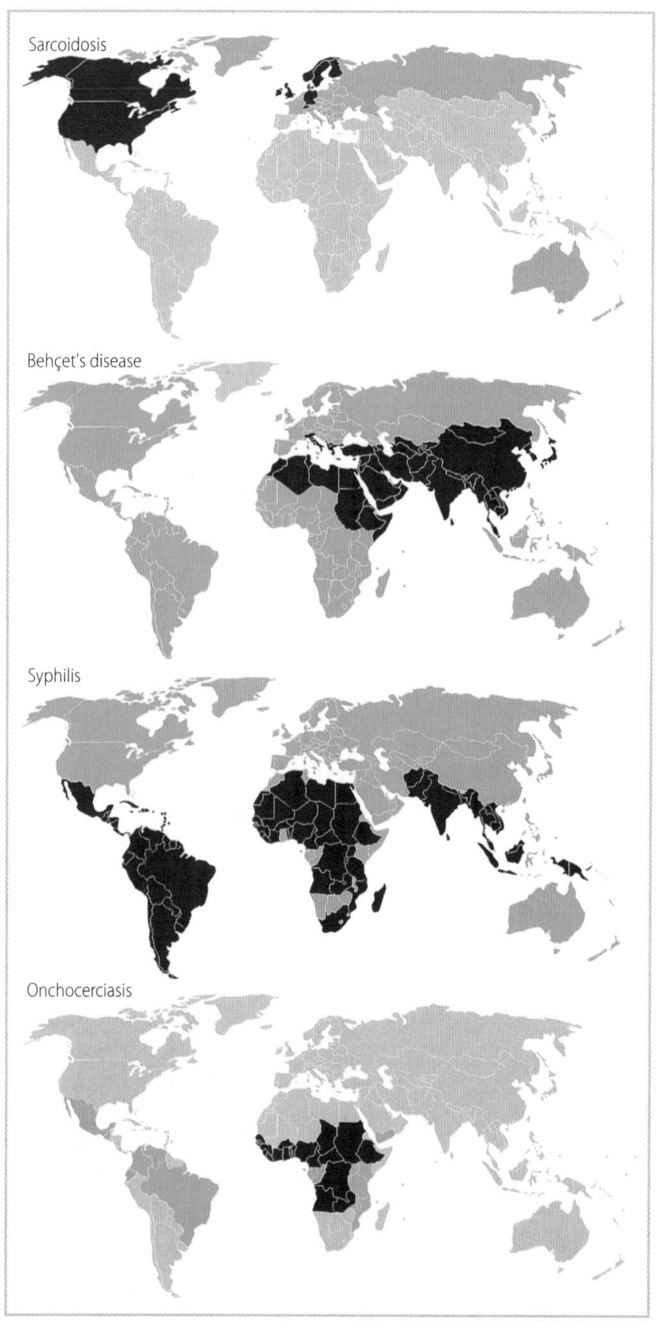

Figure 4.3 The geographical variation for several forms of uveitis.

Association with systemic disease

Many forms of uveitis are part of a more widespread inflammatory process. The identification of this is not only crucial for diagnosis, but may substantially modify future management. A complete search for systemic symptoms, and a systems review, are therefore important. The patient may perceive systemic disease to be irrelevant to the ophthalmologist and, for this reason, and sometimes (as in the case of sexually transmitted infection) because of embarrassment, questioning may need to be rigorous and persistent. The early identification of an acute illness concurrent with, or just preceding, the onset of uveitis may also be important. It is equally important to identify non-ocular physical signs, which may rarely be pathognomonic but much more frequently may strongly indicate a pathway for further investigation. The message to the ophthalmologist is therefore blunt: the patient's body does not end at the collar!

The coexistence of a systemic inflammation may be the only feature of a particular uveitis that allows diagnosis to take place. In some cases the associations are so characteristic (such as the uveitis associated with juvenile chronic arthritis) that this does not provide a practical problem. However, attempts to associate nondescript uveitis with coincident systemic disease, merely based on the fact that both are present in one body, are problematic, especially when such systemic diseases are relatively common. In the UK, sarcoidosis is a typical example. It is for this among other reasons that diagnostic criteria for specific forms of uveitis are useful if they can be agreed upon.

Etiology

It could and should be argued that a true and complete diagnosis can be reached only with a full knowledge of etiology and pathogenesis. The scarcity of such cases in clinical uveitis practice is well known. Nevertheless, a system of uveitis classification based on proven or presumed etiology has been devised by the IUSG (Deschenes et al. 2008) and, although it is confusingly described as a 'clinical' classification, it is actually etiological and is shown in **Table 4.3**. Developments in medical diagnosis over the past 25 years allow the not unreasonable speculation that, in due course, many forms of uveitis currently fitting into that large container labeled 'non-infective; no systemic disease association' will prove to be infective, or to have a proven microbiological trigger.

RECORDING A DIAGNOSIS

Accumulated information from the criteria above will allow the ophthalmologist to apply a label to the uveitis. This may include no pathogenetic or etiological information whatever (such as MEWDS),

Table 4.3 International Uveitis Study Group clinical uveitis classification

Infective	Bacterial
	Viral
	Fungal
	Parasitic
	Other
Non-infective	Known systemic disease association
	No known systemic disease association
Masquerade	Neoplastic
	Non-neoplastic

Adapted from Deschenes et al. (2008)

may contain such information at a presumptive level (such as *Toxoplasma* retinochoroiditis) or may diagnose only by association (e.g. sarcoid-associated uveitis). The quality of the information contained within the label may therefore vary widely, and the recording of any information within the above criteria, which may be relevant to diagnosis, is important. Nevertheless the patient will always appreciate the application of a diagnostic label, and this step is supplemented in this clinic by providing basic information on several of the more common diagnoses (see patient information pamphlets on the attached disk). As yet there is no such comprehensive classification system for uveitis that has been widely accepted. However, a system was devised here in Manchester 20 years ago for the recording of clinical information on all patients attending the newly formed Manchester Uveitis Clinic (**Box 4.1**). There are 24 fields to record:

The Manchester Uveitis Clinic database

1. Patient identifier
2. Surname
3. Forename
4. Postal/Zip code
5. Date of birth
6. Age at presentation to MUC
7. Racial origin
8. Date of presentation to MUC
9. Uveitis present or not (not present, eg in patients with scleritis, or for screening)
10. Age at onset of uveitis
11. Name of referring physician
12. Main anatomical location of uveitis
    Anterior
    Intermediate
    Posterior
    Panuveitis
13. Granulomatous or non-granulomatous anterior uveitis
14. Side affected
    Right
    Left
    Bilateral (not necessarily simultaneous)
15. Behavior of uveitis
    Acute single attack
    Acute recurrent attacks
    Chronic, fluctuating intensity
    Chronic, unremitting
16. Associated systemic system involvement (Y or N)
    Fever
    Joints
    Skin
    Bowel
    Chest
    Neurological
    Other
17. Main descriptor of uveitis (**Table 4.4**)
18. Etiology of uveitis (**Table 4.5**)
19. Diagnostic confidence
    CONfirmed (microbiology or histology)
    PREsumed (strong supporting evidence)
    POSsible (with no evidence of another diagnosis)
    NKU – not known
20. Ocular complications past or present (Y or N)
    Band keratopathy
    Corneal decompensation
    Occlusio
    Glaucoma
    Cataract
    Retinal neovascularization
    Retinal detachment
    Subretinal fibrosis
    Macular edema
    Phthisis
21. Methods of medical treatment past or present
    Depot steroid
    Systemic steroid
    Named immunosuppressives
    Antimicrobial
22. Methods of surgical treatment past or present:
    Cataract surgery
    Glaucoma surgery
    Vitreoretinal surgery
    Other surgery
23. Freehand: named systemic diseases, deaths etc
24. Bone densitometry status

Box 4.1 The Manchester Uveitis Clinic database.

Table 4.4 The Manchester Uveitis Clinic diagnostic database: main descriptor

Code	Description
AAU	Acute anterior uveitis
AMP	Acute posterior multifocal placoid pigment epitheliopathy
APU	Acute panuveitis
ARN	Acute retinal necrosis (includes progressive outer retinal necrosis)
BIR	Birdshot retinochoroidopathy
CAU	Chronic anterior uveitis
CPU	Chronic panuveitis
DUS	Diffuse unilateral subacute neuroretinitis
EAL	Eales' disease
FCH	Focal choroiditis
FRE	Focal retinitis
FHU	Fuchs' Heterochromic Uveitis
GEO	Geographic/serpiginous choroidopathy
INT	Intermediate uveitis
KUV	Keratitis with uveitis
MEW	Multiple evanescent white dot syndrome
MCH	Multifocal choroiditis
NER	Neuroretinitis with optic disk swelling
OTH	Other
PHA	Phakogenic/phakoanaphylactic uveitis
PSG	Posterior segment granuloma
PSS	Posner–Schlossman syndrome
PIC	Punctate inner choroidopathy
REV	Retinal vasculitis
RPE	Retinal pigment epitheliitis
SCL	Scleritis with or without uveitis
SYM	Sympathetic ophthalmia
UES	Uveal effusion syndrome
VKH	Vogt–Koyanagi–Harada syndrome

Table 4.5 The Manchester Uveitis Clinic diagnostic database: etiology of uveitis

Code	Description
A29	HLA-A29 associated
AIE	Autoimmune endotheliopathy
AIU	Autoimmune uveitis
B27	HLA-B27 associated
BEH	Behçet's disease
CAN	Candidiasis
CIN	CINCA syndrome
CMV	Cytomegalovirus uveitis
CRO	Crohn's disease associated
CSS	Churg–Strauss syndrome associated
DIA	Diabetes associated
DRU	Drug-induced uveitis
DXT	Radiotherapy-induced uveitis
GOU	Gout associated
HSV	Herpes simplex uveitis
IRU	Immune recovery uveitis
JCI	Juvenile chronic iridocyclitis
JIA	Juvenile idiopathic arthritis associated
LEP	Leprosy
LYM	Lyme disease
MAS	Malignant masquerade syndromes
NEU	Neurological disease-associated
NKU	Unknown etiology
OBA	Other bacterial uveitis
OFU	Other fungal uveitis
OPA	Other parasitic uveitis
OPR	Other protozoal uveitis
OTA	Other arthritis associated
OTB	Other bowel disease associated uveitis
OVI	Other viral uveitis
PAN	Polyarteritis nodosa associated
POH	Presumed ocular histoplasmosis syndrome
PSA	Psoriatic arthropathy associated
RED	Retinal detachment-induced uveitis
REI	Reactive arthropathy
RHA	Rheumatoid arthritis associated
SAR	Sarcoidosis
SLE	Systemic lupus associated
SUR	Surgery-induced
SYP	Syphilis
TIN	Tubulointerstitial nephritis with uveitis
TOC	Toxocariasis
TOP	Toxoplasmosis
TRA	Trauma-induced uveitis
TUB	Tuberculosis associated
VAS	Systemic vasculitis associated
ULC	Ulcerative colitis associated
VZV	Varicella-zoster virus uveitis
WEG	Wegener's granulomatosis associated
WHI	Whipple's disease associated

The database was devised to allow fairly comprehensive input at the first patient visit, with only major ephemera being recorded subsequently, such as a change in diagnosis, immunosuppressive or a surgical event. It is not a patient management record. This permits time-efficient management and the use of fields 17–19 alone identifies a rapid working diagnosis (**Table 4.6**). It also allows straightforward searches on any indexed parameter, with more detailed data being extracted from patient records for research or audit purposes where necessary. Manchester uveitis clinic-based research has been much facilitated by the database, and the use of multifaceted diagnostic parameters has permitted patient group identification for liaison with other research groups. The maintenance of a clinic database is to be strongly recommended to all clinicians with an interest in uveitis. This approach to diagnosis has served well in our clinic. By enforcing a structured approach, it minimizes the risk of speculative diagnosis and, by including a 'diagnostic confidence' section, serves to remind that the best available diagnosis at presentation may need to be revisited during the course of a uveitis, because of either changing ocular signs or the appearance of associated systemic signs.

Table 4.6 The Manchester Uveitis Clinic diagnostic database: examples of working diagnoses

	Descriptor	Etiology	Confidence
Example 1	FRE	TOP	PRE
A patient whose predominant ocular feature is a focal retinitis, presumed to be caused by toxoplasmosis on the basis of typical clinical appearance and supportive positive serology			
Example 2	AAU	B27	PRE
A patient with acute anterior uveitis, presumably related to his HLA-B27 positivity			
Example 3	MCH	SAR	CON
A patient whose predominant feature is multifocal choroiditis, where sarcoidosis has been confirmed by biopsy elsewhere			
Example 4	REV	BEH	POS
A patient whose predominant uveitis feature is occlusive retinal vasculitis, who has mouth ulcers but does not fulfill the diagnostic criteria for Behçet's disease.			
Example 5	FHU	NKU	NKU
A patient with features typical of Fuchs' heterochromic uveitis, a disease with unknown etiology			
For explanation of three-letter codes see Tables 4.4 and 4.5 and text.			

REFERENCES

Chams H, Rostami M, Mohammadi S-F, Ohno S. Epidemiology and prevalence of uveitis: review of literature. Iranian *J Ophthalmol* 2009;**21**:4–16.

Deschenes J, Murray PI, Rao N, Nussenblatt RB. International uveitis study group (IUSG) clinical classification of uveitis. *Ocular Immunol Inflamm* 2008;**16**:1–2.

Khairallah M. Are the Standardization of the Uveitis Nomenclature (SUN) working group criteria for codifying the site of inflammation appropriate for all uveitis problems? Limitations of the SUN working group classification. *Ocular Immunol Inflamm* 2010;**18**:2–4.

McCannel CA, Holland GN, Helm CJ, et al. Causes of uveitis in the general practice of ophthalmology. *Am J Ophthalmol* 1996:**121**:35–46.

Rosenbaum JT, Holland GN. Uveitis and the tower of Babel. *Arch Ophthalmol* 1996:**114**:604–5.

Sun Working Group. Standardisation of uveitis nomenclature for reporting clinical data. Results of the first international workshop. *Am J Ophthalmol* 2005;**140**:509–16.

Chapter 5 Principles of uveitis management

The management of uveitis is often complex and usually time-consuming, and may be extremely demanding of both patient and doctor. It can be a most frustrating disease which, badly managed, will blind a significant proportion of these predominantly young patients. In contrast, by using a structured and thoughtful approach, the management of even very severe chronic uveitis can be extremely rewarding. The challenges are many, the manifestations of uveitis protean and usually several are seen in an individual patient; the treatments available require careful management and may interact negatively, and are associated with potentially severe side effects; surgical intervention is rarely straightforward, and in no field of ophthalmology is the patient's ability to understand and cooperate more severely tested. Nevertheless management may be optimized: by identifying as early as possible what may be achieved by treatment; by gaining the full understanding, cooperation and support of the patient with whom the doctor must work in partnership; and by setting clear plans for management that must be monitored and regularly reappraised.

SETTING TARGETS FOR ACHIEVEMENT

Scrupulous examinations are necessary in every patient with uveitis. In those with recent-onset and straightforward uveitis, it may be a simple matter of establishing the current status and therefore the priorities for treatment. However, in some (and certainly in a high proportion of those referred to a uveitis clinic), being able to identify, from a selection of several possible causes, the main causes of visual loss and the main priorities for treatment can be challenging.

It is fundamentally important to distinguish reversible from irreversible visual loss, and to make an informed estimate of what may be achieved by treatment, e.g. it is not uncommon in our clinic to meet for the first time a patient referred with longstanding uveitis that remains active, who has formed a secondary cataract. This, together with posterior synechiae and vitreous opacification (some of which may be active inflammation, some accumulated debris), prevents an adequate view of the macula. The macula may previously have been documented as edematous, but at present it is difficult to establish whether it is either actively edematous or scarred from previous episodes, or both. The secondary glaucoma appears to be controlled medically, but the view of the disk is poor, and the low visual acuity will not allow reliable visual field testing. Would cataract extraction be useful, and if so when should it be performed? Should it be combined with intravitreal steroid injection to ameliorate or prevent postoperative macular edema, or will it worsen the glaucoma? Should it be combined with vitrectomy to avoid further surgery, or does that add too much to the surgical risk? What would be gained from enhanced anti-inflammatory treatment? In circumstances such as these the careful gathering of information, from both current examination and investigation, and a perusal of previous records (which are hopefully informative) is important.

In most circumstances it is possible to identify what can reasonably be expected from a particular form of treatment. This understanding is crucial for both doctor and patient, because the management pathway is unlikely to be straightforward, and balancing risks against benefits is constantly on the agenda. In some circumstances it may be necessary to explain to a patient that the outcome of a particular course of treatment (such as cataract surgery) is unknown, but may be useful and can be undertaken if the implications are fully understood and the risks acceptable.

GAINING PATIENT UNDERSTANDING

The issues involved in the management of some cases of uveitis are complex enough to deter most ophthalmologists, so optimizing the patient's understanding can clearly be a challenge. Nevertheless it is very important to augment understanding wherever possible. This is only fair to a patient with severe eye problems, and is essential to develop a rapport with the doctor. It will also enhance compliance and contribute to more effective management, which is rewarding for both patient and ophthalmologist.

The new patient with uveitis may describe a variety of ophthalmic symptoms, including redness, pain, photophobia, and visual disturbance or loss. Sometimes systemic symptoms are present. The patient has a lay perspective, with simple priorities: for the symptoms to abate as quickly as possible, with easily tolerable treatment that minimizes pain, inconvenience and complications, and for a speedy return to visual perfection. Very often in uveitis these expectations cannot be fulfilled; to allow unrealistic optimism to develop is to do a great disservice to a patient with severe uveitis, who may then be devastated by an unexpected outcome. It is in the early stages that the process of patient education must commence; trying to recover lost ground at a later stage is much more difficult, and often results in patient disillusionment, missed clinic visits and poorly maintained treatment; at worst, the patient's trust in the ophthalmologist may be lost and impossible to regain.

There are two important phenomena in uveitis management that the patient must understand. First, although the patient will automatically understand the need to treat inflammation where it causes symptoms, the ophthalmologist will need to explain that, in certain circumstances, inflammation, even where symptoms themselves would not justify treatment, must be treated in order to avoid the development of complications that would lead to permanent visual loss. Put simply, the treatment is not just for today, but also for tomorrow. The second concept that must be grasped is that anti-inflammatory and immunosuppressive treatment will suppress inflammation, but will not permanently remove it. Many patients use the word 'cure' when seeking better treatment for a chronic uveitis, and it is imperative that they are disabused of this notion; their expectations must be placed firmly into perspective, albeit with careful stress on the positive aspects of what can actually be achieved. The patient who is constantly, unrealistically seeking either cure from chronic inflammation or regained vision in a permanently damaged eye can only be regularly disappointed. Perhaps the most poignant patients of all are those who continue to seek the unachievable by touring many ophthalmologists, sometimes internationally – continually frustrated, continually unbelieving of the realistic advice repeated, unable to accept reality, and ultimately therefore vulnerable to the unwise and fruitless interventions that may be offered by the thoughtless or avaricious. Half an hour of honest and forthright conversation with such patients may be one of the most valuable contributions made to their care.

The successful suppression of uveitis will remove all, or almost all, signs of inflammation from the eye. For many forms of chronic uveitis, such maintenance is imperative to prevent the development of complications. After a prolonged inflammation-free period, both patient and doctor will question the need for continued treatment, at least at current levels. A careful and graded dose reduction may be appropriate, but patient compliance is imperative. A few are tempted to discontinue treatment and suffer accordingly; with proper communication such episodes can be minimized.

A patient's ability to absorb information and to understand complex explanations will clearly vary according to background, intelligence and personality. Gaining the understanding of the patient is time-consuming and must be individually tailored, but is a fundamental part of management. Doctors almost always overestimate their patients' ability to absorb information during a consultation, and this phenomenon is probably most marked at the first meeting. Gradual enhancement over several consultations is usually necessary. Some ophthalmologists believe in providing tape recordings to enable the patient to absorb by repetition. Several uveitis organizations have paper- or web-based information for patients. We have found it very useful to produce information pamphlets on several different aspects of uveitis and its management. Patients can read these in their own time at home, as the basis for more detailed discussions on their own individual status. The Manchester Uveitis Clinic patient information pamphlets are provided as a supplement to this text, in editable form, so that readers may freely use them if wished as the basis for pamphlets more appropriate for their own patients. The available pamphlets are listed in **Table 5.1** and can be found on the attached disk.

Table 5.1 Manchester Uveitis Clinic patient information pamphlets

Uveitis diagnoses	Behçet's disease and uveitis
	Birdshot retinochroidopathy
	Fuchs' heterochromic uveitis
	HLA-B27-related uveitis
	Intermediate uveitis
	Juvenile idiopathic arthritis and uveitis
	Toxoplasmosis
	Uveitis
	Viral retinitis
Uveitis complications and their treatment	Uveitis and cataract
	Uveitis and glaucoma
	Uveitis and macular oedema
	Uveitis and vitrectomy
Medical treatments	Anti-TNF-α monoclonal antibody therapy
	Azathioprine
	Ciclosporin
	Methotrexate
	Mycophenolate mofetil
	Prednisolone
	Sulfasalazine
	Tacrolimus
Others	Intraocular injection of triamcinolone or anti-VEGF antibody
	Immunosuppression, vaccination and travel abroad

See patient information pamphlets on the attached disk.

TNF, tumor necrosis factor; VEGF, vascular endothelial growth factor.

This process of regular discussion, education and cooperation is an essential part of uveitis management. In this way informed consent is genuinely obtained. It may be wise, and in some circumstances it is necessary, to obtain written consent to treatment. In contrast to some other areas of medicine using immunosuppressives or biologics (e.g. arthritis or inflammatory bowel disease) where drug manufacturers vigorously pursue licensing via funded controlled phase III trials, uveitis is very much a cinderella dependent on the continuing use of unlicensed drugs and, despite sometimes reasonably well-researched efficacy, these drugs remain 'investigational' in the treatment of uveitis (including, for instance, ciclosporin which has now been in clinical usage for over 30 years). Patients should be aware of this.

For patients with some forms of uveitis, organized patient groups have been formed to provide information and shared experience, and in some cases to support research. Some patients may benefit considerably from membership of a group, and the ophthalmologist is well placed to inform patients of their existence.

PATIENT–DOCTOR TEAMWORK

Where treatment can be complex, long term and potentially toxic, patients must play an active part in decision-making. The degree to which each will wish to do this will vary enormously. At one end of the spectrum, patients will be resistant to any attempt to involve them in decisions about their own treatment. This is often based on fear, which can be ameliorated by careful discussions at consecutive consultations. Such an approach may uncover basic misconceptions which, when properly explained, may transform a patient's attitude. It may be based on denial of any problem, which is dangerous and must be tackled head-on, or it may, particularly in teenagers, be accompanied by a general ennui because the eye problem and its treatment are perceived more as an inconvenient interference with current lifestyle than a progressive sight-threatening disorder. In getting to know patients, the ophthalmologist must tread a careful path between encouragement and reassurance, tempered by realism and diligence. Every attempt should be made to enhance cooperation.

At the other end of the spectrum are those patients who, in pedantically following their own inclination, often driven by irrelevant anecdotes obtained in social conversation or, worse, by browsing the most ill-informed that the internet has to offer, will be resistant to medical advice and may wish to follow a path that, in the view of the ophthalmologist, is unwise. With patience and persistence both of these extremes can and should be drawn inwards towards the ideal. The patient and ophthalmologist must work as a team and, although the ophthalmologist is the expert, giving advice and guidance that may be very strong, the patient must feel in control of important management decisions, especially where risk–benefit balances are under discussion. It is essential to avoid situations where patients claim that treatment has been forced upon them, or that inadequate information was given before treatment choices were made.

This process of patient–doctor teamwork and joint decision-making is a continuous one. It is enhanced by the ability to consult the same doctor on most occasions (a luxury in some busy clinics), and is rapidly destroyed by conflicting advice from different doctors. Doctors working within teams should therefore try to follow consistent approaches. Patients will be reassured by having rapid telephone access to advice where urgently needed, and the doctor will be reassured that a well-informed patient will not overuse that facility.

ESTABLISHING AND MONITORING A MANAGEMENT PLAN

Having identified realistic targets for achievement that the patient understands, a coherent plan of action will now be initiated which has either a foreseeable end-point, or predictable and regular points for reappraisal. For example, when commencing any new systemic anti-inflammatory or immunosuppressive treatment it is imperative at the outset to define criteria for success, and a timescale within which that should be achieved. Where long-term treatment is anticipated, regular reappraisal points should be identified at which time judgments on benefits versus risks will dictate future treatment.

It is important to document such plans in patient records and ensure that the patient fully understands what the targets will be. It is frustrating to encounter referred patients whose previous management does not appear to have been clearly planned, and who may have been exposed to treatment side effects but ineffective dosages or periods. The patient may already feel jaded by these approaches and the retrieval of lost ground must then precede the normal opening gambits. Such problems are largely avoidable by the formation of a management plan at the earliest opportunity, by its regular reappraisal and with the open-mindedness to change where necessary.

Careful examination and scrupulous record keeping, preferably using consistent terminology and repeatable methods of assessment of intraocular inflammation, will enable the ophthalmologist to document changes with time, and therefore to judge treatment effectiveness. Adhering to a carefully formulated management plan is much more difficult without such accurate information.

Monitoring immunosuppression safely is essential but can be mechanistic and is in several specialties delegated to specialist nurses. This is not entirely possible in ophthalmology because of the nuances of disease activity and the required skills of ocular examination. Nevertheless, the delegation of some tasks to appropriately trained support staff is logical and efficient. We have used a nurse practitioner-led health monitoring system for several years (Jones et al. 2009) and the documentation is available, with other management protocols, as Chapter 21. We can recommend such an approach.

THE TIMING OF TREATMENT

Where an eye is actively inflamed and the inflammation is causing damage, there is little question that immediate treatment is required. However, in those with chronic uveitis, and particularly where the degree of inflammation fluctuates, there are legitimate questions to be asked about the timing of treatment. Most commonly the timing of cataract surgery needs to be decided; this may be badly needed for visual reasons, but sometimes must be delayed until circumstances are favorable. The ophthalmic surgeon should never fall into the trap of operating too early on a cataract in an eye where the uveitis has not yet been brought under control. Pressure from the patient must be resisted; the visual problems resulting from badly timed cataract surgery in actively inflamed eyes are irreversible, and were once familiar in patients referred to uveitis clinics. Fortunately this is less frequent because patients are increasingly referred before surgery to the first eye is performed.

The management of surgical episodes in those with uveitis requires enhanced treatment, frequent postoperative visits and disruption of routine for several weeks. Starting some immunosuppressives requires similarly close supervision, so it is sensible to undertake treatment at a time where this intervention will cause the fewest problems for the patient. Many patients with uveitis are young adults with busy lives and essential forthcoming events: an undergraduate facing examinations; the recently employed desperate to limit time off work or needing to travel regularly; or the young woman keen to start a family and therefore wishing to defer immunosuppression. A reasonable balance must be drawn after careful discussion.

MANAGEMENT PROTOCOLS

Written guidelines for the management of common problems in uveitis, or protocols for the safe use of certain drugs, enhance consistency, efficacy and safety. They serve as a firm basis for treatment, and need not be unnecessarily proscriptive. They are of particular educational value for trainees passing through the unit, and are sometimes of interest to informed patients. They ensure consistency in teams where a patient may see different doctors. The time taken for their creation and regular updating has, in our clinic, been well spent, and the principle of written guidelines for important management problems is to be recommended. The Manchester Uveitis Clinic (MUC) patient management protocols are provided as a supplement to this text, in editable form, so that readers may freely use them if they wish as the basis for protocols more appropriate for their own clinics. The available protocols are listed in **Table 5.2** (see also the attached disk). In MUC they are available on a regional ophthalmologists' website, and all doctors about to start training or working in the MUC download all protocols on to a memory stick before starting with instructions to ensure basic knowledge of immunosuppression safety.

DEALING WITH VISUAL LOSS

Visual loss is a common accompaniment to uveitis, and visual handicap may affect a significant proportion of patients (Durrani et al. 2004). Such a disability is particularly difficult in young adults. Fortunately it is unusual for such deterioration to be rapid, and therefore the patient may be prepared in advance. It is unfair to deny the possibility of such preparation by failing to communicate a prognosis to the patient where it is clear to the ophthalmologist. Obviously such information should be given sensitively and at an appropriate time, and a gradual revelation of the possibility of permanent visual loss will allow the patient to come to terms with such devastating news.

For those at work, an inability to meet the visual standard for driving is likely to be the first problem to be encountered. Some may become unable to perform certain visual tasks at work, such as using a computer screen. Others may start to work dangerously in their manual occupation because of deteriorating vision, and sometimes those who are obliged to undergo regular employment health screening may fail because of poor eyesight. Vision may become inadequate for qualification for entry to a planned job. Those who are students may find their progress hampered by visual problems.

The ophthalmologist can and should raise such issues with the patient. Often a knowledge of deteriorating vision is suppressed by the patient, and frequently this will mean that a supervisor, teacher

Table 5.2 Manchester Uveitis Clinic management protocols

Types of uveitis	Acute anterior uveitis
	Sarcoidosis
	Toxoplasmosis
	Viral retinitis
Immunosuppressives and steroid safety	Azathioprine
	Cardiovascular disease
	Ciclosporin
	Infliximab
	Intravenous methylprednisolone
	Methotrexate
	Mycophenolate mofetil
	Prednisolone
	Tacrolimus
	Sulfasalazine
	Varicella-zoster virus and immunosuppression
Surgical treatments	Aqueous sampling
	Cataract surgery
	Intraocular bevacizumab injection
	Intraocular ganciclovir injection
	Intraocular triamcinolone injection
General management	Health review proforma and instructions
	Uveitis assessment

or employer is unaware of a visual problem. Fear of dismissal or of failure to progress with studies (usually, but not always, unfounded) may prevent the patient from discussing a visual problem at work. This is an unfortunate situation that becomes only more difficult with time. In general a properly informed employer or teacher is not only sympathetic, but also actively supportive, and can often suggest positive steps that had not been considered by the patient.

Visual handicap registration is fortunately uncommon even in those with severe and chronic uveitis, but if registration is appropriate it should not be delayed. Particularly for those at work, registration is able to generate substantial help, some of which may allow work to continue. In addition to the obvious high-resolution computer displays and large-print printers, CCTV apparatus, optical character recognition software, text-to-speech and voice recognition software may all allow continued work. In addition, there may be access to services for visually handicapped individuals from both government and charities, and sometimes financial support. The process of accurate registration also legitimately raises the profile of uveitis in blindness statistics. At present, too often the sequelae of uveitis, rather than the disease itself, are entered as the causes of visual loss.

UVEITIS IN CHILDREN

Children with uveitis are not merely a subset of a pediatric ophthalmology or uveitis practice (though they may form a significant part of either); they are in several ways qualitatively different and more challenging than adult patients. In a child presenting with uveitis the differential diagnosis is usually different, assessment is more challenging, certain treatment methods may be inadvisable, and some complications of both the uveitis and its treatment more common (Holland and Stiehm 2003).

The general ophthalmologist should have a predetermined strategy and preferably firm routes of referral for a child newly presenting with uveitis. Such patients are outside the skill range of most ophthalmologists and their care should undoubtedly be concentrated in the hands of experts, to a much greater extent than adults with uveitis. The expertise available to the generalist will of course differ with location but should be sought vigorously and quickly. Those specializing in uveitis, especially in large centers such as ours, are privileged not only to have readily accessible pediatric ophthalmology expertise, but also pediatric rheumatologists with high skills in the management of systemic inflammatory disease and uveitis in children, including the use of immunosuppressives and biologics. Close cooperation between these personnel and other ophthalmologists within the region that they serve is crucial to the long-term wellbeing of the children with whom they work. Each center will form its own model of care; our own, for example (dealing to date with over 500 children), includes a fortnightly pediatric uveitis clinic with consultants with expertise in both uveitis and pediatric ophthalmology working together. They are joined 4–6 weekly (and intermittently as required) by a pediatric rheumatologist with whom care is shared for those patients requiring oral immunosuppression, and for those with multisystem disease. New referrals are fast-tracked, there is rapid access to investigation and, where necessary, admission for urgent treatment. Access to similar levels of care undoubtedly enhances outcomes.

On encountering the new child with uveitis, it is essential to engender a firm and practical rapport with parents or carers who are naturally very concerned and who transmit this in varying degrees to their child. Their cooperation in facilitating proper examination is essential and must be sought immediately. Where this is readily forthcoming, the parent being clearly in control, their child may become a paragon of virtue, enthusiastically permitting contact tonometry and funduscopy; where lacking, and notably where the child has been allowed to perceive the parent to be the protector against the doctor, a difficult time is in store. In such situations the parent plays little or no part in facilitating examination, their contribution limited to vague expressions of sympathy and half-hearted cajoling with occasional bribes, overused and therefore not fully believed. In such circumstances a conversation with parents in the absence of the child can give the opportunity for the doctor to make clear that their active participation and leadership are important and that passivity is unhelpful. Hopefully this can be communicated in a way that is received without offence.

Sometimes slit-lamp examination is actually impossible. Some temporary measures including portable slit-lamp apparatus and non-contact tonometry may allow basic decision-making in the early stages, but neither parent nor child (especially the former) must be permitted to perceive this as an examination of acceptable standard. Repeated visits with a firm but friendly insistence on proper examination are almost always productive. The once frequently used admission of defeat was the examination under general anesthesia (itself not providing ideal conditions) but fortunately this is now needed much less often.

Every child with uveitis should undergo an assessment of general health and a physical examination. It is extremely useful for ophthalmologists dealing with such children to develop a professional rapport with a local pediatrician who understands the implications of a diagnosis of uveitis, who can examine and investigate appropriately and can contribute to future management if necessary. If a pediatric rheumatology service is available it forms the natural route of referral, first because so many children with arthritis require ophthalmological attention and vice versa, and second because of their familiarity with immunosuppression.

Many features of childhood uveitis require special thought. The risk of amblyopia may be high and should be managed aggressively. The incidence of steroid-induced glaucoma is higher in children. Band keratopathy is common. Compliance with topical medication is more difficult than for an adult patient and absolutely reliant on well-informed and supportive carers. Support by teachers and school staff in this respect varies from the superb to the totally ineffective. The removal of a cataract may be urgently needed where amblyopia is developing but must be delayed until inflammation has been adequately controlled. Intraocular lenses cannot be used as frequently as in adult uveitis and therefore a pediatric contact lens service is particularly important. Issues of consent are sometimes complex and modern approaches demand full participation from at least the older child. Considerable time and effort may be necessary and a multidisciplinary approach is preferable.

In our experience the proportion of children with uveitis being treated with oral immunosuppression is significantly higher than for our adult patients. There are several reasons for this: first many have concurrent arthritis requiring treatment; second many require such a high frequency of cataractogenic topical steroid that it is not consistently achievable by even the most diligent parent; and third and, usefully, oral immunosuppression is generally better tolerated in childhood than in adulthood. This sweeping assertion does not mean that children are free from side effects; indeed manipulating methotrexate (the usual first-choice immunosuppressive) dosage and route of administration to ensure compliance can be difficult. Nevertheless in the knowledge that most children will manage either oral or subcutaneous treatment without significant nausea or stomatitis, an early decision to commence such immunosuppression is increasingly common in children with chronic uveitis of more than mild severity.

In children, to the substantial list of acute and chronic side effects of oral steroid treatment must be added growth retardation. The avoidance of long-term systemic steroid in significant dosage is therefore of great importance and this also precipitates an early transformation to immunosuppression. Nevertheless, temporary courses of moderate- to high-dose steroids can be extremely useful at times of active disease and are generally underused. At times of severe flare-ups and as a prelude to intraocular surgery on eyes with a high risk of flare-ups, intravenous methylprednisolone should be regarded as entirely appropriate.

Some children with particularly severe uveitis cannot be adequately controlled with methotrexate with or without oral steroid. Up until 5 years ago our natural approach would be to add ciclosporin or, more recently, mycophenolate. However, the increasing availability of anti-tumor necrosis factor α (TNF-α) monoclonal antibody therapy for children with juvenile idiopathic arthritis (our largest group) has encouraged the increasing use of such treatments as second-line immunosuppression. This is described in greater detail in Chapter 8.

It is fitting to end this passage with a reference to one of the most challenging of patient groups – teenagers. In many fields of medicine the process of 'transitional care,' describing the process not only of maturation but also of transfer to a different set of doctors, is well established. There is no doubt that the typical adolescent is uncomfortable in the company of both happily screaming infants and children, and middle-aged and elderly people in the adult clinic. Those branches of medicine busy enough to establish adolescent clinics can solve part of this problem, but rarely in ophthalmology can such a format be realistic. Sometimes the uveitis specialist may have followed the young person from infancy and will continue to do so in adulthood, but on occasion these interstitial years are no less difficult for that. Every parent will recognize the paradigm: the child demands greater independence and responsibility but abuses it regularly: instilling drops only in preparation for the next clinic visit; missing that visit but telling parents that they attended. The consultation may be monosyllabic (if the earphones can be removed) and regularly diverted by the receipt of the latest text message. Attempts to maintain rapport may be challenging and management discussions difficult to portray accurately to a patient who, if fortunate enough to have retained good vision so far, assumes immortality and immunity from deterioration, or in contrast if suffering from not only the poor vision of severe chronic uveitis, but also the disfigurement of permanent joint disease, will often be introverted, depressed, and of the view that further attempts at treatment are at best irritating and at worst pointless. There is no greater challenge in an outpatient clinic but it cannot be sidestepped. The greatest reward at the end of this tunnel is a well- balanced adult who has accepted realistically and optimized his or her current visual and physical status and contributes actively to decision-making and management. Good luck.

REFERENCES

Durrani OM, Tehrani MM, Marr JE, et al. Degree, duration, and causes of visual loss in uveitis. *Br J Ophthalmol* 2004;**88**:1159–62.

Holland GN, Stiehm ER. Special considerations in the evaluation and management of uveitis in children. *Am J Ophthalmol* 2003;**135**:867–8.

Jones NP, Pickford M. Nurse-led formal health review for immunosuppressed patients with uveitis. *Eye* 2009;**23**:1400–3.

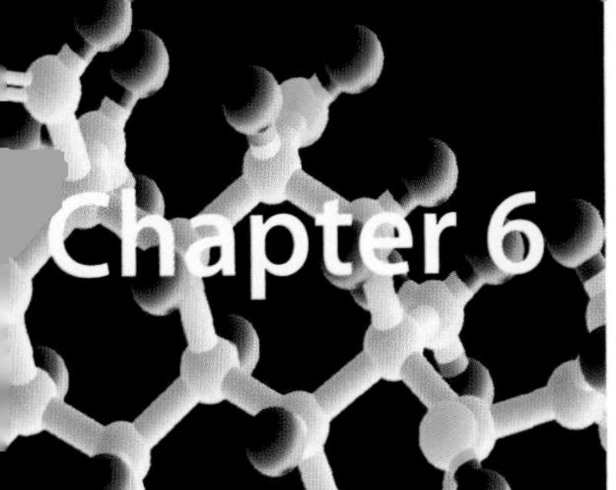

Anti-inflammatory and immunosuppressive treatment

The underlying cause of inflammation is unknown in a substantial majority of patients with uveitis. Management in this group has concentrated on modulation of the immune response. The introduction some 40 years ago of the synthetic corticosteroids for the first time allowed suppression of the immune response, albeit in a crude and generalized way. As knowledge of the human immune system has expanded, progress has been made towards understanding the immunological basis of various forms of idiopathic uveitis. This has facilitated the development of immune modulators of increasing specificity: from steroids with their crude and global effect, to cytotoxics with their more limited cellular targets; through calcineurin inhibitors with their relatively narrow action on T-cell function; and now to a rapidly increasing range of immunomodulators, especially monoclonal antibodies, their target a single protein.

Running parallel with the increasing specificity of immunosuppressive and immunomodulatory treatment have been the developing attempts to spare systemic toxicity by applying treatment directly to the end-organ – the eye. Such an approach has much to recommend it and the new methods of application are discussed here. However, uveitis, as for any immune-mediated inflammation, is a systemic process and if the holy grail of 'cure' is to be pursued, it cannot be achieved by targeting the end-organ alone.

What will this 'holy grail' be? For each specific immune-mediated disease process, it will be a treatment of absolute specificity (both functional and where necessary, anatomical), with no deleterious side effects, which will not merely suppress, but 'switch off' the stimulus to inflammation so that treatment can be discontinued and the disease cured. As immunological knowledge increases, not only do treatment targets become apparent, but often the complexity of the immunological process is gradually unraveled. This chapter now describes current usage for anti-inflammatory, immunosuppressant and immunomodulatory drugs in the management of uveitis and its complications, and discusses some recent developments in immune therapy.

CORTICOSTEROIDS

In the 1930s Edward Kendall and co-workers at the Mayo Clinic were undertaking groundbreaking, and subsequently Nobel prize-winning, work isolating substances from the adrenal glands. Identifying each compound consecutively as 'compound A,' etc. it was compound E (later named cortisone) that attracted attention because of its remarkable action against inflammation in a patient with rheumatoid arthritis. The subsequent explosion of usage of natural, and then synthetic, anti-inflammatory corticosteroids is well known. Currently used anti-inflammatory corticosteroids are synthetic analogues that have retained glucocorticoid effects but, with the exception of hydrocortisone, have been largely deprived of their mineralocorticoid potency. The steroid molecule binds to glucocorticoid α- and β-surface receptors which are present on almost all cells, the complex then migrating intranuclearly and amending gene transcription in several ways. This adjustment to protein synthesis alters cell function, but does not lead to cell lysis in humans. The multiple anti-inflammatory effects are outlined in **Table 6.1**.

The cellular-level effects shown in **Table 6.1** can be interpolated specifically to effects on intraocular inflammation. The inhibition of cyclooxygenase 2 (COX-2) will decrease the quantity of released prostaglandins and thromboxanes, thus reducing the tissue effects of these chemicals and reducing local pain including ocular ache and, to some extent, photophobia. The generation of the full inflammatory response is dependent on the ability to recruit and activate leukocytes to communicate using cytokine transmission. The effect of steroids is to suppress the ability of cells to produce and express such cytokines, thus making the inflammatory response more sluggish. Lymphocyte mobility also being reduced, this adds to the suppressive effect. The degree of intraocular cellular activity will be suppressed.

Intercellular adhesion molecules (ICAMs), integrins and selectins are crucial surface receptors expressed by vascular endothelium. They attract and then adhere activated leukocytes to vascular walls at the site of tissue inflammation, facilitating migration. Steroids inhibit ICAM action so that leukocytes are less likely to migrate into the tissues to cause their destructive effects. This, together with the steroid-induced release of neutrophils from bone marrow, explains the neutrophilia that is a constant accompaniment to oral steroid treatment. The number of cells in aqueous and vitreous is reduced.

The mode of action of glucocorticoids on passive vascular permeability is less well understood but they are believed generally to enhance vascular endothelial adhesion, probably by inhibiting the ability of zonulae occludentes to open and close. In this way not only

Table 6.1 Anti-inflammatory and immunosuppressive effects of glucocorticoids

Action	Effect
1. Inhibition of COX-2 gene transcription	Reduced prostaglandin production, analgesia
2. Inhibition of cytokine production	Reduced leukocyte recruitment, reduced pyogenesis
3. Inhibition of ICAM production	Reduced leukocyte extracellular migration
4. Increased neutrophil production (other circulating polymorphs decreased)	Neutrophilia (together with 3)
5. Decrease vascular permeability (decreased protein extravasation)	Deceased tissue swelling, less fibrinogen leakage
6. Decreased lymphocyte mobility/migration	Decreased recruitment and inhibited clonal expansion
7. Suppression of types I and IV hypersensitivity	Reduced inflammatory response

COX, cyclo-oxygenase; ICAM, intercellular adhesion molecule.

is leukocyte migration also inhibited, but passive extravasation of proteins is reduced. In the eye, aqueous flare will be reduced and the longest protein, fibrinogen, much less likely to extravasate. If applied before fibrinogen has reached the anterior chamber, adhesions can be prevented.

Steroid potency and treatment selection

A considerable array of corticosteroids of variable potency is available to the physician in various guises. When used systemically, the relative anti-inflammatory effect of the most used drugs is well established (*British National Formulary* 2010) and these are listed in **Table 6.2**. For oral administration in ophthalmology, prednisolone and prednisone are used almost exclusively; they have equivalent effect. Hydrocortisone is unsuitable for sustained systemic usage because of its mineralocorticoid effect; dexamethasone and betamethasone, although very potent glucocorticoids without significant mineralocorticoid activity, are usually reserved for shorter-term use, and rarely in ophthalmology. Deflazacort, it was hoped, would reduce steroid-induced bone loss because of its effect on osteoblast-driven bone turnover. In practice this has not led to enthusiastic uptake and the drug is little used. Methylprednisolone is suitable for high-dose intravenous infusion and has rapid effect, being therefore reserved for acute sight-threatening inflammation. Corticosteroid efficacy in non-infective intraocular inflammation will depend on a combination of factors, culminating in the intraocular drug concentration, its anti-inflammatory potency and quite possibly a dosage ceiling, above which no further beneficial effect is seen. The selection of topical steroids available makes treatment selection of interest and importance, and the penetration and potency of these drugs are discussed below.

Ocular and periocular steroid treatment

Topical steroids

A range of steroids for ocular installation is available worldwide. Each practitioner will form an experience-based assessment of the efficacy and safety of each, based largely on memorable events rather than objective assessment, and such events are likely to be failures and side effects rather than successes. In fact the paucity of reliable data on efficacy, considering the vast numbers of such prescriptions issued, is startling (Jones 2004). The effectiveness of topically instilled steroids for intraocular inflammation depends on several parameters, including the 'potency' of the steroid (usually calculated or implied from systemic usage), drug concentration in the drop, other drop components including preservatives and buffers, frequency of use, ocular contact time (prolonged for gel or ointment preparations) and ease of intraocular penetration (measured from aqueous sampling).

Assuming a degree of potency, all other parameters pale besides the need for the steroid to penetrate into the anterior chamber, and methods to achieve this have led to modifications of steroid structure. The main barrier is the corneal epithelium, its lipid components reducing the ingress of hydrophilic drugs (such as prednisolone sodium phosphate). In contrast, lipophilic preparations readily gain access; changing the phosphate component to acetate renders the drug lipophilic. Using an identical concentration and vehicle, dexamethasone sodium phosphate, prednisolone sodium phosphate and fluorometholone all produced similar anterior chamber (AC) concentrations, but using prednisolone acetate 1% produced an AC concentration 20 times greater (McGhee 1992). There must also be a ceiling above which adding further steroid has no additional anti-inflammatory effect. That threshold currently remains unknown, but clinical observation suggests that, even for potent steroids with high intraocular penetration such as prednisolone acetate 1%, increasing the frequency of administration in very severe uveitis from hourly to half-hourly appears to have an additive effect.

A steroid-induced rise in intraocular pressure (IOP) is a problem encountered in every uveitis practice. It is most commonly induced by topical steroid and there is a clear direct relationship between potency and risk. For this reason, attempts have been made for decades to create potent topical steroids with a reduced risk of ocular hypertension and glaucoma. Such drugs include fluorometholone and rimexolone. Well-designed randomized studies have shown comparable efficacy between rimexolone and prednisolone acetate, for example (Biswas et al. 2004), but the study cohorts tend to comprise those with less severe uveitis. Those with large clinical practices see, time and again, instances of simply sacrificing potency for a lowering of IOP, often exchanged between these two very drops. Most practitioners believe that the reduced tendency to cause raised IOP (which is well accepted for rimexolone, for example) is merely a result of decreased intraocular penetration and, therefore, efficacy. Some in this group therefore find their niche in the management of ocular surface disease.

It is common to encounter patients with chronic uveitis requiring long-term topical steroid who are referred to a specialist clinic for the first time. They are often referred because of advancing glaucomatous damage in the context of under-controlled inflammation. Invariably there is a history of generally inadequate control of the uveitis because the steroid-induced rise in IOP led to an exchange for a drop of lesser potency. Sometimes a roller-coaster course was induced by swapping glaucoma alternately for uveitis, but never controlling both together adequately. Over time, in such cases, to steroid-induced IOP rise can without doubt be added the irreversible effects of trabecular damage and peripheral anterior synechiae, which of course lead in any case to intractable glaucoma. The message is very clear and oft repeated, politely, in the letter of reply to the referral, and in didactic sessions to colleagues; you **must** control the uveitis and if doing so leads to steroid-induced glaucoma then you must also treat this vigorously, even if it leads to drainage tube surgery; you cannot expect success by settling for an unsatisfactory no-man's land whereby neither uveitis nor glaucoma is adequately managed. Here endeth the lesson.

The creation of lyophilized topical steroid leads to another problem – how to dispense a reliable aqueous-based product. Prednisolone

Table 6.2 Relative anti-inflammatory activity of some systemic corticosteroids

Drug	Relative potency (hydrocortisone = 1)
Hydrocortisone	1
Deflazacort	3
Prednisolone	4
Prednisone	4
Triamcinolone	5
Methylprednisolone	5
Betamethasone	25
Dexamethasone	25

Adapted (in part) from British National Formulary 2010

acetate 1% is produced in suspension, which settles over time and requires shaking. Reliable dosing is a challenge. More recently another lipophilic steroid, difluprednate, has been produced as an emulsion that, being stable in storage, more reproducible in dosing and quite possibly with enhanced intraocular penetration, has been found superior to prednisolone acetate 1% suspension, so that less frequent dosing is necessary (Foster et al. 2010). This is promising, and the effects on patients with very severe anterior uveitis will be observed with interest; any regimen that reduces drop frequency will improve compliance and efficacy.

Subconjunctival steroid injection

It is likely that most subconjunctivally injected steroid (usually betamethasone or dexamethasone) enters the eye not by local diffusion through the sclera, but by leakage through the injection puncture into the tear film, thence by diffusion through the cornea. What, then, is to be gained by submitting the patient to this uncomfortable procedure when already using, or beginning to use, topical steroid of nominally greater potency? This question has largely arisen since the introduction of prednisolone acetate drops, during which time the usage of subconjunctival injections has subsided markedly. Up to a point this is justified, but it has led to a situation where doctors consider the possibility only belatedly. This in turn means that the early subconjunctival injection of mydriatic/cycloplegic such as Mydricaine is also less commonly used, and this is unfortunate. Where frequent instillation cannot be relied upon, or in those cases where a subconjunctival mydriatic injection is to be used in any case, it seems sensible to administer subconjunctival steroid. In situations of persistent severe uveitis despite 2–3 days of intensive strong topical steroids, subconjunctival steroid injection (if necessary daily for 2–3 days) does appear to add effect. This is supported by evidence on intraocular concentrations after injection (Weijtens et al. 1999). It may be that gradual leaching from the subconjunctival bolus permits sustained corneal contact time, permitting greater intraocular penetration. In summary, strong topical steroids are as yet not a complete substitute for subconjunctival injection.

Deep peribulbar steroid injection

Deeper injections, either into the orbit floor or beneath Tenon's capsule, clearly do not suffer the same fate as subconjunctival injections because the injection track will self-seal. It is therefore possible to introduce a reservoir of steroid that will dissipate over a variable period. The dynamics of absorption into the eye from such sites is poorly understood, but it is known that the sclera is permeable to corticosteroid molecules and that substantial penetration can occur from a periocular depot. There is therefore a theoretical advantage to the administration of steroid under Tenon's capsule, rather than merely into the lower orbit. However, despite continuing arguments over the relative merits of each technique, no persuasive clinical evidence has been produced to support the superiority of sub-Tenon's injections (Ferrante et al. 2004). The injection of steroid into the orbit floor is a straightforward procedure especially when administered through the lower lid. In contrast sub-Tenon's injections require deeper surface anesthesia, more skill and more substantial patient cooperation. This procedure has been associated with a higher risk of inadvertent globe penetration and ptosis, which may require surgical correction. In the absence of clear evidence of superiority of effect, it is difficult to justify sub-Tenon's injections, especially since the introduction of intravitreal steroid injections (see below).

Methylprednisolone 40–80 mg in a depot formulation or triamcinolone 40 mg in aqueous suspension is used. There is no clear evidence to support the superiority of either, nor is there strong evidence of the claimed greater tendency of triamcinolone to raise IOP. Evidence of relative efficacy from other specialties including rheumatology is equally inconclusive.

Periocular steroid injection is an outpatient procedure in adults. Injecting the orbital floor with a steroid depot is usually followed by immediate aching, which may last for 2 hours or more and may require analgesia. Some temporary fullness of the lower lid is common. It is usually advisable to observe the patient for some time after the procedure, and to ensure that a companion is available to supervise travel. Review is normal in 4–6 weeks to judge effect.

The rationale behind local injection of steroid is the delivery of the drug to a specific target while minimizing systemic effect. However, significant systemic absorption occurs from deep periocular injections (Zakar-ur-Rab et al. 2009) and this is also well reported after local injections elsewhere. Such absorption has caused adrenal suppression and should not be under-estimated; in the uveitis clinic, anecdotes of visual improvement after intra-articular steroid injection are by no means rare, and intragluteal bolus injections can treat macular edema (Tehrani et al. 2000). Local injections of steroid are not quite so localized as has been supposed. The effectiveness of orbital injections is also unimpressive, reducing macular edema in as little as one quarter of patients (Roesel et al. 2009a).

In summary, the orbital injection of steroid is a technique that benefits from simplicity and ready availability in an outpatient setting, and has a beneficial effect in at least some patients. However, the days of repeated injections to achieve or sustain an effect on macular edema are largely gone as intraocular steroid injection and other treatments have become available.

Intraocular steroid treatment

Intravitreal steroid injection

The literature on efficacy and safety for intravitreal injection of triamcinolone acetonide (IVTA) is now fairly extensive. It is known that direct intraocular injection is more effective, and more long lasting, than orbital injection in the treatment of inflammatory macular edema (Roesel et al. 2009b). It is also known that, as with any intraocular procedure, there is a risk of both endophthalmitis and sterile pseudo-endophthalmitis. There are small risks of retinal detachment and cataract. There is a higher incidence of steroid-induced IOP rise compared with orbital injections, and this may be sustained and occasionally require drainage surgery. Uveitis carries the highest risk for IOP rise compared with other conditions requiring IVTA (Galor et al. 2007). The technique can be used in children with a similar efficacy and safety profile (Sallam et al. 2008). Indications in uveitis usually include unilateral or asymmetrical macular edema, unilateral top-up therapy for patients on long-term immunosuppression, treatment of acute unilateral flare-ups of inflammation especially in Behçet's disease, repeatedly where immunosuppression is intolerable, and as an adjunct to cataract, glaucoma or vitrectomy surgery. We use a patient information pamphlet before treatment (see patient information pamphlets on the attached disk).

The technique requires a clean room and a clean ocular surface. The procedure is normally performed under topical anesthesia, with or without subconjunctival anesthetic. Some surgeons apply pre-injection ocular pressure to reduce IOP. Povidone-iodine 5% is applied to the conjunctival sac preferably for 5–10 minutes. Most surgeons apply facial sterilizing solution and apply drapes.

Triamcinolone is in large-particle suspension that rapidly settles. Accurate dosing therefore requires rapid injection after withdrawal into a syringe. The injection is given at 3.5–4.0 mm behind the limbus, avoiding the horizontal meridian. A 27-gauge cannula is normally used (drug particles may block a 30-G cannula). The entry site is indented with a swab on withdrawal of the cannula to prevent vitreous incarceration. Ocular hemoperfusion is checked by ensuring that the patient can count fingers, by digitally checking IOP or by checking disk perfusion by ophthalmoscopy. If in doubt, AC paracentesis is required but this is unusual. Subconjunctival or topical antibiotic is administered. Review within 1 month is advisable to check IOP. The duration of action of this treatment is variable but normally 3–6 months.

The required dosage of triamcinolone to treat effectively and safely has provoked much discussion. At one end of the spectrum, we have found that 2 mg in 0.05 ml is adequate to manage macular edema in the great majority of patients and to minimize the risk of secondary glaucoma (Das-Baumik and Jones 2006). At the other end, a 25 mg 'sludge' of triamcinolone has been injected, with most practitioners settling for a middle-ground of 4 mg in 0.1 ml. Using this dosage, the rate of IOP rise is about 40%, but is effective enough to permit reduction in steroids or oral immunosuppression in about 50% (Kok et al. 2005).

The most severe complication of intraocular triamcinolone injection is postoperative inflammation. Infective endophthalmitis, in contrast to that following cataract surgery, often has a slightly delayed onset (sometimes days 3–5) and may present with less severe symptoms. In contrast sterile endophthalmitis (which may be a greater risk in patients with uveitis [Taban et al. 2007]) often presents very rapidly on days 1–2 with severe visual loss and often (though not always) ocular pain. Either may cause severe panuveitis. When the etiology is uncertain it is mandatory to treat as infective with intravitreal antibiotic injection. Sterile endophthalmitis usually responds well to intensive topical and oral steroid therapy usually with a return to pre-injection acuity after 4–8 weeks (Yoon et al. 2009). A pseudohypopyon comprising triamcinolone particles is occasionally seen, and commonly in those with aphakia (**Fig. 6.1**). It does not comprise evidence of either infective or sterile endophthalmitis. It may be associated with an increased rate of IOP rise but, in the absence of other evidence of intraocular inflammation, requires no special treatment and will dissipate in time.

The benzyl alcohol content of triamcinolone for injection has been considered the cause of sterile endophthalmitis. Those surgeons who have eliminated it, either by filtering or decanting off, or by usage of the preservative-free formulation that is now available, have noted a reduction in this complication, and this approach is now considered most appropriate (Maia et al. 2007).

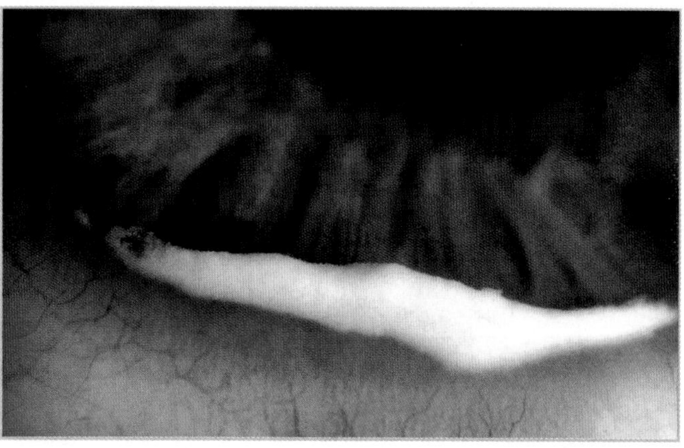

Figure 6.1 A triamcinolone pseudohypopyon in an aphakic patient. The white crystalline appearance serves to differentiate from a true inflammatory hypopyon.

Intravitreal steroid implantation

The relatively short duration of action of intravitreal steroid injection is a considerable disadvantage. In the search for longer-acting anti-inflammatory treatments that spare systemic toxicity, intraocular steroid implants have been developed and are basically of two types:

1. The sustained-release fluocinolone acetonide 0.59 mg (Retisert) implant comprises a drug pellet encased in a silicone–PVA coating and held within a polyvinyl acetate (PVA) well attached to a plate that is inserted and sutured via a pars plana incision (**Fig. 6.2a**). Drug release is regulated by its PVA coating. It has demonstrable efficacy which is possibly superior to oral immunosuppression and a duration of action of possibly more than 2 years (Jaffe et al. 2005) but causes glaucoma in about 20% and cataract in about 90% (Pavesio et al. 2010). Vitreous band formation has also been reported.
2. The injectable sustained-release dexamethasone 0.7 mg (Ozurdex) implant is a cylindrical bioerodible drug pellet that is inserted via the pars plana using an injection device (**Fig. 6.2b**). It carries a better side-effect profile than implantable fluocinolone but a fairly short duration of action for uveitis (Myung et al. 2010) in comparison to vein occlusion-related macular edema, for which it is mainly intended. Any superiority in efficacy, duration or safety profile over intravitreal triamcinolone injection has yet to be demonstrated.

Fluocinolone acetonide is also undergoing trials as an injectable polyimide-coated pellet 180 μg (Medidur), which is inserted in a similar fashion to Ozurdex. It is hoped that the method will combine the duration of action of the larger fluocinolone pellet with fewer side effects; results are awaited. A novel form of implantation has also arrived in the metallic screw, coated with surface polymers containing the active drug (I-vation), in this case triamcinolone acetonide. The device is screwed through the pars plana where it protrudes intravitreally (**Fig. 6.2c**), the external head plate stabilizing its position. Initial trials are for diabetic maculopathy but there are clear potential benefits for patients with uveitis depending upon safety profile and duration of action; more data are awaited.

Future intraocular steroid delivery systems

The above developments each represent an important step towards safely administered end-organ treatment. None as yet achieves this reliably but, in some circumstances, each may be optimal for individual patients especially where oral immunosuppression is problematic. Further developments are interesting especially in the field of in situ polymerization. The biochemistry involves the formulation of injectable (fluid) monomers, which then polymerize and coalesce, this stage being provoked by light, pH or temperature. Various polymerized gels have been devised as methods of in situ sustained drug delivery (Nirmal et al. 2010) but none is yet close to intraocular in vivo experimentation. However, the field shows great promise in pursuing easily injectable but sustained-effect drug delivery.

Iontophoresis is the technique of moving charged chemicals down an electrical gradient and is already used in some branches of dermatology. A method of using iontophoresis for intraocular drug delivery (EyeGate) is undergoing phase II trials. It requires a drug well applied to the anesthetized anterior segment, through which a current is applied for a defined period, transmitting drug into the AC. Achieving this for large-molecule drugs (such as steroids) is as yet futuristic. Further research is awaited with interest but the concept of 'non-invasive' end-organ treatment is of course very attractive.

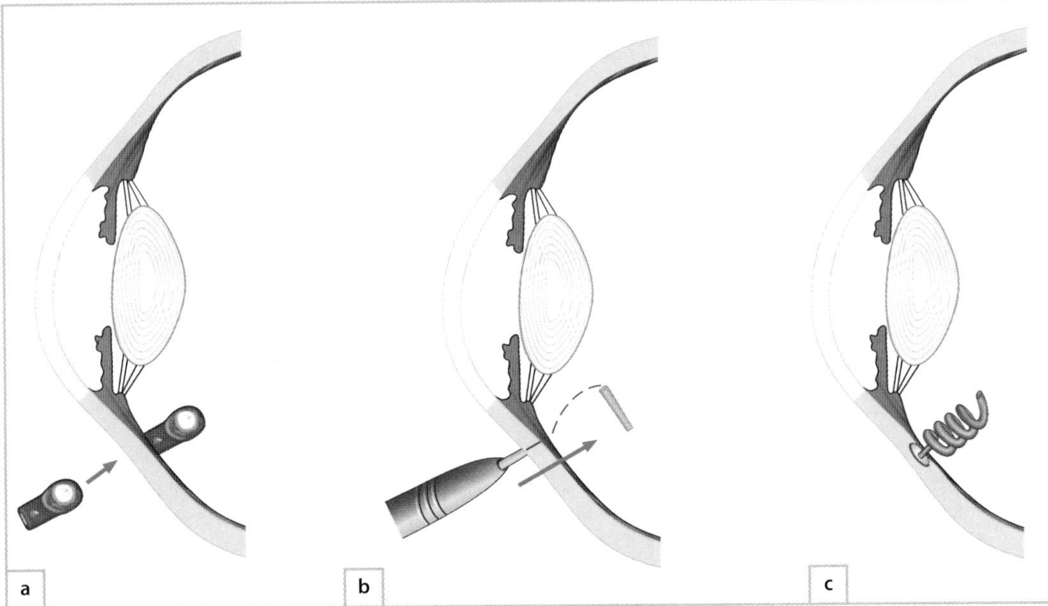

Figure 6.2 Devices for intraocular steroid implantation: (a) Retisert; (b) Ozurdex; (c) I-vation.

Oral steroid treatment

The decision to use a systemic steroid for the management of uveitis is an important threshold crossed and one that should be made only after careful reflection. The patient must be involved in this decision and must therefore be made aware of the risks versus benefits of treatment. Systemic steroid treatment for unilateral uveitis requires particularly careful justification, and is normally prescribed only after the failure of local treatment. In this clinic we use a detailed patient information pamphlet on prednisolone (see patient information pamphlets on the attached disk).

From the start, objectives must be clearly laid out for both doctor and patient. In some situations, e.g. in the management of recurrent toxoplasma retinochoroiditis or the treatment of bilateral macular edema in intermediate uveitis, a short course of systemic steroid is planned. However, some patients with chronic uveitis are likely to need continued treatment, and here the long-term implications must be considered.

It is not uncommon to encounter patients newly referred from elsewhere who are described as having failed to improve on oral corticosteroid treatment. The explanations for this are fairly consistent: the commencing dose of steroid was too low (often only 20–30 mg/day), the course was too short (often only 2–3 weeks), or the curtailment was too abrupt (e.g. reducing from 10 mg to zero), or quite often all of these. Such ineffectual approaches may have been repeated, leading to a smoldering uveitis that has lost all its characteristic diagnostic features. During this time permanent damage may have accumulated and the patient has been done a disservice.

The appropriate starting dose of steroid is the first decision to be made. Too low a dose will allow continuing inflammation while exposing the patient to side effects, and a subsequent dose increase will be less effective than starting at an adequate dose in the first place. It is not possible to stipulate a single starting dose for the management of all cases of uveitis. The patient with intermediate uveitis and bilateral macular edema does not require as high a dose as the patient with severe panuveitis. In general an adult starting dose of prednisolone 40–50 mg/day (around 0.5–0.8 mg/kg per day) will be adequate for the former, whereas 60–80 mg (approaching 1 mg/kg per day) or more is imperative for the latter. In those with particularly severe acute uveitis, intravenous methylprednisolone should be considered and this is described below.

Patients starting on high doses of steroids should be warned of the potential for acute side effects. Mood changes are frequent and, uncommonly, problematic; mild euphoria, hyperactivity and insomnia are possible, as is low mood, depression and withdrawal. Fortunately acute steroid-induced psychosis is rare. Dyspepsia is common enough to justify routine prophylaxis for doses of 40 mg/day. Increased appetite is almost universal and weight gain will follow most commonly in those who are already endomorphic or obese. Fluid retention may contribute to weight gain especially during the premenstrual week in women.

It is important to maintain the starting dose until substantial suppression of the inflammation has occurred. This will take at least 7–10 days and usually 14. In some patients, the uveitis seems genuinely to be resistant to steroid treatment, and such patients must be identified early because reinvestigation of the cause of uveitis is necessary. In those on very high doses of steroid, it is not necessary or appropriate to wait for complete quiescence before starting to reduce the dose.

Having sustained the starting dose for enough time, a tailing-off process can begin. Initially this can be quite rapid and one should think of the dose reduction curve as more exponential than linear: the lower the current dose, the slower the necessary reduction. During this dose reduction, the patient is carefully observed to ensure continued suppression of inflammation. The ability to distinguish active intraocular inflammation from the sequelae of previous inflammation is of paramount importance during this stage because any reactivation must be identified.

At any stage during this dose reduction, reactivation of inflammation may occur, requiring an increase in dose. Such an increase must be substantial in order to regain control (usually meaning at least a doubling of current dose) after which a more gentle taper can recommence (**Fig. 6.3**). Future management depends on the minimum dose at which control can be achieved. A substantial majority of cases of chronic uveitis may be controlled with dosage levels of 10 mg/day or less, but occasionally much higher doses are required; we have witnessed inflammation (sympathetic uveitis) that consistently

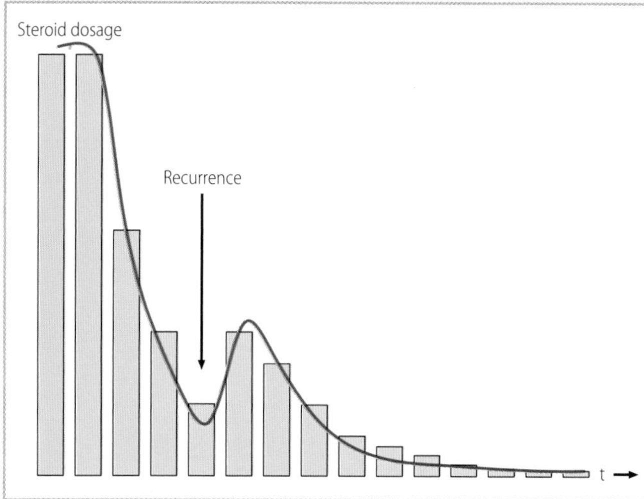

Figure 6.3 Oral steroid treatment should commence at a high enough dose that is sustained for enough time to suppress inflammation. Decrease can then initially be rapid. If uveitis recurs a substantial dose increase is required followed by a slower taper.

reactivated at less than 50 mg/day of prednisolone. In such cases the administration of steroid-sparing immunosuppression is mandatory. At lower doses of steroid the need to add an immunosuppressive is less clear, and such decisions need the input of an informed patient, who will be made aware of the potential complications of long-term steroid treatment (**Table 6.3**). Even for those patients stabilized on low-dose treatment, attempts should be made, perhaps every 6–12 months, to minimize side effects by very small reductions in dosage. The most important steroid-induced side effects are described below.

Dyspepsia

Dyspeptic symptoms are common in patients taking oral steroids, but most are only mildly affected. Generations of medical students have been taught that systemic steroid may cause peptic ulceration. Thorough meta-analysis has disproved this (Conn et al. 1994) but the misconception persists. Steroids alone do not cause peptic ulceration. However, they do cause variable dyspepsia (possibly resulting from mild gastritis) and this is a risk for compliance. It is important to understand that steroid-induced dyspepsia is a central effect following systemic absorption, not a local irritation. Those with a peptic history and those taking another drug with associated risks of peptic ulceration or gastritis (such as a non-steroidal anti-inflammatory drug [NSAID] or azathioprine) are at greater risk of dyspepsia if taking two drugs together. Unfortunately some practitioners attempt to counter the risk by using enteric-coated prednisolone. This does indeed lessen symptoms, but not because the gastric mucosa is spared any irritative effect; rather it is because systemic absorption from such preparations is unreliable and almost always incomplete, lessening the total absorbed dose. This is therefore not a logical approach. Proton pump inhibitors are excellent at preventing and treating steroid-induced dyspepsia and should be prescribed if that symptom is likely. In this clinic, patients receive non-coated prednisolone, from which absorption is more reliable. Those taking 40 mg/day or more of prednisolone, those with a history of peptic ulceration, those also taking any NSAID and those with any predisposition to or ongoing symptoms of dyspepsia are prescribed omeprazole 20 mg daily, rising to 20 mg twice daily if necessary. Persistent dyspepsia is highly unusual with this approach and compliance issues are minimized.

Table 6.3 Potential complications of systemic steroid therapy

Acute	Chronic
Mood and personality changes	Osteoporosis
Psychosis	Cushingoid features, weight gain
Increased appetite, weight gain	Myopathy, tendon ruptures
Fluid retention	Sodium/potassium imbalance, alkalosis
Nausea, dyspepsia, increased appetite	Gastritis, peptic ulcer (possibly)
Aseptic bone necrosis	Bruising, slow wound healing, thrombosis
Glaucoma	Hirsutism, hyperhidrosis
	Growth suppression in children
	Adrenal suppression
	Hypertension
	Diabetes
	Infection
	Cataract

Osteoporosis

Oral corticosteroids always lead to bone loss which is induced in several ways: doses > 10 mg/day inhibit dietary calcium absorption; suppression of androgen production depresses estrone levels and suppresses the calcitonin response, leading to increased bone resorption; osteoclasts are stimulated; and bone formation is reduced by suppression of osteoblast activity. Bone loss is inevitable during steroid therapy and starts within days of starting treatment. The rate of loss is greatest within the first 6 months, during which time typically 4–5% of bone is lost. This is partly a reflection of the starting doses used and partly metabolic. Trabecular bone is particularly affected, so effects are more marked in the spine and proximal femur (particularly the spine). Overall, the prevalence of fractures in patients treated with systemic steroids is up to 20%. There is no absolutely safe maintenance dose for oral steroid, at or below which bone density can be assumed to be unaffected. However, broadly speaking, problems are less likely to occur in doses of 5 mg/day or less.

Osteoporosis itself is asymptomatic but predisposes to low-trauma fractures. Steroid-induced osteoporosis particularly affects the spine rather than the hips and other joints. Spinal crush fractures in particular lead to considerable pain and morbidity and, sometimes, progressive deformity. There is evidence that fractures occur more readily in steroid-induced, than in postmenopausal, osteoporosis. We have found that in a uveitis population taking oral steroids nearly 50% of patients had additional underlying risk factors for bone loss (shown in **Table 6.4**) and that over 40% had either osteopenia or osteoporosis (Jones et al. 2002).

Bone densitometry

Bone density is a surrogate marker for bone quality and strength. The validity of this method is accepted as adequate for most adults, but there is evidence of a higher-than-expected rate of fracture for any given bone density in patients with steroid-induced bone loss. This indicates that bone densitometry alone may not be an adequate marker for these patients. Nevertheless there remains a clear correlation between low bone density and fracture, and no better method of assessment currently exists. Bone density may be assessed by plain radiography, quantitative computed tomography, ultrasonography or absorptiometry using photons or X-rays (Lees et al. 1998). Dual-emission X-ray absorptiometry (DXA) is the most widely used technique.

Table 6.4 Additional risk factors for osteoporosis in patients using oral steroids

Additional risk	Reason for risk
Menopause	Decreased estrogens reduces bone formation
Smoking	Accelerates bone resorption, accelerates menopause
Sarcoidosis	Abnormal Ca^{2+} metabolism, hypercalciuria (uncommon)
Inflammatory arthropathy	Low mobility – bone turnover imbalance
Pregnancy	Multifactorial
Inflammatory bowel disease	Inadequate Ca^{2+}/vitamin D uptake
Amenorrhea/oophorectomy	As for menopause
Type 1 diabetes	Unknown
Anorexia/vegan diet	Inadequate Ca^{2+}/vitamin D uptake; amenorrhea/low estrogen
High alcohol intake	Inadequate Ca^{2+}/vitamin D; reduced bone formation
Ethnic/religious	Inadequate skin exposure – reduced vitamin D
Hyperparathyroidism	Increased bone resorption
Ciclosporin treatment	Increase bone turnover + steroid effect
Hypogonadism	Reduced osteoblasts, increased osteoclasts
Heparin treatment (long-term)	Accelerates bone resorption
Genetic/familial	Multifactorial
PPI treatment	Possibly reduced Ca^{2+} absorption

In order of numerical frequency for patients in Manchester Uveitis Clinic

PPI, proton pump inhibitor.

It is rapid, taking less than 5 min per site, uses little radiation (< 1 μSv for a spine scan) and is relatively inexpensive. There are problems of reproducibility in any method of bone densitometry, both between machines and longitudinally in a single patient. Data should therefore be interpreted within these limitations. In adults the lumbar spine and femoral neck are the primary sites for assessment (**Fig. 6.4**), first because they are sites at particular risk and second because trabecular bone here is a sensitive indicator of mineral loss and gain.

Bone mineral density normally rises until early adulthood where it reaches a peak. The peak is on average higher in men than women and higher in black individuals. From around 35 years there is a slow decline, becoming more steep in postmenopausal women. Densitometry measurements are expressed objectively in g/cm^2, and clinically by comparison to age-matched, sex-matched means (Z score), or in comparison to ideal (peak) bone mass as seen in young sex-matched adults (T score). The Z score is therefore an expression of bone mass in relation to others of the same age, whereas the T score is a comparison with ideal bone mass. Those with a T score of worse than one standard deviation (1 SD) below the mean have significantly low bone mineral density (osteopenia). Those worse than –2.5 SD have osteoporosis. Those with osteoporosis who have suffered a low-impact fracture are classified as having 'established osteoporosis.'

Two examples of bone density assessment are shown in **Fig. 6.5**: the normal bone density curve for a male is shown in Fig. 6.5a,

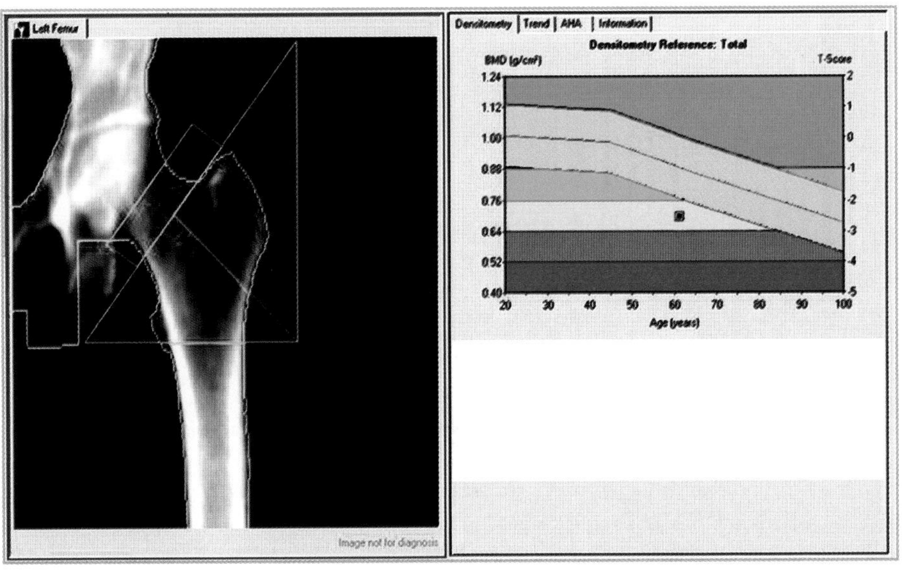

Figure 6.4 A dual-emission X-ray absorptiometry (DXA) scan of the left femur of a 62-year-old woman using oral steroid to treat uveitis. Bone density is below the acceptable range (T score –2.6 = osteoporosis).

decreasing slowly from a young adult peak. A male of age 54 using oral steroid is seen to have a bone density of Z = −0.4, *T* = −1.5. Oral bisphosphonate treatment is planned (see below). In Fig. 6.5b, the female curve commences at a lower peak mass and the age-related decrease is worsened by the menopause. A postmenopausal woman of 67 has commenced oral steroids for severe uveitis but the initial densitometry shows pre-existing osteoporosis with a T score of −2.7. An early transfer to immunosuppression is planned, together with bisphosphonate treatment.

Methods for the assessment of bone density in adults cannot be reliably extrapolated for use in children, whose bone density during growth is less easily assessed and dynamically changing. Normative values for DXA in children are incompletely understood, and fracture resistance in incompletely ossified bone is not merely a factor of bone mass. In children using long-term steroids more detailed assessment may be necessary, including carpal densitometry, and interpretation requires special expertise. The use of prophylaxis or therapeutic interventions in children for bone loss is controversial. However, steroid-induced bone changes during childhood, especially during growth spurts, may lead to permanently low bone density, which is not remediable and may induce severe adult problems.

Prevention and treatment

Those patients who are likely to need more than a short course of oral steroid therapy for uveitis should be informed of the long-term risks of bone loss and fracture. Some general lifestyle measures are useful: regular weight-bearing exercise, especially walking, should be strongly encouraged and is known to maintain bone density in weight-bearing zones. Smoking any amount, and drinking alcohol to excess are deleterious. A balanced diet with adequate calcium and vitamin D should be maintained. Strict vegetarians or vegans are at high risk of progressive bone loss.

The ophthalmologist will make every effort to minimize steroid dosage and, if long-term treatment becomes necessary, the supplementary use of immunosuppression in those at high risk should be an early priority. There is no evidence that alternate-day treatment delays bone density reduction in adults, but it may do so in children. Bone density is capable of slow recovery after treatment is stopped, or if steroid is taken in doses < 7.5 mg/day. Assuming that the patient has a normal dietary intake of calcium, adding calcium supplementation alone is not thought to be helpful. The evidence on vitamin D_3 supplementation with or without calcium remains incomplete but in most groups studied (including postmenopausal women, elderly people of both sexes, post-transplantation patients, those with inflammatory bowel disease) adding supplementation with vitamin D_3 resisted bone loss including steroid-induced effects. Whether this extrapolates to a definite effect on reduction of low-impact fracture rate is less clear but evidence for this is increasing. It is our practice to give daily fortified calcium with vitamin D_3 to all patients using oral steroid at any dose, unless there is biochemical evidence of hypercalcemia or densitometric evidence of higher-than-normal bone mass.

In addition to calcium and vitamin D supplementation, several forms of treatment have been shown to have a beneficial effect on bone density. The optimal prophylaxis and management of osteopenia and osteoporosis are the subject of continued research and may differ significantly between different risk groups, age ranges and sexes. There is now extensive experience of the increasing range of bisphosphonate therapies and in almost all adult risk groups a bisphosphonate is the first recommended therapy for prevention and treatment.

Bisphosphonates

The bisphosphonates are a group of small-molecule drugs comprising two phosphate groups linked by a variable core. A list of available bisphosphonates with their mode of delivery is given in **Table 6.5**. The non-nitrogenous bisphosphonates act by inhibiting osteoclast ATP and inducing apoptosis. The nitrogenous group may have a more complex effect on osteoclasts, inhibiting cell genesis, bone matrix metabolism and cell death.

During the early years of bisphosphonate usage the potential for adverse effects including osteomalacia were a concern. Low-dose etidronate was for some years the preferred drug, being administered for only 2 weeks in quarterly cycles, with calcium supplementation. The drug was only approved initially for use in postmenopausal women

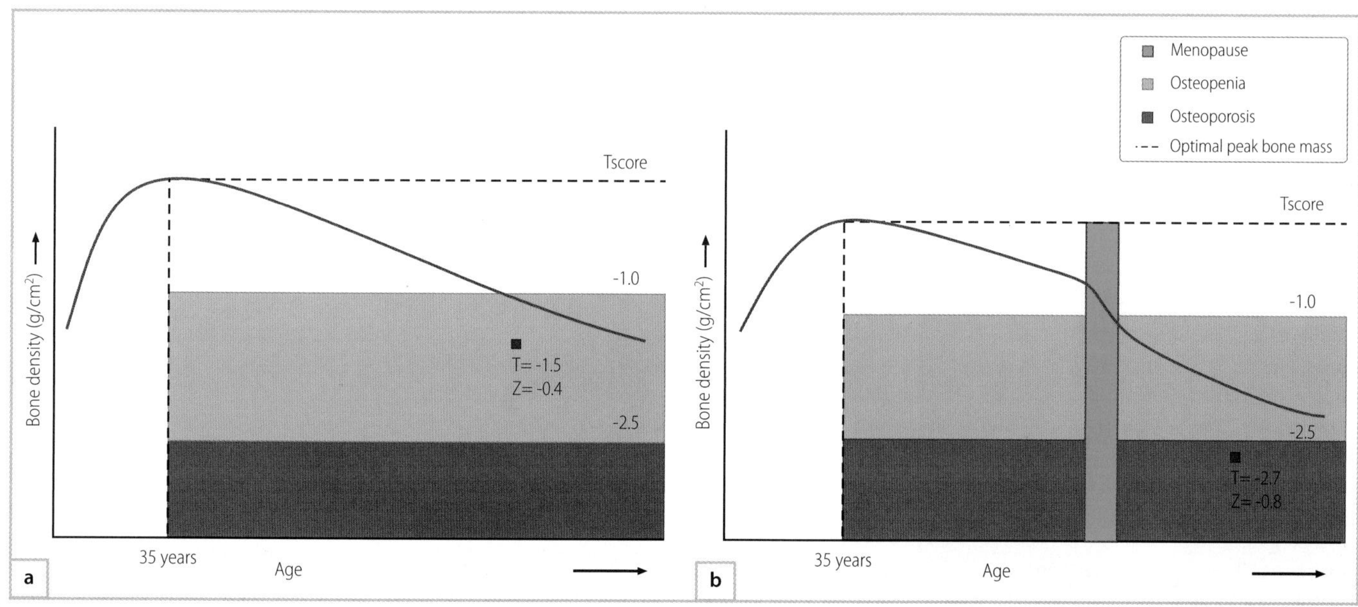

Figure 6.5 Two examples of bone densitometry assessment compared to sex-matched bone density curves. (a) A man aged 54, (b) a woman aged 67. The results are discussed in the text.

Table 6.5. Bisphosphonate types and mode of delivery

Non-nitrogenous	
Etidronate	Oral, cyclical
Tiludronate	Oral, daily
Nitrogenous	
Ibandronate	Oral, daily
Alendronate	Oral, weekly or daily
Risedronate	Oral, monthly or weekly
Pamidronate	Intravenous infusion up to monthly
Zolendronate	Intravenous infusion, yearly

but, as fears subsided, treatment was extended to other groups and the superiority of alendronate was rapidly established leading to its pre-eminent position as the most commonly used prophylaxis and treatment of bone loss. It is of proven efficacy in steroid-induced bone loss (Sambrook et al. 2003). All nitrogenous bisphosphonates have the potential to cause substantial esophagitis (less commonly esophageal ulceration and rarely, as a complication, esophageal cancer) and the oral types must be taken with particular care to avoid this. However, only a small number are unable to tolerate oral administration. Our current practice is to prescribe alendronate 70 mg weekly to all adults on oral steroid at any dose whose T score falls below −1.5. We do not prescribe, as some do, to any patient without assessment of bone density. Other side effects of bisphosphonates include myalgia and arthralgia, osteonecrosis of the jaw (a rare but exaggerated problem almost exclusive to elderly people with poor dentition receiving intravenous pamidronate) and, ironically, uveitis (anecdotal but again most common in those using pamidronate, less so risedronate).

Patients with more difficult problems of bone loss are better managed by an expert in bone metabolism, if available. Our practice is to refer all young men with osteoporosis for further investigation, and all women with established osteoporosis, those in need of but unable to tolerate oral bisphosphonate treatment and children on long-term steroid. Currently the most common alternative in adults is 6-monthly intravenous pamidronate. The use of bisphosphonates in children is not common practice but intravenous pamidronate or alendronate has been used with acceptable tolerability and efficacy. There is previous experience of bisphosphonates in osteogenesis imperfecta, where the prognosis has been markedly improved. Where bisphosphonates are inadequate or unsuitable in adults, there are other alternatives.

Hormone replacement therapy

Previously the first-choice method of treatment for postmenopausal osteoporosis, hormone replacement therapy (HRT) has been supplanted by bisphosphonates, but there remains a role for HRT in some patients and it can substantially reduce the risk of osteoporotic fracture. It is most effective during the ten years immediately following the menopause. There are risk factors associated with HRT and decisions on treatment and duration should be made by the patient and general practitioner.

Calcitriol and alfacalcidol

Calcitriol is a highly active metabolite of vitamin D, and it acts by increasing calcium and phosphate absorption and decreasing calcium excretion. It also paradoxically increases calcium loss from bone, but overall its effect on bone calcification is positive. It may be taken orally in a dose of 0.25 μg twice daily. Its effect is dependent on an adequate dietary intake of calcium, but further calcium supplementation is undesirable; hypercalcemia is possible and it is necessary to monitor serum calcium and creatinine levels at 1, 3 and 6 months and 6-monthly thereafter. There is debate over any superiority of calcitriol over simple vitamin D, but both are inferior to alendronate (Sambrook et al. 2003).

Alfacalcidol is a vitamin D analog that has a smaller direct effect un calcium metabolism but a more potent effect on parathyroid hormone. It is usually given orally in a dose of 1 μg. It is not as potent as alendronate (De Nijs et al. 2006). A meta-analysis of trials of these two vitamin D metabolites has shown efficacy in enhancing spinal bone density (including steroid patients) and decreasing fracture rate (not including steroid patients), but the evidence base is weak and neither was clearly superior (Richy et al. 2004).

Calcitonin

The hormone calcitonin inhibits parathyroid hormone and therefore osteoclasts, stimulates osteoblasts and reduces calcium excretion. It is given by daily subcutaneous or intramuscular injection of 100 units (usually with supplementary calcium 500–600 mg/day) or may be administered orally or more often today by intranasal spray. Salmon calcitonin is more potent than the human form and its synthetic forms are mostly used. Concomitant administration of vitamin D may also be necessary. Only one specific study in steroid-induced bone loss has been performed (in heart transplant recipients), finding that intranasal calcitonin was good at the early prevention of bone loss in patients on high-dose steroids but that the benefit of long-term usage was less clear (Emmanouil et al. 2005).

Human parathyroid hormone and teriparatide

Paradoxically one primary action of parathyroid hormone (PTH) is to enhance osteoclasis and release calcium from bone. However, in doing so it is able to improve skeletal microarchitecture and thus enhance bone strength and fracture resistance. It is currently primarily considered a treatment for severe postmenopausal or established steroid-induced osteoporosis, or in those with a high fracture risk. Treatment is limited to 2 years or less. Teriparatide is a shortened recombinant human PTH with a similar action and therapeutic profile. Calcium monitoring and limitation of intake is necessary. Teriparatide may be superior to alendronate in treating steroid-induced osteoporosis (Saag et al. 2009). Currently it is not considered safe to combine the two but the effect of PTH appears not to be maintained after cessation; following PTH treatment, alendronate has been effective (Black et al. 2005). The place of PTH or teriparatide in prophylaxis is not yet established.

Strontium ranelate and others

The strontium salt of ranelic acid has a dual effect on bone modeling, first by accelerating osteoblast formation and action and second by inhibiting osteoclasis. It is proven effective in reducing vertebral and non-vertebral fractures in postmenopausal osteoporosis, and in prevention. Comparisons with alendronate are as yet incomplete and specific studies into steroid-induced osteoporosis have not been performed.

Other systemic side effects

Hormonal effects and weight gain

The mineralocorticoid side effects of synthetic steroids include sodium and water retention, potassium loss and systemic hypertension. Glucocorticoid effects include raised blood sugar and diabetes. All patients using oral steroids should have regular urinalysis and, if glycosuria is found, fasting blood sugar analysis. In this clinic, all patients have weight, blood pressure and urinalysis recorded at each visit. An aggressive approach to weight control is imperative at the outset; an explanation to the patient of steroid-induced changes to both appetite and metabolism will enhance compliance with weight maintenance. Access to a dietician is helpful.

Steroid myopathy

Two forms of myopathy can occur in those using oral steroid and women are more at risk. The least uncommon (seen much less in prednisolone users than in those using fluorinated steroid such as dexamethasone) is a chronic, indolent, progressive problem usually affecting those on very long-term drug use, and the risk is dose related. It manifests as weakness primarily affecting proximal limb muscles, especially quadriceps, and neck flexors. Myalgia may also occur. It is probably a slow atrophy provoked by the catabolic effect of the glucocorticoid. More rarely an acute-onset severe myopathy with rhabdomyolysis presents as sudden generalized weakness some days after commencing high-dose steroids. Dose reduction for the former, and discontinuation for the latter, is therapeutic.

Avascular bone necrosis

Infarction of the end-arteriole supply (avascular or aseptic bone necrosis, osteonecrosis) may in theory affect any bone, but predominantly steroid-induced necrosis affects the head of femur, knee or shoulder. There may be signs of involvement in several joints simultaneously. It is fortunately a rare complication of oral steroid treatment and is almost confined to those with pre-existing bone or joint disease. It leads untreated to collapse of the affected bone and destruction of an affected joint surface, resulting in substantial morbidity and pain. Joint replacement or resurfacing may be required. Presentation is with focal deep pain, and in steroid-treated patients a high degree of suspicion is required. Diagnosis is optimal with magnetic resonance imaging (MRI). Early diagnosis may permit surgical decompression or other less interventional techniques. If suspected, urgent referral to an orthopedic surgeon is required. If possible the cessation or rapid reduction of high-dose steroid may be beneficial.

Skin

Many younger patients will develop steroid-induced acne, especially on higher doses, and this predominates on the shoulders and back. It is reversible but requires dose reduction. Very long-term usage always leads to subepidermal atrophy and vascular fragility, showing as translucent skin with highly visible underlying structures, multiple bruises provoked by minimal trauma and poor wound healing. Skin tearing can be induced by such minor trauma as the removal of a self-adhesive ECG electrode.

Infection

Risks of intercurrent infection are not high unless steroids are used in very high doses, or in combination with immunosuppression. Varicella is a particular risk in these circumstances; it may develop into a fulminating, fatal infection. Non-immune patients at risk should avoid contact with those affected by chickenpox or shingles. If knowingly exposed, immunization with varicella-zoster immunoglobulin is required, preferably within 3 days. Patients on steroid treatment should not receive live vaccines, and should always carry a steroid treatment card with them.

Growth suppression in children

Growth suppression occurs in children using systemic steroids. It is important to measure height and weight from a baseline and to record this using standardized child height/weight charts. Alternate-day steroid regimens are known to alleviate the problem of growth suppression.

Adrenocortical suppression

In those taking oral steroid treatment for many months or years, adrenocortical atrophy can be profound. Rapid cessation of treatment may therefore be fatal. In this clinic, for those who are chronic users, steroid dosages are reduced in increments no larger than 2.5 mg/day per month from 10 mg to 5 mg, and then no more than 1 mg/day per month thereafter. At these dosage levels, the uveitis itself may in any case be exquisitely sensitive to small changes. Patients who complain of unexplained tiredness and weakness when attempting discontinuation of long-term oral steroid should be treated with care. There may also be dizziness, disorientation, postural hypotension, hypoglycemia and weight loss. If the diagnosis is clear or if in doubt, the previous dose of steroid should be restored immediately and an endocrinological opinion sought. An ACTH stimulation test (usually a short Synacthen test) will be performed. On occasion it is necessary to maintain very low-dose (usually prednisolone 2.5 mg/day or less) treatment for life to prevent adrenal crisis.

Ocular side effects

Ophthalmologists are acutely aware of the potential for ocular side effects in those on local or systemic steroid treatment. Induction of glaucoma occurs in a significant minority of those using topical steroids, especially those with high rates of penetration. It is imperative at the outset, where glaucoma arises in a patient with uveitis who is using topical steroid treatment, to diagnose the etiology of the glaucoma. In some cases it is obvious that steroid induction is the cause; in others the uveitis or its sequelae are the cause, but quite frequently it is in doubt; with the passage of time this distinction becomes only more difficult. It may therefore be necessary temporarily to modify topical treatment in order to provoke change, e.g. administering very asymmetrical dosages while observing IOP responses. Systemic steroid-induced glaucoma is very uncommon, by comparison. However, cases of very severe glaucoma have arisen after depot injections of steroid and, rarely, the need to remove the depot surgically has been reported. The best approach to this problem is prevention; steroid responders can be identified by their response to topical medication, and there are very few situations where periocular depot injections are required before this can be ascertained.

Cataract is a common and highly significant complication of both uveitis and steroid treatment, and in an individual patient the relative effect of each component may be difficult to judge. Patients may be legitimately concerned about the development of cataract as a complication of steroid usage (as stated on their drug information sheet). However, it can be said with confidence that, in the patient with uveitis, the visual consequences of inadequate systemic steroid treatment are far greater, and far more likely to be irremediable.

In a small number of patients using either topical or oral steroid treatment, herpetic corneal ulceration occurs. This may be challenging, first because a geographic ulcer may develop before presentation, and second because a reduction in steroid dosage may be difficult to achieve safely. The use of both topical and systemic aciclovir is recommended in this situation.

INTRAVENOUS METHYLPREDNISOLONE INFUSION

Where a rapid potent anti-inflammatory effect is required, intravenous infusion of high-dose methylprednisolone is the treatment of choice. The effect of a single dose may last for up to 1 week. This management technique is most useful in situations of fulminating sight-threatening uveitis, as may occur, for instance, in Behçet's disease, sympathetic uveitis and occasionally in very severe Vogt–Koyanagi–Harada syndrome, in scleritis with severe pain, and preoperatively or perioperatively in patients with severe unstable uveitis undergoing intraocular surgery. Methylprednisolone is administered by slow intravenous infusion over 1–2 h, in adult dosages from 500 mg to 1 g. Doses may be repeated, or 'pulsed' at intervals of 24–48 h, three doses usually being the maximum for a course. In children with severe uveitis associated with juvenile idiopathic arthritis, in addition to baseline immunosuppression it is our practice to administer 2 pulses of intravenous methylprednisolone in the 3 days before cataract or glaucoma surgery.

The effect of this mode of treatment can be rapid and dramatic. Severe scleritic pain can be removed within 6 h and uveitis responds significantly within 48 h. The effect may be short-lived but in severe uveitis there are clear advantages to initial rapid control, which can then be maintained by oral steroids with or without immunosuppression.

High-dose intravenous steroids are not without risk. Patients are exposed to the side effects normally associated with high-dose systemic therapy, including hypokalemia and mood changes, and sometimes euphoria or insomnia. Cutaneous flushing and sweating are sometimes seen. Anaphylaxis is rare. Although cardiovascular toxicity is very uncommon, a variety of arrhythmias can result including supraventricular tachycardia, atrial fibrillation and flutter, severe bradycardia, any of these possibly leading to circulatory collapse and death. Side effects are reduced by the avoidance of rapid infusion, but nevertheless cardiac monitoring should be readily available and blood pressure checked during infusion. It is our practice to admit patients to hospital for such treatment on the first two occasions. If pulsed therapy has been repeated without incident, it can then be administered in the outpatient clinic.

NON-STEROIDAL ANTI-INFLAMMATORY DRUGS

A wide variety of NSAIDs are used in many inflammatory diseases. Topically they are considered useful in the management of routine postoperative inflammation after cataract surgery, and in the management of mild ocular surface inflammation. Their use in uveitis has not been thoroughly investigated but current opinion is that this drug group adds little to uveitis management generally, either systemically or topically. All act by inhibition of the COX pathway, which is responsible for prostaglandin formation. The initial claimed advantages of the COX-2 inhibitors have been overshadowed by problems of cardiovascular risk and no superiority has been effectively demonstrated for any ocular inflammation.

Several topical NSAIDs are available. In comparison with topical steroid they do not cause glaucoma or cataract, encourage viral keratitis or affect wound healing. In theory they are attractive alternatives to topical steroids in situations where only low anti-inflammatory activity is required, but they have not demonstrated adequate potency in the management of significant uveitis.

Continuous oral NSAID may reduce the frequency of attacks of anterior uveitis (Fiorelli et al. 2010). Although oral NSAID has been found effective in the management of some forms of macular edema (particularly after cataract surgery), efficacy is thought inadequate for uveitic macular edema. Intravitreal diclofenac has been injected in the management of a small heterogeneous group of macular edemas with some sign of efficacy (Soheilian et al. 2010) but this requires further study in the context of uveitis. In summary, for future topical or systemic NSAID to prove of interest to most uveitis practitioners, a substantial increase in efficacy without a worsening of side-effect profile would be necessary.

IMMUNOSUPPRESSIVES

The development of therapeutic immunosuppression is an interesting mixture of inspiration, hard work and serendipity, liberally sprinkled with Nobel prizes. The extremely unpleasant characteristics of sulfur mustard, initially created in the nineteenth century but used first as a weapon of war in 1917, led to further military experimentation to pursue increased toxicity. Fortunately the resultant, even more repulsive nitrogen mustards were used as weaponry only on a few occasions, but knowing of the marrow suppressive effect, experimentation in human cancer began in the 1940s. In 1953 it was discovered that the aromatization of chlorinated mustard (creating **chlorambucil**) decreased toxicity, and in 1958 the addition of phenylalanine (creating **cyclophosphamide**) enhanced cell uptake. The drugs acted by alkylating DNA cross-links, preventing cell replication and inducing cell death.

The pterins are folate analogs discovered initially in butterfly wing pigment. In 1947, at Boston Children's hospital, Farber and co-workers began to use the folate antagonist aminopterin in lymphoblastic leukemia but its very high toxicity was problematic. In 1950 the derivative amethopterin (subsequently named **methotrexate**) was synthesized by Subbarao but despite the obvious effectiveness of the drug it was not until 1988 that it received US Food and Drug Administration (FDA) approval in the management of rheumatoid arthritis.

The pioneering work of Hitchings and Elion at the Wellcome Laboratories in 1953 was based on the concept that the synthesis of analogs of the bases constituting DNA could be used to counteract DNA synthesis. The first useful analog, developed in 1953, was 6-mercaptopurine and soon afterwards the drug underwent trials in the leukemias. The drug is highly toxic, but the development in 1959 of its prodrug, **azathioprine**, permitted a much better therapeutic ratio. In the meantime the groundbreaking work of Peter Medawar had identified the basis of tissue rejection, and Roy Calne was the first to introduce 6-mercaptopurine and then azathioprine in the prophylaxis of kidney transplant rejection, starting a new era in the management of organ failure.

Since the introduction of effective microscopy, various dedicated mycologists have concentrated their efforts on the discovery and classification of the enormous worldwide number of fungi, many of which undoubtedly remain undiscovered. In Italy in 1896, Gosio discovered *Penicillium brevicompactum* as a soil saprophyte, and its production of mycophenolic acid was immediately identified (also produced by *P. stoloniferum*). Florey discovered its antifungal properties in 1946 at a time when the therapeutic antibiotic potential of fungal secretions was the subject of intensive study. As has happened for other potential fungus-produced antibiotics, this function never reached clinical usefulness but a degree of immunosuppressive property was identified. The prodrug **mycophenolate mofetil** was initially introduced, and following this the salt **mycophenolate sodium**. FDA approval followed in 1995 and both remain in current use.

In the continuing search for useful microorganisms, *Streptomyces hygroscopicus* was first discovered on Rapa Nui (Easter Island) in 1965. The antifungal/immunosuppressant macrolide rapamycin (or **sirolimus**) was isolated from it and was discovered to block IL-2 response. After trials it came into approved clinical use in 1999. A similar story follows in Wisconsin in 1970, where *Tolypocladium inflatum* was found to produce cyclosporin A, now renamed **ciclosporin**. The drug, also produced by other fungi and bacteria, was found to inhibit the calcineurin cycle, responsible for the maintenance of effective IL-2 secretion and reception by lymphocytes. Once more a failed antifungal became a prominent immunosuppressive, and the first human trials in transplant rejection started again by Roy Calne in 1978. Finally on the misty slopes on Mount Tsukuba, on Honshu, Japan in 1984, *S. tsukubaensis* was found to secrete the inappropriately named Fujimycin (FK506), subsequently renamed **tacrolimus**. FDA approval followed in 1994.

The above immunosuppressives have been the mainstay of antirejection management and the treatment of severe autoimmune disease for up to half a century. Although there is much current interest in biologic therapies for these purposes, the use of oral immunosuppression has transformed the prognosis for many patients with uveitis and remains of great importance. The individual drugs are discussed below, but some of the generic issues of immunosuppression are discussed mainly in the section on ciclosporin.

Calcineurin inhibitors and macrolides

Ciclosporin

Ciclosporin (previously cyclosporine or cyclosporin A, marketed as Neoral and others) is now synthesized for use as an immunosuppressive. Extensive experience has accumulated over the past 25 years on its use in ocular inflammatory disease, and it is part of the standard armamentarium in uveitis. It should, however, be used according to a strict protocol.

Ciclosporin has a narrow effect on the immune system. It depresses CD4+ (T-helper or Th) lymphocyte function by blocking both expression and reception of IL-2. It achieves this by inhibiting the action of intracellular calcineurin. Calcineurin is essential in the pathway that activates nuclear factor of activated T cells (NFAT). NFAT is essential for the nuclear synthesis of IL-2. The suppression of these IL-2 pathways inhibits replication and recruitment of CD4+ cells. In addition in uveitis, dendritic cell function, IL-12 and interferon-γ production are all suppressed. The effect appears to spare CD8+ (Ts) lymphocytes. It does not affect phagocytosis or (usually) hemopoiesis.

Ciclosporin should be used with care but the problem of renal toxicity is much reduced by modern low-dose regimens. The drug is lipophilic and insoluble in water. It is now administered in capsules containing emulsified drug, which has reduced some problems of variable absorption in previous preparations. Nevertheless, monitoring of trough plasma levels is a routine part of early management. After absorption, the compound is concentrated in tissues with high fat content, including liver, kidney, spleen and lymph nodes. About 40% of the plasma concentration is found in aqueous humor. Metabolism occurs in the liver, and drugs that interfere with the liver cytochrome P450 microsomal enzyme system may substantially modify ciclosporin metabolism. In the past this phenomenon was used by the co-prescription of ketoconazole, which, as a P450 inhibitor, led to enhanced ciclosporin effect.

Selection of patients for therapy

Ciclosporin is most commonly used as a second-line agent in the patient with severe uveitis, in whom the dose of corticosteroid required to control the inflammation leads to unacceptable side effects. This steroid dosage varies from patient to patient, but it is unusual to regard a dose of > 10 mg/day as acceptable in the long term. The aim in introducing any immunosuppressive is to maintain quiescence on a lower dose of systemic steroids, and a reduction of 50% or more is usually possible. This treatment combination has now been used with success in various forms of uveitis. Ciclosporin is sometimes used as a first-line agent, particularly in the management of severe Behçet's disease.

Informed consent from the patient is required for this as for any immunosuppressive. This clinic uses a patient information pamphlet (see patient information pamphlets on attached disk). The possible complications and side effects of the drug may appear fearsome (**Table 6.6**), and indeed a majority of patients experience one or more of these (Matthews et al. 2010). However, carefully and sensitively managed, ciclosporin is associated with considerably less morbidity in the long term than systemic corticosteroids. The onset of ciclosporin effect takes 2 weeks or more, and it is therefore used in long-term suppression and maintenance, not in the immediate management of acute uveitis.

It may be necessary to consider the combination of two immunosuppressives for a patient with particularly severe disease. Two drugs both acting on the same site (e.g. ciclosporin and tacrolimus) cannot safely be combined. Ciclosporin should not be combined with the cytotoxic drugs chlorambucil or cyclophosphamide, or used within 1 month of stopping these drugs. It may be usefully combined with azathioprine, mycophenolate or methotrexate. Renal tubular toxicity will be worsened if NSAIDs are combined with ciclosporin; the combination is best avoided. Several other drugs interfere with ciclosporin metabolism and should be used only with caution. Grapefruit and its juice interfere with metabolism and increase toxicity. A summary of drug interactions is given in **Table 6.7**. There is extensive experience of the drug in pregnancy and it is considered non-mutagenic and non-teratogenic. It is often better tolerated in children than in adults where until recently it has been added to methotrexate as a second immunosuppressive. However, this function is being increasingly replaced by anti-tumor necrosis factor (TNF-α) monoclonal antibodies.

Table 6.6 Potential complications and side effects of ciclosporin therapy

Renal tubular damage, reduced glomerular filtration rate, raised creatinine
Systemic hypertension, ankle edema
Hypercholesterolemia, hypomagnesaemia, hyperuricemia, hyperkalemia
Gingivitis, gum hypertrophy, caries
Hirsutism
Normochromic anemia
Headache, light-headedness, dysphoria
Fatigue, loss of libido
Paraesthesiae of extremities, burning sensations, tremor
Central neurotoxicity: confusion, aphasia, dystonia, fits, catatonia, coma
Nausea, dyspepsia, abdominal cramps
Palpitations, acute arrhythmias
Warts, thrush, other infections
Lymphoma

Table 6.7 Drugs interacting with ciclosporin

1. Drugs with an independent risk of renal toxicity, e.g. aminoglycosides, non-steroidal anti-inflammatory drugs
2. Drugs that increase plasma concentrations of ciclosporin, e.g. ketoconazole, erythromycin, verapamil, oral contraceptives
3. Drugs that decrease plasma concentrations of ciclosporin, e.g. phenytoin, carbamazepine, rifampicin, sulfadiazine
4. Nifedipine and ciclosporin together may cause severe gingival swelling
5. Cyclophosphamide or chlorambucil should not be used with ciclosporin

Preliminary investigations

The side effects of ciclosporin are predictable and mostly dose-related (see Table 6.6). Of particular significance is renal tubular damage. When ciclosporin was used in doses up to 10 mg/kg per day, over a long period, irreversible tubular damage was sometimes sustained and therefore regular renal biopsy was required in patients on treatment. However, low-dose regimens (5mg/kg per day or less) do not lead to irreversible damage if creatinine levels and blood pressure are normal. Those with pre-existing abnormal renal function are unsuitable for ciclosporin treatment, and a serum creatinine level > 130 μmol/l is a contraindication.

Systemic hypertension commonly occurs in patients using ciclosporin. Pre-existing hypertension is a relative contraindication to treatment, but ciclosporin should not be used if the systolic blood pressure is > 140 mmHg, or the diastolic > 95 mmHg. Abnormal liver function is also a contraindication to treatment. In this clinic, full blood count (FBC), urea and electrolytes (U&Es), liver function tests (LFTs), blood pressure (BP), weight and urinalysis are assessed before commencing treatment. Borderline renal function requires estimated glomerular renal function (GFR) before a final decision on treatment.

The questions to be answered on starting any patient on a new immunosuppressive for uveitis are fairly straightforward, but each must be answered with a definite 'yes' before further treatment is justified:

- Is the drug tolerated by the patient in terms of symptomatic side effects?
- Are the monitoring parameters within acceptable limits?
- Is the treatment working?

The time taken to answer these questions varies depending upon the drug. An approximate onset delay for each is given in **Table 6.8**.

Trial of therapy

A trial period, usually of 3 months, is set with clear aims in mind: achieving or maintaining quiescence of uveitis, despite a set reduction in steroid dosage preferably by at least 50% and preferably to 10 mg/day or less, and maintenance or improvement in visual acuity. The effect of ciclosporin usually takes 2 weeks to start. During the trial period (and thereafter), the improvements achieved must be judged against the problems associated with the drug. The decision to stop or continue with the drug is made jointly with the patient, having set further aims over the next 6–12 months. If the drug is stopped, this should take several weeks of dose reduction, which will need to be covered by enhanced steroid dosage. A rebound inflammation will otherwise be experienced.

Table 6.8 How long does it take to work? The approximate speed of onset of effect for corticosteroids and immunosuppressives used for uveitis

Drug	Usual onset delay
Intravenous methylprednisolone	6 h
Prednisolone	2–3 days
Ciclosporin	10–14 days
Tacrolimus	2 weeks
Mycophenolate	2 weeks to months (very variable)
Azathioprine	3–6 weeks
Methotrexate	10–12 weeks

Our current choice of starting dose has overall decreased with time. If uveitis is severe and clearly requiring early immunosuppression, we may commence with 5 mg/kg per day, but in less demanding circumstances, usually 3 mg/kg per day. Daily intake is divided into two, which gives lower peak plasma levels and reduces renal toxicity. Most patients start on 100–200 mg twice daily. Patient compliance must be assured to allow a proper judgment of effect, and drug absorption for the individual patient must be monitored. On the morning of each visit the usual dose of ciclosporin is delayed to allow trough serum levels to be measured, until a satisfactory response is reached.

The most common adverse symptoms experienced by patients early in the course of treatment are headache, paraesthesiae, burning sensations in the fingers, tremor and dyspepsia. Occasionally they are immediately severe and the drug must be abandoned. Often they improve after 48 h and, with dose reduction often followed later by gentle reinstatement, it can be tolerated.

Maintenance and monitoring

Regular assessment of safety parameters is essential when monitoring ciclosporin treatment, as for all immunosuppression. Each center will have different methods of collection of laboratory results, and acquiring all of these in a timely fashion may be frustrating to the clinician trying to maintain safety. Our previous approach was to create a paper flowchart, but this has now been replaced by a screen-based flowchart where sequential blood test results can be compared, and therefore changing trends and abnormalities identified at a glance. Patients settled on ciclosporin treatment are then assessed 6-weekly, but, if demonstrably stable after some months, we permit 8-weekly assessment as a maximum. At each visit, blood pressure, weight urinalysis, FBC, U&Es and LFTs are performed. After the trial period, trough ciclosporin level is assessed as described below. Consecutive diastolic pressures > 95 mmHg require action; a 25% dose reduction should be made. If this does not lead to a reduction in BP, then antihypertensive medication is required or the use of the drug should be reconsidered. The appropriate antihypertensive is not as important as thought previously; nifedipine was once considered preferable but in fact predisposes to gingival hyperplasia. The initial choice of most general practitioners will be an angiotensin-converting enzyme (ACE) inhibitor and this is acceptable.

A rise in creatinine level is not uncommon. However, a rise above 130 μmol/l or more than 30% above the baseline measurement is unacceptable. Dose reduction by 25% should follow. Hyperkalemia, hyperuricemia or hypomagnesemia is associated with ciclosporin treatment. The last seems very closely associated with the severity of side effects, and patient symptoms are therefore a good surrogate marker. We no longer assess serum magnesium.

In the long term, ciclosporin may be reasonably well tolerated by the uncomplaining patient yet problems do arise. Hirsutism in women is tolerated and often not noticed by the male ophthalmologist because of facial waxing. Chronic warts are not uncommon. Dental supervision is essential if there is significant gingival hyperplasia, and gingivitis with gum bleeding or caries may require discontinuation of the drug.

In contrast to some other inflammatory diseases, there is no clear relationship between trough serum drug levels and control of uveitis; there is no 'therapeutic range' to aim for. After assessing initial absorption, trough levels are mainly used to check compliance. A slow taper of ciclosporin, usually reducing by 50 mg/day every 3 months or more, is often possible while maintaining suppression of inflammation. Trough serum levels are reported as undetectable below 25 U, yet doses as low as 50 mg once daily, with undetectable trough plasma levels, sometimes continue to be therapeutic; in a few patients we have mistakenly considered such doses no longer necessary, only to be confronted immediately by disease flare after discontinuation.

There are some concerns about the combined effect of ciclosporin and corticosteroid on bone metabolism. Ciclosporin has a neutral effect on bone but does accelerate bone turnover. When given with systemic steroid (which causes bone loss), the effect of ciclosporin may therefore be to steepen the slope of bone density loss. Ironically the main reason for introducing ciclosporin (to reduce steroid dosage and therefore steroid-induced side effects) may not be achieved in some patients despite achieving a steroid dose reduction. Data on this are incomplete; the effect if any on fracture rate is unknown (Mazzantini et al. 2007) and has not been studied in patients with uveitis, but is a source of concern.

There is much experience now on the long-term safety of ciclosporin. The irreversible renal tubular atrophy and interstitial fibrosis that followed some early treatments are now known to be related to high starting dosage, high creatinine levels and higher age. With a starting dosage of 5 mg/kg per day or less and strict monitoring of creatinine, damage is most unlikely despite continuous treatment for many years. Long-term follow-up studies are available, showing no progressive nephrotoxicity.

Ciclosporin is considered by some ophthalmologists to be an unpleasant drug for their patients, not often used. In our experience, especially when used in low dose in combination with a second immunosuppressive, it is usually well tolerated in the long term. However, there remains an extensive side-effect profile (Matthews et al. 2010) and, since the introduction of mycophenolate immunosuppression, we have used much less ciclosporin than previously.

Ciclosporin is now available in topical preparations but intraocular absorption is negligible and its use is therefore confined to ocular surface disorders. Both deep lamellar scleral and intraocular implantation of bioerodible ciclosporin devices have been used in animal models of uveitis with some success, but devices available for human use are not yet close.

Finally in relation to ciclosporin and other immunosuppressives used for the treatment of uveitis, the subject of drug-related cancer should be discussed. Anecdotes of cancers in patients with uveitis on immunosuppression have been published, and the carcinogenic profile for azathioprine and others either after organ transplantation or in systemic autoimmune disease are well reported. It was on the basis of the latter that we tended to include in our drug information a small but significant cancer risk, followed by a detailed explanation of the likely tumors involved (skin cancer or lymphoma), the high cure rate especially for the former and the small relative risk compared with normal lifetime risks of cancer. However, anecdotally the risk of immunosuppression-associated cancer for patients with uveitis has been very much less than reported in other specialties, and the publication of a recent study (Kempen et al. 2008) has given great reassurance that the risk of cancer in uveitis patients as a result of using ciclosporin and other calcineurin inhibitors, azathioprine, methotrexate and mycophenolate is zero or negligible. The data for anti-TNF-α monoclonal antibodies is less clear, and cyclophosphamide is associated with some risk if used for longer than 18 months. We have now removed the cancer risk from drug information where appropriate and have discontinued our previously introduced skin cancer early diagnosis system, though we retain that information for patients if necessary.

Tacrolimus and pimecrolimus

Tacrolimus (Prograf and others) is a macrolide that exerts a similar but not identical suppressive mechanism on the calcineurin pathway to ciclosporin. The drug is very similar to ciclosporin in its profile of toxicity and side effects but there are additional possibilities of gastrointestinal effects, neurological problems, pruritus, cardiomyopathy and diabetes. This clinic uses a patient information pamphlet (see patient information pamphlets on attached disk). However, there are enthusiasts for the drug who consider it to be as effective as ciclosporin while reportedly carrying a reduced incidence of toxicity (Murphy et al. 2005) and it is said to remain tolerable and effective in the longer term (Hogan et al. 2007). It has replaced ciclosporin in the management of graft rejection in many centers. Dosages for uveitis are in the range of 0.05–0.15 mg/kg per day with averages of 2–6 mg/day. Trough serum levels are more important for tacrolimus, and levels under 20 ng/ml must be maintained. Dosing is perhaps more difficult to achieve safely than with ciclosporin and users should be sufficiently familiar with the possible toxic effects to ensure early diagnosis and management. Most users of calcineurin inhibitors concentrate expertise on, and favor one or other of, ciclosporin or tacrolimus. There are anecdotes of successful management of uveitis with tacrolimus where ciclosporin has failed, but failure of tacrolimus is highly unlikely to be followed by success with ciclosporin.

Pimecrolimus (Elidel) is a further calcineurin inhibitor with similarities to tacrolimus. It is used topically in dermatoses and is not used systemically. The interest to uveitis practitioners is that, when applied to genital ulcers in Behçet's disease, it speeds healing and decreases pain (Kose et al. 2009).

Sirolimus

Although sirolimus (Rapamune) is a macrolide similar to tacrolimus, it does not act on the calcineurin pathway although it does affect the afferent rather than the efferent loop of IL-2 reception/activation. It can therefore be synergistic with both ciclosporin and tacrolimus, as has been seen in experimental uveitis (Martin et al. 1995), and in human uveitis it has been used alone with some degree of success (Shanmuganathan et al. 2005). However, despite being a fairly old drug it has not yet found a firm place in the treatment of uveitis and is unlikely to do so.

Voclosporin

A new calcineurin inhibitor designed with the specific intention of pursuing licensing for uveitis, voclosporin has shown clear effect in an animal model (Cunningham et al. 2009). Disappointingly, therefore, having undergone the LUMINATE phase III human trials with inconclusive results, further trials are now underway. Results are awaited.

Cytotoxic immunosuppressives

The alkylating agents chlorambucil and cyclophosphamide have been used as cytotoxic agents for many years, and there is also considerable experience of their use in autoimmune inflammation. Experience is also prolonged for both the purine analog antimetabolite azathioprine and the folate antagonist methotrexate. All of these drugs have substantial toxicity profiles and require strict monitoring, but with appropriate usage and stringent supervision have been found to cause less morbidity than long-term systemic corticosteroid treatment (Tamesis et al. 1996).

Azathioprine

Azathioprine (Imuran and others) is a synthetic thiopurine that interferes with purine and therefore DNA synthesis, and has a degree of selectivity for CD4+ T cells. It is a prodrug that is converted in the liver to its active metabolites, 6-mercaptopurine, 6-thioiosinic acid and 6-thioguanine. There is long experience of its efficacy in ocular inflammatory disease. It is used as a second- or third-line steroid-sparing agent for patients with difficult uveitis, and alone or in combination for Behçet's disease (Yazici et al. 1990). This clinic uses a patient information pamphlet (see patient information pamphlets on attached disk).

Azathioprine is taken orally in doses ranging from 1 mg/kg per day to 2.5 mg/kg per day, divided twice daily, usually starting at the lower end of this range and, if necessary and tolerated, increasing later. The usual adult starting dose is 75–100 mg/day. The drug takes 3–6 weeks to take effect; any therapeutic trial must allow adequate time, and steroid dosage should not be reduced until after this period. If no effect has been seen after 6 weeks, the dose may be increased with care. If the patient is taking allopurinol, the effect of azathioprine is increased and a dose reduction is necessary. The trial targets are set as described in the section on ciclosporin. Progress is assessed at appropriate times, and azathioprine discontinued if it has failed to achieve its effect within 3 months of commencement or dosage increase. Abrupt discontinuation may lead to rebound inflammation which will require increased steroid treatment.

Careful safety monitoring is required, especially in the first few weeks. The greatest potential problem is bone marrow depression, mainly of white cells. In this clinic, all patients have baseline liver and renal function, blood counts and differentials. FBC and differential are then repeated weekly for the first 4 weeks, fortnightly for 4 weeks, if satisfactory monthly for the succeeding 3 months, and 3-monthly thereafter. Renal and liver functions are assessed 4-weekly at first, and then 3-monthly. The most common initial side effect is nausea and dyspepsia, with or without abdominal pain and diarrhea. Alopecia may occur early or late.

Azathioprine has predictable dose-related effects on the blood, or less predictable effects on blood or liver. Efforts to improve predictability and reduce acute adverse events are constantly pursued. Lymphopenia is predictable and probably necessary for effect; for those with a pre-existing normal lymphocyte count a drop within a few weeks to 0.6–0.8 can be considered therapeutic. Caution should be taken with lower counts. Occasionally azathioprine is used in those with pre-existing mild lymphopenia, and the count may drop only slightly from such levels. For counts < 0.6, many physicians would prescribe prophylactic antibiotic cover in the form of co-trimoxazole 960 mg three times weekly. For uveitis patients without associated systemic inflammatory disease, the infection risk appears substantially lower and such prophylaxis is not routinely used.

In time, azathioprine frequently causes red-cell macrocytosis. If pronounced this will go on to cause a degree of hemolysis and subsequent anemia. Our practice is to observe macrocytosis carefully in the presence of normal hemoglobin levels, but to reduce dosage if hemoglobin has fallen below normal levels and falls further on a second occasion. Liver enzymes are occasionally disturbed but, as for other drug-induced liver problems, a doubling of enzyme levels is normally considered necessary for concern to be raised. For smaller rises, close observation is adequate.

In unusual circumstances azathioprine usage can be associated with rapid deterioration in hematological parameters, resulting in either agranulocytosis or aplasia. Such events may occur even after a considerable period of stability and are potentially fatal. The ability to predict and therefore avoid such idiosyncrasy may be possible using a detailed knowledge of azathioprine metabolism:

The metabolic pathways of azathioprine are shown in **Fig. 6.6**. Both 6-mercaptopurine and 6-thioiosinic acid are converted to inactive

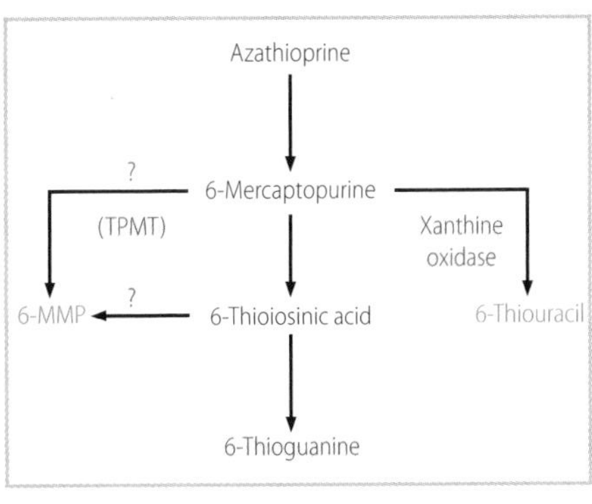

Figure 6.6 Azathioprine is ultimately transformed to its active metabolite, 6-thioguanine. During the metabolic process a proportion is transformed to the inactive metabolites, 6-methylmercaptopurine and 6-thiouracil. The former pathway is more important and it requires enough thiopurine methyltransferase to counter the toxicity of 6-thioguanine.

6-methylmercaptopurine by the enzyme thiopurine methyltransferase (TPMT), and 6-mercaptopurine is converted to inactive 6-thiouracil by xanthine oxidase. Drug potency and toxicity are therefore achieved by a balance between these three pathways. Of these, TPMT has the greatest importance in preventing the accumulation of toxic metabolites.

There is a genetic basis for variability in individual TPMT activity, and this is measurable. High secretors metabolize and inactivate azathioprine products easily; low secretors allow them to accumulate. About 1 patient in 300 is homozygous for absent TPMT activity, with a risk of profound and sudden toxicity. The use of TPMT assays before or during azathioprine treatment is becoming more frequent and is to be encouraged (Ford and Berg 2010); however, the prescription of azathioprine itself stimulates TPMT, so that assays performed after commencing medication give a less accurate measure of secretor limitation. A failure to assay TPMT where the test is available is now becoming difficult to defend medicolegally. However, a normal assay does not guarantee a toxicity-free course. The other metabolites are assayable and studies on this may in future permit more accurate dosing. The near future brings possibility of tailored dosage for individual patients with a much-reduced complication rate and probably enhanced efficacy.

Methotrexate

Methotrexate is an analog of folic acid that disrupts the tetrahydrofolate pathway. This is necessary for both purine and pyrimidine synthesis and therefore methotrexate interferes with both DNA and RNA synthesis, inhibiting both G1- and S-phases of the cell cycle. The drug also inhibits the release of histamine. It is used in high doses in the treatment of malignancy, and rheumatologists have considerable experience of its use in both adult and juvenile arthritis.

Methotrexate is the immunosuppressive of first choice in the management of children with juvenile idiopathic arthritis and, although a controlled trial is lacking, it is considered helpful also for the uveitis associated with this disease (Foeldvari and Wierk 2005). This subject, and methotrexate in children in general, is considered in detail in Chapter 8. It is usually well tolerated in both children and adults, but in general methotrexate is considered the least potent of the immunosuppressives available to treat uveitis and is certainly the least rapidly acting (**Table 6.8**). Nevertheless there seems to be a useful place for it in adult uveitis, where not only has it been found useful in the management of chronic uveitis with relative steroid resistance in adults (Samson et al. 2001) but also in the prevention of relapses of recurrent acute anterior uveitis (Munoz-Fernandez et al. 2009). This clinic uses a patient information pamphlet (see patient information pamphlets on attached disk).

Methotrexate may be injected intraocularly in the management of either intraocular lymphoma (see above) or uveitis. An injection of 400 μg in 0.1 ml was effective in reducing intraocular inflammation during exacerbations of adult uveitis and was apparently still working at 6 months (Taylor et al. 2009).

Low-dose oral methotrexate in adults is taken weekly and is usually commenced at 7.5–10 mg/week, rising if tolerated to 10–20 mg/week. Early side effects if experienced include nausea and vomiting, gastrointestinal disturbance, angular stomatitis or mouth ulcers. For any given dose such symptoms are ameliorated by transferring to subcutaneous injections. Side effects are lessened by the use of folic acid, given 5 mg weekly (usually 3 days after the methotrexate dose). A greater dose of folic acid may counteract the methotrexate effect. The main toxicity concern is liver dysfunction which may progress to fibrosis or cirrhosis. Bone marrow suppression, renal damage or alopecia is an unusual problem. Sterile pneumonitis is a very unusual but life-threatening complication, and patients with chronic cough, chest pain or hemoptysis should be urgently investigated. It may cause infertility, which is usually reversible. Liver, renal and marrow functions are normally assessed monthly. Historically, methotrexate has been considered to carry a high risk of teratogenicity whether used by the father or the mother, and current recommendations are that conception should not be permitted until 6 months after stopping the drug (by either parent). More recent analysis considers the risk to be exaggerated, but, in the absence of more concrete data, contraception should be carefully observed. In the case of inadvertent pregnancy discovered within the first trimester, it is recommended that the drug be stopped immediately and obstetric advice sought.

Our practice is to consider methotrexate in adults with uveitis where the frequency of topical steroid for anterior uveitis is problematic, where mild chronic uveitis of any type nevertheless requires immunosuppression and after an inability to tolerate azathioprine or ciclosporin. It is not an immunosuppressive of first choice for most patients. If it is not tolerated at standard doses we do not persist with supportive measures, but switch to another drug.

Cyclophosphamide and chlorambucil

Cyclophosphamide (Endoxan and others) is a nitrogen mustard derivative, an alkylating agent that is activated by liver metabolism. It interferes with guanine and therefore DNA synthesis. It interferes non-specifically with all stages of the cell cycle including mitosis. At low doses, cellular immunity is most affected, but B lymphocytes are also affected at higher doses. It is standard therapy for some life-threatening autoimmune diseases including systemic vasculitis, particularly Wegener's granulomatosis, where the prognosis for survival has been transformed. Its place in the management of necrotizing scleritis is also well established. It has been used as 'rescue' treatment for both ophthalmic and other severe manifestations of Behçet's disease (Davatchi et al. 2004).

Cyclophosphamide has also been used in uveitis, but is limited to very severe cases unresponsive to other immunosuppressives, because of its potentially severe side effects. The drug can be administered orally as continuous or intermittent (pulsed) regimens, or pulsed intravenously, most frequently using the Birmingham Vasculitis Protocol, which minimizes toxicity. In a mixed cohort of patients with various ocular inflammatory diseases, cyclophosphamide was found to be effective if tolerated for a full course of treatment for up to 1 year (Pujari et al. 2010). Importantly, unlike other immunosuppressives, there is clear evidence that cyclophosphamide can induce long-term remission of inflammation in some patients.

A metabolite of cyclophosphamide (acrolein) is concentrated in urine, and is toxic to uroepithelium. If no precautions are taken a sterile cystitis is common, which may be severe and hemorrhagic. The condition predisposes to bladder carcinoma. To minimize this risk, cyclophosphamide is administered only in the morning, with a supervised oral fluid push, and MESNA (2-mercaptoethanesulfonate) is routinely administered, which neutralizes acrolein within the bladder. Generalized (usually reversible) alopecia is more common with oral regimens. Mild anemia is usual. Infections may occur but this is uncommon. The drug is teratogenic. Decreased fertility is usual, but permanent azoospermia and testicular atrophy, or ovarian failure, may occur, so sperm or egg banking should be offered if there is the opportunity before treatment.

Oral dosages are in the range of 1 mg/kg per day, a typical starting dose being 100 mg/day. This is taken as a single morning dose. At least 3 l of fluid per day should be taken. Leukopenia, or more specifically lymphopenia, is intrinsic to the activity of cyclophosphamide. In the management of uveitis, a predominant aim is to lower the lymphocyte count to between 0.6 and 1.0 x 10^9/l. The neutrophil count should not drop below 2.0 x 10^9/l and the total white cell count should not fall below 3.5 x 10^9/l. Baseline and twice-weekly FBC and differential counts should be used for the first 2 or 3 weeks, then fortnightly. The drug is rarely used for longer than 1 year, mainly because of risks of malignancy, and it is standard practice for patients with chronic autoimmune disease to transfer to azathioprine or another immunosuppressive.

Despite its potentially severe toxicity profile, cyclophosphamide has retained a place in the management of very severe uveitis, not least because of its ability to induce long-term remission. However, infliximab (see below) since its introduction has gradually been assuming this role and the future of cyclophosphamide in this patient group is uncertain. Doubtless it will retain some usefulness for a few patients.

Chlorambucil (Leukeran) is an aromatic derivative of phosphoramine mustard with similar actions to cyclophosphamide. It was for a time widely used for the treatment of Behçet's disease and severe uveitis and, similar to cyclophosphamide, is capable of inducing long-term remission. However, it is a potent drug with a toxicity profile similar to, but generally more profound than, cyclophosphamide. For this reason, after the development of the above immunosuppressives, it has become largely superseded in this field. If uveitis is severe enough to warrant an alkylating agent, cyclophosphamide is almost always now used in preference.

Leflunomide

As azathioprine inhibits purine synthesis, so leflunomide (Arava) inhibits the synthesis of the DNA pyrimidines cytosine and thiamine, and uracil in RNA. It is a derivative of isoxazole used clinically as a disease-modifying anti-rheumatic drug (DMARD) in arthritis, but was investigated briefly and found probably effective in experimental uveitis (Robertson and Lang 1994), but this has led to only anecdotal usage in human uveitis. Further studies are required.

Mycophenolate

Mycophenolate is the esterified precursor of mycophenolic acid, which inhibits inosine monophosphate dehydrogenase. This is important in the primary guanine synthesis pathway, which is therefore disrupted, mostly in rapidly dividing cells including activated T and B cells. It is more selective than azathioprine. It is available as the more commonly used prodrug mycophenolate mofetil (CellCept) or the salt mycophenolate sodium (Myfortic).

There is now considerable experience of mycophenolate in both transplantation and autoimmune disease. In the field of uveitis it is most commonly prescribed to patients in whom azathioprine has been either intolerable or ineffective, but it is sometimes prescribed as a first-line immunosuppressive. It is used for various manifestations of Behçet's disease with mixed results. It may be used with care together with calcineurin inhibitors, but not with azathioprine or alkylating agents. A large retrospective series found mycophenolate to be effective in about half the patients treated, but there was often a delay in efficacy of more than 6 months (Daniel et al. 2010). A similar report found a higher success rate (Teoh et al. 2008). Our experience in over 70 patients is that occasionally there is a dramatic response within 2 weeks, more usually a slower-developing response over a few months. This clinic uses a patient information pamphlet (see patient information pamphlets on the attached disk).

Most patients tolerate mycophenolate well but very occasionally there is early and severe intolerance. For this reason we normally start mycophenolate mofetil in adults at 500 mg twice daily and observe for 2 weeks before aspiring to 1 g twice daily, raising to 1.5 g twice daily after some months if well tolerated but inadequately ineffective. Early intolerance usually includes severe malaise, diarrhea, dizziness and insomnia. Later problems may include gastrointestinal upset, myalgia, rash, headache, tremor and dose-related myelosuppression. We monitor FBC, U&Es and LFTs 2-weekly for 6 weeks, then 6-weekly, reducing to 8-weekly if reliably tolerant. The drug is also useful in children as second-line immunosuppression and is usually well tolerated (Doycheva et al. 2007) but of course must be supervised by an expert.

Mycophenolate is not safe for use in pregnancy – a specific syndrome of teratogenicity has been identified that may affect up to a quarter of pregnancies. This rate far outweighs the risk of methotrexate teratogenicity and stringent precautions to avoid pregnancy should be taken. Both oral and depot contraception can be rendered ineffective by mycophenolate and so barrier methods are necessary. In the case of inadvertent pregnancy discovered within the first trimester, obstetric advice should be sought immediately to offer counseling on termination.

MONOCLONAL ANTIBODIES AND OTHER BIOLOGIC THERAPIES

The concept of highly specific treatment, initially for infection, was that of Paul Ehrlich a century ago, whose excellent work led to the subsequently much over-used and over-enthusiastic term 'magic bullet.' However, it was investigation into the peculiar paraprotein-producing characteristics of myeloma cells in the 1970s that provoked interest in cell lines actually capable of specific antibody production. Hybridoma technology came into existence: the ability to create a cell line by fusing myeloma cells (the 'antibody factory' component) with a specific antibody-producing cell (normally created in mice spleen by immunizing with the specific antigen), the resultant culture being capable of vigorous production of a specific antibody from this single cell clone. A series of complex steps are then required to produce a pure product. These first 'monoclonal' antibodies (MAbs) were chimeric, meaning that elements of mouse protein were necessarily included. This was paradoxically likely to induce an immune response in the recipient, which remains a substantial disadvantage in these drugs. The subsequent development of recombinant technology in the 1980s allowed either viruses or yeasts to become the antibody factory component. This permitted cloning and molecular manipulation on a scale previously impossible, so that bespoke antibody design became a reality. In the meantime genetically engineered murine cells have been produced that exclude the mouse element from the antibodies produced. This technique, or bacteriophage-generated antibodies, now permits fully humanized protein constituents, eliminating the risks associated with chimeric drugs. There is justifiably immense excitement as new MAbs are progressively produced. Already a large number are available not only for the treatment of cancers and inflammatory diseases, but also for laboratory use. The very high research and development (R&D) investment in producing such drugs leads to the eye-watering costs of prescription; as new treatment opportunities arise, so healthcare organizations are increasingly challenged by the expense of provision. There is therefore no current field of medicine more in need of controlled trials to create a firm evidence base. The MAbs discussed here include those currently in use or in development for uveitis, or used in inflammatory diseases with an ophthalmic component, or with potential use in uveitis. The MAbs are summarized in **Table 6.9**, and an approximate cost comparison of systemic treatment for uveitis is shown in **Table 6.10**.

Anti-TNF-α monoclonal antibodies

Tumor necrosis factor α is a multifunctional cytokine with central roles in the induction of inflammation and the generation of the acute phase reaction. It also inhibits viral replication and suppresses embryonic tumor development. It has a central role in several forms of

Table 6.9 Monoclonal antibodies, a summary of their cell or cytokine targets and their current usage

Monoclonal antibody	Target	Clinical usage
Adalimumab	TNF-α	Arthritis, IBD, JIA, uveitis
Alemtuzumab	CD52	Leukemias, severe autoimmune disease
Anakinra	IL-1R	Rheumatoid arthritis, CAPS syndromes
Bevacizumab	VEGF	Bowel cancer, SNVM
Canakinumab	IL-1β	CAPS syndromes
Daclizumab	IL-2Rα (CD25)	Organ transplantation, ?MS, ?uveitis
Enlimomab	ICAM-1 (CD54)	? burn injuries, ? autoimmune diseases
EOL4G8	ICAM-2 (CD102)	? anti-cancer, ? autoimmune diseases
Etanercept	TNF-α	Arthritis, JIA, psoriasis
Infliximab	TNF-α	Arthritis, severe autoimmune disease including Behçet's disease, uveitis
Ofatumumab	CD20	Rheumatoid arthritis, autoimmune disease
Pegsunercept	TNF-α	Arthritis, ? other autoimmune disease
Rituximab	CD20	Lymphomas, JIA with uveitis, scleritis

CAPS. cryopyrogen-associated periodic syndromes; CD, cluster of differentiation; IBD, inflammatory bowel disease; ICAM, intercellular adhesion molecule; IL, interleukin; JIA, juvenile idiopathic arthritis; SNVM, subretinal neovascular membrane; TNF, tumor necrosis factor; VEGF, vascular endothelial growth factor.

Table 6.10 The approximate direct costs of some systemic treatments for uveitis, based on one year of treatment in the UK. Includes drug costs only; excludes costs of hematological monitoring, day-case admission or management of complications.

Drug	Cost (UK £)
Prednisolone 10 mg once daily	25
Methotrexate 15 mg weekly oral	35
Azathioprine 50 mg twice daily	100
Mycophenolate mofetil 1 g twice daily	2500
Interferon-α2a 3 MU alternate days	2500
Ciclosporin 150 mg twice daily	3000
Infliximab (weeks 0, 2 ,6, 8-weekly 3 mg/kg)	7000 (+ cost of immunosuppressive)
Adalimumab 40 mg 2-weekly	9000

inflammatory arthropathy, for which treatments were first developed. However, these drugs have gradually found a much wider role in the management of autoimmune disease:

Etanercept and pegsunercept

Although etanercept (Enbrel) is a TNF-α inhibitor, it does not act as a monoclonal antibody but as a soluble dimeric decoy receptor, effectively mopping up soluble TNF and reducing activity. Pegsunercept is a similar drug currently in development. Etanercept is administered by weekly (usually 50 mg in adults) or twice-weekly (usually 25 mg) subcutaneous injection, and may be self-administered at home. It has been extensively used in inflammatory arthropathies including ankylosing spondylitis and juvenile idiopathic arthritis (JIA), for which it can be very useful (Lovell et al. 2003). However, the effect of etanercept on the uveitis associated with JIA has been the subject of much debate, the current opinion being that it is probably not helpful (Smith et al. 2005), and possibly unhelpful (Schmeling and Homeff 2005). A number of reports of uveitis occurring anew in patients using etanercept have not reached statistical significance but this remains a concern.

Currently our approach for children with JIA and uveitis is to proceed directly to adalimumab if methotrexate is inadequate (less commonly now with ciclosporin or mycophenolate as an intermediate treatment). Patients using etanercept for any reason who present with new uveitis are treated topically as required, and if the uveitis becomes difficult or unresponsive our advice to their physician is that a substitute should be sought for the etanercept.

Infliximab

This anti-TNF-α MAB is chimeric, containing both human- and mouse-derived protein. It therefore induces antibody formation against its murine element and, in order to reduce the risk of future immune reactions to it, concurrent immunosuppression is required, usually but not necessarily in the form of methotrexate. Nevertheless it remains antigenic in humans and antinuclear antibodies (ANAs) are usually formed, drug-induced lupus sometimes being seen. First developed for use in rheumatoid arthritis, its toxicity profile is now well defined: pre-existent unidentified tuberculosis may reactivate, typically in an aggressive and antibiotic-resistant form with a high mortality rate; multiple sclerosis can be substantially worsened; other serious infections may occur; infusion reactions are sometimes severe; blood dyscrasias are not uncommon; and malignancy may be provoked (although the risk of this is poorly defined).

Infliximab (Remicade) is administered by intravenous infusion over 1–2 h, traditionally as 3 mg/kg in adult rheumatological disorders but often at 5 mg/kg for severe uveitis. During infusion, headache, dizziness, rash, sweating and flushing are quite common. Occasionally, severe infusion reactions are experienced. Administration therefore must always take place under medical supervision. If tolerated and effective, doses are given at weeks 0, 2 and 6, and normally 8-weekly thereafter.

Despite the significant risk profile of infliximab, the drug has provoked great interest, having been shown to be effective in controlling recalcitrant uveitis, and inadequately responsive to conventional immunosuppression, in a significant proportion of patients (Suhler et al. 2009). Particular attention has been paid to its use in various manifestations of Behçet's disease including uveitis, where not only can it be rapidly effective during a hyperacute flare-up (Marchomikelakis et al. 2011) but also used in the longer-term management of immunosuppressant-resistant disease (Tugal-Tutkun et al. 2005). It has partially replaced cyclophosphamide as a rescue drug for patients with particularly difficult disease. Resistance to the drug is not uncommon and studies on long-term efficacy show significant failure rates. The subsequent introduction of the humanized analog, adalimumab, has led to comparative studies, and adalimumab is partially replacing infliximab in its turn. This clinic uses a basic patient information pamphlet on anti-TNF MAb treatment (see patient information pamphlets on attached disk). The physicians with whom we liaise to administer treatment take more detailed informed consent.

Infliximab has been used intravitreally in attempts to treat both age-related and diabetic maculopathy, with unpromising results and a substantial complication rate. It seems unlikely that this will progress to become useful in the management of uveitis.

Adalimumab

This almost-fully humanized anti-TNF-α MAb has the advantage over infliximab of only uncommonly generating an immune response in the recipient but, nevertheless, concurrent methotrexate is usual. The two MAbs are not otherwise identical and, anecdotally, clinically different responses have been observed on switching from one to the other. The risks of treatment are otherwise similar to infliximab. It is given by subcutaneous injection, an adult dose being 40 mg every 2 weeks, and is supplied in pre-filled syringes or injector pens that can be self-administered at home. The evidence base for efficacy is sparse but increasing. Adalimumab (Humira) seems to reduce the frequency of flare-ups of uveitis in patients with ankylosing spondylitis (Rudwaleit et al. 2009) and is effective in controlling chronic refractory uveitis in the majority of patients (Diaz-Llopis et al. 2008).

There has been particular interest in the usage of adalimumab in children with JIA-related uveitis. It has been claimed superior to infliximab over 1 year or more (Simonini et al. 2010) and perhaps, as expected, over etanercept (Biester et al. 2007). The drug is considerably more attractive than infliximab for use in children owing to the decreased risks and because intravenous infusion is not necessary, but should nevertheless be used under stringent supervision.

Adalimumab, similar to infliximab, has been administered intravitreally, and the sparse evidence to date suggests that it is ineffective in the management of uveitic macular edema (Androudi et al. 2010). The results of current prospective trials are awaited with interest; TNF-α blockade clearly has a place in uveitis, albeit not such a central one as in inflammatory arthropathy, and evidence on patient selection would aid decision-making in this costly field.

Anti-VEGF antibodies

The MAbs against vascular endothelial growth factor (VEGF) include bevacizumab (Avastin) which is used systemically as an anti-angiogenic treatment of vascularized cancers, and off-label intravitreally, and ranibizumab (Lucentis), developed specifically for intraocular injection. They are both now well known to ophthalmologists. Neither is used systemically in the management of uveitis or other autoimmune disease, so they are dealt with in Chapter 7.

Anti-ICAM antibodies

The intercellular adhesion molecules (ICAMs) are surface proteins expressed by leukocytes and endothelial cells which facilitate adhesion. They bind to leukocyte adhesion protein LFA-1, also expressed on leukocytes, making cells 'sticky' to each other. In particular ICAM-1 (CD54) is an important contributor to leucocyte migration. It is expressed by vascular endothelium at the site of extravascular inflammation and, together with selectins and integrins, attracts and captures passing leukocytes so that they can migrate extravascularly. Inhibition of ICAM-1 therefore prevents leukocytes reaching the site of inflammation and downregulates the acute phase response. It was hoped that enlimomab, a murine anti-CD54 MAB, would limit post-ischemic inflammatory damage in acute stroke, and be an anti-rejection agent. It failed on both counts but was found of some use in limiting post-burn dermal injury. ICAM-2 (CD102) is also expressed by leukocytes and facilitates interaction during the inflammatory response. The anti-ICAM-2 MAb EOL4G8 shows some promise as an anti-tumor drug but is in the early stages of investigation. Whether this group has a role in autoimmune inflammation remains unclear.

Other anti-cytokine antibodies

As the complexity of the immune response becomes deciphered for more autoimmune diseases, MAbs tailored to inhibit selective targets are found to be of clinical use in a variety of settings:

Daclizumab

Daclizumab (Zenapax) is a fully humanized MAb that inhibits CD25 (the α-subunit of the IL-2 receptor on T cells), and was developed primarily for use in organ transplantation. However, there are clear reasons for its potential use in autoimmune disease including uveitis. In particular, the recent identification of a population subset of steroid-resistant T cells in some patients with uveitis (Lee et al. 2009) may permit a degree of patient selectivity. It is given by intravenous infusion, typically 1 mg/kg every 2 weeks. Initial studies reveal some efficacy in patients with recalcitrant uveitis (Bhat et al. 2009). Although some success has been demonstrated in difficult birdshot retinochoroidopathy (Sobrin et al. 2008,) it is not yet known whether this disease has a particular affinity for anti-CD25 treatment.

Anakinra and canakinumab

This anti-IL-1 receptor antagonist is used mainly as a biological response modifier in rheumatoid arthritis. However, anakinra (Kineret) may be encountered in the management of the rare pediatric multisystem diseases sometimes causing uveitis, including the cryopyrin-associated periodic syndromes (CAPS – CINCA syndrome and Muckle–Wells syndrome) and chronic granulomatous disease where it has been used with some success (Neven et al. 2010). Canakinumab (Ilaris) is a humanized anti-IL-1β MAb that may induce sustained remission in CAPSs.

Anti-lymphocyte antibodies

Individual immune cell-selective markers are capable of global inhibition and MAbs targeting such markers are obviously capable of profound effect on the immune system. Such treatments are available against both B and T lymphocytes:

Rituximab and ofatumumab

Rituximab (Rituxan and others) is a chimeric anti-CD20 MAb, CD20 being found predominantly as a B-cell marker. It is therefore a profoundly potent anti-B-cell drug, inducing apoptosis, and was developed initially for the management of lymphomas. However, it is active against neoplastic, activated and normal passive B cells, and globally suppresses the capability of antibody production. Its side effects include those of all chimeric MAbs and it is liable to predispose to severe infection. Its use in a variety of autoimmune inflammatory diseases is expanding. There are anecdotes of its use in refractory adult uveitis, Behçet's disease and particularly scleritis, and a small case series claiming effective rescue therapy in severe JIA with uveitis (Heiligenhaus et al. 2011). Ofatumumab (Arzerra) is a fully humanized alternative but targets a slightly different component of CD20. It is in the early stages of human trials for autoimmune disease including rheumatoid arthritis.

Alemtuzumab

The surface marker CD52 is expressed on all mature lymphocytes and this anti-CD52 MAb, initially chimeric but then humanized (Campath-1H), was initially introduced in the management of lymphocytic leukemias. It causes massive lymphocyte depletion and has a high complication rate of lethal infections, major infusion reactions and cardiotoxicity. It has been used anecdotally as last-ditch therapy for blinding uveitis with some at least short-lived success, but with a substantial mortality rate. Better MAbs are now available.

Abatacept

Not strictly an MAb, this chimeric protein is a recombinant construct of immunoglobulin and CTLA-4, a surface marker binding to HLA-B7. The molecule was specifically designed to inhibit T-cell activation by interfering with one stage of the process; normally activation commences with a T cell (via its surface receptor) interacting with the antigen-presenting cell (APC), via its MHC marker; however, a co-stimulatory process is also necessary for full activation, the T-cell CD28 marker also binding to the APC's HLA-B7. Abatacept (Orencia) binds to the APC's HLA-B7 and therefore blocks the second stage of the process. Initially devised to treat rheumatoid arthritis, data on its efficacy are conflicting. However, it has shown initial promise in the management of the most difficult of children with JIA and uveitis, who are already resistant to immunosuppression and anti-TN-Fα MAb (Zulian et al. 2010). It may therefore have a legitimate role in the management of this tiny but unfortunate group of children. No hard data on its use in adult uveitis are yet available.

INTERFERONS

The interferons (IFNs) are a group of cytokines produced by lymphocytes and have a range of functions including being antiviral, anti-tumor and pyrogenic. A substantial number have been used therapeutically, including IFN-α2a to treat hepatitis B and C, IFN-α2b to treat neurofibromatosis and recurrent melanoma, and IFN-β1a and IFN-β1b to treat multiple sclerosis. The drug is injected subcutaneously, usually around 3 MU on alternate days. For intraocular inflammation, attention has focused on the IFN-α group; there is clear evidence of efficacy in patients with Behçet's disease, enabling the cessation of immunosuppression (Stubinger et al. 2001), and in some cases leading to prolonged remission (Sobaci et al. 2010). Mainly used as a tertiary treatment in patients with difficult uveitis, it may become a primary treatment in selected patients.

The success of IFN-α in Behçet's disease led to its use in other forms of severe uveitis, also with significant success but rather less than for Behçet's disease (Bodaghi et al. 2007). Used specifically to treat recalcitrant uveitic macular edema, again it has been successful (Deuter et al. 2009). Therapeutically, this treatment has shown clear evidence of efficacy and if tolerated may spare patients immunosuppression.

The tolerability of IFN treatment is, unfortunately, the substantial downside. To a variable extent all IFNs cause pyrexia, myalgia, tiredness, lethargy and depression; some studies find that symptoms decline after a few months of treatment, but the side effects can at worst be debilitating and should not be under-estimated; despite visual success, depression has led to a suicide attempt (Piskova et al. 2007). In addition, alopecia, skin rashes and lymphopenia are frequently seen. Unfortunately most of the adverse effects are intrinsic to interferon functions; separating these biochemically from therapeutic effects may be a laboratory challenge too far.

IMMUNOSUPPRESSION, BIOLOGICS AND INFECTION RISK

The risks versus benefits of immunosuppression or biologics must be addressed by the patient and doctor before commencement, and this risk will include infection. Carefully addressed, the risks are manageable and appear to be substantially less for patients with isolated uveitis, in comparison with those suffering from multisystem inflammatory disease or with significant comorbidity. There is an exception with the use of alkylating agents which are associated with substantially higher risk. Most patients on immunosuppression will say that they seem to acquire infections somewhat more readily than before, and that they seem to persist longer than before; in practice this means more courses of antibiotics for patients with upper respiratory and urinary infections. However, in 20 years of using immunosuppression in this clinic, treating approaching 400 patients with more than 2000 patient-years of cumulative exposure, only one patient with isolated uveitis has required hospital admission with bacterial infection. A few deaths from infection have occurred, entirely in those using heavy immunosuppression in the management of severe multisystem inflammatory disease, mainly lupus and systemic vasculitis. There are, however, other risks that should be specifically addressed:

Varicella-zoster virus and immunosuppression

Acquiring varicella-zoster virus (VZV) while immunosuppressed is life threatening mainly because of the risk of meningoencephalitis. Exposure to VZV should therefore be regarded as a medical emergency. Patients undertaking immunosuppression should have herpesvirus serology checked to ascertain previous exposure. Immune patients are not at risk. Those not previously exposed should be warned that if they contact a person with chickenpox or shingles they should take same-day medical advice. If this clinic is contacted, serology is re-checked on the same day. If positive, close observation is adequate with oral antiviral being prescribed with symptoms. If negative, VZV immunoglobulin is administered. Immunosuppression should be discontinued temporarily if overt disease develops, and a high-dose antiviral used.

Tuberculosis, measles and immunosuppression

Before starting immunosuppression it should be ascertained that the patient has no prior history of tuberculosis (TB) or contact with the disease. Immunization with BCG should be recorded. If at potential risk, chest radiograph, tuberculin testing and interferon-γ testing should be arranged. If positive, advice on treatment should be obtained from an expert physician before starting treatment. TB can reactivate and become miliary in immunosuppressed individuals. The risk is small but should not be ignored.

Measles can be lethal in immunosuppressed individuals. In the UK, herd immunity has fallen significantly in the last 10 years following inappropriate concern about combined immunizations. A history of immunization should be taken. If immunized there is no significant risk. If not, patients should be advised to report immediately any contact with the disease.

Immunosuppression, immunization and travel abroad

Patients using 40 mg or more of prednisolone, using any oral immunosuppressive in any dose, having received either of these within the last 3 months or having received an alkylating agent within the past 6 months are all considered at greater risk from live vaccines. Patients undergoing immunization schedules should always make their physician aware of their immune status. Live vaccines are unsafe; sometimes alternatives are available, sometimes not. Travel abroad is a greater risk, not least because effective immunization cannot be relied upon where a patient is less able to produce a response to a vaccine. Some countries refuse entry without certain immunization certificates.

Annual influenza immunization is, in contrast, to be recommended for all immunosuppressed patients, and pneumococcal vaccine should be administered if non-immune. We produce an information pamphlet on the subject of immunization for our uveitis clinic patients (see patient information pamphlets on attached disk).

Immunosuppression, lymphopenia and neutropenia

Lymphopenia is a characteristic feature of azathioprine treatment and is sometimes seen in mycophenolate, methotrexate, ciclosporin or tacrolimus treatment. Physicians treating systemic inflammatory disease usually prescribe prophylactic co-trimoxazole 960 mg three times weekly to patients with lymphocyte counts < 0.6. It is not our practice to do so as we do not believe it necessary in patients with isolated ocular inflammatory disease and no other risk factors. Indeed, azathioprine may be used with caution in patients with pre-existing lymphopenia if there is no sign of progressive deterioration in parameters.

Neutropenia on immunosuppression is different; it places the patient at substantially greater risk. It is not an expected or acceptable manifestation of oral immunosuppression, with the exception of alkylating agents which should be administered only by those expert in their use, and in which a neutrophil count dip is expected and managed carefully. Any unexpected neutropenia should be managed urgently and with care; prophylactic antibiotic is essential and occasionally granulocyte colony-stimulating factor needed. The advice of a hematologist should be urgently sought and the immunosuppressive immediately stopped.

REFERENCES

Androudi S, Tsironi E, Kalegoropoulos C, et al. Intravitreal adalimumab for refractory uveitis-related macular edema. *Ophthalmology* 2010;**117**:1612–6.

Bhat P, Castaneda-Cervantes RA, Doctor PP, Foster CS. Intravenous daclizumab for recalcitrant ocular inflammatory disease. Graefes Arch Clin *Exp Ophthalmol* 2009;**247**:687–92.

Biester S, Deuter C, Michels H, et al. Adalimumab in the therapy of uveitis in childhood. *Br J Ophthalmol* 2007;**91**:319–24.

Biswas J, Ganeshbabu TM, Raghavendran SR, et al. Efficacy and safety of 1% rimexalone versus 1% prednisolone acetate in the treatment of anterior uveitis – a randomized triple masked study. *Int Ophthalmol* 2004;**25**:147–53.

Black DM, Bilezikian JP, Ensrud KE, et al. One year of alendronate after one year of parathyroid hormone (1–84) for osteoporosis. *N Engl J Med* 2005;**353**:555–65.

Bodaghi B, Gendron G, Wechsler B, et al. Efficacy of interferon alpha in the treatment of refractory and sight threatening uveitis: a retrospective monocentric study of 45 patients. *Br J Ophthalmol* 2007;**91**:335–9.

British National Formulary, vol 59 London: British Medical Association/Royal Pharmaceutical Society 2010: 427.

Conn HO, Poynard T. Corticosteroids and peptic ulcer: meta-analysis of adverse events during steroid therapy. *J Intern Med* 1994;**236**:619–32.

Cunningham MA, Austin BA, Li Z, et al. LX211 (voclosporin) suppresses experimental uveitis and inhibits human T-cells. *Invest Ophthalmol Vis Sci* 2009;**50**:249–55.

Daniel E, Thorne JE, Newcomb CW, et al. Mycophenylate motefil for ocular inflammation. *Am J Ophthalmol* 2010;**149**:423–32.

Das-Baumik R, Jones NP. Low-dose intraocular triamcinolone for refractory uveitis and macular oedema. *Eye* 2006;**20**:934–7.

Davatchi F, Shahram F, Chams H, Akbarian M. Pulsed cyclophosphamide in ocular manifestations of Behcet's disease: a double-blind crossover study. *Arch Iranian Med* 2004;**7**:201–5.

De Nijs RN, Jacobs JW, Lems WF, et al. Alendronate or alfacalcidol in glucocorticoid-induced osteoporosis. *N Engl J Med* 2006;**355**:675–84.

Deuter CM, Kotter I, Gunaydin I, et al. Efficacy and tolerability of interferon alpha treatment in patients with chronic cystoid macular oedema due to non-infectious uveitis. *Br J Ophthalmol* 2009;**93**:906–13.

Diaz-Llopis M, Garcia-Delpech S, Salom D, et al. Adalimumab therapy for refractory uveitis: a pilot study. *J Ocul Pharmacol Ther* 2008;**24**:351–61.

Doycheva D, Deuter C, Stuebiger N, et al. Mycophenolate mofetil in the treatment of uveitis in children. *Br J Ophthalmol* 2007;**91**:180–4.

Emmanouil K, Athanassios A, Theofani A, et al. Effect of long-term calcitonin administration on steroid-induced osteoporosis after cardiac transplantation. *J Heart Lung Transplant* 2005;**24**:526–32.

Ferrante P, Ramsey A, Bunce C, Lightman S. Clinical trial to compare efficacy and side-effects of injection of posterior sub-Tenon triamcinolone versus orbital floor methylprednisolone in the management of posterior uveitis. *Clin Exp Ophthalmol* 2004;**32**:563–8.

Fiorelli VM, Bhat P, Foster CS. Non-steroidal anti-inflammatory therapy and recurrent acute anterior uveitis. *Ocular Immunol Inflamm* 2010;**18**:116–20.

Foeldvari I, Wierk A. Methotrexate is an effective treatment for chronic uveitis associated with juvenile idiopathic arthritis. *J Rheumatol* 2005;**32**:362–5.

Ford LT, Berg JD. Thiopurine S-methyltransferase (TPMT) assessment prior to starting thiopurine drug treatment; a pharmacogenetic test whose time has come. *J Clin Pathol* 2010;**63**:288–295.

Foster CS, DaVanzo R, Flynn TE, et al. Durezol (difluprednate ophthalmic emulsion 0.05%) compared with PredForte 1% ophthalmic suspension in the treatment of endogenous anterior uveitis. *J Ocul Pharmacol Ther* 2010;**26**:475–83.

Galor A, Margolis R, Brasil OM, et al. Adverse events after intravitreal triamcinolone in patients with and without uveitis. *Ophthalmology* 2007;**114**:1912–18.

Heiligenhaus A, Miserocchi E, Heinz C, et al. Treatment of severe uveitis associated with juvenile idiopathic arthritis with anti-CD20 monoclonal antibody (rituximab). *Rheumatology* 2011;Epub.

Hogan AC, McAvoy CE, Dick AD, Lee RW. Long-term efficacy and tolerance of tacrolimus for the treatment of uveitis. *Ophthalmology* 2007;**114**: 1000–6.

Jaffe GJ, McCallum RM, Branchaud B, et al. Long-term follow-up results of a pilot trial of a fluocinolone acetonide implant to treat posterior uveitis. *Ophthalmology* 2005;**112**:1192–8.

Jones NP. Anterior uveitis. In: Wormald R, Smeeth L, Henshaw K (eds), *Evidence-based Ophthalmology*. London: BMJ Books, 2004: 191–4.

Jones NP, Anderton LC, Cheong FM. Corticosteroid-induced osteoporosis in patients with uveitis. *Eye* 2002;**16**:587–93.

Kempen JH, Gangaputra S, Daniel E et al. Long-term risk of malignancy among patients treated with immunosuppressive agents for ocular inflammation: a critical assessment of the evidence. *Am J Ophthalmol* 2008;**146**:802–12.

Kok H, Lau C, Maycock N, et al. Outcome of intravitreal triamcinolone in uveitis. *Ophthalmology* 2005;**112**:1916e1–7.

Kose O, Dinc A, Simsek I. Randomized trial of pimecrolimus cream plus colchicine tablets versus colchicine tablets in the treatment of genital ulcers in Behçet's disease. *Dermatology* 2009;**218**:140–5.

Lee RW, Schewitz LP, Nicholson LB, et al. Steroid refractory CD4+ T cells in patients with sight-threatening uveitis. *Invest Ophthalmol Vis Sci* 2009;**50**:4273–8.

Lees B, Banks LM, Stevenson JC. Bone mass measurements. In: Stevenson JC, Lindsay R (eds), *Osteoporosis*. London: Chapman & Hall, 1998: 137–55.

Lovell DJ, Giannini EH, Reiff A, et al. Long-term efficacy and safety of etanercept in children with polyarticular-course juvenile rheumatoid arthritis: interim results from an ongoing multicenter, open-label, extended-treatment trial. *Arthrit Rheum* 2003;**48**:218–26.

McGhee CN. Pharmacokinetics of ophthalmic corticosteroids. *Br J Ophthalmol* 1992:**76**:681–4.

Maia M, Farah ME, Belfort RN, et al. Effects of intravitreal triamcinolone acetonide injection with and without preservative. *Br J Ophthalmol* 2007;**91**:1122–4.

Markomichelakis N, Delicha E, Masselos S, et al. A single infliximab infusion vs corticosteroids for acute panuveitis attacks in Behçet's disease: a comparative 4-week study. *Rheumatology* 2011;**50**:593–7.

Martin DF, DeBarge LR, Nussenblatt RB, et al. Synergistic effect of rapamycin and cyclosporin A in the treatment of experimental autoimmune uveoretinitis. *J Immunol* 1995;**154**:922–927.

Matthews J, Matthews D, Jones NP. Long-term ciclosporin for sight-threatening uveitis: efficacy and tolerability. *In J Ophthalmol* 2010;**58**:55–58.

Mazzantini M, Di Munno O, Sinigaglia L, et al. Effect of cyclosporine A on bone density in female rheumatoid arthritis patients: results from a multicenter, cross-sectional study. *Clin Exp Rheumatol* 2007;**25**:709–15.

Munoz-Fernandez S, Garcio-Aparicio AM, Hidalgo MN, et al. Methotrexate: an option for preventing the recurrence of acute anterior uveitis. *Eye* 2009;**23**:1130–3.

Murphy CC, Greiner K, Plskova J, et al. Cyclosporine vs tacrolimus therapy for posterior and intermediate uveitis. *Arch Ophthalmol* 2005;**123**:634–41.

Myung JS, Aaker GD, Kiss S. Treatment of noninfectious posterior uveitis with dexamethasone intravitreal implant. *Clin Ophthalmol* 2010;**4**:1423–6.

Neven B, Marvillet I, Terrada C, et al. Long-term efficacy of the interleukin-1 receptor antagonist anakinra in ten patients with neonatal-onset multisystem inflammatory disease/chronic infantile neurologic, cutaneous, articular syndrome. *Arthrit Rheum* 2010;**62**:258–67.

Nirmal HB, Bakliwal SR, Pawar SP. In-situ gel: new trends in controlled and sustained drug delivery system. *Int J Pharm Tech* Res 2010;**2**:1398–408.

Pavesio C, Zierhut M, Bairi K, et al. Evaluation of an intravitreal fluocinolone acetonide implant versus standard systemic therapy in noninfectious posterior uveitis. *Ophthalmology* 2010;**117**:567–75.

Piskova J, Greiner K, Forrester JV. Interferon-α as an effective treatment for noninfectious posterior uveitis and panuveitis. *Am J Ophthalmol* 2007;**144**:55–61.

Pujari SS, Kempen JH, Newcomb CW, et al. Cyclophosphamide for ocular inflammatory diseases. *Ophthalmology* 2010;**117**:356–65.

Richy F, Ethgen O, Bruyere O, Reginster J-Y. Efficacy of alfacalcidol and calcitriol in primary and cotricosteroid-0induced osteoporosis: a meta-analysis of their effects on bone mineral density and fracture rate. *Osteopor Int* 2004;**15**:301–10.

Robertson SM, Lang LS. The efficacy of leflunomide in S-antigen-induced autoimmune uveitis. *Inflamm Res* 1994;**41**(suppl 2):C274–5.

Roesel M, Gutfleisch M, Heinz C, et al. Orbital floor triamcinolone acetonide injections for the management of active non-infectious uveitis. *Eye* 2009a;**23**:910–14.

Roesel M, Guttfleisch M, Heinz C, et al. Intravitreal and orbital floor triamcinolone acetonide injections in non-infectious uveitis: a comparative study. *Ophthal Res* 2009b;**42**:81–6.

Rudwaleit M, Rodevand E, Holck P, et al. Adalimumab effectively reduces the rate of anterior uveitis flares in patients with active ankylosing spondylitis: results of a prospective open-label study. *Ann Rheum Dis* 2009;**68**:696–701.

Saag KG, Zanchetta JR, Adler RA, et al. Effects of teriparatide versus alendronate for treating glucocorticoid induced osteoporosis: thirty-six month results of a randomized, double-blind, controlled trial. *Arthrit Rheum* 2009;**60**:3346–55.

Sallam A, Corner RM, Chang JH, et al. Short-term safety and efficacy of intravitreal triamcinolone acetonide for uveitic macular oedema in children. *Arch Ophthalmol* 2008;**126**:200–5.

Sambrook PN, Kotowicz M, Nash P, et al. Prevention and treatment of glucocorticoid-induced osteoporosis: a comparison of calcitriol, vitamin D plus calcium, and alendronate plus calcium. *J Bone Mineral Res* 2003;**18**:919–24.

Samson CM, Waheed N, Baltatzis S, Foster CS. Methotrexate therapy for chronic noninfectious uveitis. *Ophthalmology* 2001;**108**:1134–9.

Schmeling H, Horneff G. Etanercept and uveitis in patients with juvenile idiopathic arthritis. *Rheumatology* 2005;**44**:1008–11.

Shanmuganathan VA, Casely EM, Raj D, et al. The efficacy of sirolimus in the treatment of patients with refractory uveitis. *Br J Ophthalmol* 2005;**89**:666–9.

Simonini G, Taddio A, Cattalini M, et al. Prevention of flare recurrences in childhood refractory chronic uveitis: an open-label comparative study of adalimumab versus infliximab. *Arthrit Care Res* 2011;**63**:612–8.

Smith JA, Thompson DJ, Whitcup SM, et al. A randomized, placebo-controlled, double-masked clinical trial of etanercept for the treatment of uveitis associated with juvenile idiopathic arthritis. *Arthrit Care Res* 2005;**53**:18–23.

Sobaci B, Erdem U, Durukan AH, et al. Safety and effectiveness of interferon alpha-2a in treatment of patients with Behçet's uveitis refractory to conventional treatments. *Ophthalmology* 2010;**117**:1430–5.

Sobrin L, Huang JJ, Christen W, et al. Daclizumab for treatment of birdshot chorioretinopathy. Arch *Ophthalmol* 2008;**126**:186–91.

Soheilian M, Karimi S, Ramezani A, Peyman GA. Pilot study of intravitreal injection of diclofenac for treatment of maculae edema of various etiologies. *Retina* 2010;**30**:509–15.

Stubinger N, Kotter I, Deuter C, Zierhut M. Behçet's disease: uveitis-therapy with interferon alpha2a – prospective clinical study in 33 patients. *Klin Monatsbl Augenheilkd* 2001;**218**:768–73.

Suhler EB, Smith JR, Giles TR, et al. Infliximab therapy for refractory uveitis: 2-year results of a prospective trial. *Arch Ophthalmol* 2009;**127**:819–22.

Taban M, Singh RP, Chung JY, et al. *Am J Ophthalmol* 2007;**144**:50–4.

Tamesis RR, Rodriguez A, Christen WG, et al. Systemic drug toxicity trends in immunosuppressive therapy of immune and inflammatory ocular disease. *Ophthalmology* 1996;**103**:768–75.

Taylor SR, Habot-Wilner Z, Pacheco P, Lightman S. Intraocular methotrexate in the treatment of uveitis and uveitic cystoid macular edema. *Ophthalmology* 2009;**116**:797–801 .

Tehrani NN, Saeed T, Murray PI. Deep intramuscular methylprednisolone for the treatment of cystoid macular oedema in uveitis. *Eye* 2000;**14**:691–4.

Teoh SC, Hogan AC, Dick AD, Lee RW. Mycophenolate mofetil for the treatment of uveitis. Am J Ophthalmol 2008;**146**:752–60.

Tugal-Tutkun I, Mudun A, Urgancioglu M, et al. Efficacy of infliximab in the treatment of uveitis that is resistant to treatment with the combination of azathioprine, cyclosporine and corticosteroids in Behçet's disease: an open-label trial. *Arthrit Rheum* 2005;**52**:2478–84.

Weijtens O, Feron EJ, Schoemaker RC, et al. High concentration of dexamethasone in aqueous and vitreous after subconjunctival injection. *Am J Ophthalmol* 1999;**128**:192–7.

Yazici H, Pazarli H, Barnes CG, et al. A controlled trial of azathioprine in Behçet's syndrome. *N Engl J Med* 1990;**322**:281–5.

Yoon SJ, Rhee DY, Marz JL, et al. Anatomic and visual outcomes of noninfectious endophthalmitis after intravitreal triamcinolone. *Am J Ophthalmol* 2009;**147**:1031–6.

Zakar-ur-Rab S, Mahmood S, Shukla M, et al. Systemic absorption of triamcinolone acetonide after posterior subTenon injection. *Am J Ophthalmol* 2009;**148**:414–19.

Zulian F, Balzarin M, Falcini F, et al. Abatacept for severe tumour necrosis factor alpha refractory juvenile idiopathic arthritis-related uveitis. *Arthrit Care Res* 2010;**62**:821–5.

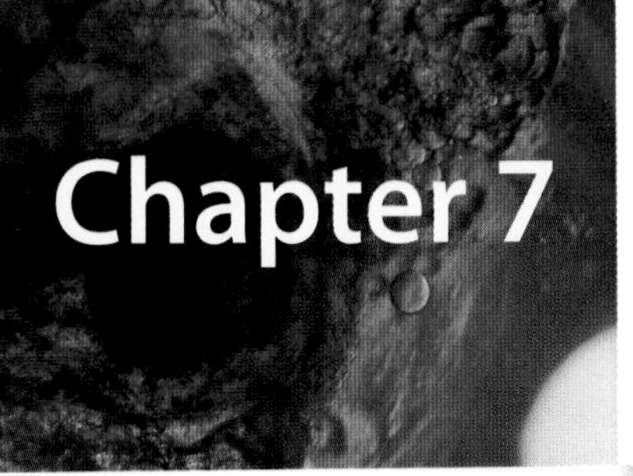

Chapter 7 Complications of uveitis and their management

Acute or chronic inflammation can lead to a variety of sequelae within the eye, especially related to fibrosis; some of these may be permanent and all can damage vision. To prevent or minimize such changes is the main aim of anti-inflammatory and immunosuppressive treatment as described in Chapter 6. Despite such treatment, complications are frequent in uveitis and their management can be very challenging, yet fundamental to the retention of useful vision.

ANTERIOR SEGMENT COMPLICATIONS

Band keratopathy

Band keratopathy is a degenerative accumulation of calcium salts, in the form of hydroxyapatite, in the corneal epithelial basement membrane, in Bowman's membrane and sometimes in the anterior stroma (**Fig. 7.1**). It is not uncommon in chronic anterior uveitis, but typically is limited to the corneal periphery at the 3 o'clock and 9 o'clock positions. More profound band keratopathy, with progression across the visual axis, is most common in children with uveitis and juvenile chronic arthritis, where it tends to be a particular feature in those with early onset and severe inflammation, and it is among the important causes of visual loss (Woreta et al. 2007). At its most severe, corneal epithelial erosions may occur, with recurrent pain and possible superinfection. In the uveitis clinic the most common reasons to treat band keratopathy are to enhance vision and sometimes to prevent amblyopia in the affected child, and for comfort in the adult who usually has longstanding poor vision.

Traditionally band keratopathy has been removed by the application of a dilute solution of disodium ethylenediamine tetraacetate (EDTA) to the exposed calcium salts, which chelates and removes the opacities. Solutions from 0.4% to 2% have been used. Following epithelial debridement, pledgets dipped in EDTA are wiped repeatedly across the affected area, combined with surface scraping. The method is time-consuming, and for more dense deposits must be combined with more vigorous physical removal, either with a blade or a large-diameter corneal burr. As most uveitis-associated band keratopathy occurs in children, this procedure requires general anesthesia. Postoperative pain can be substantial and intravenous and/or oral diclofenac is usually effective. Recently the application of amniotic membrane after debridement has been found to enhance comfort, facilitate epithelialization and reduce the rate of band recurrence (Anderson et al. 2001).

The excimer laser may also be used to remove band keratopathy. The method is rapid and effective and is tolerated by adults under topical anesthesia. There is a significant hypermetropic shift averaging +1.4 D after treatment (O'Brart et al. 1993). Reaccumulation of calcium salts is not uncommon in those with chronic uveitis, but re-treatment gives cumulative refractive change, usually limiting excimer treatment to two episodes.

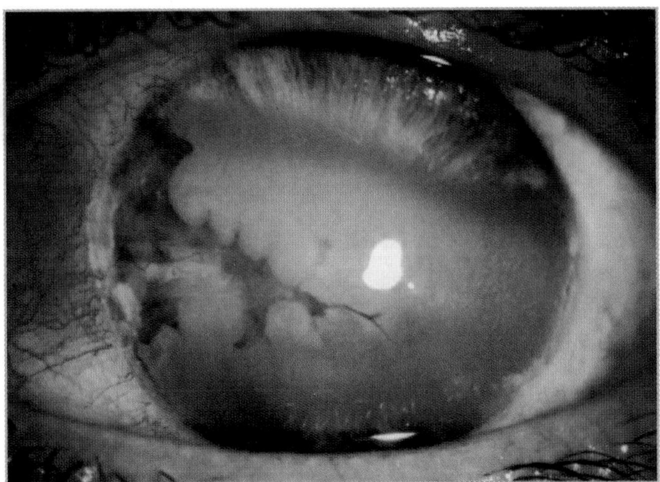

Figure 7.1 Severe band keratopathy in a patient with lupus-associated chronic uveitis.

Corneal decompensation

The corneal endothelium in the region of keratic precipitates (KPs) in acute anterior uveitis is known to be deranged, albeit temporarily, and doubtless recurrent attacks will lead to a degree of endothelial cell loss. However, there are no firm data on the longitudinal behavior of a corneal endothelium in chronic or severe recurrent uveitis, and in clinical practice it is perhaps surprising that corneal decompensation is so uncommonly seen.

In our experience corneal decompensation in patients with uveitis is rare, but is least uncommon in very chronic uveitis, usually sympathetic uveitis or Fuchs' heterochromic uveitis. It is rarely seen in corneal endotheliitis and in herpetic keratouveitis and is a well-recognized feature of chronic cytomegalovirus (CMV) anterior uveitis. As expected the histology of cornea in sympathetic uveitis often shows not only endothelial but Bowman's membrane disruption and calcification (Shankar et al. 2010). The cornea may be involved in heterochromic uveitis in various ways, and localized peripheral decompensation with edema may be seen (Jones 1991) despite an apparently normal central endothelial cell count. Large corneal endothelial plaques are a feature in a few patients, and occasionally frank endothelial dystrophy develops (**Fig. 7.2**). This may be a coincidence of two separate diseases, but is therefore rather surprising in a patient's fifth decade. In a cohort of over 300 patients with heterochromic uveitis here in Manchester, 4 patients have undergone penetrating keratoplasty and a further 7 show a degree of decompensation.

The survival of corneal grafts in patients with uveitis is poorly studied, although newly acquired uveitis has been reported to lead to graft failure. Endothelial survival is known to be compromised in those with herpetic keratouveitis (Lee and Kim 2009). Uveitis can only be a deleterious presence to endothelium after keratoplasty, and stringent control of inflammation before and after surgery is clearly required.

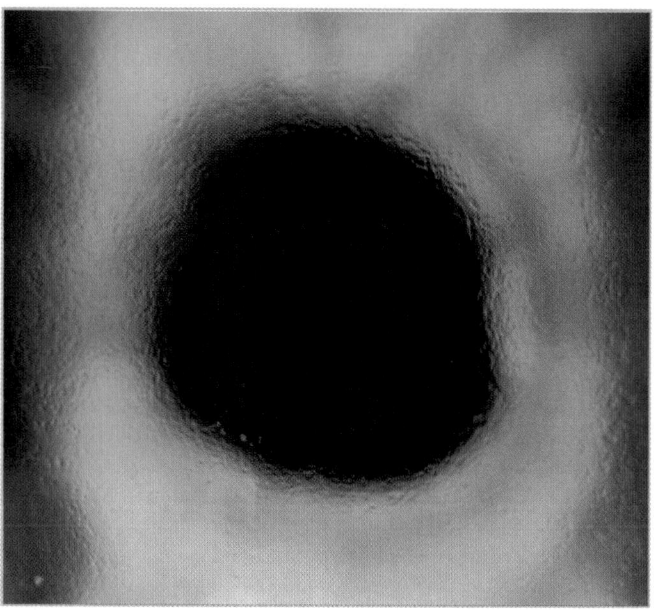

Figure 7.2 Frank endothelial dystrophy in a 45-year-old patient with Fuchs' heterochromic uveitis, showing a few keratic precipitates in addition to endothelial changes.

Anterior segment fibrosis and adhesions

The release of fibrinogen into the anterior chamber (AC), with consequent adhesion formation, is a common accompaniment to recurrent acute anterior uveitis, and the need to prevent cicatricial synechiae by the use of both mydriatics and topical steroids is well recognized. Less well appreciated is the insidious formation of adhesions in any patient with chronic anterior uveitis where there is a significant breakdown of the blood–ocular barrier. The progressive formation of posterior synechiae gradually occludes the pupil, may form a fibrotic pupillary membrane *(***Fig. 7.3***)* and may go on to close all aqueous flow, causing iris bombé and acute glaucoma *(***Fig. 7.4***)*. The gradual formation of peripheral anterior synechiae is an important cause of secondary glaucoma, especially in chronic anterior uveitis *(***Fig. 7.5***)*. For this and other reasons it is important not to under-treat those with apparently mild chronic anterior uveitis, and the continued use of regular mydriasis, although inconvenient, may also be important.

Some patients with chronic uveitis develop posterior synechiae not only at the pupil margin, but over a considerable part of the posterior iris surface. This phenomenon is particularly seen in the uveitis associated with juvenile idiopathic arthritis (JIA). In these circumstances classical iris bombé is not possible, but, following occlusio, peripheral, sectoral or irregular iris bowing demonstrates

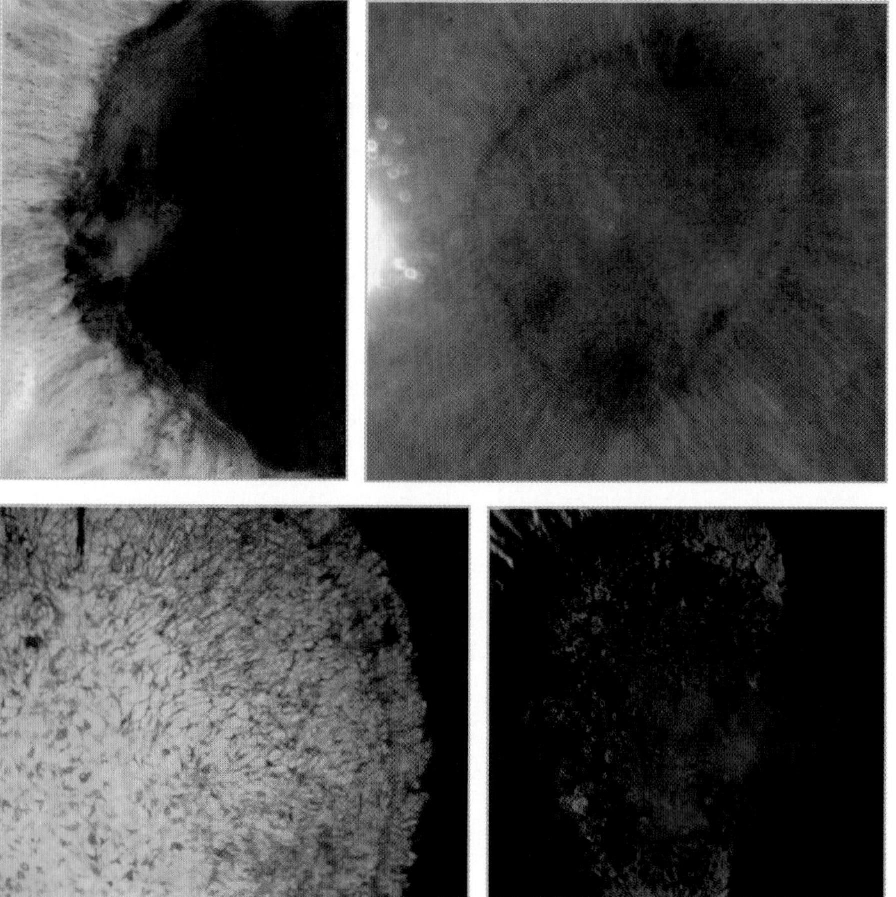

Figure 7.3 A selection of pupils compromised by chronic uveitis, causing posterior synechiae, pupil membrane formation and occlusio.

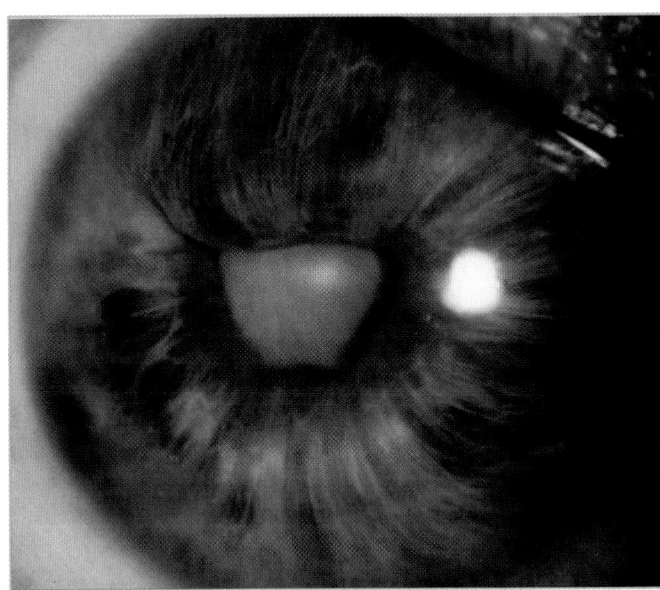

Figure 7.4 Iris bombé following progressive posterior synechia formation in chronic anterior uveitis. (Courtesy of Mr E O'Donoghue.)

the location of wide posterior synechiae. Primary or secondary angle closure may still follow, and it may be necessary to create iridotomies in selected locations to permit aqueous flow. In these circumstances, making a judgment on the relative contributions to secondary glaucoma may be a challenge. To attempt to prevent all of these anterior segment fibrotic complications, adequate and sustained anti-inflammatory treatment, with adequate mydriasis where necessary, must be given.

Mydriasis and cycloplegia

There is a range of potency and duration for the anticholinergic mydriatics, but the usefulness of a sympathomimetic should not be overlooked. For those with acute iridocyclitis and ocular pain, both cycloplegia and mydriasis are essential; in contrast, those with mild chronic uveitis may need intermittent mydriasis, but daytime cycloplegia is an inconvenience that can be minimized. For maximal mydriasis to break posterior synechiae, both cholinergic sphincter paralysis and sympathomimetic dilator stimulation are required.

All of the anticholinergic mydriatics cause cycloplegia, and in those with acute uveitis this is an essential combination. Atropine 1% is the most potent and long lasting; the effect of a single drop may last for 2 weeks, but this is not usually a disadvantage in such eyes. The exception is the eye with a rather shallow anterior chamber, where posterior synechiae may form even with the pupil dilated; in this situation an early decision must be made (once having broken any synechiae) to retain pupil mobility to prevent adhesion formation. In those with a normal depth AC, full mydriasis will completely clear the pupil of the lens surface and adhesions in this circumstance will be exceptional. For less severe acute uveitis, cyclopentolate 1% is frequently substituted, probably too often; when seeing referred patients with non-settling severe anterior uveitis our first action is often to administer more potent mydriasis. Phenylephrine 2.5% enhances mydriasis when used in combination with an anticholinergic. In situations where very potent mydriasis is necessary, Mydricaine subconjunctival injection (atropine, epinephrine and procaine) is excellent, especially for those attending for the first time with severe anterior uveitis. The following mydriatic and cycloplegic regimens are examples of the techniques used for patients attending this clinic:

Acute painful unilateral anterior uveitis with fibrin deposition

Treatment if with immediate mydriasis using atropine 1% and phenylephrine 2.5%, with local heat. The patient is observed for at least 30–60 min to attempt to break incipient posterior synechiae. If unsuccessful, the drops are repeated. If still unsuccessful, and for those with particularly severe fibrinous uveitis, subconjunctival Mydricaine is helpful, usually combined with betamethasone. Atropine 1% four times daily is prescribed for at least 1 week, changing to cyclopentolate 1% four time daily and reducing the dose in tandem with recovery.

Mydriasis for clinical examination

Tropicamide 1% alone is usually adequate for posterior pole examination, with phenylephrine 2.5% added for comprehensive funduscopy, or in patients with diabetes, or in those with deeply pigmented irides. The combination acts rapidly and gives more effective mydriasis (especially important for those requiring peripheral fundal examination).

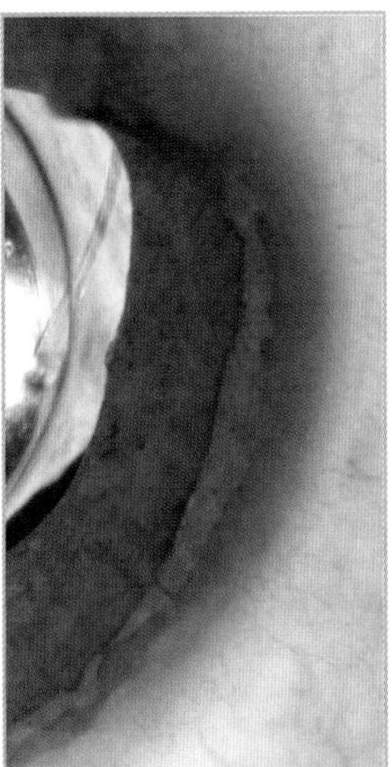

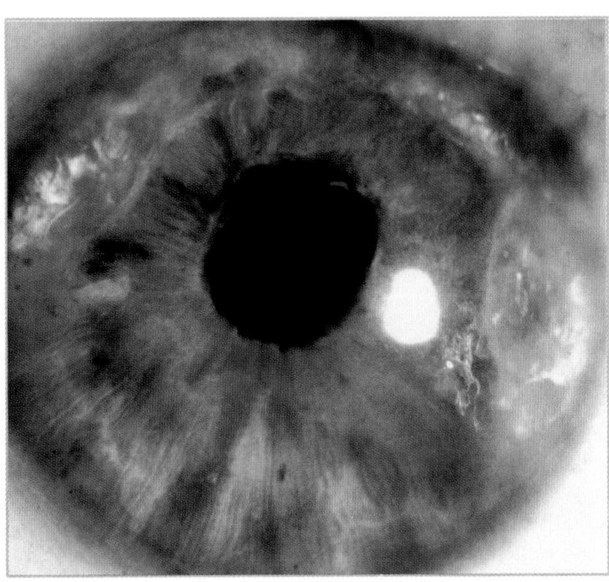

Figure 7.5 Two eyes with chronic uveitis demonstrating extensive peripheral anterior synechiae; the eye on the left from 1 o'clock to 6 o'clock (40% of angle), the eye on the right from 9 o'clock to 5 o'clock (65% of angle).

For regular attenders who do not require pre-dilation tests at the next visit and who understand the effect of the drops, it is useful to give single-dose applicators for self-instillation before attendance. The enhanced speed of consultation is often welcome to both patient and doctor.

Mydriasis for cataract surgery

Cyclopentolate 1% and phenylephrine 2.5% are first instilled 60–90 min before surgery, and instilled again after 15 or 30 min if the pupil is not fixed and dilated. It remains useful to instill mydriatics in those with fixed posterior synechiae, as dilator tension will permit some dilation during surgery after dividing the adhesions. Phenylephrine should not be applied more than twice preoperatively because corneal epithelial opacification will follow and compromise surgical visibility.

Mydriasis in chronic anterior uveitis

We aim for the minimum safe level of mydriasis, sparing daytime cycloplegia if possible. Theoretically, a sympathomimetic would be ideal, but most ophthalmologists would be unhappy to prescribe phenylephrine for regular instillation because of the possibility of systemic effects, especially after inadvertent overdosage. All anticholinergics cause cycloplegia, but it may be possible to minimize their effect. For those patients with chronic uveitis who are felt to be at risk of posterior synechia formation, cyclopentolate 0.5% or 1% at bedtime may be adequate. This will still lead to a degree of cycloplegia early the following morning, and this can sometimes be a problem for children at school. If this is the case, then bedtime tropicamide 1% may prove adequate. In some situations the inconvenience of cycloplegia must be tolerated in order to prevent posterior synechia formation, and compliance will be enhanced if the patient fully understands this principle; if necessary reading glasses must be provided for those with ongoing cycloplegia.

Iridotomy and iridectomy

The introduction of the neodymium:yttrium–aluminium–garnet (Nd-YAG) laser has rendered surgical peripheral iridectomy, once a common procedure, virtually redundant in patients with narrow-angle glaucoma. However, in patients with chronic uveitis, over half the laser iridotomies performed become closed by adhesions and fibrosis (Spencer et al. 2001) and this may occur at any time after treatment, with a tendency towards recurrent acute glaucoma. It is our practice to instill four times daily or more topical steroid for 3 days before laser treatment and four time daily to 2-hourly afterwards for some days.

If closure of an iridotomy has already occurred once, the risk at a second attempt may be reduced by combining Nd-YAG iridotomy with argon laser applications to the iris surface; some suggest gentle diffuse argon to precede YAG, whereas others apply rather more argon near the edge of the YAG-created iridotomy, which causes clear immediate widening of the ostium. Despite this, repeated closure may occur. If acute glaucoma recurs after Nd-YAG iridotomy in chronic uveitis, it is preferable to perform surgical peripheral iridectomy, which is less likely to become occluded. Sometimes such problems precipitate lens extraction, which is itself curative.

Glaucoma

Glaucoma is a common secondary feature of uveitis, affecting almost 20% of patients in our clinic, and causes are multifactorial, often in a single patient. It may be a chronic open-angle glaucoma caused by progressive trabecular sclerosis, as is common in Fuchs' heterochromic uveitis, herpetic uveitis and some others. Chronic glaucoma may also develop as a result of progressive peripheral anterior synechiae. Intermittent pressure rises may accompany exacerbations of some forms of uveitis, classically in the Posner–Schlossman syndrome, but also where inflammatory exudate compromises angle drainage, e.g. in typical granulomatous sarcoid uveitis. Ciliary body swelling or ciliochoroidal effusion may lead to glaucoma by shallowing the peripheral anterior chamber, and this may be the mechanism in several conditions including the uveal effusion syndrome and the acute phase of the Vogt–Koyanagi–Harada (VKH) syndrome. Glaucoma may be lens induced. Many uveitic eyes undergoing cataract surgery appear more prone to postoperative glaucoma. Acute glaucoma may arise because of iris bombé. Topical steroids themselves may cause glaucoma. Some etiological forms of uveitis have been associated with a higher risk of glaucoma, but the reasons for these associations may be diverse. Each case of glaucoma should be diagnosed and managed on the basis of individual findings rather than a presumed generic association.

Identifying the mechanism of glaucoma in these patients is challenging and, if not approached carefully at the outset, becomes more difficult with time. It is particularly important to identify, at the first opportunity, those who are true steroid responders. We enhance patient explanation in this clinic by the use of an information pamphlet (see patient information pamphlets on the attached disk).

Steroid-induced glaucoma

The rise in intraocular pressure (IOP) seen in a substantial minority of patients after topical steroid administration is caused by reduced trabecular outflow. A significant rise in IOP may be detected in up to a third of patients receiving topical steroid treatment, but a substantial rise is much less common. It is known that glucocorticoids can induce myocilin within the cells of the trabecular meshwork and canal of Schlemm (Clark et al. 2001) and, although the precise mechanism of this protein complex is not fully understood, recent advances have been well summarized (Kersey and Broadway 2006).

Steroid-induced glaucoma in patients with uveitis is most commonly caused by topical steroids, because first they are the most commonly used form of treatment, and second they have a greater effect on outflow facility than the systemically administered drug. However, some of the most dramatic pressure rises have occurred after the administration of peribulbar or intraocular steroid injections, and these techniques should be used with caution if at all in those with known steroid-induced pressure rise, or where treatment for raised IOP is already being administered. Indeed it has been suggested that the risk of severe IOP rise after intravitreal steroid injection can be minimized by selecting patients following a provocative trial of topical prednisolone acetate (Hollands et al. 2010).

The great majority of patients who develop steroid-induced glaucoma do so within 4–6 weeks of starting topical steroid treatment, although a very small proportion may develop it at any stage thereafter and, even when developing very late, a pressure rise may be dramatic. For this reason, there is never a 'safe' period after which IOP monitoring becomes unnecessary. If it is possible to discontinue steroid treatment, IOP almost always returns to normal within days or weeks, but in a few patients may remain permanently raised.

It may be difficult to determine the cause of glaucoma in a patient with uveitis. In a patient who develops it only after starting steroid treatment, the cause should be established as soon as possible, with careful gonioscopy and, if possible, amendment of steroid dosage. It is rarely possible merely to discontinue steroid treatment in a patient with uveitis, and a balance must be drawn between the risks and benefits of a reduction in steroid dosage. It is not acceptable to reduce steroid frequency or potency, or to choose a steroid with less intraocular penetration, if this allows an unacceptable level of intraocular inflammation; the long-term sequelae of this approach are likely to be worse than the immediate problem of steroid-induced glaucoma. An approach to this dilemma is discussed in Chapter 6.

For many reasons it is always the aim of the ophthalmologist to keep steroid treatment, however administered, to the minimum safe level. If this approach alone cannot reverse steroid-induced glaucoma, the condition usually responds well to standard topical anti-glaucoma medication. In only a few patients has formal drainage surgery proved necessary but sometimes it has been necessary to apply emergency cycloablation. Almost all uveitis patients proceeding to trabeculectomy have other causes of glaucoma.

Medical treatment of glaucoma

As shown above, there are many mechanisms of secondary glaucoma in uveitis. An appreciation of the underlying mechanism of glaucoma in the individual patient is vital, and will ensure appropriate treatment. Those with raised pressure as a direct result of intraocular inflammation will require anti-inflammatory treatment. However, most patients will, either temporarily or long term, require topical anti-glaucoma medication. Currently available drugs include the following.

Topical β blockers

Topical timolol was first introduced in 1978, and there are now several alternatives. The drugs act by reducing aqueous secretion, and seem to have no effect on aqueous outflow. The pharmacology, topical and systemic effects, and drug compatibility are admirably dealt with in many sources. The drugs are extremely effective in the management of secondary open-angle glaucoma in uveitis. There are well-documented systemic advantages to the use of the β_1-selective drug betaxolol in open-angle glaucoma in elderly people, but for younger patients timolol is more commonly used. Granulomatous uveitis has been reported as a complication of high-dose metipranolol treatment, but this drug is now largely historic.

Adrenergics

Apraclonidine is an α_2-adrenergic agonist which appears to increase aqueous outflow and to decrease episcleral venous pressure (Toris et al. 1995). It has a rapid onset of action and therefore has most often been used in single doses to counteract pressure rises following intraocular surgical or laser procedures, but it has also been used for longer periods in combination with other topical anti-glaucoma medication with significant pressure-lowering effect, at least in the early stages. The effect may diminish over a period of months and this, together with the fairly high rate of late-onset allergy, leads to its cessation in at least half the patients within a year (Araujo et al. 1995). However, the drug (at either 0.5 or 1%) often proves useful in the short term as additional topical treatment in particularly difficult uveitic glaucoma, especially where attempts are being made to control intraocular inflammation rather better before formal drainage surgery is performed.

The older topical adrenergics tended to be poorly tolerated by patients with active anterior uveitis, frequently provoking irritation with conjunctival hyperemia. In addition to this, the well-documented problems of conjunctival fibrosis and bleb failure after trabeculectomy, in patients using topical adrenergics preoperatively, merely added to the already high risks of surgical failure in those with uveitis who do proceed to drainage surgery. Apraclonidine may also provoke adverse reactions but remains invaluable in some patients in the short term.

Brimonidine is another clonidine analog, with enhanced α_2-adrenergic selectivity compared to apraclonidine, which appears also to enhance uveoscleral outflow (Wilensky et al. 1996). No published studies assess either brimonidine or apraclonidine in patients with uveitis, but in primary glaucoma the two drugs have very similar effect (Maus et al. 1999). Anecdotally brimonidine has been reported to cause granulomatous uveitis, but there are no published suggestions that pre-existing intraocular inflammation is worsened by either drug, and that reflects our own experience.

Miotics

Pilocarpine is a cholinergic miotic that reduces IOP by movement of the scleral spur, enhancing aqueous drainage. Although highly effective, it is often poorly tolerated in the ageing primary glaucoma group, and much less well tolerated in the generally young group of patients with uveitis. The accompanying miosis is often unacceptable for several reasons: accommodative and darkening effects may be disabling; posterior synechia formation may be provoked; the drug provokes the release of inflammatory enzymes; and iris- or ciliary body-induced discomfort is likely to be enhanced in those with anterior uveitis of any degree of severity. The drug is only rarely appropriate in the patient with uveitis.

Carbonic anhydrase inhibitors

There will be occasions in the management of uveitic glaucoma when medical control becomes extremely difficult, yet there is a legitimate need to delay surgical intervention, perhaps because of increased intraocular inflammation. In these circumstances, oral acetazolamide can be extremely useful. Difficult uveitic glaucoma is one of the few permissible indications for longer-term treatment with acetazolamide despite its potential side effects, including renal calculus formation. It is often very well tolerated in children. It is our practice to give acetazolamide 250 mg three times over 18 h after cataract surgery in uveitis, when a postoperative pressure spike is anticipated, e.g. after long-lasting surgery or where a high phako power has been used.

The topical carbonic anhydrase inhibitors dorzolamide and brinzolamide inhibit ciliary body carbonic anhydrase and thus reduce aqueous secretion, but systemic side effects as seen with acetazolamide are avoided. However, tachycardias, dyspnea and allergies are sometimes seen. It is not usually appropriate as a first-line treatment in uveitic glaucoma but is often added in combination with timolol. No studies exist specifically for uveitic glaucoma, but the beneficial effect on both ocular blood flow and visual field preservation has been demonstrated for eyes with primary glaucoma, of combined timolol and topical carbonic anhydrase inhibitor (Gugleta 2010), dorzolamide being regarded as superior to brinzolamide.

Prostaglandins

The introduction of latanoprost, a prostaglandin $F_{2\alpha}$, in the 1990s gave an important new choice of treatment for the primary glaucomas. Theoretically the application of a drug with potential proinflammatory effect to an eye with pre-existing inflammation was a source of concern, and its first tentative usage in uveitis led to a succession of anecdotal reports of exacerbated anterior uveitis, induced granulomatous uveitis or macular edema. Our own few experiences of treatment-resistant macular edema following soon after the introduction of latanoprost led to a period of caution, since overcome by greater experience; latanoprost is probably not responsible for an increased incidence of inflammatory events in those with uveitic glaucoma (Marchomikelakis et al. 2010).

Prostaglandin analogs may demonstrate measurable disruption of the blood–ocular barrier. In comparison with latanoprost, neither travoprost nor bimatoprost disrupts the blood–ocular barrier as much, at least in eyes with primary glaucoma (Cellini et al. 2004), and are therefore theoretically a better option in inflamed eyes. No clinical advantage over latanoprost has been demonstrated, however. As for latanoprost, bimatoprost seems well tolerated in eyes with uveitis (Fortuna et al. 2008). There are few comparative data for unoprostone and no information on its use in uveitis.

Prostaglandin analogs some years ago replaced topical β blockers as the first-line choice of topical hypotensive agent for primary open-angle glaucoma and ocular hypertension, and many management guidelines are now encouraging an early move to drainage surgery after the failure of only this single agent. The management of uveitic glaucoma, however, remains more complex and difficult, many young patients remaining on several topical medications for a considerable period before surgery, with its high failure and complication rate, is attempted. Our summative choice of topical treatments in order of preference (contraindications excepted) is currently: β blocker → dorzolamide → travoprost → apraclonidine → acetazolamide. We prefer to avoid using prostaglandins unilaterally, and the order may differ in children. The deleterious effects of topical hypotensive agents and their co-constituents on conjunctiva are well reported (Broadway and Chang 2001). However, it is also understood that topical steroid treatment ameliorates some of these effects (Broadway et al. 1996) and therefore the risk balance is not well understood for those patients with uveitis. At some stage, however, the decision may be made to intervene with laser or surgery, and these techniques are discussed below.

Selective laser trabeculoplasty

Argon laser trabeculoplasty was in vogue for the management of primary open-angle glaucoma during the 1980s, but had largely been dismissed as a temporizing measure that merely delayed the decision to perform formal drainage surgery. It had been used to manage uveitic glaucoma with disappointing results. Interest has been regenerated by the introduction of selective laser trabeculoplasty (SLT), a relatively minor modification of the original technique, the superiority in efficacy of which is not universally accepted. The mode of action remains unclear for either method. Although SLT applied over 180–360° can be effective for a period, a degree of induced anterior uveitis is usual (Nagar et al. 2005), and the potential for peripheral anterior synechia formation in eyes with pre-existing inflammation is a source of concern. No formal studies have examined the potential for SLT in eyes with uveitis, and we have to date avoided its use in these eyes.

Cyclodestruction

Eyes with chronic uveitis and glaucoma may have, in addition to a reduced outflow facility, reduced aqueous secretion because of ciliary body damage. Surgical methods to reduce aqueous secretion may therefore have a very narrow therapeutic window, and cyclodestructive procedures have always been associated with a high rate of postoperative phthisis. Historically, cyclocryotherapy was associated with postoperative uveitis, and was a most unattractive procedure in those with pre-existing intraocular inflammation. High-power Nd-YAG cyclodestruction caused sympathetic uveitis in some eyes (Lam et al. 1992). The cyclodiode lasers are by no means benign methods free of induced inflammation, but in comparison have crossed the border of acceptability for eyes with uveitic glaucoma in well-defined circumstances.

In eyes with uveitic glaucoma, cyclodestruction is usually confined to the emergency management of intractable raised IOP. The trend is towards longer, lower-energy applications. The avoidance of 'pops' reduces post-treatment inflammation. We have no objection to the application of 24 burns over 360° as a single application in most uveitic eyes but regard repeat applications as carrying a high risk of induced phthisis, especially in very longstanding uveitis. The risk is not necessarily immediate; phthisis may occur earlier than would otherwise have been the case, at any future date. In practice, therefore, each cyclodiode treatment applied only in urgent situations tends to be followed whenever safe by a formal drainage procedure. We tend to use oral steroid in addition to subconjunctival injection to manage post-laser inflammation.

Glaucoma drainage surgery

Trabeculectomy

Trabeculectomy has a high failure rate in patients with inflammatory glaucoma, possibly the highest failure rate of any risk group (Noble et al. 2007). The use of anti-metabolites goes some way towards prolonging efficacy and fairly high success rates have been claimed (Towler et al. 2000) but others assert that failure rates remain at a level which should encourage primary drainage tube implantation in this group. The higher risk of complications associated with the use of mitomycin C (MMC) or implantation devices makes this a difficult choice for the individual, usually a young patient, with uveitis. Whichever surgical approach is used, it is universally agreed that, as for cataract surgery, stringent control of inflammation before and after surgery enhances success rates and minimizes subsequent failure and recurrent inflammation.

Most experience has accrued with 5-fluorouracil (5FU), which is applied to the conjunctiva and sclera for 2–3 min during surgery and also if necessary as a repeated postoperative subconjunctival injection. For higher-risk glaucomas there has been a substantial trend away from 5FU and towards MMC. It may offer better protection against bleb failure in uveitic glaucomas (Prata et al. 1994) and typically results in an avascular bleb (**Fig. 7.6**) but is associated with a significant complication rate including postoperative hypotony, choroidal detachment, macular edema, cataract, bleb leakage and endophthalmitis. In this clinic, primary trabeculectomy in patients with uveitis uses 5FU as the anti-metabolite and our postoperative IOP control and bleb survival results (Chawla et al. 2012) are comparable with published studies of either MMC-enhanced trabeculectomy or primary drainage tube implantation.

The problems of bleb failure in uveitic glaucoma are not limited to the immediate postoperative period, because inflammatory mediators

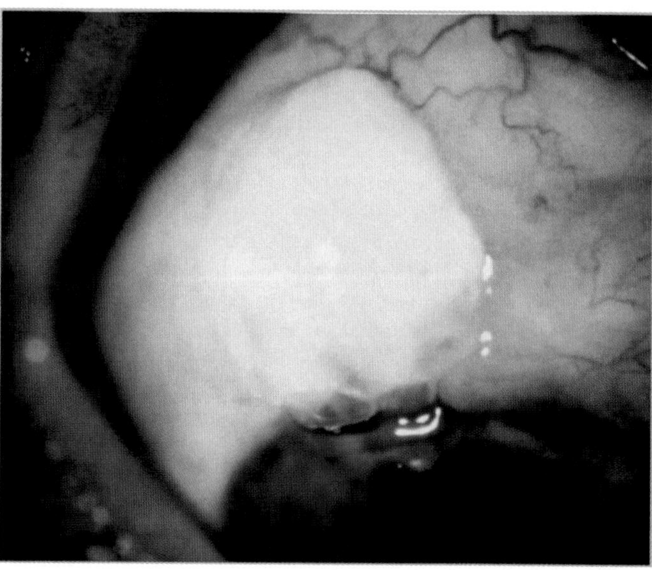

Figure 7.6 An avascular trabeculectomy bleb following the use of mitomycin C.

and cells are constantly present in those with chronic uveitis. Early success rates in drainage surgery may not be maintained over time, and a continual attrition rate is to be expected. This is very problematic in a group of patients who are on average 30–40 years younger than most patients undergoing drainage surgery. Bleb needling with subconjunctival 5-FU or MMC injection is a well-accepted method for re-establishing drainage (Broadway et al. 2004); although there are few data on success rates specifically for patients with uveitis, it remains a valid intervention in this group, and one that is used regularly in this clinic.

Repeated trabeculectomy progressively uses available AC angle and sclera and is recognized as a poor option after primary failure, even in primary open-angle glaucoma. It is not performed in this clinic for patients with uveitis, who undergo drainage tube implantation as a second procedure if necessary.

Deep sclerectomy and other forms of drainage surgery

Non-AC-penetrating deep sclerectomy carries a potential advantage in patients with uveitis, in that no direct intraocular trauma is sustained, and in particular no iris is abscised. It may offer equivalent efficacy to trabeculectomy in such patients (Dupas et al. 2010) and the reduced incidence of complications may suggest it as a valid alternative (Auer et al. 2004). The use of scleral collagen or other implantation has not been specifically studied in patients with uveitis. A brief early foray into trabeculodialysis for uveitic glaucoma failed to displace trabeculectomy as a first-choice procedure in these patients. Viscocanalostomy has been suggested as a possible alternative to open drainage (Miserocchi et al. 2004) but has few adherents.

Glaucoma drainage implants

Despite the use of anti-metabolite enhancement during trabeculectomy for uveitic glaucoma, there is a substantial long-term failure rate. The evolution of glaucoma drainage devices has encouraged some to recommend their usage during a primary procedure in uveitic glaucoma. It is our current practice to use primary drainage devices in children with uveitic glaucoma and sometimes in young adults with additional risk factors. For others with uveitic glaucoma, if enhanced trabeculectomy has failed despite needling with 5FU, then a drainage device (**Fig. 7.7**) is implanted.

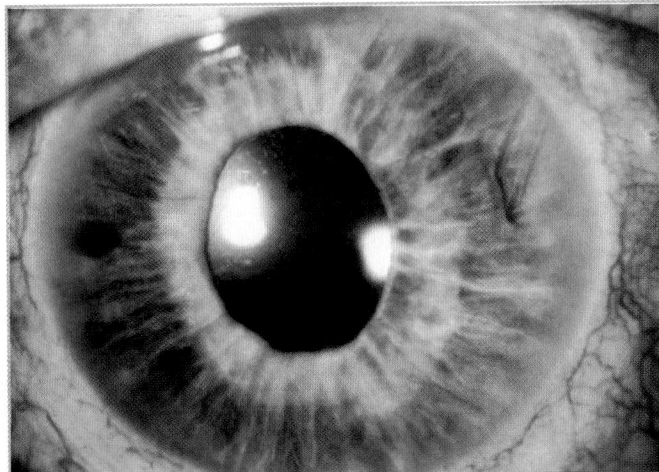

Figure 7.7 The intracameral end of a single-plate Molteno drainage implant in seen in this pseudophakic eye with chronic uveitis.

Since the introduction of the first Molteno tube in the 1960s, a well-recognized range of complications has accompanied such devices, including hypotony, choroidal effusion, cystoid macular edema, corneal decompensation, conjunctival erosion and endophthalmitis. Nevertheless, their use in high-risk glaucomas is well accepted. The Molteno tube itself had some success (Hill et al. 1993) but later devices including the Baerveldt implant permit a reasonable success rate in uveitic glaucoma (Ceballos et al. 2002) with fewer complications. The Ahmed valve has also been used with reasonable results, although replacement is more often necessary in those with chronic inflammation (Rachmiel et al. 2008), with valve occlusion being, predictably, the most common reason for failure (Ozdal et al. 2006). Added topical medications often remain necessary (Papadaki et al. 2007). The advent of mini-shunts is of future interest but their usefulness in actively inflamed eyes is likely to be limited by occlusive tendencies.

The surgical management of uveitic glaucoma evolves gradually into better outcomes with a realization that aggressive intervention in association with exemplary medical control of inflammation is paramount. In the meantime studies into the effectiveness of additional perioperative treatments are under way; although studies into anti-transforming growth factor β (TGF-β) monoclonal antibody (MAb) have been disappointing, work with anti-vascular endothelial growth factor (VEGF) MAb is more promising, and work on the anti-fibroblast activity of tetrandrine is interesting. The results of their efficacy in uveitic glaucoma require further study.

Uveitis–glaucoma–hyphema syndrome

During the 1970s and 1980s the majority of intraocular lenses (IOLs) were fixated to the iris by closed loops with or without suturing, necessitating chronic iris touch. A small minority of such eyes developed chronic, usually mild uveitis with associated recurrent hyphema, ranging from microscopic to florid and persistent, and associated with raised IOP; the appropriately named uveitis–glaucoma–hyphema (UGH) syndrome came into being. It was recognized that chronic iris trauma by IOL material was the provocation. Although the syndrome was by no means unique to eyes with pre-existing uveitis, such eyes had the capability of generating aggressive and sight-threatening problems (**Fig. 7.8**). Lens explantation was necessary and such experiences contributed to the then prevalent view that IOL implantation was unsafe for eyes with uveitis. Following the move to sulcus-fixated IOLs, the UGH syndrome became much less common and, although now rare when endocapsular IOL fixation is initially achieved, ultrasound biomicroscopy clearly demonstrates that subsequent haptic migration with chronic trauma to posterior iris or pars plicata is a constant feature (Piette et al. 2002). It has been argued that the implantation of sulcus-fixated large-optic IOLs in eyes with uveitis minimizes the risk of iris/IOL entrapment and posterior synechiae, but the risk of frequent posterior iris touch and occasional UGH syndrome almost certainly outweighs this advantage. Endocapsular fixation clearly minimizes the risk; it is also likely that the lesser force expressed on the capsule equator by one-piece injectable acrylic IOLs reduces the possibility of erosion and subsequent uveal touch.

Cataract

Cataract may be caused either by intraocular inflammation or its treatment (most frequently both), and is a common and important complication of uveitis. It has been a privilege to witness developments over the last 25 years that have transformed the outlook from

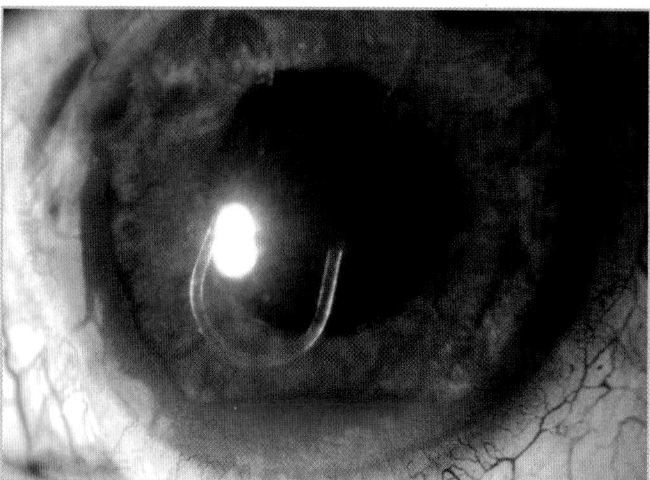

Figure 7.8 The implantation of an iris-loop intraocular lens in an eye with chronic uveitis has led to worsened uveitis, glaucoma and hyphema (UGH) syndrome with associated rubeosis. Removal of the IOL was necessary.

surgery. In the 1980s, complications were often severe and virtually universal, IOL implantation usually being disastrous. These problems have been progressively tempered by developments in surgical technique, instrumentation and IOL design. A proper appreciation of the risk factors involved, and an understanding of the crucial importance of controlling inflammation pre- and perioperatively, has transformed the prognosis. As a result, cataract surgery is undertaken earlier in the individual patient and IOL implantation is almost always safe (Rahman and Jones 2005). Nevertheless, chronic uveitis is more likely than any other preoperative risk factor to lead to a problematic inflammatory response after cataract surgery. Within the broad field of 'uveitis' there is a wide spectrum, ranging from the relatively benign Fuchs' heterochromic uveitis at one end (in which phakoemulsification and IOL implantation are almost always safe) to severe intractable uveitis at the other with permanent breakdown of the blood-ocular barrier, including some eyes with uveitis in association with juvenile chronic arthritis, in which IOL implantation is dangerous and the complication rate high.

Many publications on the results of cataract surgery in patients with uveitis have concentrated on single disease entities; however, such studies have limited usefulness as each will report variability in outcomes reflecting that the basic risk factors are largely not disease dependent but process dependent and current status dependent. The preoperative factors that predict a difficult postoperative period and may modify the surgical approach are: inadequately controlled preoperative anterior segment inflammation; chronic aqueous flare implying permanent blood-ocular barrier breakdown releasing fibrinogen; dense or broad-based posterior synechiae, pupillary membrane or sphincter fibrosis necessitating significant iris manipulation; dense cataract necessitating higher phako power; corneal opacity compromising the surgical view; coexistent difficult glaucoma; and lens instability. Above all, strict perioperative control of inflammation is fundamental to the success of surgery.

In many patients with uveitis, the decision to remove a cataract, the timing of surgery, the choice of operation, the need for perioperative treatment changes and expectations of visual improvement in the context of other intraocular problems are complex issues that may require a considerable degree of preparation and patient discussion. It is rarely necessary to make a precipitate decision regarding surgery, but, in some patients, occasions will arise that must be used promptly as 'windows of opportunity.' It is wise to have prepared the ground in anticipation of such events.

Preparation for surgery

Several parameters will affect the outcome of cataract surgery in uveitis for the individual patient, and an appreciation of these by both surgeon and patient is important. This clinic supplies patient information pamphlets on the subject of uveitis and cataract that deal with generic issues, and we have found such an approach to be a useful preliminary to a more detailed discussion of the individual patient's particular problem (see patient information pamphlets on attached disk). The following are the main issues.

Type of uveitis

Some forms of uveitis are characterized by an expected response to intraocular surgery. Although each type will have an unique expression in the individual patient, such broad diagnostic groups do serve to allow a degree of planning and prognostication, and overall it is useful to place patients into risk groups dependent on the type of uveitis that they have, e.g. we now realize that modern cataract surgery with lens implantation in patients with Fuchs' heterochromic uveitis is usually well tolerated, but in contrast surgery in those with uveitis associated with juvenile chronic arthritis has been fraught with difficulty. Those with recurrent anterior uveitis respond well to surgery performed between attacks, with only rare postoperative flares of inflammation which may well be stress induced rather than surgically provoked. Those with chronic anterior uveitis need special management, whereas those with chronic panuveitis can be extremely challenging. The greater the degree of inflammation, the higher the risk. To some degree, the choice of surgery will depend un these factors.

Expectations of improvement of vision

The patient with uveitis may have several causes of visual loss, of which a cataract is only one. Expectations of visual improvement must be tempered by an appreciation of established coexisting lesions, which will limit visual improvement even in the absence of postoperative complications. Macular scarring after previous macular edema, epiretinal membrane (ERM) formation, vitreous opacification, visual field loss caused by glaucoma or focal posterior segment scarring, and amblyopia are the most important of these, and overall macular scarring is predominant (Rahman and Jones 2005). In many patients the relative contributions of such lesions to the whole visual problem are difficult to quantify; in such cases, it is important that the patient does not develop unreasonable expectations.

To this concept of limited expectation, even at best, must be added the different, but equally important, possibility of operative or postoperative complications, especially worsened inflammation, macular edema or glaucoma, any of which may worsen the final visual outcome.

The timing of surgery

Many patients are referred to this clinic specifically with a request to manage cataract in the context of uveitis, and arrive with an expectation of early surgery. They are disappointed to learn that more effective anti-inflammatory treatment is often necessary not only to prevent future complications generally but also to permit safe cataract surgery in particular. This will delay their cataract removal by weeks if not months, and no remonstration should persuade the surgeon to compromise this safety-first approach. Some patients with uveitis have a stormy course requiring heavy immunosuppression in addition to systemic steroid treatment. In such individuals, periods of relative quiescence should be regarded as 'windows of opportunity' for cataract surgery. In others with more stable courses, we usually allow the patient to choose the appropriate time for surgery, balancing their own visual loss against the fully understood implications of surgery.

Informed consent

A good understanding of the implications of surgery is important for the patient, in order to avoid unreasonable expectations and to enhance compliance with treatment. General written information for the patient is supplemented by a discussion of the individual's situation. In particular, the presence of other causes of visual loss (which may be irremediable) must be understood, as must the potential for postoperative complications, the possible need for prolonged anti-inflammatory treatment and the small possibility of the need for further surgery.

In this predominantly young age group, IOL implantation is optimal, but in a few this is an unrealistic goal. Where IOL implantation is not intended, we assess contact lens tolerance by a preoperative trial, bearing in mind that the use of soft contact lenses may be compromised by the need for frequent topical medication. We continue to be disappointed by the proportion of young uveitic patients with unilateral aphakia who, for various reasons, choose to discard their contact lens and function monocularly; there is therefore a constant drive towards IOL implantation even in high-risk eyes. Such a preference must always be tempered by a realistic appraisal of risks.

We always explain the principles of postoperative presbyopia to our young patients; this phenomenon is not easily understood but in practice rarely causes problems, and those with unilateral IOL implantation usually choose to read only with their other eye until natural presbyopia supervenes. We are not aware of any reported experience of multifocal IOL implantation in uveitic eyes.

Perioperative control of inflammation

It is now generally understood that strict preoperative control of intraocular inflammation is of fundamental importance in ensuring an optimal outcome from surgery. Clearly the treatment required to achieve this will vary immensely. Having reached this point a decision is required on the need for additional treatment just before or during surgery. Our approach to this has been published (Suresh and Jones 2001) and a modified form is shown in **Table 7.1**, which takes into account more recent experience with intravitreal steroid injection and intravenous methylprednisolone.

Patients with recurrent anterior uveitis, who are free of inflammation without treatment at the time of surgery, do not appear to be at increased risk of postoperative uveitis and require no preoperative preparation. In patients with controlled chronic anterior or Fuchs' heterochromic uveitis, it is our practice to administer Pred Forte drops four to six times daily for 1 week before surgery. Where significant posterior segment inflammation is present, or where chronic anterior uveitis is particularly recalcitrant, systemic steroid cover is advisable. In this clinic, adults not already taking systemic steroids are prescribed 20–30 mg/day of prednisolone for 1 or 2 weeks preoperatively; those already using prednisolone will usually receive significantly higher doses perioperatively, 40 mg/day being average.

Background immunosuppression is not increased just before surgery, because it achieves nothing. Higher-risk patients will benefit from intravenous methylprednisolone on the day of surgery, and/or intravitreal triamcinolone. We have not been persuaded by the findings of some others that intravenous pulsed steroid is an adequate replacement for 1 week of enhanced oral steroid.

The operation

Phakoemulsification with endocapsular IOL implantation is the aim in the vast majority of patients. Indeed, in younger adults phakoaspiration is frequently possible as the nucleus is usually soft. Anterior segment scarring interferes with standard-approach surgery; those with band keratopathy or herpetic corneal scarring have a compromised view (**Fig. 7.9**). Peripheral anterior synechia formation is frequent but it is usually possible to avoid these by selecting an angle and plane of approach, even in those few with very anterior iridocorneal adhesions (**Fig. 7.10**). In a small minority a pars plana approach may be preferable.

Many patients with a uveitic cataract have posterior synechiae (**Fig. 7.11**). Usually these can be easily detached by sweeping a Rycroft cannula gently underneath the iris toward the center of the pupil; if there are few and narrow adhesions, adequate dilation can then often be achieved without mechanical pupil manipulation. However, extensive posterior synechiae are usually associated with peripapillary iris surface and sphincter fibrosis, often with pupil membrane formation (**Fig. 7.12**), which may require careful dissection and excision before iris hooks can be inserted (**Fig. 7.13**). Vitreous scissors of varying curvature are excellent for this purpose. Iris hooks are then usually required and are preferable to simple mechanical dilation

Table 7.1 The Manchester Uveitis Clinic preoperative preparation protocol

Type of uveitis	Normal treatment	Preoperative treatment
1. Quiescent anterior uveitis	Nil	Nil
2. Fuchs' heterochromic uveitis	Nil	Pred Forte drops four to six times daily for 1 week
3. Chronic anterior uveitis	Topical steroid	Topical treatment enhanced to at least the above, with prednisolone 20–30 mg for 1 week in high-risk cases
4. Chronic panuveitis – stable	Topical steroid + prednisolone	Topical treatment enhanced to at least the above. Prednisolone dosage usually unchanged
5. Chronic panuveitis – unstable	Topical steroid + prednisolone	Topical treatment enhanced to at least the above. Prednisolone dosage increased to at least 20 mg, or doubled, whichever is the higher dose
6. Any uveitis with permanent blood-ocular barrier breakdown	Topical steroid ± prednisolone	As for 5. With additional intravenous methylprednisolone 0.5–1 g on day
A. Any of 3–6 above with active or significant risk of macular edema	As above	Intravitreal triamcinolone 4 mg at surgery

[a]Patients also using immunosuppression maintain the same dosage throughout. Preparation may be modified if the patient is known to be a steroid 'responder'. (Modified from Suresh and Jones 2001.)

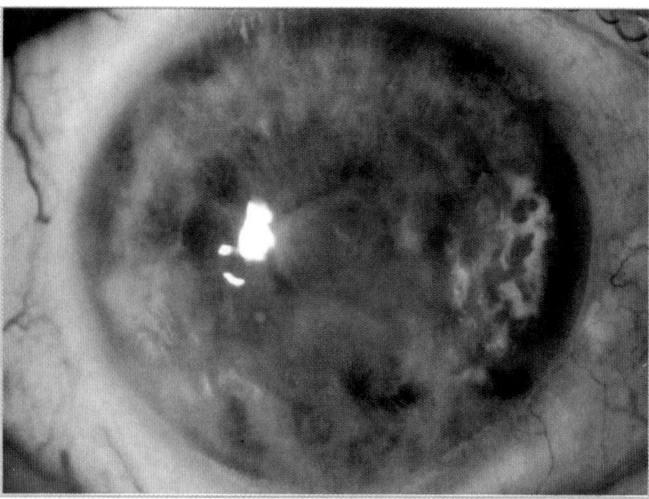

Figure 7.9 Band keratopathy and subepithelial corneal scarring provide an interesting variation in this uveitic eye awaiting cataract surgery.

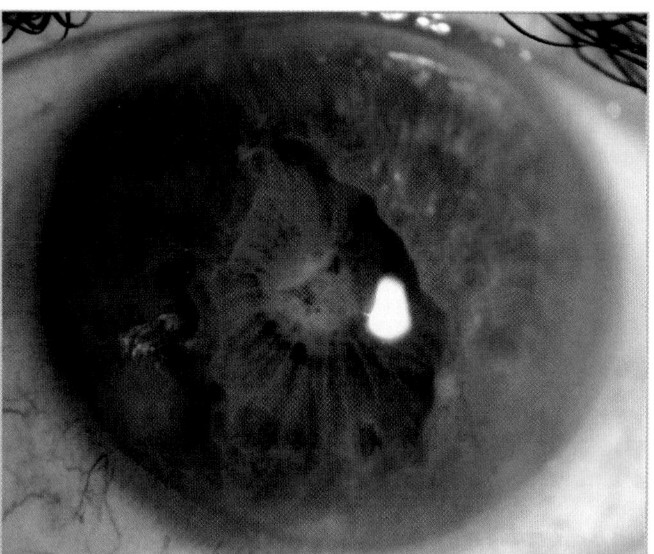

Figure 7.10 Extremely anterior peripheral anterior synechiae provide a great challenge to anterior-approach cataract surgery.

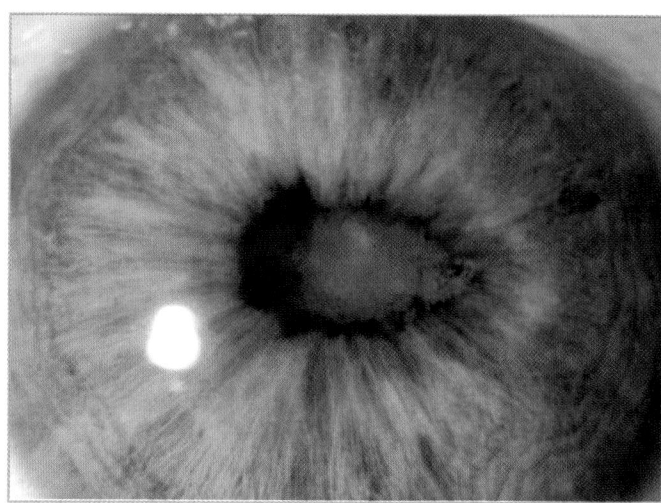

Figure 7.11 Subtotal posterior synechiae with pupillary fibrosis – a common barrier to lens access in uveitic cataract surgery.

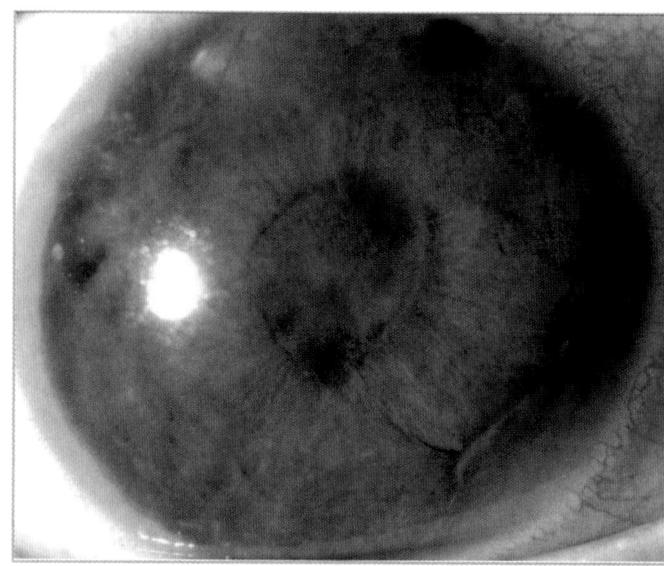

Figure 7.12 A fibrinous pupillary membrane associated with complete posterior synechiae in an eye with severe recurrent anterior uveitis, requiring surgical iridectomy. There are also PAS visible inferolaterally.

because they ensure a taut pupil margin and avoid accidental iris phako damage. Sphincter rupture is common with the use of hooks but cannot be avoided if adequate exposure is sought. Postoperatively most pupils are cosmetically quite acceptable despite this trauma. Iris manipulation may lead to hemorrhage; minor bleeding into the AC angle, occasionally also from the iris surface, is also a consistent feature in those with Fuchs' heterochromic uveitis.

In the 1990s one-piece polymethylmethacrylate (PMMA) IOLs were the preferred option for eyes with uveitis, heparin surface modification providing some additional benefit. As foldable and injectable IOLs have developed, it has become clear over the past decade that the choice of IOL material remains important for eyes with uveitis. Silicone has been felt to be less well tolerated than acrylics (Alio et al. 2002) but the sharp-edged configuration of any foldable IOL appears to minimize posterior capsule opacification (Abela-Formanek et al. 2011).

Perhaps the most difficult group of patients in which to perform cataract surgery are those youngsters with uveitis associated with juvenile chronic arthritis. In these, and some others with chronic uveitis, a permanent substantial breakdown of the blood–ocular barrier is shown by chronic aqueous and vitreous flare. These eyes are particularly likely to be problematic after surgery; increased inflammation, heavy fibrinous reaction, cyclitic membrane formation and phthisis are all well recognized. Much recent argument has revolved around the safety of IOL implantation in this group, with no clear consensus. Historically the clear message was that IOL implantation was always unsafe, with later explantation frequently being necessary. In the last 10 years, these children have been managed with a greater willingness to use oral immunosuppression and anti-tumor necrosis factor (TNF) treatment, creating the ocular environment where IOL implantation may be acceptable in selected children. In a direct comparison of aphakic and pseudophakic eyes in this group, no long-term disadvantage was attributed to IOLs and better visual results were obtained (Sijssens et al. 2010). A string of recent papers all advocate IOL implantation in this group. However, all correctly identify

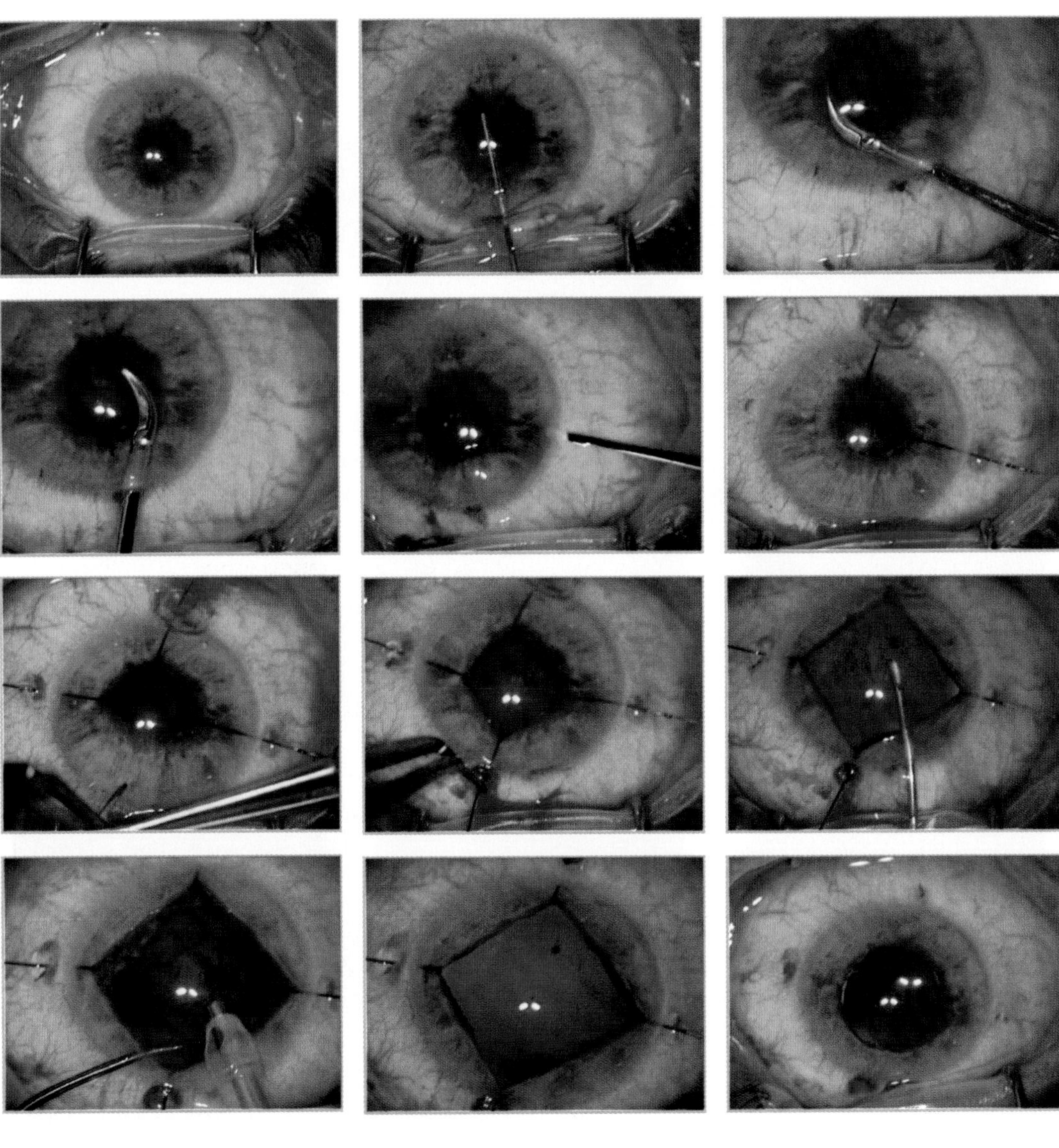

Figure 7.13 A montage of images from a cataract operation in a patient with chronic uveitis. After dislocation of posterior synechiae, a pupillary membrane is abscised with vitreous scissors. Sclerotomies for iris hook insertion are made just anterior to the iris plane to avoid anterior traction of the pupil. One hook is placed between keratome incision and side-port, the remainder at 90°, which gives good visibility at the phako tip and avoids iris chafe superiorly. A sphincter rupture has occurred at the 1 o'clock hook (coinciding with the only non-fibrosed point of the pupil margin. Nevertheless the pupil once released reforms adequately and this is usually maintained or improved post-operatively.

stringent perioperative control of inflammation as mandatory, and most discuss a significant rate of postoperative complications. This group of vulnerable patients should be managed with the greatest care and circumspection, and IOL implantation performed only if the eye is very well controlled on treatment.

Postoperative management and potential complications

Postoperative inflammation

Worsened intraocular inflammation after surgery is the main risk in patients with uveitis. It is the mark of successful preoperative preparation (and of careful surgery) that such inflammation is minimized, if possible, to the level expected after routine cataract surgery. We identify an expected level of inflammation from the preoperative status and the surgery performed. The highest-risk patients use hourly Pred Forte drops for the first few days after surgery, together with cyclopentolate 1% two to four times daily and chloramphenicol four times daily. All patients with uveitis in this clinic are reviewed on the first day after surgery, and again on day 5 routinely (earlier if necessary). On day 5, topical steroid dose reduction is commenced if the eye is 'well behaved', and if possible mydriasis is discontinued. The aim is to be completely intolerant of inflammation; it is far easier to maintain this status by over-treating than to attempt to retrieve it having once allowed inflammation to gain ground. We normally then review patients on day 12 and, subsequently, less frequently if all is well. It is necessary to maintain topical steroid treatment at higher levels and for significantly longer in patients with uveitis. Those undergoing routine cataract surgery usually discontinue their topical steroid treatment within 3 weeks, whereas those with uveitis will need them for about 8–12 weeks before a return to 'baseline' treatment (that level used preoperatively). Those patients who are given systemic steroids are usually maintained on the same dose for 1 week postoperatively; having demonstrated a satisfactory postoperative course it is then possible to reduce this treatment quite rapidly, with careful observation. It is usually possible to discontinue (or return to preoperative dosage) within 6–8 weeks of surgery.

Sometimes despite apparently stringent preparation, an eye becomes substantially inflamed early in the postoperative period. The experience of such episodes should always be used to reassess risk levels for future patients and to amend protocols if necessary. In witnessing severe postoperative uveitis an initial decision is needed on diagnosis; fortunately the incidence of postoperative endophthalmitis is now so low with the use of intracameral antibiotics during surgery that this is not often a serious consideration. A fibrinous response (**Fig. 7.14**) is almost always uveitis rather than infective. It should not be allowed to persist, and aggressive additional treatment is required,

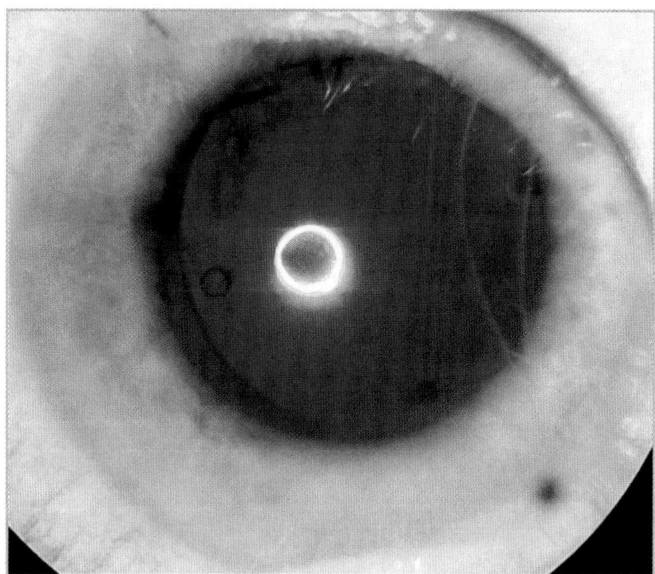

Figure 7.14 Fibrinous uveitis on the first day after cataract surgery in a patient with chronic anterior uveitis. A fibrin web has formed within the anterior chamber with curved strands visible across the pupil.

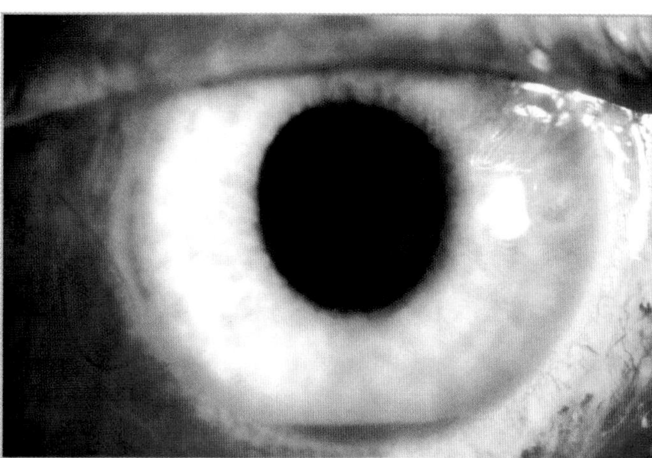

Figure 7.15 A small hyphema on the first postoperative day after routine cataract surgery in an eye with heterochromic uveitis; the intraocular pressure was > 40 mmHg.

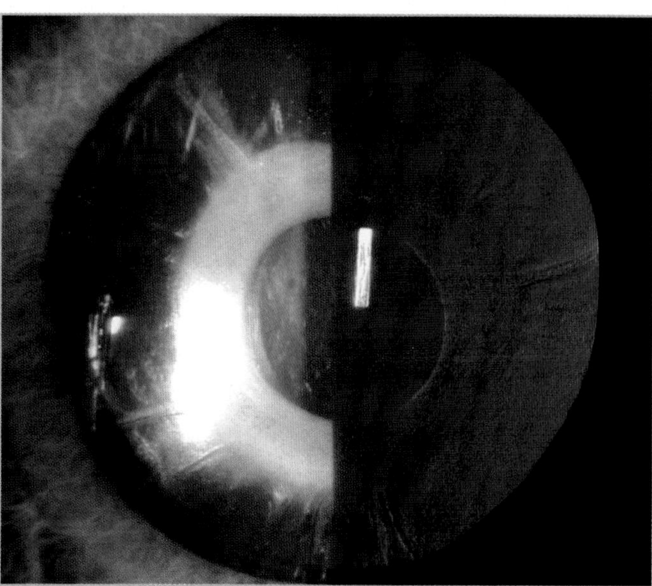

Figure 7.16 Substantial anterior capsulorrhexis phimosis several months after routine phakoemulsification surgery. The edge intruded within the pupil, necessitating surgical excision of the fibrotic band.

usually with daily supervision. Initially, immediate mydriasis with both anticholinergic and sympathomimetic (sometimes as a subconjunctival injection of Mydricaine), together with subconjunctival steroid injection and topical steroid of increased frequency, is often adequate. If unimproved the following day, then high-dose oral steroid or intravenous methylprednisolone should be added. It is not uncommon for a fibrinous web involving internal section, IOL and pupil to persist for several days after all cells are eliminated from the AC.

In our experience it is only rarely necessary to consider the use of intracameral tissue plasminogen activator; although fibrin will dissolve very rapidly afterwards, there is a risk of hyphema and it should be used only with great care, in a dose of 12.5 μg at maximum. We would consider its use only if the fibrinous reaction were severe enough to cover the IOL and occlude the pupil.

Raised intraocular pressure

Raised IOP on the first postoperative day is frequent but unpredictable; the diligent removal of viscoelastic at the end of surgery is helpful, but nevertheless a significant proportion of patients require treatment for glaucoma in the first few days after surgery. Patients with Fuchs' heterochromic uveitis often show minor bleeding into the angle during surgery; only occasionally is this significant and only very uncommonly does it remain on the first postoperative day (**Fig. 7.15**), when it may cause a significant IOP rise. Those requiring substantial phako power and any prolonged operation also have increased risk of first-day IOP rise. It is our practice to administer three doses of oral acetazolamide 250 mg to all patients in these risk groups before their first-day review. Any subsequent problem is managed as required. We do not discontinue prostaglandin analog drops postoperatively if they were required before surgery, but we avoid starting them anew to control a postoperative rise in pressure because of the risk of macular edema.

Anterior capsule fibrosis and phimosis

Continuous circular capsulorrhexis during phakoemulsification surgery makes possible the capsule contraction syndrome, or capsular 'phimosis,' by providing an aperture that is at risk of shrinkage; the remnant lens epithelial cells adherent to the edge of the capsulorrhexis undergo fibrotic changes and cause contraction (**Fig. 7.16**). This effect may be more common in uveitic eyes, although in practice treatment is rarely necessary. We have in two patients applied an 'episiotomy' – one or more radial lines of Nd-YAG laser to the fibrosed area. This has been ineffective and reoperation to remove the stricture has been necessary but successful. Rarely, total contracture of the anterior capsule to obliterate the capsulorrhexis is seen. Although anecdotally reported in eyes with silicone IOLs, our single patient had a foldable acrylic implanted (**Fig. 7.17**). Surgical reintervention was again necessary.

The best treatment of capsular phimosis is prevention – the larger the capsulorrhexis, the less likely it is to occur. However, the technical problems of producing a safe, large capsulorrhexis in a difficult capsule behind a pupil dilated only by the use of iris hooks are significant. As endocapsular (not sulcus) IOL implantation is a very high priority in uveitic eyes, 'losing' the capsulorrhexis would be a serious complication; it is safer to create a small-to-moderate capsulorrhexis, if necessary enlarging this after the IOL is implanted. If residual lens epithelial cells can safely be aspirated from the anterior capsule then this will reduce risk.

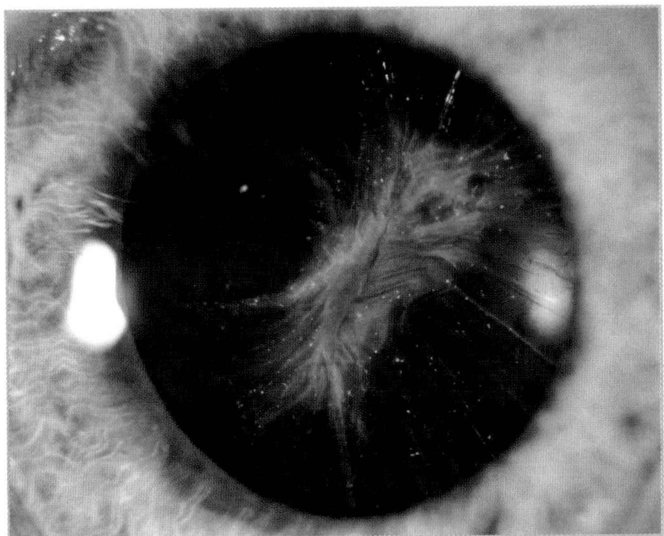

Figure 7.17 Complete stenosis of the anterior capsulorrhexis, occluding it entirely. Surgical excision of the fibrotic mass was required.

If capsule fibrosis and shrinkage does occur, there is a theoretical risk of deformation of a foldable or injectable IOL so that gross astigmatism is induced. In practice we have not witnessed this and presume that the capsule shrinkage would have to be severe enough to deform the optic at 5.75–6.25 mm diameter; at this level of shrinkage, total dislocation would presumably be a greater risk.

Giant cell accumulation on IOL implants

Giant cell accumulation on the surface of an implanted IOL is not uncommon in uveitic eyes but in our experience is far more likely in eyes with Fuchs' heterochromic uveitis. The majority of affected patients have one or two cells present at any time which are of no clinical significance. Those few with enough to affect vision almost inevitably have Fuchs' heterochromic uveitis (**Fig. 7.18**). In this circumstance a course of semi-intensive topical steroid treatment usually removes most cells, but there is a tendency for them slowly to reaccumulate. They can usually be kept at bay by long-term low-dose topical steroid and this is one of the few indications for such treatment in heterochromic uveitis.

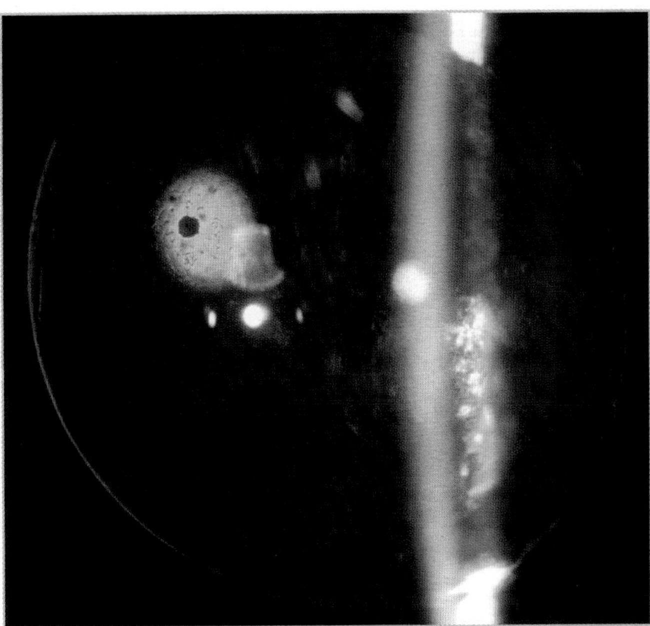

Figure 7.18 Widespread giant cell deposition on the anterior surface of a heparin surface-modified PMMA intraocular lens in a patient with Fuchs' heterochromic uveitis.

Posterior synechiae to capsule and iris entrapment

An iris with an imperfect pupillary margin is capable of rapid adhesion, not to the IOL but to exposed capsule. The edge where posterior synechiae have been released, pupil margin tears by iris hooks and areas exposed by the removal of a pupillary membrane all have small blood vessels that release fibrinogen and are at risk of forming adhesions. Affected irides are also relatively atonic and, if the sphincter has been disrupted, extremely so. Once an area is adherent it is virtually impossible to remove with topical mydriasis and surgical reintervention is unjustified. At best a small adhesion is a minor problem (**Fig. 7.19**); at worst a significant area of iris becomes entrapped behind the IOL, inducing chronic rub, IOL subluxation (**Fig. 7.20**) and sometimes permanently enhanced inflammation, requiring more topical steroid than preoperatively.

The best strategy to avoid this problem is a matter of debate. Some argue that atropine is too long lasting and once administered cannot be modified rapidly enough; some advocate avoiding mydriasis altogether in some circumstances, to permit iris movement and therefore avoid adhesion. It has been argued that it is better to implant large-optic (7 mm) PMMA IOLs into the sulcus to physically prevent iris from reaching the posterior capsule, but, as a proportion of these patients develop chronic iris rub anyway, it is clearly not a generic solution. In principle, minimizing operative iris trauma and postoperative inflammation is imperative, but in practice a few will develop permanent adhesions no matter what efforts are made to avoid it.

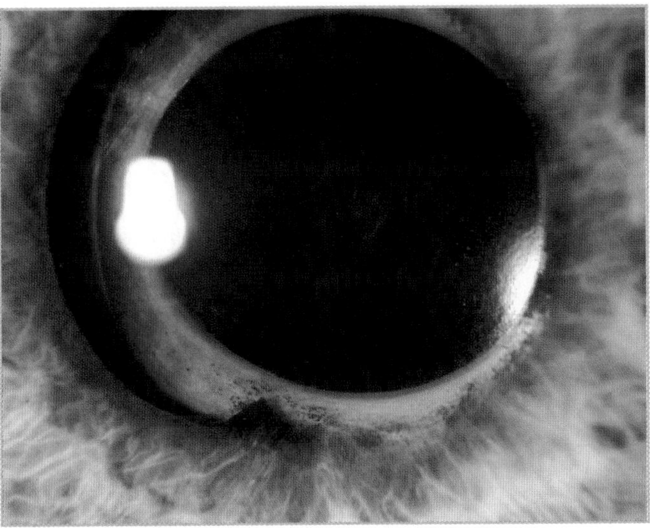

Figure 7.19 Posterior synechiae to the capsulorrhexis edge in a patient with chronic anterior uveitis.

Posterior capsule opacification and lens epithelial proliferation

Posterior capsule opacification is common in patients with uveitis after cataract surgery (Rahman and Jones 2005) but modern square-edge foldable IOLs appear to reduce this risk. Unfortunately Nd-YAG capsulotomy is associated with some increased risk for patients with uveitis, and the procedure must be undertaken with this in mind; worsened inflammation, raised IOP and macular edema are the main risks.

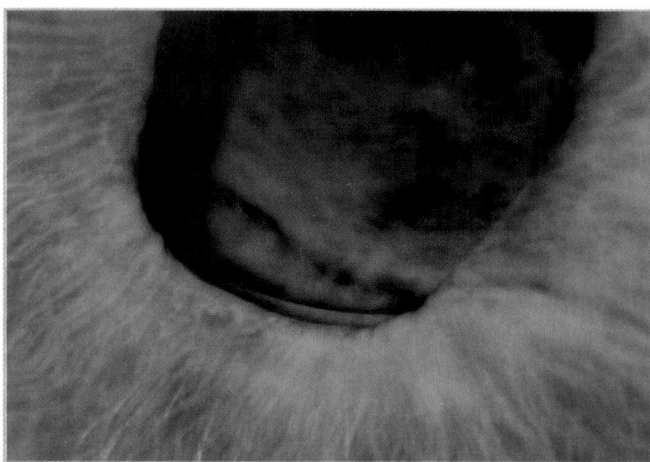

Figure 7.20 More substantial iris–capsule adhesions have contracted to cause intraocular lens (IOL) subluxation. The chronic iris–IOL touch has necessitated long-term topical steroid treatment.

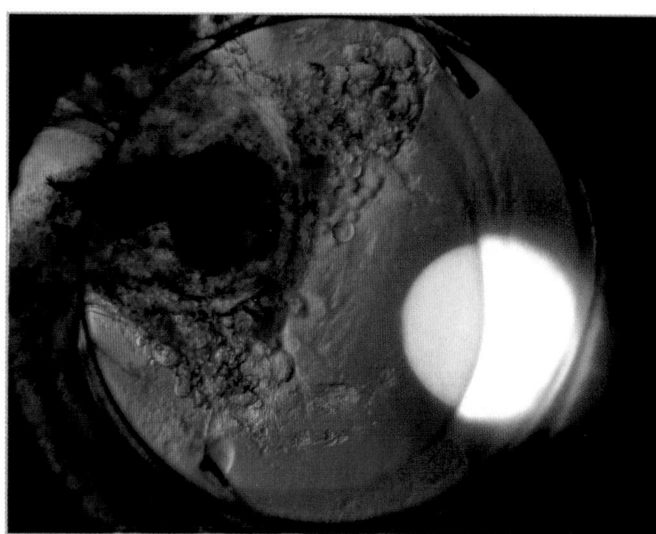

Figure 7.21 Substantial lens epithelial cell proliferation behind an intraocular lens in a patient with chronic uveitis.

In some patients, particularly those with Fuchs' heterochromic uveitis, a raised IOP may be sustained and problematic. It is our practice to give enhanced topical steroid for 3 days pre-laser, to measure IOP afterwards, and to administer apraclonidine 0.5% and review within 1 week. Patients should be made aware of the somewhat increased risk before choosing the timing of the procedure.

A few patients with uveitis develop substantial lens epithelial proliferation, sometimes before (**Fig. 7.21**) but more usually after (**Fig. 7.22**) YAG capsulotomy. This phenomenon has been described in a number of diseases, each of which probably expresses posterior segment cytoproliferative cytokines (Jones et al. 1995). In these situations Elschnig pearls bulge into the visual axis and surgical removal rather than repeated laser capsulotomy is necessary. Fortunately the complication is uncommon but the possibility should be added to those already recognized for eyes with uveitis undergoing posterior capsulotomy.

Macular edema

Postoperative macular edema is a common and potentially severe problem in eyes with uveitis undergoing cataract surgery. Its treatment generally is discussed below. However, it is appropriate here to reiterate that a pre-emptive approach is important and rarely regretted; injecting triamcinolone into the vitreous at the time of cataract surgery prevents most episodes in those at high risk.

POSTERIOR SEGMENT COMPLICATIONS

Vitreous opacification and vitrectomy

Vitreous opacification is a common feature in posterior uveitis, the component of intermediate uveitis that most frequently causes symptoms (**Fig. 7.23**) and common in Fuchs' heterochromic uveitis. Recurrent or chronic vitreous involvement may lead to opacities, which are permanent, and these often become suddenly more problematic after posterior vitreous detachment, which may be an early phenomenon in uveitic eyes. In some cases pars plana vitrectomy is justified solely to remove opacities, and outcomes have been generally satisfactory.

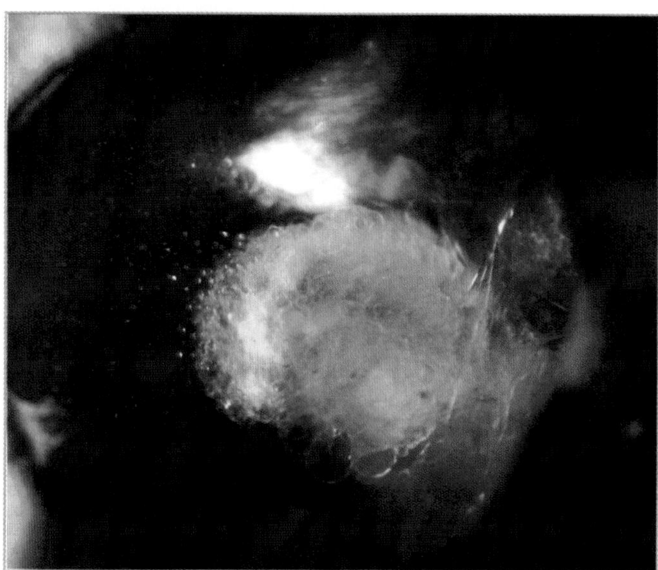

Figure 7.22 Massive lens epithelial proliferation forming Elschnig pearls, after Nd-YAG capsulotomy in a patient with chronic uveitis.

The procedure has been used here in a number of patients with Fuchs' heterochromic uveitis, with uniformly good results (Waters et al. 2000).

Vitrectomy has been advocated by some not merely to clear opacities from the posterior segment, but to improve macular edema or intraocular inflammation. In a cohort of patients with intermediate uveitis, vitrectomy was superior to immunosuppression on several parameters (Quinones et al. 2010). It has been found capable of reducing the necessary immunosuppressive medications in children (Giuliari et al. 2010) and may improve macular edema (Tranos et al. 2006). Overall the evidence base for a therapeutic effect from vitrectomy is poor (Becker and Davis 2005). However, decisions are made in the context of an individual patient with a combination of manifestations, each of which may be affected differently by surgery. The most important task is to identify preoperatively those who will be likely to benefit. In this clinic, surgical decisions are made on pragmatic grounds with a careful calculation of risk versus benefit. Patients without a pre-existing

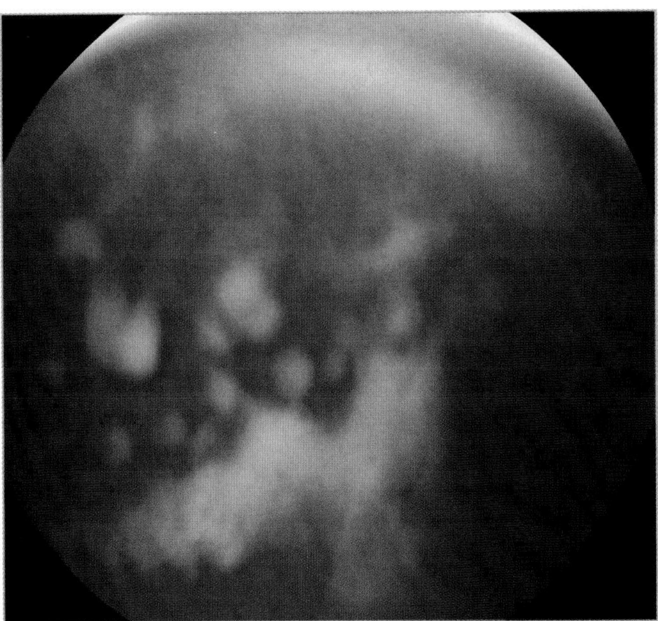

Figure 7.23 Substantial vitreous opacification in a 15-year-old boy with intermediate uveitis.

posterior vitreous detachment are appraised with this additional risk in mind. Those with unilateral or asymmetrical vitreous opacification are more likely to be managed with surgery rather than immunosuppression. Those who are already pseudophakic, already have a high risk of uveitis-induced cataract or can undergo combined vitrectomy with cataract extraction are more likely to undergo vitrectomy.

Overall there are three main indications for therapeutic vitrectomy in uveitis. The first is vitreous opacification. Some patients even with relatively high visual acuity are quite adamant that their vitreous floaters are very problematic and wish to pursue surgery despite the associated risks. The great majority are highly satisfied with the visual result. Those with relatively opaque vitreous have a demonstrable improvement in visual acuity which symptomatically is even better owing to enhanced contrast acuity. A subset of this group is the patient with recurrent or recalcitrant vitreous hemorrhage in which removal is importantly combined with internal search and endolaser where necessary. The two other main indications are in the management of macular edema and ERM, which are dealt with below. Diagnostic vitrectomy for cytology is discussed in Chapter 20. An information pamphlet on vitrectomy is provided in this clinic (see patient information pamphlets on attached disk).

Enzymatic vitrectomy

Interesting work is under way to identify biochemical methods to disrupt vitreous and hyaloid architecture. It is known that cortical collagen does not adhere directly to retina, but via a gluey extracellular matrix, the precise structure of which is poorly understood. Constituents are, however, known to include heparan sulfate, chondroitin sulfate, opticin, fibronectin and laminin. It is possible to inject an enzyme to promote vitreolysis and, more importantly, to induce posterior vitreous detachment. Studies on various enzymes have focused attention currently on microplasmin, which is a recombinant protein similar in action to plasmin but more stable for storage and administration. A phase II trial specifically to examine the effect of intravitreal microplasmin injection to facilitate posterior vitreous detachment before surgical vitrectomy (Benz et al. 2010) found significant effect and, importantly for those patients with vitreomacular traction, the potential to avoid surgery entirely. When aimed specifically to remove vitreomacular traction without surgery, a substantial cure rate was observed (Stalmans et al. 2010) using 125 μg, if necessary repeated up to three times. Phase III trial results are awaited with interest but are showing great promise.

Enzymatic vitrectomy has not yet been trialed specifically for patients with active intraocular inflammation, but there are a number of clear potential indications, not least the management of ERM formation and macular traction. Current management of this frequent complication of uveitis is discussed below.

Macular edema

Macular edema is the scourge of the uveitis clinic, and overall is responsible for more irreversible visual loss than any other phenomenon in uveitis patients (Durrani et al. 2004). It may occur as a complication of uveitis which is otherwise solely anterior, usually in severe HLA-B27-associated uveitis; in this instance it usually settles spontaneously as the anterior uveitis is treated with topical steroids. More recalcitrant macular edema is extremely common in intermediate uveitis and is a very significant feature in a high proportion of patients with posterior uveitis or retinal vasculitis. Left untreated, persistent or recurrent macular edema will cause insidious and progressive derangement of the retinal architecture and pigment epithelium, with granular scarring and loss of visual acuity. It may also lead to acute macular pseudo-hole or true hole formation and sudden visual loss.

In the context of uveitis, macular edema can be discussed in three morphological forms (Markomichelakis et al. 2004): first, classic cystoid macular edema (**Fig. 7.24**) is centered on the fovea with variable retinal elevation and degree of cyst coalescence and is a common feature, e.g. in intermediate uveitis; second, diffuse macular or posterior pole edema, as commonly seen, for instance, in birdshot retinochoroidopathy (**Fig. 7.25**) is more widespread and often less pronounced in elevation but can progress to widespread permanent retinal damage; last, fluid accumulation substantial enough to cause serous retinal elevation (**Fig. 7.26**) is usually a feature of severe acute posterior uveitis including VKH syndrome, sympathetic uveitis or acute posterior multifocal placoid pigment epitheliopathy (APMPPE). These forms may require somewhat different approaches to treatment.

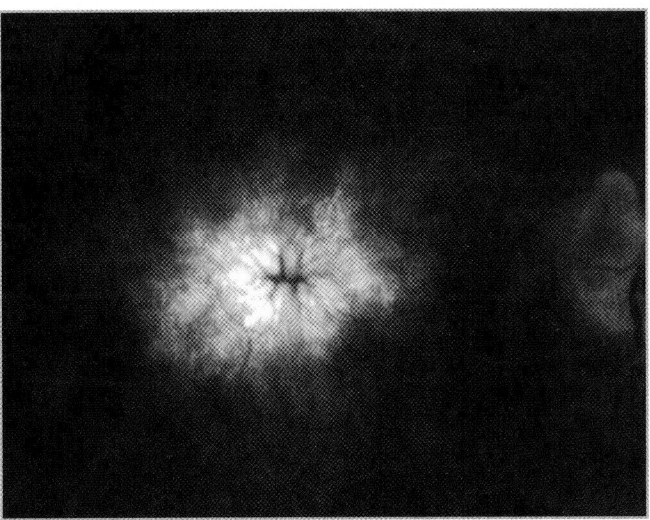

Figure 7.24 Classical cystoid macular edema.

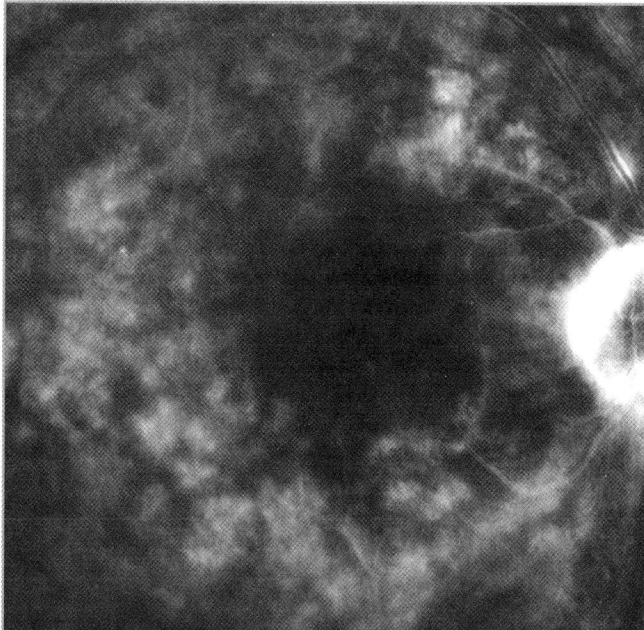

Figure 7.25 Widespread diffuse macular edema in a patient with birdshot retinochoroidopathy.

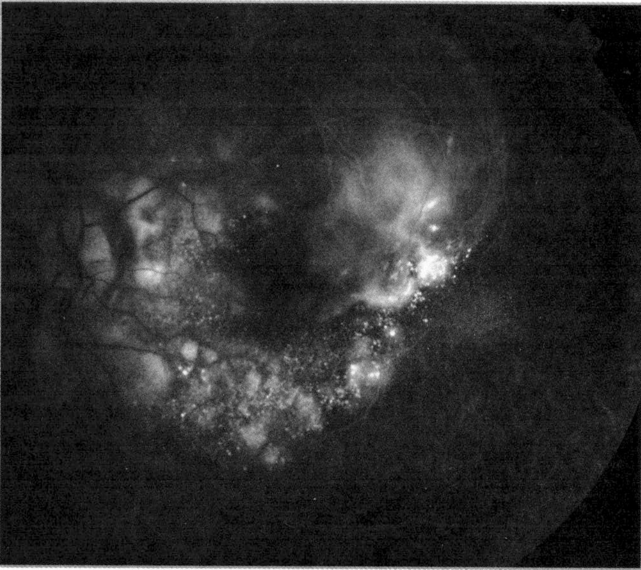

Figure 7.26 Massive macular edema with serous detachment in an eye with acute Vogt–Koyanagi–Harada syndrome.

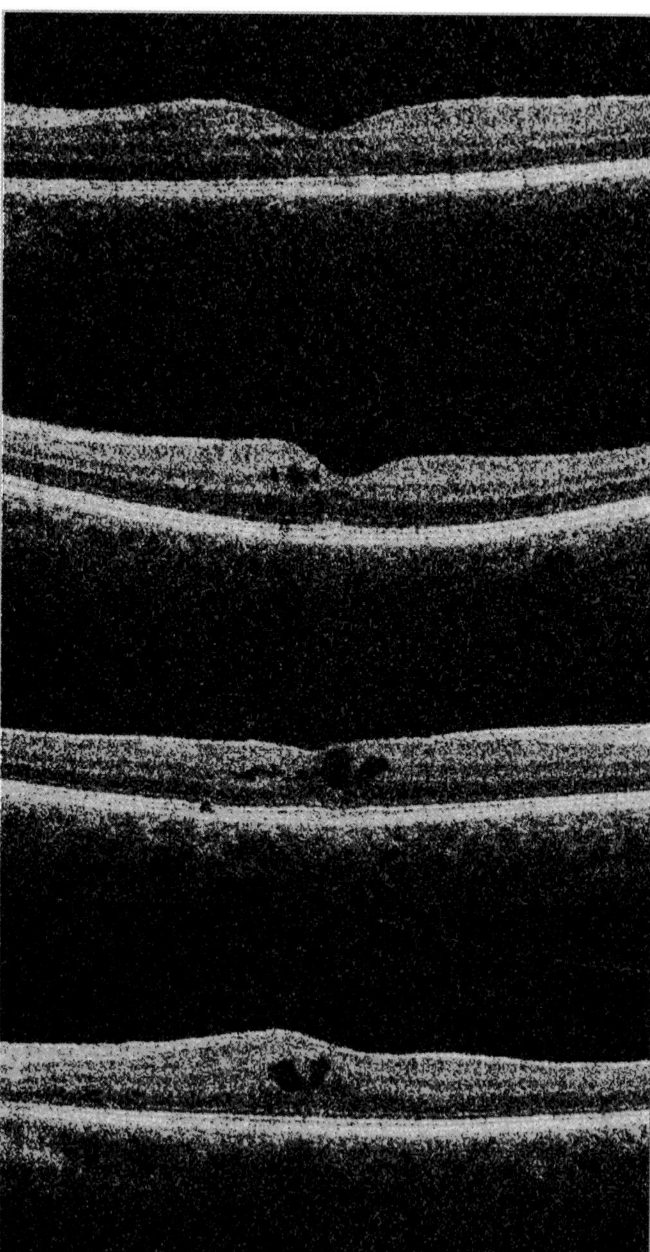

Figure 7.27 Four examples of mild cystoid macular edema with visual acuities of 6/6, 6/5, 6/6 and 6/9 respectively – treatment required?

Since the introduction of ocular coherence tomography (OCT), the management of uveitic macular edema has been much more closely scrutinized both in the clinic and in research. In particular the easy identification of mild cystic change in a macula thought to be 'dry' on clinical examination (**Fig. 7.27**), and commonly with a high visual acuity, has provoked much thought on the optimal management of a condition that may not be causing current visual loss but which left untreated may inexorably do so. Thresholds for treatment have been lowered significantly and therefore the search for low-risk but effective treatment continues. The ability to identify associated serous foveal elevation (**Fig. 7.28**) has explained the lower acuity in this subgroup (Ossewaarde-can Norel et al. 2011).

Sometimes macular edema is untreatable. This situation is normally found either after a patient has presented late or where edema has remained under-treated for a period of many months. Such eyes were partly identifiable using fluorescein angiography, which tends to show a clearly defined honeycomb pattern (**Fig. 7.29**), often in association with an enlarged foveal avascular zone. The introduction of OCT has facilitated the identification of such cases, confirming the permanent disruption of retinal architecture by very long-standing edema (**Fig. 7.30**). Where doubt exists as to the usefulness of treating very long-standing macular edema, a therapeutic trial is essential; for bilateral changes we would use high-dose oral steroid, for unilateral intravitreal steroid injection.

The research base for uveitic macular edema is weak, and the optimum management remains contentious. Several patient variables

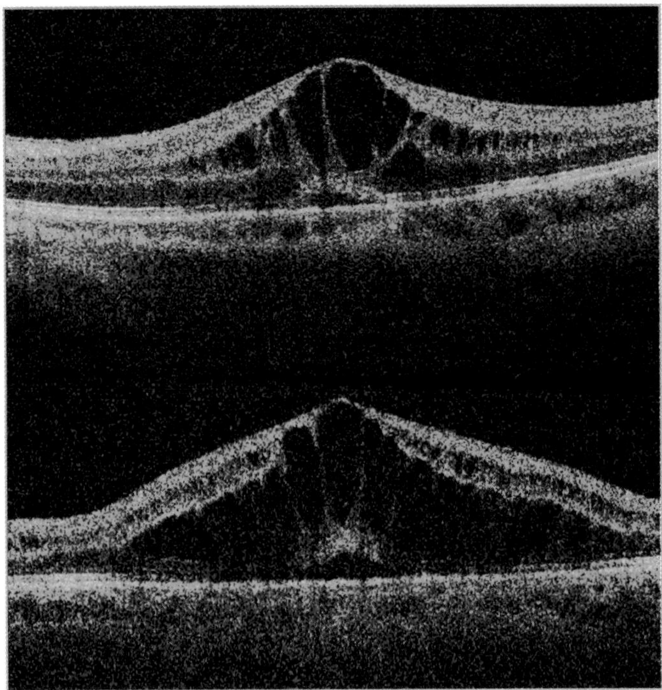

Figure 7.28 **Two patients with gross uveitic macular edema**, accompanied by underlying serous foveal elevation.

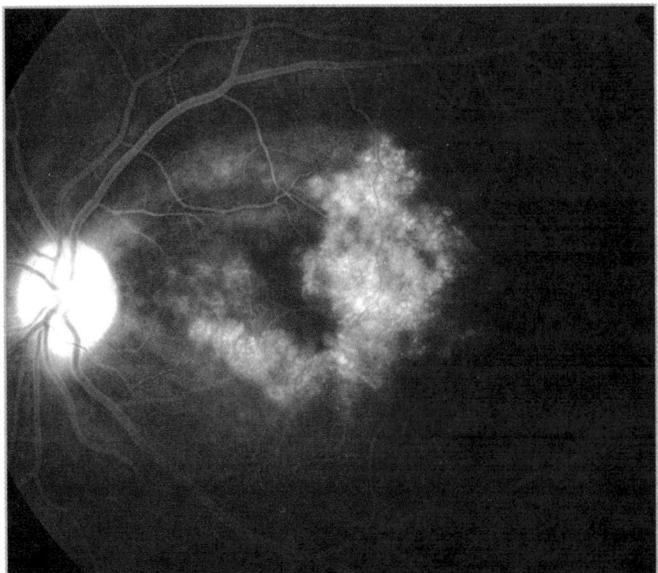

Figure 7.29 **Honey-comb pattern of late macular edema** – a poor prognostic indicator.

will modify the individual approach, including a history of steroid-induced IOP rise, the degree, location and chronicity of intraocular inflammation, the age of the patient and the laterality of uveitis. In many eyes the macular edema is a reflection of the intensity of the uveitis, and management decisions are made in tandem for both. Such general approaches are discussed in Chapter 6. To assist our patients' understanding we provide an information pamphlet on the subject (see patient information pamphlets on attached disk). This section will deal specifically with the management of macular edema as the predominant active problem.

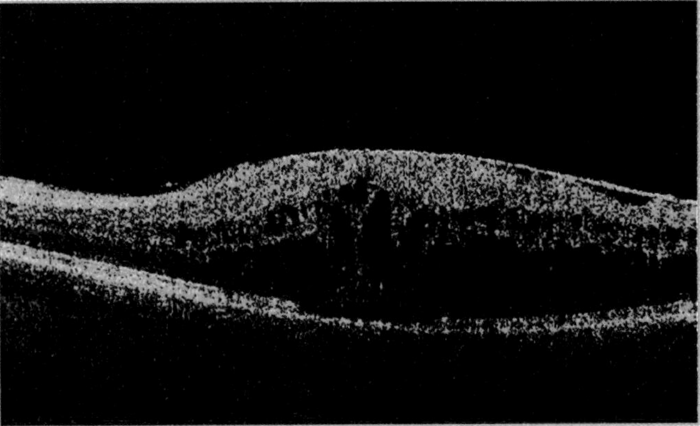

Figure 7.30 **Permanent disruption of intraretinal architecture** is the consequence of very chronic untreated macular edema. Visual improvement will not accompany any anatomical improvement after treatment.

In the great majority of patients, macular edema is rapidly responsive to systemic steroids in adequate doses. However, the side effects of such medication mean that its continued use, for this indication alone, is unsatisfactory. Deep periocular injections of either triamcinolone or methylprednisolone are effective in a substantial minority, the positioning of bolus and the preferred drug being the source of much unresolved argument. The approach in this clinic has been to use methylprednisolone in the perception that induced IOP rise is less common, and to inject into the orbit floor because the evidence for a better effect from posterior sub-Tenon's injection has not been convincing enough to justify the somewhat increased risk. Before the introduction of intraocular steroid injection it was common practice to administer up to three consecutive orbital injections 4–6 weeks apart before abandoning the procedure as unsuccessful. The approach now in this clinic is to administer a single injection and to use the treatment again later only if it has been substantially effective, moving on to intravitreal steroid injection if it fails.

The usefulness of acetazolamide for inflammatory macular edema is a contentious issue, with no hard evidence for its effect when used alone (Whitcup et al. 1996). Although not directly researched, there is a body of opinion that supports its use in combination with periocular steroid injection, suggesting enhanced effect, and we agree with this concept. However, acetazolamide is intolerable to some patients, and is barely tolerated by many more. Its long-term use is no more acceptable in the management of macular edema than it is in chronic glaucoma.

Systemic non-steroidal anti-inflammatory drugs (NSAIDs) are able to reduce macular edema after cataract surgery, but their usefulness in uveitic macular edema is more contentious. Effect has been claimed as both sole treatment and somewhat better in combination with depot steroid injection (Rojas et al. 1999), but few have been persuaded to use this regimen. Similarly, topical NSAIDs have been found useful in post-surgical macular edema, but this has not been extrapolated to the treatment of inflammatory edema. Vitrectomy may reduce inflammatory macular edema (Stavrou et al. 2001) but only in a minority, although visual improvement may result from vitreous removal itself. The usefulness of laser grid photocoagulation to treat non-inflammatory macular edema is well reported, but its use in uveitis is poorly investigated and rarely used.

The introduction of intravitreal triamcinolone injection for inflammatory macular edema added a substantial new form of management, its superiority over orbital injection being clearly demonstrated (Roesel et al. 2009). Its usefulness in the short term is undisputed, and the risks well recognized. The choice of dose has varied from 2 mg to 25 mg or more, with 2 mg being adequate as a first procedure for most patients (Das-Bhaumik and Jones 2006). The initial enthusiasm for this technique in the years immediately following its introduction has been tempered by the realization that its effect may be maintained for only 3–6 months, sometimes less. Attention has therefore turned to the steroid implants discussed in Chapter 6; there are no direct comparison studies as yet available, but injectable sustained-release dexamethasone may prove to have a duration of action no longer than intravitreal triamcinolone injection; the fluocinolone implant has a substantially better duration of action but with a higher side-effect profile. Further studies are required.

For patients who are steroid responders, a very high IOP can follow within 3–6 weeks of intravitreal steroid. The usefulness of anti-VEGF MAbs has been studied in uveitis; both bevacizumab (Mackensen et al. 2008) and ranibizumab (Acharya et al. 2009) have been used with some effect. However, frequent injections may be necessary and, in the absence of any intrinsic anti-inflammatory effect, concomitant treatment of the uveitis is of course mandatory (Gulati et al. 2011). The optimal intraocular treatment for uveitic macular edema has clearly yet to be devised.

Investigation into alternative methods of treatment for inflammatory macular edema is under way. Subcutaneous injections of anti-CD11A MAb have been used; CD11a is an adhesion molecule cofactor that interacts with intercellular adhesion molecule 1 (ICAM-1) to facilitate leukocyte migration. Mild-to-moderate improvement in visual acuity and macular thickness is reported (Faia et al. 2011). Intraocular methotrexate has been used, also with moderate effect lasting for about 4 months (Taylor et al. 2009). Intraocular adalimumab, in contrast, has not been effective. The diversity of methods attempted attests to the complex and incompletely understood pathogenesis of inflammatory macular edema. In most patients without vitreomacular traction, the basics remain unchanged: control the intraocular inflammation and then add treatment as appropriate for the macular edema, using local methods if possible. The added complexity of vitreomacular traction is discussed below.

Epiretinal fibrosis and vitreomacular traction

Any chronic uveitis, anterior, intermediate or posterior, can lead to ERM formation, surface wrinkling and vitreomacular traction. One particular dilemma in the uveitis clinic is to choose the level of appropriate therapeutic aggression for a patient with otherwise minimal signs of ongoing inflammation who, if untreated, may develop this complication. An example is the patient with mild non-occlusive retinal vasculitis with a few vitreous cells, no anterior segment inflammation and visual acuity of 6/5. Is long-term oral immunosuppression justified? If the answer is 'no', then one sometimes looks back after 10 years when visual acuity is 6/12 because of epiretinal maculopathy, wondering whether surgery is justified and whether treatment should have been more aggressive.

Early signs of ERM formation include small patches of reflection from retinal surface, probably commencing in Müller cell end-plates, which coalesce gradually to form irregular sheets. Gradual aggregation and shrinkage lead to surface wrinkling (**Fig. 7.31**) and potentially to massive retinal folding (**Fig. 7.32**). As for macular edema, the OCT has greatly facilitated diagnosis, showing a range of surface retinal traction, varying from the subtle to the profound (**Fig. 7.33**) and greatly enhancing surgical decision-making.

Surgery for surface wrinkling and vitreomacular traction requires careful decision-making, taking into account the visual acuity and degree of metamorphopsia, level of active inflammation, presence or absence of cataract, degree of vitreous opacification and vitreoretinal attachment, age of the patient and, clearly, degree of tractional macular damage being accrued. In some cases, despite the clear removal of tractional edema and the resolution of hole or pseudo-hole, visual recovery is disappointing. There is a paucity of data on appropriate choice of patient, and no modern studies for uveitic surgery in particular. The avoidance of three-port vitrectomy in such patients is attractive, hence the considerable interest in enzymatic vitrectomy (see earlier) which may relieve vitreomacular traction without conventional surgery. Further studies are awaited, leaving the ophthalmologist currently to make surgical decisions on an individual basis. For this

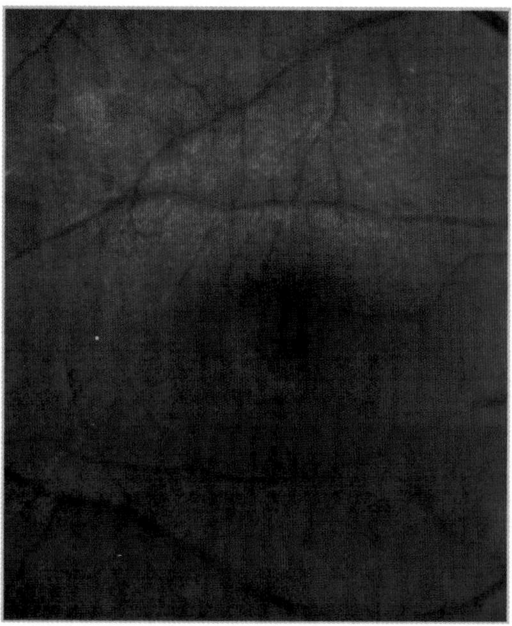

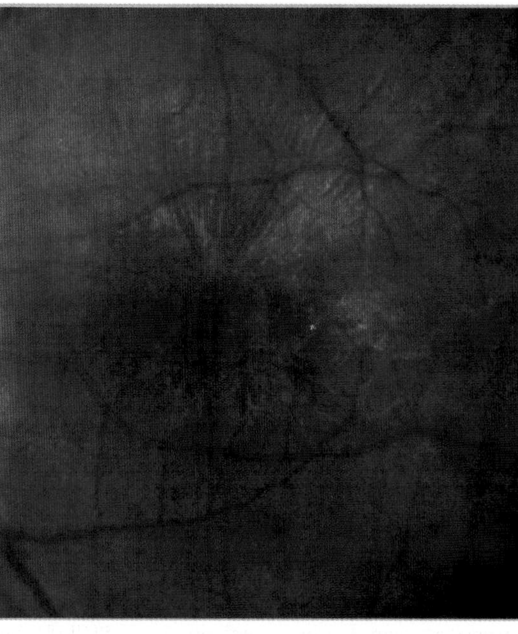

Figure 7.31 A patient with mild chronic retinal vasculitis and vitritis. The right macula (shown left) demonstrates patchy epiretinal membrane formation; the left shows more substantial change with surface wrinkling and adjacent retinal traction folds.

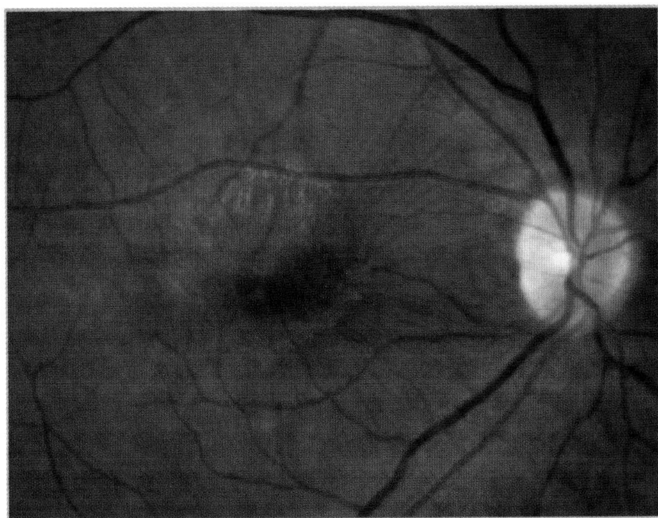

Figure 7.32 A macular epiretinal membrane has contracted to cause a classic 'cellophane maculopathy' with radial retinal traction folds and substantial visual distortion.

complication of uveitis, perhaps more than any other, prevention is definitely better than the cure.

Retinal traction, detachment and retinoschisis

Vitreoretinal traction is of course not unique to the macula. Intermediate uveitis, in particular, may cause peripheral pars plana and retinal gliosis, and this may induce traction, causing retinal elevations that are characteristically self-limiting (Jalil et al. 2010). Only if combined with macular traction does rhegmatogenous change tend to supervene. Morphologically such elevations are difficult to diagnose as detachments or 'schises' (see Fig. 15.10), although both probably occur. Tractional change is a particular feature of progressive toxocariasis. Any substantial posterior uveitis may modify hyaloretinal adhesion, either inducing patchy or total posterior vitreous detachment, or forming gliotic adhesions that may induce traction during the vitreous detachment process (**Fig. 7.34**). Retinal vasculitis has a tendency to produce such adhesions specifically along the line of large retinal vessels, which may be considerably distorted by tractional change. Rhegmatogenous detachment may supervene if traction is adequate and may affect perhaps 3% of patients with uveitis (Kerkhoff et al. 2003). The incidence of proliferative vitreoretinopathy is substantially increased in uveitic detachments, with consequently lower reattachment rate and a higher vitrectomy rate.

Exudative retinal detachment is typically a feature of very severe choroidal involvement in, for example, sympathetic uveitis or VKH syndrome, lupus choroidopathy (**Fig. 7.35**), uveal effusion syndrome and posterior scleritis. It is also typical in temporary and localized form for any severe macular focus of inflammation. It has been reported specifically in association with syphilis. Management is predominantly with aggressive anti-inflammatory treatment, which often leads to rapid resolution. However, recurrence or chronicity typically leads to retinal pigment epithelium (RPE) derangement, characteristically with concentric tidemarks and leopard-spot pigmentation (**Fig. 7.36**) and permanent loss of function. In patients with recalcitrant detachment, surgical drainage has been performed (Galor et al. 2008) with claimed success.

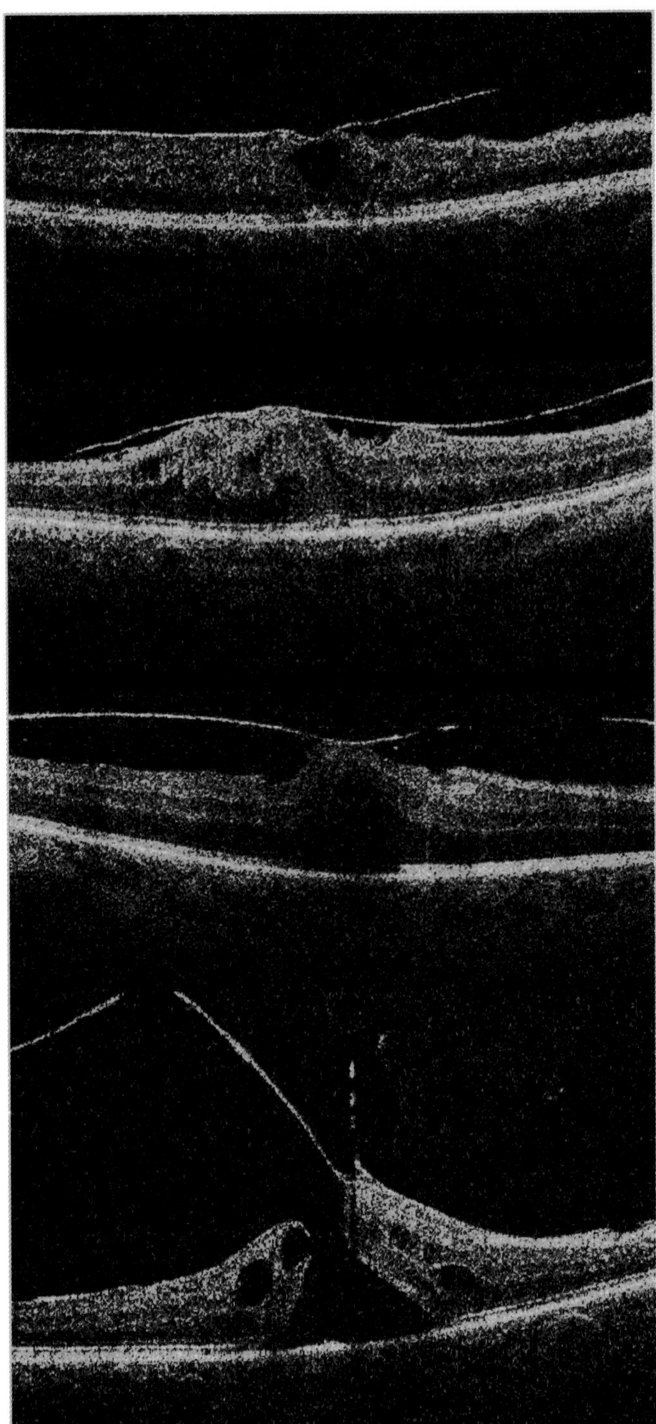

Figure 7.33 Vitreomacular traction in a series of eyes with epiretinal membrane formation ranging from subtle surface wrinkling to tractional retinal hole formation.

The principles of retinal detachment prevention and management are essentially unchanged for patients with uveitis, but, with the knowledge that some forms of inflammation may carry a higher risk, that complex surgery is more likely, and outcomes are modified not only by retinal structural changes and proliferative vitreoretinopathy (PVR) risk, but by ongoing inflammation and epiretinal fibrosis. Skilled management is necessary and such patients are not ideal for intervention by surgical trainees.

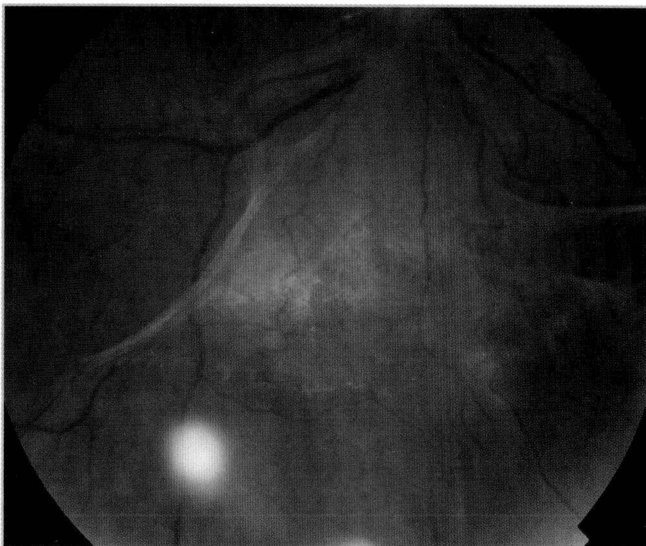

Figure 7.34 A gliotic sheet has formed on the posterior hyaloid with retinal adhesion producing some tractional change.

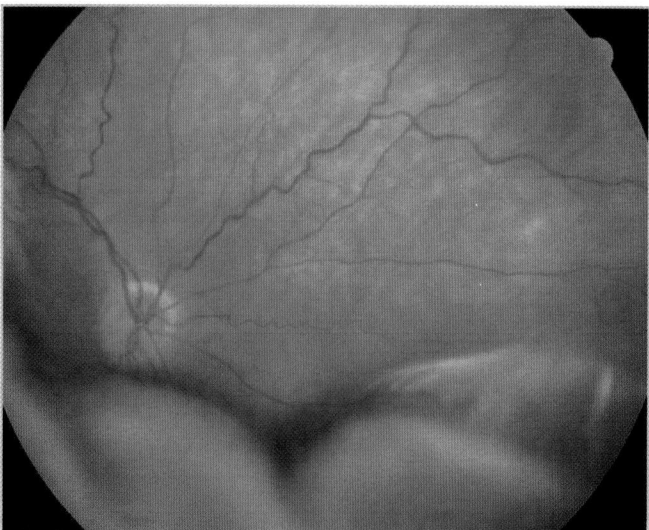

Figure 7.35 The inferior retina is elevated by shifting fluid in a patient with end-stage lupus and necrotizing choroidopathy.

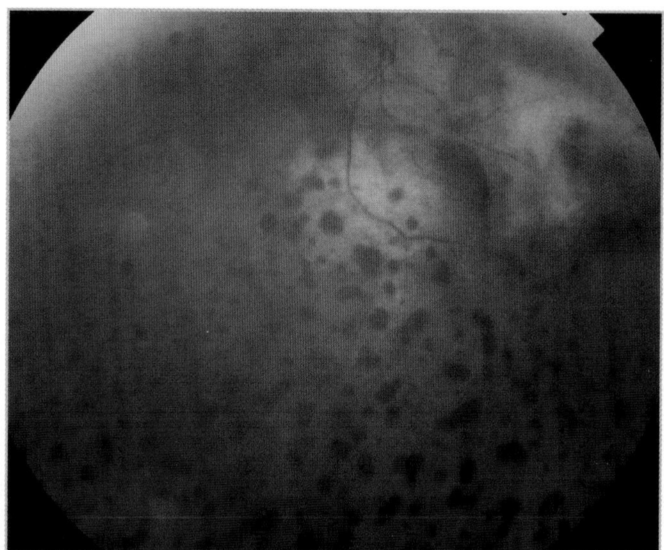

Figure 7.36 Leopard-spot or thrush-breast pigmentation is the characteristic appearance of retina chronically or recurrently detached by serous elevation.

Retinal ischemia and neovascularization

Many forms of intraocular inflammation affect retinal circulation, either primarily or secondarily, and this may involve vascular occlusion. The specific syndromes are discussed in their individual chapters, particularly Chapter 18 for retinal vasculitis. The general principles are discussed here. Ischemia requires occlusion and this may either be substantial and stepwise, as is characteristically seen in Behçet's disease, or slow and insidious. The former variety is usually symptomatic and consequent examination and imaging identify risk factors and provoke anti-inflammatory and retinal laser treatment as necessary. It is probably an over-generalization, but nevertheless true for most patients with uveitis, that retinal neovascularization does not seem to occur with the readiness that might be seen, for example, after an equivalent area of ischemia in diabetic retinopathy, despite the high levels of VEGF that have been detected in some intraocular inflammations. Further, it is often found that only light peripheral retinal laser ablation is often adequate in combination with adequate anti-inflammatory treatment. This is not to say that management can be complacent; vitreous hemorrhage during monitoring indicates a failure of supervision.

A far greater challenge exists in the prevention of creeping ischemia, which may not cause neovascularization at all. Some patients with low-grade occlusive retinal vasculitis could be reliably monitored only with serial Goldmann visual fields and standard angiography. However, the introduction of wide-field fluorescein angiography (**Fig. 7.37**) has massively improved the clinician's ability to supervise, to identify creeping change and therefore to amend immunosuppression levels. This will facilitate (but never completely prevent, because some patients appear completely unresponsive to treatment) profound shrinkage of the retinal vascular tree with consequent blindness (**Fig. 7.38**).

A subset of patients with either retinal vasculitis or uveitis appears to be capable of forming optic disk and peripapillary new vessels without any angiographic evidence of retinal ischemia (**Fig. 7.39**). In the limited experience of this clinic, widespread retinal capillaritis may be present; the pathogenesis of this process is not understood, but fortunately the vessels are often steroid responsive (Sanisio et al. 2000), sometimes exquisitely so. The longer-term management seems, however, to require fairly heavy immunosuppression.

Macular ischemia is a consequence of chronic macular inflammation or edema presumably affecting the capillary bed. It has long been recognized as a cause of a failure to improve vision after eliminating chronic edema (Bentley et al. 1993). It is irreversible and recognized as an enlarged foveal avascular zone on angiography (**Fig. 7.40**). Ischemia is one possible cause of foveal atrophy (Forooghian et al. 2009) which can be identified on high-resolution OCT. Such atrophy is often multifactorial, other causes including RPE and choriocapillaris dysfunction or serous macular detachment. Prevention is the only treatment; perhaps high-resolution imaging, in identifying an at-risk photoreceptor layer, will provoke more aggressive immunosuppression in some patients.

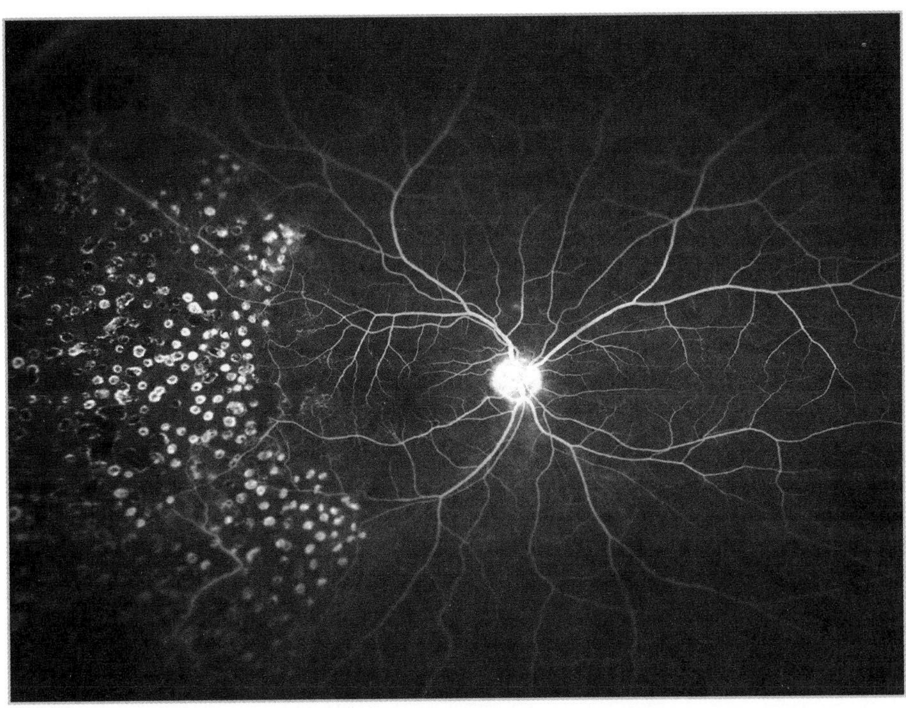

Figure 7.37 Widefield fluorescein angiography in a patient with occlusive primary retinal vasculitis.

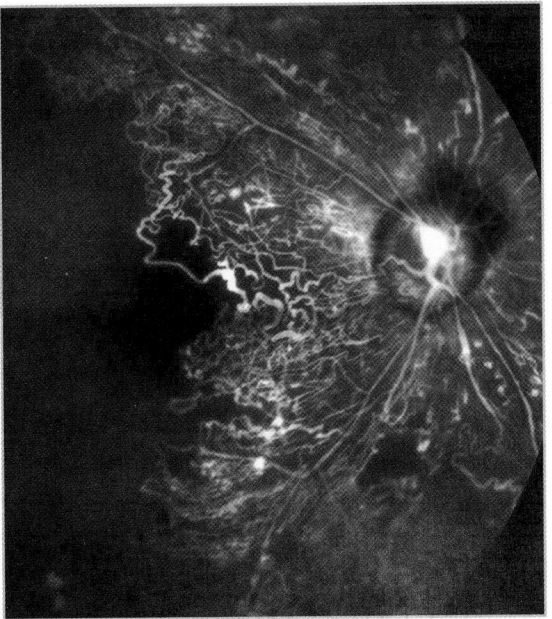

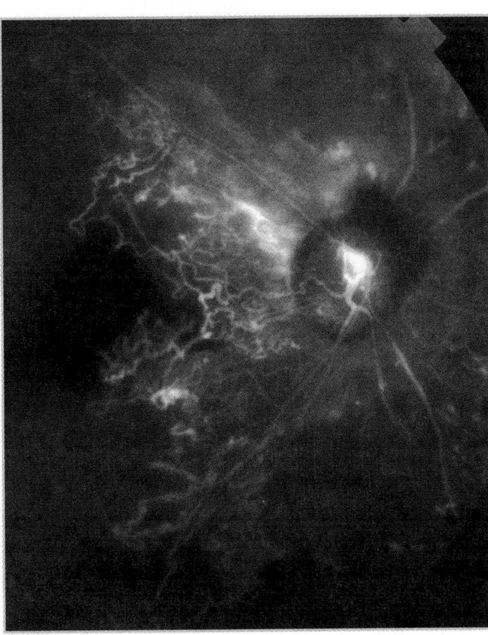

Figure 7.38 Progression of occlusive retinal vasculitis in Mantoux-positive Eales' disease despite anti-tuberculous therapy and immunosuppression. The angiograms were taken 2 years apart.

Choroidal neovascularization

A choroidal neovascular membrane (CNM) may occur adjacent to any post-inflammatory outer retinal or subretinal scar. In practice the complication is uncommon in uveitis, being found in only 2% recently (Perentes et al. 2005), but has a particular predilection for the presumed ocular histoplasmosis syndrome, punctate inner choroidopathy (**Fig. 7.41**) and persistent placoid maculopathy, which are discussed in the relevant chapters. CNM may also occur in Behçet's disease, sympathetic ophthalmia, VKH syndrome, serpiginous choroiditis and toxoplasma retinochoroiditis, and anecdotes appear in a variety of other forms of uveitis causing focal chorioretinal scarring.

Most post-inflammatory membranes are completely or predominantly classical, and fluorescein angiography is therefore excellent for diagnosis and monitoring (Kotsolis et al. 2010). Fifteen years ago the management of such membranes was confined to systemic steroid administration (as most such membranes are at least partially responsive) and traditional ablative argon laser if not subfoveal; using these methods many membranes could be adequately arrested. However, the burgeoning development of new treatments driven by age-related macular degeneration has proven serendipitous for uveitic patients with these similar complications. Nevertheless for small extramacular membranes, standard argon ablation remains an entirely valid treatment method.

Verteporfin-assisted photodynamic therapy (PDT) for wet age-related macular degeneration (AMD) seems to have passed through its evolution to virtual extinction in the blink of an eye, driven by the superior efficacy of anti-VEGF injections. However, for inflam-

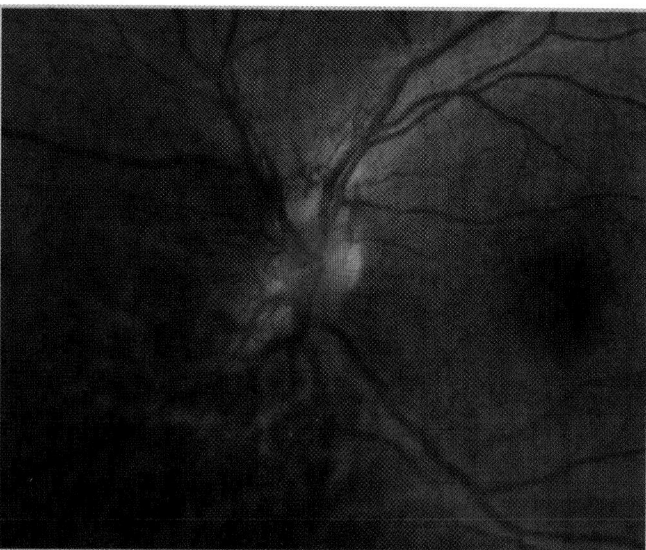

Figure 7.39 Florid disc and peripapillary retinal neovascularization in a patient with non-occlusive retinal vasculitis and no angiographic evidence of retinal ischemia.

matory CNM, PDT appeared to produce better results than in AMD (Wachtlin et al. 2003) and in some cases in our experience has proved to be remarkably successful. The invasive nature of repeated intravitreal injections may yet suggest a place for PDT, although a small recent comparative study between PDT and anti-VEGF treatment for patients with multifocal choroiditis felt that bevacizumab was superior (Parodi et al. 2010). There are no data on the combination of these treatments for inflammatory CNM. As for age-related membranes, bevacizumab demonstrates significant effect albeit often necessitating multiple injections (Arevalo et al. 2011, Julian et al. 2011), and similar results are found for ranibizumab (Rouvas et al. 2011). The surgical removal of post-inflammatory CNM has been successfully achieved, with visual improvement in some. However, the availability of more successful interventions as above has rendered this form of management very uncommon for this group of patients.

In this rapidly changing field the current approach in this clinic, on encountering a patient with clear clinical evidence of a perifoveal CNM in association with active or previous chorioretinitis (and also for patients with punctate inner choroidopathy [PIC], sudden-onset deterioration of visual acuity but no clear membrane) is immediately to initiate moderate-dose oral steroid treatment, confirm diagnosis with angiography and arrange an intravitreal bevacizumab injection within 7–14 days. Patients with membranes two or more disc diameters from the fovea may be adequately treated with argon ablation instead. Steroid treatment is slowly tapered and further bevacizumab administered if required following repeat angiography.

Optic nerve involvement

The optic nerve head is potentially affected in uveitis by direct inflammation, such as by an optic nerve granuloma, papillitis (**Fig. 7.42**) or neuroretinitis, by reactive swelling as in pediatric intermediate uveitis, by papilledema in patients with intracranial disease, by ischemic change in those with vasculitis (particularly by acute ischemic optic neuropathy in patients with systemic vasculitis) and, most commonly, by secondary glaucoma. In the complexity of ocular assessment for a patient with uveitis, the optic nerve manifestations are sometimes given inadequate attention, but examination and assessment of the optic disc are essential in every patient.

In children and young adults with recurrent or chronic anterior uveitis, or more commonly with intermediate uveitis, optic nerve head swelling (**Fig. 7.43**) is quite a common phenomenon, and appears to be a marker of activity, disappearing as the inflammation subsides. It is difficult to dismiss optic nerve head swelling, especially when bilateral, as being merely a manifestation of intraocular inflammation and, despite the absence of focal neurological signs, intracranial imaging is often recommended by a neurologist. However, in all patients under our care such imaging has proved normal and we are unlikely to proceed to neurological investigation if the association with the degree of uveitis is obvious and there are no focal neurological signs. To over-generalize, children with intermediate uveitis may develop disc swelling whereas adults develop macular edema.

The optic nerve head may be damaged by secondary glaucoma or show neovascularization in those with ischemic changes, especially in severe intermediate uveitis or occlusive retinal vasculitis

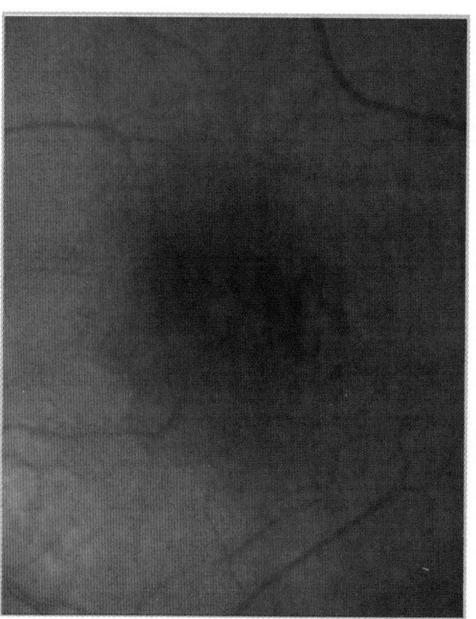

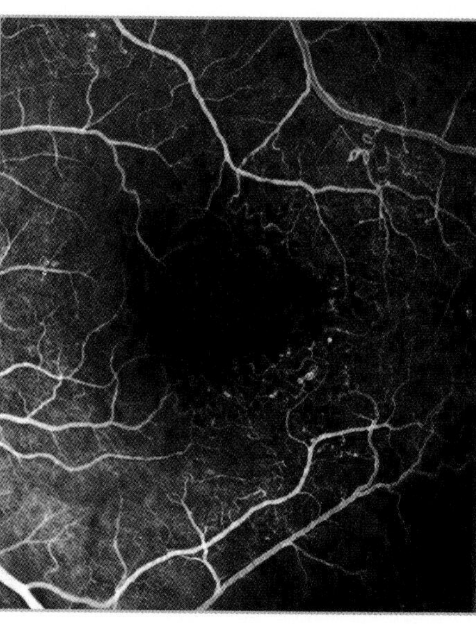

Figure 7.40 Macular ischemia in chronic posterior uveitis. The foveal avascular zone is enlarged with temporal perifoveal telangiectasis and edema.

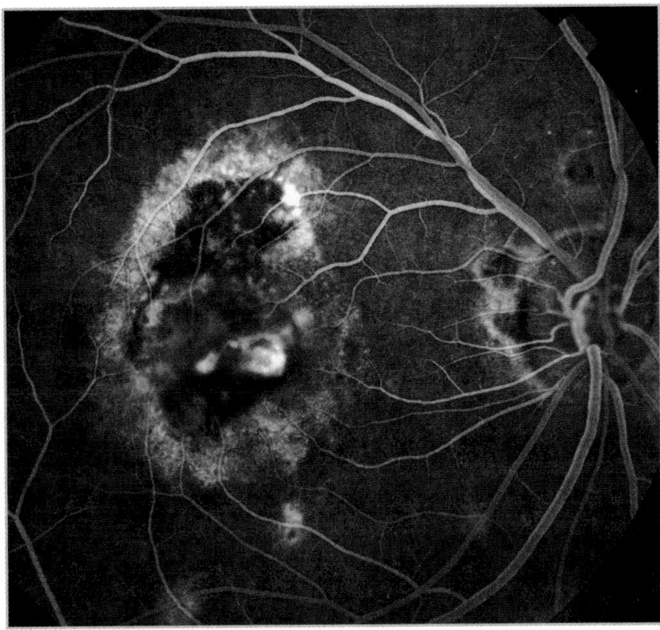

Figure 7.41 Choroidal vascular membrane as a complication of punctate inner choroidopathy.

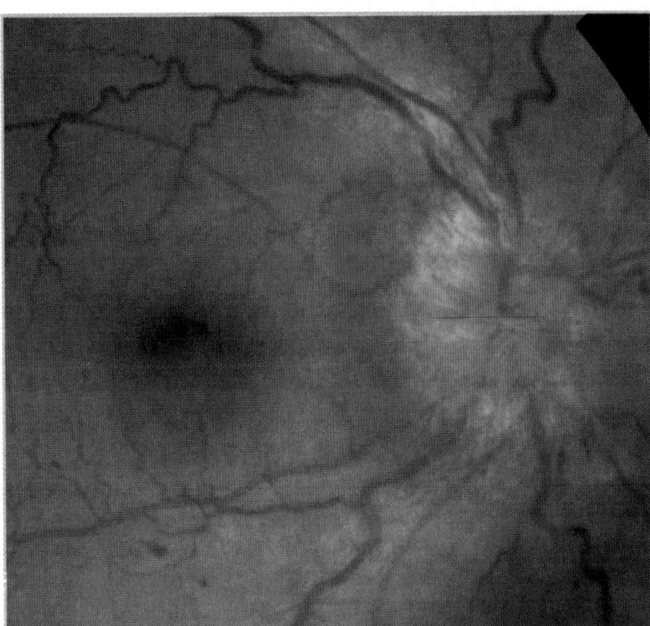

Figure 7.42 Papillitis in a patient with ocular tuberculosis.

including Behçet's disease. Direct inflammatory involvement of the optic nerve head is most common in toxoplasmosis (see Fig. 13.3) and such focal inflammation usually leads to substantial nerve fiber bundle defects and, often, permanently reduced central vision. Optic nerve head granulomas may be a feature of sarcoidosis, especially in neurosarcoidosis. Neuroretinitis with uveitis is most commonly caused by toxoplasmosis (see Fig. 13.26), but should also raise the possibility of other infections including bartonellosis (**Fig. 7.44**), borreliosis or syphilis.

Peripapillary inflammation with subsequent scarring is a typical feature of PIC and the presumed ocular histoplasmosis syndrome. Peripapillary edema is a common feature of sympathetic uveitis and VKH syndrome, and appears to be a sensitive marker of ongoing inflammation in some patients with the former.

Inflammation at or near the optic nerve head leads to scarring and/or atrophy. Gliotic scars overlying the optic nerve head are not uncommon in uveitis of several types and is in itself not an important sign ,although if severe it may be associated with peripapillary fibrosis and retinal traction (**Fig. 7.45**). Optic atrophy in contrast is a marker of permanent damage in some patients with severe uveitis or retinal vasculitis, and of course indicates untreatable visual loss (**Fig. 7.46**). In a few patients, subtle pallor of the optic nerve head may be the only clinical indicator of progression in an otherwise quiet eye, and sensitivity to such changes should be acute.

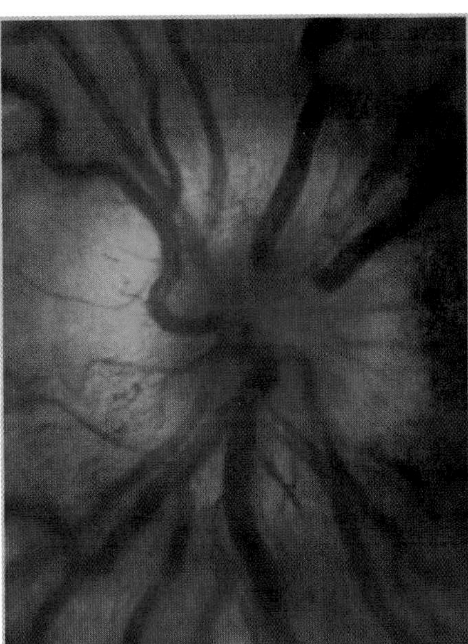

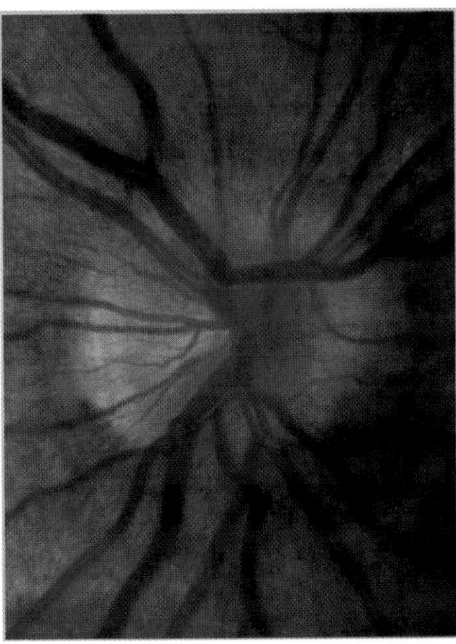

Figure 7.43 Bilateral optic nerve head swelling in a child with chronic intermediate uveitis.

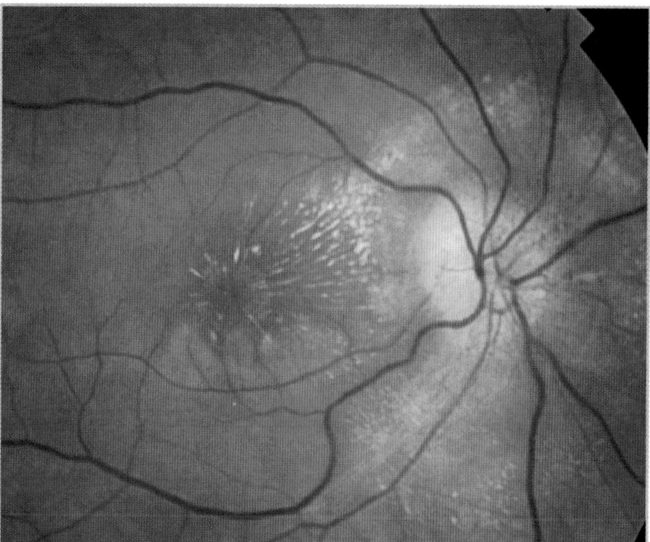

Figure 7.44 Neuroretinitis in a patient with bartonellosis.

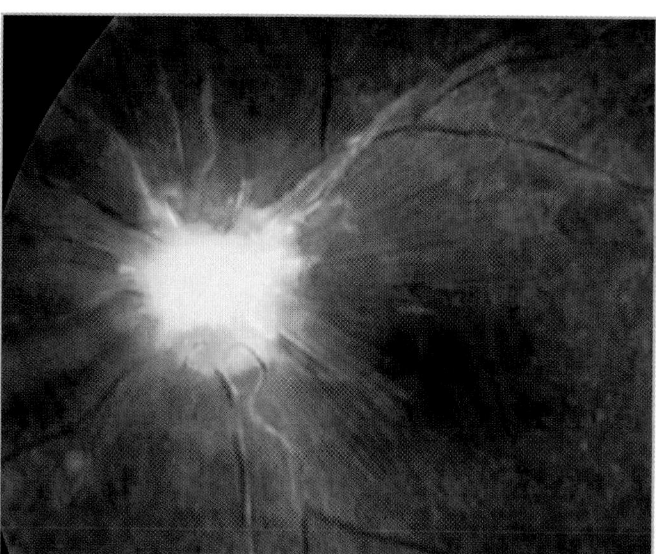

Figure 7.45 Massive pre- and peripapillary gliosis with retinal traction in a patient with Behçet's disease.

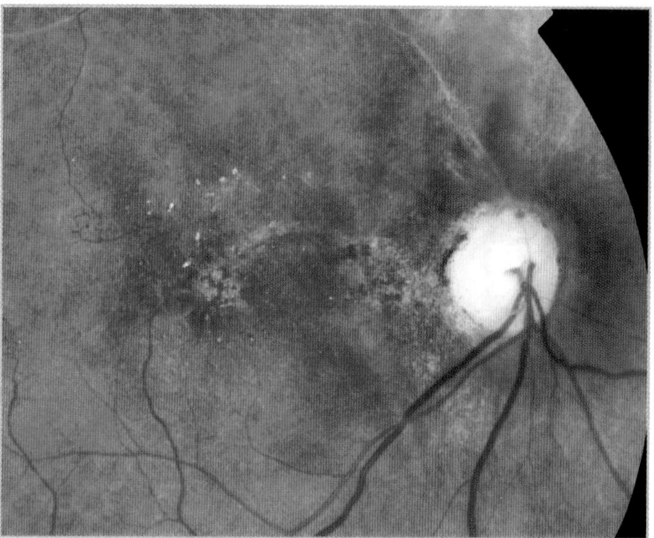

Figure 7.46 Optic atrophy superiorly in tandem with superior retinal infarction – end-stage Behçet's disease.

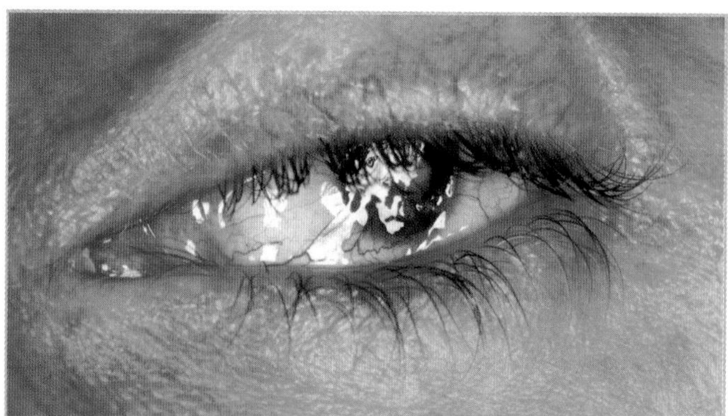

Figure 7.47 Phthisis. The intraocular pressure is unmeasurable, the eye is shrunken leading to enophthalmos and pseudoptosis, and the anterior segment is disorganized with corneal shrinkage. The eye is blind and intermittently aches.

Phthisis

The dreaded word. The end of the line. The failure of treatment. Blindness. Most likely to be encountered in JIA-associated uveitis, sympathetic uveitis or severe HLA-B27-associated uveitis (**Fig. 7.47**). Unlike some complications of uveitis, there is usually a long deterioration to this point, during which all aspects should be thoroughly investigated. As IOPs hover around the 2–6 mmHg mark, any residual inflammation should be eradicated if possible. The possibility of cyclitic membrane and ciliary body distraction should be considered; surgery may be effective (Yu et al. 2007). For those with clearly deteriorating vision and intraocular pressures of 0–2 mmHg, it is feasible to perform vitrectomy with silicone oil injection, which does lift IOP by a slight amount. However, it is the experience in this clinic and of others (Kapur et al. 2010) that the effect is not long lasting and that top-up silicone oil injections are often given but are of limited value. Some have found that where ciliary processes are not visibly atrophic, the removal of surface membranes from this area can restore function (Gupta et al. 2009).

Large-dose intravitreal steroid injection and/or intensive topical steroid has not been found by us to have sustained effect. The injection of dense sodium hyaluronate, either alone or in the anterior segment on top of silicone oil, although claimed to be successful in some cases (Kucukerdonmez et al. 2009), in our experience is short lasting and requires frequent repetition. In addition to hypotonic maculopathy, globe shape change, especially where inflammation is present, can induce bizarre posterior segment changes (**Fig. 7.48**) which are irreversible. Eyelid movement on a hypotonous eye induces massive fluctuating astigmatism, and our efforts to control this with haptic contact lenses have failed. In short, most efforts at management of the pre-phthisical state fail in the short to moderate term. In those in whom this is the only eye, reactions in the patient vary from stoicism to panic. We have found it fruitful to begin, at an early stage, the process of explanation and education into non-visual methods of functioning, to arrange meetings with those similarly affected and to ensure contact with the relevant social services. Total blindness is fortunately rare in patients with uveitis but must be encountered occasionally by the specialist. Managing the situation with a combination of responsible intervention tempered with sympathetic pragmatism is a challenge in itself.

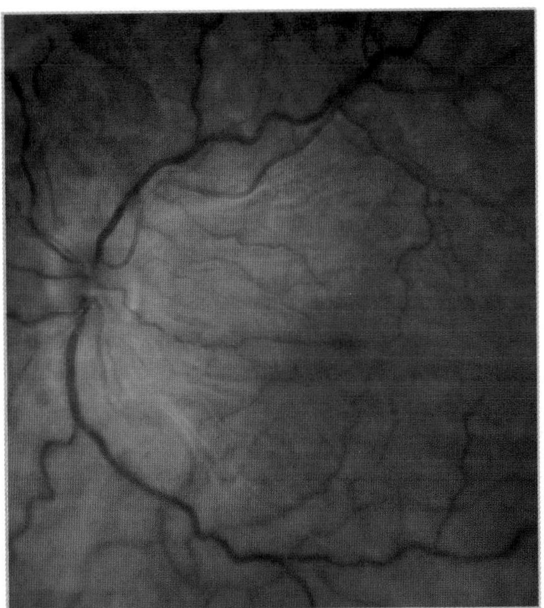

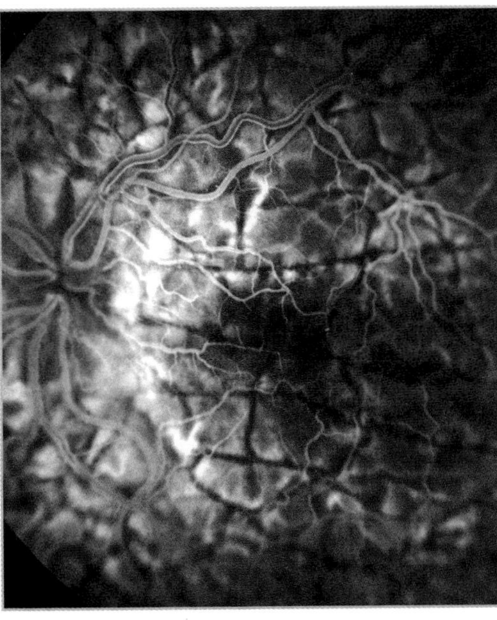

Figure 7.48 Chronic ocular hypotony in uveitis: choroidal folding has become adherent with fibrosis, the changes being more starkly seen on angiography.

REFERENCES

Abela-Formanek C, Amon M, Kahraman G, et al. Biocompatibility of hydrophilic acrylic, hydrophobic acrylic, and silicone intraocular lenses in eyes with uveitis having cataract surgery: long-term follow-up. *J Cataract Refract Surg* 2011;**37**:104–12.

Acharya N, Hong K, Lee S. Ranibizumab for refractory uveitis-related macular edema. *Am J Ophthalmol* 2009;**148**:303–9.

Alio JL, Chipont E, BenEzra D, et al. Comparative performance of intraocular lenses in eyes with cataract and uveitis. *J Cataract Refract Surg* 2002;**28**: 2096–108.

Anderson DF, Prabhasawat P, Alfonso E, Tseng SC. Amniotic membrane transplantation after the primary surgical management of band keratopathy. *Cornea* 2001;**20**:354–61.

Araujo SV, Bond JB, Wilson RP, et al. Long term effect of apraclonidine. *Br J Ophthalmol* 1995;**79**:1098–101.

Arevalo JF, Adan A, Berrocal MH, et al. Intravitreal bevacizumab for inflammatory choroidal neovascularisation: results from the Pan-American Collaborative Retina Study Group at 24 months. *Retina* 2011;**31**:353–63.

Auer C, Mermoud A, Herbort CP. Deep sclerectomy for the management of uncontrolled uveitic glaucoma: preliminary data. *Klin Monatsbl Augenheilkd* 2004;**221**:339–42.

Becker M, Davis J. Vitrectomy in the treatment of uveitis. *Am J Ophthalmol* 2005;**140**:1096–105.

Bentley CR, Stanford MR, Shilling JS, et al. Macular ischaemia in posterior uveitis. *Eye* 1993;**7**:411–14.

Benz MS, Packo KH, Gonzales V, et al. A placebo-controlled trial of microplasmin intravitreous injection to facilitate posterior vitreous detachment before vitrectomy. *Ophthalmology* 2010;**117**:791–7.

Broadway DC, Grierson I, Sturmer J, Hitchings R. Reversal of topical antiglaucoma medication effects on the conjunctiva. *Arch Ophthalmol* 1996;**114**:262–7.

Broadway DC, Chang LP. Trabeculectomy; risk factors for failure and the preoperative state of the conjunctiva. *J Glaucoma* 2001;**10**:237–49.

Broadway DC, Bloom PA, Bunce C, et al. Needle revision of failing and failed trabeculectomy blebs with adjunctive 5-fluorouracil: a survival analysis. *Ophthalmology* 2004;**111**:665–73.

Ceballos EM, Parrish RK, Schiffman JC. Outcome of Baerveldt glaucoma drainage implants for the treatment of uveitic glaucoma. *Ophthalmology* 2002;**109**:2256–60.

Cellini M, Caramazza R, Bonsanto D, et al. Prostaglandin analogs and blood-aqueous barrier integrity: a flare cell meter study. *Ophthalmologica* 2004;**218**:312–17.

Chawla A, Mercieca K, Fenerty CH, Jones NP. Outcomes and complications of trabeculectomy enhanced with 5-fluorouracil in adults with glaucoma secondary to uveitis. *J Glaucoma* 2012; in press.

Clark AF, Steely HT, Dickerson JE, et al. Glucocorticoid induction of the glaucoma gene MYOC in human and monkey trabecular meshwork cells and tissues. *Invest Ophthalmol Vis Sci* 2001;*42*:1769–80.

Das-Bhaumik RG, Jones NP. Low-dose intraocular triamcinolone injection for intractable macular oedema and inflammation in patients with uveitis. *Eye* 2006;**20**:934–7.

Dupas B, Fardeau C, Cassoux N, et al. Deep sclerectomy and trabeculectomy in uveitic glaucoma. *Eye* 2010;**24**:310–14.

Durrani OM, Tehrani NN, Marr JE, et al. Degree, duration and causes of visual loss in uveitis. *Br J Ophthalmol* 2004;**88**:1159–62.

Faia LJ, Sen HN, Li Z, et al. Treatment of inflammatory macular edema with humanized anti-CD11a antibody therapy. *Invest Ophthalmol Vis Sci* 2011;Epub.

Forooghian F, Yeh S, Fafa LJ, Nussenblatt RB. Uveitic foveal atrophy: clinical features and associations. *Arch Ophthalmol* 2009;**127**:179–86.

Fortuna E, Cervantes-Castaneda R, Bhat P, et al. Flare-up rates with bimatoprost therapy in uveitic glaucoma. *Am J Ophthalmol* 2008;**146**:876–82.

Galor A, Lowder CY, Kaiser P, et al. Surgical drainage of chronic serous retinal detachment associated with uveitis. *Retina* 2008;**28**:282–88.

Giuliari GP, Chang PY, Thakuria P, et al. Pars plana vitrectomy in the management of pediatric uveitis: the Massachusetts Eye Research and Surgery Institution experience. *Eye* 2010;**24**:7–13.

Gugleta K. Topical carbonic anhydrase inhibitors and visual function in glaucoma and ocular hypertension. *Curr Med Res Opin* 2010;**26**:1255–67.

Gulati N, Forooghian F, Lieberman R, Jabs D. Vascular endothelial growth factor inhibition in uveitis : a systematic review. *Br J Ophthalmol* 2011;**95**:162–5.

Gupta P, Gupta A, Gupta V, Singh R. Successful outcome of pars plana vitreous surgery in chronic hypotony due to uveitis. *Retina* 2009;**29**:638–43.

Hill RA, Nguyen QH, Baerveldt G, et al. Trabeculectomy and Molteno implantation for glaucomas associated with uveitis. *Ophthalmology* 1993;**100**:903–8.

Hollands H, Seif G, Hollands S, Gale J. A trial of topical prednisolone acetate before intravitreal triamcinolone acetonide decreases intraocular pressure spikes. *Can J Ophthalmol* 2010;**45**:484–8.

Jalil A, Dhawahir-Scala F, Jones NP. Non-progressive tractional inferior retinal elevations in intermediate uveitis. *Ocul Immunol Inflamm* 2010;**18**:60–63.

Jones NP. Fuchs' heterochromic uveitis: a reappraisal of the clinical spectrum. *Eye* 1991;**5**:649–61.

Jones NP, McLeod D, Boulton ME. Massive proliferation of the lens epithelial remnants after Nd-YAG capsulotomy. *Br J Ophthalmol* 1995;**79**:261–263.

Julian K, Terrada C, Fardeau C, et al. Intravitreal bevacizumab as first local treatment for uveitis-related choroidal neovascularisation: long-term results. *Acta Ophthalmol* 2011;**89**:179–84.

Kapur R, Birnbaum AD, Goldstein DA, et al. Treating uveitis-associated hypotony with pars plana vitrectomy and silicone oil injection. *Retina* 2010;**30**:140–5.

Kerkhoff FT, Lamberts QJ, van den Biesen PR, Rothova A. Rhegmatogenous retinal detachment and uveitis. *Ophthalmology* 2003;**110**:427–31.

Kersey JP, Broadway DC. Corticosteroid-induced glaucoma: a review of the literature. *Eye* 2006;**20**:407–16.

Kotsolis AI, Killian FA, Ladas ID, Yanuzzi LA. Fluorescein angiography and ocular coherence tomography concordance for choroidal neovascularisation in multifocal choroiditis. *Br J Ophthalmol* 2010;**94**:1506–8.

Kucukerdonmez C, Beutel J, Bartz-Schmidt KU, Gelisken F. Treatment of chronic ocular hypotony with intraocular application of sodium hyaluronate. *Br J Ophthalmol* 2009;**93**:235–9.

Lam S, Tessler HH, Lam BL, et al. High incidence of sympathetic ophthalmia after contact and noncontact neodymium:YAG cyclotherapy. *Ophthalmology* 1992:**99**:1818–1822.

Lee HS, Kim MS. Influential factors on the survival of endothelial cells after penetrating keratoplasty. *Eur J Ophthalmol* 2009;**19**:930–5.

Mackensen F, Carsten H, Becker M, Heilegenhaus A. Intravitreal bevacizumab (Avastin) as a treatment for refractory macular edema in patients with uveitis: a pilot study. *Retina* 2008;**28**:41–5.

Markomichelakis NN, Halkiadakis I, Pantelia E, et al. Patterns of macular edema in patients with uveitis: qualitative and quantitative assessment using optical coherence tomography. *Ophthalmology* 2004;**111**:946–53.

Markomichelakis NN, Kostakou A, Halkiadakis I, et al. Efficacy and safety of latanoprost in eyes with uveitic glaucoma. *Graefes Arch Clin Exp Ophthalmol* 2010;**247**:775–80.

Maus TL, Nau C, Brubaker RF. Comparison of the early effects of brimonidine and apraclonidine as topical ocular hypotensive agents. i 1999;117:586–91.

Miserocchi E, Carassa RG, Bettin P, Brancato R. Viscocanalostomy in patients with glaucoma secondary to uveitis: preliminary report. *J Cataract Refract Surg* 2004;**30**:566–70.

Nagar M, Ogunyomade A, O'Brart DP, et al. A randomized, prospective study comparing selective laser trabeculoplasty with latanoprost for the control of intraocular pressure in ocular hypertension and open angle glaucoma. *Br J Ophthalmol* 2005;**89**:1413–7.

Noble J, Derzko-Dzulynsky L, Rabinovitch T, Birt C. Outcome of trabeculectomy with intraoperative mitomycin C for uveitic glaucoma. *Can J Ophthalmol* 2007;**42**:89–94.

O'Brart DP. Gartry DS, Lohmann CP, et al. Treatment of band keratopathy by excimer laser phototherapeutic keratectomy: surgical techniques and long-term follow-up. *Br J Ophthalmol* 1993;**77**:702–8.

Ossewaarde-van Norel J, Berg EM, Sijssens KM, Rothova A. Subfoveal serous retinal detachment in patients with uveitic macular edema. *Arch Ophthalmol* 2011;**129**:158–62.

Ozdal PC, Vianna RN, Deschenes J. Ahmed valve implantation in glaucoma secondary to chronic uveitis. *Eye* 2006;**20**:178–83.

Papadaki TG, Zacharopoulos IP, Pasquale LR, et al. Long-term results of Ahmed glaucoma valve implantation for uveitic glaucoma. *Am J Ophthalmol* 2007;**144**:62–9.

Parodi MB, Iacono P, Kontadakis DS, et al. Bevacizumab vs photodynamic therapy for choroidal neovascularisation in multifocal choroiditis. *Arch Ophthalmol* 2010;**128**:1100–3.

Perentes Y, Van Tran T, Sickenberg M, Herbort CP. *Ocul Immunol Inflamm* 2005;**13**:219–24.

Piette S, Canlas OA, Tran HV, et al. Ultrasound biomicroscopy in uveitis-glaucoma-hyphema syndrome. *Am J Ophthalmol* 2002;**133**:839–41.

Prata JA, Neves RA, Minckler DS, et al. Trabeculectomy with mitomycin C in glaucoma associated with uveitis. *Ophthalmic Surg* 1994:**25**:616–620.

Quinones K, Choi JY, Yilmaz T, et al. Pars plana vitrectomy versus immunomodulatory therapy for intermediate uveitis: a prospective randomized pilot study. *Ocul Immunol Inflamm* 2010;**18**:411–7.

Rachmiel R, Trope GE, Buys YM, et al. Ahmed glaucoma valve implantation in uveitic glaucoma versus open-angle glaucoma patients. *Can J Ophthalmol* 2008;**43**:462–7.

Rahman I, Jones NP. Long-term results of cataract extraction with intraocular lens implantation in patients with uveitis. *Eye* 2005;19:191–7.

Roesel M, Gutfleisch M, Heinz C, et al. Intravitreal and orbital floor triamcinolone acetonide injections in noninfectious uveitis: a comparative study. *Ophthalmic Res* 2009;**42**:81–6.

Rojas B, Zafirakis P, Christen W, et al. Medical treatment of macular edema in patients with uveitis. *Doc Ophthalmol* 1999;**97**:399–407.

Rouvas A, Petrou P, Douvali M, et al. Intravitreal ranibizumab for the treatment of inflammatory choroidal neovascularisation. *Retina* 2011;**31**:871–9.

Sanisio SR, Lowder CY, Kaiser PK, et al. Corticosteroid therapy for optic disc neovascularisation secondary to chronic uveitis. *Am J Ophthalmol* 2000;**130**:724–31.

Shankar V, Roberts F, Ramaesh K. Histopathological changes of cornea in long-term sympathetic ophthalmitis. *Cornea* 2010;**29**:1287–90.

Sijssens KM, Los LI, Rothova A, et al. Long-term ocular complications in aphakic versus pseudophakic eyes of children with juvenile idiopathic arthritis-associated uveitis. *Br J Ophthalmol* 2010;**94**:1145–9.

Spencer NA, Hall AJ, Stawell RJ. Nd:YAG laser iridotomy in uveitic glaucoma. *Clin Exp Ophthalmol* 2001;**29**:217–9.

Stalmans P, DeLaey C, de Smet M, et al. Intravitreal injection of microplasmin for treatment of vitreomacular adhesion: results of a prospective, randomized, sham-controlled Phase II trial (MIVI-IIt trial). *Retina* 2010;**30**:1122–7.

Stavrou P, Baltatzis S, Letko E, et al. Pars plana vitrectomy in patients with intermediate uveitis. *Ocul Immunol Inflamm* 2001;**9**:141–51.

Suresh P, Jones NP. Phacoemulsification with intraocular lens implantation in patients with uveitis. *Eye* 2001;**15**:621–8.

Taylor SR, Habot-Wilner Z, Pacheco P, Lightman S. Intraocular methotrexate in the treatment of uveitis and uveitic cystoid macular edema. *Ophthalmology* 2009;**116**:797–801.

Toris CB, Tafoya ME, Camras CB, et al. Effects of apraclonidine on aqueous humor dynamics in human eyes. *Ophthalmology* 1995:**102**:456–461.

Towler HM, McCluskey P, Shaer B, Lightman S. Long-term follow-up of trabeculectomy with intraoperative 5-fluorouracil for uveitis-related glaucoma. *Ophthalmology* 2000;**107**:1822–8.

Tranos P, Scott R, Zambarajki H, et al. The effect of pars plana vitrectomy on cystoid macular oedema associated with chronic uveitis: a randomized, controlled pilot study. *Br J Ophthalmol* 2006;**90**:1107–10.

Wachtlin J, Heimann H, Behme T, Foerster MH. Long-term results after photodynamic therapy with verteporfin for choroidal neovascularisations secondary to inflammatory chorioretinal diseases. *Graefes Arch Clin Exp Ophthalmol* 2003;**241**:899–906.

Waters FM, Goodall K, Jones NP, McLeod D. Vitrectomy for vitreous opacification in Fuchs' heterochromic uveitis. *Eye* 2000;**14**:216–18.

Whitcup SM, Csaky KG, Podgor MJ, et al. A randomized, masked crossover trial of acetazolamide for macular edema in patients with uveitis. *Ophthalmology* 1996;**103**:1054–62.

Wilensky JT. The role of brimonidine in the treatment of open-angle glaucoma. *Surv Ophthalmol* 1996;**41**(suppl):3–7.

Woreta F, Thorne JE, Jabs DA, et al. Risk factors for ocular complications and poor visual acuity at presentation among patients with uveitis associated with juvenile idiopathic arthritis. *Am J Ophthalmol* 2007;**143**:647–55.

Yu EN, Paredes I, Foster CS. Surgery for hypotony in patients with juvenile idiopathic arthritis-associated uveitis. *Ocul Immunol Inflamm* 2007;**15**:11–17.

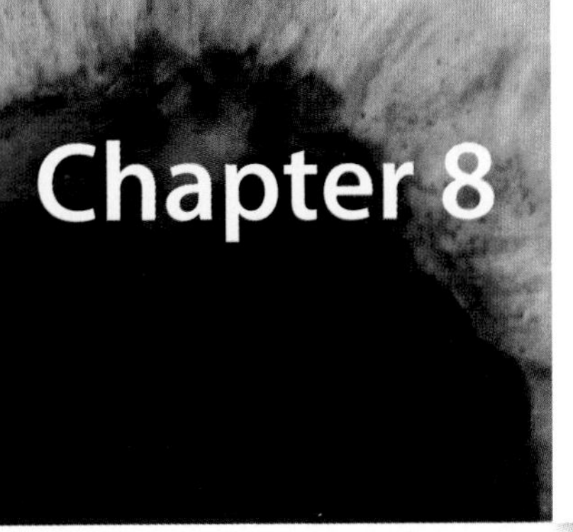

Chapter 8 Uveitis associated with HLA-B27, arthritis and inflammatory bowel disease

HLA-B27-ASSOCIATED UVEITIS, SERONEGATIVE ARTHRITIS AND INFLAMMATORY BOWEL DISEASE (box 8.1)

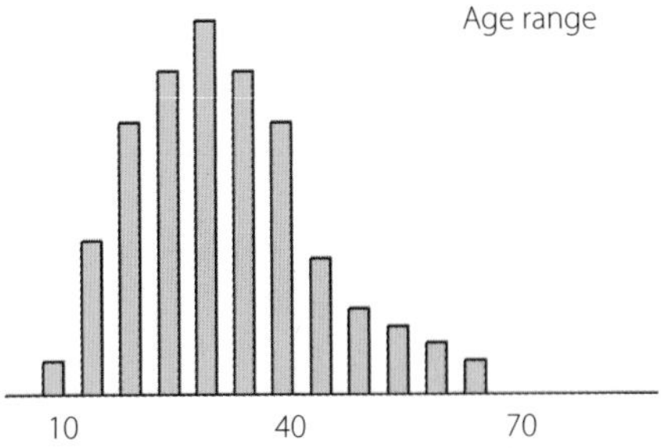

Age range

10 40 70

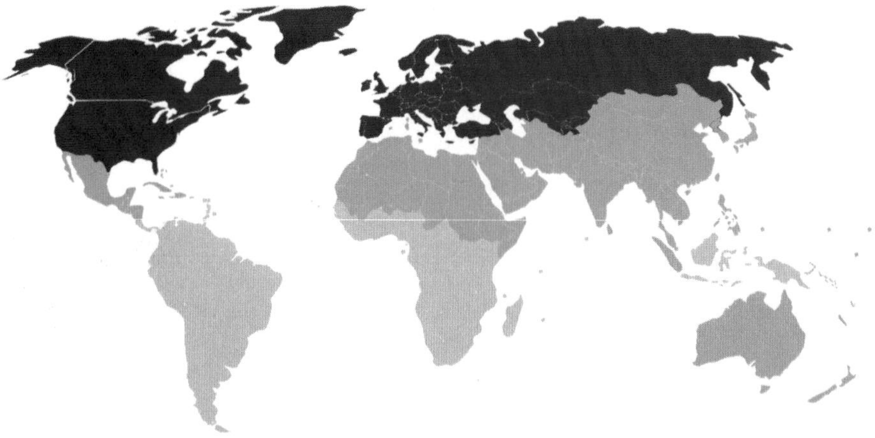

Cause	HLA-B27 positivity, followed by one or more unknown triggers for the onset of uveitis
Sex, age, race, geography	M:F 1.5:1
Systemic disease	Ankylosing spondylitis, reactive arthritis, psoriatic arthropathy, inflammatory bowel disease are all associated
Ocular disease	Typically, acute recurrent unilateral non-granulomatous anterior uveitis
Differential diagnosis	If typical, pathognomonic. If not, other causes of non-granulomatous uveitis
Investigation	HLA-B27 assessment if in doubt
Management	Intensive topical and periocular steroids and mydriatics. Systemic steroid for severe inflammation. Identification and management of associated disease
Prognosis	With prompt and vigorous management, good. Synechiae, glaucoma and cataract can occur. May become chronic. If severe may lead to phthisis

Box 8.1 HLA-B27-associated uveitis

Introduction

The association between acute anterior uveitis (AAU) and the human leukocyte antigen HLA-B27 is the most common known etiological association in the field of uveitis . HLA-B27 is also associated with a number of systemic inflammatory diseases in which arthropathy is a prominent factor. The possession of HLA-B27 not only increases the likelihood of developing these diseases, but also seems to modify their clinical attributes; HLA-B27-associated uveitis tends to exhibit certain characteristic features, and HLA-B27-associated arthropathy tends to involve the axial skeleton. Many subtypes of HLA-B27 have been identified, and it is suggested that B*2705 is associated with a higher incidence of both anterior uveitis (Konno et al. 1999) and ankylosing spondylitis (AS) (Cipriani et al. 2003). This subtype also has a higher preponderance in males, which may in part explain the higher incidence of these diseases in men. The geographical distribution of HLA-B27 reflects in part a racial distribution, but pockets of rarity and frequency exist (Pavesio et al. 2009). Although HLA-B27 is the only class I allele associated with AAU, more subtle associations among class II and other MHC (major histocompatibility complex) genes have recently been described in an overview (Martin et al. 2011).

The precise role of HLA-B27 in the pathogenesis of uveitis remains the subject of investigation. In a white population in the UK, 6–8% are HLA-B27 positive, yet the lifetime risk of AAU for these is still only 0.4%. Substantial evidence has gathered that enteric infection with some Gram-negative bacteria, or chlamydial urethritis, may act as a trigger to induce inflammation including AAU, arthropathy and reactive arthritis; this includes serological evidence of exposure to these organisms, and the demonstration of bacterial components in synovial fluid in those with a sterile arthropathy. The mechanism(s) of this association between AAU and infections in HLA-B27 positive people remains unclear, although suggestions of molecular mimicry by homologous regions of the epitope of HLA-B27 and bacterial receptors are attractive (Feltkamp et al. 1996).

Systemic disease

A substantial proportion of patients with HLA-B27-associated anterior uveitis have associated systemic disease (Monnet et al. 2004), over half of whom may have, or may develop, spondyloarthropathy. Some of these patients will already be aware of this. For the remainder, the early identification of such disease, particularly the arthropathies, may substantially affect the long-term outcome. The ophthalmologist therefore has an important role in identifying or suspecting associated systemic disease, and arranging appropriate referral.

As for anterior uveitis, the possession of HLA-B27 is not mandatory for these diseases to occur. However, HLA-B27 makes the onset of such diseases more likely (the relative risk of HLA-B27 for ankylosing spondylitis is about 90%), and may modify the clinical picture, especially of the associated reactive arthropathy, which then preferentially involves the axial skeleton.

Ankylosing spondylitis

Ankylosing spondylitis is a chronic axial arthropathy affecting predominantly the lower spine and sacroiliac joints. Affected males outnumber females by 5:1. The symptomatic onset is usually in the teens or 20s, with intermittent buttock or lower back pain, typically worse in the morning and evening and relieved by exercise. The discomfort is exacerbated by rest and may radiate into the thigh, sometimes mimicking sciatica. Spinal stiffness, if untreated, may progress into an inability to flex, and ultimately a thoracic kyphosis (**Fig. 8.1**). Unrecognized and untreated, the disease may, in those worst affected, progress to complete spinal fusion and severe disability (**Fig. 8.2**). The association between HLA-B27 and AS is striking, over 95% of AS patients being HLA-B27 positive. About a quarter of patients with AS experience AAU at some stage.

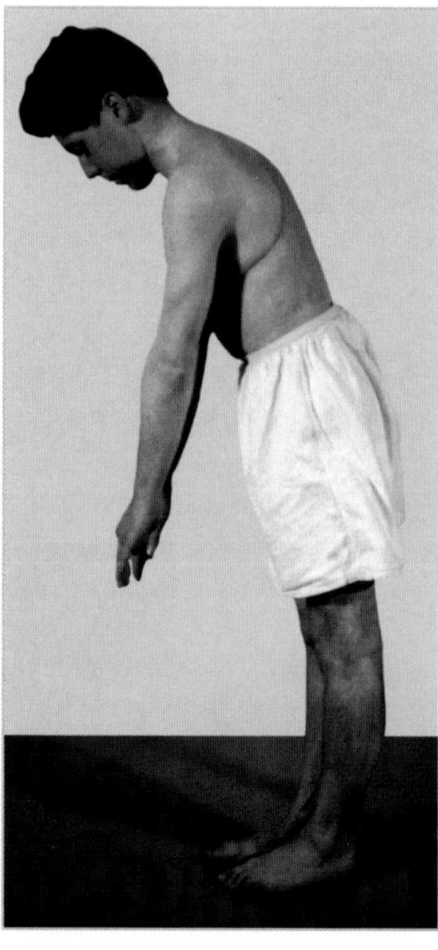

Figure 8.1 Spinal fusion causing an inability to flex the spine in a man with ankylosing spondylitis.

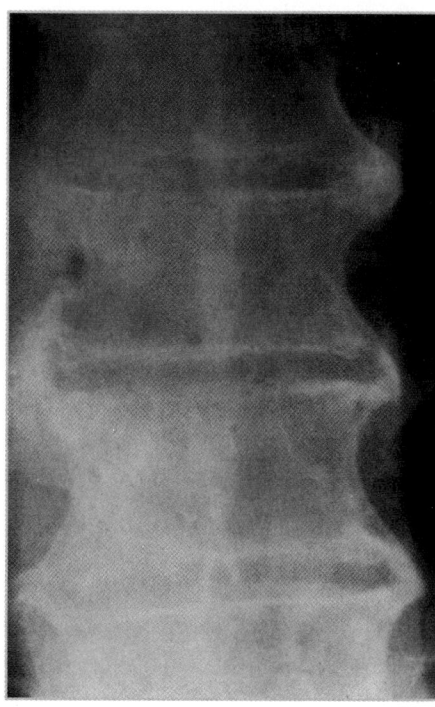

Figure 8.2 Complete spinal fusion ('bamboo spine') in advanced ankylosing spondylitis.

As symptoms of AS may precede radiological evidence by some years, it is our practice to enquire about symptoms suggestive of AS in any patient presenting with anterior uveitis. Many symptomatic patients have not been seen by a rheumatologist, and we refer for expert opinion all those with suspicious symptoms. As radiological evidence should not be a prerequisite for rheumatological referral, we do not consider it appropriate that the ophthalmologist should request such radiological investigations. They should be requested if considered necessary by a rheumatologist after referral and interpreted in the context of expert examination.

The ophthalmologist, in facilitating AS diagnosis, may improve prognosis; early recognition allows instruction in appropriate regular exercise, which if correctly performed greatly improves the outlook. Non-steroidal anti-inflammatory drugs (NSAIDs) are used during intermittent flare-ups of activity. In the one-third of patients who develop peripheral joint disease, local steroid injection or the use of sulfasalazine or cytotoxic agents may be necessary. Oral immunosuppression may be necessary and there is a trend towards earlier anti-tumor necrosis factor α (TNF-α) monoclonal antibody treatment.

Reactive arthritis (Brodie's syndrome)

This multisystem disease was originally named after a physician who was later convicted of war crimes after the deaths of hundreds of prisoners during medical experimentation at Buchenwald and elsewhere. It is appropriate that his name has been expunged from the medical literature. As for so many eponymous diseases, earlier claims exist in any case. A good description of reactive arthritis and its accompanying syndrome was made 100 years earlier in 1818 by Sir Benjamin Brodie PRS (Sheldrake 2008), in his acclaimed treatise *Pathological and Surgical Observations on the Diseases of the Joints*, in which he introduced pain scoring and conservation rather than amputation. As the term 'reactive arthritis' is very inadequate to describe a sometimes complex multisystem syndrome of inflammation, it is here proposed that Brodie is a worthy bearer of the eponym.

Brodie's syndrome (BS) appears to be a reactive multifocal inflammation in predisposed individuals (most being HLA-B27 positive) exposed to infection with certain organisms. The predominant site of infection is genitourinary or enteric, and there is a particular association with chlamydial urethritis, or dysentery caused by some *Salmonella* and *Yersinia* species, *Shigella flexneri* and *Campylobacter jejuni*. Reactive arthritis alone may follow the above infections whether or not the patient is HLA-B27 positive, but positivity makes more widespread manifestations more likely. Nevertheless, BS is a very uncommon sequel to dysentery, affecting fewer than 1% of cases. In some the association between the causative infection and the subsequent reactive syndrome is obvious because of microbiological diagnosis and a rapid onset of BS; in others the primary infection may have been asymptomatic or forgotten.

Brodie's syndrome is rare in women. The classic triad of signs includes urethritis (either chlamydial or sterile), conjunctivitis and, later, arthritis. The last occurs in almost all patients, but conjunctivitis is seen in only a minority. In addition a variety of other features may be seen, including oral ulceration (**Fig. 8.3**), painless circinate balanitis (**Fig. 8.4**), keratoderma blenorrhagicum (red hyperkeratotic or pustular lesions on the soles of the feet, rarely on the palms, sometimes resembling acute pustular psoriasis or pompholyx eczema – **Fig. 8.5**) and onycholysis. In some, a generalized psoriasiform rash develops.

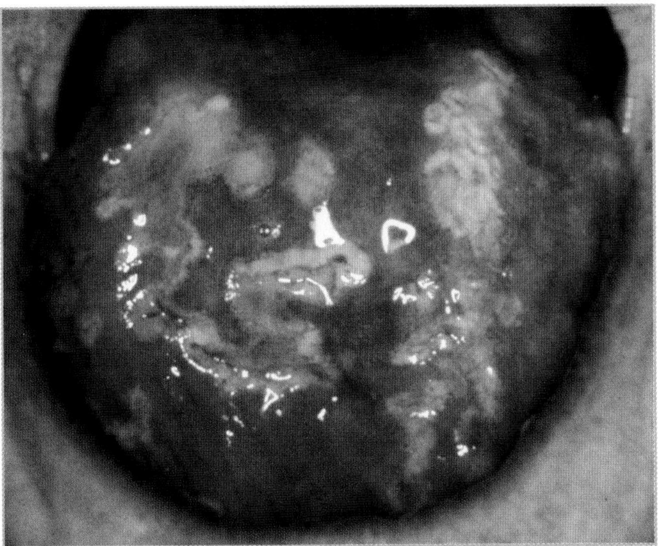

Figure 8.3 Severe confluent ('geographic') ulceration of the tongue in association with reactive arthritis (Brodie's syndrome). (Courtesy of the late Dr PJ Holt.)

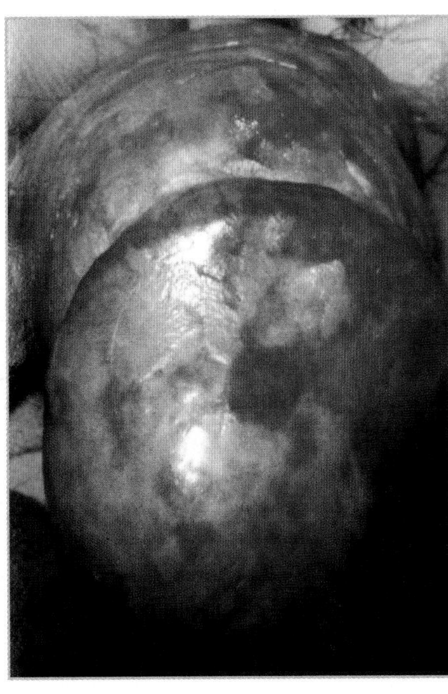

Figure 8.4 Circinate balanitis in association with reactive arthritis (Brodie's syndrome). (Courtesy of Dr K Haye.)

Arthritis is usually most marked in the lower limbs and hands, and is usually asymmetrical and pauciarticular, but occasionally a polyarthropathy ensues. In most cases the arthropathy is mild, but in some the disease is persistent and in a few can become severely disabling. Some go on to develop AS. In some patients the features of BS are protean and, although usually acute and clustered together, may occur independently over a long period. A diagnostic dilemma exists in some cases which is reminiscent of a similar problem in Behçet's disease and lupus, not only in principle but also in the context of symptoms and signs.

Acute anterior uveitis may occur at any stage during or after the acute phase of the disease. It is usually typical of HLA-B27-associated uveitis; indeed those patients with BS who go on to develop anterior uveitis are almost invariably HLA-B27 positive. In a few patients a nummular keratitis may develop. A significant minority of BS patients develop a more severe and chronic uveitis and they can be among the most difficult to manage in this group.

Psoriatic arthritis

Psoriasis is a common disease, affecting up to 2% of the population. A seronegative psoriatic arthritis (PSA) affects some 7% of these patients. The predominant component of the arthritis is usually peripheral, with diffuse swelling of affected fingers (dactylitis), but the disease is often focal or asymmetrical, and distal interphalangeal joints may be particularly affected (**Fig. 8.6**). Psoriatic nail changes are present in almost all patients with PSA, including pitting, onycholysis (separation of the nail from its bed) and abnormal ridging. There is no correlation between the severity of a psoriatic rash and the accompanying PSA. The onset of PSA may precede a rash and in a few patients a typical arthropathy occurs in isolation with no evidence of skin involvement. A proportion of patients with PSA have axial skeleton involvement, including spondylitis and sacroiliitis. Such patients are almost always HLA-B27 positive (Paiva et al. 2000).

Some 5% or more of patients with peripheral PSA develop anterior uveitis, which may be acute recurrent or chronic. In contrast, those with axial PSA who are HLA-B27 positive have approaching a 30% chance of developing anterior uveitis, the pattern usually being

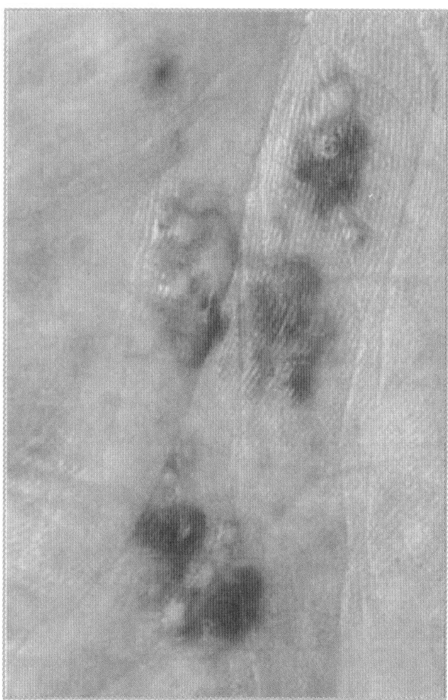

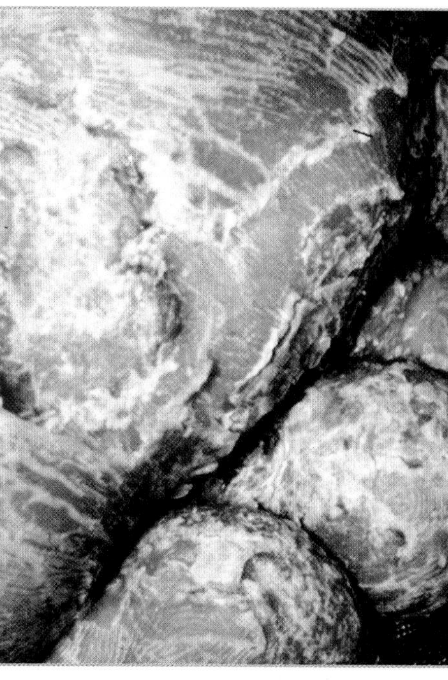

Figure 8.5 Keratoderma blenorrhagicum of the feet in Brodie's syndrome. Milder forms as seen on the left can resemble pustular psoriasis, pompholyx eczema or tinea. Severe and widespread involvement as shown on the right leads to desquamating hyperkeratotic lesions. (Courtesy of the late Dr PJ Holt.)

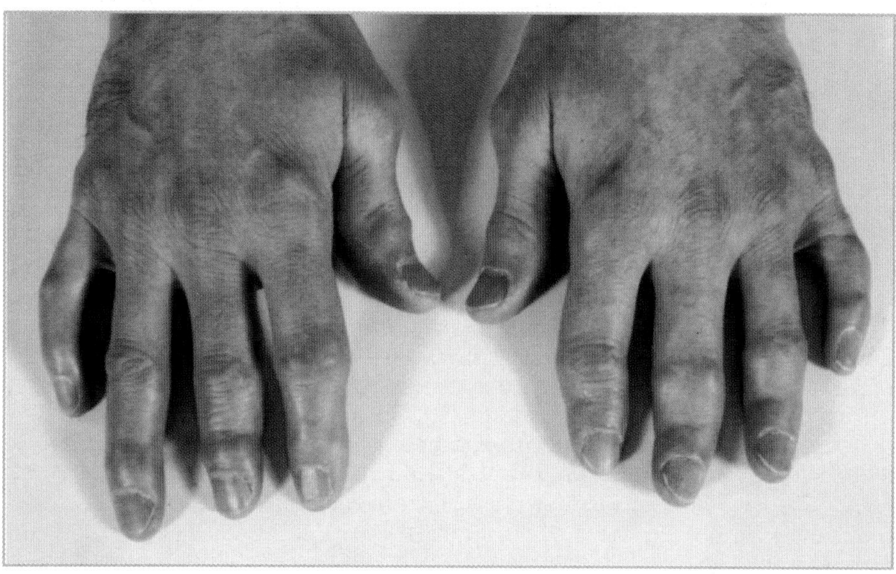

Figure 8.6 Destructive psoriatic arthritis has a tendency to affect more distal interphalangeal joints with subsequent deformity.

typical of HLA-B27 positivity. Some have an indolent chronic form with posterior segment involvement and bilateral simultaneous inflammation is common (Queiro et al. 2002). The management of the uveitis is usually straightforward but some go on to develop severe chronic disease requiring immunosuppression.

Inflammatory bowel disease

Both ulcerative colitis and Crohn's disease may exhibit numerous extraintestinal manifestations and may be associated with uveitis, but from the perspective of an ophthalmologist the association is uncommon. In this clinic it is found in only 1.1% of patients. Uveitis appears to be particularly associated with colonic inflammation, being more often seen in ulcerative colitis than in Crohn's disease, and being seen in the latter condition only rarely when the colon is uninvolved. Ulcerative colitis is a chronic inflammatory disease limited to the large bowel, whereas Crohn's disease is granulomatous and may affect any part of the gastrointestinal tract. A significant degree of genetic susceptibility for both diseases has been clarified, being linked to CARD15, IRGM and others (Henckaerts et al. 2008). However, further triggers are clearly necessary. Environmental factors are unclear although oral contraceptives may contribute to the risk, as does smoking. Originally considered an autoimmune disease, it is now possible that Crohn's disease may result from a breakdown in control systems of the innate immunity system. Interest had previously centered on evidence of microorganisms within affected bowel, but currently this is considered to represent opportunistic infection within disordered mucosas rather than a causative trigger.

There are geographical variations in incidence especially for ulcerative colitis, which is particularly common in northern Europe. This may be related to differences in diet. Both diseases have a familial incidence, but the sexes are equally affected. It is most unusual for a symptomatic undiagnosed patient to present with uveitis, but the ophthalmologist should be aware that, although the presentations of these two diseases tend to differ, any of the following may be suggestive: persistent diarrhea, with or without mucus or fresh or changed blood, aching abdominal pain, tenesmus, colic, weight loss, malaise, lassitude, anorexia or anemia. Extraintestinal manifestations may occur in both conditions: aphthous ulceration may be seen in both, whereas perianal and perineal ulceration is a feature only of Crohn's disease; both signs may simulate Behçet's disease. Glossitis and angular stomatitis (reflecting anemia) may also occur. Cutaneous complications include erythema nodosum, pyoderma gangrenosum and nail abnormalities.

An arthropathy may occur in up to 10% of patients with ulcerative colitis or Crohn's disease. The pattern of disease tends to reflect the patient's HLA-B27 status, negative patients tending to develop an asymmetrical lower limb arthritis which may settle as the bowel disease is treated, and positive patients developing axial arthropathy, some going on to develop typical ankylosing spondylitis, which may persist despite resolution of the enteritis.

Ocular disease

Conjunctivitis, episcleritis, scleritis or keratitis may occur in association with either Crohn's disease or ulcerative colitis. Those who are HLA-B27 positive may develop a typical acute anterior uveitis. However, other forms of uveitis may occur which include posterior segment involvement and, rarely, retinal vasculitis. Those HLA-B27-negative patients with peripheral arthropathy more often tend to develop a chronic bilateral uveitis, in contrast to the HLA-B27-positive patients with axial arthropathy. Anecdotes describing subclinical enteritis in association with anterior uveitis suggest that the association may be more common than is normally diagnosed.

The proportion of patients with anterior uveitis who are HLA-B27 positive is difficult to quantify, as most studies have as their base population a group of pre-selected patients. Percentages as high as 81% HLA-B27 positivity have been obtained for a population with unilateral AAU. Although figures of this order are probably unrepresentative, it is likely that more than half of such patients are HLA-B27 positive.

The clinical appearance of anterior uveitis tends to depend on the HLA-B27 status. There are no absolute boundaries and there may be considerable overlap for individual signs, but the trends are highly significant. The paradigm for HLA-B27-associated uveitis is a young male, possibly with associated systemic disease, with very acute unilateral AAU (possibly recurrent) causing moderate pain and severe photophobia, widespread conjunctival congestion, fibrinous exudate or non-liquid hypopyon in the anterior chamber, and posterior synechiae (**Fig. 8.7**). The clinical appearance of the uveitis seems more dependent on the HLA-B27 status than on the presence or absence of associated arthropathy or inflammatory bowel disease.

A study of 148 patients with HLA-B27-associated uveitis (Tay-Kearney et al. 1996) found that only 7% of patients had simultaneous bilateral uveitis; the remainder had either completely unilateral (56%) or asynchronous bilateral (37%) disease. The inflammation was acute in 87%, with posterior synechiae in 55%. A previous study of 144 patients (Rothova et al. 1987) had identified six criteria which, if all present, had a 100% correlation with HLA-B27 positivity and, for four or more criteria, 88% (**Table 8.1**). It is therefore clear that towards this end of the spectrum of AAU, HLA-B27 positivity is virtually assured; the young patient with recurrent acute unilateral fibrinous uveitis can almost be guaranteed to be HLA-B27 positive.

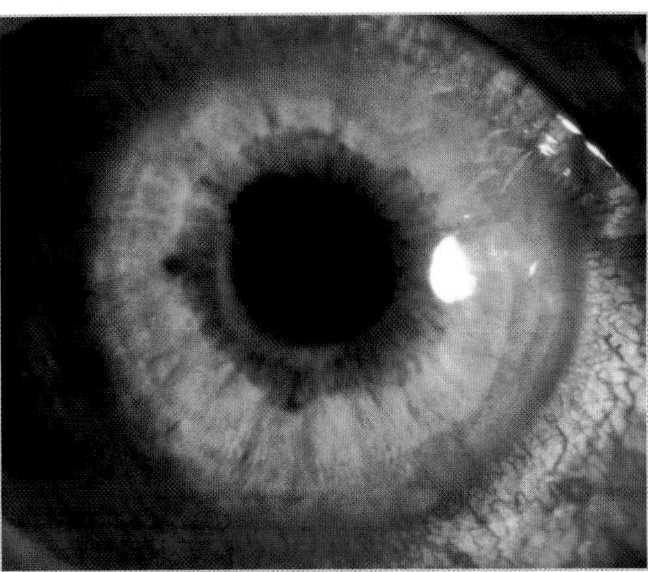

Figure 8.7 Acute HLA-B27-related anterior uveitis showing ciliary congestion, exudate in the anterior chamber and posterior synechiae.

Table 8.1 Criteria indicative of HLA-B27 positivity in anterior uveitis

1. Unilateral acute anterior uveitis
2. Fibrin or 3+ cells in the anterior chamber
3. Recurrent disease
4. Age at onset < 40 years
5. Absence of mutton-fat keratic precipitates
6. Concurrent ankylosing spondylitis or Reiter's syndrome
Adapted from Rothova et al. (1987).

Macular edema is not uncommon in association with HLA-B27-associated uveitis and usually settles along with the anterior segment inflammation. If recalcitrant a single orbital depot steroid injection usually suffices. Active posterior segment inflammation is not normally seen (although anterior vitritis accompanying iridocyclitis is common). However, severe posterior segment manifestations are occasionally seen, including severe vitritis, papillitis, retinal vasculopathy and pars planitis. In a small but significant minority, systemic steroid is required. Rarely an HLA-B27-associated hyperacute unilateral hypotensive panuveitis can be so severe as to mimic endophthalmitis (Merceica et al. 2010), precipitating intraocular sampling for microbiological diagnosis and requiring high-dose oral steroid treatment. Such patients often develop seclusio with glaucoma and cataract, and may require immunosuppression to prevent explosive recurrences. An aphakic pre-phthisical eye may result.

Some patients with troublesome frequent recurrences of uveitis go on to develop chronic fluctuating disease, often in both eyes together. The prognosis in such eyes can be as poor as any patient with a chronic uveitis, and the confinement of inflammation to the anterior segment should not dissuade the ophthalmologist from using oral immunosuppression. Such patients are often those with severe arthropathy or bowel inflammation and liaison with the relevant physician over the choice of immunosuppressive can be very helpful for the patient.

Diagnosis

In a patient with uveitis typical of HLA-B27 positivity, no investigation is necessary. Where associated systemic symptoms are demonstrated, proving HLA-B27 positivity may be important. The test is inexpensive; if positive in a fit patient with nothing to suggest a different etiology, it may spare the patient further investigation.

Management

In a patient with recurrent HLA-B27-associated AAU, frequently the first attack is the most severe and prolonged, often because of misdiagnosis by the patient's general practitioner. Subsequent attacks are invariably self-diagnosed and present earlier. Vigorous early intervention minimizes the severity and timescale of each attack and, cumulatively, the long-term prognosis.

Intensive (hourly, sometimes more frequently) topical steroid treatment is essential in the early stages. If compliance with this very frequent regimen cannot be guaranteed or is inadequate after 48 h, subconjunctival steroid injection of betamethasone or dexamethasone is helpful, repeated daily if necessary, two or three times. With such a vigorous approach over the first 3 days to 1 week the duration of the attack is likely to be greatly shortened.

The importance of vigorous mydriasis cannot be overstressed. The progressive accumulation of synechiae (**Fig. 8.8**) over several attacks can be pernicious and should be resisted energetically. Every effort should be made, for those patients who present with a new attack, to cause maximal mydriasis at the first visit by any reasonable means, initially by the use of topical anticholinergics and phenylephrine and, if unsuccessful, by the use of subconjunctival agents such as Mydricaine. The use of local heat, once part of routine management in such instances but latterly disregarded, should be encouraged; with successful mydriasis and cycloplegia the patient leaves with greatly reduced discomfort, and a better outlook.

Phenylephrine is generally under-used in the acute attack. Its ability to rip off incipient synechiae (especially assisted by local heat) should not be under-estimated (**Fig. 8.9**). It is, however, rarely necessary to continue that prescription once adhesions are detached. Both mydriasis and cycloplegia are analgesic and by reducing movement probably enhance recovery. However, opinions differ as to the required potency and duration of treatment. With the exception of those few patients with shallow anterior chambers who are at risk of peripheral posterior synechia formation, the preference in this clinic is for atropine over cyclopentolate, the latter being used only in milder attacks.

Most patients with such acute forms of AAU have a reduced intraocular pressure (IOP) on presentation. However, a minority with exudative uveitis have secondary glaucoma. Although the IOP often settles very quickly after steroid treatment, some will require anti-glaucoma medication, usually in the form of topical β blockers, occasionally with additional treatment.

The patient with recurrent anterior uveitis soon learns that early presentation greatly speeds and enhances recovery; such an approach should be energetically encouraged and facilitated, and this educational aspect of management is important for long-term prognosis. The more self-reliant patient will request a stock of topical steroid to self-administer if an attack is suspected. In our clinic this is encouraged for those patients who have demonstrated reliability in symptomatic self-diagnosis, but never replaces ophthalmological diagnosis and supervision, which should still be sought within a day of the attack. A few patients develop the impression that repeated self-treatment of any sore red eye with topical steroid, with no attempt to consult their ophthalmologist, is acceptable; they should be disabused of this notion.

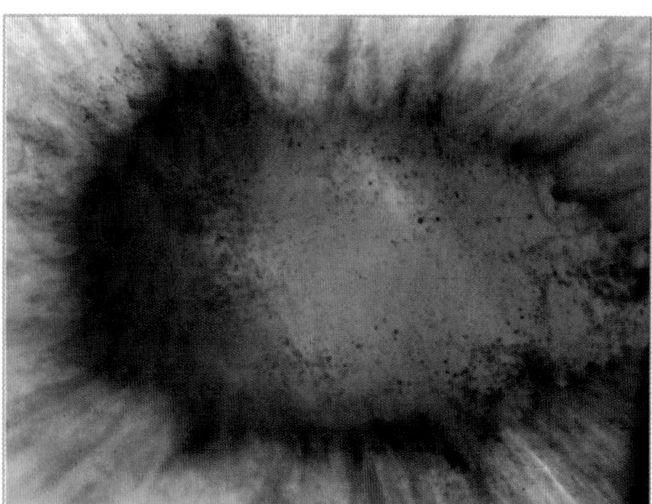

Figure 8.8 Allowing posterior synechiae to accumulate leads to progressive pupillary occlusion with potential for acute glaucoma.

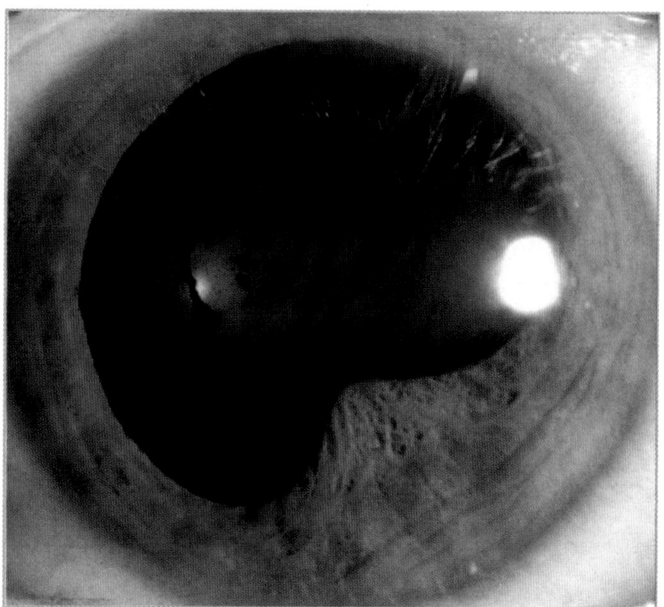

Figure 8.9 The use of maximal mydriasis and local heat to break incipient posterior synechiae is essential. The remaining adhesion at 5 o'clock is being detached by sympathomimetic drops. The pigment residue of adhesions already broken can also be seen.

JUVENILE IDIOPATHIC ARTHRITIS AND UVEITIS (box 8.2)

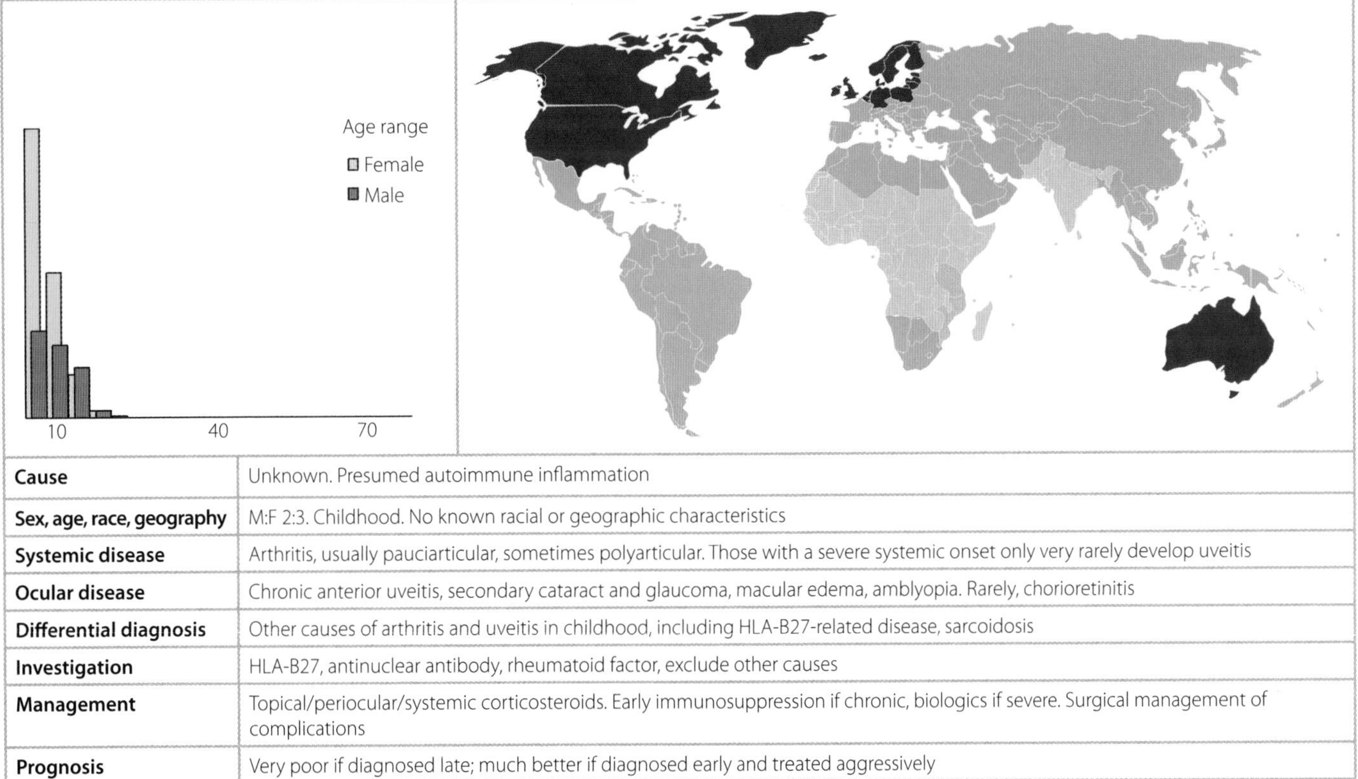

Cause	Unknown. Presumed autoimmune inflammation
Sex, age, race, geography	M:F 2:3. Childhood. No known racial or geographic characteristics
Systemic disease	Arthritis, usually pauciarticular, sometimes polyarticular. Those with a severe systemic onset only very rarely develop uveitis
Ocular disease	Chronic anterior uveitis, secondary cataract and glaucoma, macular edema, amblyopia. Rarely, chorioretinitis
Differential diagnosis	Other causes of arthritis and uveitis in childhood, including HLA-B27-related disease, sarcoidosis
Investigation	HLA-B27, antinuclear antibody, rheumatoid factor, exclude other causes
Management	Topical/periocular/systemic corticosteroids. Early immunosuppression if chronic, biologics if severe. Surgical management of complications
Prognosis	Very poor if diagnosed late; much better if diagnosed early and treated aggressively

Box 8.2 Juvenile idiopathic arthritis and uveitis

Introduction

Chronic arthritis in children (juvenile idiopathic arthritis or JIA) was once considered a rare disease; enhanced diagnosis and possibly increasing incidence have latterly established a wide variation between populations, with an annual incidence of 3–15/100 000 per year and a prevalence of 15–400/100 000. The highest rates have been reported from Scandinavia and Australia, with the lowest from India. Affected children should preferably be referred to a pediatric rheumatologist with expertise in managing JIA. Uveitis in association with the arthritis is common. Ophthalmological screening and uveitis management is essential and is the latter is preferably performed in a specialist center.

Systemic disease

Juvenile idiopathic arthritis is now defined as an arthritis starting before the age of 16 years and lasting for 6 weeks or more. This group of inflammations is clinically heterogeneous, and terminology of its classification has changed and remains inconsistent and confusing. Although not universally accepted, the International League of Associations for Rheumatology (ILAR) has defined the various subsets (Petty et al. 2001) and these are shown in **Table 8.2**. The terms used within this book are shown in bold within the table. In the UK and in most other countries, the term 'juvenile chronic arthritis' was previously used but that term has now been abandoned. The term 'juvenile rheumatoid arthritis' (JRA) is reserved here for the small minority who are rheumatoid factor (RhF) positive. Confusingly, in the USA, the historical term JRA has been retained also for those who are seronegative (in other words JRA can be synonymous with JIA). This is unhelpful and anachronistic.

The variation in presentation and development of the JIA subtypes may differ but the principles of management are similar: untreated arthritis leads to effusion, scarring and reduced mobility; if severe and prolonged, it leads to fixed flexion deformity, growth retardation and permanent disablement. Early and effective control of inflammation by anti-inflammatory medication and intra-articular steroid injection, combined with physiotherapy, may suffice; for more severe disease immunosuppression and if necessary biologic treatment is important.

For the ophthalmologist, the classification of the arthritis is only of interest in defining risk factors for the development of uveitis, defining whether the uveitis will be symptomatic or not, and predicting clinical variability in intraocular inflammation. Patients only at risk of symptomatic uveitis rarely need to participate in a screening program. First, therefore, the types of arthritis not requiring ophthalmological screening are described.

HLA-B27-positive and enthesitis-related juvenile arthritis

Although HLA-B27+ arthritis does not exist as a separate category within the ILAR definitions, it is recognized that a subset of children with JIA who are HLA-B27+, almost always boys presenting over 6 years of age, is a significantly different group. There may be evidence of early onset spondyloarthropathy, or the arthritis may be polyarticular

Table 8.2 International League of Associations for Rheumatology (ILAR) definitions in juvenile idiopathic arthritis (JIA)[a]

Name	Definition	Exclusion criteria
Oligoarticular JIA	Arthritis in one to four joints for up to 6 months[b]	Psoriasis (personal or family history)
(Persistent)	No more than four joints are affected during the entire course of disease	HLA-B27+ male > 6 years
(Extended)	After the first 6 months, more than four joints are effected	AS, ERA, IBD, RhF+
Polyarticular JIA	Arthritis in five or more joints during the first 6 months of disease	Psoriasis (personal or family history)
(Polyarthritis RhF–)		HLA-B27+ male > 6 years
		AS, ERA, IBD, RhF+
Systemic JIA[c]	Arthritis in one or more joints preceded by fever of > 2 weeks duration, including at least 3 successive days of fever, together with one or more of:	Psoriasis (personal or family history)
	Evanescent erythematous rash	HLA-B27+ male > 6 years
	Lymphadenopathy, hepatomegaly, splenomegaly	AS, ERA, IBD, RhF+
	Serositis	
Juvenile rheumatoid arthritis	Arthritis in five or more joints during the first 6 months of disease	Psoriasis (personal or family history)
(Polyarthritis RhF+)	RhF+	HLA-B27+ male > 6 years
		AS, ERA, IBD, RhF+
Psoriatic Arthritis	Arthritis with skin psoriasis or arthritis with at least two of:	HLA-B27+ male over 6yrs
	Dactylitis	AS, ERA, IBD, RhF+
	Nail pitting or onycholysis	
	Psoriasis in a first-degree relative	
Enthesitis related arthritis	Arthritis with enthesitis, or either together with two or more of:	Psoriasis (personal or family history)
	Sacroiliac pain, HLA-B27+, male with onset > 6 years, AAU or history of any of these in first-degree relative	Systemic JIA
		RhF+
Undifferentiated juvenile arthritis	Any arthritis not consistent with the above groups	None

AS, ankylosing spondylitis; ERA, enthesitis-related arthritis; IBD, inflammatory bowel disease; RhF, rheumatoid factor; enthesitis = inflammation of the insertion of tendons or ligaments into bones.

[a]The names in bold are those used in this text. Those in parentheses are those of the ILAR. The definitions and exclusion criteria have been slightly abbreviated.

[b]To be classified as oligoarticular, no more than four joints must be affected **for the first 6 months**, otherwise it should be classified as polyarticular.

[c]Traditionally known as Still's disease.

in childhood, developing later into ankylosing spondylitis. HLA-B27 positivity may also be associated with psoriasis or inflammatory bowel disease. If these children develop uveitis, it is a symptomatic acute unilateral uveitis, as for adults with HLA-B27, and therefore screening is not required for this group. About 10% of children have enthesitis-related arthritis (ERA). If uveitis develops, again it will also be symptomatic and therefore screening is not required.

Juvenile rheumatoid factor-positive arthritis

These children are considered to be RhF+ if two assessments, at least 3 months apart, are both positive for IgM RhF. Only about 2% of children with JIA fall into this category. The development of uveitis is rare, and the risk probably approaches zero (Saurenmann et al. 2007). Ophthalmological screening is not required.

Inflammatory bowel disease-related and psoriatic arthritis in children

The ILAR classification excludes both juvenile psoriatic arthritis and inflammatory bowel disease-related arthritis (IBDA) from the umbrella of JIA. However, psoriatic arthritis carries a risk of uveitis commensurate with numbers of joints involved as for JIA (Butbul et al. 2009) and such patients should be screened for uveitis. The risks for IBDA are poorly understood but undoubtedly exist and, similarly, such children should be screened.

Systemic JIA

George Still described JIA 100 years ago, but in the past 50 years the eponymous term 'Still's disease' was reserved for this subset of JIA, which affects some 10–15% of those with JIA. Presentation is typically acute with high swinging pyrexia, macular rash, hepatosplenomegaly, lymphadenopathy and arthralgia. Other complications may occur, and a pauciarticular or polyarticular arthritis may subsequently develop, usually within weeks. The risk of development of uveitis is very low indeed, almost certainly below 1%, and probably most of these have uveitis at presentation. Ophthalmological screening is not justified.

Polyarticular JIA

This form, affecting some 20% of patients with JIA, usually symmetrically involves large and small joints of the hands and wrists, especially the interphalangeal joints. The knees, ankles, cervical spine and temporomandibular joints are also frequently involved. About 15% of patients develop uveitis at some time.

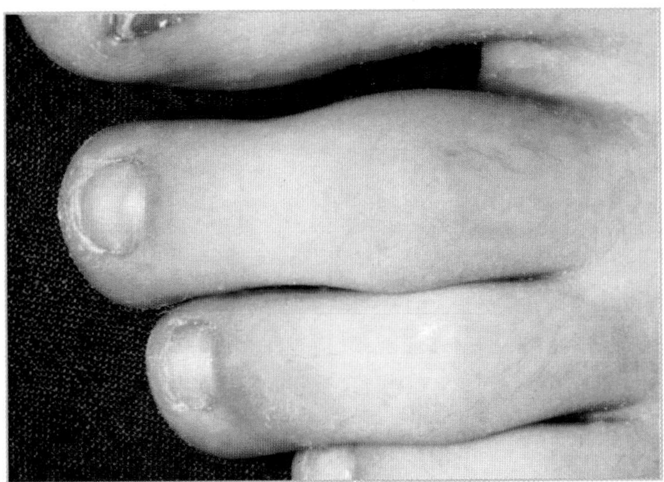

Figure 8.10 Monoarticular arthritis in juvenile chronic arthritis: there is fusiform swelling of the second proximal interphalangeal joint. (Courtesy of the late Dr PJ Holt.)

Oligoarticular JIA

By far the largest subset of JIA, about 40–50% of children fall into this category, which involves four joints or fewer (**Fig. 8.10**) within the first 6 months of onset. The term 'pauciarticular' was previously used. The large joints of the lower limbs, especially the knees, are most frequently affected, often asymmetrically, then ankles, elbows and other joints. Those three-quarters who remain with fewer than five joints affected (about 30% of all cases of JIA) are known as 'persistent oligoarticular' whereas those who progress to a polyarthritis ('extended articular') account for the remaining quarter (about 10% of all cases of JIA). Oligoarticular arthritis carries the greatest risk, among JIA types, of developing uveitis, at about 20–25%, but those with extended oligoarthritis have the highest risk of all at about 30%. However, as those who develop uveitis almost always do so before the oligoarthritis extends, the subset cannot be used as a risk marker; rather it is the development of uveitis in an oligoarticular patient that may be a marker for extended joint involvement.

Ocular disease

The uveitis associated with JIA is characteristically a chronic, indolent, non-granulomatous anterior uveitis, either unilateral or more often bilateral. Keratic precipitates are usually fine and inferior but if severe they may be large or confluent. Despite this the eyes are characteristically white or minimally injected (**Fig. 8.11**). Acute monophasic and acute intermittent anterior uveitis are sometimes seen (although rarely with substantial inflammation) and the posterior segment may be involved, sometimes with macular edema or optic disk swelling, less often with active vitritis and rarely with chorioretinitis. Posterior synechiae form readily and band keratopathy is a very common long-term sequel (**Fig. 8.12**). Histologically, the uveitis is usually an iridocyclitis with infiltration predominantly of lymphocytes and plasma cells, and with some giant cells. Although sequential involvement of the second eye does occur, this is unusual after more than a year has elapsed. The onset is almost always asymptomatic, and even in eyes where substantial anterior chamber (AC) cellular activity is detected, there is typically no discomfort and no photophobia. AC flare may be a major component, and is sometimes profound in eyes with very chronic inflammation.

The severity and chronicity of the uveitis vary markedly. A minority have very mild, self-limiting uveitis which requires only short-term topical steroid. This may or may not recur. However, about three-quarters develop chronic inflammation and perhaps a quarter of these have disease of challenging severity with a high incidence of cataract and glaucoma (**Fig. 8.13**). Those with severe uveitis at onset (usually younger children) or those in whom the uveitis predates the arthritis, going untreated for a period, have the worst prognosis. It is in this group that amblyopia is most common and disabling, and its treatment difficult.

Many eyes with JIA-related uveitis develop chronic AC flare, indicating permanent structural breakdown of the blood–ocular barrier. In the absence of AC cells, it does not denote active inflammation and does not itself require steroid treatment. However, the presence of flare during active inflammation is a risk factor for synechia formation and mydriasis is necessary. Many eyes with burnt-out uveitis retain marked AC flare for life. The duration of the uveitis in JIA varies enormously, but usually outlives the arthritis itself by a number of years. A small

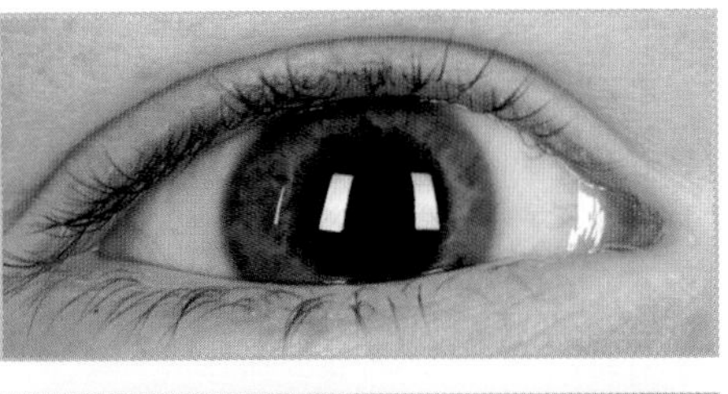

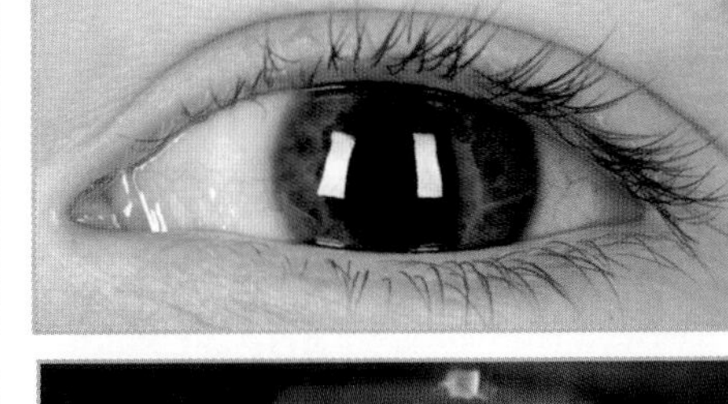

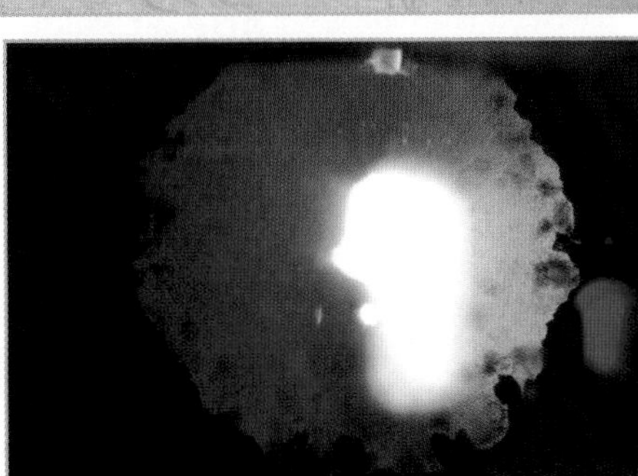

Figure 8.11 A child with juvenile idiopathic arthritis presenting with white painless eyes demonstrating severe chronic bilateral anterior uveitis with extensive posterior synechia formation. Each pupil is shown magnified below.

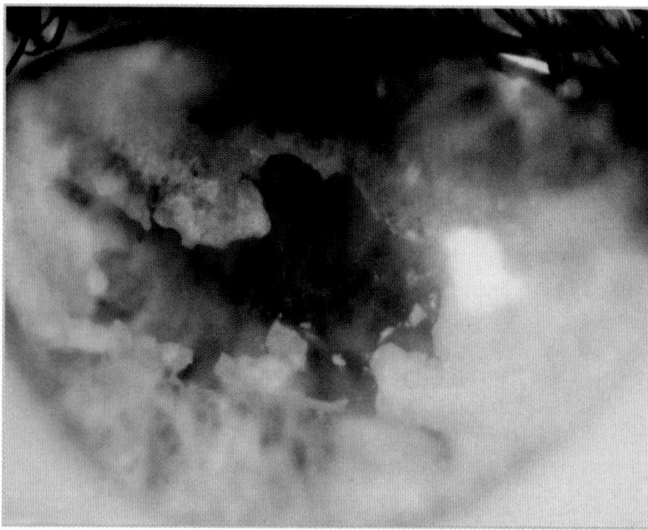

Figure 8.12 Band keratopathy in juvenile idiopathic uveitis.

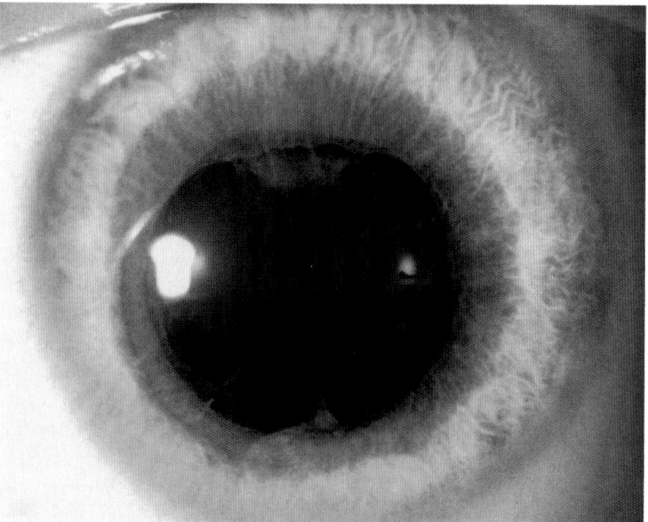

Figure 8.13 Chronic anterior uveitis in juvenile idiopathic arthritis. Iris atrophy, ectropion uveae, posterior synechiae, secondary cataract and amblyopia.

but significant subset of children has inflammation that persists into adulthood.

Diagnosis

The great majority of children with JIA have been diagnosed by the pediatrician or pediatric rheumatologist, being referred to the ophthalmologist for screening. The arthritis subtype and the HLA-B27 and antinuclear antibody (ANA) status should have been determined and this information included in the referral letter to facilitate risk calculations. On occasion the arthritis and uveitis are simultaneously diagnosed, and in these cases childhood sarcoidosis, reactive arthritis, psoriatic arthropathy and inflammatory bowel disease must be considered in the differential diagnosis.

Uveitis in association with JIA is usually insidious in onset, and can be progressive and visually damaging. Although no controlled trial has reported statistically on the value of early diagnosis and treatment, the evidence overwhelmingly suggests that aggressive management markedly improves the outcome (Foster et al. 1993). As the uveitis is asymptomatic, there is clear justification for a screening program for those children at significant risk. Occasionally a child will present to an ophthalmologist without JIA, but with evidence of chronic anterior uveitis. A few parents recall a previous minor episode of monoarthritis that went undiagnosed and resolved spontaneously. Some of these children (usually girls) with no active arthritis will go on to develop JIA. Others (see below, juvenile chronic iridocyclitis without arthritis) will not.

RISK FACTORS FOR UVEITIS AND THE EVIDENCE BASE FOR SCREENING PROGRAMS

About 15% of children with JIA develop uveitis (Saurenmann et al. 2007). A very small proportion of these do so before the diagnosis of JIA and are therefore unreachable by a screening program. A significant minority has active uveitis on first diagnosis of JIA. It is therefore imperative for the ophthalmologist to examine the eyes of newly diagnosed children quickly. For this reason, this clinic permits the direct booking, by our pediatric rheumatologists, of such children into the next available pediatric ophthalmology clinic.

The remaining children with a form of JIA that places them at risk of asymptomatic uveitis should be screened regularly to enable diagnosis and treatment. There are no surrogate markers for those individuals who will develop uveitis and so slit-lamp examination is necessary. As many affected children are often called upon to travel considerable distances in the management of their disease, such a program must balance effectiveness with parental acceptance. The identification of risk factors is therefore of importance so that a program is reasonably effective, practical and cost-effective. However, clarifying risk factors within this heterogeneous group is not easy even when very large cohorts are studied; some risk factors, once considered to be independent, are now thought to be age or sex related, newly defined diagnostic subsets carry separate risks so that studies of older cohorts cease to be relevant, and the change of risk with age, JIA duration and sex may show surprising results.

There is clear geographical disparity between populations. In addition, data collection may be tertiary clinic based, multicenter or population based, each producing a group of children with a different disease mix; the elimination of selection bias is difficult. Despite these difficulties, some aspects of risk are gradually being clarified. The large Toronto studies, with a group of more than 1000 children with JIA (Saurenmann et al. 2007, 2010), are important in this respect and their results are preferentially used here. The perceived risk factors that may be used to design screening programs are discussed individually:

Increased risk of uveitis for low age at onset of JIA?

Early age is undoubtedly a risk factor for uveitis, relative risk (RR) 2–3 depending on JIA subset (highest for polyarticular JIA). However, the relationship is not linear and differs between the sexes. For boys, there is no significant change in uveitis risk for any age at onset of JIA. For girls, however, the highest risk is for JIA onset at 1–2 years, with a substantial decrease in risk until the age of 6–7, after which it decreases very slowly (**Fig. 8.14a**).

Increased risk of uveitis for girls?

Before the separate analysis of JIA subtypes, female sex was considered an independent risk factor overall. However, it now appears to be a risk

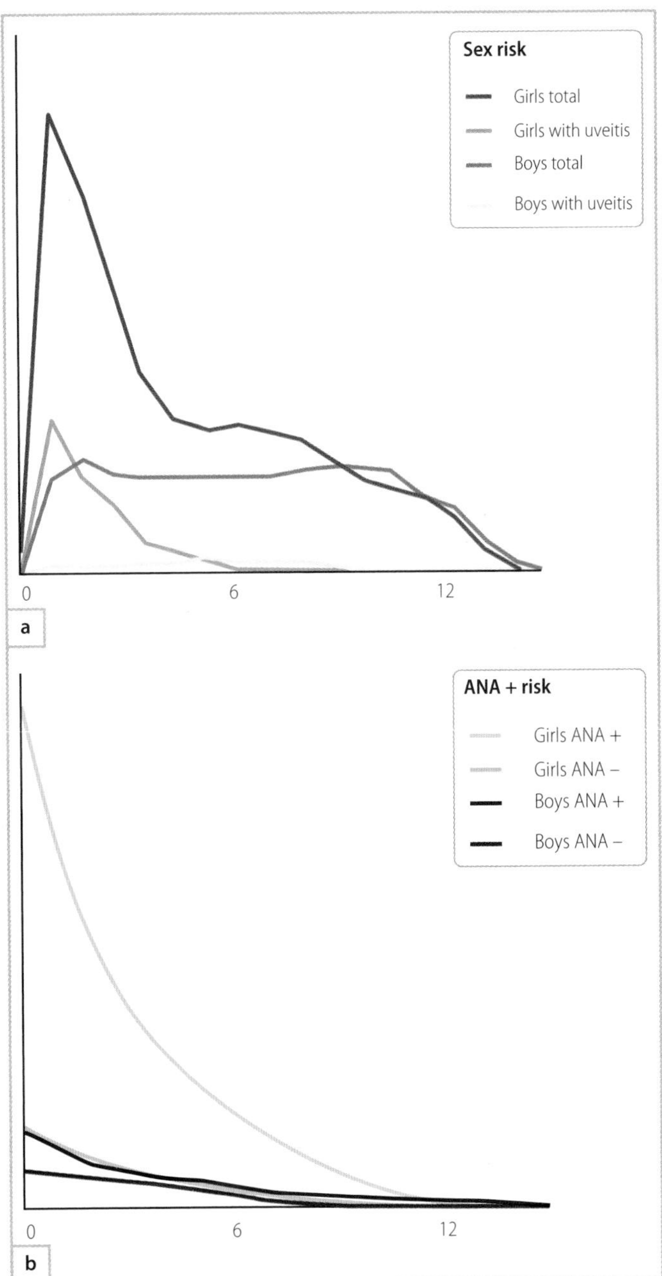

Figure 8.14 (a) Early age at onset of juvenile idiopathic arthritis is a substantial risk factor for the development of uveitis in girls until the age of 6–7, but for boys the spread is much smoother and the overall rate lower. (b) ANA positivity is a substantial risk factor in young girls, much less so for boys. (Adapted from Saurenmann et al. 2010.)

factor for oligoarthritis (RR 2.2), particularly persistent oligoarthritis (RR 2.5) but not other subgroups.

Increased risk of uveitis for children who are ANA positive?

There is an RR of 2.77 for ANA positivity in all cases of JIA. However, multiple regression analysis shows that the RR is not similar for JIA subtypes; it is highest at 4.0 for polyarticular JIA and is also significant for persistent oligoarthritis, but is not an independent risk factor for extended oligoarthritis. It is also a substantial risk factor for girls, but not for boys (**Fig. 8.14b**). Overall around 80% of those who develop uveitis will be ANA positive.

Increased risk of uveitis for oligoarticular arthritis?

Oligoarthritis undoubtedly carries the highest risk of uveitis, approaching 25% over time. In addition, being the most common subset, oligoarthritis produces about 60% of all cases of uveitis in JIA.

Decreasing risk of uveitis with duration of JIA since diagnosis?

The highest rate of diagnosis of uveitis takes place within 1 year of diagnosis of JIA, and that rate progressively declines thereafter, more rapidly at first, then more slowly (**Fig. 8.15**). Some 90% of those who develop uveitis have done so within 7 years of the onset of the arthritis, yet a very small risk persists for 20 years or more.

Who should be screened, how often, and for how long?

Much heated debate has circulated on this topic over several decades, and currently there are several screening protocols available worldwide, each with differences that vary from the subtle to the substantial. At one end of the argument hinges the claim that, as it is accepted that delay in treatment worsens the prognosis, frequent screening up to 8-weekly is required at least for some patients. The occasional discovery of severe uveitis at screening supports such a view (Chia et al. 2003). At the other extreme is the claim that low risks do not justify screening at all and are not cost-effective. The pragmatist also knows that, even with excellent parent education and communication, persuading frequent attendance for years can be impossible to attain and that, with a less stringent program, adherence is more likely. Others have argued that relative risks should be ignored because they do not affect the severity of uveitis should it occur, so all included subtypes of

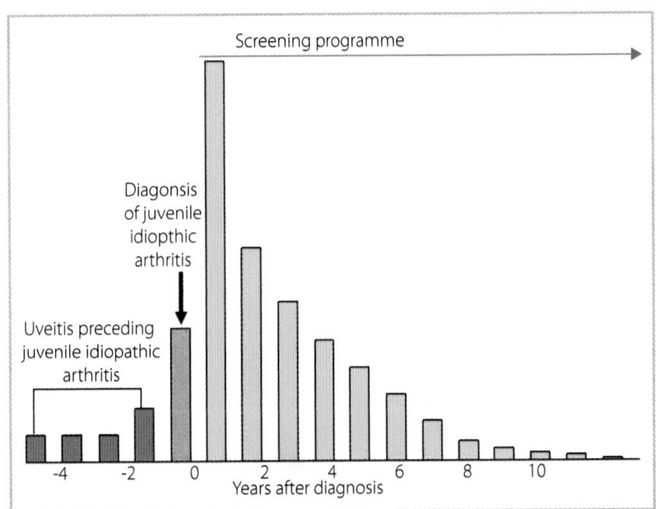

Figure 8.15 Duration of juvenile idiopathic arthritis (JIA) following diagnosis as a risk factor for uveitis. A proportion (orange columns) has uveitis diagnosed before the JIA; a further subset (buff column) has uveitis on diagnosis of JIA; only those developing uveitis subsequently (yellow columns) can be screened. Of these, the rate of uveitis diagnosis is highest in the year after diagnosis of JIA, declining rapidly over subsequent years. (Adapted from Saurenmann et al. 2007.)

JIA should be screened at the same interval. What principles should be used here?

Unlike some medical screening programs, there is no risk of false positivity and the adverse effects (except for cost and inconvenience) are minimal; there is no invasive investigation. There should be no selection bias. There is no lead-time bias as outcomes are different for those diagnosed earlier. The 10 WHO criteria for screening are all fulfilled. Although statistical models of cost efficiency are well established in medical screening generally (Preston 2001), they have not been established for uveitis. Guidelines are therefore as much empirically as evidence based, preferring to err on the side of caution but usually with no description of the method of calculation (if any) of screening frequency (British Society for Paediatric and Adolescent Rheumatology/Royal College of Ophthalmologists 2006).

The above estimates of relative risk for the five parameters derived from the Toronto studies would permit the development of an individualized screening program for each child, if one were to calculate frequency of examination as a time interval giving the same risk of development of uveitis. However, such complexity is surely unnecessary, and screening children in broad groups of risk is appropriate. The approach in this clinic is to examine, once, every child referred with JIA of any subtype. Thereafter, for those without uveitis, those in the following subtypes are not screened: systemic JIA, RhF positives, HLA-B27+ enthesitis-related arthritis, HLA-B27+ boys > 6 years. All others are screened including those with psoriatic arthritis, inflammatory bowel disease-related and undifferentiated arthritis. The screening program used in this clinic has evolved over 20 years to reflect available evidence. New evidence on risk factors will doubtless lead to change in due course, but a widespread consultation on new evidence is now overdue and a coherent strategy from the uveitis community worldwide would be welcomed.

Juvenile chronic iridocyclitis without arthritis

In some children, especially antinuclear factor (ANF)-positive girls, a uveitis is diagnosed that resembles and behaves in a way typical of the chronic uveitis associated with JIA, but without any history or subsequent development of arthropathy. These patients may or may not have had a subclinical arthropathy at some time, and it is likely that they represent one end of a disease spectrum. The uveitis and its complications are generally managed to the same principles as JIA-associated uveitis.

Management of JIA-related uveitis and its complications

Uveitis

The uveitis associated with JIA, although varying in behavior, is on average a very chronic process requiring frequent visits to both ophthalmologist and pediatric rheumatologist. Both visual loss and time lost from school may affect the child's education. The rationale of treatment is to control inflammation rapidly but safely to prevent permanent visual loss and physical disablement. Approaches have evolved enormously in recent years, with earlier introduction of immunosuppression and effective biologics becoming available.

Topical steroid is required for all patients and the frequency of administration may initially need to be high. Unlike symptomatic acute uveitis, posterior synechiae if present are usually established; however, an immediate attempt should be made to detach them with mydriasis. For those with any AC cells and/or with heavy flare, at least nocturnal mydriasis is necessary. For those with less severe uveitis, tropicamide 1% is adequate, otherwise cyclopentolate 1% is used despite its morning 'hangover' for blurred near vision. Those children with severe bilateral uveitis requiring atropine treatment will of course require spectacles for reading. The past 20 years has seen a revolution in the approach to uveitis in JIA. Previously a concern over both long-term systemic steroid and oral immunosuppression in children left many on inadequate but frequent topical regimens, with a high rate of cataract and glaucoma.

There is sparse evidence on the relationship between topical steroid frequency and duration, and the development of cataract. Our approach is a pragmatic one; a three times daily regimen of prednisolone acetate is regarded as a threshold, because this regimen can be reasonably given by parents for schoolchildren without necessitating administration at school (which can be problematic). There is some evidence to suggest that this is a reasonable approach in terms of cataract risk (Thorne et al. 2010). If this is inadequate to control uveitis, whether unilateral or bilateral, we use methotrexate whether or not the child has active arthritis.

The long-term use of oral steroid as the sole systemic agent is unacceptable; they may cause growth retardation in addition to the ocular and systemic problems that affect the adult, and the combination of active arthritis and corticosteroid is a potent cause of osteoporosis. However, some children present with a severe uveitis and others develop a substantial flare intermittently. The use of judicious short-term oral steroid in such circumstances is entirely appropriate. For those children with very severe uveitis at onset or with a severe flare, two or three pulses of intravenous methylprednisolone is also appropriate.

The efficacy of methotrexate for most children with uveitis associated with JIA is now beyond dispute (Foeldvari et al 2005, Heiligenhaus et al. 2007). The drug, if administered and monitored carefully, is safe with only few discontinued because of systemic toxicity. Younger children can use liquid rather than tablets. Nausea is not uncommon. The addition of an antiemetic or conversion to subcutaneous injection is usually helpful at a given dose and the latter also tends to increase efficacy. Stomatitis, bowel upset or liver dysfunction is much less common and sterile pneumonitis is rare. Nevertheless a minority of children cannot tolerate methotrexate and about a quarter of those treated do not respond adequately. The administration of any immunosuppressive to a child requires expert supervision and the ophthalmologist, even if an experienced uveitis practitioner prescribing immunosuppression to adults, cannot safely do so in children. Large medical centers such as our own have the benefit of clinics combining the expertise of both uveitis ophthalmologist and pediatric rheumatologist. Elsewhere, developing a professional relationship with an interested and expert pediatrician is essential. The uveitis relapse rate of children discontinuing methotrexate is substantial (Kalinina et al. 2011) and therefore such children should be screened as if presenting anew.

It has until recently been our practice to add ciclosporin, or less frequently mycophenolate mofetil, to methotrexate where the latter, together with topical steroid, has been inadequate to control inflammation. Both drugs are usually well tolerated in children, ciclosporin in particular being generally much less problematic than in adults. The success rate of these combinations is greater than methotrexate alone, controlling about half of patients (Sobrin et al. 2008, Tappeiner et al. 2009). Others have used azathioprine with efficacy in over 60% (Goebel et al. 2011). Although we still use combined immunosuppression in some children, practice has evolved towards the earlier prescription of biologics in children with difficult uveitis. There are three anti-TNF-α monoclonal antibody treatments available, and data on relative efficacy are gradually evolving. The details of individual drugs are given in Chapter 6.

The value of etanercept for the arthritis of JIA is established. Its efficacy in JIA-related uveitis is unimpressive. In a large cohort treated with etanercept, continuing uveitis continued in a significant subset of those who discontinued the drug (Southwood et al. 2011). Concerns about induced uveitis in JIA patients on etanercept are not convincing, but anecdotes of optic neuropathy are reported. Infliximab is more effective (Foeldvari et al. 2007) but requires intravenous infusion with a significant incidence of infusion reactions, occasional anaphylaxis and induced intolerance. Although adalimumab is not fully humanized, it induces far less immune reaction, is administered subcutaneously and the current (as yet inadequate) evidence suggests that it may be the most effective drug for uveitis in JIA, being superior to infliximab in direct comparison (Simonini et al. 2011). A success rate approaching 90% has been reported (Biester et al. 2007) but this is not representative of the wider literature. For those residual groups of children with severe disease who have been refractory to the above immunosuppressive and biologic regimens, abatacept has been used with favorable outcomes (Zulian et al. 2010) and this drug may become established as rescue therapy in such cases.

In contrast to traditional oral immunosuppression, anti-TNF-α monoclonal antibodies carry a risk of cancer. After the identification of 48 childhood malignancies worldwide after such treatment, concern has been expressed about this group but it has been argued that the evidence for etanercept being carcinogenic is much weaker. More evidence is needed, but currently the possibility of malignancy is an important element in the risk–benefit calculations made by the prescribing physician, parent and child in these more severe, sight-threatening cases of uveitis.

Band keratopathy can be problematic in some patients, for visual or cosmetic reasons or because of intermittent pain and inflammation. Debridement and chelation, and excimer phototherapeutic keratectomy, are both temporarily effective. In a small minority of children, often those who have required multiple operations, eyes still become blind and phthisical (**Fig. 8.16**) and the management of these complications is discussed in Chapter 7.

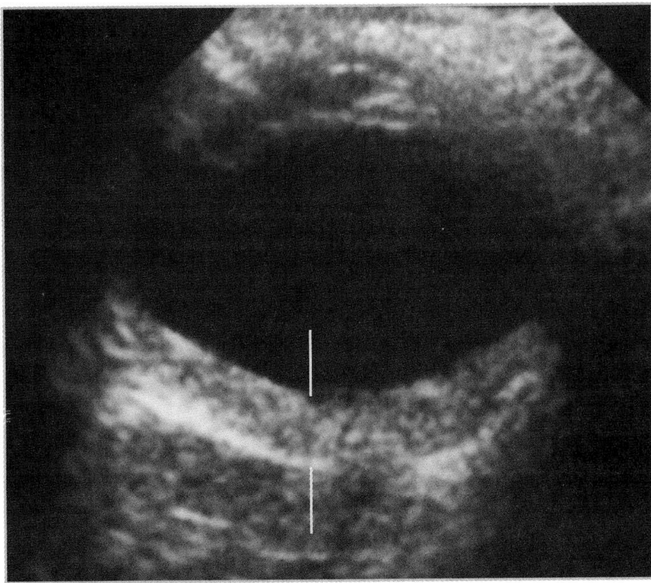

Figure 8.16 Phthisis in a child with juvenile idiopathic arthritis and uveitis. The globe is collapsed and the posterior coats grossly thickened, as defined by the yellow lines.

Cataract

Modern immunosuppressive treatment regimens that both enhance control and spare the use of topical and systemic steroids undoubtedly reduce the incidence of secondary cataract in JIA. Nevertheless the need for cataract surgery will arise. The management of cataract surgery in JIA is difficult. A young child at risk of amblyopia may develop or present with a dense cataract in an eye with inadequately controlled inflammation. To operate too early is to precipitate wildfire inflammation, cyclitic membrane and phthisis. The use of intraocular lenses (IOLs) in uveitis patients generally, assuming control of inflammation, is now almost universal. Improving results in adults and immunosuppression-enhanced disease control in children have persuaded some to use IOLs in JIA; there is now a number of publications claiming low complication rates (Grajewski et al. 2011). However, there is undoubted publication bias and reports should therefore be treated with caution; the need to explant IOLs from damaged eyes (Adan et al. 2009) is undoubtedly under-represented in the literature. Comparisons of aphakic versus pseudophakic children may claim superior outcomes for the latter (Sijssens et al. 2010), but surgical selection bias cannot be reliably excluded. The majority of the uveitis community still regard the use of IOLs in children with JIA-associated uveitis as dangerous in any child with inflammation requiring treatment, whether controlled or not. The formation of a fibrinous IOL cocoon or a vascularized cyclitic membrane, with tractional cyclodialysis and phthisis, is well recognized. A reliable pediatric contact lens service is therefore essential. In the child > 6 years with unilateral cataract, there is a clear option of deferring surgery in the hope of future quiescence, which will permit safer IOL implantation.

The optimal surgical technique for cataract removal in JIA is debatable. The removal of the entire lens capsule and anterior vitreous was considered to be necessary until recently. However, the retention of capsule as a template for future secondary IOL implantation is attractive if safe. Even those reporting success after IOL implantation have performed posterior capsulorrhexis and anterior vitrectomy. Whatever surgical technique is used the operation should be preceded by complete and reliable control of intraocular inflammation, and probably accompanied by a short course of systemic steroid treatment; it is our current practice to precede surgery with two pulses of intravenous methylprednisolone at days 3 and 1 preoperatively.

Glaucoma

The incidence of glaucoma in JIA-associated uveitis approaches 40% (Sijssens et al. 2006), either as a response to steroid treatment or secondary to the uveitis, and it can be problematic. Long-term medical control is achieved in only a minority, and the use of long-term systemic acetazolamide, although often well tolerated in children, is potentially complicated and children are not immune from renal calculi. In those who develop, or who are at risk of, iris bombé, surgical peripheral iridectomy may be necessary; in any eye with chronic uveitis, especially with AC flare, a laser iridotomy is likely to occlude repeatedly. Cyclodiode laser may be used for urgent treatment but outcomes are poorer than in adults with glaucoma (Heinz et al. 2006) and there is a substantial risk of future phthisis. Goniotomy has its adherents for a variety of childhood uveitides (Ho et al. 2004) but the procedure is less appropriate for secondary than for primary pediatric glaucomas, and is unlikely to be adequately effective alone. There is also a concern that such procedures may precipitate or worsen PAS formation and compromise future management. Unenhanced glaucoma drainage surgery in any young person with uveitis will fail, and enhancement with mitomycin C carries a substantial progressive failure rate.

There is substantial agreement that a primary drainage device is the current best option where surgery is required electively, despite its associated risks. Most current literature on the use of implants in children focuses on primary glaucoma and Sturge-Weber syndrome and there is a paucity of data on uveitis of any type in children. However, experience is accumulating; although some centers favor the Ahmed valve (Kafkala et al. 2005) there is a greater trend towards the Baerveldt device (van Overdam et al. 2006). As for cataract surgery, whichever method is used, stringent perioperative control of inflammation is mandatory.

Macular edema and other posterior segment manifestations

The uveitis associated with JIA may manifest primarily as an anterior uveitis, but posterior segment involvement may lead to substantial visual loss. The introduction of ocular coherence tomography (OCT) has substantially improved the approach to such children by providing a non-invasive technique for macular assessment. Macular edema is the most common posterior segment manifestation (Ducos de Lahitte et al. 2008) but epiretinal membrane formation, papillitis and, much less commonly, chorioretinitis, retinal vasculitis and retinal detachment are all reported (Paroli et al. 2010). The principle here is that the posterior segment of affected children must be included in the supervision process, treatment being enhanced where indicated.

CRYOPYRIN-ASSOCIATED PERIODIC SYNDROMES

The cryopyrin-associated periodic syndromes (CAPSs) are a related group (or possibly a continuum) of rare, inherited, autoimmune inflammations. There is an abnormality in the production and interaction of the proinflammatory marker cryopyrin, which cascades into an over-production of the interleukin IL-1β. The mutations causing CAPSs are within the gene NLRP3. The multisystem signs include recurrent rash, fevers, polyarthropathy and sometimes include uveitis, and are thus in the differential diagnosis of polyarticular/systemic JIA and juvenile sarcoidosis. They are, in ascending order of severity, as follows:

Familial cold autoinflammatory syndrome

Familial cold autoinflammatory syndrome (FCAS; previously called familial cold urticaria) is the least rare form of CAPSs, comprising cold-induced maculopapular rash, fever and arthralgia with raised inflammatory markers, usually subsiding within 48 h but readily recurrent. Rarely organ failure can ensue, e.g. after renal amyloidosis.

Muckle–Wells syndrome

Muckle-Wells syndrome (MWS) is similar to FCAS and often triggered by cold but also appears recurrently and spontaneously, less acutely and lasting for longer periods. It may be associated with sensorineural deafness and frequent renal amyloidosis.

Chronic infantile neurological cutaneous and articular syndrome (CINCA)

This, by far the most severe of the CAPS group, is also known as neonatal-onset multisystem inflammatory disease (NOMID). In addition to the features of FCAS/MWS there is frequent central nervous system (CNS) involvement with sterile meningoencephalitis and optic neuropathy, often with chronic papilledema. Uveitis is common (Dollfus et al. 2000), usually in the anterior segment but sometimes with posterior segment involvement. There may be delayed development, hepatosplenomegaly, organ failure and structural joint deformity.

Traditional anti-inflammatory and immunosuppressive therapy for the CAPSs has been disappointing. A better-targeted biologic treatment is canakinumab, an anti-IL-1 monoclonal antibody, which has shown promise (Toker and Hashkes 2010).

Relapsing polychondritis

This is a very rare (prevalence probably 0.3/100 000), idiopathic, presumed autoimmune vasculitis. It is least rare around the Mediterranean, the Middle East and Silk Route countries. It affects both articular and non-articular cartilage, predominantly the latter. The nose and pinnae become intermittently inflamed and painful, eventually becoming deformed due to replacement by fibrous tissue; the larynx and trachea may collapse causing stridor. Arthropathy is common, and heart valves may be affected. Characteristic involvement of nose or ears with a raised erythrocyte sedimentation rate (ESR) or C-reactive protein (CRP) is diagnostic. A significant minority develops systemic vasculitis or a myelodysplastic disorder. The mortality rate is less than 10% at 10 years, most deaths being caused by tracheobronchial collapse, heart failure or blood dyscrasia. Systemic steroid therapy is usually necessary and oral immunosuppression common. A variety of anecdotal reports of success with most currently available biologics has failed to clarify the preferred choice of treatment.

Episcleritis is the most common ocular complication but anterior uveitis occurs in some, probably the minority overall. but possibly in most of those with more severe disease (Jimenez-Balderas et al. 2011), and on rare occasions an exudative retinopathy simulating Coats' disease has been described. Management of ocular inflammation is likely to be secondary to the systemic need for disease suppression.

REFERENCES

Adan A, Gris O, Pelegrin L, et al. Explantation of intraocular lenses in children with juvenile idiopathic arthritis-associated uveitis. *J Cataract Refract Surg* 2009;**35**:603–5.

Biester S, Deuter C, Michels H, et al. Adalimumab in the therapy of uveitis in childhood. *Br J Ophthalmol* 2007;**91**:319–24.

British Society for Paediatric and Adolescent Rheumatology/Royal College of Ophthalmologists. *Guidelines for screening for uveitis in juvenile idiopathic arthritis (JIA)*. London: British Society for Paediatric and Adolescent Rheumatology/Royal College of Ophthalmologists, 2006.

Butbul YA, Tyrrell PN, Schneider R, et al. Comparison of patients with juvenile psoriatic arthritis and nonpsoriatic juvenile idiopathic arthritis: how different are they? *J Rheumatol* 2009;**36**:2033–41.

Chia A, Lee V, Graham EM, Edelsten C. Factors related to severe uveitis at diagnosis in children with juvenile idiopathic arthritis in a screening programme. *Am J Ophthalmol* 2003;**135**:757–62.

Cipriani A, Rivera S, Hassanhi M, et al. HLA-B27 subtypes determination in patients with ankylosing spondylitis from Zulia, Venezuela. *Hum Immunol* 2003;**64**:745–9.

Dollfus H, Hafner R, Hoffman HM, et al. Chronic infantile neurological cutaneous and articular/neonatal onset multisystem inflammatory disease syndrome: ocular manifestations in a recently recognised chronic inflammatory disease of childhood. *Arch Ophthalmol* 2000;**118**:1386–92.

Ducos de Lahitte G, Terrada C, Tran TH, et al. Maculopathy in uveitis of juvenile idiopathic arthritis: an optical coherence tomography study. *Br J Ophthalmol* 2008;**92**:64–9.

Feltkamp TEW, Khan MA, Lopez de Castro JA. The pathogenic role of HLA-B27. *Immunol Today* 1996;**17**:5–8.

Foeldvari I, Wierk A. Methotrexate is an effective treatment for chronic uveitis associated with juvenile idiopathic arthritis. *J Rheumatol* 2005;**32**:362–5.

Foeldvari I, Nielsen S, Kummerle-Deschner J, et al. Tumour necrosis factor-alpha blocker in treatment of juvenile idiopathic arthritis-associated uveitis refractory to second-line agents: results of a multinational survey. *J Rheumatol* 2007;**34**:1146–50.

Foster CS, Barrett F. Cataract development and cataract surgery in patients with juvenile rheumatoid arthritis-associated iridocyclitis. *Ophthalmology* 1993;**100**:809–817.

Goebel JC, Roesel M, Heinz C, et al. Azathioprine as a treatment option for uveitis in patients with juvenile idiopathic arthritis. *Br J Ophthalmol* 2011;**95**:209–13.

Grajewski RS, Zurek-Imhoff B, Roesel M, et al. Favourable outcome after cataract surgery with IOL implantation in uveitis associated with juvenile idiopathic arthritis. *Acta Ophthalmol* 2011;Epub.

Heiligenhaus A, Mingels A, Heinz C, Ganser G. Methotrexate for uveitis associated with juvenile idiopathic arthritis: value and requirement for additional anti-inflammatory medication. *Eur J Ophthalmol* 2007;**17**:743–8.

Heinz C, Koch JM, Heiligenhaus A. Transscleral diode laser photocoagulation as primary surgical treatment for secondary glaucoma in juvenile idiopathic arthritis: high failure rate after short-term follow-up. *Br J Ophthalmol* 2006;**90**:737–40.

Henckaerts L, Figueroa C, Verniere S, Sans M. The role of genetics in inflammatory bowel disease. *Curr Drug Targets* 2008;**9**:361–8.

Ho CL, Wong EY, Walton DS. Goniosurgery for glaucoma complicating childhood chronic uveitis. *Arch Ophthalmol* 2004;**122**:838–44.

Jimenez-Balderas FJ, Fernandez-Arrieta G, Camargo-Coronel A, et al. Uveitis in adult patients with rheumatic inflammatory autoimmune diseases at a tertiary-care hospital in Mexico City. *J Rheumatol* 2011;**38**:325–30.

Kafkala C, Hynes A, Choi J, et al. Ahmed valve implantation for uncontrolled pediatric uveitic glaucoma. *J Am Assoc Pediatr Ophthalmol Strabismus* 2005;**9**:336–40.

Kalinina AV, van de Winkel EL, Rothova A, de Boer JH. Relapse rate of uveitis post-methotrexate treatment in juvenile idiopathic arthritis. *Am J Ophthalmol* 2011;**151**:217–22.

Konno Y, Numaga J, Tsuchiya N, et al. HLA-B27 subtypes and HLA class II alleles in Japanese patients with anterior uveitis. *Invest Ophthalmol Vis Sci* 1999;**40**:1838–44.

Martin TM, Rosenbaum JT. An update on the genetics of HLA B27-associated acute anterior uveitis. *Ocul Immunol Inflamm* 2011;**19**:108–14.

Merceica K, Sanghvi C, Jones NP. Very severe HLA B27-associated uveitis mimicking endophthalmitis: a case series. *Ocul Immunol Inflamm* 2010;**18**:139–41.

Monnet D, Breban M, Hudry C, et al. Ophthalmic findings and frequency of extraocular manifestations in patients with HLA-B27 uveitis. *Ophthalmology* 2004;**111**:802–9.

Paiva ES, Macaluso DC, Edwards A, Rosenbaum JT. Characterisation of uveitis in patients with psoriatic arthritis. *Ann Rheum Dis* 2000;**59**:67–70.

Paroli MP, Spinucci G, Fabiani C, Pivetti-Pezzi P. Retinal complications of juvenile idiopathic arthritis-related uveitis: a microperimetry and ocular coherence tomography study. *Ocul Immunol Inflamm* 2010;**18**:54–9.

Pavesio C, Jones NP. Uveitis related to HLA-B27 and juvenile arthritis. In: Yanoff M, Duker JS (eds), *Ophthalmology*, 3rd edn. London: Elsevier 2009; 838–43.

Petty RE, Southwood TR, Manners P, et al. International league of associations for rheumatology classification of juvenile idiopathic arthritis second revision, Edmonton 2001. *J Rheumatol* 2004;**31**:390–2.

Preston AJ. Disease screening designs: sensitivity and screening frequency. *Proc Ann Am Stat Assoc* 2001;5–9.

Queiro R, Torre JC, Belzunequi J, et al. Clinical features and predictive factors in psoriatic arthritis-related uveitis. *Semin Arthrit Rheum* 2002;**31**:264–70.

Rothova A, van Veenendaal WG, Linssen A, et al. Clinical features of acute anterior uveitis. *Am J Ophthalmol* 1987;**103**:137–45.

Saurenmann RK, Levin AV, Feldman BM, et al. Prevalence, risk factors and outcomes of uveitis in juvenile idiopathic arthritis: a long-term follow-up study. *Arthrit Rheum* 2007;**56**:647–57.

Saurenmann RK, Levin AV, Feldman BM, et al. Risk factors for development of uveitis differ between boys and girls with juvenile idiopathic arthritis. *Arthrit Rheum* 2010;**62**:1824–8.

Sheldrake JS. Sir Benjamin Collins Brodie (1783–1862). *J Med Biography* 2008;**16**:84–8.

Sijssens KM, Rothova A, Berendschott TT, de Boer JH. Ocular hypertension and secondary glaucoma in children with uveitis. *Ophthalmology* 2006;**113**: 853–9.

Sijssens KM, Los LI, Rothova A, et al. Long-term ocular complications in aphakic versus pseudophakic eyes of children with juvenile idiopathic arthritis-associated uveitis. *Br J Ophthalmol* 2010;**94**:1145–9.

Simonini G, Taddio A, Cattalini M, et al. Prevention of flare recurrences in childhood-refractory chronic uveitis: an open-label comparative study of adalimumab versus infliximab. *Arthritis Care Res* 2011;**63**:612–8.

Sobrin L, Christen W, Foster CS. Mycophenolate mofetil after methotrexate failure or intolerance in the treatment of scleritis and uveitis. *Ophthalmology* 2008;**115**:1416–21.

Southwood TR, Foster HE, Davidson JE, et al. Duration of etanercept treatment and reasons for discontinuation in a cohort of juvenile idiopathic arthritis patients. *Rheumatology* 2011;**50**:189–95.

Tappeiner C, Roesel M, Heinz C, et al. Limited value of cyclosporine A for the treatment of patients with uveitis associated with juvenile idiopathic arthritis. *Eye* 2009;**23**:1192–8.

Tay-Kearney M-L, Schwam BL, Lowder C, et al. Clinical features and associated systemic diseases of HLA-B27 uveitis. *Am J Ophthalmol* 1996;**121**:47–56.

Thorne JE, Woreta FA, Dunn JP, Jabs DA. Risk of cataract development among children with juvenile idiopathic arthritis-related uveitis treated with topical corticosteroids. *Ophthalmology* 2010;**117**:1436–41.

Toker O, Hashkes PJ. Critical appraisal of canakinumab in the treatment of adults and children with cryopyrin-associated periodic syndromes (CAPS). *Biologics* 2010;**25**:131–8.

van Overdam KA, de Faber JT, Lemij HG, de Waard PW. Baerveldt glaucoma implant in paediatric patients. *Br J Ophthalmol* 2006;**90**:328–32.

Zulian F, Balzarin M, Falcini F, et al. Abatacept for severe anti-tumour necrosis factor alpha refractory juvenile idiopathic arthritis-related uveitis. *Arthrit Care Res* 2010;**62**:821–5.

Chapter 9 Fuchs' heterochromic uveitis and other anterior uveitis syndromes

Some patients with uveitis exhibit forms of inflammation that predominantly affect the anterior segment, tend to present with subacute rather than hyperacute symptoms (in contrast to HLA-B27-associated anterior uveitis) and often demonstrate signs that are either pathognomonic or highly suggestive of the particular diagnosis. These forms of uveitis are included here. Herpetic anterior uveitis might usefully be described here, but for pathogenic clarity it is instead placed with other viral forms of uveitis in Chapter 11. Some non-inflammatory conditions may masquerade as anterior uveitis but these are also dealt with elsewhere, with other malignant or non-malignant masquerades, in Chapter 20.

FUCHS' HETEROCHROMIC UVEITIS (box 9.1)

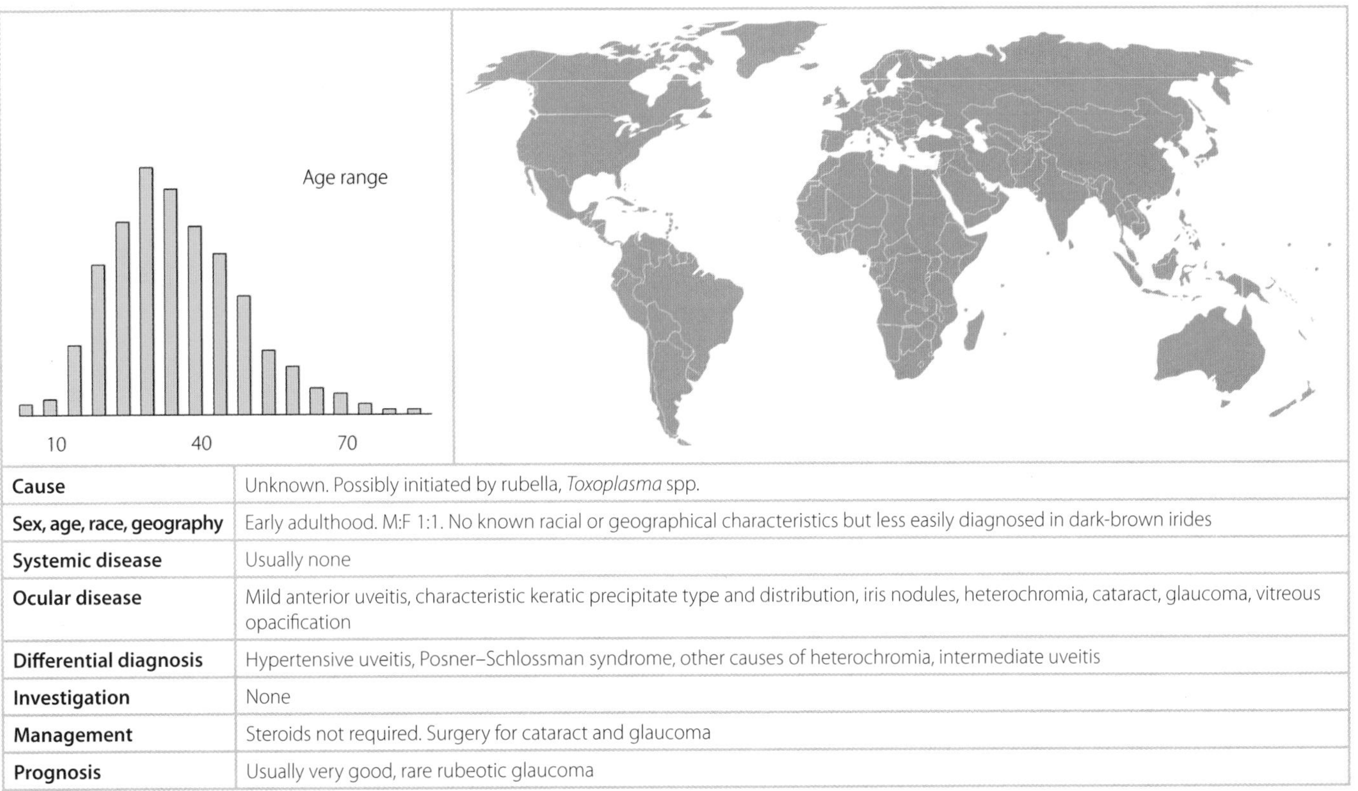

Cause	Unknown. Possibly initiated by rubella, *Toxoplasma* spp.
Sex, age, race, geography	Early adulthood. M:F 1:1. No known racial or geographical characteristics but less easily diagnosed in dark-brown irides
Systemic disease	Usually none
Ocular disease	Mild anterior uveitis, characteristic keratic precipitate type and distribution, iris nodules, heterochromia, cataract, glaucoma, vitreous opacification
Differential diagnosis	Hypertensive uveitis, Posner–Schlossman syndrome, other causes of heterochromia, intermediate uveitis
Investigation	None
Management	Steroids not required. Surgery for cataract and glaucoma
Prognosis	Usually very good, rare rubeotic glaucoma

Box 9.1 Fuchs' heterochromic uveitis

Introduction

In 1906 a group of 38 patients with similar features were reported by Ernst Fuchs. Although previously reported in the nineteenth century by several other authors, the condition that Professor Fuchs so comprehensively described is now known as Fuchs' heterochromic uveitis (FHU). The syndrome is not uncommon, accounting for up to 5% of uveitis in some populations. In its classic form it is unmistakable, but a spectrum of appearances remains compatible with the diagnosis (Jones 1991a). Historically linked to a variety of underlying systemic disorders (Jones 1993), its cause or causes remain elusive. However, much recent interest has resulted from the finding by several groups of local intraocular IgG antibody production against rubella virus in FHU eyes, and much less often its DNA has been detected by polymerase chain reaction (PCR) on aqueous specimens (Quentin and Reiber 2004). Some have asserted that those with FHU have not undergone rubella immunization and it has been recorded that the falling incidence of the disease in the USA is related to a changed immunization program (Birnbaum et al. 2007). The validity of the Goldman–Witmer method in claiming intraocular antibody production is discussed in Chapter 3. However, evidence is mounting for an association between FHU and rubella virus.

Systemic disease

Thousands of cases of FHU have now been reported in the literature. Despite many attempts to identify any associated systemic disease, the epidemiology suggests that this is a purely ocular disorder. However, reports of associations with the Parry–Romberg syndrome of hemifacial atrophy have been made, although the pathogenic connection between these two conditions is unknown.

Ocular disease

Introduction and symptoms

Characteristically FHU is unilateral. However, the incidence of bilateral disease is up to 8%. In these cases macroscopic heterochromia is absent, but other typical signs will aid diagnosis. Patients with bilateral disease appear to develop inflammation simultaneously in the two eyes; sequential involvement of the second eye has not been observed in our large cohort, and patients with unilateral disease may be reassured with confidence that their other eye is not at risk of developing FHU.

Most patients with FHU present in early to mid-adulthood but it is clear on presentation that their disease is chronic and it is highly likely that most cases have their true onset in childhood or adolescence. Indeed, there is persuasive evidence of congenital or early onset disease in some (including the presence of 'congenital' heterochromia or amblyopia). The most common reasons for presentation include floaters (because of vitreous opacification) and blurred vision (because of cataract). The heterochromia itself is only occasionally noticed; most are unaware of their heterochromia until noticed by an acquaintance, or an ophthalmologist. In some cases, ocular discomfort is experienced, and overall a significant subset of patients develop a chronic intermittent periocular aching, which may radiate to give unilateral headache, and which appears unrelated to either the degree of intraocular inflammation or to the intraocular pressure (IOP). It may, however, be secondary to anterior segment ischemia.

The anterior chamber

Ciliary injection and vigorous anterior uveitis are not features of FHU. However, it seems in some cases that the pattern of inflammation at the onset of the disease may differ, and an apparent acute anterior uveitis, or an intermediate-type uveitis, may over a period of time develop features typical of FHU. The number of anterior chamber (AC) cells may fluctuate, but only occasionally exceeds 1+. Flare, representing protein leakage, is not usually a significant feature and therefore the absence of protein, including fibrinogen from the aqueous humor, would explain the consistent absence of cicatricial synechiae in this condition. Some eyes may pass through periods without detectable cells in the AC, and eventually some appear to reach a 'burnt-out' stage where inflammation is no longer seen. Interestingly, this is most likely to be observed after the cataract has been removed. A few patients seem to exhibit an 'aggressive' form of FHU that does cause flare, and more cells in the AC than usual. Such patients should be managed with great care if coming to cataract surgery (see below).

The cornea

Keratic precipitates (KPs) are typically numerous, moderate but variable in size, translucent and grayish, and characteristically scattered over the whole corneal endothelium. Although a greater concentration of KPs is usually seen inferiorly, it is their widespread distribution that is the most reliable sign of the disease, being so different from other forms of uveitis (**Fig. 9.1**). Morphologically, most KPs are rounded, but under higher magnification (**Fig. 9.2**) it can be seen that some have extensions almost like 'pseudopodia,' giving the KPs a stellate appearance, and over the intervening endothelium is sometimes a meshwork of very fine fibrillary structures, some of which appear to interconnect the KPs. Mutton-fat KPs, or an inferior spindle of very fine KPs, is not a feature of FHU and should suggest another diagnosis. The appearance and distribution of KPs are so individual that it must indicate a particular cellular immune behavior as yet unexplained; previous findings of a corneal autoantigen (which could not be replicated by others) or another phenomenon may explain the non-thermal KP distribution.

There are two other corneal features that have each affected several patients in our large cohort. First, large corneal endothelial 'plaques' are occasionally seen, cell bare on specular microscopy and

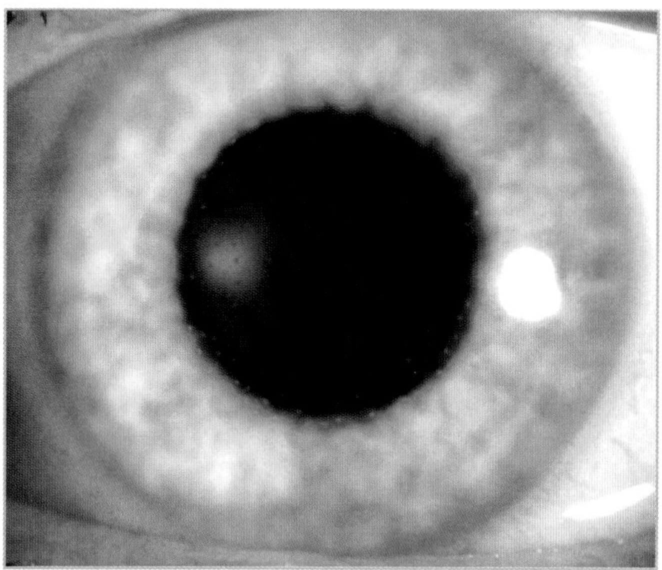

Figure 9.1 Multiple keratic precipitates spread over the whole corneal endothelium in an eye with Fuchs' heterochromic uveitis.

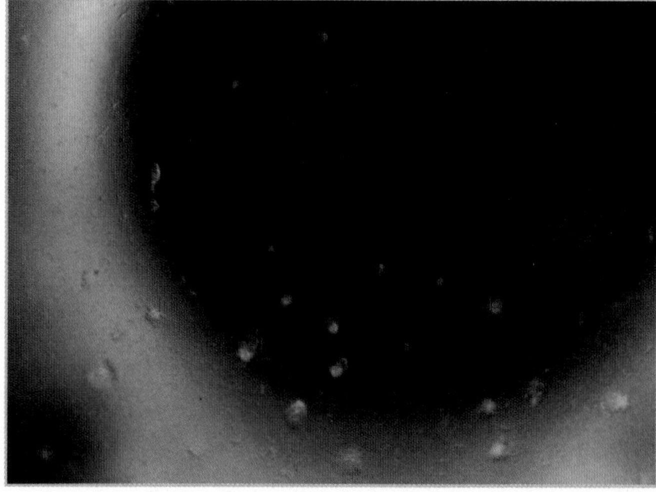

Figure 9.2 Under higher magnification most keratic precipitates are milky translucent, some showing 'stellate' extensions almost like pseudopodia. In between are tiny fibrillary deposits.

sometimes with KPs at their edges, which may represent areas of destroyed Descemet's membrane (**Fig. 9.3**). Second, a few patients have endothelial dystrophy and sometimes persistent localized corneal decompensation, usually inferiorly, not dissimilar to the appearance of corneal endotheliitis (**Fig. 9.4**). Rarely total decompensation has necessitated corneal grafting.

The iris

Iris nodules are an important feature of some patients with FHU but are frequently missed or misinterpreted. Actually, FHU is probably the most common cause of inflammatory iris nodules. In this disease, the nodules are always most predominant on the pupillary side of the colarette (**Fig. 9.5**). They are small, domed and translucent, therefore being almost diaphanous on a blue iris. Those impinging on the pupil margin are more easily seen in silhouette. They also occur on the posterior iris surface. Koeppe and Busacca originally described 'ectodermal nodules' on the pupil margin and 'mesodermal floccules' on the anterior iris surface, respectively, in an era where granulomatous disease was common, and described nodules that were larger, fewer and more irregular in shape, iris position and appearance. There is no suggestion that nodules at the pupil edge or on the anterior iris surface in an eye with FHU have a different pathogenesis; these two venerable eponyms thus have no relevance to modern diagnosis, in FHU or any form of uveitis.

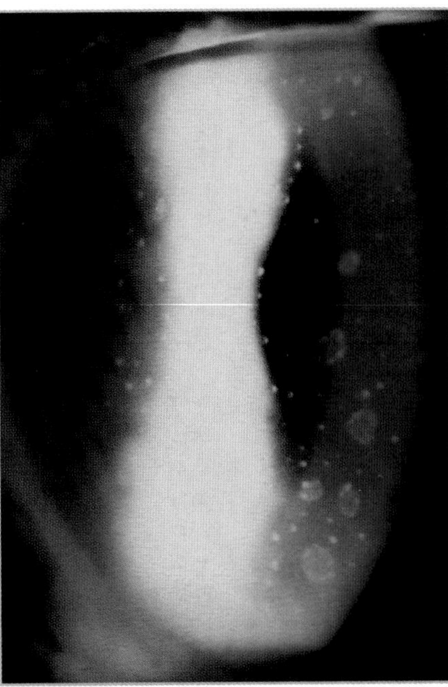

Figure 9.3 Corneal endothelial plaques in Fuchs' heterochromic uveitis, with active keratic precipitates at their edges and in between.

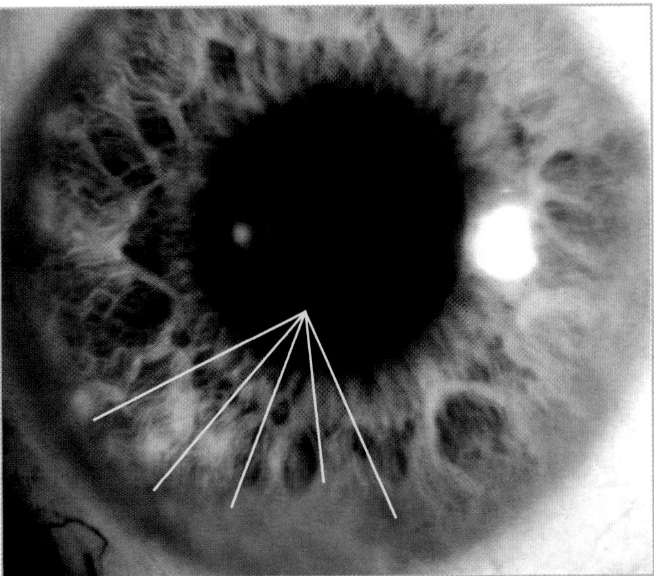

Figure 9.4 Localized peripheral corneal decompensation in Fuchs' heterochromic uveitis, the edge of the edematous area highlighted. No associated trabeculitis. Central endothelial cell count normal.

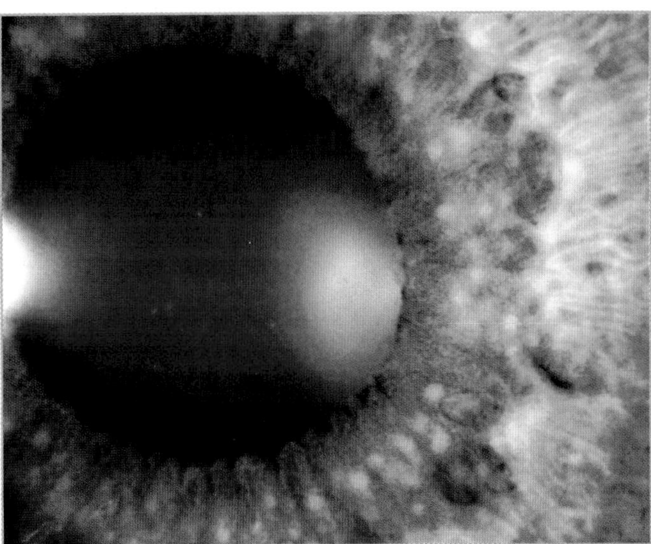

Figure 9.5 Small round translucent iris nodules in Fuchs' heterochromic uveitis are all on the pupillary side of the collaret or on the pupil margin.

The heterochromia (a difference in color between the irides) is the most well-known feature of FHU, and rarely it is striking, but in a majority of patients it is only a subtle feature. Also, FHU is not the only form of uveitis that may be accompanied by heterochromia. It is therefore important to be aware of the structural iris changes that occur in FHU, heterochromia being only an end-stage manifestation of this chronic progressive atrophy; the pupillary pigment ruff becomes patchy, breaks up and may eventually disappear; the anterior border layer of iris stroma appears particularly liable to depigmentation and atrophy; the resultant heterochromia is most striking in eyes with an orange anterior border layer over a blue stroma (**Fig. 9.6**). Iris nevi may also depigment. In irides that are blue, significant heterochromia will not occur and observations of stromal atrophy become diagnostically important. Only in rare cases does stromal atrophy become so profound that the (brown) pigmented epithelium becomes visible anteriorly. This is the explanation of so-called 'inverse heterochromia', where the affected blue iris paradoxically appears to turn brown (**Fig. 9.7**). Where the original iris color is deep brown (because of a thick stroma packed with pigment-containing cells), even profound stromal atrophy leads to little or no macroscopic heterochromia. However, the structural changes of stromal atrophy are visible on the slit-lamp, so that radial fibers and sphincter pupillae (always invisible in a normal brown iris) become exposed (**Fig. 9.8**).

Cicatricial posterior synechiae are not seen in FHU, except sometimes after intraocular surgery. However, rarely a part of the pupil is seen to be adherent to the anterior lens surface, and such a point always coincides with a visible iris nodule. Such phenomena presumably occur rather more often, however, as in many patients dilation of the pupil will

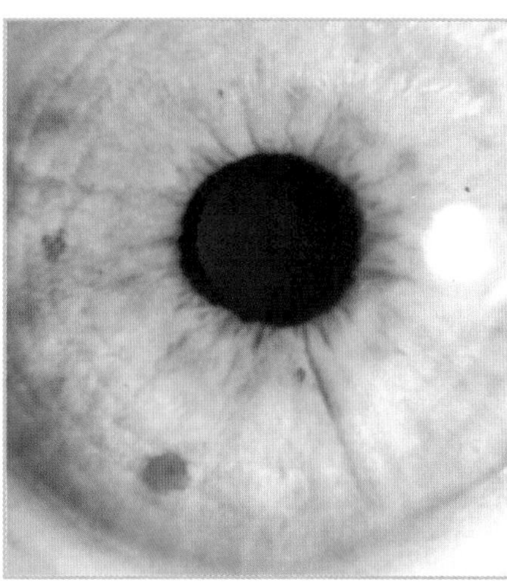
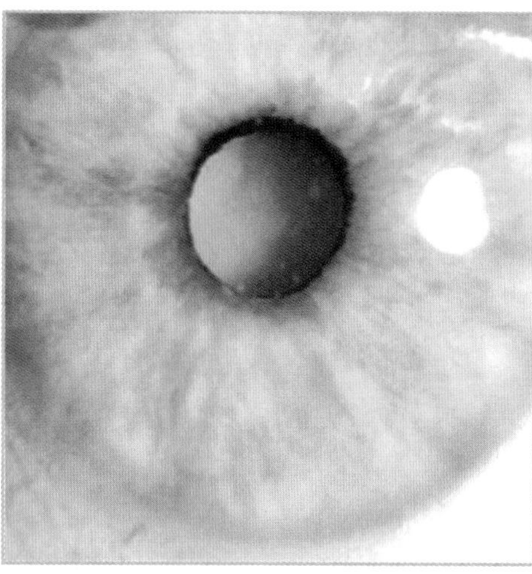

Figure 9.6 The affected left eye of a patient with Fuchs' heterochromic uveitis has entirely depigmented the anterior border layer (the colarette is white) and lost stromal pigment. There is also a cataract.

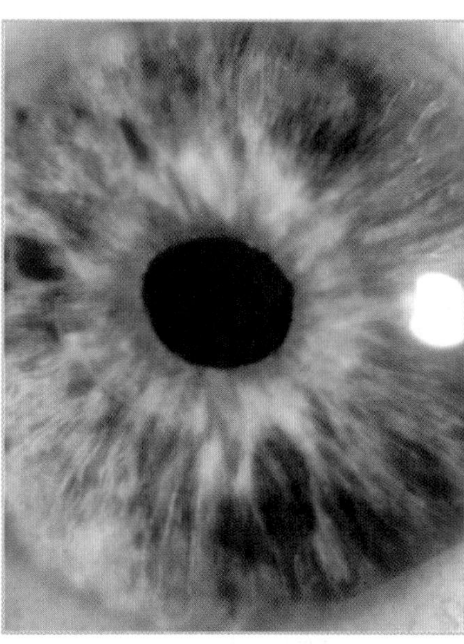
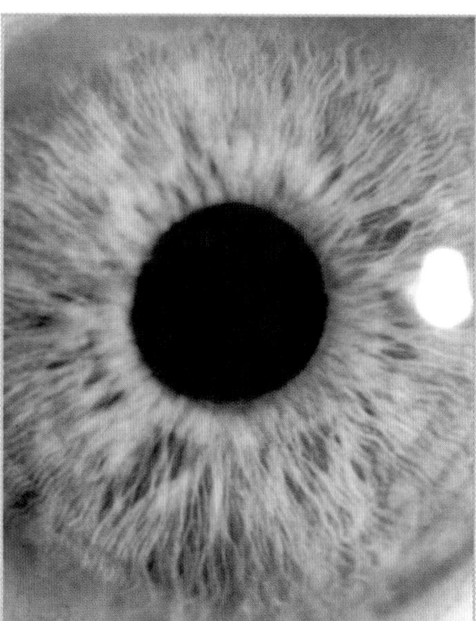

Figure 9.7 The affected right eye shows profound iris stromal atrophy, exposing the pigment epithelium to direct observation and leading to so-called 'inverse heterochromia'.

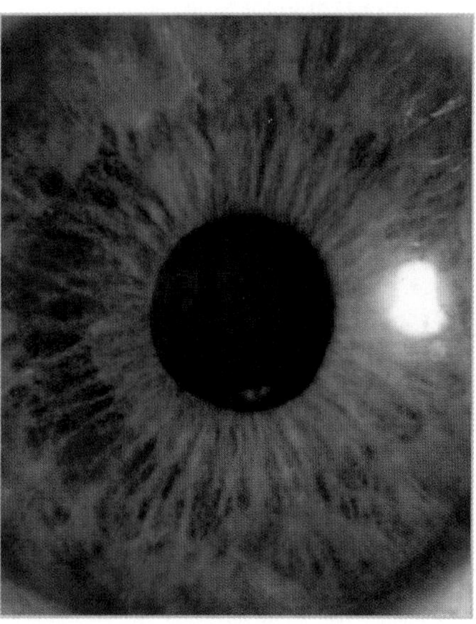
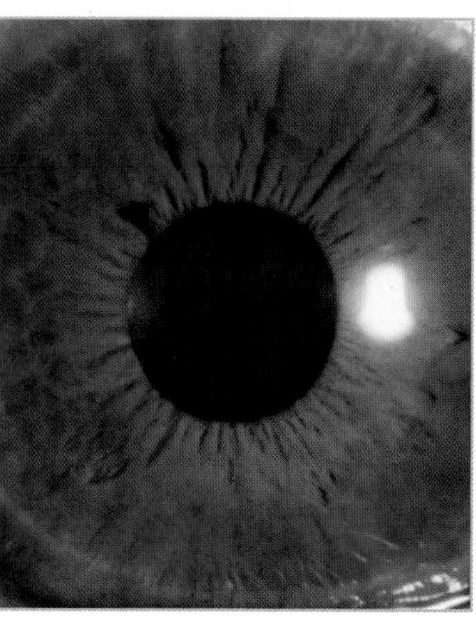

Figure 9.8 The right iris of an African–Caribbean patient with Fuchs' heterochromic uveitis shows gross erosion of stromal tissue with exposure of sphincter pupillae and radial fibers. In the normal left iris this architecture remains covered by dense stromal pigment.

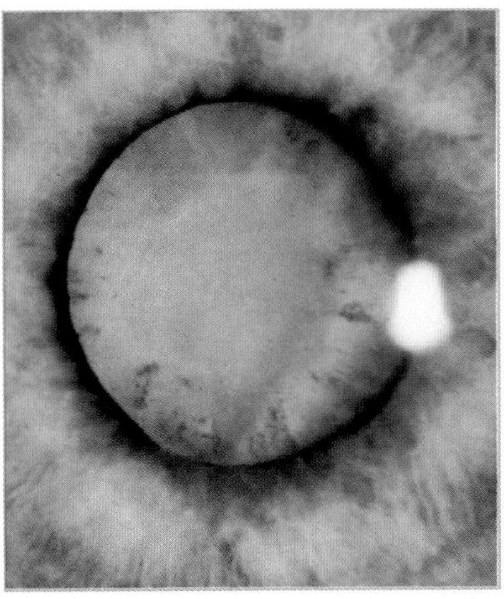
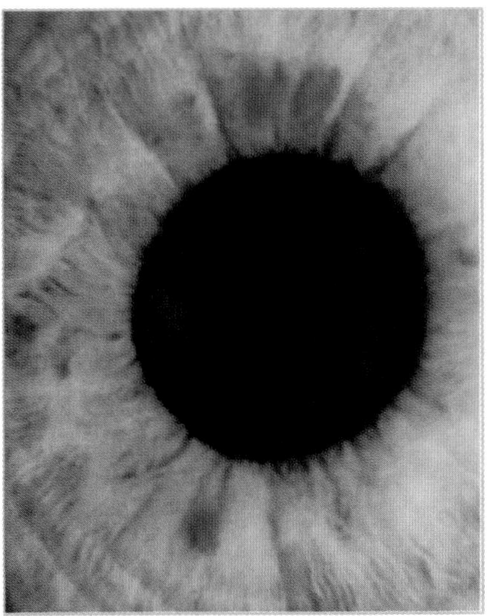

Figure 9.9 The affected right eye has radial smears of pigment on the anterior lens surface. Note also the complete depigmentation of the anterior border layer in contrast to the unaffected left eye.

reveal radial lines of iris pigment on the anterior lens surface (**Fig. 9.9**). These probably represent previous lines of contact with posterior iris surface nodules that have 'smeared' pigment on to the lens.

Anterior segment vasculature

An abnormality of anterior segment vasculature is an important, perhaps a key, feature of FHU. The ultrastructural cause is as yet unidentified, but the abnormality causes vascular fragility and an increased tendency to bleed. Minor bleeding into the AC angle (known as Amsler's sign, first described as an outpatient provocative test using paracentesis [Amsler 1948]) was a reliable accompaniment to intraocular surgery in the era of extracapsular cataract extraction (**Fig. 9.10**) - not troublesome, but confirmatory of the diagnosis of FHU. The phenomenon is less often seen during modern small-incision surgery because of better-maintained IOP. Hyphema on the first postoperative day is very uncommon. Recurrent 'spontaneous' hyphema is occasionally recorded, and minor trauma including gonioscopy or even applanation may also cause bleeding. It is highly likely that trivial day-to-day trauma such as eye rubbing or wiping may cause repeated microscopic hyphema in FHU eyes. More rarely, significant vitreous hemorrhage or even blood-filled iris pigment epithelial cysts have been observed.

Iris neovascularization is only rarely seen in FHU. AC angle rubeosis, once thought quite common, is misdiagnosed because iris root atrophy has rendered the normal vasculature abnormally visible. Nevertheless true neovascularization, demonstrated on iris angiography (**Fig. 9.11**), does occur, and a few eyes have been enucleated because of intractable rubeotic glaucoma. No evidence of posterior segment ischemia accompanies such changes and rubeosis seems entirely induced by the underlying anterior segment ischemic vasculopathy.

Glaucoma

Glaucoma is the most problematic feature of FHU, and is common, affecting about a quarter of eyes (Jones 1991b). It is usually present when the patient first presents to the ophthalmologist, but may develop at any time, the most likely precipitant being cataract surgery.

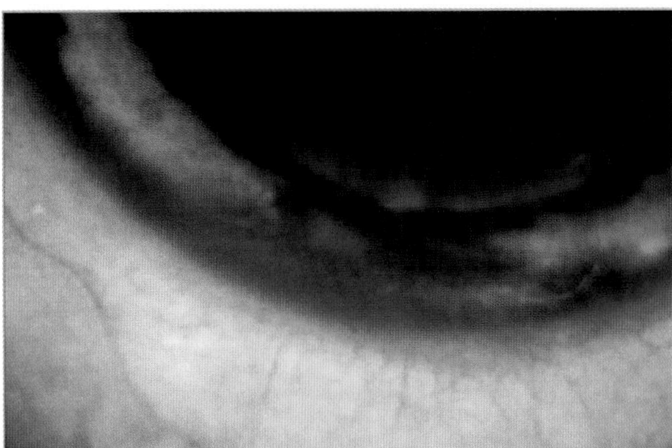

Figure 9.10 Bleeding into the anterior chamber angle during cataract surgery is characteristic of eyes with FHU. (Reproduced with permission from Jones 1996.)

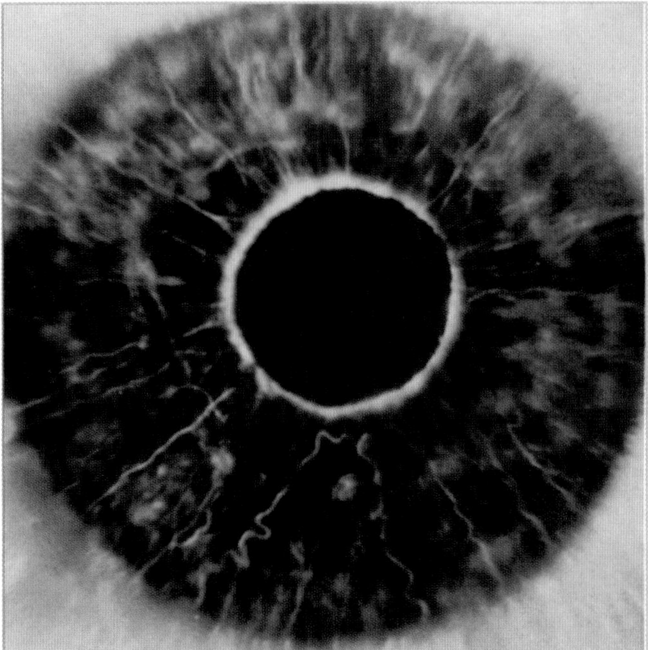

Figure 9.11 Iris fluorescein angiography in Fuchs' heterochromic uveitis shows multiple leaking neovascular tufts from the iris stroma, and significant pupillary margin leakage.

It results from progressive trabecular sclerosis. Usually quite responsive to medical treatment, only a minority needs surgical drainage.

The lens and vitreous

Posterior subcapsular cataract can be expected in a great majority of patients with FHU, although some appear immune to this complication. Vitreous opacification, contrary to the expectation of most ophthalmologists, can be highly significant (**Fig. 9.12**) in FHU and is quite consistent with the diagnosis. The opacities are usually widespread and fibrillary, but small inferior snowballs may be seen or there may be large swirling condensations. This may resemble intermediate uveitis, but pars plana exudate is not seen. The vitreous element may be a significant part of the patient's visual problem and vitrectomy is entirely justified for some. Many patients with FHU develop early posterior vitreous detachment, and the sudden worsening of vitreous floaters at this point is a not uncommon reason for presentation.

The retina

Macular edema is rare in FHU, even after cataract surgery and in some cases its presence serves to differentiate FHU from intermediate uveitis. Focal chorioretinal scarring, or macular coloboma which suggests previous *Toxoplasma* infection, is seen in a significant minority (Jones 1991b). It has been suggested that toxoplasmosis may cause some cases, and active *Toxoplasma* chorioretinitis and FHU have coexisted, either in the same eye or in fellow eyes. The association seems too well reported for mere coincidence. Retinitis pigmentosa is occasionally reported in association with FHU, but its relevance is unknown.

It can be seen that the original term 'cyclitis' is very inadequate to describe a form of inflammation that regularly affects an eye from cornea to retina. Even the term 'uveitis' does not encompass all possibilities, but it embraces rather more and has long been the preferred term of this author.

Diagnosis

The etiology of FHU is unknown and there is no diagnostic test. Classic cases are striking and should not be missed. Less typical or bilateral disease requires a more careful observation of iris structural changes, and misdiagnosis is not infrequent. The Posner–Schlossman syndrome, also causing heterochromia and glaucoma in the presence of mild uveitis, can be a challenging differential diagnosis, and unilateral intermediate uveitis may occasionally lead to heterochromia. Non-inflammatory causes of heterochromia should not present a problem, although eyes with burnt-out FHU may occasionally confuse. The diagnosis of FHU is probably more often missed than any other in the field of uveitis. This is not merely an academic problem; such patients are sometimes extensively over-investigated and over-treated and these are avoidable issues.

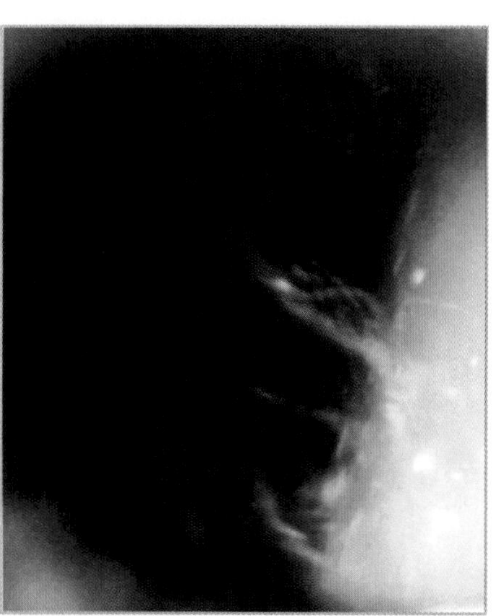

Figure 9.12 Substantial vitreous opacification is not uncommon in Fuchs' heterochromic uveitis. (Reproduced with permission from Jones 1996.)

Management

Uveitis

The frequent misdiagnosis of FHU leads to the automatic use of topical steroid treatment in many patients. This is usually unnecessary and probably undesirable. The mild degree of inflammation does not cause characteristic uveitic pain and the absence of protein in aqueous humor means that synechiae are not a potential problem. A significant proportion of young patients are steroid responders and long-term steroid treatment may accelerate cataract formation. Unnecessary topical treatment is to be avoided.

It is therefore our practice to use topical steroids only in specific circumstances: first where a particularly dense accumulation of KPs or precipitates on the posterior lens surface is affecting vision; second in those rare cases where genuine flare-ups of inflammation are seen; third in preparation for, and for an extended period after, intraocular surgery; and fourth to clear away giant cell deposition from intraocular lenses (IOLs – see below).

Cataract

The majority of patients with FHU require cataract surgery, most often around the age of 40, but sometimes much earlier. In the early years of IOL development much angst surrounded the advisability of IOL implantation and, if so, the appropriate IOL to use. This temerity was entirely justified; early reports of success were too often followed by ultimate failure, e.g. with the appropriately named UGH (uveitis–glaucoma–hyphema) syndrome (**Fig. 9.13**). When extracapsular surgery was the method, in the context of a degree of IOL–iris touch, heparin

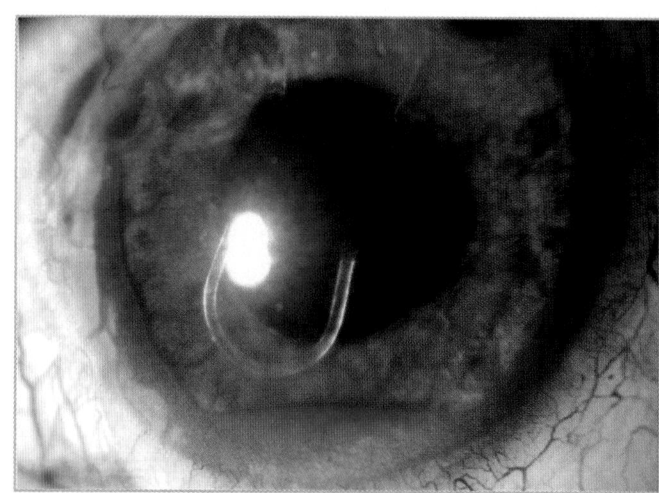

Figure 9.13 An early disaster of inappropriate intraocular lens implantation in an eye with Fuchs' heterochromic uveitis, 1980: chronic uveitis, intractable raised intraocular pressure and rubeosis with hyphema (uveitis–glaucoma–hyphema syndrome); the eye was enucleated.

surface modification was undoubtedly beneficial (Jones 1995), but it was the introduction of endocapsular fixation inherent in the phakoemulsification technique that has allowed us to implant IOLs with confidence in almost all eyes (Jones 1996). Indeed, a period followed of secondary IOL implantation in FHU eyes that had initially been left aphakic (Jones 2002). The excellent tolerance of foldable acrylic IOLs was a further advance. Despite the overall reliability of modern IOLs in such eyes, a degree of caution should be retained in some circumstances: those eyes with profound iris atrophy, more than usual preoperative inflammation (especially with significant flare), and pre-existent glaucoma or iris neovascularization are at much greater risk of postoperative problems including intractable uveitis and glaucoma.

The Manchester sliding scale for preoperative preparation of patients with uveitis including FHU (Suresh et al. 2001) is discussed in detail in Chapter 7, but, in summary, topical steroid for 1 week preoperatively (usually prednisolone acetate four to six times a day) will reduce intraocular inflammation to a minimum. At the time of surgery periocular or intraocular steroid is injected and postoperatively intensive (2-hourly) topical steroid is used at least for the first few days, together with mydriasis. In the great majority of eyes that settle quickly and uneventfully after surgery, this cautious approach has not been detrimental; in those few that become quite inflamed after surgery, it has been most helpful. Topical steroid treatment is titrated downwards according to response, discontinuing after 6–8 weeks. Only a few require more vigorous treatment, but the capacity of FHU to cause postoperative problems including fibrinous uveitis is often underestimated.

After discontinuing topical steroid postoperatively a proportion of FHU eyes begin to deposit giant cells on the IOL. This phenomenon affects eyes with FHU more than any other form of uveitis. The use of intensive topical steroid for a few weeks has been helpful in reducing their number, although slow re-accumulation has been the rule. Very uncommonly, high visual acuity is maintained only by long-term topical steroid.

Posterior capsule opacification does not appear to be a particular problem in FHU eyes in comparison with age-matched patients, but laser capsulotomy has been followed by the onset of glaucoma in a small number of patients, and by substantial worsening of pre-existing glaucoma in others. As for other patients with uveitis, laser capsulotomy should be used only when clearly necessary and preceded and followed by a few days of topical steroid.

Glaucoma

Some patients with FHU will have glaucoma at presentation. For those who develop it while under supervision, it is typical for several spikes of raised IOP to precede a sustained rise (Jones 1991b). Occasionally these pressure spikes can be so high as to cause either symptomatic pain or temporary amaurosis on standing up. Sometimes the uninflamed eye also develops glaucoma. Medical management of the glaucoma is usually straightforward. Some will require drainage surgery. The failure rate of such surgery in FHU is higher as for all eyes with uveitis. Enhanced surgery is required.

Vitreous opacification

Many patients with FHU find their vitreous floaters troublesome and this should not be underestimated by the ophthalmologist: about 10% in our cohort have requested vitrectomy, which has been entirely successful with significant improvement in acuity (Waters et al. 2000), although pre-existing posterior vitreous detachment, itself not uncommon in young adults with FHU, is a reassurance for the surgeon although not a prerequisite.

OTHER ANTERIOR UVEITIS SYNDROMES

Posner–Schlossman syndrome

Posner and Schlossman (Posner and Schlossman 1948) described nine patients with intermittent unilateral acute glaucoma and mild anterior uveitis, and their syndrome (PSS) is also known as glaucomatocyclitic crisis. The condition is actually rare but the term is sometimes mistakenly used to describe any acute anterior uveitis with secondary glaucoma, and is overused generally. Presentation of true PSS is actually quite distinctive, typically with mild ocular discomfort and blurred vision in one eye. On examination the IOP is raised, often to more than 40 mmHg. Mild corneal edema may be present. The AC depth is normal. KPs are usually seen, are characteristically few and may be located peripherally or centrally (**Fig. 9.14**). Occasionally only a single precipitate is seen, and this has been described as a 'sentinel' KP. The KPs may be moderate in size, but are not of the large mutton-fat variety. A mild anterior uveitis is present, and there may be a few cells in the vitreous. No synechiae are present. The AC angle is open and there is no plateau iris, but there may be an abnormal 'fluffy' white appearance to the trabecular meshwork, with overlying precipitates, and it has been suggested that a trabeculitis is the primary cause of the syndrome. Anterior ischemic optic neuropathy has been anecdotally reported in attacks of PSS, presumably secondary to raised IOP, but strangely no vein occlusions.

Topical steroid therapy was not available when Posner and Schlossman and others described early cases. The glaucoma was treated, but the uveitis was noted to be self-limiting, recurrent and unilateral. Three of the original nine cases demonstrated iris heterochromia but in fact, with careful observation, it is probable that, after several attacks, subtle heterochromia can be seen in most cases (**Fig. 9.15**). Recurrences may be frequent for a period but tend to become less so, although the disease typically lasts for several years. With prompt treatment of attacks, cumulative glaucomatous damage can be prevented. Although loss of corneal endothelial cells has been demonstrated, progression to frank corneal decompensation does not seem to occur.

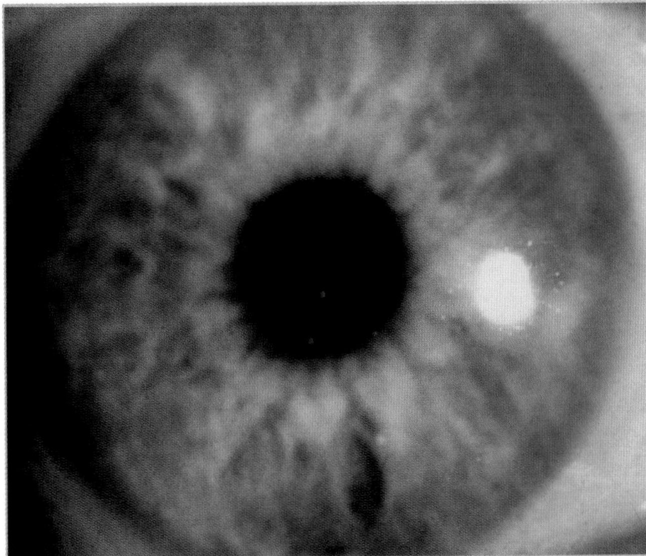

Figure 9.14 A small cluster of medium-sized keratic precipitates is seen on the central endothelium during an attack of Posner–Schlossman syndrome.

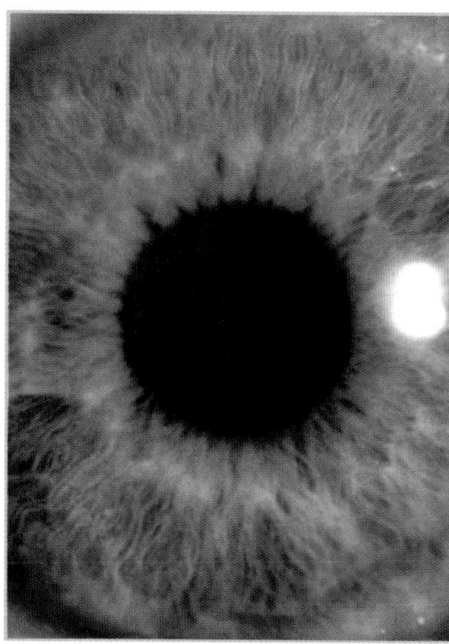

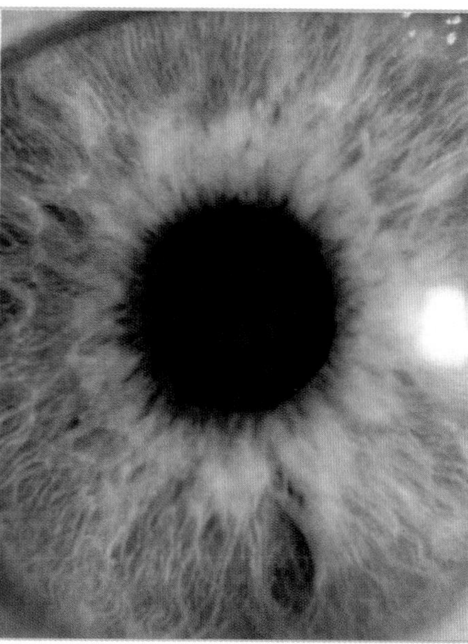

Figure 9.15 The affected left eye of a patient with Posner–Schlossman syndrome has lost anterior border layer pigment after several attacks, causing subtle heterochromia.

The mild uveitis is usually very sensitive to topical steroid treatment. Although this alone tends to shorten each attack and thereby reduce the IOP, most patients also require topical anti-glaucoma medication at the onset, usually topical apraclonidine 1%, and only occasionally systemic acetazolamide. Mydriasis is unnecessary. The IOP returns to normal after each attack. Repeated attacks may cause progressive glaucoma damage and occasionally patients develop chronic mild uveitis better suppressed with long-term topical steroid. Monitoring of IOP and serial visual fields is preferred.

The combination of heterochromia, mild anterior uveitis and raised IOP is common to both PSS and FHU. However, the KP number and distribution, the occurrence of cataract in the latter, the different temporal behavior and the different iris architecture indicate that they are separate entities. Earlier findings of herpes simplex virus DNA in the aqueous humor of a few PSS patients was temporarily distracting, this and the common clinical identification of trabeculitis suggesting to many that PSS was merely a form of herpetic anterior uveitis. More recently the finding of cytomegalovirus (CMV) DNA in the aqueous of some patients has been interesting (Chee et al. 2008). Some patients have therefore been treated with ganciclovir or valganciclovir with apparent clinical response but relapse after treatment cessation. The etiology of PSS clearly requires further investigation but, even if proven to be related to CMV intraocular infection, it would be difficult to justify long-term anti-CMV treatment where current simple topical measures suffice.

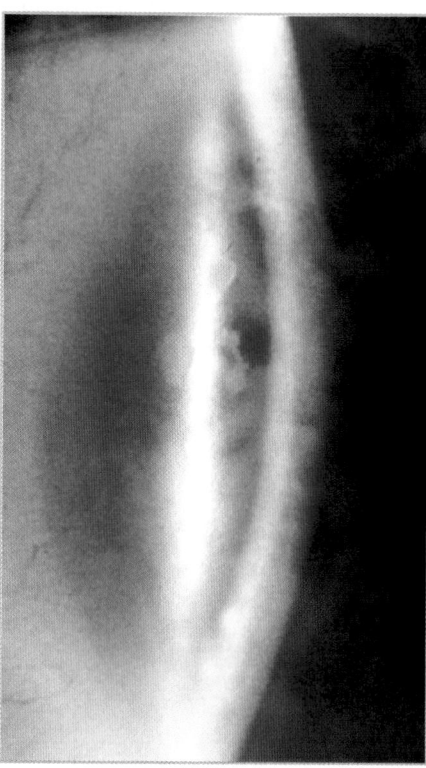

Figure 9.16 Peripheral endotheliitis affecting the temporal cornea, with grouped large keratic precipitates, and a well-demarcated zone of affected endothelium.

Peripheral corneal endotheliitis

The primary focus of inflammation in this condition (peripheral corneal endotheliitis or PCE), initially thought to be autoimmune (Khodadoust et al. 1982), appears to be the corneal endothelium, but a significant anterior uveitis is usual. Patients present with unilateral or bilateral blurring of vision. The central cornea is usually clear, but a variable area of the corneal periphery may be edematous. Underlying this a white infiltration of deep cornea may be seen (**Fig. 9.16**), and the border between this and apparently normal endothelium may be seen as a distinct line, resembling the Khodadoust line of corneal rejection after corneal transplantation. Usually large KPs underlie the abnormal area, and gonioscopy may reveal that these occupy most of the AC angle within the affected sector. A few cases are associated with intermediate uveitis (Khodadoust et al. 1986).

Disciform corneal endotheliitis is a well-known manifestation of herpetic inflammation and several other viruses including mumps, varicella-zoster virus (VZV), human herpesvirus 7 (HHV7) and rhabdovirus can also affect the endothelium. However, there is increasing recognition of CMV as a cause of corneal endotheliitis, both primarily (Chee et al. 2007) and after corneal grafting, with focal endothelial lesions and linear accumulations of KPs being characteristic (Koizumi et al. 2008). It is not known whether PCE is one subset of such infections.

Both the corneal changes and the uveitis respond to topical steroid medication (which may need to be intensive at first), as does any associated secondary glaucoma, which nevertheless may also require temporary treatment. Untreated, progressive corneal inflammation and decompensation may ensue. The condition is typically recurrent, often frequently so, and usually bilateral, although recurrences in each eye are often independent of each other. Chronic glaucoma may result from repeated episodes of inflammation. There is no evidence on the usefulness of antiviral treatment.

Lens-induced uveitis

The induction of uveitis and glaucoma by components of the crystalline lens may occur either by trauma or surgery to the lens capsule, or where a hypermature intumescent cataract disrupts its own capsule. It appears that at least two distinct mechanisms are involved, but the old terminology of lens-induced uveitis was confusing, the terms 'phakoanaphylactic,' 'phakoantigenic,' 'phakogenic,' 'phakolytic,' 'phakoallergic' and 'phakotoxic' all being used to describe what in many cases was similar pathology. Nevertheless, forms of uveitis at different ends of this spectrum appear to be substantially different, both in presentation and in cytology, and presumably in immunology.

Phakolysis is a process that occurs in hypermature cataracts where cortex has liquefied. It can be microscopic, in which instance lens proteins are able to pass through what appears biomicroscopically to be an intact lens capsule; the accompanying inflammatory response is usually mild, with a few AC cells (mostly macrophages) and usually few or absent KPs, but larger refractile lens protein particles (**Fig. 9.17**). Raised IOP is very common, presumably because lens fragments block trabecular meshwork. Macroscopic changes mean that the lens has visibly ruptured so that the anterior chamber fills with flocculent lens material (**Fig. 9.18**). Removal of the offending lens is necessary as soon as possible, but, in those cases accompanied by significant anterior uveitis, a short period of intensive topical steroid therapy should precede this. The rarity of advanced cataract in the western world in the twenty-first century means that these forms of lens-induced uveitis are now almost unknown.

Equally rare, but with a different form of inflammation, is phakoanaphylactic uveitis, an acute granulomatous inflammation that was occasionally seen after extracapsular surgery with retained lens matter, or after unrepaired lens trauma. It is less rare in microphthalmic eyes, in which it was reported as occurring spontaneously (Thach et al. 1991). This inflammation may be severe and, although it may rarely arise after months or years, usually follows within days of trauma, at a time when infective endophthalmitis is the main differential diagnosis. Mutton-fat KPs are usual and a severe AC reaction is frequent, possibly with synechiae or hypopyon. Either glaucoma or hypotony is compatible with the diagnosis. A focal white accumulation of inflammatory debris around retained lens material is typical, although such appearances are also consistent with *Propionibacterium acnes* infection. Inflammation may also involve the posterior segment and, importantly, in some cases the fellow eye.

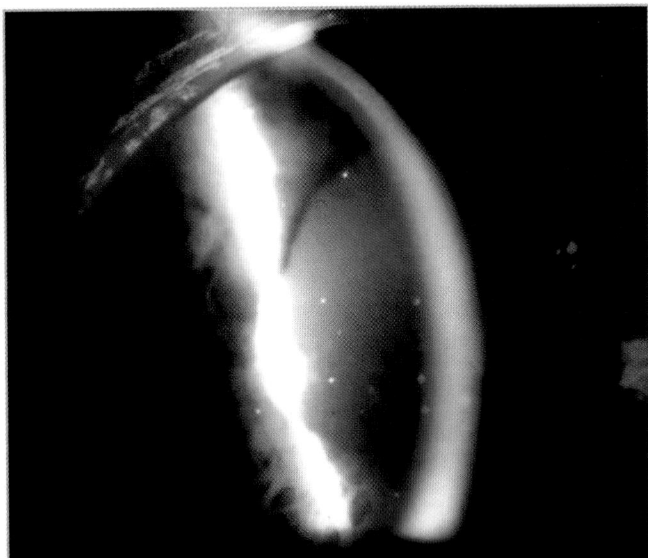

Figure 9.17 Refractile lens particles within the aqueous humor in lens-induced uveitis/glaucoma. A morgagnian cataract is seen.

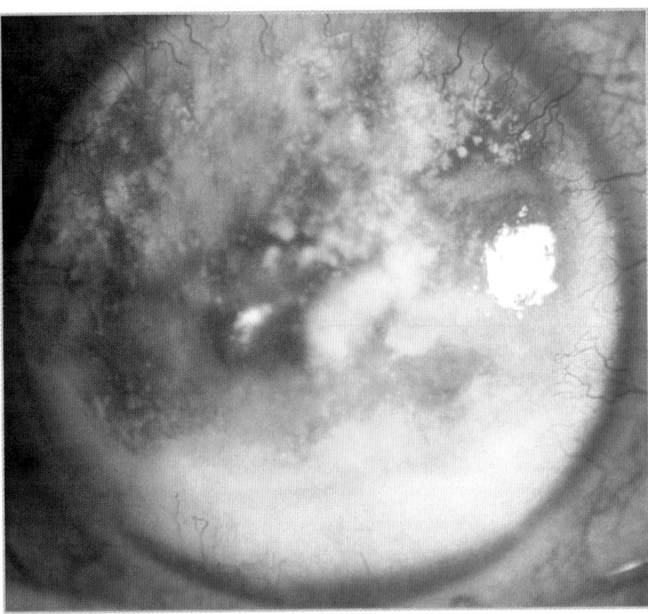

Figure 9.18 A hypermature cataract has burst, releasing flocculent cortical lens material into the anterior chamber causing uveitis and glaucoma.

The occurrence of a bilateral granulomatous uveitis after penetrating trauma or surgery should also suggest sympathetic uveitis, but sympathetic and phakoanaphylactic uveitis may occur together (Allen 1987). Whether this represents a spectrum in sympathizing uveitis, or an association between two distinct forms of inflammation with a common etiology, is unclear.

If infective uveitis is part of the differential diagnosis, then paracentesis for cytology and microbiology is urgent. Biopsy of a focus of inflammation can provide confirmatory pathology of phakoanaphylactic uveitis. Intensive topical, and sometimes high-dose systemic, steroid treatment is justified, but not adequate in itself; the surgical removal of all retained lens matter is necessary and this will include capsule and IOL. If this is not achieved, chronic uveitis may progress to cause severe sequelae including cyclitic membrane formation, chronic glaucoma or phthisis. Similar to phakolysis, phakoanaphylaxis is much rarer in the western world now than 20 years ago and this is mainly a reflection of modern methods of cataract surgery.

Uveitis, glaucoma and hyphema syndrome

In the era of iris-supported, and to some extent sulcus-fixated or AC, IOLs, chronic IOL–iris touch would induce in some patients (and reliably in those with uveitis) a chronic anterior segment inflammation associated with glaucoma and recurrent hyphema (see Fig. 9.13), the UGH syndrome. It was recognized that chronic IOL rub, especially to the iris pigment epithelium, induced the problem and the widespread transfer to endocapsular IOL placement has rendered the complication rare in the twenty-first century. Nevertheless cases do still occur and IOL misplacement with iris touch has been proven biomicroscopically in such cases (Piette et al. 2002). IOL implantation has evolved enormously in the last two decades and the complications so common after widespread iris-supported IOL usage are now merely a dull but uncomfortable memory. It is therefore ironic that such a retrograde step as AC implants inserted for mere cosmetic reasons should be reported only recently (Arthur et al. 2009) as a modern cause of UGH syndrome. Large numbers of iris claw lenses for phakic or aphakic high ametropia have now been used, with no significant incidence of UGH syndrome. However, a new trend for retropupillary fixation, permitting IOL contact with iris pigment epithelium, may be counterproductive and follow-up studies are awaited with interest.

Tubulointerstitial nephritis and uveitis

The association of tubulointerstitial nephritis with uveitis (TINU) was first described in 1975 (Kikkawa et al. 1975) and is uncommon. This unusual form of nephritis appears particularly likely to follow treatment with non-steroidal anti-inflammatory agents or certain antibiotics, and is more common in young women or children with a median age at presentation of 15 and a 3:1 female:male ratio (Mandeville et al. 2001). Familial cases have been reported. There is a particularly strong association with HLA-DRB1*0102 with a huge relative risk of 167 (Levinson et al. 2003) and less strongly with HLA-DQA1*01, DQB1*05 and DRB1*01, all of which are in linkage disequilibrium. Diagnosis is usually straightforward on renal biopsy, but histology may show granulomatous features, and in this circumstance sarcoidosis must be excluded. The renal disease precedes the uveitis in 80% of cases, sometimes by more than 1 year, presenting with fatigue, weight loss, proteinuria, anemia, hypertension, Fanconi's syndrome or non-oliguric renal failure. The uveitis is usually acute onset, bilateral and non-granulomatous, and TINU should be considered in the differential diagnosis of this presentation in any young patient; in one series (Mackensen et al. 2007) a third of all patients under 20 with acute bilateral anterior uveitis were diagnosed with TINU. Where granulomatous features are seen, again sarcoidosis should be considered. Retinal capillary leakage, macular edema, papillitis and neuroretinitis have been reported. The renal component usually requires systemic steroid treatment, and complete resolution within months with restoration of normal kidney function is the rule, whereas the accompanying anterior uveitis, although responsive to topical steroids, becomes recurrent or chronic in over half the cases. On occasion oral immunosuppression has proved necessary. Despite occasional difficult cases the management of TINU is rarely troublesome for the ophthalmologist.

REFERENCES

Allen JC. Sympathetic uveitis and phacoanaphylaxis. *Am J Ophthalmol* 1987;**103**:63–83.

Amsler M. New clinical aspects of the vegetative eye. *Trans Ophthalmol Soc UK* 1948;**68**:45–74.

Arthur SN, Wright MM, Kramarevsky N, et al. Uveitis-glaucoma-hyphaema syndrome and corneal decompensation in association with cosmetic iris implants. *Am J Ophthalmol* 2009;**148**:790–3.

Birnbaum AD, Tessler HH, Schultz KL, et al. Epidemiological relationship between Fuchs heterochromic iridocyclitis and the United States rubella vaccination program. *Am J Ophthalmol* 2007;**144**:424–8.

Chee SP, Bacsal K, Jap A, et al. Corneal endotheliitis associated with evidence of cytomegalovirus infection. *Ophthalmology* 2007;**114**:798–803.

Chee SP, Bacsal K, Jap A, et al. Clinical features of cytomegalovirus anterior uveitis in immunocompetent patients. *Am J Ophthalmol* 2008;**145**:834–40.

Fuchs E. Über Komplicationen der Heterochromie. *Z Augenheilkd* 1906;**15**: 191–212.

Jones NP. Fuchs' heterochromic uveitis: a reappraisal of the clinical spectrum. *Eye* 1991a;**5**:649–61.

Jones NP. Glaucoma in Fuchs' heterochromic uveitis: aetiology, management and outcome. *Eye* 1991b;**5**:662–7.

Jones NP. Major review: Fuchs' heterochromic uveitis: an update. *Surv Ophthalmol* 1993;**37**:253–72.

Jones NP. Cataract surgery using heparin surface-modified intraocular lenses in Fuchs' heterochromic uveitis. *Ophthal Surg* 1995;**26**:49–52.

Jones NP. Cataract surgery in Fuchs' heterochromic uveitis: past, present and future. *J Cataract Refract Surg* 1996;**22**:261–8.

Jones NP. Secondary intraocular lens implantation in Fuchs' heterochromic uveitis. *Eye* 2002;**16**:494–6.

Khodadoust AA, Attarzadeh A. Presumed autoimmune corneal endotheliopathy. *Am J Ophthalmol* 1982;93:718–22.

Khodadoust AA, Karnama Y, Stoessel KM, et al. Pars planitis and autoimmune endotheliopathy. *Am J Ophthalmol* 1986;**102**:633–9.

Kikkawa Y, Sakurai M, Mano T, et al. Interstitial nephritis with concomitant uveitis. Report of two cases. *Contrib Nephrol* 1975;**4**:1–11.

Koizumi N, Suzuki T, Uno T, et al. Cytomegalovirus as an aetiologic factor in corneal endotheliitis. *Ophthalmology* 2008;**115**:292–7.

Levinson RD, Park MS, Rikkers SM, et al. Strong associations between specific HLA-DQ and HLA-DR alleles and the tubulointerstitial nephritis and uveitis syndrome. *Invest Ophthalmol Vis Sci* 2003;**44**:653–7.

Mackensen F, Smith JR, Rosenbaum JT. Enhanced recognition, treatment and prognosis of tubulointerstitial nephritis and uveitis syndrome. *Ophthalmology* 2007;**114**:995–9.

Mandeville JT, Levinson RD, Holland GN. The tubulointerstitial nephritis and uveitis syndrome. *Surv Ophthalmol* 2001;**46**:195–208.

Piette S, Canlas OA, Tran HV, et al. Ultrasound biomicroscopy in uveitis–glaucoma–hyphema syndrome. *Am J Ophthalmol* 2002;**133**:839–41.

Posner A, Schlossman A. Syndrome of unilateral recurrent attacks of glaucoma with cyclitic symptoms. *Arch Ophthalmol* 1948;**39**:517–33.

Quentin CD, Reiber H. Fuchs heterochromic cyclitis: rubella virus antibodies and genome in aqueous humor. *Am J Ophthalmol* 2004;**138**:46–54.

Suresh P, Jones NP. Phakoemulsification with intraocular lens implantation in patients with uveitis. *Eye* 2001;**15**:621–628.

Thach AB, Marak GE, McLean IW, et al. Phacoanaphylactic endophthalmitis: a clinicopathological review. *Int Ophthalmol* 1991;**15**:271–279.

Waters F, Goodall K, Jones NP, McLeod D. Vitrectomy for vitreous opacification in Fuchs' heterochromic uveitis. *Eye* 2000;**14**:216–18.

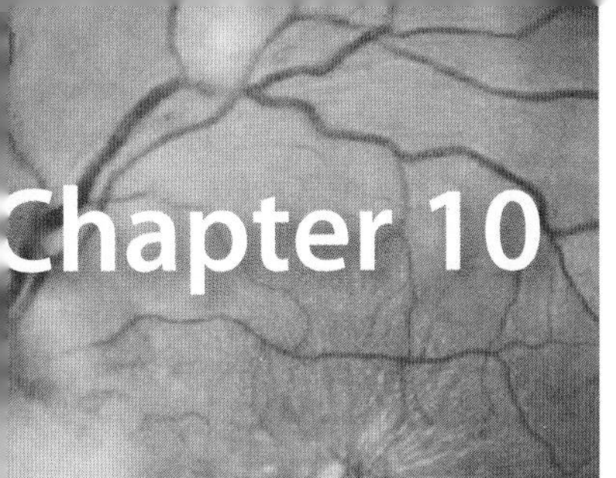

Chapter 10 Bacterial infection

The diagnosis of bacterial uveitis is crucial because specific antibiotic therapy is usually indicated, and systemic anti-inflammatory treatment given alone may be damaging. Prompt diagnosis and treatment may be important not only for sight, but also for an associated systemic inflammation. The mycobacteria and spirochetes appear prominently here, with a resurgence of both tuberculosis (TB) and syphilis in many countries. Microbial evolution may lead to new human disease; recent examples causing uveitis include borreliosis and bartonellosis. Some manifestations of posterior segment involvement in these bacterial infections may be infective, others due to immune hypersensitivity, whereas any associated anterior uveitis is usually non-infective and may become chronic.

Blood-borne endogenous endophthalmitis, fortunately very uncommon, is caused by more pathogenic bacteria. It is therefore more rapidly progressive and may be fulminating. Its diagnosis and management are included here. The diagnosis and therapy of post-surgical and post-traumatic exogenous infection are different from endogenous bacterial uveitis and are well described in other sources. Exogenous bacterial infection is therefore not included in this text.

TUBERCULOSIS (box 10.1)

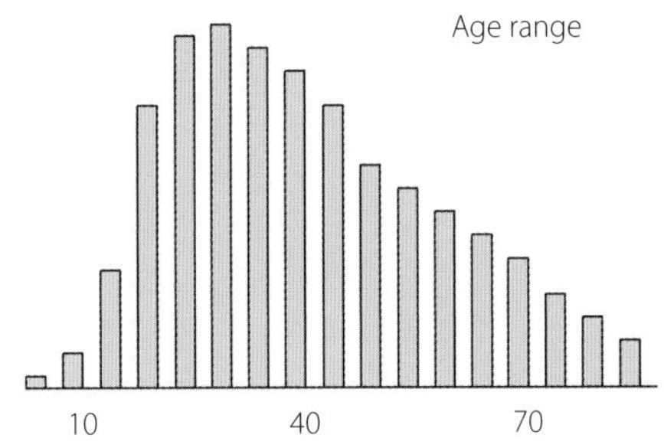

Age range

10 40 70

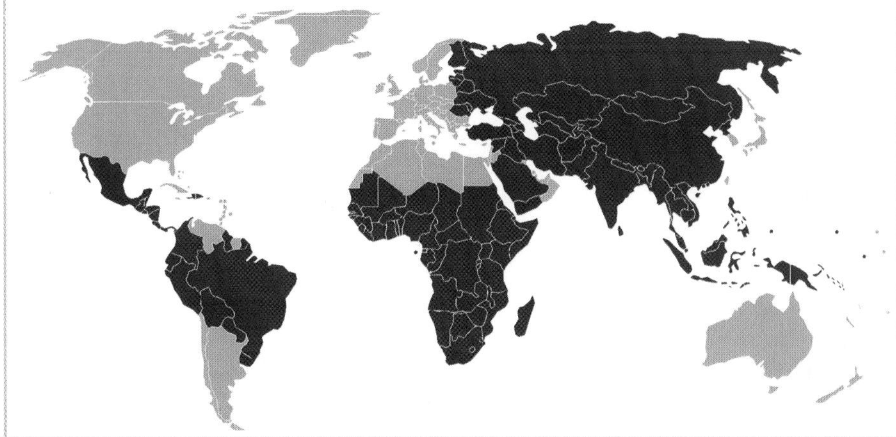

Cause	*Mycobacterium tuberculosis, an acid-fast bacillus; rarely, M. bovis*
Sex, age, race, geography	M:F 2:1, any age. Endemic in parts of Asia. In the west, highest incidence in immigrants from Indian subcontinent, Africa and Russia. Common in AIDS patients
Systemic disease	If present, pulmonary or extrapulmonary TB, sometimes miliary. Ocular TB may be sole manifestation
Ocular disease	Choroidal tubercles, subretinal abscess, retinal periphlebitis, placoid retinochoroiditis, granulomatous anterior uveitis
Differential diagnosis	Sarcoidosis, other causes of multifocal choroiditis and placoid retinochoroiditis, granulomatous uveitis
Investigation	Tuberculin skin-testing, gamma-interferon testing, chest radiograph, PCR of intraocular fluid
Management	Standard anti-mycobacterial therapy, more in resistant cases. Judicious use of steroids
Prognosis	Depends on site of ocular lesion

Box 10.1 Tuberculosis

Introduction

Mycobacterium tuberculosis, its south Indian subtype, and its related subspecies *M. bovis* and *M. africanum* can all cause human TB. In addition the genus *Mycobacterium* has many environmental saprophytic members, and some with primary hosts that are non-mammalian; some of these may cause opportunistic human infection. The curved bacilli of *M. tuberculosis* (**Fig. 10.1**) are Gram positive and acid fast (retaining carbol fuchsin dye despite attempted decolorization by mineral acids).

The incidence of TB during the latter half of the twentieth century showed a clear and consistent decline in the western world, and a more patchy and less profound fall elsewhere. However, the disease is again rising in frequency, a phenomenon due in part to the AIDS epidemic. On average, the immunocompetent host infected by *M. tuberculosis* has a 10% chance of active symptomatic TB developing at some stage during life (half of this risk manifesting within 2–3 years of acquisition, followed by a profound fall in risk thereafter to as low as 0.1% per annum). In immunodeficient individuals, the risk rises

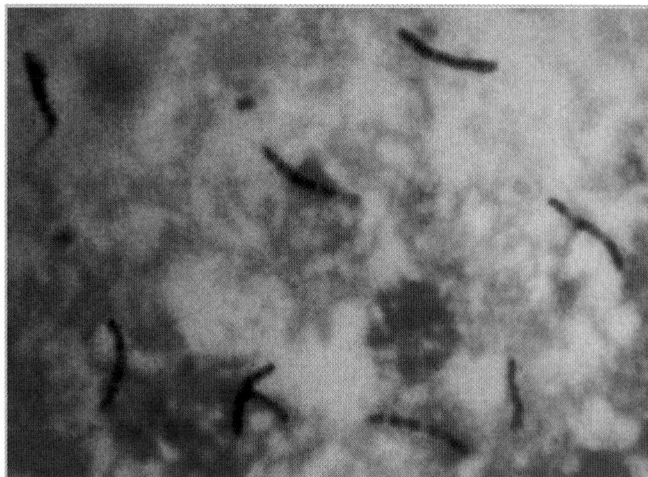

Figure 10.1 Acid-fast *Mycobacterium tuberculosis* bacilli seen under Ziehl–Neelsen stain. (Modified from Centers for Disease Control, Public Health Image Library.)

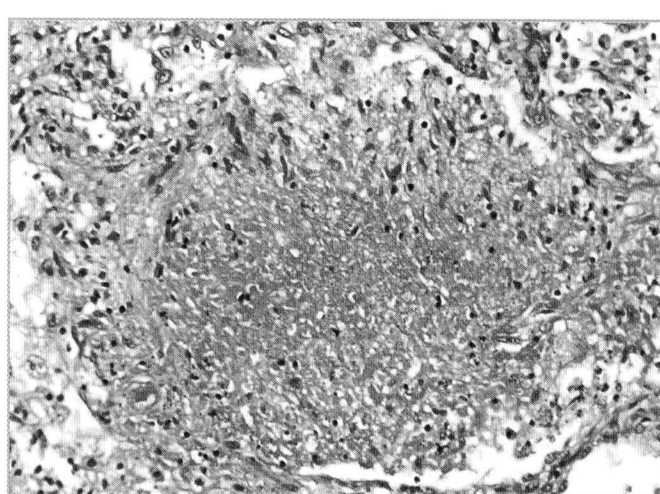

Figure 10.2 Caseating granuloma formation in tuberculosis. (Courtesy of Dr R Bonshek.)

precipitately to some 8% per annum, so that the incidence of TB in AIDS patients is 500 times greater than that in the general population. Up to half the patients in some TB clinics are HIV infected. Other disease states may lower resistance to reactivation, including malnutrition, diabetes, malignancy or immunosuppression. There is a particular risk during treatment with anti-tumor necrosis factor α (TNF-α) monoclonal antibodies.

Tuberculosis is more common in developing countries and in poorer socioeconomic groups in western countries. The disease is common in the Indian subcontinent and in parts of Asia, and emigrants from these countries carry with them a high rate of infection. More recently those from eastern Europe and Russia also have a higher prevalence, as do those from sub-Saharan Africa, where drug resistance is particularly important. In the USA, TB is generally more common in non-white individuals. In the UK, indigenous white individuals contract TB at a rate of 5/100 000 per annum, compared with 500/100 000 in recent immigrants from the Indian subcontinent. Overall in the UK the incidence is 14/100 000 with 36% of patients originating in India or Pakistan and 24% from Africa (Anderson et al. 2008). Pulmonary TB is more common in men.

Systemic disease

Primary TB causes a granulomatous lesion at the site of implantation. Usually spread by exhaled droplets, the most common site of implantation is in the lung parenchyma. Secondary lesions develop in the regional lymph nodes draining the area of the primary lesion (usually the hilar nodes), and together these are known as a Ghon focus. Wider dissemination at this stage is rare. The primary complex heals and calcifies, remaining as a radiological marker of past infection. The much rarer infection with *M. bovis* is by ingestion of infected milk, the primary site being alimentary.

Postprimary TB may result from reactivation, or by reinfection. Parenchymal lung disease is most common, usually in the upper lobes, often with multiple caseating, necrotic tuberculomas (**Fig. 10.2**), which may cause cavitation, scarring, lobe collapse or pleurisy. Lesions may discharge infected contents into a bronchus, allowing rapid mycobacterial proliferation. Such a patient with 'open' TB expectorates large numbers of organisms and is highly infective. Swallowed mycobacteria may cause gut lesions. Extrapulmonary dissemination is unusual, but is more common in Asian immigrants and in immunocompromised individuals. Manifestations include lymphadenitis, arthritis, meningitis, pericarditis and lupus vulgaris.

Some patients with active pulmonary infection are symptom free. Others may present with non-specific malaise, anorexia and weight loss, swinging pyrexia, night sweats, morning cough, hemoptysis or dyspnea. Late-presenting patients may be cachectic. Often abnormal auscultatory sounds are evident, but often less profound than might be suggested by signs on a chest radiograph; bronchial breathing, reduced breath sounds and rhonchi may be heard.

Ocular disease

Ocular TB may occur in a fit person with no evidence of active systemic TB. It may occur in the presence of active post-primary pulmonary TB, or rarely as a component of miliary dissemination, with or without meningoencephalitis. It may occur in combination with other active extrapulmonary lesions including cervical lymphadenopathy, spinal infection, psoas abscess, lupus vulgaris and others. Primary extraocular TB, although extremely rare, has been reported. However, it is assumed that intraocular TB is spread hematogenously from post-primary infection elsewhere, almost always pulmonary.

Until the 1960s, TB was considered to be a common cause of uveitis, but almost certainly the disease was overdiagnosed, partly because of the much higher prevailing incidence of TB and partly because of inadequate knowledge of other causes of intraocular inflammation including toxoplasmosis. Despite the increasing incidence, TB remains a very uncommon cause of intraocular inflammation in the west, and uncommon in endemic countries.

Intraocular inflammation is usually unilateral or asymmetrical, but manifestations are widely varied. Anterior uveitis may be granulomatous with iris nodules (**Fig. 10.3**) or nondescript, and may occur alone, but is less common than posterior segment involvement, where the most likely manifestations of direct infection are choroidal tubercles. These lesions are usually cream colored and ill defined (**Fig. 10.4**), and if smaller than disk size may not be significantly raised. They are most often found near the posterior pole, and may be multiple or single. Associated papillitis is common (**Fig. 10.5**). Large single lesions are sometimes seen (**Fig. 10.6**), and rarely a subretinal abscess with hypopyon may appear (**Fig. 10.7**), as may intraretinal hemorrhage

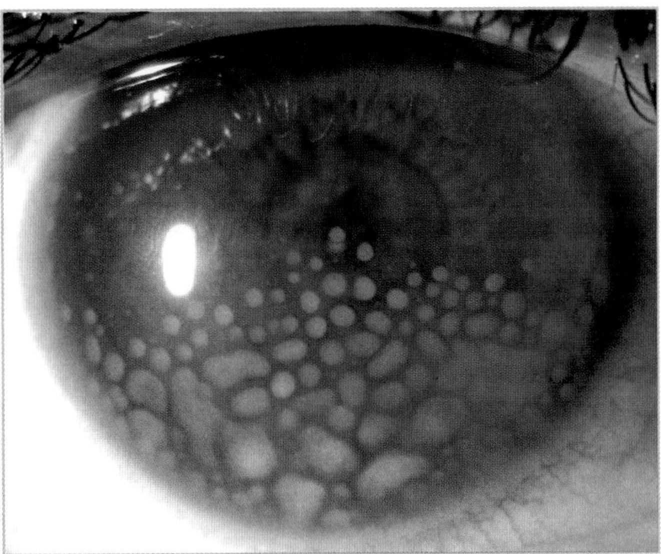

Figure 10.3 Large mutton-fat keratic precipitates with posterior synechia formation in a patient with ocular tuberculosis.

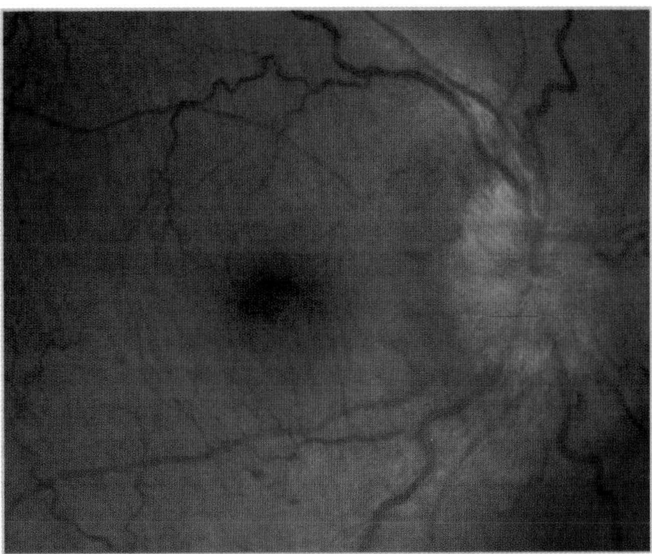

Figure 10.5 Severe papillitis in ocular tuberculosis.

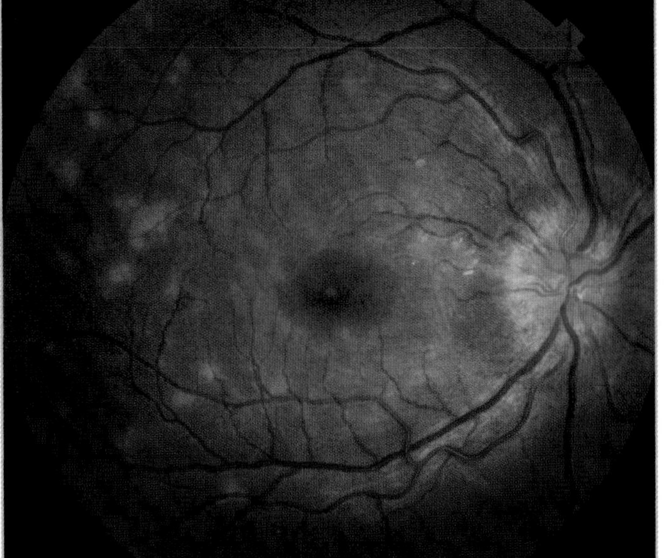

Figure 10.4 Multifocal choroidal lesions and papillitis in a patient with tuberculosis.

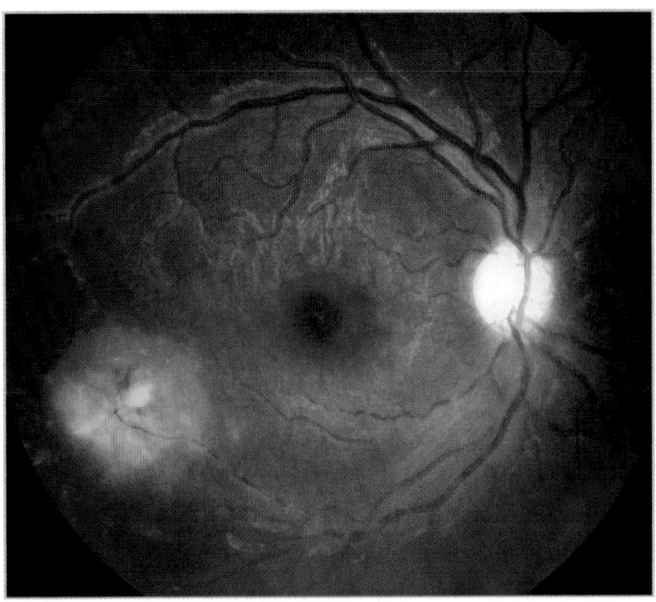

Figure 10.6 A large solitary chorioretinal granuloma in association with periphlebitis in a patient with tuberculosis.

and associated serous detachment. Very rarely a subretinal focus will burst through into the vitreous cavity, causing endophthalmitis. Endogenous infection by other bacteria should be considered in this form of presentation; although most will cause a much more rapid presentation, some bacteria such as *Nocardia* (see below) also rarely cause subretinal abscess.

Recent evidence has shown that TB can be associated with outer retinal and/or inner choroidal inflammations, initially described as 'serpiginous-like' choroiditis (Gupta et al. 2003) but encompassing a variety of multifocal or contiguous choriocapillaropathies of the 'placoid' or 'serpiginous' group (**Figs 10.8** and **10.9**). Mycobacteria have been identified in the retinal pigment epithelium (Rao et al. 2006), but the paucity of organisms in contrast to the degree of inflammation is notable and, in some patients with PCR positivity, no organisms are seen on microscopy (Wroblewski et al. 2011). Any patient with an inexorable placoid-like or rapidly progressive serpiginous choroidopathy should be investigated for TB and treated appropriately if evidence is supportive.

Tuberculosis is recognized as a disease associated with retinal vasculitis, specifically that subset of occlusive phlebitis with vitreous hemorrhage traditionally known as Eales' disease; many such patients are Mantoux positive (**Fig. 10.10**). The pathogenesis of the vasculitis was until recently assumed to be indirect, the vasculitis being a result of autoimmune inflammation induced by *M. tuberculosis* elsewhere in the body. However, there is accumulating evidence of the presence of mycobacterial DNA within the vitreous of, or epiretinal membranes removed from, such eyes (Gupta et al. 2001) and it may be that the relationship between *M. tuberculosis* and retinal vasculitis is more direct. Traditionally Eales' disease has been treated with retinal photocoagulation, with systemic steroid treatment for those

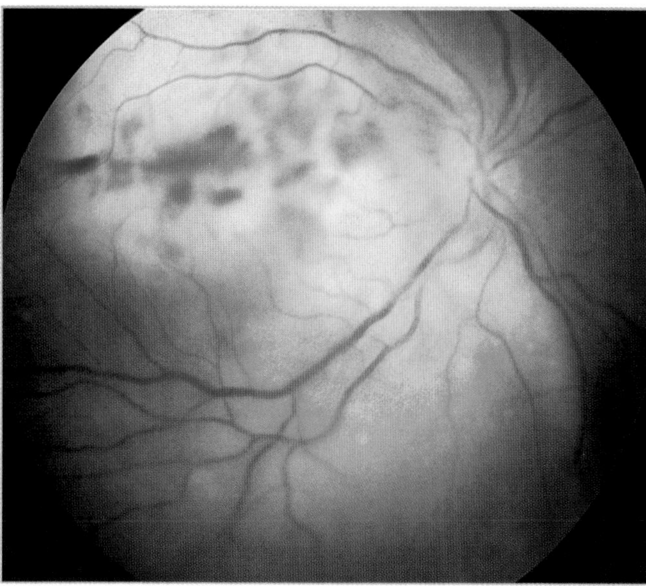

Figure 10.7 Subretinal abscess formation secondary to a large choroidal tubercle; the lesion settled rapidly on anti-tuberculous chemotherapy.

with substantial intraocular or perivascular inflammation, with variable results. However, the accumulating evidence of direct infection together with the small risk of dissemination strongly suggests that antibiotic treatment should be used in such eyes and this may enhance outcomes (El-Asrar and Al-Kharashi 2002). Fortunately only a small minority of patients goes on to develop profound and progressive retinal ischemia (**Fig. 10.11**).

Although intraocular TB has a particular tendency to show the above clinical appearances, it can manifest in any way and for a progressive or indolent steroid-refractory uveitis it is essential to exclude TB. When evidence of TB is suggestive but not confirmatory, the administration of a therapeutic course of antibiotics will support the diagnosis if the uveitis responds (Sanghvi et al. 2011).

Diagnosis

The weight of evidence supporting a diagnosis of intraocular TB, or of intraocular inflammation in association with TB, is variable in the individual but rarely reaches the level of a culture-positive intraocular specimen. Diagnosis in the individual is therefore almost always based on an accumulation of circumstantial evidence, often supported retrospectively by resolution of the inflammation after treatment. For any patient with inflammation suggestive of TB, or with systemic or other features raising the risk of that disease, further investigation is mandatory. The patient born in an endemic area, whether or not BCG (bacille Calmette–Guérin) immunization has taken place, is at risk and this is increased by repeated visits back to that country. Any patient who has a history of exposure to TB, usually within the family, should be further investigated even if, at the time, a course of prophylactic treatment was given; such courses are usually limited to 3 months of treatment with two antibiotics, which cannot guarantee disease eradication.

Close questioning of the patient presenting with undiagnosed uveitis may reveal systemic symptoms and signs suggestive of past or present tuberculosis. Some may recall a discharging cervical node

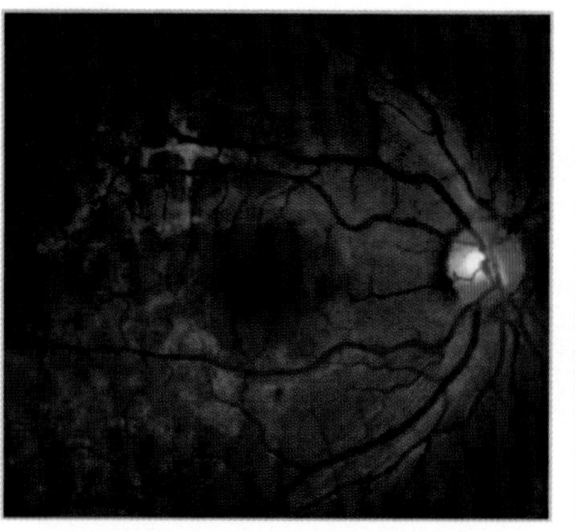

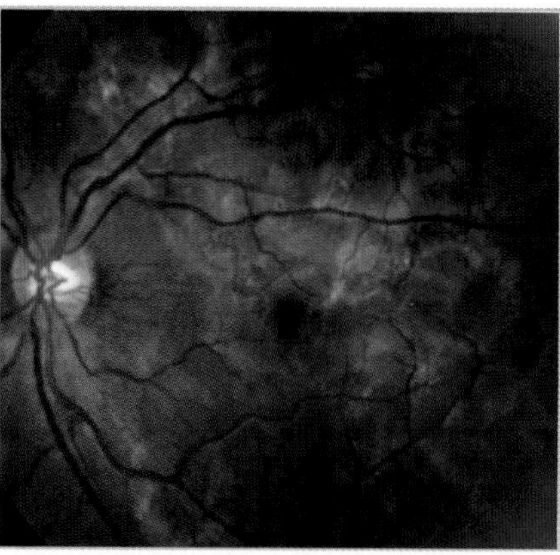

Figure 10.8 Confluent irregular atypical placoid-like retinochoroidopathy in a patient with tuberculosis.

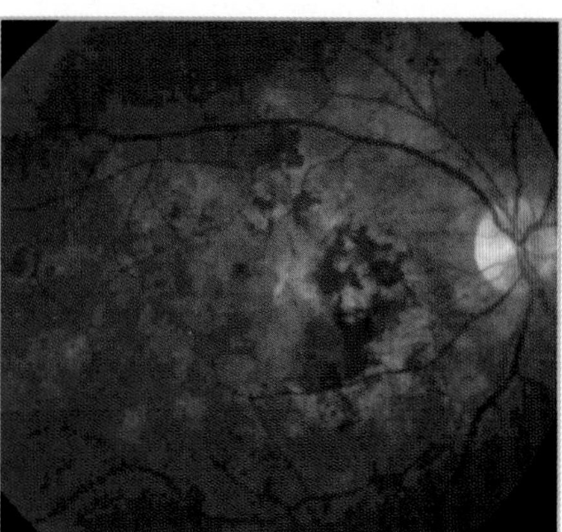

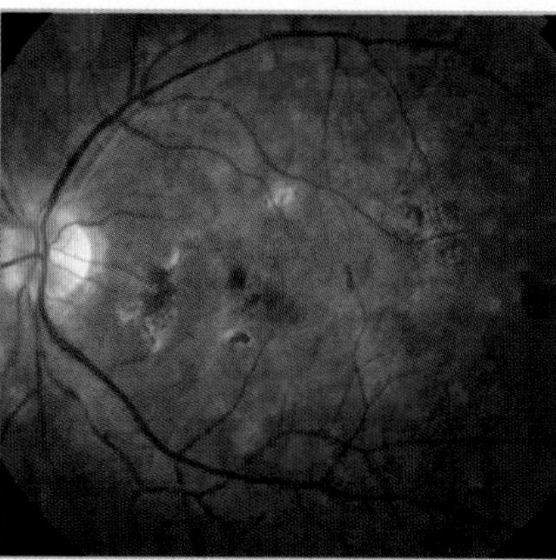

Figure 10.9 Irregular contiguous retinochoroidopathy with recurrent lesions in a patient with tuberculosis.

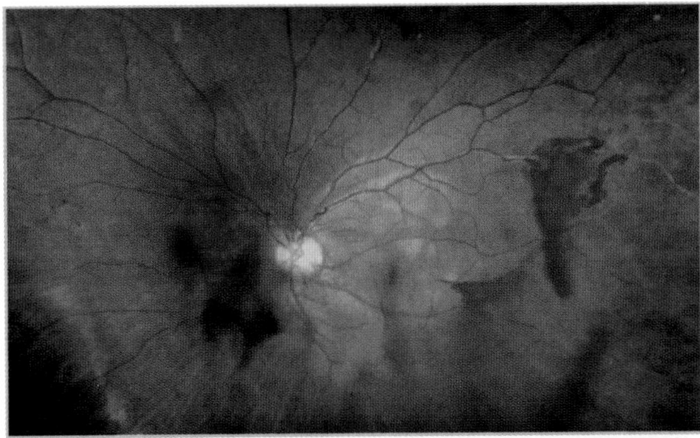

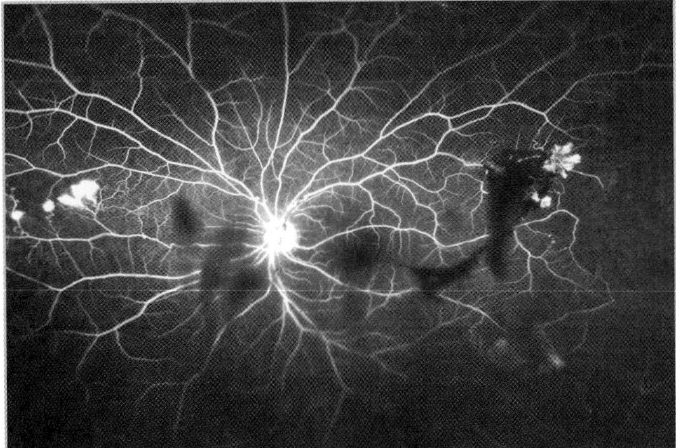

Figure 10.10 Eales' disease in a patient with tuberculosis; there is patchy widespread ischemic vasculitis with fresh vitreous hemorrhage secondary to neovascularization.

or may have active focal neck swellings that can be biopsied. Others may have focal axial arthropathy or loin swelling. Associated malaise, fatigue, unexplained weight loss or night sweats must be investigated.

Chest radiograph

The great majority of patients with intraocular TB will not have active pulmonary TB. Nevertheless the differential diagnosis of qualifying uveitis mandates a chest radiograph. Old primary infection characteristically leads to a Ghon focus, which heals to leave a calcified pulmonary nodule in association with calcified hilar lymph nodes. Active pulmonary TB may have many features, including multifocal parenchymal nodules, especially in the upper lobes, and hilar lymphadenopathy (**Fig. 10.12**). Broadly speaking, bilateral symmetrical lymphadenopathy is more supportive of sarcoidosis whereas unilateral or asymmetrical involvement is more suggestive of TB. Later, areas of consolidation may appear, and these may cavitate (**Fig. 10.13**) or fibrose, typically with lung collapse and linear shadowing in the upper zones. Pleural effusion may be seen. Miliary lesions, rarely encountered, are small and extremely numerous throughout the lung fields (**Fig. 10.14**); affected patients are very ill or moribund, frequently with associated meningoencephalitis, and a high proportion are HIV positive.

Tuberculin skin testing

The interpretation of tuberculin skin testing (TST) is complex and dependent on several factors of which the interpreting physician must be aware. The field is contentious to the extent that a substantial minority of chest physicians practices largely without TST in diagnosis. However, doctors dealing with extrapulmonary TB have an added disadvantage in that they are deprived of sputum for culture and usually of the more characteristic pulmonary symptoms and signs. The ophthalmologist cannot make the diagnosis in most patients without TST.

The intradermal injection of antigens derived from *M. tuberculosis* usually, in a patient previously exposed to the organism, or currently having TB, raises an erythematous skin weal of significant size. The antigens are contained in a solution of PPD (purified protein derivative), which is injected intradermally. Two different modes of injection are used: the Mantoux test and, much less commonly now, the Heaf test. The former has always been preferred in the USA and several other countries; the latter was the preferred method in the UK until 2005 when it was abandoned owing to lack of acceptable supplies. The interpretation of the reaction to the Heaf test is probably easier and the window of opportunity wider. However, the Mantoux test is moving toward the universal standard.

The Mantoux test

Usually 5 or 10 tuberculin units (TU) of PPD in 0.1 ml is injected to raise an intradermal blister of 5–10 mm (**Fig. 10.15**). It must not be injected subcutaneously or the test will fail. The diameter of the area

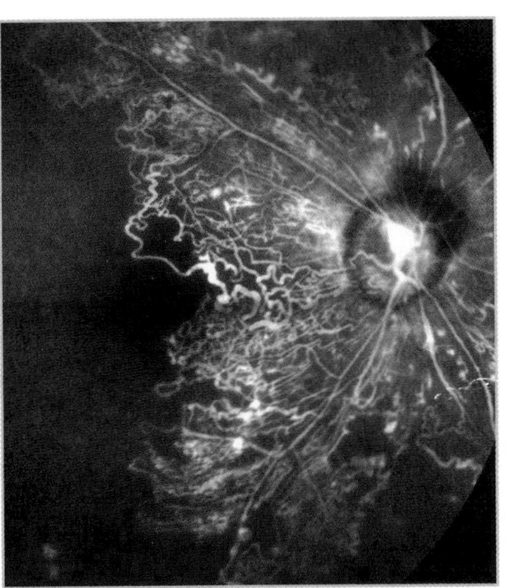

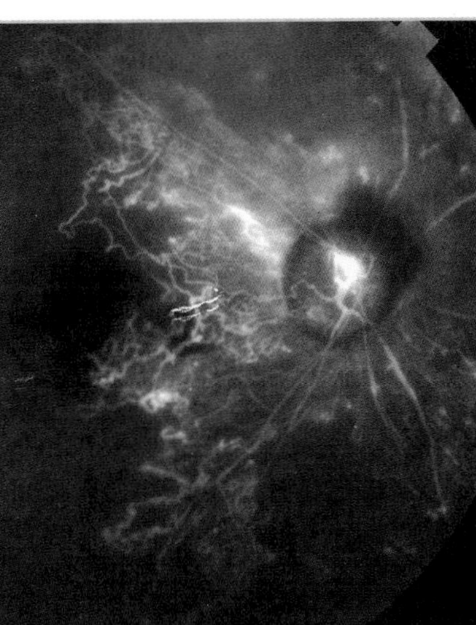

Figure 10.11 Inexorable vascular closedown in a patient with occlusive vasculitis secondary to tuberculosis; two angiograms taken a year apart show increasing ischemia with residual eccentric vision in this only eye.

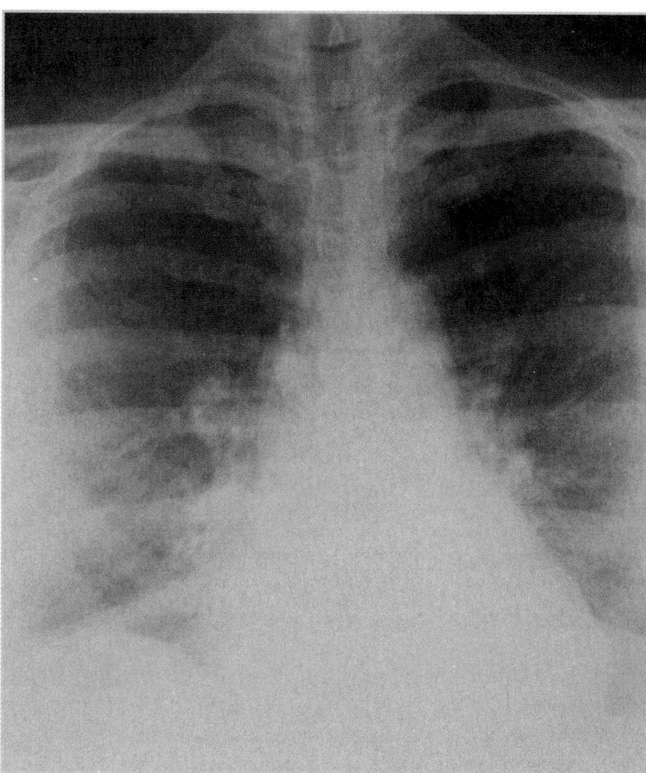

Figure 10.12 Bilateral hilar lymphadenopathy and lung parenchymal nodules in active pulmonary tuberculosis. (Courtesy of Dr C Hardy.)

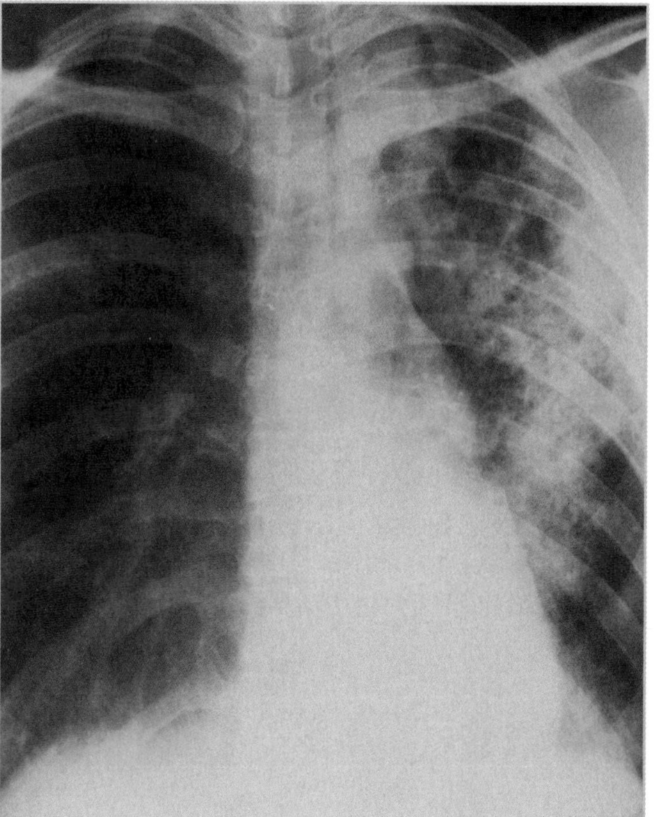

Figure 10.13 Left upper lobe consolidation and cavitation in advanced pulmonary tuberculosis. (Courtesy of Dr C Hardy.)

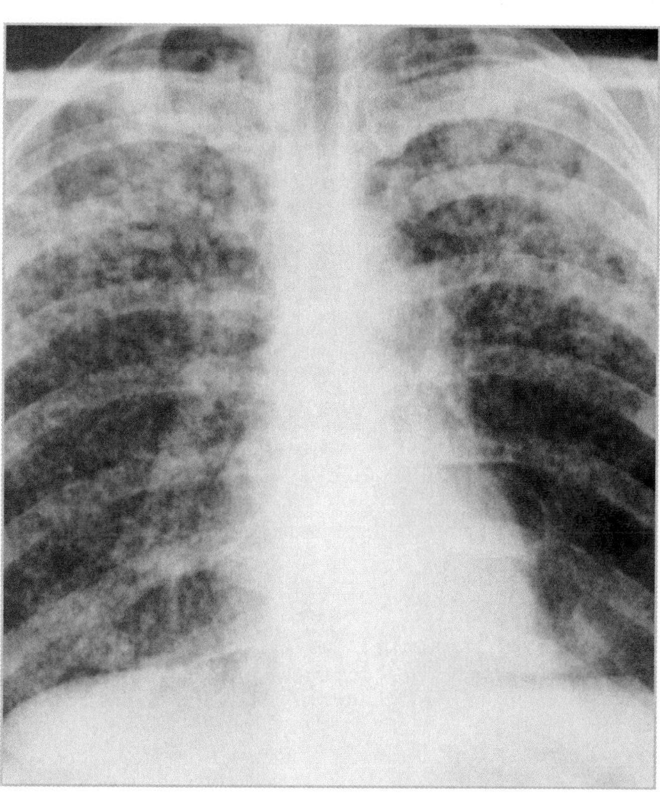

Figure 10.14 Miliary tuberculosis showing widespread granular opacification of lung fields. (Courtesy of Dr C Hardy.)

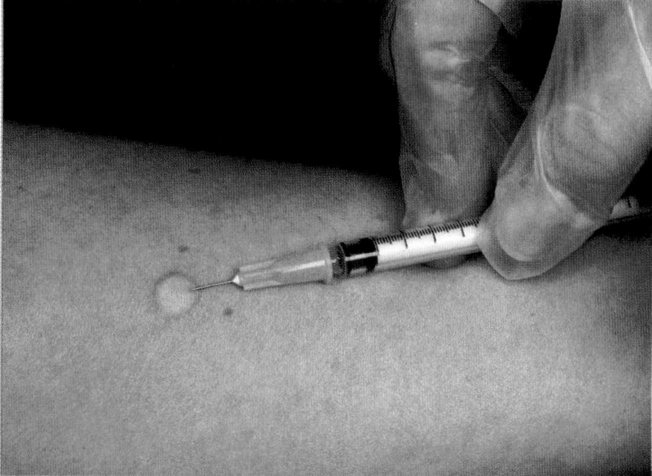

Figure 10.15 The Mantoux test requires the intradermal injection of tuberculin antigen to raise a blister. (Modified from Centers for Disease Control, Public Health Image Library.)

of induration in millimeters (not the degree of erythema [which is wider] or any overlying cutaneous reaction) is measured 48–72 h later. Higher concentrations of PPD are available if subsequent re-testing is thought necessary for those testing negative.

The Heaf test (Sterneedle test)

A drop of undiluted PPD (100 000 TU/ml) is applied to the skin surface and a six-tine gun is triggered which introduces this intradermally. The degree of reaction is measured 3–11 days after the test and is graded

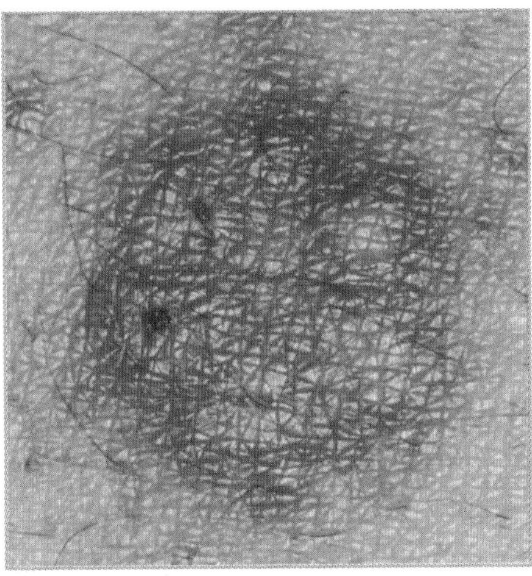
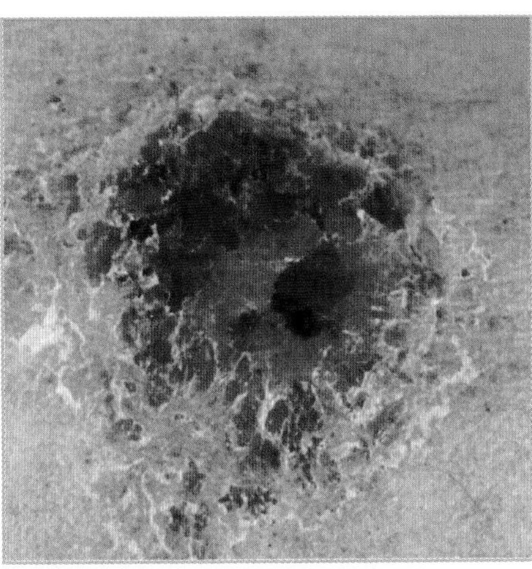

Figure 10.16 Two Heaf test responses: grade 3 at left; grade 4+ at right. Both are considered positive.

Table 10.1 Comparative readings of the Heaf and Mantoux tests

Heaf test	Mantoux test (using 10 TU)
Grade 0 (no reaction)	< 5 mm induration
Grade 1 (4 or more papules)	5–9 mm
Grade 2 (confluent ring of papules)	10–14 mm
Grade 3 (indurated disk)	15–19 mm
Grade 4 (disk > 10 mm, or blistering)	> 20 mm

depending on appearance (**Fig. 10.16**). The agreed equivalence levels for Mantoux and Heaf tests are shown in **Table 10.1**.

The measurement of TST reactions is objective, but interpretation is not. There are no universally agreed dimensions of the Mantoux reaction, which are regarded as negative or positive for the patient with normal immunity, and the results are modified by both the immune status, by previous immunization and paradoxically by the severity of active disease. The test may be negative in a patient who does have TB, either because of incorrect testing or owing to the presence of anergy, sarcoidosis, renal failure or viral infection. It may also be negative in patients using systemic steroid medication, and paradoxically in those with miliary TB. Overall, the rate of false negativity is as high as 17%, but this increases with age, and only a third of AIDS patients with TB are skin test positive. In the absence of other supportive information and where an initial TST is inconclusive, a second test performed within 1–6 weeks may show a greater reaction. In this circumstance the result of the second test is considered more accurate.

The test may be positive in a patient who does not have TB. The most common cause of such a reaction is previous BCG immunization. BCG was derived from *M. bovis* and TST contains antigens common to *M. tuberculosis*, *M. bovis* and other mycobacteria, including environmental saprophytes. Mantoux testing often therefore induces significant induration and interpretation is required. Some sources have recommended ignoring previous BCG immunization in the assessment of TST response, but most use a dimensional cut-off below which the reaction is attributed to previous immunization. Similarly, previous exposure to environmental mycobacteria does not usually produce a strong response, but there is substantial geographical variation in the prevalence of such organisms.

The development of different national standards for interpretation of TST reflects both the variable atypical mycobacterial exposure risk and the current or previous health policy for BCG immunization. Immunization has never provided high protection against pulmonary TB and health policies have differed accordingly. Although most countries have administered BCG to all children, the USA and the Netherlands never had a nationwide BCG immunization policy; the UK did so until recently, abandoning it in favor of a targeted policy.

In geographical areas where TB is endemic, TST is certainly less discriminatory for active pulmonary or focal extrapulmonary TB. However, positivity in the context of qualifying uveitis should be regarded as significant unless another clear cause of uveitis is identified.

In a patient undergoing a Mantoux test with no prior identified risk of TB and with a normal immune system, most countries use a minimum of 14 mm or 15 mm induration as positive for TB (latent or active; TST alone cannot differentiate, although the greater the reaction the higher the likelihood of active TB). For those with underlying conditions that might predispose to TB and whose immune reaction might be compromised, a minimum of 10 mm may be used. This includes patients using systemic steroid treatment, people with diabetes, and those with leukemias or renal failure. Indeed for those with uveitis already using oral steroid treatment, interpretation can be difficult and for those on a high dose (e.g. 1 mg/kg per day) a reaction of 5-mm induration may be significant. Those who undertake the test from a position of high risk (including immunodeficient individuals, especially HIV-positive patients, immunosuppressed individuals including transplant recipients), and those with a clear recent history of contact with TB or clear signs of previous TB infection should also use a lower threshold such as 5 mm. Individual national guidelines will differ millimeter by millimeter according to differing interpretations of risk, but in a patient with unexplained sight-threatening uveitis and no other identified cause, any measurable TST reaction should be considered carefully in the context of known factors affecting the result, and TB treatment should be carefully considered on the balance of risks.

In the UK it is current policy that any person with a significant TST response aged < 35 years should undergo a 3-month course of two-drug treatment/prophylaxis. Extrapolating this logically, the policy in this clinic is that those with such a response and unexplained uveitis should almost certainly receive a full 6-month therapeutic course (Sanghvi et al. 2011).

One weakness of the TST is the confounding effect of previous BCG immunization and environmental mycobacteria. However, interferon-γ blood tests do not suffer from this problem and are now commonly used in conjunction with TST to provide additional evidence:

Interferon-γ testing

In a patient previously exposed to wild *M. tuberculosis*, exposing that patient's lymphocytes to antigens specific to *M. tuberculosis* will stimulate the production of interferon-γ and this response is detectable and measurable. The antigens are ESAT-6 and CFP-10, and importantly they do not occur in *M. bovis* and only uncommonly in environmental mycobacteria. The test therefore has high specificity for *M. tuberculosis* and is not affected at all by previous BCG immunizations.

There are two currently available interferon-γ assays that use different methods. The first and more widely used is the QuantiFERON-TB Gold In Tube which uses an enzyme-linked immunosorbent assay (ELISA) to measure the total production of interferon-γ from whole blood exposed to the antigens. The second, T-SPOT TB, uses an immunospot assay to identify by staining individual secreting lymphocytes.

Evidence is accumulating that these assays are superior to TST in diagnosing latent or active TB, but none can alone reliably distinguish between the two. Although these assays are to some extent quantifiable, this cannot currently be used reliably to differentiate active from latent TB; specificities are impressive at up to 99% but sensitivities are still under 90% (Diel et al. 2010).

In this clinic, which deals predominantly with those previously BCG immunized, the policy is to perform both Mantoux and QuantiFERON-TB Gold in patients suspected of uveitis related to TB. The combination is particularly useful where Mantoux reactions are moderate (5–12 mm), so that the positive or negative interferon-γ assay serves to provide useful additional evidence where the Mantoux diameter alone is insufficient to support the diagnosis. Further evidence on efficacy for interferon-γ assays may lead to the abandonment of TST in due course, but as yet that stage has not been reached.

Intraocular sampling

Positive microscopy and culture for acid-fast bacilli from intraocular fluid is rare. However, PCR methods have been useful in a widening group of patients. In general both sensitivity and specificity of TB PCRs are currently inferior to those available for herpes viral detection. Testing on extrapulmonary specimens using the primers devR and IS6110 produced a claimed sensitivity of 94% and a specificity of 88% (Chakravorty et al. 2005). However, for those with tuberculous uveitis, aqueous sampling using IS6110, 219bp and 123bp produced a sensitivity of only 77% (Ortega-Larrocea et al. 2003). In due course the optimal combination of primers will doubtless enhance efficacy but currently PCR testing on intraocular fluid must be regarded as only one component of a diagnostic sequence.

In summary, the diagnosis of intraocular TB, or uveitis in association with TB, usually remains a matter of judgment based on a combination of supportive evidence; suggestive uveitis in a patient with a clear risk of having acquired TB, who has evidence supporting either latent or active disease, should be presumed to be TB associated if no other cause has been identified after thoughtful investigation. In uncertain cases a good response to treatment will provide further support for the working diagnosis. The assistance of a chest physician with a TB interest who understands the implications of sight-threatening uveitis is invaluable. We are fortunate in this clinic to have a close association with a regional TB service which assists us in diagnosis and management. We recommend forging such a relationship if possible.

Management

Intraocular inflammation may be the sole manifestation of reactivated TB, or less commonly may be part of pulmonary or multifocal extrapulmonary TB. It is therefore necessary to use systemic anti-tubercular medication in all patients with presumed ocular TB.

It is current standard practice to treat active TB (excluding neurological, drug-resistant or special cases) with a 6-month course of drugs, the first 2 months with four drugs, the following 4 months with two drugs. In the absence of contraindications the normal drugs are 2 months of isoniazid, rifampicin, pyrazinamide and ethambutol, followed by 4 months of isoniazid and rifampicin. It has been claimed that 9 months or more of treatment reduces uveitis recurrence (Ang et al. 2011) but it is arguable that recurrences after 6 months of treatment are in fact non-tubercular (Sanghvi et al. 2011).

Ethambutol may cause optic neuropathy. For patients with pre-existing uveitis, the question arises whether its use is safe, for two reasons: first, are those with pre-existing inflammation at greater risk of optic nerve involvement?(the answer is probably 'no') and second does the uncommon risk of optic neuropathy, in a patient who already has compromised vision, justify its use? The current consensus is that, in order to achieve the usual 98% TB cure rate for the standard regimen, the benefits outweigh the risks for those with uveitis.

All anti-TB drugs are potentially hepatotoxic and must be monitored. Pyrazinamide is the drug most frequently not tolerated and discontinued; the physician should decide whether a temporary replacement is necessary. Rifampicin may color urine, sweat and tears pale orange and patients should be informed of this. Isoniazid may cause mono- or polyneuritis and simultaneous pyridoxine is given to reduce this risk. Other side effects of treatment include malaise, nausea, rashes, gout, pyrexia, dizziness and bone pains. In short, treatment should be prescribed and monitored by physicians and nurse specialists dealing regularly with such treatment, not by the ophthalmologist.

Drug resistance in TB is an increasing problem worldwide. In multidrug-resistant TB (MDR-TB) the organism is resistant to both isoniazid and rifampicin. In extensively resistant TB (XDR-TB) there is, in addition to this, resistance to quinolones and also to one of amikacin, kanamycin or capreomycin. There is great concern over the spread of XDR-TB, to the extent that some authorities consider enforced isolation for those with open pulmonary disease. In numerical terms the current likelihood of resistant organisms causing uveitis is low, but should be considered during the appraisal of treatment efficacy where organisms have not been available for culture and sensitivity. Although the incidence of TB in general is highest in sub-Saharan Africa, it is the former Soviet Union, eastern Europe and the Caucasus that generate most patients with MDR-TB.

The need for systemic steroid in patients with TB-associated uveitis will vary but, in some circumstances, they are mandatory. Some diagnoses will be made only after further investigation of a steroid-resistant uveitis. In theory there is a risk of systemic reactivation of TB in such patients but fortunately such problems are rare. The concurrent usage of both oral steroid and anti-tuberculous chemotherapy will inhibit interpretation of antibiotic efficacy, but the ability to discontinue both treatments without recurrence will support the diagnosis.

Mycobacterium avium complex and other mycobacteria

Many mycobacteria exist as environmental saprophytes, *M. avium* and *M. intracellulare* being two of the most important in human infection. They are closely related and in the context of human infection are grouped with a few others as the *Mycobacterium avium-intracellulare* complex (MAC). Pulmonary infection resembling TB may occur in healthy people, but more usually in those with previous lung damage such as bronchiectasis or industrial lung disease, or in immunosuppressed individuals. Disseminated MAC infection is not uncommon in AIDS patients and was frequently lethal until the introduction of highly reactive anti-retroviral treatment (HAART).

In immunosuppressed individuals with MAC, clarithromycin or azithromycin is usually combined with two of rifabutin, clofazimine, ciprofloxacin or ethambutol, and a combination regimen may be necessary for life. In patients on treatment for MAC who present with ocular inflammation, two main possibilities exist. First, MAC itself may rarely cause multifocal choroiditis. Much more commonly, rifabutin can cause uveitis ranging from mild vitritis to severe, sometimes fibrinous, hypopyon panuveitis, especially when combined with clarithromycin. This is dealt with in Chapter 20.

There is a very large number of environmental mycobacteria that are capable of causing infection predominantly in immunodeficient individuals, sometimes causing multifocal subcutaneous nodules, an abscess, lymphadenopathy or focal indurated dermatitis. Uveitis is possible but rare and arranging skin biopsy may be very helpful. The least rare organism is *M. chelonae* and there are anecdotes of other organisms. Treatment requires microbiological advice.

SYPHILIS (box 10.2)

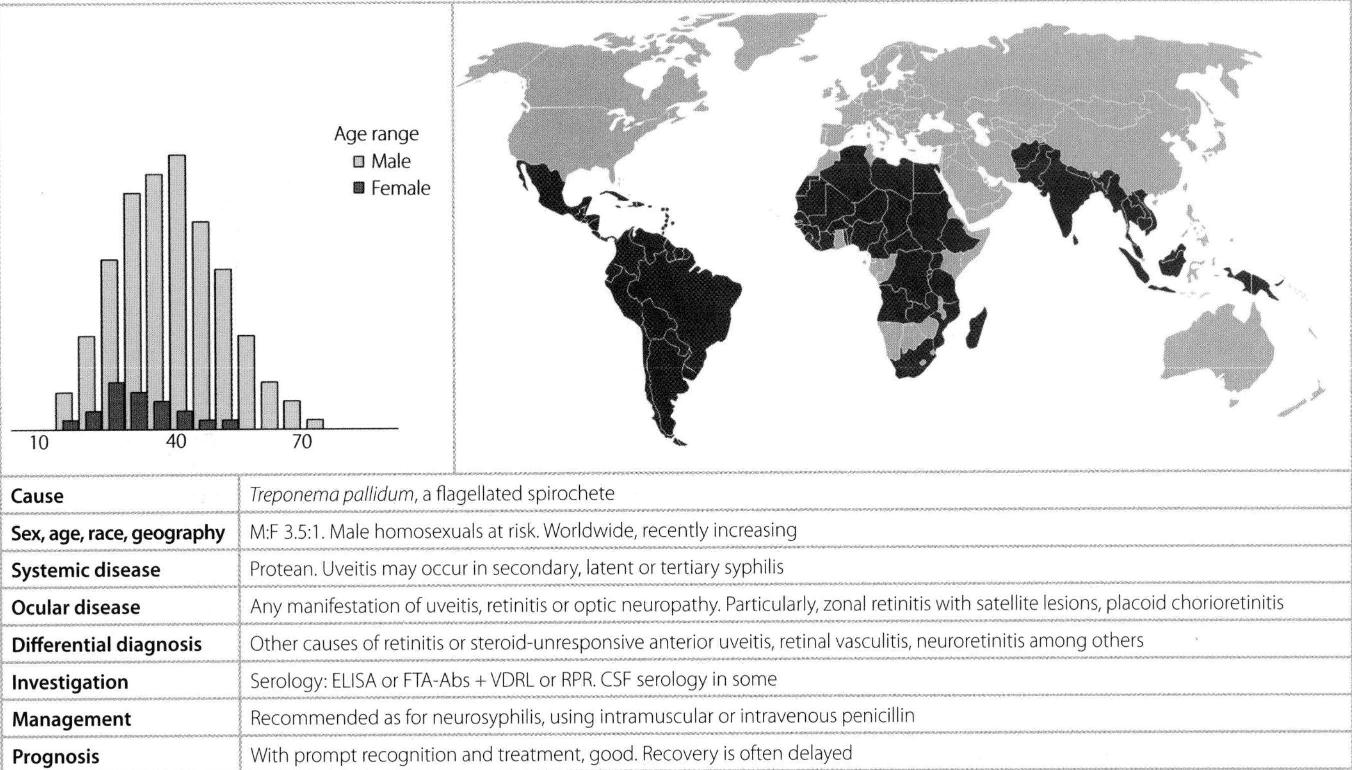

Cause	*Treponema pallidum*, a flagellated spirochete
Sex, age, race, geography	M:F 3.5:1. Male homosexuals at risk. Worldwide, recently increasing
Systemic disease	Protean. Uveitis may occur in secondary, latent or tertiary syphilis
Ocular disease	Any manifestation of uveitis, retinitis or optic neuropathy. Particularly, zonal retinitis with satellite lesions, placoid chorioretinitis
Differential diagnosis	Other causes of retinitis or steroid-unresponsive anterior uveitis, retinal vasculitis, neuroretinitis among others
Investigation	Serology: ELISA or FTA-Abs + VDRL or RPR. CSF serology in some
Management	Recommended as for neurosyphilis, using intramuscular or intravenous penicillin
Prognosis	With prompt recognition and treatment, good. Recovery is often delayed

Box 10.2 Syphilis

Introduction

Treponema pallidum is the small, helical, flagellated spirochete bacterium (**Fig. 10.17**) that is responsible for syphilis. Transmission is almost always venereal, by direct contact with active mucocutaneous lesions of primary or secondary syphilis. Infection is also possible from those with early latent disease, but after some 2 years the person is no longer infective. The spirochete can penetrate intact mucosae, but only abraded skin. Vertical transmission is possible as *T. pallidum* is small enough to cross the placenta. Parenteral infection is possible but uncommon. In time, exposure generates a partial immunity to future infection, except for those with congenital syphilis. However, rapid and effective treatment prevents the development of immunity. Reinfection is therefore possible on subsequent exposure, and quite frequent in promiscuous individuals.

The worldwide incidence of syphilis had progressively reduced during the latter half of the twentieth century after the introduction of effective antibacterials, but over the last 10–15 years a substantial re-emergence has been seen in the west, particularly in metropolitan areas of the USA and Europe, because of a fall in the use of barrier protection.

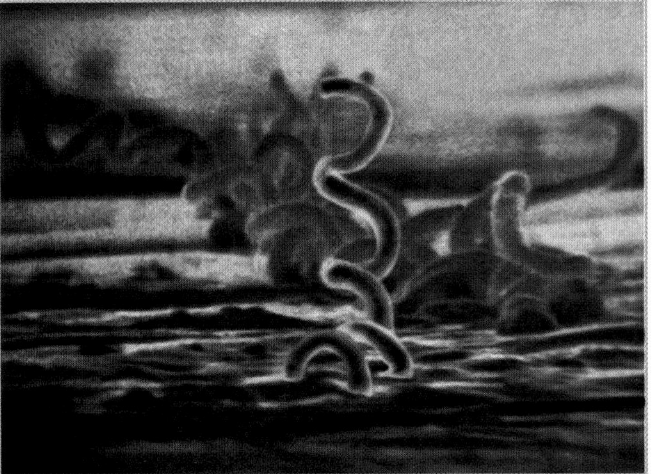

Figure 10.17 ***Treponema pallidum***, the syphilis spirochete, seen under scanning electron micrography. (Modified from Centers for Disease Control, Public Health Image Library.)

The introduction of HAART during the 1990s has transformed the prognosis for HIV infection such that it has changed, if treated optimally, from a lethal disease to a manageable chronic problem. This news was accompanied by a perception of decreased risk from unprotected sex and resultant complacency; the recent syphilis epidemic is one of the results (Simms et al. 2005). The particular rise in syphilis seen in male homosexuals has led to increasing polarity of the sex ratio, which has changed from a male:female ratio of about 3:1 during the 1990s to about 5:1 now.

Systemic disease

Although syphilis has classically been described as a three-stage disease, these stages may overlap, and not all will be discernible. A high index of suspicion may therefore be necessary to suggest the diagnosis. A painless, ulcerated chancre forms at the site of initial penetration. This is usually genital but other sites may be affected, including the conjunctiva. Vaginal, rectal and some oropharyngeal chancres are occult. Dissemination does occur in this primary stage but systemic symptoms are unusual. The chancre usually heals within a month or so of initial ulceration. Ocular involvement does not occur during the primary phase and the chancre will not therefore be seen by the ophthalmologist (at least not in a professional capacity).

The great majority of untreated patients then go on to develop symptomatic secondary syphilis within 4–12 weeks of infection. Pyrexia, malaise and lymphadenopathy are typical, but the most characteristic feature is a widespread non-irritating maculopapular rash (**Fig. 10.18**), most commonly involving the trunk. Centrifugal spread to involve the face, hands and feet is highly suggestive of syphilis (**Fig. 10.19**). Secondary lesions involving mucosae or in intertriginous areas typically enlarge into fleshy discoid lesions termed 'condylomata lata.' These and the 'snail-track' lesions of oral (**Fig. 10.20**) and genital mucosae shed spirochetes liberally and are highly infectious. The symptoms last for several weeks, sometimes months, and occasionally recur. It is in this active secondary stage of the disease that ocular involvement is most likely.

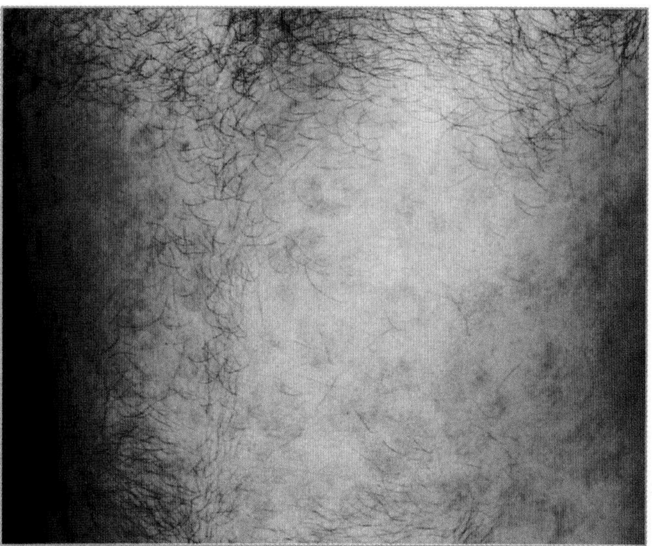

Figure 10.18 Widespread maculopapular rash in a man with secondary syphilis and uveitis.

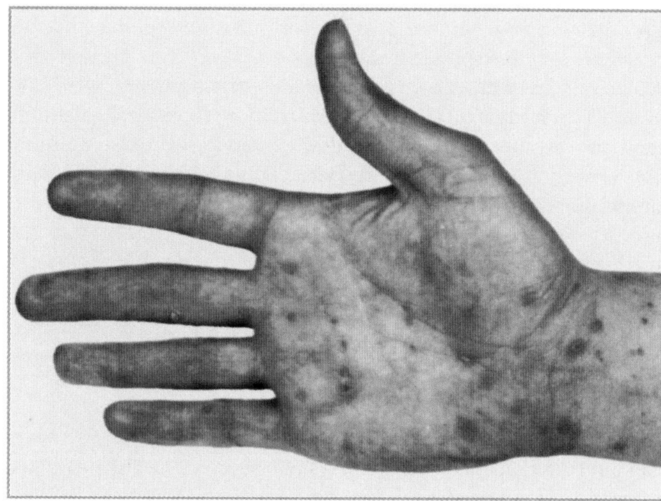

Figure 10.19 Maculopapular eruption on the palm and forearm in a young man with secondary syphilis. The soles of the feet were also affected. (Courtesy of Dr K Haye.)

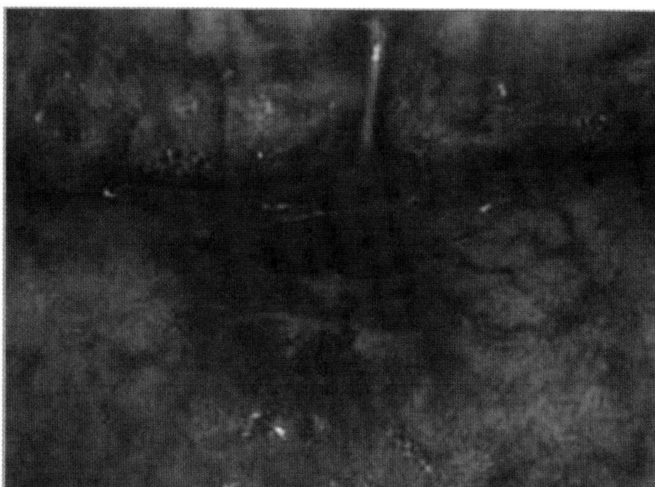

Figure 10.20 A snail-track ulcer of the buccal mucosa in secondary syphilis.

Untreated, tertiary manifestations with focal inflammation (gumma) will affect 40% of patients, and may occur in any location. Three subtypes of tertiary syphilis are defined: first, benign tertiary syphilis usually involves gummatous inflammation of skin, but gummas can involve any tissue, including the eye; second, cardiovascular syphilis may lead to aortic problems including aneurysms and valvular disease; and third, neurosyphilis affects about a third of patients, and may include aseptic meningitis, Argyll Robertson pupils, cranial nerve palsies, optic neuropathy, tabes dorsalis, dementia or psychosis. With better detection and treatment, new cases of tertiary syphilis are now rare, but the recent upsurge in new cases of acquired syphilis may lead to a future resurgence.

Syphilis is common in homosexual AIDS patients and, although in this context the disease is more difficult to diagnose and treat, usually the systemic manifestations are as seen in immunocompetent individuals. There appears to be a tendency for AIDS patients to develop more rapidly progressive syphilis with a higher incidence of neurological and ocular involvement.

Ocular disease

Periocular chancres are rare, but conjunctivitis, sometimes with episcleritis or scleritis, may be seen in secondary syphilis. Interstitial keratitis is almost always a manifestation of congenital rather than acquired syphilis. Modern ophthalmologists observe late corneal interstitial scarring less now than 20 years ago, but are likely once more to encounter acute interstitial keratitis in youngsters as the incidence of congenital syphilis rises again. Acute inflammation may resemble marginal keratitis, but, unlike the latter, both anterior uveitis and deep stromal corneal vascularization are present (see Fig. 2.7). Argyll Robertson pupils may rarely be seen in association with early syphilitic meningoencephalitis, but more usually are a feature of tertiary neurosyphilis.

Syphilitic uveitis occurs most commonly during the secondary stage and is usually associated with systemic signs of the disease (Doris et al. 2006). However, if it presents late in the secondary stage, or later during the latent phase, it may be the only overt manifestation of syphilis. The spectrum is protean; any form of uveitis may be expressed but iridocyclitis (both non-granulomatous [**Fig. 10.21**] and granulomatous with iris nodules) may occur alone. Posterior segment involvement is, however, more usual. Vitritis varies from mild to dense but does not cause cell clumping; retinitis (**Fig. 10.22**) can have a very typical appearance, with affected areas anywhere in the fundus characteristically associated with overlying or adjacent fluffy punctate lesions, which appear to be on the surface of the retina (**Fig. 10.23**) and have been described as 'punctate inner retinitis' (Wickremasinghe et al. 2009). Retinal vasculitis (**Fig. 10.24**), papillitis (**Fig. 10.25**), neuroretinitis, panuveitis and multifocal choroiditis have all been described. Syphilitic chorioretinitis may lead to extensive retinal edema or even serous detachment, and characteristic late changes include 'salt-and-pepper' retinal pigment epithelium (RPE) pigmentary changes not dissimilar to a tapetoretinal degeneration (**Fig. 10.26**). Subretinal fibrosis may be a feature, and late neovascular membranes may appear.

A form of placoid chorioretinitis virtually pathognomonic of syphilis (and usually in those with concurrent HIV infection) has been described (Gass et al. 1990). The affected (usually single) plaque in these eyes is very large and may occupy the whole macula (**Fig. 10.27**),

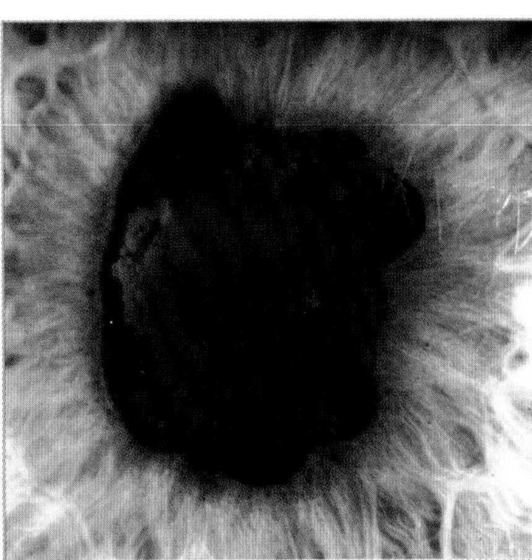
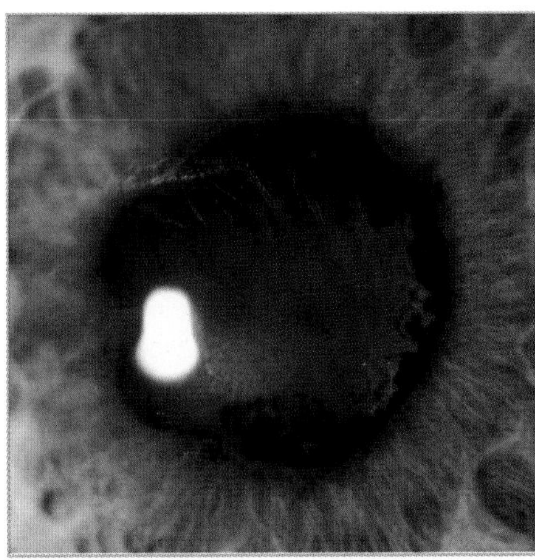

Figure 10.21 Bilateral non-granulomatous anterior uveitis as the sole manifestation of syphilitic uveitis.

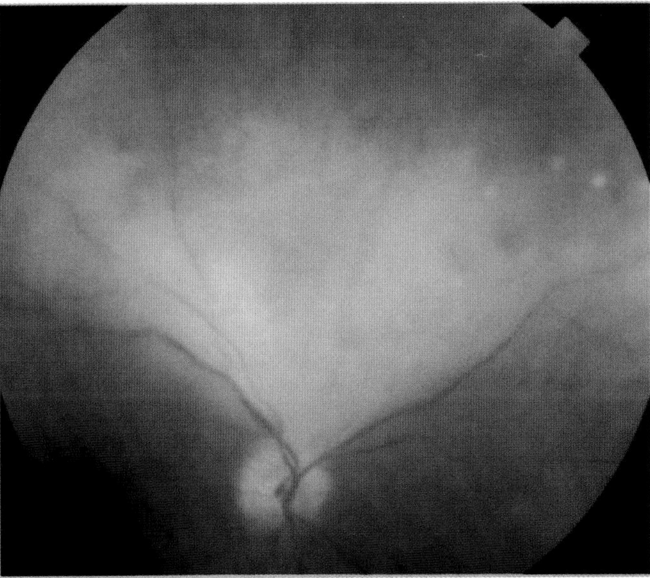

Figure 10.22 Unilateral zonal retinitis in a patient with secondary syphilis including maculopapular rash and headache. There is also vitritis, arteriolar caliber changes and punctate satellite lesions. The visual acuity was reduced to Hand Movements. (Reproduced from Doris et al. 2006.)

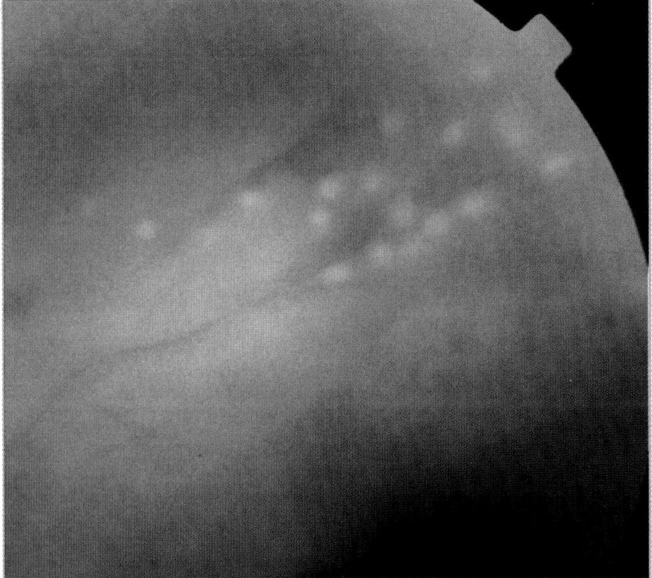

Figure 10.23 Multifocal satellite lesions adjacent to zonal retinitis is a characteristic sign of syphilitic inflammation.

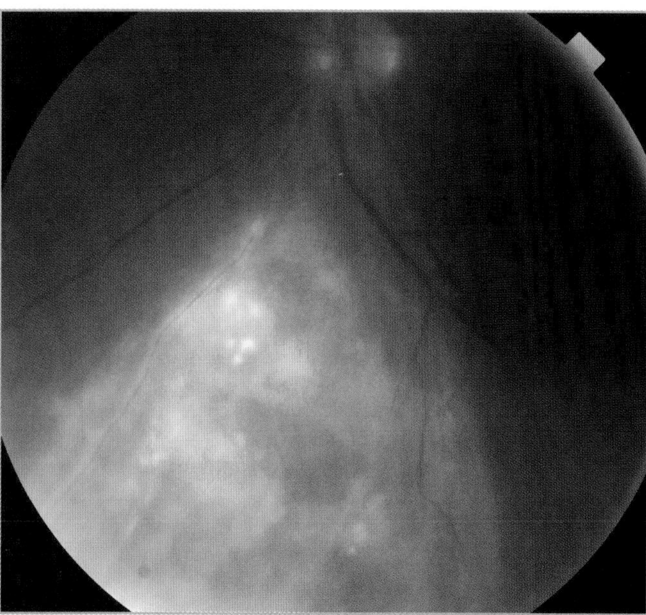

Figure 10.24 Arteriolar cuffing and narrowing indicate vasculitis associated with retinitis and satellite lesions.

in contrast to typical placoid pigment epitheliopathy. Necrotizing retinitis resembling acute retinal necrosis has also been observed, again typically in those with HIV infection (**Fig. 10.28**).

Several case reports have appeared describing intraocular syphilis as being 'unmasked' after the intraocular injection of triamcinolone to manage undiagnosed uveitis. The inflammation has included placoid chorioretinitis and vascular occlusion. Unfortunately, despite belated recognition and treatment, outcomes have been poor (Song et al. 2008).

Intraocular inflammation is considered to be a risk factor for the presence of asymptomatic neurosyphilis; positive cerebrospinal fluid (CSF) serology is found in 20% of those with uveitis. The ophthalmologist should liaise closely with the genitourinary medicine (GUM) physician and arrange investigation including CSF serology in appropriate cases.

Diagnosis

T. pallidum is invisible using direct light microscopy but may be seen using the dark-field technique, which can be used on fluid from active mucocutaneous lesions before serological tests become positive. In practice, however, serology is the most important means of diagnosis, of both active and latent syphilis.

Some serological tests (the treponemal tests) specifically detect antibody against treponemal antigens, whereas non-treponemal tests detect antibodies to cardiolipin–lecithin–cholesterol antigen. Sensitivity and specificity vary depending on the stage of disease and other factors. Patients with AIDS and syphilis cannot mount a normal immune response, and therefore tend to develop positive serology late, if at all, and revert to negative sooner after treatment. The use of dark-field microscopy of fluid from lesions therefore assumes a greater significance in this group.

It is necessary when performing syphilis serology to perform both a treponemal and a non-treponemal test. The former is a much more specific and reliable method of detecting the antigen but the result cannot reliably be quantified. The latter (rapid plasmin reagin [RPR] or Venereal Disease Reference Laboratory [VDRL]) may be falsely positive in a number of conditions, but is titratable and therefore is an indicator of activity, differentiating between current active syphilis and previously treated, inactive disease. Although the treponemal tests are specific for *T. pallidum*, this also includes its subspecies *T. pertenue* and others so that, in endemic areas, false positivity can occur (see below for other treponemal infections). Cross-reactivity with *Borrelia burgdorferi* antigens may also give false positive results, especially with fluorescent treponemal antibody absorption (FTA-Abs), but less so with RPR and VDRL. A simplified summary of the interpretation of serology reactions is shown in **Fig. 10.29**. Diagnostic decisions should always be made with the advice of the local microbiology service; most will recommend confirmation with a second treponemal test and/or an IgM assay.

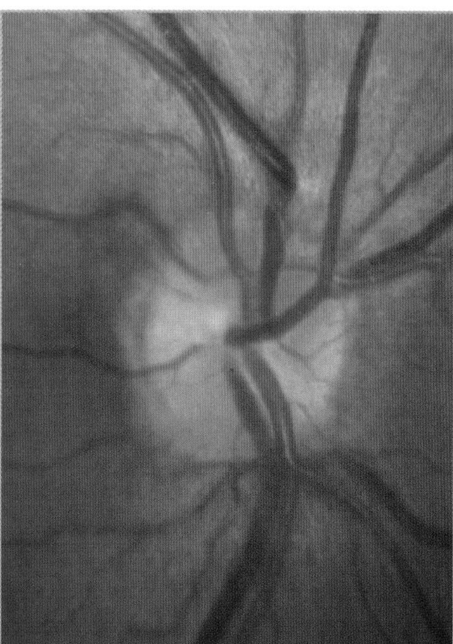

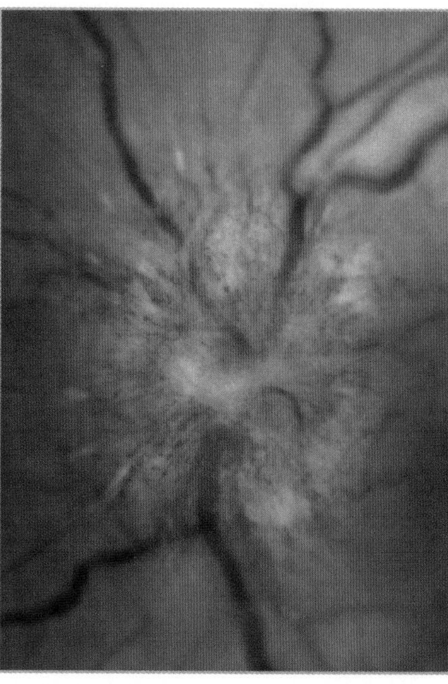

Figure 10.25 Left papillitis in ocular syphilis.

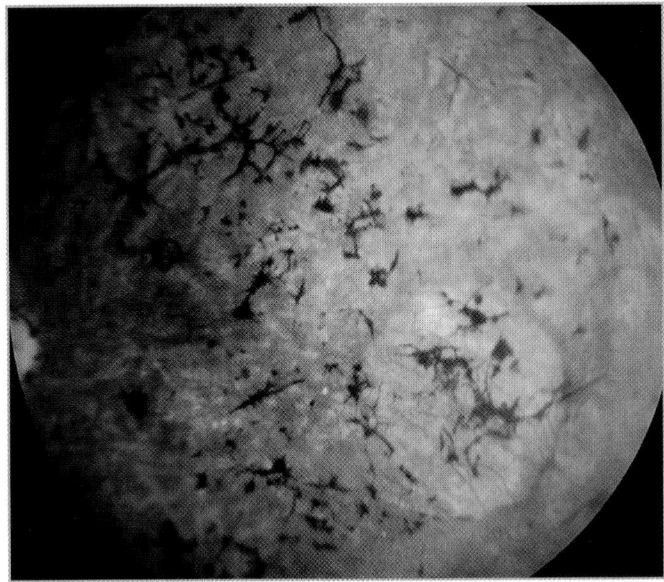

Figure 10.26 Post-inflammatory syphilitic scarring resembles a pigmentary dystrophy.

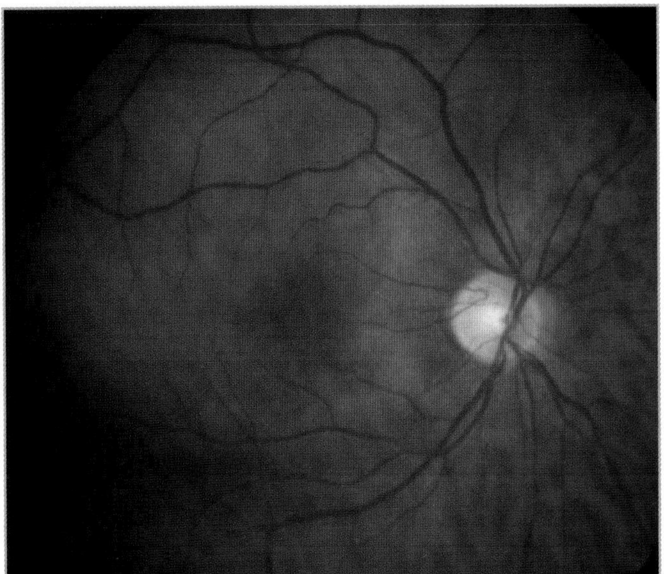

Figure 10.27 A large pale placoid lesion occupies the whole macular area; syphilitic placoid chorioretinitis.

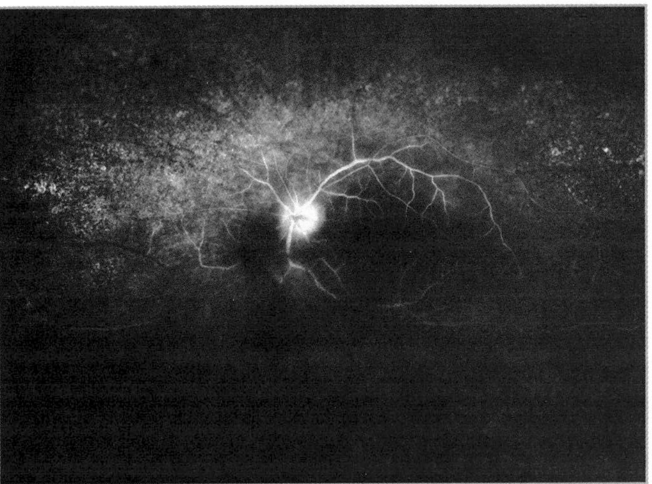

Figure 10.28 Severe vascular occlusion with widespread necrotizing retinopathy in ocular syphilis.

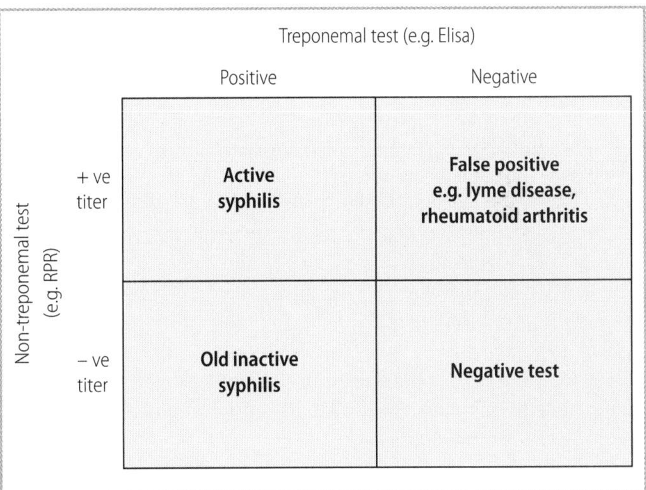

Figure 10.29 A simplified interpretation of syphilis serology for a patient with qualifying uveitis. Confirmation and treatment requires liaison with local microbiologist and genitourinary medicine physician.

Treponemal tests

All these tests remain positive for life after acquisition of syphilis, whether treated or not. They therefore cannot be used to differentiate active from old disease. They are also positive for other *T. pallidum* subspecies, which is of relevance in those small areas endemic for these diseases. They may cross-react with *Borrelia* spp. The main causes of false positivity in both treponemal and non-treponemal serology are summarized in **Table 10.2**. In practice serology is complex and expert interpretation is necessary (Ratnam 2005).

ELISAs

During the last 10 years ELISAs have been gradually replacing the older tests requiring whole bacteria as substrate. Being automated they are more cost-effective and the various commercial kits compete at very high levels of both sensitivity and specificity. They are being increasingly recognized as superior to the previously assumed 'gold standard' of FTA-Abs in the secondary and later stages. Immunoblotting is sometimes used for confirmation.

FTA-Abs test

The FTA-Abs is an indirect fluorescence technique using a lyophilized suspension of whole killed *T. pallidum* as antigen. It was considered the most sensitive diagnostic test for syphilis but some ELISAs are now better. It becomes positive earlier in the course of the disease than other tests.

Other treponemal-specific tests for syphilis include the *T. pallidum* particle agglutination (TPPA) tests, which include the *T. pallidum* hemagglutination (TPHA) and microhemagglutination (MHA) variants. All of these have approximately the same characteristics as the FTA-Abs test, but in general both the latter and ELISAs are superior and all except the ELISAs are personnel intensive and complex to

Table 10.2 The main causes of false positivity (marked Y) in syphilis serology

Cause	Treponemal tests	Non-treponemal tests
Advancing age	Y	Y
Bacterial endocarditis		Y
Bejel, pinta, yaws	Y	Y
Brucellosis	Y	Y
Cirrhosis	Y	
Chickenpox		Y
Drug addiction	Y	Y
Glandular fever	Y	Y
Hepatitis		Y
Immunization (recent)	Y	Y
Leprosy	Y	Y
Malaria	Y	
Malignancy		Y
Measles, mumps		Y
Rheumatoid arthritis		Y
Rickettsial infection		Y
Systemic lupus erythematosus	Y	Y
Systemic vasculitis		Y
Thyroiditis	Y	Y
Tuberculosis		Y
Ulcerative colitis		Y

Adapted from Ratnam (2005).

perform. The TPI (*T. pallidum* immobilization) test probably has higher specificity than FTA-Abs but its complexity and expense has precluded its routine use.

Non-treponemal tests

VDRL test

VDRL is a microflocculation screening test that requires microscopy. It is quantitative and useful in detecting responsiveness to treatment. However, it has up to a 40% incidence of false-positive results caused by a variety of circumstances shown in Table 10.2. False-positive results are often of low titer (< 1:8) in comparison to most true positives (> 1:8), which in active secondary syphilis are usually > 1:32.

VDRL usually reverts gradually to 'negative' (titer < 1:8) after successful treatment of syphilis, and even in untreated syphilis titers will fall in time. A third of those with tertiary syphilis are VDRL negative. The test is therefore not a reliable indicator of past infection, whether treated or untreated, and *Treponema*-specific tests should be used for this purpose. VDRL is the only non-treponemal test that may reliably be used on CSF specimens to diagnose neurosyphilis. CSF testing is unnecessary if the serum ELISA or FTA-Abs is negative.

RPR (rapid plasma reagin) test

The RPR is a rapid-performance flocculation test using charcoal particles that can be read with the naked eye. It is essentially a simplified version of the VDRL test and, like it, positivity is a titer > 1:8. It is mainly used for screening but is adequate for clinical diagnosis together with a treponemal test, and is the method of choice in our laboratory. It is inadequate for CSF serology.

The quantitative nature of the VDRL and RPR tests mean first that current disease activity can be diagnosed by a high titer, second that treatment efficacy can be monitored by following reducing titers, and third that failed treatment or reinfection can be diagnosed by titers rising again. However, these linear interpretations require the serial performance of the same test (VDRL and RPR titers are not interchangeable) and preferably by the same laboratory. Most treated patients show a fourfold decline in titers within 3 months and eightfold within 6 months. Some take longer but slower falls may indicate treatment failure. As reversion may be a slow process, treated patients should be followed with serology for at least 2 years.

Intraocular sampling

The potentially confusing presentation of some patients with ocular syphilis, especially in AIDS where the differential diagnosis will include necrotizing herpetic retinopathies, toxoplasmosis and TB (or indeed where infections may be recurrent), aqueous or vitreous sampling for PCR can be crucial. Microscopy of intraocular fluid is not helpful.

Management

The ophthalmologist will manage syphilitic uveitis in consultation with a GUM or infectious diseases physician, and HIV serology if unknown must always be tested; management plans will be modified by HIV positivity and over half of such patients are undiagnosed before the ocular involvement (Tucker et al. 2011). In the immunocompetent patient, syphilis within the primary or secondary stage, or within 1 year of this, will usually respond to a single intramuscular injection of benzathine benzylpenicillin. However, the patient with uveitis is normally considered to have neurosyphilis which requires extended treatment. Although this may be anatomically correct, the point has been argued that uveitis itself has not been proven to necessitate the treatment recommended for involvement of the brain or spinal cord. Nevertheless it is the practice in this uveitis clinic and in most others to consider uveitis as neurosyphilis and to treat accordingly.

Many patients with secondary syphilis and uveitis have concurrent, sometimes severe, headache. However, in the absence of focal neurological symptoms or signs and in the knowledge that an antibiotic course appropriate for neurosyphilis will in any case be administered, it seems reasonable to argue that neither central nervous system (CNS) imaging nor CSF analysis is necessary. Opinions differ and the argument will doubtless continue because a controlled trial of simple versus prolonged antibiotic therapy for uveitis is highly unlikely to appear.

The recommendations for neurosyphilis treatment differ depending on the country of origin but most are similar. In the UK the recommendation of the Association of Genitourinary Medicine is for 17 consecutive days of intramuscular procaine benzylpenicillin 1.8–2.4 MU, enhanced with probenecid. Several alternative regimens are used including intravenous penicillins and cephalosporins. All regimens use the parenteral route. In immunocompetent individuals, 3-monthly VDRL assessments will confirm treatment efficacy by gradually decreasing titers. Using the above regimens, about three-quarters of those with secondary syphilis revert to negative serology within 1 year.

Concurrent with antibiotic treatment, anterior uveitis is treated with topical steroid as required. There is no consensus on the advantage of oral steroid therapy, but our impression has been that it is advantageous for those with severe vitritis and retinitis or papillitis, and enhances resolution. Many patients with syphilitic uveitis have a visual acuity that is lower than might be expected from signs on examination. Our experience is that this depressed acuity can persist for weeks during apparently effective treatment, with a belated and sometimes profound improvement then following, except where direct macular involvement was seen. Extensive retinitis is followed by extensive scarring (**Fig. 10.30**) and substantial reduction of visual field. Nyctalopia is sometimes experienced.

The Jarisch–Herxheimer reaction

The sudden release of large amounts of treponemal endotoxin after treatment may, especially in the treatment of early syphilis, lead to a reaction including malaise, fever, flushing and increased redness of secondary cutaneous lesions. The reaction is usually minor and self-limiting. Much less commonly, in late neurosyphilis rapid disease progression may occur. It is therefore usual to precede penicillin treatment by moderate-dose oral steroids for a day, tailing off over a few days, in order to reduce a reaction should it occur.

Other treponemes: bejel, pinta and yaws

Subspecies of *T. pallidum* are responsible for three human diseases affecting well-defined geographical areas. All are serologically indistinguishable. Bejel (non-venereal endemic syphilis or sahel) is caused by *T. endemicum* and occurs in the eastern Mediterranean, Middle East and West Africa. It is a chronic skin disease with raised eroded lesions. There is a significant incidence of uveitis or optic neuropathy. Pinta (*T. carateum*) is a Central and South American disease with similar skin lesions but often late-stage widespread hyper- and depigmentation. Yaws (*T. p. pertenue*) is a widespread disease of the tropics (see **Fig. 10.39b**), a classic staged spirochetosis which, similar to syphilis, can cause late extensive tissue destruction including skin, bones and joints. Chorioretinal involvement with extensive scarring has been seen, and neuro-ophthalmological sequelae are problematic. All these treponematoses are treated in a similar way to syphilis.

LYME BORRELIOSIS (box 10.3)

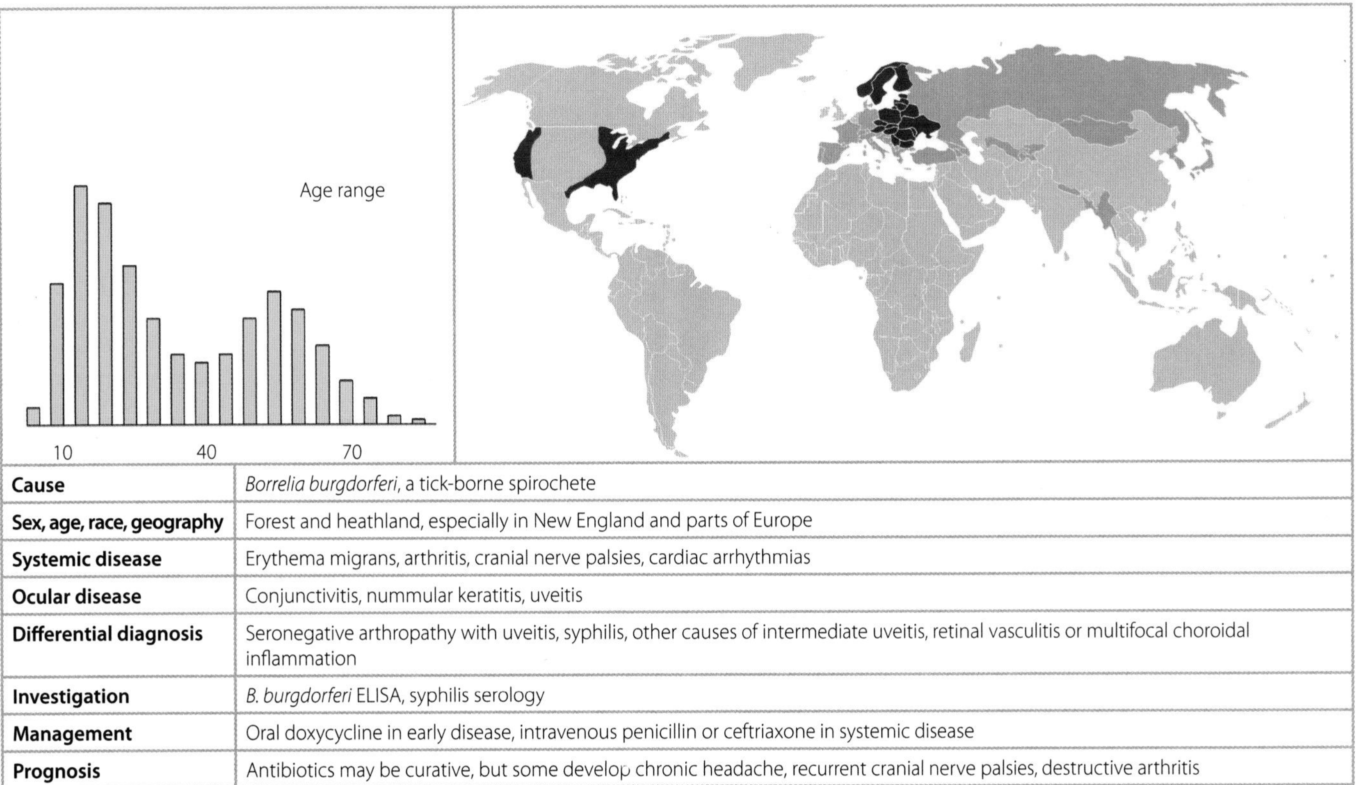

Cause	*Borrelia burgdorferi*, a tick-borne spirochete
Sex, age, race, geography	Forest and heathland, especially in New England and parts of Europe
Systemic disease	Erythema migrans, arthritis, cranial nerve palsies, cardiac arrhythmias
Ocular disease	Conjunctivitis, nummular keratitis, uveitis
Differential diagnosis	Seronegative arthropathy with uveitis, syphilis, other causes of intermediate uveitis, retinal vasculitis or multifocal choroidal inflammation
Investigation	*B. burgdorferi* ELISA, syphilis serology
Management	Oral doxycycline in early disease, intravenous penicillin or ceftriaxone in systemic disease
Prognosis	Antibiotics may be curative, but some develop chronic headache, recurrent cranial nerve palsies, destructive arthritis

Box 10.3 Lyme borreliosis

Introduction

Lyme borreliosis is a tick-borne bacterial infection. The disease is named after Old Lyme, Connecticut, where in 1975 a cluster of cases of arthritis and skin rash was encountered and, subsequently proved to be transmitted by ticks of the genus *Ixodes*. However, some 7 years were to pass before the organism carried by the ticks, a previously unknown spirochete, was identified and named *Borrelia*. In due course up to 40 distinct species have been identified and, within those, quite marked strain diversity. Collectively those *Borrelia* species causing Lyme disease and its variants are grouped together under the 'specific' name *B. burgdorferi*. The bacteria are helical (**Fig. 10.31**), and their rotational motility is achieved by two spiral rows of flagella. Lyme borreliosis is probably a relatively new disease in humans, although there is retrospective evidence of sporadic cases over several decades in the eastern USA. In Europe, erythema chronicum migrans, sometimes with systemic manifestations (the neurological type being known as Bannwarth's syndrome),

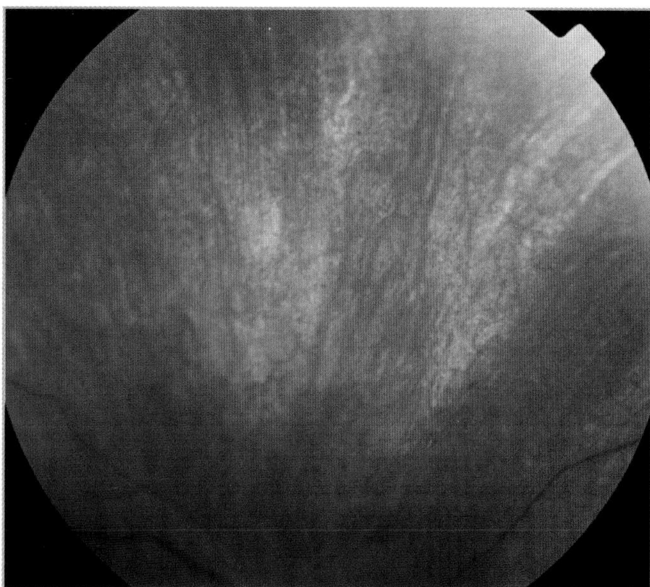

Figure 10.30 Same patient as Figure 10.22, after treatment showing widespread retinal pigment epithelium atrophy and vascular occlusion in the affected area but visual acuity recovered to 6/9. (Reproduced from Doris et al. 2006.)

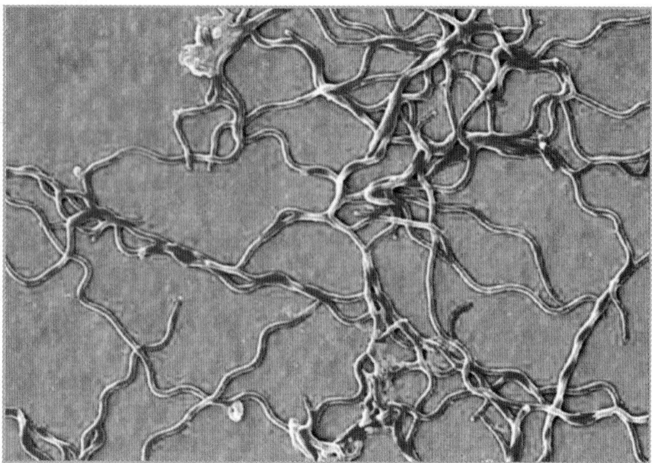

Figure 10.31 A group of *Borrelia burgdorferi*, the Lyme disease spirochete. (Modified from Centers for Disease Control, Public Health Image Library.)

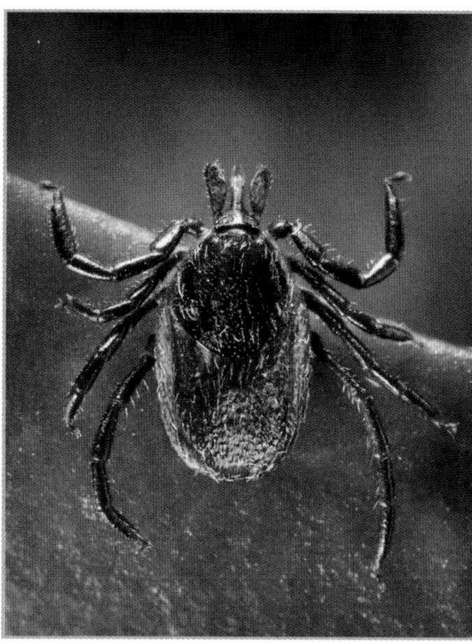

Figure 10.32 *Ixodes pacificus*, a North American tick. Other *Ixodes* spp. spreading borreliosis are similar. (Modified from Centers for Disease Control, Public Health Image Library.)

has occurred for a century or more (Burgdorfer and Schwan 1996), and the isolation of *B. burgdorferi* from European ticks has now confirmed the etiology of this form of the disease. The different species within *B. burgdorferi* are associated with different forms of the disease; European borreliosis is caused by *B. garinii* and *B. afzelii*, and American Lyme disease by *B. burgdorferi sensu stricto*. Similar to other spirochetal disease, protean manifestations have been described affecting several systems.

Cases of Lyme disease or erythema chronicum migrans occur throughout the USA at a rate of about 5000 per year, with cases being concentrated in New England, where the vector appears to be *Ixodes scapularis*. This tick also carries the disease in the mid-west USA, and *I. pacificus* (**Fig. 10.32**) is responsible on the western seaboard. The disease is much less common, although widespread, in Europe, the vector being *I. ricinus*. Most cases here have been reported from the forests of Scandinavia, and eastern and middle Europe. Lyme disease causes about 4% of uveitis in Finland (Mikkila et al. 1997). The disease is so far uncommon in the UK, but may be acquired in any rural area; the ticks are mainly resident in woodland and heathland, and may parasitize any mammal (including rodents, deer, sheep and horses) in which the spirochetal life cycle may be maintained. Domestic dogs may bring the infected insects into close human contact.

Human tick bites are seasonal, peak incidences occurring in late spring and autumn, but, in areas with mild climates, activity may be year round. The prevalence of infected ticks varies markedly, but may be very high in some localities. Tiny and unnoticed before a bite, a tick swells with blood and becomes pea sized if allowed to complete its meal, which may take 3 days. Transmission of *Borrelia* spp. is much more likely the longer the tick remains attached and removal within 24 hours usually prevents infection. Workers in endemic rural areas have been found to have high rates of seropositivity, but most infections were acquired asymptomatically.

Systemic disease

Asymptomatic infection by *B. burgdorferi* is not uncommon, and some patients may present with complications of the disease (including ocular involvement) but no recollection of a primary skin lesion. However, classic Lyme disease follows a three-stage form as seen with other spirochetal infections. *B. burgdorferi* is inoculated via a tick bite, which leaves a small papule. The most common sites are the thigh, groin or axilla, presumably reflecting the fact that ticks hidden in flexures more often remain for days as they are often missed. After a period varying from 3 days to 3 weeks, the typical primary lesion, erythema chronicum migrans, commences as a slowly expanding, erythematous rash, characteristically associated with intense itching or sometimes pain. If untreated the lesion may reach a considerable diameter, with erythema and induration at its edge and center, giving it a target appearance (**Fig. 10.33**). Vesiculation or even necrosis and ulceration of the center may occur, but is unusual. Eventually the center clears to leave an annular erythema which will ultimately fade.

If untreated, second-stage disease may develop. Some 60% develop recurrent pauciarticular arthritis within a few months of infection.

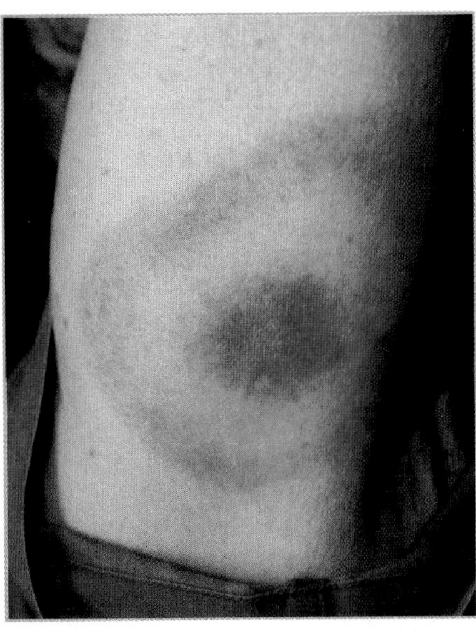

Figure 10.33 A typical advanced erythema chronicum migrans with a target appearance – the tick bite reaction is at centre and there is a spreading margin with internal clearance. (Modified from Centers for Disease Control, Public Health Image Library.)

Flitting recurrent musculoskeletal pains, radiculoneuritis or acute arthritis with pain, swelling and redness may occur, especially affecting the knees, but capable of involving any joint, large or small. In a few, the arthritis becomes chronic and destructive.

Headache with mild symptoms of meningism are common, but perhaps 15% will develop definite neurological involvement, including isolated cranial nerve palsies (particularly facial palsy, but paralysis of cranial nerves III, IV and VI are well known), meningitis or peripheral neuropathy. Cardiovascular involvement may also occur, sometimes early in the course of the disease. Atrioventricular block (presenting as dizziness or faints), myocarditis and pericarditis (causing retrosternal chest pain), and cardiomegaly have all been reported. In general, manifestations of the European form of the disease are more diverse than that of the American form, which more predictably causes acute, then chronic arthritis as its most common feature.

Only a minority will pass into third-stage chronic disease (or 'late persistent infection'), but progressive arthritis is common, particularly in the knees. Neurological complications affect about 5% and include peripheral polyneuropathy and encephalopathy or encephalomyelitis, characteristically with cognitive abnormalities, gait disorder and sometimes psychosis. Cord involvement may cause permanent paralysis. In Europe, patches of acrodermatitis atrophicans may appear as purple discoloration on the hands or feet, changing slowly to mimic vitiligo.

Ocular disease

Patients tend to present with ocular inflammation 3 months to 3 years after their erythema migrans, if recollected. A stromal, nummular keratitis may be seen and tends to leave permanent scarring. Intraocular inflammation is seen in up to 5% of cases (Huppertz et al. 1999), but if present usually arises with second-stage disease. Of those with uveitis, a majority will have other manifestations of the disease. Inflammation is usually bilateral, but no specific type of uveitis is suggestive of Lyme disease as such. Anterior uveitis is regularly reported, and may be granulomatous. Intermediate uveitis, choroiditis, papillitis and neuroretinitis all occur; retinal vasculitis is fairly common (Mikkila et al. 2000) and vascular occlusions have been seen. In HLA-A29-positive patients, birdshot chorioretinopathy has been seen in association with *B. burgdorferi* seropositivity, and acute posterior multifocal placoid pigment epitheliopathy (APMPPE) has been mimicked.

It should be noted that most cases of ocular involvement have been described in association with the American version of Lyme disease, which seems to differ from the European in respect of its systemic manifestations. Uveitis in association with *B. burgdorferi* seems much less common in the UK and Europe despite localized high rates of seropositivity in those at risk. Both the incidence and manifestations of ocular involvement may differ in Europe and the USA.

Diagnosis

Typical erythema migrans is unique and this rash alone can be used to diagnose Lyme disease. However, skin lesions may be atypical or pass unnoticed. In these cases the ophthalmologist should suspect Lyme disease where chronic anterior uveitis, intermediate uveitis or retinal vasculitis is seen in association with risk factors or manifestations such as arthropathy, facial or other cranial nerve palsy, palpitations, paraesthesiae or chronic fatigue. An ELISA test is available for *B. burgdorferi*. This has high sensitivity for those with arthritis (approaching 100%) but the various ELISAs are designed for continent-specific species and travelers may not produce reactive serum. Specificity is poor because of cross-reactivity with other spirochetes, notably *Treponema pallidum*, which may give a false-positive result. Cross-reactivity with the FTA-Abs test is high, whereas the non-treponemal RPR or VDRL tests produce less confusion. False-positive results may also occur in those who are positive for rheumatoid factor or antinuclear factor, and for those with glandular fever or cytomegalovirus (CMV) infection. The ELISA test should be combined with serological tests for syphilis (VDRL, RPR and FTA-Abs) to clarify the situation. If ELISA is positive, Western blotting is recommended as a more specific confirmatory test. Serology during the primary, erythema migrans phase is characteristically positive in only a third of patients, whereas if performed 1 month later this rises to two-thirds (Steere et al. 2008). Bacteria may be isolated from skin biopsy specimens, blood or synovial fluid, but its culture requirements are fastidious and it is very slow growing; culture is not used generally in diagnosis. The submission of clinical samples to PCR is increasingly performed but positivity rates are as low as 15% on CSF in patients showing typical signs of neuroborreliosis. PCR may be positive on urine but opinions differ as to the validity of the method. In this context, PCR on intraocular fluid is not proven to be diagnostically useful.

Seropositivity to *B. burgdorferi* is more common than Lyme disease itself. As some causes of false positivity may be associated with inflammatory disease that may mimic some components of Lyme disease, care should be taken in the interpretation of serological results. It is currently thought that most cases unresponsive to antibiotic therapy were initially misdiagnosed.

A variety of diagnostic criteria for Lyme disease have been proposed in various parts of the world. These should be treated with caution, first as manifestations differ internationally according to the *Borrelia* sp. involved and second because the symptoms and signs of later disease may be consistent with a wide range of diagnoses. There seems to be general agreement that erythema chronicum migrans witnessed by a physician is the strongest indicator of disease, positive serology alone without symptoms or disease should not lead to treatment, and diagnosis is made by a combination of history, current symptomatology and signs, and supportive laboratory diagnosis. The ophthalmologist should therefore be aware that positive serology in the presence of undifferentiated uveitis, but without any other history, symptoms or signs, is not diagnostic of Lyme disease-associated uveitis.

Management

In the late 1990s a Lyme disease vaccine was introduced in the USA, having demonstrated adequate protection in three-quarters of adults and approaching 100% of children. Within 2 years a large number of claims of vaccine-induced side effects led to federal investigation, which found no such link. Despite this reassurance, adverse publicity led to poor uptake and withdrawal of the vaccine. Others may be in development.

Current treatment recommendations for Lyme disease depend on the disease stage and manifestations. Erythema migrans in adults usually responds to oral doxycycline for 2–3 weeks, and amoxicillin can be used in children. For those with significant stage 2 involvement of organ systems and in those with uveitis, the use of intravenous antibiotics is recommended, usually ceftriaxone for 3 weeks. The effect on intraocular inflammation may be slow, but continued improvement may be observed over a period of months. Argument has been vigorous over the usefulness of prolonged antibiotic treatment, owing to the frequent persistence of symptoms despite apparent eradication of organisms. The current consensus is that nothing is added by prolonged treatment. However, persistent or recurrent symptoms of arthralgia, myalgia and headache are extremely common after treatment is finished. For those with late-stage disease, intravenous ceftriaxone for at least 4 weeks has been advocated and, for those with neuroborreliosis, to this may be added minocycline, which has good penetration across the blood–brain barrier.

BARTONELLOSIS (box 10.4)

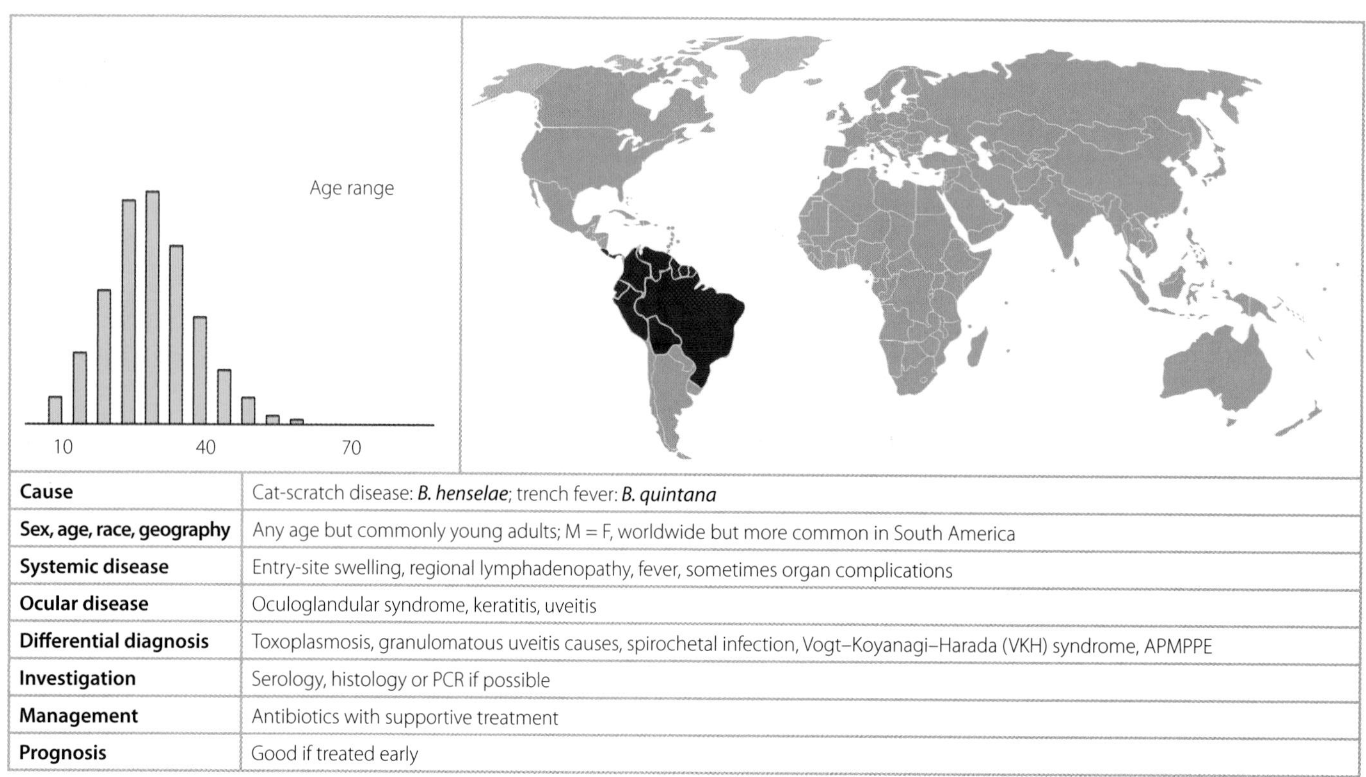

Cause	Cat-scratch disease: *B. henselae*; trench fever: *B. quintana*
Sex, age, race, geography	Any age but commonly young adults; M = F, worldwide but more common in South America
Systemic disease	Entry-site swelling, regional lymphadenopathy, fever, sometimes organ complications
Ocular disease	Oculoglandular syndrome, keratitis, uveitis
Differential diagnosis	Toxoplasmosis, granulomatous uveitis causes, spirochetal infection, Vogt–Koyanagi–Harada (VKH) syndrome, APMPPE
Investigation	Serology, histology or PCR if possible
Management	Antibiotics with supportive treatment
Prognosis	Good if treated early

Box 10.4 Bartonellosis

Introduction

In the late nineteenth century the French ophthalmologist Henri Parinaud described his 'oculoglandular syndrome' comprising unilateral follicular conjunctivitis and ipsilateral lymphadenopathy. The condition can be caused by several infections, one of which can be initiated by a cat scratch. More generally, cat-scratch disease has been recognized for almost a century as regional lymphadenopathy and malaise with or without other symptoms, following a scratch. In the 1950s it was discovered that the cat was the natural reservoir of the disease and subsequently that various species of *Bartonella*, a small facultative intracellular bacterium, were the cause. The most commonly involved in human infection is *B. henselae* (**Fig. 10.34**). The bacteria are spread among cats by fleas and thence to humans through scratches, often by kittens. However, in many cases a history of cat scratch, or indeed contact with cats, is not reported. It is now known that humans can contract the disease directly from cat-flea feces, and also through the bites of ticks and sandflies. All cats whether domesticated or feral can harbor the bacteria, and in the USA about 30% of domestic cats do so, more so in warmer states where the prevalence rises above 50%. A similar organism, *B. quintana*, is spread by human lice and, being the scourge of troops in the First World War, was known as trench fever; there are some clinical similarities to cat-scratch disease and there may be similar ocular involvement.

Systemic disease

At the site of entry of *B. henselae* a papulopustular reaction forms which histologically shows necrosis. Pyrexia then develops together with regional lymphadenopathy. The severity of this phase is variable. Some pass on to develop complications including endocarditis, hepatitis with or without abscess formation, and more rarely glomerulonephritis, meningoencephalitis and anemia. *B. quintana* causes a different syndrome known as trench fever. Spread is via lice and causes cyclic fever with lymphadenopathy, and sometimes endocarditis and other complications.

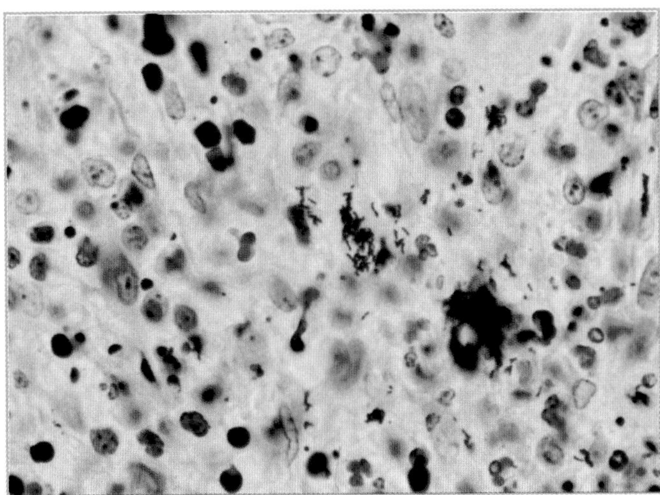

Figure 10.34 ***Bartonella henselae*** **organisms** within a lymph node. (Courtesy of Dr D Ramnani, WebPathology.com.)

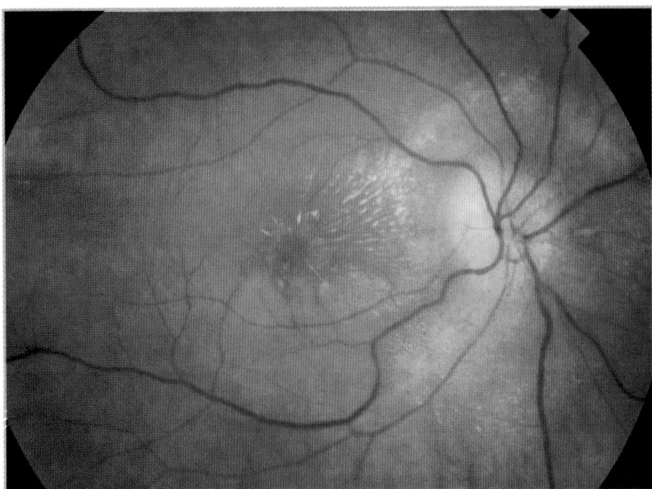

Figure 10.35 Neuroretinitis with branch artery occlusion in bartonellosis. There is substantial disk swelling, a macular star and inferotemporal retinal pallor in the ischemic area.

Ocular manifestations tend to be similar to those seen in cat-scratch disease. Carrion's disease is a fortunately uncommon but sometimes lethal disease confined to parts of South America and caused by *B. bacilliformis*. Abrupt fever with severe hemolytic anemia and hepatosplenomegaly will, if survived, lead on to chronic widespread verrucous skin lesions with multiple organ complications. Uveitis has not been reported.

Ocular disease

About 5% of those infected with *B. henselae* will develop oculoglandular syndrome and this is thought to arise from contaminated hand-to-eye infection. This clinical syndrome has also been reported with *B. quintana* infection. Intraocular inflammation is rather less common, but the majority presenting with uveitis have associated fever or lymphadenopathy. If anterior uveitis appears it may or may not be granulomatous. The most well-reported manifestation is neuroretinitis incorporating disk swelling with partial or complete macular star formation (Kalogeropoulos et al. 2011). It has been suggested that *Bartonella* spp. may be the most common cause of neuroretinitis (Suhler et al. 2000). There may also be branch retinal artery occlusion, and these two manifestations together are highly supportive of the diagnosis (**Fig. 10.35**). There may be apparently focal disk involvement, and lesions may cause significant serous retinal elevation. As for any neuroretinitis, macular exudates may persist for months (**Fig. 10.36**), and optic nerve head damage with resultant permanent neuropathy may result in some (**Fig. 10.37**). Some patients develop retinitis, which is characteristically unifocal or involving several foci (**Fig. 10.38**), sometimes each with serous detachment. This may statistically be the most common posterior segment manifestation (Curi et al. 2010). An intermediate uveitis type with cell clumping may be seen and occasionally there is panuveitis. Retinal vasculitis is often seen peripherally, sometimes centrally. The vasculitis may manifest as angiomatous lesions, sometimes peripapillary, or resembling peripheral nodular telangiectasis. If untreated these intraocular manifestations may be self-limiting and relatively benign unless severe optic disc or macular inflammation is seen. However, active treatment is usually recommended.

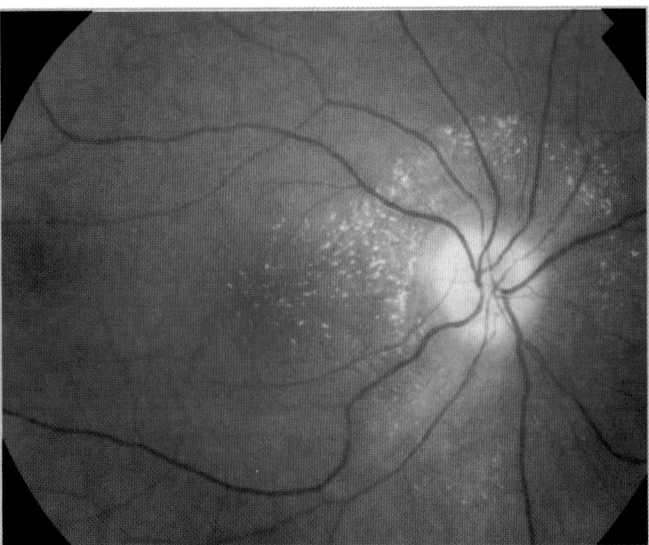

Figure 10.36 Same eye as 10.35 after 8 weeks showing further peripapillary exudate and substantial optic nerve head pallor. The swelling resolved to leave permanent optic atrophy.

Diagnosis

The clinical presentations of *Bartonella* infections are various; new species are regularly identified and culture of the fastidious bacteria, even in liquid media, is prolonged and technical. Material for culture may not be readily available. Serological methods are of high importance but the antigenicity of, for instance, *B. henselae* and *B. quintana* is very similar, with definite cross-reactivity. Current ELISA methods suffer from a low sensitivity (< 70%) if specificity is lifted to above 90% and vice versa. Studies into age-dependent variations in antibody responses and the combined usage of IgG and IgM ELISAs may lift predictive values. In areas where the organisms are commonly found in cats, human population seroprevalence is high especially in those such as farmers and veterinary surgeons who work closely with animals. The predictive value of serology is therefore low using standard cut-off titers for positivity in IgG and it may be more useful to use IgM titers only in diagnosis (Vermeulen et al. 2007). Molecular methods are improving and likely to prove of greater use in the future (Agan et al. 2002). Currently a variety of PCR primers is used, and combined PCR and immunohistochemistry may be necessary.

In summary the diagnosis of cat-scratch disease in patients with uveitis requires a summation of relevant clinical and laboratory information, in the knowledge that none of these has excellent predictive value. In sight-threatening uveitis of qualifying form, if supporting information is inconclusive, empirical treatment is justified.

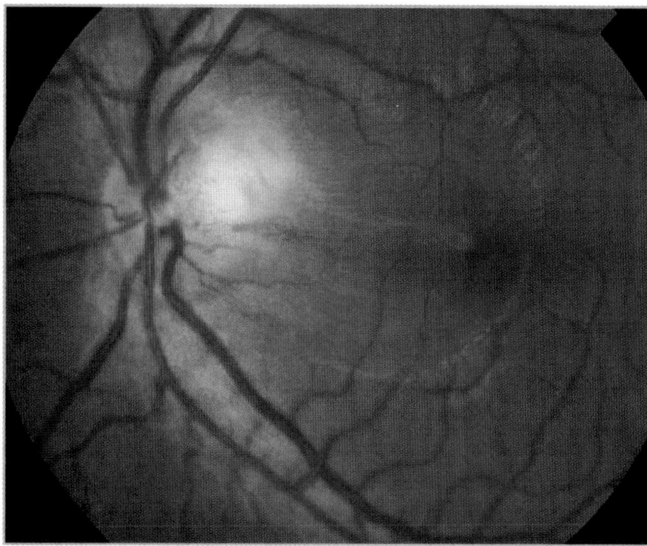

Figure 10.37 Focal optic nerve head involvement with adjacent serous retinal elevation in *Bartonella* infection. (Courtesy of Dr A Curi.)

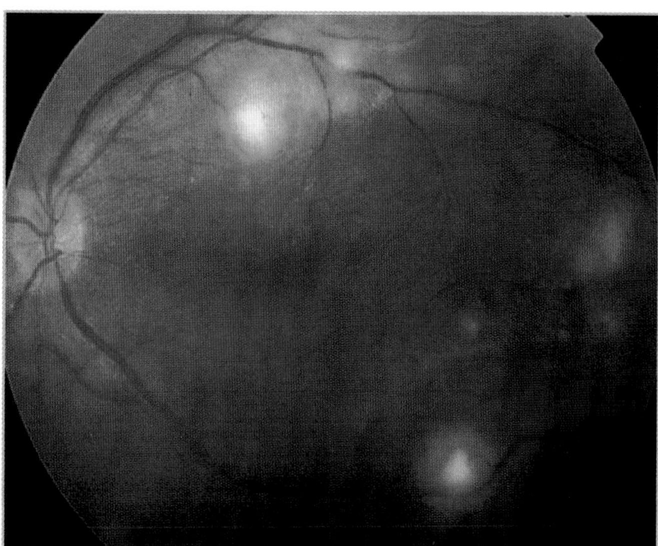

Figure 10.38 Multifocal retinitis and periphlebitis in a patient with cat-scratch disease. The foci are associated with local serous retinal elevation. (Courtesy of Dr A Curi.)

Management

Patients with mild cat-scratch disease can be observed without treatment. Those with severe lymphadenopathy or pyrexia will require antibiotic treatment. The organism is sensitive to a variety of antibiotics including tetracyclines (typically doxycycline), and aminoglycosides including azithromycin, rifampicin and co-trimoxazole. Those with uveitis involving the posterior pole should be treated. Topical steroid is helpful where required but the use of oral steroid is uncertain. Pragmatically the addition of prednisolone to antibiotic treatment, where optic disk swelling or retinal edema is substantial, seems logical and is probably helpful in shortening the episode and possibly in limiting scarring. Data are insufficient to make clear recommendations. The differential diagnosis of those with neuroretinitis and/or focal retinitis includes toxoplasmosis and therefore the use of co-trimoxazole or another antibiotic with dual efficacy is reasonable. Most immunocompetent patients recover good vision.

ENDOGENOUS BACTERIAL ENDOPHTHALMITIS (box 10.5)

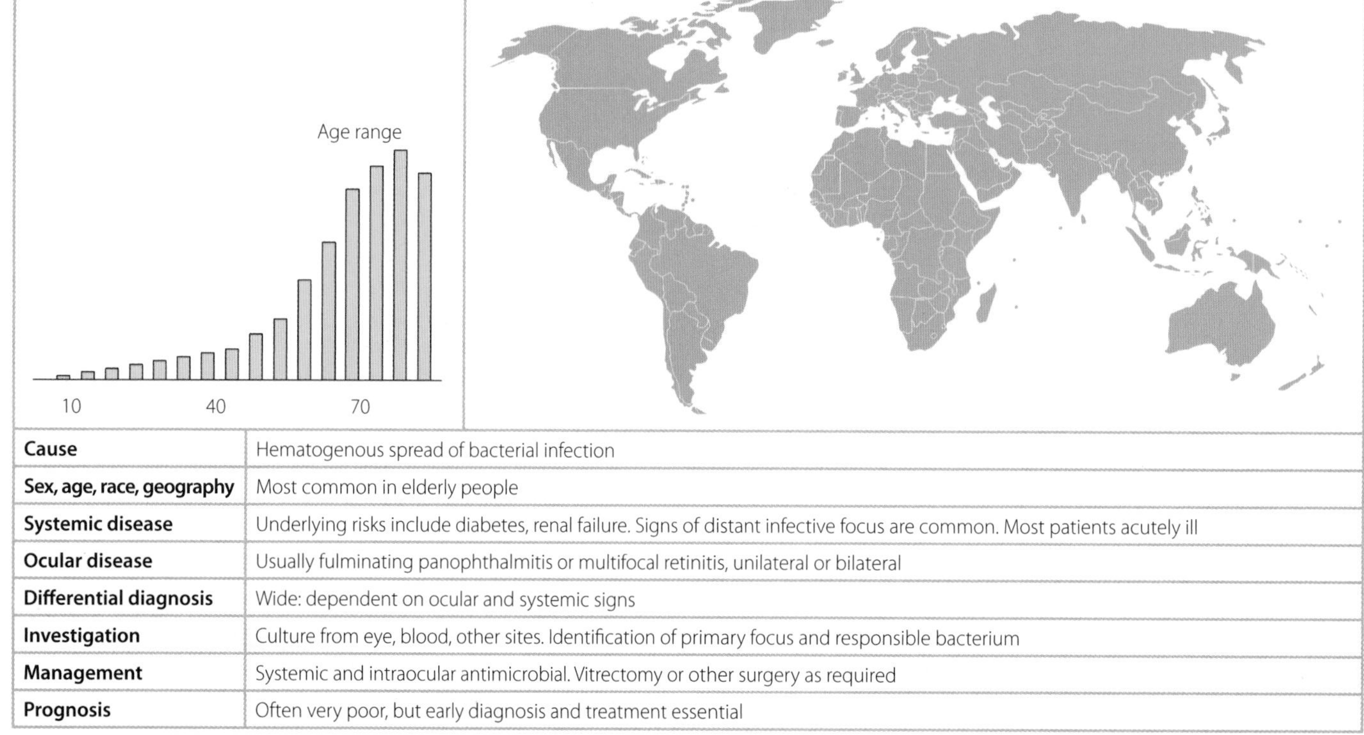

Cause	Hematogenous spread of bacterial infection
Sex, age, race, geography	Most common in elderly people
Systemic disease	Underlying risks include diabetes, renal failure. Signs of distant infective focus are common. Most patients acutely ill
Ocular disease	Usually fulminating panophthalmitis or multifocal retinitis, unilateral or bilateral
Differential diagnosis	Wide: dependent on ocular and systemic signs
Investigation	Culture from eye, blood, other sites. Identification of primary focus and responsible bacterium
Management	Systemic and intraocular antimicrobial. Vitrectomy or other surgery as required
Prognosis	Often very poor, but early diagnosis and treatment essential

Box 10.5 Endogenous bacterial endophthalmitis

Introduction

Endogenous endophthalmitis (i.e. intraocular infection acquired by hematogenous spread of infection elsewhere in the body) is rare, accounting for only a small proportion of cases of endophthalmitis, most of which follow intraocular surgery or trauma. Up to half of all cases are fungal in origin, particularly in intravenous drug abusers or where indwelling catheters are used. These are discussed in Chapter 12, the section here being limited to bacterial infection. Both ophthalmologist and physician require a high degree of suspicion if early diagnosis and treatment are to prevent blindness.

As a result of its rarity, the general features of endogenous bacterial endophthalmitis are difficult to rationalize; individual experience of the disease is usually anecdotal, and this is reflected in the preponderance of isolated case reports in the literature. However, certain general trends are apparent, which will be helpful in diagnosis.

Systemic disease

The pre-existence of certain underlying systemic problems predisposes to a greater likelihood of hematogenous spreading infection, and therefore to endophthalmitis. Diabetes is of particular importance and is overwhelmingly the most common underlying feature in reported cases. Blood dyscrasias, renal impairment, any neoplasia, some connective tissue disorders, and immunodeficiency or immunosuppression, are also important, as is advancing age. In addition, foreign bodies that may introduce or encourage bacterial proliferation include prosthetic heart valves and indwelling venous or urinary catheters. Bacteremia may be provoked by recent surgery, including dental surgery and splenectomy, especially where local sepsis is involved, and of course can be introduced during intravenous drug abuse (Connell et al. 2011) or renal dialysis.

The source of infection is most likely to be the urinary tract, endocardium, meninges or localized sepsis including wound infections, although many other sites have been implicated. Certain bacteria are associated with particular systemic features; *Streptococcus viridans* is typically associated with endocarditis, *Staphylococcus aureus* with cutaneous sepsis, and clostridia with bowel neoplasia; *Bacillus cereus* has recently been associated with intravenous drug injection; Gram-negative bacteria such as *Klebsiella* spp., *Escherischia coli* and *Pseudomonas* spp. are commonly seen in urinary tract infections and *Klebsiella* spp. have a particular affinity for the hepatobiliary system; either *Neisseria meningitis* or *Haemophilus influenzae* may cause meningitis or septicemia.

The systemic manifestations associated with bacterial endophthalmitis can vary widely depending on the affected sites and the diagnostic delay. At worst the patient may already be moribund from a fulminating septicemia; at the other end of the spectrum, there may be minimal, or even no, symptoms or signs of an infective focus in a patient presenting with ocular inflammation (Shankar et al. 2009). Overall, most patients presenting to the ophthalmologist with apparent endogenous endophthalmitis will already have a diagnosed systemic infection, and some will be acutely ill. A proportion of patients present a difficult management problem in that they are severely ill with septicemia and reside, sometimes sedated or unconscious, on high-dependency units where visual symptoms may not present, and ocular signs may pass unnoticed, at least in the early stages of infection. Such locations also hamper ophthalmic examination and treatment. The ophthalmologist therefore has a role in reminding physician colleagues of the possibility of intraocular involvement in disseminated infection, and of the consequences of late diagnosis. Less often the endophthalmitis is the presenting feature of the systemic infection, and in these circumstances the identification of the primary source is urgent. The identification of risk factors such as those described above, followed by immediate investigation, is necessary.

Ocular disease

Endophthalmitis may be unilateral or bilateral. The right eye is more commonly involved than the left, and this has been attributed to blood supply asymmetry. Some organisms appear more likely to cause bilateral involvement (*Neisseria meningitidis, Escherichia coli, Klebsiella* spp.). Appearance and progress may differ markedly. Fulminating infection may present with rapid visual loss and pain, red eye, hypopyon and a dense vitritis preventing a view of the posterior segment. Sometimes panophthalmitis or orbital cellulitis follows. Less virulent progress may lead to multifocal posterior segment lesions such as Roth's spots, retinitis or retinal vasculitis, with less dramatic vitritis, or occasionally, nodular iritis. The eye in these cases may be white. On occasion relatively localized vitreous or chorioretinal inflammation in children has simulated endophytic retinoblastoma. Hypopyons of peculiar color may indicate infection with either *Serratia* or *Listeria* spp.

Diagnosis

The ophthalmologist will wish to involve a physician in diagnosis and management. On occasion the source of infection is obvious, but this does not preclude vigorous investigation. Cultures from blood, urine and stool are paramount, together with an organ function screen, chest radiograph and echocardiography. White cell count and differential and erythrocyte sedimentation rate (ESR) or C-reactive protein (CRP) may be useful. Specific signs may suggest the need for lumbar puncture or liver ultrasonography. Any indwelling catheter should be removed, the tip cultured and replaced if necessary.

Where the responsible organism is not already identified, urgent intraocular sampling is required. This should precede the commencement of systemic antibiotics. Vitreous biopsy is more likely to provide positive results and can be combined with the intraocular injection of antibiotics. Many patients will be unfit for travel to an ophthalmic theatre and bedside surgery under the naked eye may be enforced; pars plana vitreous tap may be performed with topical and subconjunctival local anesthesia using a 21-G cannula to aspirate 0.2 ml of liquid vitreous from a site 3 mm posterior to the limbus. Intraocular sampling is not necessary if an organism has been isolated from blood culture.

Management

In the absence of bacteriological diagnosis, intraocular vancomycin 1 mg in 0.1 ml, and ceftazidime 2.25 mg in 0.1 ml, should be administered intravitreally at the time of vitreous tap. Systemic antibiotics, preferably intravenous, should also be commenced. In contrast to postoperative or post-traumatic endophthalmitis, endogenous infection may respond well to intravenous administration. Before culture and sensitivity, a combination of aminoglycoside and vancomycin is most common, but microscopy results may modify this choice. The advice of the microbiologist should be sought at all stages.

The role of formal pars plana vitrectomy in the management of exogenous endophthalmitis has been clarified substantially over the past decade; this is not the case for endogenous endophthalmitis. In the context of endogenous infection, there will in any case be a proportion of patients who are unfit to submit to formal surgery. If visual loss is profound and no fundal view is achieved, pars plana vitrectomy and intraocular antibiotic injection should be considered as a first procedure, if feasible.

It is unsurprising that endogenous endophthalmitis is, in those patients who survive, associated with a worse visual prognosis than that for exogenous endophthalmitis. Diagnosis is more difficult and may be delayed, more obscure organisms may be involved and management may be compromised by circumstances. Nevertheless, prompt recognition and treatment may prevent blindness.

OTHERS

Brucellosis

Brucellosis is a zoonosis caused by one of four bacterial species of the genus *Brucella*, namely *B. abortus* (from cattle). *B. suis* (from pigs), *B. canis* (from dogs) and *B. melitensis* (from sheep and goats), the last being the most important worldwide cause of the disease. The disease is endemic in many countries, and only mainland Canada, the UK, Scandinavia, parts of northern Europe and Australasia are disease free (**Fig. 10.39d**). The disease may be transmitted by droplet infection, or by drinking unpasteurized milk or cheese, venereally or parenterally.

After an incubation period of 1–3 weeks, malaise, fever (especially in the evening, with rigors and sweats), myalgia, headache, anorexia, abdominal symptoms and, occasionally, a macular rash or polyarthritis will develop. Carditis may be seen and hilar lymphadenopathy may develop. Abscess formation affecting joint, bone, lung, spleen, kidney or mesenteric nodes is uncommon. Diagnosis is by ELISA for *Brucella* antigens, or by positive blood or tissue culture (which may take 8 weeks or more and which is uncommonly performed – the organisms are a danger to laboratory staff).

The eyes are involved in about 20% of cases (Sungur et al. 2009) and the diagnosis should be considered in any patient with uveitis and a pyrexia of unknown origin with known risk factors such as travel to an endemic area, consumption of untreated foods or occupation (abattoir workers or veterinary surgeons). Anterior uveitis or multifocal choroiditis are the most common manifestations, and less commonly panuveitis, hemorrhagic retinopathy and optic neuritis.

Uveitis usually responds well to systemic antibiotic treatment. Systemic treatment is warranted for any patient with uveitis and significant *Brucella* serology with a recent pyrexial illness and no other demonstrable cause of uveitis. Combined antibiotic treatment is necessary because the organisms are facultative intracellular parasites; current optimal treatment for brucellosis requires the combination of a tetracycline (usually doxycycline) and an aminoglycoside, preferably streptomycin by intramuscular injection. After 1 month of combined treatment, the aminoglycoside is replaced by either rifampicin 600 mg/day or co-trimoxazole 960 mg twice daily, for a further 1 or 2 months. Shorter treatment courses are associated with high relapse rates.

Leprosy

Leprosy is a chronic inflammatory disease caused by infection with *Mycobacterium leprae*. It is common, with an estimated total of over 10 million people affected worldwide. It is predominantly a tropical disease (**Fig. 10.39c**) but is occasionally seen in temperate areas. It is associated with poverty and overcrowding and is probably droplet spread. It has a very long incubation period of up to 20 years. A wide variability in disease severity is based on differing host cell-mediated immunity. The mildest form, tuberculoid leprosy, is usually localized and extremely chronic, whereas lepromatous leprosy is progressive, leading to widespread dermal nodular infiltrates and causing the typical 'leonine' facies. Progressive dermal anesthesia and laryngeal swelling occur. If untreated, lepromatous leprosy leads eventually, through progressive deformity, to death from intercurrent infection, laryngeal obstruction or renal failure.

Ocular involvement is most common in the lepromatous form, and up to a third develop some form of ocular complication. Lagophthalmos,

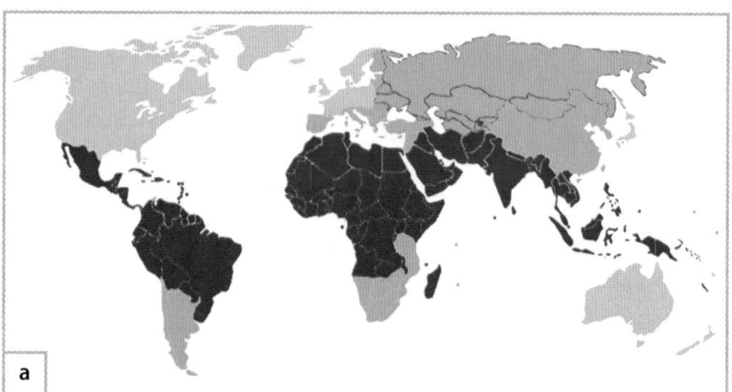

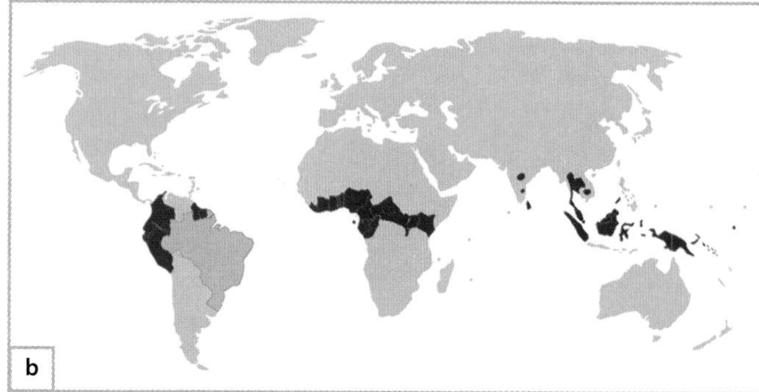

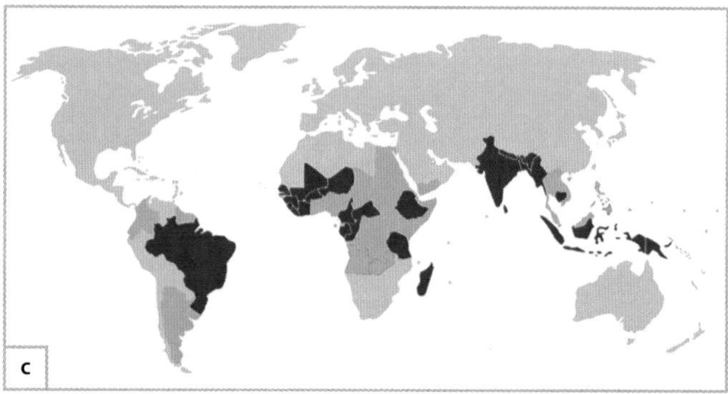

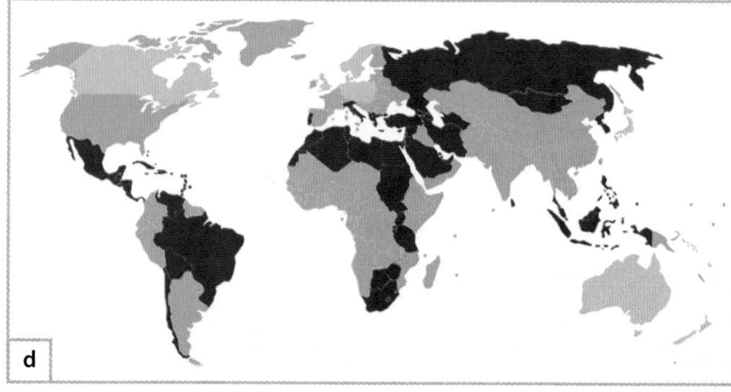

Figure 10.39 World distribution maps for some bacterial diseases involving uveitis: (a) leptospirosis; (b) yaws; (c) leprosy; and (d) brucellosis.

exposure keratopathy and corneal ulceration are common; chronic iridocyclitis affects up to 10% (Jawadhi et al. 2009). Uveitis and its sequelae or corneal problems are the most common cause of visual loss (Nepal and Shrestha 2004). Extreme miosis, iris atrophy, posterior synechiae and corectopia are typical. Secondary glaucoma or macular edema may occur. Iris pearls are tiny, round, white granulomas resting on the iris surface near to the pupil, or falling into the bottom of the anterior chamber. They are pathognomonic of leprosy.

Vitiligo, cutaneous mycosis, discoid lupus, lupus vulgaris, psoriasis and cutaneous sarcoidosis should all be considered in the differential diagnosis. Thickened peripheral nerves are pathognomonic of leprosy and corneal nerve beading is visible on the slit-lamp. The organism has not been cultured in vitro; diagnosis is by microscopy of a skin biopsy. Treatment is given according to the bacterial number seen; paucibacillary leprosy is treated usually with a 6-month course of rifampicin and dapsone and multibacillary with the above plus clofazimine for 12 months. These regimens are usually curative.

Leptospirosis

Leptospirosis is a worldwide zoonotic infection caused by the spirochete *Leptospira interrogans* and occasionally others in the genus. Although many mammals can act as the reservoir of infection, rats are the most important. Infection is by direct contact with an infected animal or with areas contaminated by its excreta and urine, within which *L. interrogans* may survive for weeks. The disease is most common and year round in the tropics, but peaking in the wet seasons in temperate areas (**Fig. 10.39a**). Those most at risk include farmers, slaughterhouse workers and sewerage workers. Swimming in stagnant water is also a risk. The disease presents in most as a pyrexia with malaise, severe myalgia and headache with a macular skin rash. Renal malfunction of some degree is usual. Conjunctivitis, sometimes with petechiae, is common. In this early stage, bacteremia is present. Most will recover gradually, but severe forms (Weil's disease) may develop into meningitis, cholestatic jaundice, renal failure and a bleeding diathesis. Differential diagnosis includes dengue and hemorrhagic fevers, malaria and typhoid.

Uveitis affects up to half of patients, usually starting after the acute bacteremic stage. Mild, bilateral, non-granulomatous, anterior uveitis is most common (Pappachan et al. 2007), but vitritis and retinal infiltration have been reported. Most cases are mild and self-limiting, but troublesome and prolonged cases have been reported. Blood culture is usually positive for the first 10 days and thereafter urine culture or serology is used. PCR for leptospirosis is now available and has been used on intraocular fluid (Merien et al. 1993). Antimicrobials are effective only if commenced within 1 week of disease onset. Usually, benzylpenicillin is given intravenously for 1 week. However, uveitis is not considered to be directly infective and, similar to other second-stage manifestations of the disease, does not respond to antimicrobial therapy but to topical corticosteroids.

Mycoplasma, Ureaplasma and Chlamydia infections

All of these primitive bacteria lack cell walls. The mycoplasmas are the least sophisticated of bacteria, containing the smallest genome. *Mycoplasma pneumoniae* is the important human pathogen but, in addition to causing atypical pneumonia, it is known to cause acute arthralgia, rash and fever without lung involvement. Acute bilateral anterior uveitis is reported anecdotally and mycoplasmas should be considered in the differential diagnosis of young patients with an acute illness with rash and arthralgia. A reported association between *Ureaplasma hominis* and acute anterior uveitis was not supported by further data. The chlamydiae very uncommonly cause mild uveitis during acute conjunctivitis. All of this group of organisms are capable of inducing a reactive arthritis with uveitis (Brodie's syndrome) which is discussed in Chapter 8. Macrolides are the antibiotics of choice when required but the efficacy for related uveitis is unproven.

Nocardiosis

Nocardia spp. are filamentous actinomycetes bacteria and widespread soil saprophytes. *N. asteroides* or *N. farcinica* infection is well recorded in patients who are immunodeficient, and may cause endophthalmitis or subretinal abscess (**Fig. 10.40**); although subretinal abscess is rare, *Nocardia* spp. may be its most common bacterial cause (Harris et al. 2000). Nocardia infection may present with ocular involvement, but at least one other site is invariably affected, often lung or brain.

The differential diagnosis of subretinal abscess includes infection by *Klebsiella* spp., *Pseudomonas* spp., *M. tuberculosis*, *Staph. aureus* and *Strep. viridans*. Microscopy of *Nocardia* spp. requires Ziehl–Neelsen or Gomori's methenamine silver staining, but identification may be difficult. Culture requires 10% carbon dioxide. Antibiotic sensitivity is variable, but staples include co-trimoxazole, amikacin, ampicillin, cefotaxime, vancomycin and linezolid. Combination treatment is usual, continuing for 1 year to avoid recrudescence.

Rickettsia, Orientia and Coxiella infections

These microorganisms share the characteristics of being very small, pleomorphic, Gram-negative coccobacilli which are obligate intracellular bacteria. Some rickettsias cause arthropod-borne human infection including the typhus group and spotted fevers. Disease tends broadly to cause severe pyrexia and malaise with rash and a necrotic black-centered

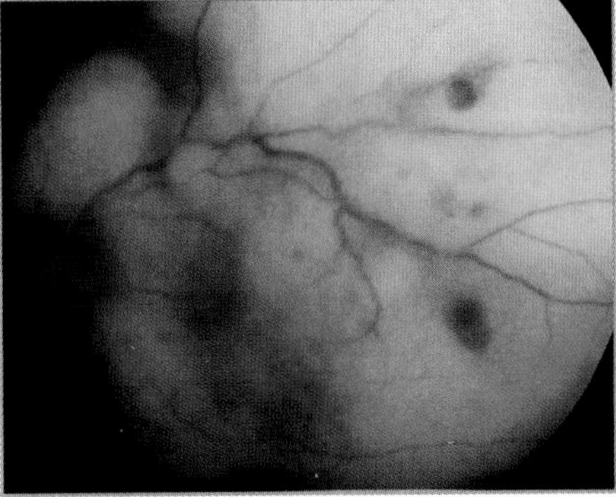

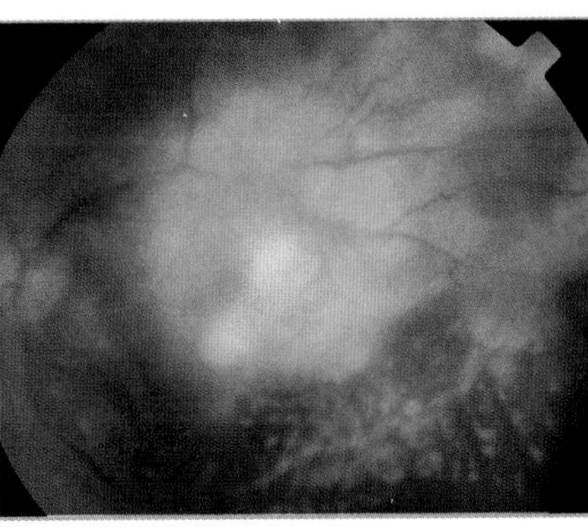

Figure 10.40 Subretinal abscess caused by *Nocardia asteroides*, on presentation (left) and after 2 weeks of treatment (right). The patient also had cavitating lesions in liver, lung and brain. (Reproduced in part from Jones, 2010.)

tick bite known as the 'tache noir.' The literature on ocular involvement is sparse and largely anecdotal but has been reported in typhus, murine typhus, and Mediterranean and Rocky Mountain spotted fevers (**Fig. 10.41**) and Queensland typhus (Khairallah et al. 2009). There is a definite tendency to retinal involvement with multifocal retinitis or vasculitis. Vascular occlusion and optic neuropathy may occur. Endophthalmitis is rare. Diagnosis is by serology and early treatment of systemic disease is preferably by doxycycline or alternatively chloramphenicol or macrolides. The antibiotic of choice for those with ocular involvement is unknown but fluoroquinolones have better ocular penetration. Concurrent topical or systemic steroid therapy may be required for intraocular inflammation. Most episodes are self-limiting after some weeks and resolution of posterior segment lesions with return to good vision is usual.

Orientia tsutsugamuchi causes scrub typhus and in the acute phase conjunctival hemorrhage, limbitis, anterior uveitis, posterior uveitis, papillitis, retinal hemorrhage and exudate can be seen. Intraocular involvement is uncommon. *Coxiella burnetii* causes Q-fever, in which uveitis or optic neuropathy is anecdotal. Tetracyclines or chloramphenicol are effective for both diseases.

Whipple's disease

This rare (approximate incidence 0.1/100 000 per year) multisystem disease, usually presenting in middle-aged white men (almost 90% of patients are male) with a malabsorption syndrome, is caused by infection by a recently identified actinomycetes bacillus, *Tropheryma whippeli* (Dutly and Altwegg 2001), which is now known to be a very common environmental organism. Weight loss, diarrhea, centrifugal arthropathy, skin pigmentation, finger clubbing and edema may all be seen, as may pleurisy, pericarditis and CNS manifestations, most commonly early onset dementia, headache or epilepsy. Jejunal biopsy demonstrates abnormal macrophages and, usually, abundant Gram-positive bacilli, but culture is extremely difficult. If bacteria are not found on biopsy, PCR techniques have been used with some success but are not yet entirely validated. Ocular involvement is unusual and reports are only anecdotal. Inflammation usually causes vitritis with chorioretinitis and may cause a hemorrhagic and exudative retinal vasculitis. Untreated Whipple's disease is ultimately fatal but diagnosis is usually delayed for years and sometimes decades. Current treatment is usually with co-trimoxazole or alternately penicillin or tetracycline. A 2-year course is required for eradication.

Post-streptococcal disease

The group A β-hemolytic streptococci (*Strep. pyogenes*) are common causes of bacterial pharyngitis with or without rash, and less severe forms are often dismissed as viral infection. It is long established that these infections can induce, within 2 weeks or so, a constellation of presumed autoimmune responses, especially if passing untreated. In addition to poststreptococcal glomerulonephritis (which can affect up to 3% of those infected), arthritis and rheumatic fever (1%), a variety of CNS disorders can ensue, including dystonias and neuropsychiatric syndromes. The organisms produce an extensive range of exotoxins and it may be one or more of these that can induce such reactions.

In cases of uveitis after sore throat or tonsillitis, especially in children between 5 and 15 years, poststreptococcal inflammation should be considered, and is probably much more common than is suggested by the published literature. Significantly raised anti-streptolysin-O (ASO) titers support the diagnosis and convalescent serological changes can be confirmatory. The majority of patients develop only non-granulomatous anterior uveitis which is usually self-limiting. A substantial minority develops vitritis or panuveitis (Tinley et al. 2011) and in the most severe cases multifocal chorioretinitis and/or retinal vasculitis can occur, with or without disk swelling (De Smet 2009) (**Fig. 10.42**). Rarely visual loss can be severe and inflammation recalcitrant.

For the majority a course of topical steroid is all that is required. Most pediatricians recommend penicillin V treatment until ASO titers have returned to normal. Severe posterior segment inflammation may require oral steroid treatment.

In conclusion, many patients with uveitis currently remain undiagnosed yet occasionally a pathogen is suggested to be relevant to specific forms of inflammation. Many bacteria are poorly understood and resistant to culture. Such fastidious, often low-grade pathogens may be increasingly found to be causative in some patients with uveitis and diligent microbiological investigation may prove to be key in future (Bodaghi et al. 2009).

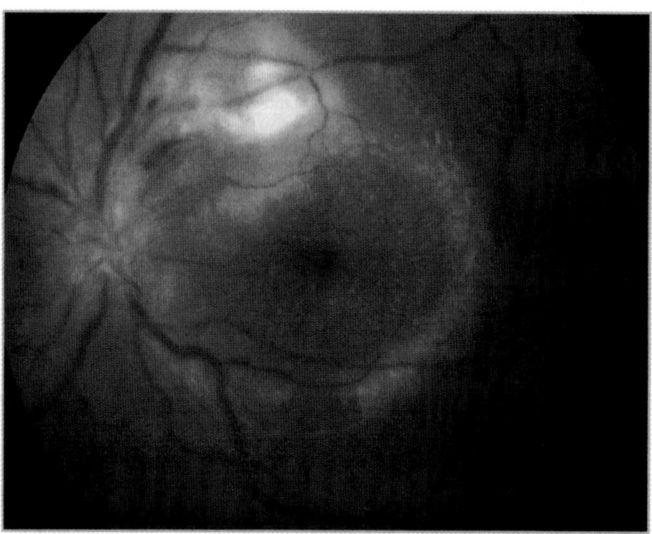

Figure 10.41 A focus of retinitis is accompanied by serous retinal detachment in Mediterranean spotted fever. (Reproduced from Khairallah et al. 2009.)

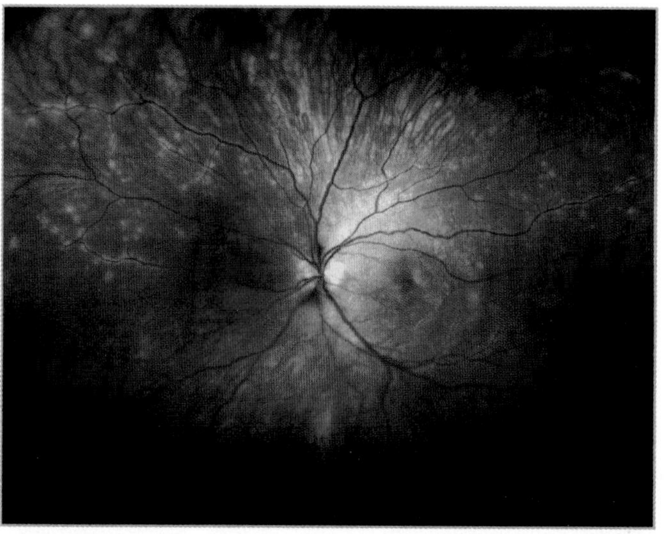

Figure 10.42 Bilateral widespread multifocal chorioretinitis, patchy non-occlusive periphlebitis, papillitis and severe macular edema in an 11-year-old girl with poststreptococcal uveitis. Visual acuity on presentation was HM in both eyes.

REFERENCES

Agan BK, Dolan MJ. Laboratory diagnosis of Bartonella infections. *Clin Lab Med* 2002;**22**:937–62.

Anderson C, Moore J, Kruijshaar M, Abubakar I. *Tuberculosis in the UK*: annual report on *tuberculosis surveillance in the UK 2008*. London, Health Protection Agency Centre for Infections, 2008.

Ang M, Hedayatfar A, Wong W, Chee SP. Duration of antitubercular therapy in uveitis associated with latent tuberculosis: a case control-study. *Br J Ophthalmol* 2011;**96**:332–6.

Bodaghi B, Drancourt M, Cassoux N, et al. Uveitis caused by fastidious bacteria. *Acta Ophthalmol* 2009;**87**:s244p0.

Burgdorfer W, Schwan TG. Lyme disease. In: Weatherall DJ, Ledingham JG, Warrell DA (eds), *Oxford Textbook of Medicine*, 3rd edn. Oxford: Oxford University Press, 1996: 689–92.

Chakravorty S, Sen MK, Tyagi JS. Diagnosis of extrapulmonary tuberculosis by smear, culture and PCR using universal sample processing technology. *J Clin Microbiol* 2005;**43**:4357–62.

Connell PP, O'Neill EC, Fabinyi D, et al. Endogenous endophthalmitis: 10-year experience at a tertiary referral centre. **Eye** 2011;25:66–72.

Curi AL, Machado D, Heringer G, et al. Cat-scratch disease: ocular manifestations and clinical outcome. *Int Ophthalmol* 2010;**30**:553–8.

De Smet MD. Papillophlebitis and uveitis as a manifestation of post-streptococcal uveitis syndrome. *Eye* 2009;**23**:985–7.

Diel R, Loddenkemper R, Nienhaus A, et al. Evidence-based comparison of commercial interferon-γ release assays for detecting active TB: a meta-analysis. *Chest* 2010;**137**:952–68.

Doris JP, Saha K, Jones NP, Sukthankar A. Ocular syphilis: the new epidemic. *Eye* 2006;**20**:703–5.

Dutly F, Altwegg M. Whipple's disease and '*Tropheryma whippeli*'. *Clin Microbiol Rev* 2001;**14**:561–83.

El-Asrar AM, Al-Kharashi SA. Full panretinal photocoagulation and early vitrectomy improve prognosis of retinal vasculitis associated with tuberculoprotein hypersensitivity (Eales' disease). *Br J Ophthalmol* 2002;**86**:1248–51.

Gass JDM, Braunstein RA, Chenoweth RG. Acute syphilitic posterior placoid chorioretinitis. *Ophthalmology* 1990:**97**:1288–97.

Gupta A, Gupta V, Arora S, et al. PCR-positive tubercular retinal vasculitis: clinical characteristics and management. *Retina* 2001;**21**:435–44.

Gupta V, Gupta A, Arora S, et al. Presumed tubercular serpiginous-like choroiditis: clinical presentations and management. *Ophthalmology* 2003;**110**:1744–9.

Harris EW, D'Amico DJ, Bhisitkul R, Priebe GP, Petersen R. Bacterial subretinal abscess: a case report and review of the literature. *Am J Ophthalmol* 2000;**129**:778–85.

Huppertz HI, Munchmeier D, Lieb W. Ocular manifestations in children and adolescents with Lyme arthritis. *Br J Ophthalmol* 1999;**83**:1149–53.

Jawadhi S, Das H, Agrawal S. Pattern and determinants of ocular complications in leprosy patients in eastern Nepal. *Nepal J Ophthalmol* 2009;**1**:2–8.

Jones NP. Disseminated *Nocardia* infection with subretinal abscess. *Eye* 2010;**24**:187–8.

Kalogeropoulos C, Koumpoulis I, Pappa C, et al. *Bartonella* and intraocular inflammation: a series of cases and review of the literature. *Clin Ophthalmol* 2011;**5**:817–29.

Khairallah M, Jelliti B, Jenzeri S. Emergent infectious uveitis. *Middle East Afr J Ophthalmol* 2009;**16**:225–38.

Merien F, Perolat P, Mancel E, et al. Detection of Leptospira DNA by polymerase chain reaction in aqueous humor of a patient with unilateral uveitis. *J Infect Dis* 1993;**168**:1335–6.

Mikkila HO, Seppala IJ, Leirisalo-Repo M, et al. The etiology of uveitis: the role of infections with special reference to Lyme borreliosis. *Acta Ophthalmol Scand* 1997;**75**:716–9.

Mikkila HO, Seppala IJ, Viljanen MK, et al. The expanding clinical spectrum of ocular Lyme borreliosis. *Ophthalmology* 2000;**107**:581–7.

Nepal BP, Shrestha UD. Ocular findings in leprosy patients in Nepal in the era of multidrug therapy. *Am J Ophthalmol* 2004;**137**:888–92.

Ortega-Larrocea G, Bobbadilla-del-Valle M, Ponce-de-Leon A, et al. Nested polymerase chain reaction for mycobacterium tuberculosis DNA detection in aqueous and vitreous of patients with uveitis. *Arch Med Res* 2003;**34**: 116–q9.

Pappachan JM, Mathew S, Thomas B, et al. The incidence and clinical characteristics of the immune phase eye disease in treated cases of leptospirosis. *Indian J Med Sci* 2007;**61**:441–7.

Rao NA, Saraswathy S, Smith RE. Tuberculous uveitis: distribution of *Mycobacterium tuberculosis* in the retinal pigment epithelium. *Arch Ophthalmol* 2006;**124**:1777–9.

Ratnam S. The laboratory diagnosis of syphilis. *Can J Infect Dis Med Microbiol* 2005;**16**:45–51.

Sanghvi C, Bell C, Woodhead M, Hardy C, Jones NP. Presumed tuberculous uveitis: diagnosis, management and outcome. *Eye* 2011;**25**:475–80.

Shankar K, Gyanendra L, Hari S, Narayan SD. Culture proven endogenous bacterial endophthalmitis in apparently healthy individuals. *Ocul Immunol Inflamm* 2009;**17**:396–9.

Simms I, Fenton KA, Ashton M, et al. The re-emergence of syphilis in the United Kingdom: the new epidemic phases. *Sex Transm Dis* 2005;**32**:220–6.

Song JH, Hong YT, Kwon OW. Acute syphilitic posterior placoid chorioretinitis following intravitreal triamcinolone acetonide injection. *Graefes Arch Clin Exp Ophthalmol* 2008;**246**:1775–8.

Steere AC, McHugh G, Damle N, et al. Prospective study of serologic tests for Lyme disease. *Clin Infect Dis* 2008;**47**:188–95 .

Suhler EB, Lauer AK, Rosenbaum JT. Prevalence of serologic evidence of cat scratch disease in patients with neuroretinitis. *Ophthalmology* 2000;**107**: 871–6.

Sungur GK, Hazirolan D, Gurbuz Y, et al. Ocular involvement in brucellosis. *Can J Ophthalmol* 2009;44:598–601.

Tinley C, Van Zyl L, Grotte R. Poststreptococcal syndrome uveitis in South African children. *Br J Ophthalmol* 2011;Epub.

Tucker JD, Li JZ, Robbins GK, et al. Ocular syphilis among HIV-infected patients: a systematic analysis of the literature. *Sex Transm Infect* 2011;**87**:4–8.

Vermeulen MJ, Herremans M, Verbakel H, et al. Serological testing for Bartonella henselae infections in the Netherlands: clinical evaluation of immunofluorescence assay and ELISA. *Clin Microbiol Infect* 2007;**13**:627–34.

Wickremasinghe S, Ling C, Stawell R, et al. Syphilitic punctate inner retinitis in immunocompetent gay men. *Ophthalmology* 2009;**116**:1195–200.

Wroblewski KJ, Hidayat AA, Neafie RC, et al. Ocular tuberculosis: a clinicopathologic and molecular study. *Ophthalmology* 2011;**118**:772–7.

Chapter 11 Viral infection

The viruses are transmissible agents ranging from 20 nm to 250 nm in size, having a variable structure with some consistent features. The DNA or RNA genome may be single or double stranded, and is contained and protected within the proteinaceous capsid, the shape of which usually has geometric symmetry. This layer offers some protection against temperature and pH changes. Some virions also have a lipoprotein envelope, acquired by budding from the host cell membrane but incorporating viral elements that assist adhesion to, and penetration of, other host cells.

The classification of viruses is a source of regular discussion and change. Taxonomic methods use DNA versus RNA core, shape, symmetry, main host target, vectors and methods of replication, and are used side by side by different expert groups. The complexity is therefore daunting to the clinician. The International Committee on the Taxonomy of Viruses is attempting to bring cohesion to this difficult area. Except where generic structure or function is important to the ophthalmologist, viruses are discussed here as species, their higher groupings being mentioned only where necessary.

There are reports of intraocular inflammation occurring in virtually every human pathogenic virus. However, overwhelmingly in the field of uveitis it is the DNA herpesviruses that are most important, both numerically and in potential severity. The human herpesviruses (HHVs) include herpes simplex virus type 1 (HSV-1, also known as HHV-1), herpes simplex virus type 2 (HSV-2, HHV-2), varicella-zoster virus (VZV, HHV-3), Epstein–Barr virus (EBV, HHV-4) and cytomegalovirus (CMV, HHV-5). These are the only DNA viruses with high importance to the ophthalmologist. Of the RNA viruses, the picornaviruses (Coxsackievirus), togaviruses (rubella virus), flaviviruses (dengue fever, West Nile virus), paramyxoviruses (mumps virus, measles virus) and retroviruses including HTLV-I and HIV are also important. The occurrence of uveitis as a side issue in viral illnesses with high mortality, including rabies and Ebola fever, is not discussed here. The behavior of viruses characteristically evolves by mutation so that new and changing diseases affect humans with each passing decade. The emergence of West Nile virus is important, and this and other viral forms of uveitis are discussed here.

Viral intraocular inflammation may have protean manifestations, but there are certain general trends. The herpesviruses are overwhelmingly the most common cause of viral uveitis and retinitis. Primary infection may be asymptomatic, or cause a cutaneous blistering disease or an infectious mononucleosis. Herpesviruses then become permanently resident in latent form and may cause recurrent disease, either predominantly in the anterior segment, such as herpes simplex keratouveitis and zoster uveitis, or in the retina, the latter being a greater risk in immunodeficient individuals and probably also in those with a genetic predisposition.

All the DNA herpesviruses have, with greater or lesser frequency, been associated with retinitis. The vocabulary of such pathology has been confusing and sometimes misleading, partly because of an inconsistency of terminology, partly because the viruses responsible for some forms of retinitis have only recently been identified. Retinitis caused by herpesviruses may occur in both immunocompetent and immunodeficient individuals but the clinical presentation will vary depending on immune status. The immunocompetent patient developing zoster herpetic retinitis usually presents with acute retinal necrosis (ARN), whereas the grossly immunodeficient patient will develop progressive outer retinal necrosis (PORN). There are intermediate and variable forms so that the wider term of 'necrotizing herpetic retinopathy' has been introduced. For this chapter it is felt most useful to consider recognized syndromes separately even though there may be clinical overlap. First the common and well-recognized HSV and VZV uveitis is discussed, followed by ARN which is the usual presentation of necrotizing retinitis in immunocompetent individuals. The human immunodeficiency virus (HIV) is then be inserted to introduce immunodeficiency, followed by those syndromes most important in this group: CMV retinitis and PORN. Other, mostly RNA viruses also important in human uveitis are discussed at the end.

HERPES SIMPLEX UVEITIS AND KERATOUVEITIS (box 11.1)

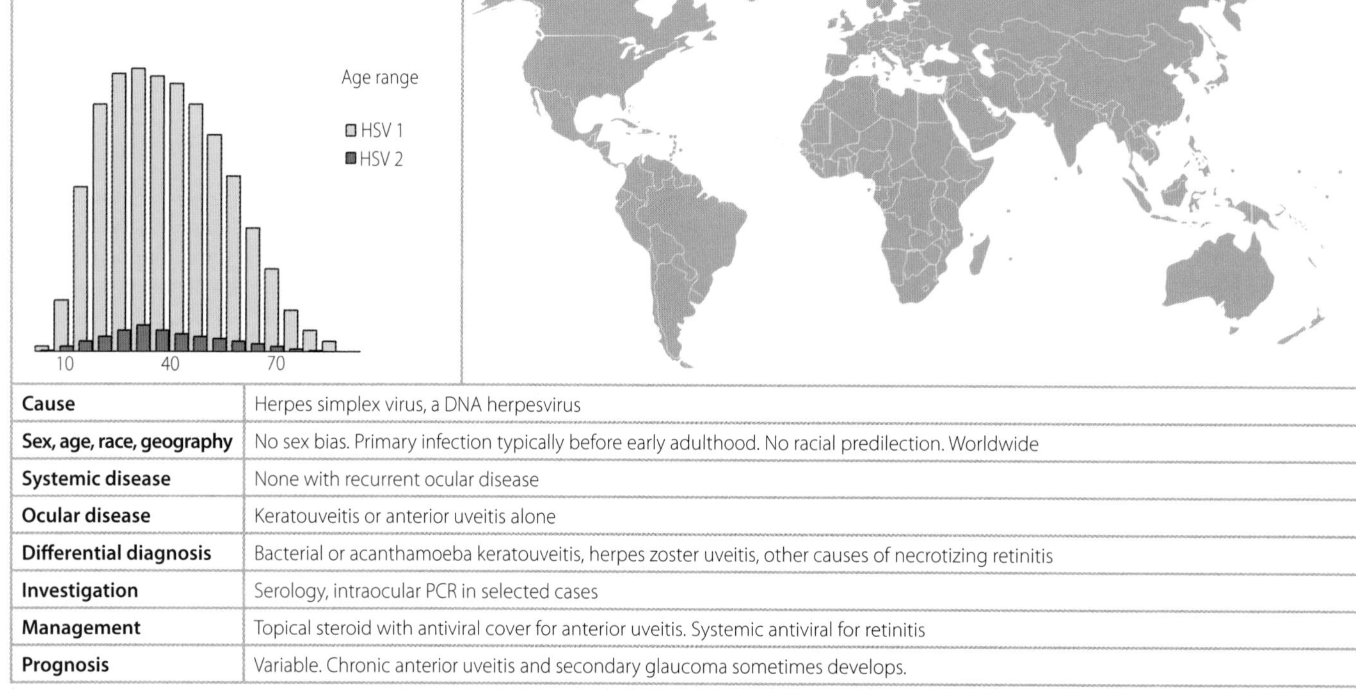

Cause	Herpes simplex virus, a DNA herpesvirus
Sex, age, race, geography	No sex bias. Primary infection typically before early adulthood. No racial predilection. Worldwide
Systemic disease	None with recurrent ocular disease
Ocular disease	Keratouveitis or anterior uveitis alone
Differential diagnosis	Bacterial or acanthamoeba keratouveitis, herpes zoster uveitis, other causes of necrotizing retinitis
Investigation	Serology, intraocular PCR in selected cases
Management	Topical steroid with antiviral cover for anterior uveitis. Systemic antiviral for retinitis
Prognosis	Variable. Chronic anterior uveitis and secondary glaucoma sometimes develops.

Box 11.1 Herpes simplex uveitis and keratouveitis

Introduction

Herpes simplex virus is a DNA virus comprising an icosahedral capsid surrounded by a spiked lipid envelope (**Fig. 11.1**). It is an obligate human parasite in two forms, HSV-1 being much more commonly responsible for ocular infection, and HSV-2 more commonly responsible for genital herpes. Infection is by direct contact with infected secretions and over 80% are asymptomatic. In others a blistering mucocutaneous eruption occurs which heals within 2 weeks. Latent virus resides in affected areas including regional nerves, frequently in the trigeminal ganglion. Recurrent corneal epithelial disease is typical, at which time virus is shed and may infect others. Although both types 1 and 2 may infect either oral or genital sites, oral recurrences are much more common if HSV-1 is involved and genital if HSV-2 is responsible. Population prevalence has decreased in high socioeconomic groups over the past 40 years, although infection by the virus remains extremely common.

Systemic disease

Congenital infection is fortunately very uncommon, but usually involves HSV-2 acquired during birth. Dermatological manifestations may resemble adult disease, but encephalitis in this group, presenting with neurological signs, fits and pyrexia, is usual and serious; untreated disease may progress to multiorgan dissemination and fatality.

If the primary infection is oral and (in a minority) symptomatic, pyrexia and pharyngitis are usual. Painful vesicular lesions may appear in the oral mucosa, and uncommonly a severe ulcerative gingivostomatitis may ensue. Future perioral recurrences (cold sores) affect a third of seropositive individuals, triggers including sunlight, stress, pyrexia and menstruation. Rarely, primary infection in the adult leads to severe disease. This may include disseminated infection with encephalitis. Immunosuppressed individuals are more at risk, but overall more cases occur in immunocompetent individuals. Systemic manifestations are not seen with recurrent HSV keratouveitis.

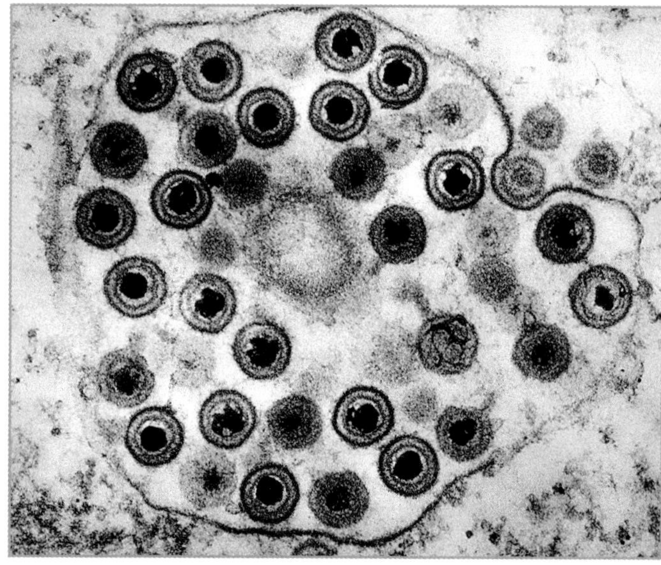

Figure 11.1 A cluster of herpes simplex virions. (Modified from Centers for Disease Control, Public Health Image Library.)

Ocular disease

Primary infection may involve the eye, in which case unilateral follicular conjunctivitis or vesicular blepharitis is seen. Corneal ulceration is unusual at this stage. However, the dendritic epithelial keratitis typical of subsequent recurrent HSV infection (**Fig. 11.2**) is well known to ophthalmologists. Despite this familiarity the diagnosis should always be confirmed during the first clinical attack by conjunctival swabs.

Herpetic keratouveitis or uveitis is almost always unilateral. Stromal disciform keratitis (**Fig. 11.3**) may accompany, or occur independently of, recurrent epithelial keratitis. There is usually a mild uveitis, but commonly a group of large keratic precipitates (KPs) is clustered behind the affected area of cornea (**Fig. 11.4**). Sometimes a severe uveitis ensues, characteristically painful and causing extreme photophobia and marked ciliary injection. There are usually myriad fine KPs but occasionally a granulomatous appearance. Posterior synechiae may occur, and there is a high incidence of acute secondary glaucoma, probably as a result of trabeculitis. Rubeosis may develop. Sectoral iris atrophy with transillumination is historically considered typical of VZV uveitis, but molecular methods have increasingly found evidence of HSV in affected eyes with no evidence of past or present keratitis, and it is clear that HSV is also capable of such damage (**Fig. 11.5**).

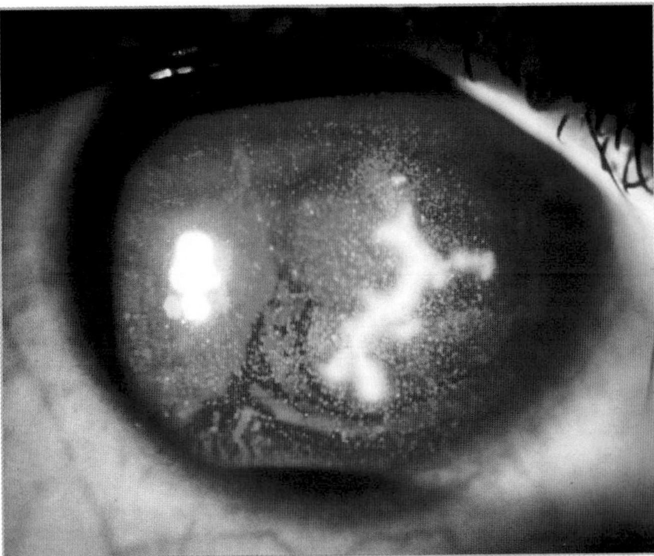

Figure 11.2 Typical herpes simplex keratitis showing a fluorescein-stained dendritic corneal ulcer.

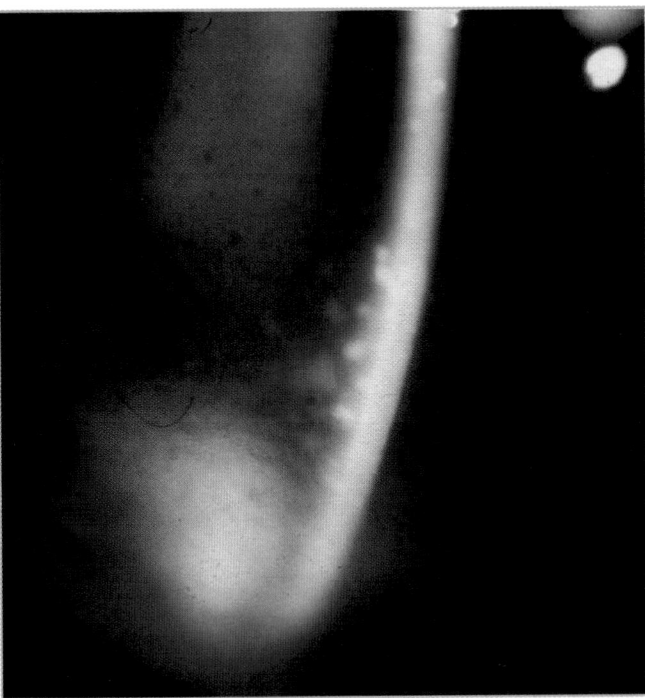

Figure 11.4 A cluster of large keratic precipitates is grouped under an area of active herpetic stromal keratitis.

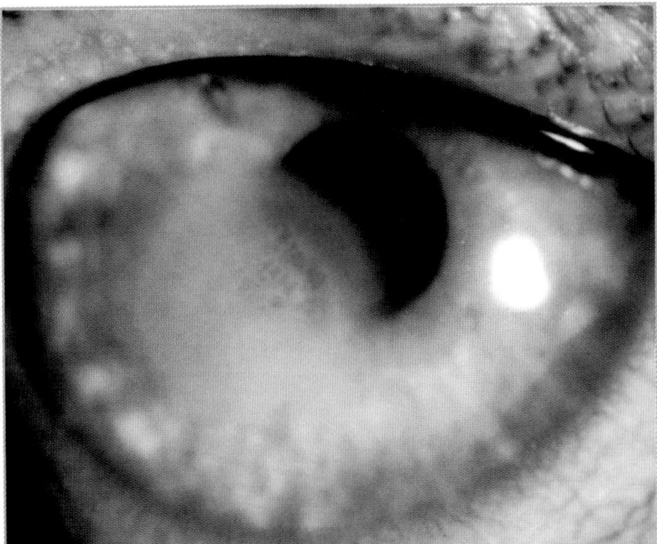

Figure 11.3 Herpetic stromal disciform keratitis.

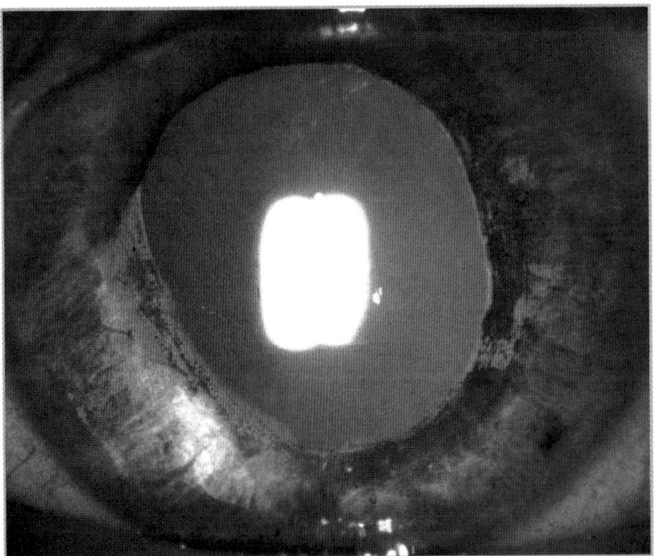

Figure 11.5 Widespread sectoral iris transillumination in chronic herpes simplex uveitis.

A proportion of patients go on to develop permanent and severe fixed mydriasis. In some cases evidence of stromal scarring supports the diagnosis, but in others such evidence is lacking. Corneal hypoesthesia is a sign supportive, but by no means diagnostic, of previous herpetic involvement. It has become clear that HSV-associated anterior uveitis can occur without corneal involvement (van der Lelij et al. 2000). In chronic uveitis, secondary glaucoma is quite common and may affect more than half of patients (Miserocchi et al. 2002). The virus has been isolated from aqueous humor but it is unclear whether the uveitis represents direct uveal invasion, or a secondary immune response. Retinitis caused by HSV is discussed with acute retinal necrosis.

Diagnosis

Where past or present corneal involvement is seen, the clinical diagnosis of HSV-associated keratouveitis is usually straightforward. The confirmation of HSV infection in epithelial keratitis will serve as a future marker in patients who subsequently present again with a less clear diagnostic picture. As HSV serology is very commonly positive in the general population, positivity is never diagnostic for HSV-associated uveitis. However, negativity can be helpful and, as both VZV and CMV are known to cause a similar clinical picture, serology for all herpesviruses may be useful in differential diagnosis. In some cases aqueous humor has been tapped and polymerase chain reaction (PCR) techniques have identified HSV DNA. The pathogenic association in these cases is unproven.

Management

The management of stromal keratouveitis is more generally agreed than that of uveitis alone. Most ophthalmologists will use topical steroid for stromal keratouveitis in combination with a course of oral aciclovir or valaciclovir. Those attacks that are self-limiting will leave no residual uveitis and require no long-term treatment. However, for those with frequent recurrences or in those with accumulating corneal scarring, the long-term prescription of maintenance aciclovir 400 mg twice daily is increasingly used, with mixed evidence as to efficacy. For those with HSV-associated uveitis without corneal involvement, with rare exceptions lifelong topical steroid treatment is necessary. There is a huge variation in the dosage required to maintain quiescence, varying from four time daily Pred Forte to once-weekly prednisolone 0.5%. In such cases, after some months or years an overenthusiastic trainee or a bored patient will attempt discontinuation of treatment. Within days or weeks a recurrence will reliably appear, in some cases of a high severity, requiring intensive treatment that will take months to titrate downwards to the previous maintenance dose. Hopefully the lesson will have been learned. Very occasionally cessation of treatment is possible but only in a small minority. Those on long-term topical steroid rarely develop recurrent corneal epithelial ulceration, but such cases require an urgent high-dose oral antiviral. Much discussion has centered around the usefulness of systemic antiviral treatment for those with chronic HSV-associated anterior uveitis. No firm evidence of efficacy has been demonstrated and treatment does not permit the cessation of topical steroid.

HERPES ZOSTER OPHTHALMICUS (box 11.2)

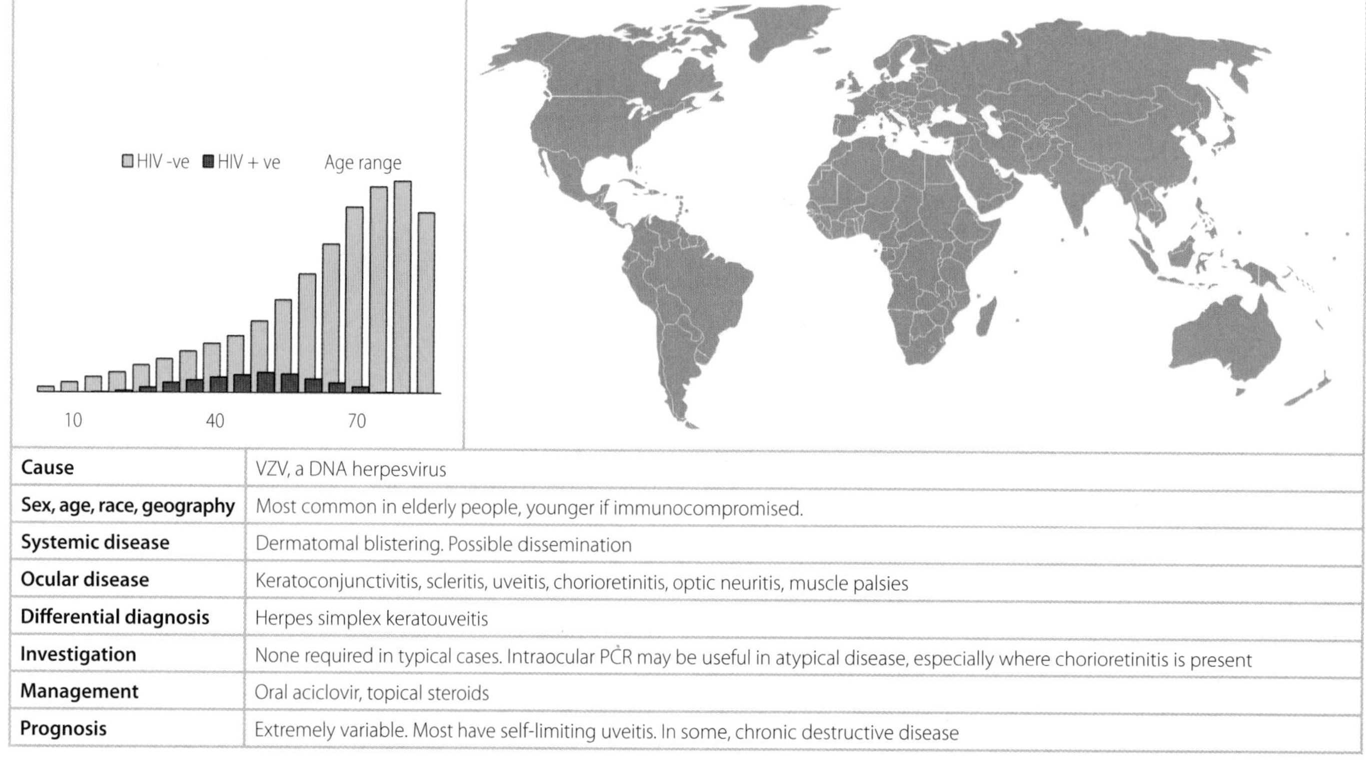

Cause	VZV, a DNA herpesvirus
Sex, age, race, geography	Most common in elderly people, younger if immunocompromised.
Systemic disease	Dermatomal blistering. Possible dissemination
Ocular disease	Keratoconjunctivitis, scleritis, uveitis, chorioretinitis, optic neuritis, muscle palsies
Differential diagnosis	Herpes simplex keratouveitis
Investigation	None required in typical cases. Intraocular PCR may be useful in atypical disease, especially where chorioretinitis is present
Management	Oral aciclovir, topical steroids
Prognosis	Extremely variable. Most have self-limiting uveitis. In some, chronic destructive disease

Box 11.2 Herpes zoster ophthalmicus

Introduction

Varicella-zoster virus (VZV, HHV-3) is a DNA herpesvirus, sharing the familial features of an icosahedral core and lipid envelope. The virus is transmitted by inhalation of droplets. Primary infection may be asymptomatic but usually leads to generalized vesiculopustular varicella. During primary infection the virus migrates up sensory axons and becomes latent within dorsal root and cranial nerve sensory ganglia, but more commonly within the trigeminal ganglion than at any other site. Shingles may occur due to reactivation of latent virus, or also after reinfection from a contact with either varicella or shingles. There is evidence that reactivation within sensory ganglia is actually quite frequent but that intact cell-mediated immunity aborts the majority of such events, which therefore pass without symptoms. More substantial reactivation leads to an acute inflammation of the sensory ganglion, which is followed by both centrifugal and centripetal spread of the virus, the former down sensory axons to lead to cutaneous dermatomal infection, the latter down the sensory root to damage the sensory nucleus.

A VZV live-attenuated vaccine has been undergoing trials for some years. It provides substantial protection against varicella. Immunization is now routine in some countries including the USA where it is also offered to the over-60s. Varicella is occasionally severe and rarely lethal and these cases are substantially reduced by immunization. However, the phenomenon of immune boosting of adults previously VZV infected by occasional exposure to children or others with varicella is known to protect against future shingles; the removal of such boosting by immunization may increase the zoster rate for several decades. These conflicting facts have led other countries including the UK to decide not to aim for population immunization.

Systemic disease

Reactivation of latent VZV within sensory ganglia to cause the typical dermatomal involvement known as shingles is common. Its incidence increases with age and with immunodeficiency, in which it tends to occur younger and sometimes on several occasions. Up to a quarter of all cases of shingles involve all or part of the ophthalmic division of the trigeminal nerve which is therefore the most commonly affected, but involvement of maxillary or mandibular divisions is much less common.

In herpes zoster ophthalmicus (HZO) symptoms usually precede the development of cutaneous signs. An unpleasant burning cutaneous discomfort, paraesthesiae and hyperesthesia may precede the development of rash by several days. The rash usually starts with erythema, on which blisters appear within 2 or 3 days (**Fig. 11.6**). The severity of this blistering eruption varies markedly, as does the level of associated pain that at worst may be disabling. During the stage of erythema and blistering the patient is highly contagious. Within 2 weeks, discharge and crusting of the lesions occur, gradual resolution leading to a variable degree of cutaneous scarring and hair loss. Permanent cutaneous sensation changes are usual, ranging from mild numbness to a debilitating and depressing postherpetic neuralgia.

Although intraocular inflammation is considered to be a particular risk when the cutaneous distribution of the nasociliary branch of the ophthalmic division is involved (**Fig. 11.7**), involvement is common in any case, occurring in half the affected cases, and ophthalmological examination should be part of the management of every patient with HZO.

Disseminated VZV infection may occur during an episode of shingles. In immunocompetent individuals, such signs are usually mild, with a few scattered varicelliform vesicles. In the severely immunocompromised or immunosuppressed individual, dissemination is more likely and is sometimes fatal. Recurrent shingles is most unusual in immunocompetent individuals, but may be troublesome in AIDS patients, as may the involvement of multiple dermatomes in a single attack.

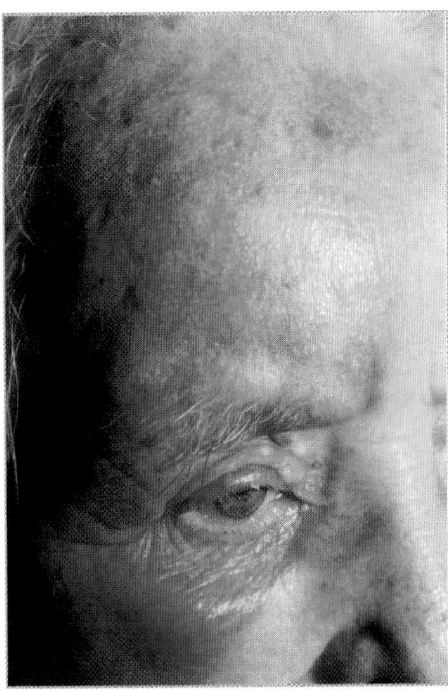

Figure 11.6 Early shingles shows erythema occupying the ophthalmic division of the trigeminal nerve. A few blisters are starting and the rash is already causing substantial pain.

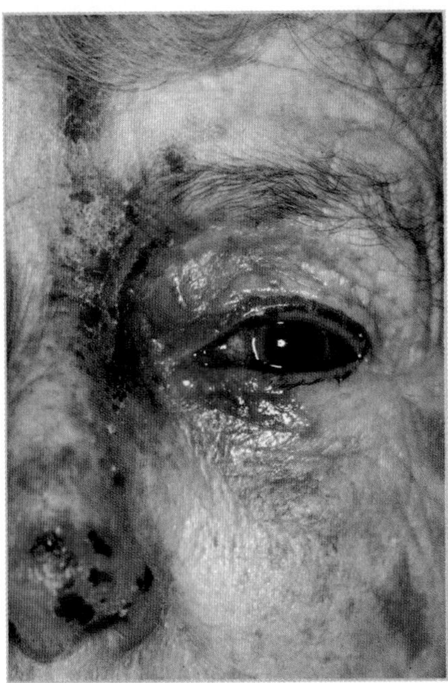

Figure 11.7 The involvement of the external nasal cutaneous branch of the nasociliary nerve is well defined here, together with keratouveitis which is most common when this nerve is inflamed.

Ocular disease

Conjunctivitis and blepharitis are common accompaniments to HZO, as is microdendritic or punctate keratitis (**Fig. 11.8**). Episcleritis is common and scleritis rare. Uveitis may start early or may be delayed by 1 week or more. Mild self-limiting uveitis is usual, but a minority

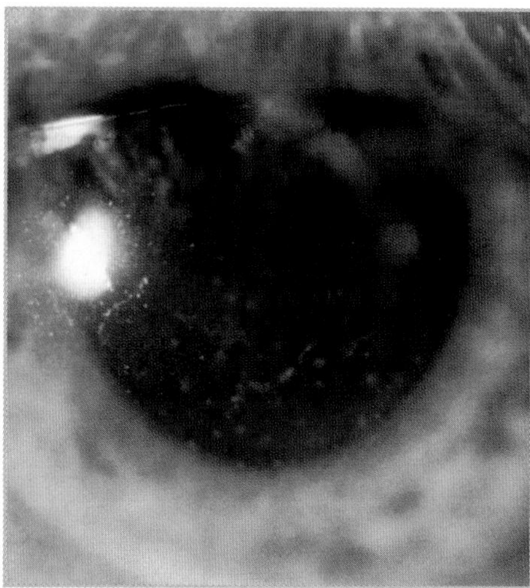

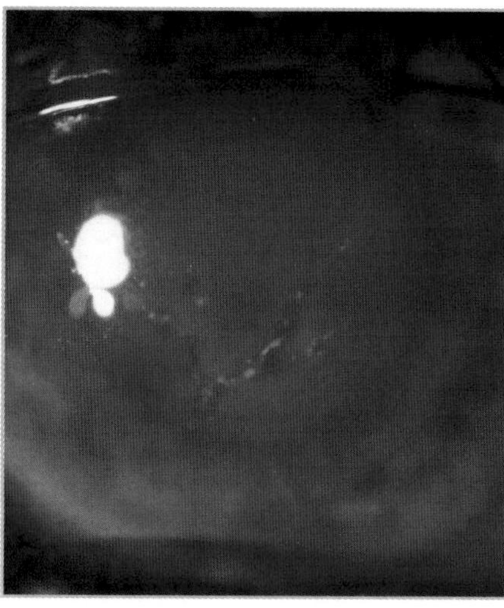

Figure 11.8 Microdendritic keratitis during ophthalmic shingles, under direct and blue illumination. (Courtesy of Mr AB Tullo.)

of patients develops severe uveitis with large KPs and posterior synechiae. Hypopyon may be seen, and if present is often associated with hyphema. The inflammation is essentially a vasculitic process, and it is now considered that ischemic changes contribute to the severity of the uveitis. Rarely, ischemic anterior segment necrosis may supervene. Glaucoma occurs in a significant minority and may be very troublesome, usually being caused by a trabeculitis. In the most severely inflamed eyes, phthisis may ensue. In general uveitis of any degree of severity is a marker of visual loss in those with HZO (Nithyanandam et al. 2010). Shingles without skin rash ('zoster sine herpete') is well described and can involve the ophthalmic nerve. Zoster DNA has been isolated from aqueous humor in these cases (Kido et al. 2008) and the degree of iris damage seems to correlate with viral load. In patients presenting with uveitis and raised intraocular pressure, with either retrobulbar pain or ophthalmic dermatomal symptoms but no skin signs, zoster sine herpete should always be considered and empirical antiviral treatment is reasonable.

Posterior segment involvement during HZO is very uncommon but may include zonal necrotizing retinitis, occlusive retinal arteriolitis (**Fig. 11.9**) or optic neuropathy. Extraocular muscle palsy or orbititis is very unusual. It is very unusual to develop necrotizing VZV retinitis during acute HZO, but it may follow soon after in a tiny minority, and this is discussed in the section on ARN below. A significant minority of patients, particularly those presenting with severe uveitis, goes on to develop chronic inflammation, possibly exacerbated by anterior segment ischemia. After a time, sectoral iris atrophy and denervation may develop in about 20%, causing corectopia and transillumination (**Fig. 11.10**). In this group glaucoma is common and cataract often develops. Lifelong topical steroid is likely to be necessary.

Diagnosis

The clinical diagnosis of typical HZO is straightforward. Occasionally, especially in young patients, the cutaneous manifestations are so mild and scattered within the dermatome that primary herpes simplex infection is considered. Uveitis is rare in primary simplex infection. As shingles is a marker for AIDS, HIV testing should be considered in a patient within a risk group, especially with severe, disseminated or recurrent zoster. PCR can be used if necessary on

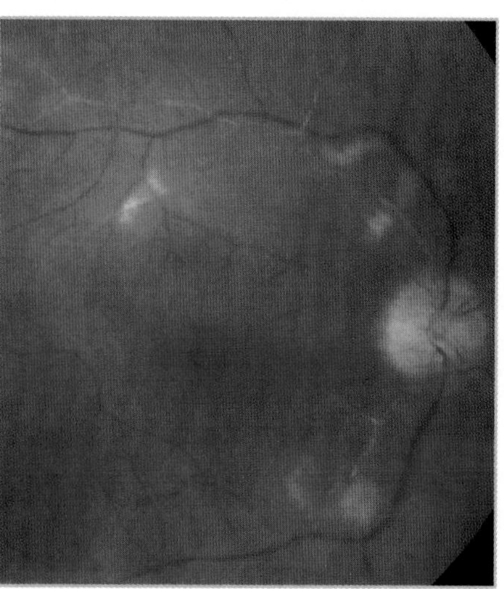

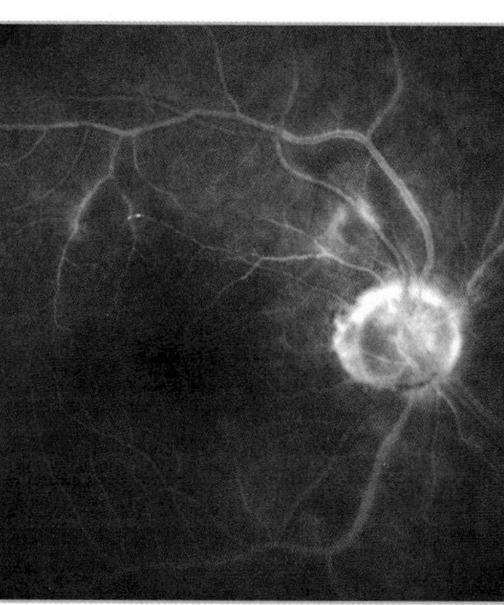

Figure 11.9 Occlusive retinal arteriolitis during acute ophthalmic zoster. Arteriolar attenuation and occlusion, with cotton-wool spots, can be seen.

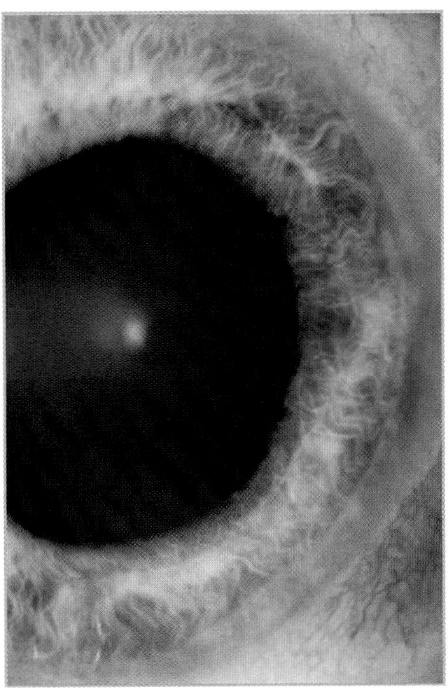

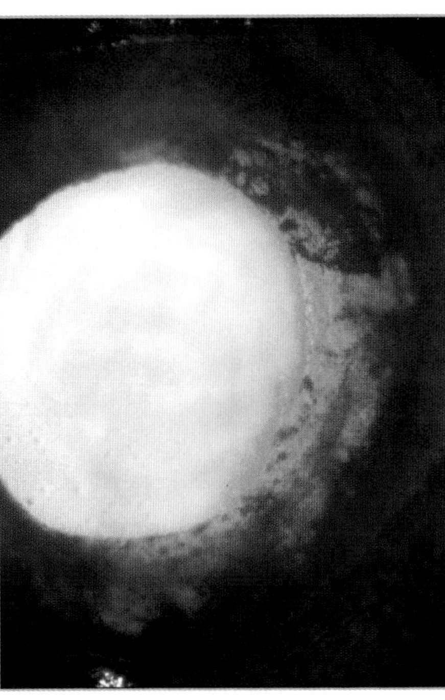

Figure 11.10 Iris atrophy with an irregular pupil and transillumination in chronic VZV anterior uveitis.

cutaneous blisters and, in cases of uveitis without clear diagnosis, aqueous PCR is also useful. An attack of herpes zoster in any dermatome affects about 5% of those seropositive for VZV at a median age of 64 years. About 5% of these will develop a second attack and it is recommended that this group be investigated for cellular immune deficiency.

Management

The evidence base for the management of zoster in general has been recently reviewed (Dworkin et al. 2007). Oral antiviral treatment commencing as early as possible after the diagnosis of HZO (within 3 days at most of the appearance of the rash) has been shown to have a beneficial effect in reducing acute pain and rash duration; the probability of and duration of postherpetic neuralgia is also reduced by a modest amount. Aciclovir 800 mg five times a day for 7–10 days was the first drug so used; the prodrug valaciclovir (1 g three times daily for 7 days) has similar, possibly slightly superior, action but less frequent administration; famciclovir (250–500 mg three times daily for 7 days) may share that benefit and both of these achieve higher serum levels. All of these drugs are in general well tolerated, a minority developing nausea and headache. Dosages should be reduced in renal failure. The usefulness of oral steroid during acute zoster has been debated; a Cochrane review found no evidence that it prevented postherpetic neuralgia (Chen et al. 2010) but it may contribute to acute pain reduction.

Analgesia during acute HZO is frequently necessary, especially in the over-50s. Simple non-steroidal analgesia may suffice but in more severe cases gabapentin or opiates may be necessary. Capsaicin cream may be administered to the skin after the blistering phase. The effectiveness of carbamazepine, or amitriptyline and other antidepressants, is unproven. In severe and chronic cases transcutaneous electrical nerve stimulation (TENS) or rhizotomy may be used. The management of zoster in immunodeficient patients may be difficult. Aciclovir resistance is possible and supplementary treatment with intravenous foscarnet or cidofovir may be necessary.

When treating acute HZO with an oral antiviral, topical antivirals add nothing. Those with epithelial disruption should receive topical antibiotic prophylaxis to prevent superinfection. Early reports suggested that, for those with associated uveitis, topical steroid usage in the early stage was detrimental in prolonging inflammation; evidence for this view has not been forthcoming. Zoster uveitis undoubtedly responds to topical steroid treatment and in the acute phase severe inflammation mandates intensive treatment. Worsening of microdendritic keratitis does not appear to be a risk. Very severe uveitis, possibly including anterior segment ischemia, may justify oral steroid treatment. As for herpes simplex uveitis, the inflammation may become chronic or relapsing and may require a variable topical steroid dose to control it, sometimes as little as one drop of weak steroid per week. A significant minority needs lifelong topical steroid treatment.

ACUTE RETINAL NECROSIS (box 11.3)

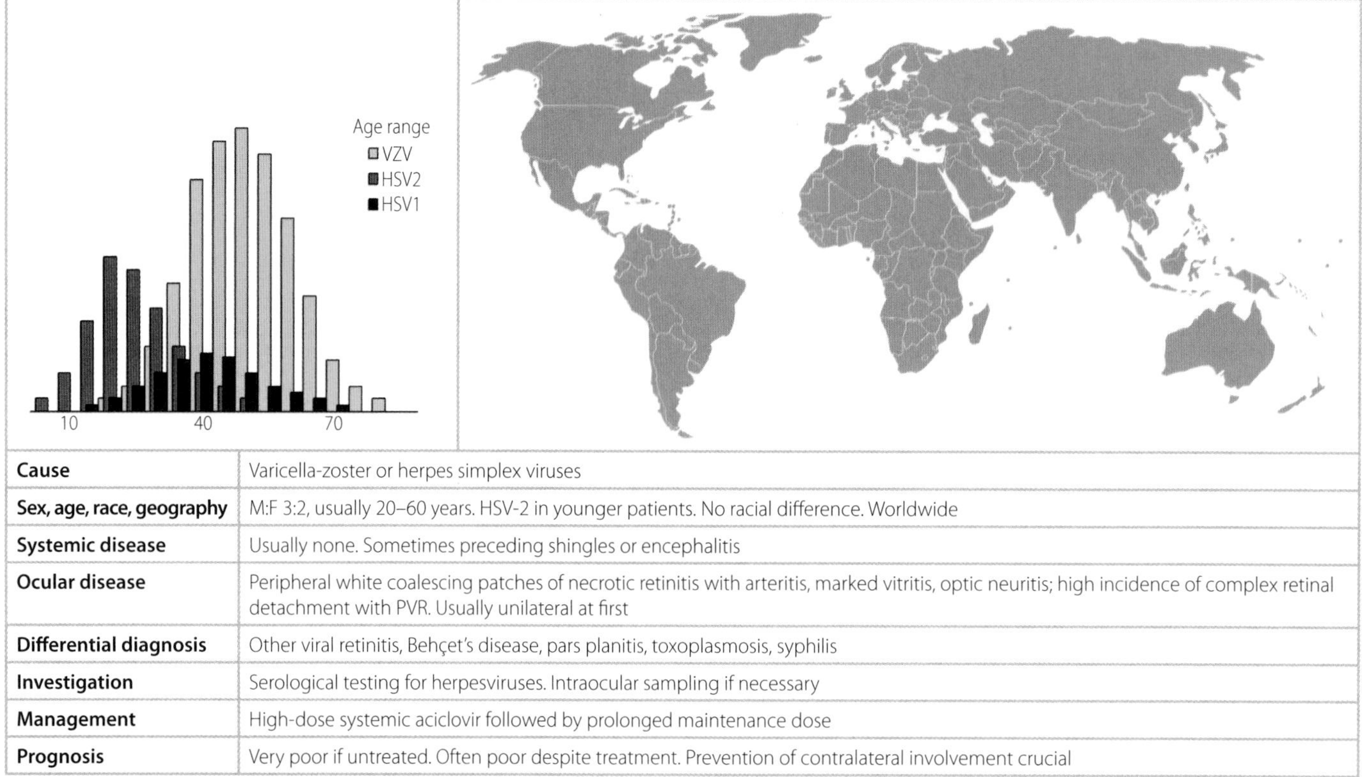

Cause	Varicella-zoster or herpes simplex viruses
Sex, age, race, geography	M:F 3:2, usually 20–60 years. HSV-2 in younger patients. No racial difference. Worldwide
Systemic disease	Usually none. Sometimes preceding shingles or encephalitis
Ocular disease	Peripheral white coalescing patches of necrotic retinitis with arteritis, marked vitritis, optic neuritis; high incidence of complex retinal detachment with PVR. Usually unilateral at first
Differential diagnosis	Other viral retinitis, Behçet's disease, pars planitis, toxoplasmosis, syphilis
Investigation	Serological testing for herpesviruses. Intraocular sampling if necessary
Management	High-dose systemic aciclovir followed by prolonged maintenance dose
Prognosis	Very poor if untreated. Often poor despite treatment. Prevention of contralateral involvement crucial

Box 11.3 Acute retinal necrosis

Introduction

The first description of the rare, aggressive retinal infection now known as acute retinal necrosis (ARN) is 40 years old (Urayama et al. 1971), and the disease is presumed to be new; there are no convincing earlier reports of this characteristic and destructive retinopathy. It is now known that VZV is the causative agent in about half the patients, HSV-2 in about 30%, (especially in children and young adults), HSV-1 in about 15% and CMV in about 5%. The latter diagnosis is largely descriptive - CMV has a greater tendency to cause a rather specific form of necrotizing retinitis that is different in presentation to ARN and the above statistic is probably a diagnostic overlap phenomenon. It is presumed that reactivation of latent virus, rather than new infection, is responsible for most cases of ARN.

A slight male preponderance has been noted, but no racial preference has been identified. Most affected patients are between 20 and 60 years of age and the bimodal age distribution, with peaks at around 20 and 50 years, reflects the peak incidences of HSV and VZV infection, respectively.

Systemic disease

Most patients have no concurrent systemic disease. However, about 40% of patients have had shingles within the previous year (in any dermatome). There is a significant association between HSV-induced ARN and meningoencephalitis (**Fig. 11.11**); some patients will give a history of undiagnosed or presumed viral encephalitis during the previous year; rarely the comatose patient regains consciousness to find severe visual loss. Retinal examination should be mandatory and urgent in any patient with undiagnosed meningoencephalopathy. Some patients will manifest signs of immune deficiency, such as chronic warts (**Fig. 11.12**) or recurrent infection, and all patients presenting with ARN should be investigated for cellular immune deficiency because this will modify long-term management.

Ocular disease

There is a spectrum of severity in ARN. Not all patients fulfill the characteristic appearances and the variability has led some to suggest the more generic term 'necrotizing herpetic retinopathy' to include the manifestations of both CMV retinopathy and outer retinal necrosis. However, the manifestations of typical disease within these well-described areas remain individually useful for diagnostic purposes and they are discussed separately here. Typical ARN will be presented first, followed by examples of variability.

Classic ARN is fortunately almost always unilateral at onset, but about a third of patients develop sequential involvement of the second eye if untreated, often after a delay of several weeks and, rarely, several years later. When severe it is a dramatic disease, presenting with visual loss that deteriorates over a period of days, which may be profoundly reduced at presentation and which is often painful. However, the onset may be more insidious with only minimal loss of acuity. Any patient presenting with an 'anterior' uveitis should have the fundus examined quickly to exclude posterior segment inflammation. Particular urgency should be given to those with visual loss or periocular pain inconsistent with anterior segment findings.

All patients will have anterior chamber inflammation, usually with KPs, which may be quite large. The intraocular pressure (IOP) is often

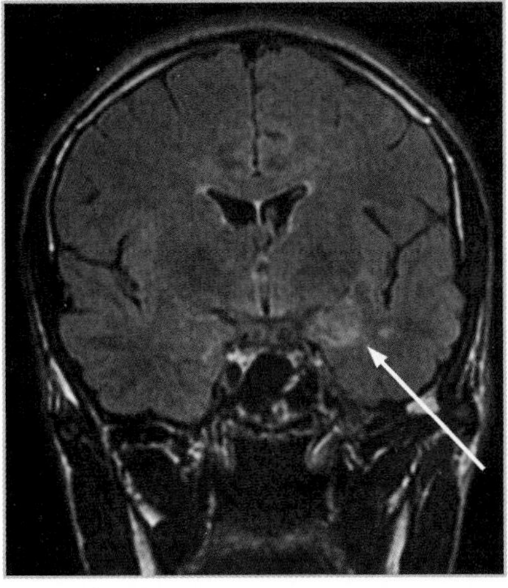
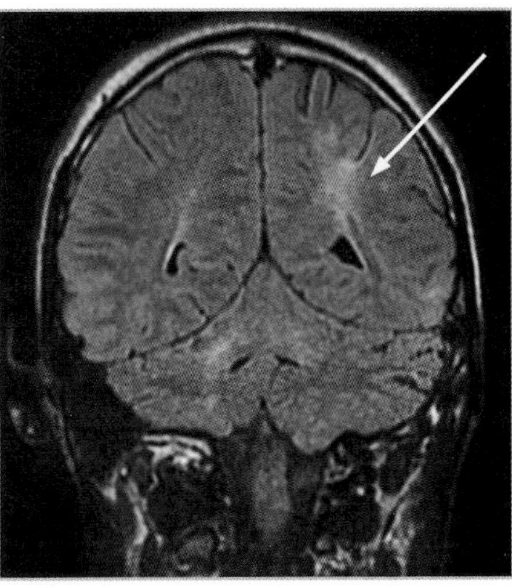

Figure 11.11 Foci of herpes simplex virus 2 encephalitis in a patient subsequently presenting with acute retinal necrosis.

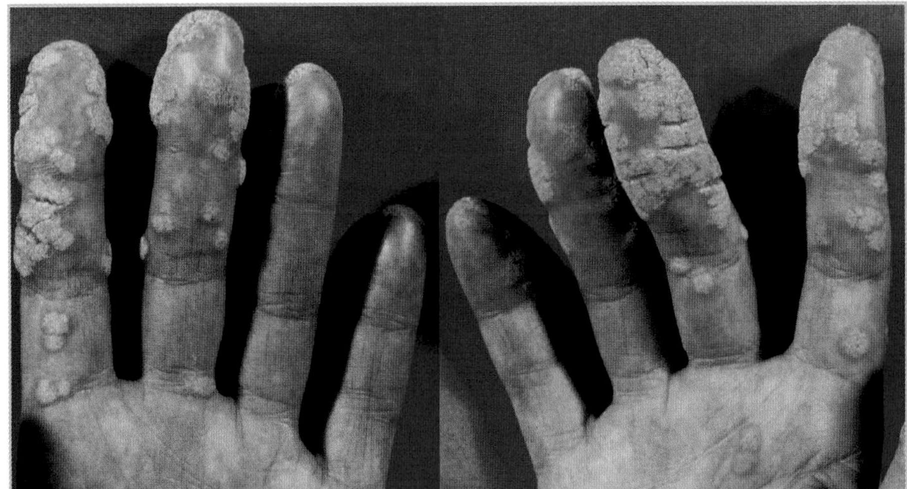

Figure 11.12 Chronic warts in a patient with immunodeficiency.

raised, in contrast to many eyes with anterior uveitis. Both ciliary injection and localized episcleritis may occur, and much less commonly scleritis is present, often posteriorly (**Fig. 11.13**). There may even be facial swelling. In immunocompetent individuals the cornea is normal, but evidence of viral keratitis may coexist if the patient is immunodeficient, and some of the latter group may have had recent ophthalmic shingles. Vitreous involvement is essential for the diagnosis of ARN. In the early stages this may be no more than moderate, but in late-presenting or progressive untreated disease it may be so marked that retinal visualization is difficult even with the indirect ophthalmoscope.

Necrotic peripheral retina is visible through hazy vitreous as a whitened area, usually showing a well-defined posterior border with normal retina (**Fig. 11.14**). These areas may initially be multifocal, but in time coalesce and become confluent circumferentially (**Fig. 11.15**), and progress posteriorly, often by focal extensions at the apex of which is usually a retinal arteriole (**Fig. 11.16**). An occlusive retinal vasculitis, predominantly an arteriolitis, is an important component of ARN, both within areas of necrotic retina and further posterior (**Fig. 11.17**), and there may be significant perivascular retinal hemorrhage (**Fig. 11.18**), which raises the possibility of CMV retinitis. However, the more aggressive behavior of ARN normally makes the diagnosis clear. Optic nerve head swelling and sometimes frank optic neuritis may be seen, as may secondary macular edema. Resolution of the retinitis leads to a reduction in retinal whitening and ultimately retinal pigment epithelium (RPE) scarring underlying previously inflamed areas, which become grossly atrophic and, similar to CMV retinitis, prone to multiple breaks, especially just anterior to the junction with normal retina. Retinal detachment is very common (**Fig. 11.19**), sometimes with multiple or large breaks, and proliferative vitreoretinopathy (PVR) often follows (**Fig. 11.20**). Herpes viral retinitis may present in unfamiliar patterns that do not fulfill the criteria of ARN. Retinitis may be patchy and not peripheral (**Fig. 11.21**), sometimes with multifocal satellite lesions (**Fig. 11.22**), or more hemorrhagic than usual.

Rare histopathology specimens reveal complete destruction of retinal architecture within necrotic areas, with widespread perivascular (particularly periarterial) inflammation, especially in the retina but also involving the choroid and sclera. The cell infiltrate is predominantly lymphoid. Electron microscopy may identify herpes virions within the retina. Broadly speaking, VZV-induced ARN is more severe than HSV ARN.

Diagnosis

The differential diagnosis of ARN may be challenging. Patients presenting with severe contiguous mutton-fat KPs will have a very poor fundal view, as will those with severe vitritis. The 'headlight in the fog' appearance will raise the possibility of toxoplasmosis and this is probably the most important differential diagnosis (Balansard et al. 2005). A high degree of suspicion and early re-examination is

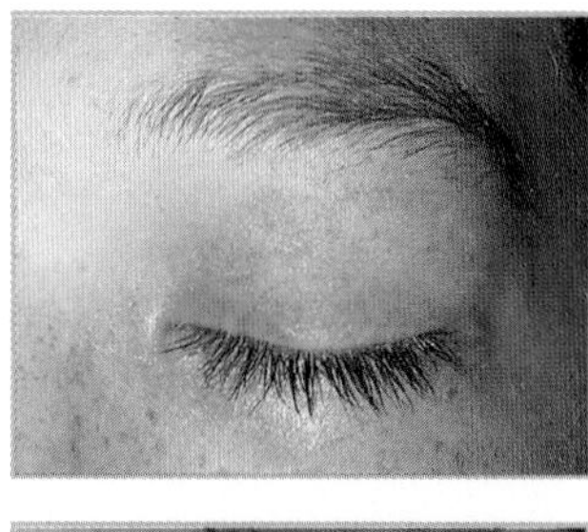

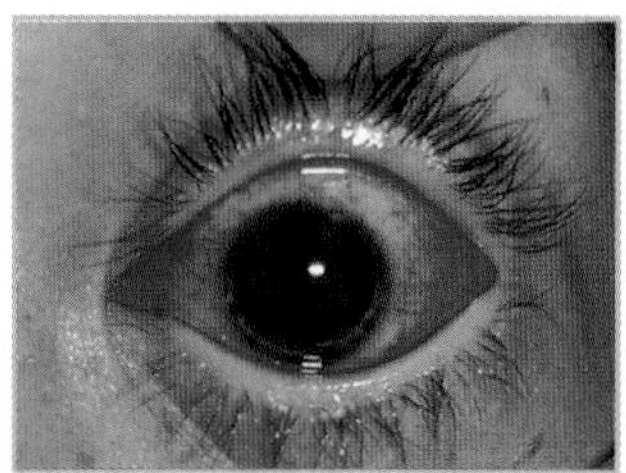

Figure 11.13 A teenager presenting with unilateral periocular pain and swelling with visual loss exhibits posterior scleritis and acute retinal necrosis.

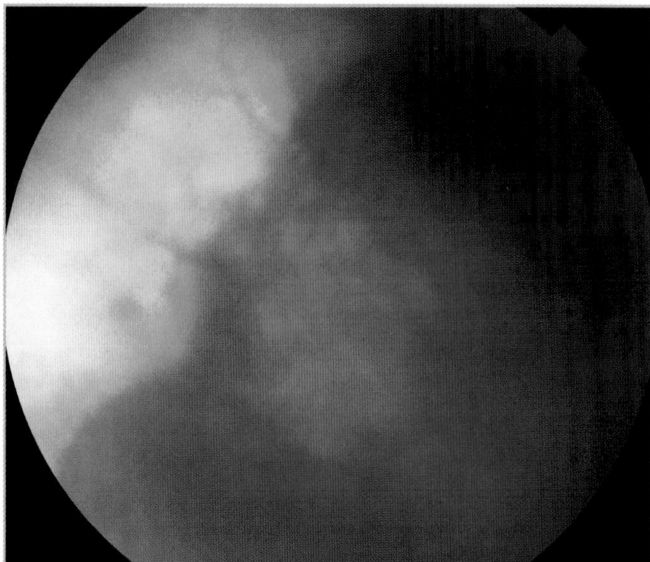

Figure 11.14 A large area of necrotizing retinitis is seen through hazy vitreous. There is nevertheless a well-defined posterior border.

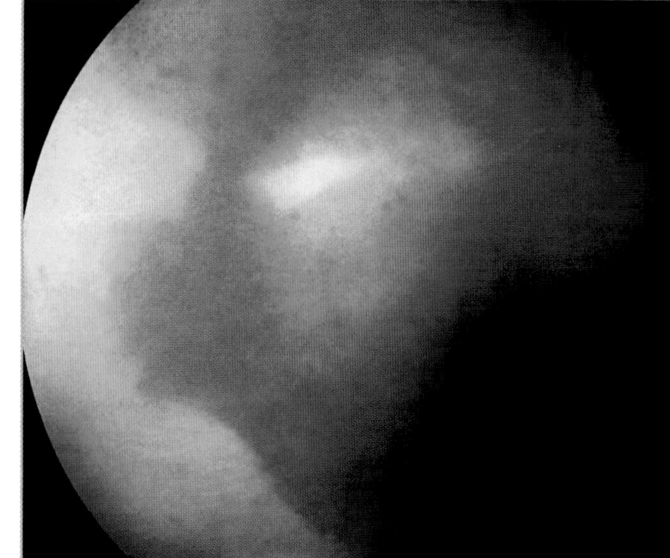

Figure 11.16 A posterior extension of retinitis follows the line of a retinal arteriole, occluded.

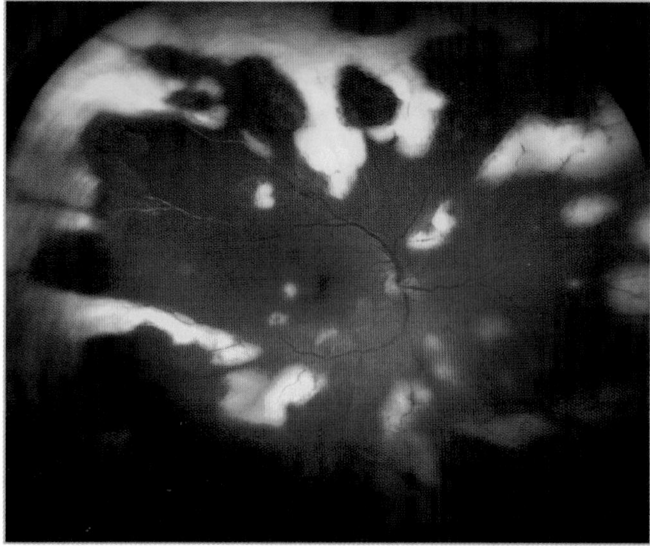

Figure 11.15 Wide-field photography of circumferential acute retinal necrosis with multiple posterior extensions and occlusive arteriolitis.

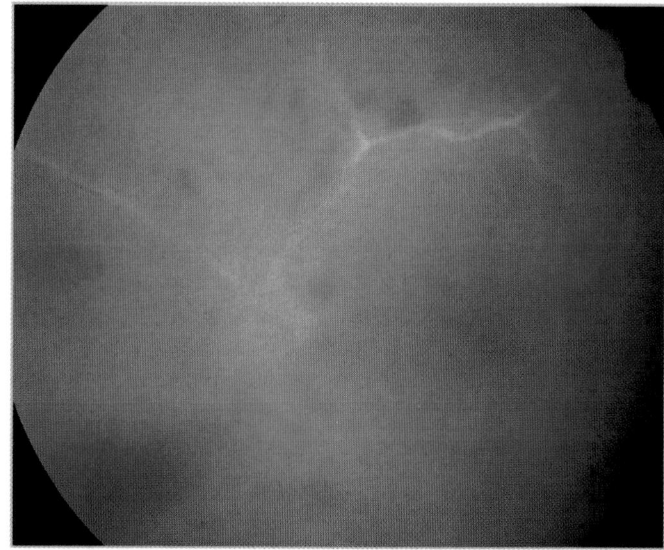

Figure 11.17 Widespread occlusive arteriolitis seen through dense vitritis during acute retinal necrosis.

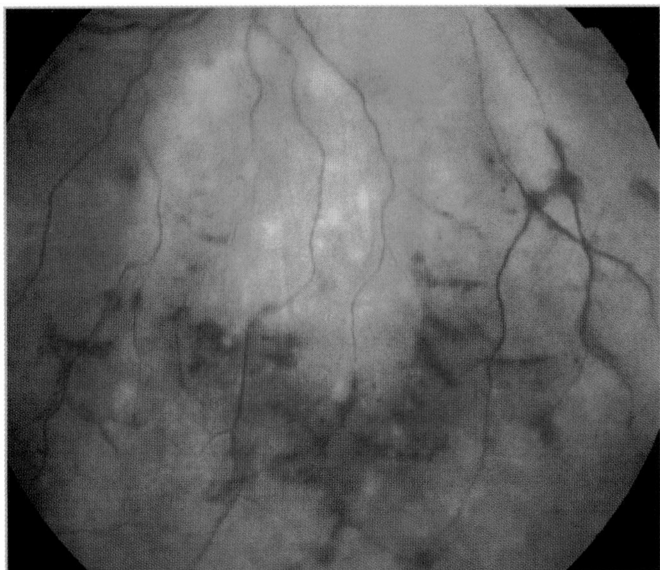

Figure 11.18 Less striking retinal whitening and more hemorrhage than usual may mimic cytomegalovirus retinitis.

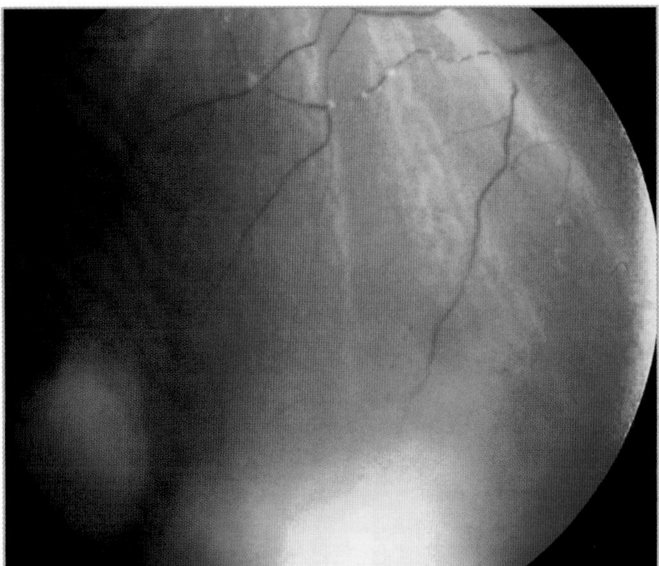

Figure 11.19 Early retinal detachment during acute retinal necrosis. There is still active retinitis within the detached retina, together with patchy vasculitis.

mandatory. The difference between typical ARN and CMV retinitis is clear, but on occasion ARN is associated with a severe retinal periphlebitis, and in this case substantially more retinal hemorrhage may be visible (**Fig. 11.23**). Multifocal retinal whitening or branch vessel occlusion may also be seen, and therefore Behçet's disease may enter the differential diagnosis. Syphilis may cause retinal whitening, arteritis and vitritis. Large-cell lymphoma can occasionally cause widespread necrotizing change. Severe pars planitis may show substantial peripheral retinal whitening through opacified vitreous, but the prolonged history and the quality of vitreous involvement usually serve to differentiate. Even sarcoidosis can rarely cause necrotizing retinopathy.

The diagnosis of ARN can be equivocal. The American Uveitis Society defined minimal diagnostic criteria (Holland 1994), which include:

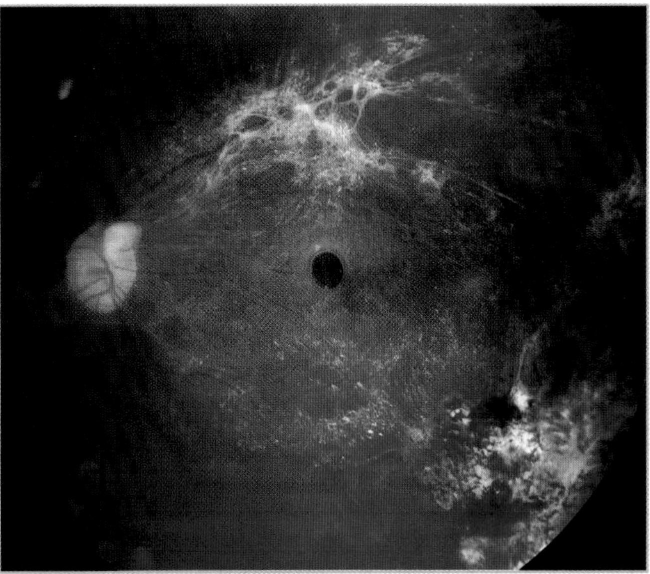

Figure 11.20 Total inoperable retinal detachment with proliferative vitreoretinopathy and secondary macular hole following two failed vitrectomies in acute retinal necrosis.

focal, well-demarcated areas of retinal necrosis outside the major vascular arcades, progressing rapidly if untreated; occlusive retinal vasculitis; and significant vitreous and anterior chamber inflammation. The diagnosis may be made regardless of the patient's immune status.

At its most typical, the diagnosis of ARN is made clinically. Nevertheless serological tests for VZV, HSV-1 and -2 and CMV should be requested to confirm previous exposure. Intraocular sampling to confirm the herpesvirus type involved does not influence management if the diagnosis of ARN is already clear. However, in those instances where diagnosis is not clear, intraocular sampling for PCR is imperative. It is sensible to start systemic antiviral therapy while the results are awaited because ARN is the most aggressive and destructive of those on the differential diagnosis list.

Should aqueous or vitreous humor be taken for PCR? There is some evidence that sensitivity is increased in vitreous specimens, but the diagnostic rate from aqueous humor is now very high. Obtaining a sample is straightforward and carries low risk; in contrast, generating possible vitreal traction from sampling in an eye with necrotizing retinal damage, and a high risk of rhegmatogenous detachment, persuade us that the vitreous should not be sampled unless as part of formal three-port vitrectomy.

The diagnosis of ARN is 95% clinical and 5% laboratory based. For those providing a specialist uveitis service it is a source of regular concern that patients are diagnosed and referred late, and this is very detrimental to outcome. The main reason for this is mundane; patients with suggestive symptoms in association with anterior uveitis do not have their fundi examined adequately until the disease is advanced. Patients are typically referred to this clinic 10–14 days after presentation. For those very few who have had empirical oral steroid prescribed in the interim, the outcome can be disastrous, and we have seen bilateral blindness ensue.

Management

ARN is a self-limiting process with a relatively short course, which does not tend to recur. Its spectrum of severity, and therefore resultant damage, may vary significantly, with limited forms occasionally

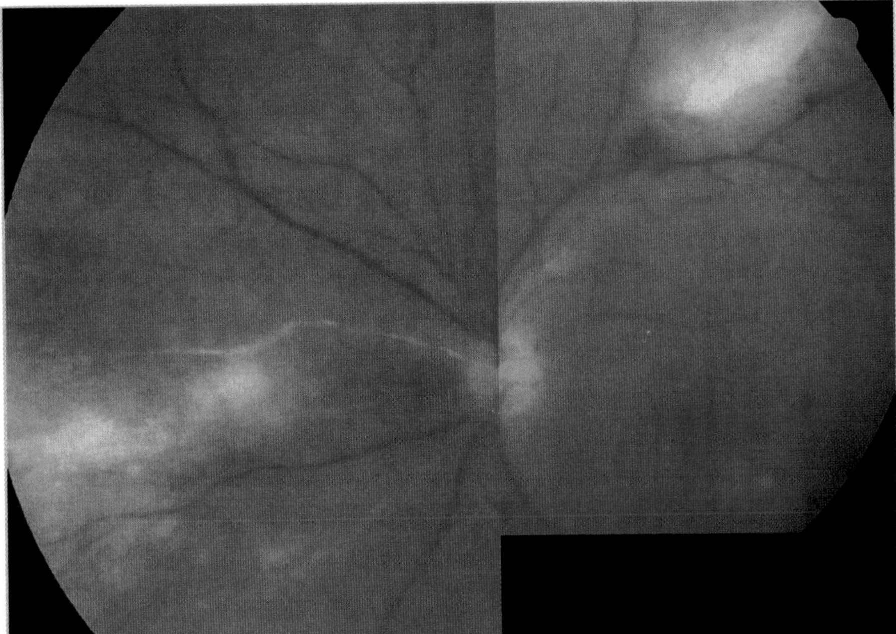

Figure 11.21 Polymerase chain reaction-confirmed herpes simplex 1 necrotizing retinitis in a middle-aged man undergoing chemotherapy for myelomatosis.

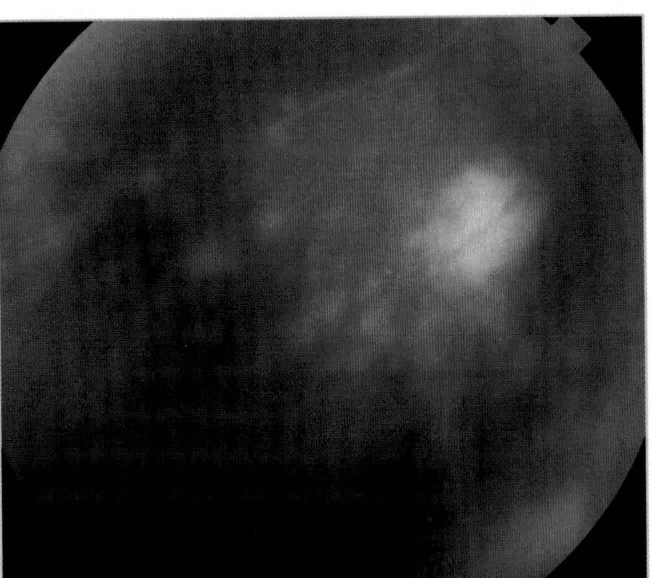

Figure 11.22 Multifocal retinitis as satellite lesions posterior to contiguous retinitis in acute retinal necrosis.

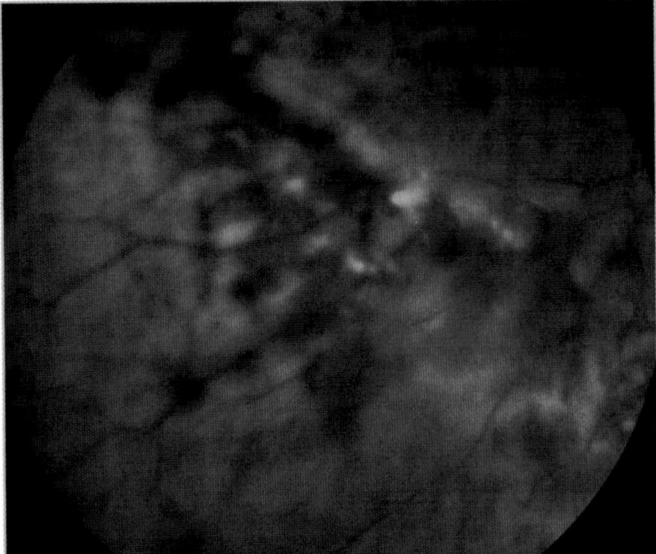

Figure 11.23 Severe and hemorrhagic acute retinal necrosis.

described. However, in general if eyes are untreated the prognosis is extremely poor and consequent involvement of the second eye common; unilateral blindness is usual and bilateral blindness possible. It is accepted that early and vigorous treatment is associated with a better visual prognosis and fewer complications for the affected eye, and that involvement of the second eye can almost always be prevented.

Traditionally, treatment of ARN required high-dose intravenous aciclovir (for an adult of average weight, 800 mg infused over 1 hour, three times daily) until the retinal inflammation is clinically resolved. A response is usually detectable within 72 hours, but at least 10 days of treatment is required. After this, conversion to oral aciclovir treatment at a dose of 400–800 mg five times per day is made, reducing to a maintenance dose of 400 mg twice daily for a period of debatable length.

The emergence of the prodrug valaciclovir raised the possibility of oral induction treatment giving equal or superior bioavailability to intravenous aciclovir, and thus permitting outpatient management. Other oral antivirals including famciclovir (which can also achieve adequate virustatic levels in vitreous) have appeared and intraocular administration is also possible. There is no consensus on the optimum regimen in these patients and studies have not tended to show a clear advantage of one treatment protocol (Tibbetts et al. 2010). Oral administration without intravenous induction may be adequately effective (Aizman et al. 2007) but there may be inadvertent selection bias and currently the evidence base is poor. Our current approach is to insist on intravenous treatment for those with extensive retinitis because it also facilitates daily reassessment.

The additional use of intraocular antiviral injections has been studied, suggesting that intravitreal foscarnet may lessen the retinal detachment rate (Wong et al. 2010). Both HSV and VZV are, very uncommonly, aciclovir resistant. Using intravitreal ganciclovir as an early adjunct to systemic aciclovir or ganciclovir aided control of inflammation (Guo et al. 2007). Our approach is to consider intravenous ganciclovir first for those with clearly aggressive disease.

The usefulness of systemic steroid treatment in conjunction with an antiviral has been a matter for debate. Such treatment undoubtedly aids clearance of vitreous opacification, and will therefore facilitate effective laser treatment if it is considered. However, such treatment may also facilitate viral replication. For those with severe vitritis we commence moderate-dose prednisolone treatment several days after intravenous aciclovir has been commenced, tapering rapidly after 1 week and aiming to discontinue within 6 weeks. Topical steroids are indicated for the associated anterior uveitis.

Retinal vaso-occlusive disease is a significant component of ARN and the use of either anticoagulation or anti-platelet drugs has been advocated. Warfarinization has not been justified, but the use of aspirin 75–300 mg/day seems reasonable, because increased platelet aggregation has been demonstrated in ARN. There is currently no evidence base for the efficacy of this.

Retinal detachment is a common sequel to ARN and may occur early. The usefulness of prophylactic laser treatment applied as a barrage behind the posterior edge of involved retina is debatable; an early study claiming a marked reduction in detachment rate has not been replicated by others. In cases where vitreous opacification is marked, weeks of aciclovir therapy may be necessary before this is possible. The management of established retinal detachment in ARN patients is a particular challenge, in view of the extensive areas of necrotic retina, the high incidence of vitreous organization and the predisposition to PVR. The outcomes of vitrectomy remain unsatisfactory and the reoperation rate is high (Usui et al. 2010). The high retinal detachment rate and difficult consequent surgery in ARN have led some to suggest prophylactic vitrectomy in these patients. A recent study found that, in those with primary posterior pole involvement, rhegmatogenous detachment was inevitable and not prevented by vitrectomy; however, for those with midperipheral retinitis, vitrectomy prevented detachment (Ishida et al. 2009).

When should antiviral treatment be stopped? Consecutive involvement of the other eye has been reported years after presentation, and immunodeficient or immunosuppressed patients are at greater risk. Few now discontinue antivirals after 6 weeks as suggested in the early days of ARN; our approach is to exclude cellular immune deficiency in all patients; those with intact immune systems continue on aciclovir maintenance at 400 mg twice daily for 1 year; immunodeficient or immunosuppressed patients continue for life.

In summary, the evidence base for a variety of treatment parameters in ARN is meager and the published results vary markedly, reflecting possible selection bias or varying disease presentations internationally. The approach of various uveitis specialists has therefore differed more on personality than evidence. The aggressive ophthalmologist will wish to intervene with intravenous induction and, if the retinal surgeon colleague cannot be persuaded to undertake prophylactic vitrectomy, he or she will use steroids to clear vitritis so that laser barrage is possible. Aspirin and omeprazole will be added to this and supervision will be intense. At the other end of the spectrum, some ophthalmologists have been depressed by the poor outcomes even after vigorous intervention and may follow a laissez-faire pathway, using antiviral and managing retinal detachment if it occurs, in the knowledge that at least consecutive involvement of the second eye is unlikely. There is little strong evidence to suggest that either should change direction. Despite the complexity of this disease, multicenter comparative studies are urgently needed.

HUMAN IMMUNODEFICIENCY VIRUS AND AIDS (box 11.4)

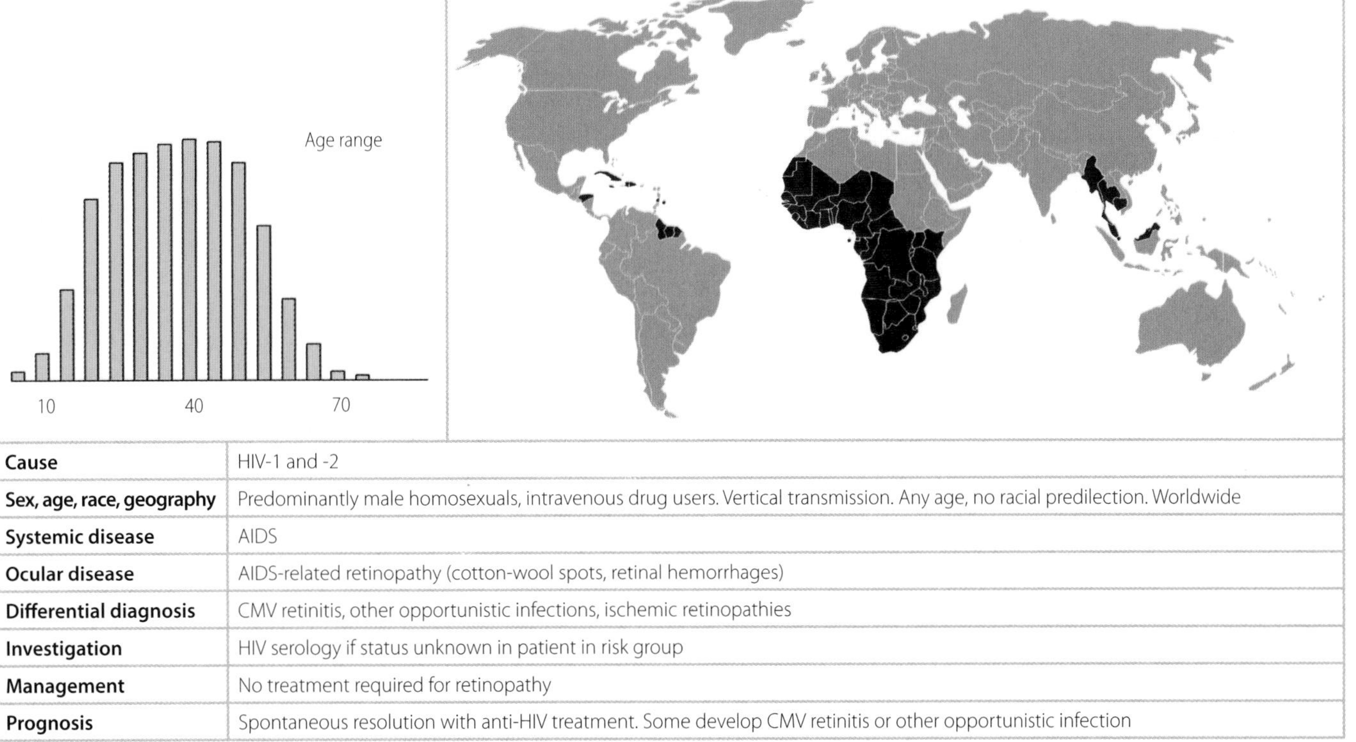

Cause	HIV-1 and -2
Sex, age, race, geography	Predominantly male homosexuals, intravenous drug users. Vertical transmission. Any age, no racial predilection. Worldwide
Systemic disease	AIDS
Ocular disease	AIDS-related retinopathy (cotton-wool spots, retinal hemorrhages)
Differential diagnosis	CMV retinitis, other opportunistic infections, ischemic retinopathies
Investigation	HIV serology if status unknown in patient in risk group
Management	No treatment required for retinopathy
Prognosis	Spontaneous resolution with anti-HIV treatment. Some develop CMV retinitis or other opportunistic infection

Box 11.4 Human immunodeficiency virus and AIDS

Introduction

HIV-1 and HIV-2 are RNA retroviruses, both of which may cause the acquired immune deficiency syndrome (AIDS) in humans. HIV-2, which is less easily transmissible and less pathogenic, is mainly limited to West Africa, but HIV-1 is responsible for a worldwide pandemic. Infection by HIV is either venereal or parenteral. Outside Africa, early spread in the 1980s was mainly in the male homosexual community, with intravenous drug abusers the second risk group. With increasing prevalence (and in some sub-Saharan countries population seroprevalence now exceeds 40%), heterosexual spread has become more common and vertical transmission (which is seen in 25% of children of infected mothers) therefore occurs in rapidly increasing numbers.

After infection by HIV, antibody develops usually within 3 months. Infection is often asymptomatic. HIV binds specifically to CD4 lymphocytes, and also macrophages and microglia. Using reverse transcriptase, the viral RNA is converted to DNA and the host nucleus is used to modify intracellular metabolism, so that endoplasmic reticulum forms viral components which, via Golgi apparatus, creates large numbers of HIV virions per cell by surface budding (**Fig. 11.24**), ultimately leading to death of the host cell. Over a period of years, the CD4 lymphocyte population becomes depleted to the extent that opportunistic infection or other manifestations of AIDS become apparent, usually when the count falls <200/µl. The immunodeficiency caused by HIV infection allows characteristic opportunistic infections to intervene, some of which affect the eye. These infections are separately discussed under their microbiological headings, and include CMV retinitis, PORN, tuberculosis, *Mycobacterium avium* choroiditis, syphilis, toxoplasmosis, Pneumocystis choroiditis, cryptococcal choroiditis and other fungal infections.

Systemic disease

Some patients develop a mild flu-like illness with lymphadenopathy within 2–4 weeks of exposure but the symptoms are non-specific and usually pass without medical attention. During the subsequent latent years of HIV infection, the carrier is asymptomatic but there may be mild chronic lymphadenopathy. A very few patients pass into AIDS within only weeks of initial infection, but the majority will take at least several years, and sometimes more than 20 years, to do so. AIDS may be diagnosed if an HIV-positive individual has a CD4 count <200/µl, or where one or more AIDS-indicator diseases have occurred, including various opportunistic infections, Kaposi's sarcoma, and non-Hodgkin's or primary cerebral lymphoma. Some 50% of HIV-positive patients will develop AIDS within 10 years of infection, and 90% within 15 years.

The possible manifestations of AIDS are protean and complex; malignancies are common, Kaposi's sarcoma and lymphoma being prominent. Gastrointestinal problems are frequent, with *Candida* spp. and cryptosporidia being common pathogens. Hepatitis may be seen. Opportunistic infections by many organisms, including those mentioned above, may also cause multisystem disease such as pneumonitis, meningitis and encephalitis.

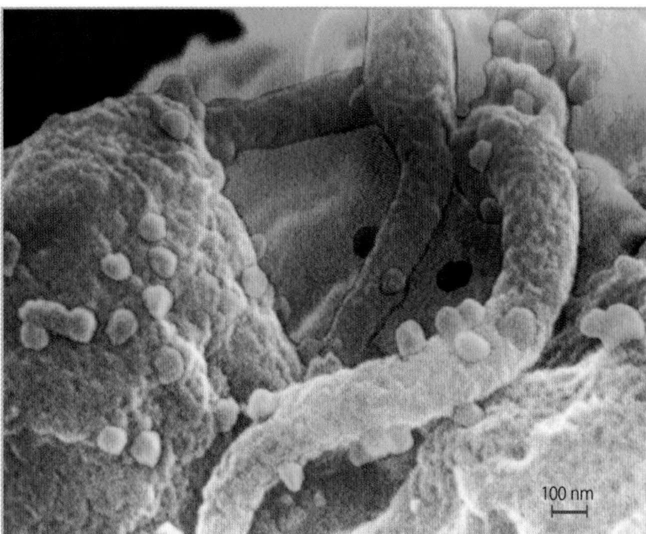

Figure 11.24 HIV virions are seen budding off the cell membrane of a CD4 lymphocyte. False-color scanning electron microscopy. (Modified from Centers for Disease Control, Public Health Image Library.)

Ocular disease

The eye is not affected by early HIV infection. However, an HIV-related retinopathy may become manifest as the patient develops AIDS, and most patients show a retinopathy at some stage. Characteristically, scattered cotton-wool spots are seen. These are almost always symptomless and there is no evidence of associated retinal ischemia. They are evanescent, one disappearing over a few weeks as another appears. Cotton-wool spots in AIDS patients are said to lie more eccentrically about the nerve fiber layer axes than do cotton-wool spots in people with diabetes. Retinal hemorrhages, both deep and superficial, may also be seen. The absence of any underlying ischemic cause of cotton-wool spots in an otherwise normal fundus should arouse suspicion of HIV-related retinopathy. This concurrence of cotton-wool spots and retinal hemorrhage (**Fig. 11.25**) sometimes causes confusion among physicians with the diagnosis of CMV retinitis. The ophthalmologist is usually able to reassure, but, if in doubt, a period of observation over 2–3 weeks will clarify the situation; the HIV-related lesions will fade, whereas CMV (**Fig. 11.26**) will spread and worsen. Occasionally the ophthalmologist may be asked to see a patient by an optometrist who has located abnormality on routine examination. In this circumstance the need for further investigation, including serology for HIV and syphilis, must be approached with sensitivity. The need for pre-test counseling is crucial, and the expertise of those who perform this task regularly should be sought.

Diagnosis

Within 3 months of infection antibody to viral envelope protein is detectable, and remains for life. The ELISA (enzyme-linked immunosorbent assay) test for this antibody is highly specific and sensitive; those reacting positive are re-tested, and confirmation may be made by western blot analysis. Equivocal cases are re-tested within weeks.

Management

The history of anti-HIV treatment is one of hard-won progressive improvement over 30 years. The first drugs to have antiretroviral action were the reverse transcriptase inhibitors, including zidovudine introduced in the mid-1980s. The first protease inhibitors such as ritonavir (which disrupt intracellular viral assembly) emerged in 1994, and there is now a wide range of both groups available. In 2003 the first HIV fusion inhibitor was introduced, which made entry of the

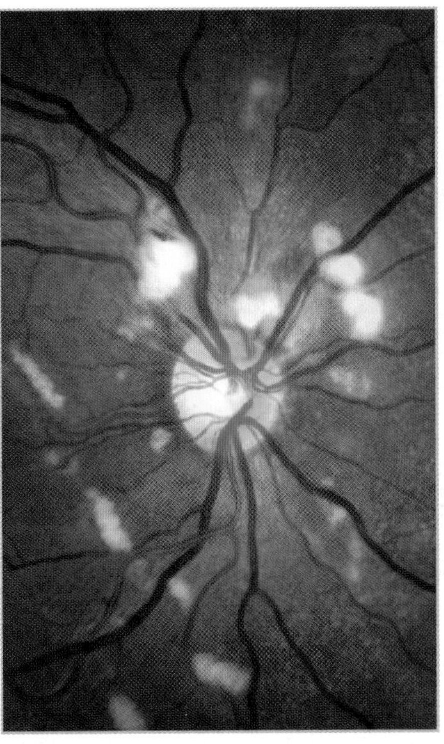
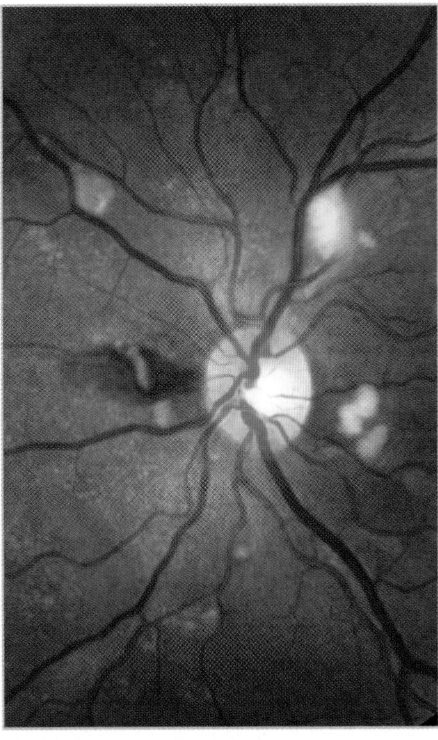

Figure 11.25 A young African woman newly diagnosed with AIDS shows HIV-related retinopathy with multiple cotton-wool spots around the discs, and two flame-shaped hemorrhages.

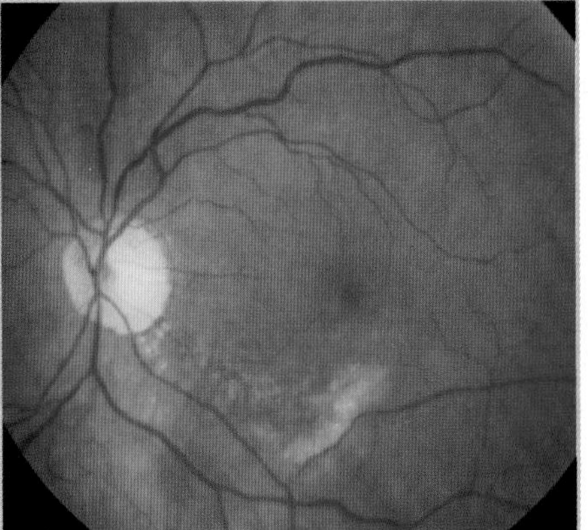
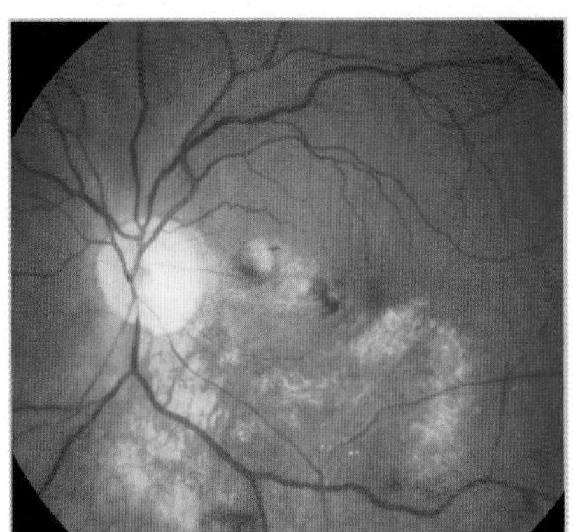

Figure 11.26 Early cytomegalovirus (CMV) retinitis (left) can occasionally be mistaken for HIV retinopathy. Progression within 10 days (right) makes it clear that this is CMV retinitis.

virus into the CD4 cell more difficult. Also in this decade, interferon-α was discovered to inhibit virion capsid maturation and others with similar action are under investigation. More are in development to target a variety of stages in the viral lifecycle. There is therefore now a substantial armament of drugs that can be used in combination in patients with AIDS.

HIV has a high mutation rate and therefore develops resistance to single drugs with singular ease. The ability to give tolerable drug combinations reduces this risk, increases efficacy and has transformed outcomes for many patients. This highly active antiretroviral treatment (HAART), which implies three or four drugs (usually one reverse transcriptase inhibitor, two protease inhibitors and one other), are sometimes available in fixed-dose combinations and can at best convert AIDS from a disease usually lethal within 1–2 years to a chronic but sustainable illness. Current recommendations are that antiretroviral treatment should be initiated for all patients with either an AIDS-defining illness or a CD4 count <350/µl, and it is recommend for HIV-positive individuals with counts of 350–500/µl. Treatment may be started earlier but opinion is divided.

The retinopathy associated with HIV infection is asymptomatic and requires no treatment. However, several associated opportunistic infections are highly significant and are dealt with in their relevant sections.

CMV RETINITIS AND UVEITIS (box 11.5)

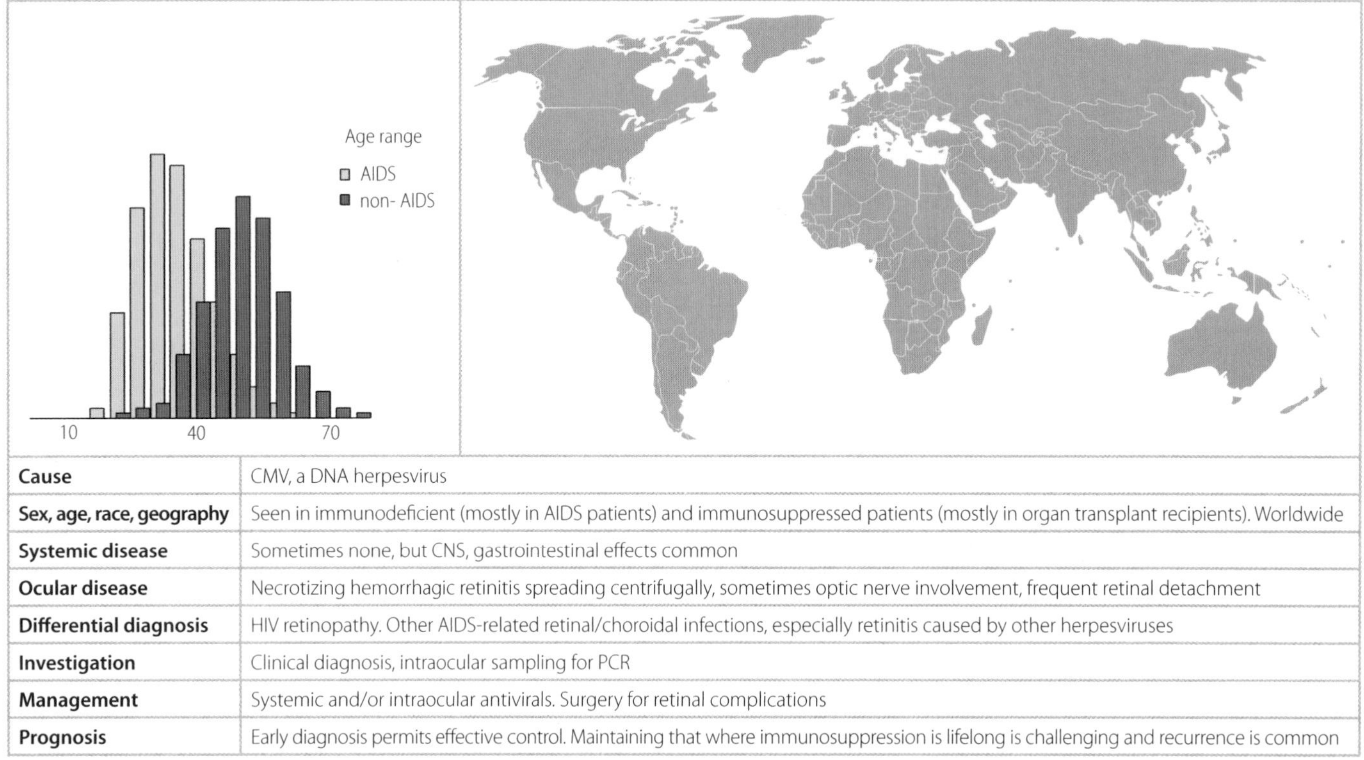

Cause	CMV, a DNA herpesvirus
Sex, age, race, geography	Seen in immunodeficient (mostly in AIDS patients) and immunosuppressed patients (mostly in organ transplant recipients). Worldwide
Systemic disease	Sometimes none, but CNS, gastrointestinal effects common
Ocular disease	Necrotizing hemorrhagic retinitis spreading centrifugally, sometimes optic nerve involvement, frequent retinal detachment
Differential diagnosis	HIV retinopathy. Other AIDS-related retinal/choroidal infections, especially retinitis caused by other herpesviruses
Investigation	Clinical diagnosis, intraocular sampling for PCR
Management	Systemic and/or intraocular antivirals. Surgery for retinal complications
Prognosis	Early diagnosis permits effective control. Maintaining that where immunosuppression is lifelong is challenging and recurrence is common

Box 11.5 CMV retinitis and uveitis

Introduction

Cytomegalovirus (CMV, HHV-5) is a DNA herpesvirus, named because of the typical enlargement of infected cells caused by viral disruption of cytoarchitecture and cell swelling. Infected cells typically contain both nuclear and cytoplasmic inclusion bodies. Infection is by direct contact with body fluids and is most commonly venereal. The virus may also be transmitted in utero, perinatally or via transfused blood products.

In immunocompetent patients, CMV is commonly acquired subclinically or as a mild pyrexial illness. Only a small minority develops significant problems; a syndrome similar to infectious mononucleosis may be seen. However, acquisition during pregnancy may lead to a spectrum of congenital sequelae for newborn babies. Seropositivity indicating previous infection increases with age at a variable rate, overall 1–3% per annum, but with higher rates during adolescence. There is marked variation both regionally and internationally, but on average 50% of young adults and over 90% of homosexual men are seropositive. Antigenic variants of CMV may cause further episodes of primary infection.

Similar to all herpesviruses, CMV remains latent once acquired but a normal immune system is able to suppress it so that no symptomatic inflammation occurs. In immunodeficient individuals, particularly in the AIDS population, it is permitted to replicate, becoming an important pathogen, and gives rise to multisystem infection including retinitis. In AIDS patients, the CD4 lymphocyte count is usually <100 cells/μl before disease activation occurs. The virus is also important in those who have received organ transplantation, particularly bone marrow, where lifelong immunodepression may allow CMV to recur frequently and require regular or chronic intervention.

Systemic disease

In post-transplantation patients and other immunosuppressed groups without AIDS, the manifestations of primary systemic CMV are variable but may include pyrexia, myalgia, hepatosplenomegaly, marrow suppression and pneumonitis. In AIDS patients, pneumonitis, gastrointestinal involvement including mucosal ulceration, esophagitis, colitis, central nervous system (CNS) involvement and, particularly, retinitis are prominent. However, CMV retinitis may present without systemic symptoms.

Ocular disease

CMV retinitis

Before the AIDS epidemic, CMV retinitis (CMVR) was a rare complication after organ transplantation and in other heavily immunosuppressed patients such as those undergoing cancer chemotherapy. In AIDS patients during the 1980s and 1990s, the disease was extremely common, affecting up to half of these patients. Effective antiretroviral treatment has reduced the incidence substantially in the west. Most patients presenting for the first time to an ophthalmologist have established AIDS and are aware of the implications of their disease and its prognosis. However, in a small proportion of patients CMVR is the AIDS-defining illness in a patient who may or may not be known to be HIV positive. The ophthalmologist should be prepared to deal with the impact of this event on the patient.

The symptomatology of CMVR will depend on the area of retina involved. Some patients present with visual loss. Others, asymptomatic, are diagnosed on funduscopy by their AIDS physician, who will often screen those with CD4 counts <100/μl.

The hallmark of CMVR is a necrotizing retinitis that in its early stages may be confused with the evanescent cotton-wool spots of HIV retinopathy. However, the appearance of contiguous areas of white necrosis and retinal hemorrhage will clarify the diagnosis (**Fig. 11.27**), and thus careful observation is required in the patient with equivocal signs. Multifocal or bilateral presentations are possible, but some two-thirds will start with a unilateral focus.

CMVR lesions have tendency to begin in retinal midperiphery and spread more rapidly towards the retinal periphery than towards the posterior pole. However, slow creepage of the posterior border is inevitable if untreated. Due to this spread pattern, areas of retinitis are characteristically sectoral (**Fig. 11.28**). The spreading edge of the lesion is most active and looks pale, the expansion therefore being compared with a 'brush-fire' (**Fig. 11.29**). Outside the apparent edge of the area of retinitis, there may be small white satellite lesions and perivenous cuffing (**Fig. 11.30**). Within the lesion there is usually a substantial associated retinal vasculitis (**Fig. 11.31**), and widespread vascular occlusion is common. Usually detectable change in a lesion takes a week or two, rather than days. The appearance of this typical combination of exudate, retinal necrosis, edema and hemorrhage in advanced CMVR has been likened to a pizza, and the description, although hardly epicurean, is accurate.

Some patients may present late with CMVR because they notice their visual field defect encroaching centrally (**Fig. 11.32**). Unusually, the macula may be primarily involved (**Fig. 11.33**), and visual loss may be subacute. It may also become edematous due to the proximity of an active lesion. Where the optic nerve head is involved (**Fig. 11.34**), catastrophic visual loss may ensue. Occasionally there is pronounced perivenous exudation in association with CMVR. In some cases part of the vascular tree develops a 'frosted branch' appearance (**Fig. 11.35**). In rare cases the appearance can be most florid (**Fig. 11.36**).

The degree of overlying vitreous and anterior chamber activity is variable, although never profound and most commonly low; detectable vitreous cells are usual, but vitreous clouding should suggest a different diagnosis. Anterior chamber activity is not typical, but cells, fine KPs and minimal photophobia are consistent with the diagnosis. Pain and ciliary injection, however, are not.

Untreated, CMVR will, over a period of several weeks involve the entire retina and lead to blindness. Rarely, patients present at this stage (**Fig. 11.37**). Treatment, discussed below, is virustatic and will halt progression of the disease. After treatment the affected retina will slowly change in appearance, with resolution of edema, exudate and hemorrhage to leave subtle retinal atrophy and fine underlying RPE scarring. Choroidal scarring and pigmentary clumping are generally not seen.

Having undergone initial treatment the patient will revert to maintenance treatment. The diagnosis of recurrent CMVR in those patients on maintenance is more difficult than for the patient presenting anew; new areas may become inflamed as on initial presentation, but usually a more subtle reactivation at the leading edge of the retinal scar is seen. There is gradual enlargement of the affected area of retina and its

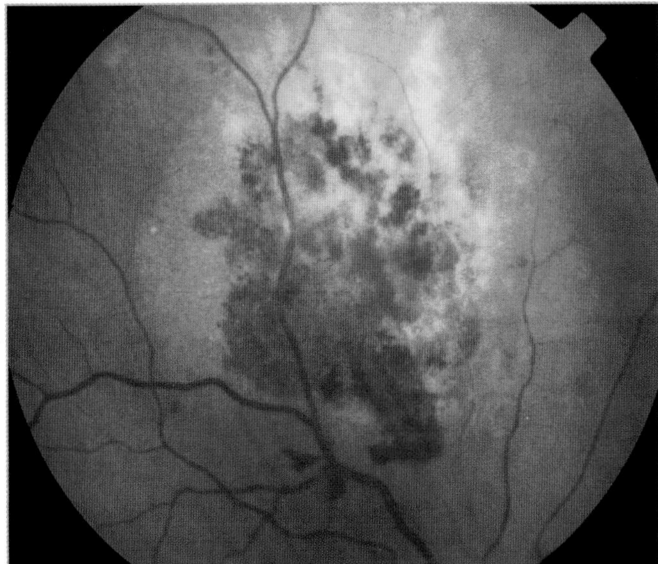

Figure 11.27 A single focus of cytomegalovirus retinitis in a patient with sarcoma treated with bone marrow transplantation. Pale necrotizing retinitis and associated hemorrhage are typical. The lesion is midperipheral.

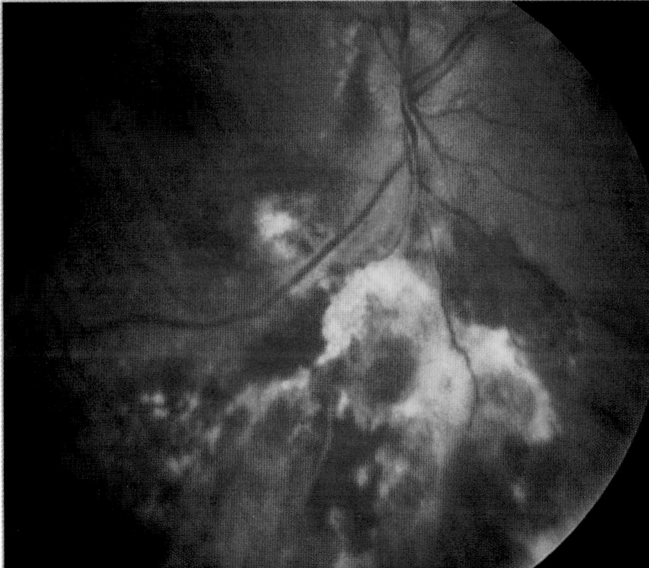

Figure 11.28 A characteristic sectoral area of cytomegalovirus retinitis in a young man with AIDS.

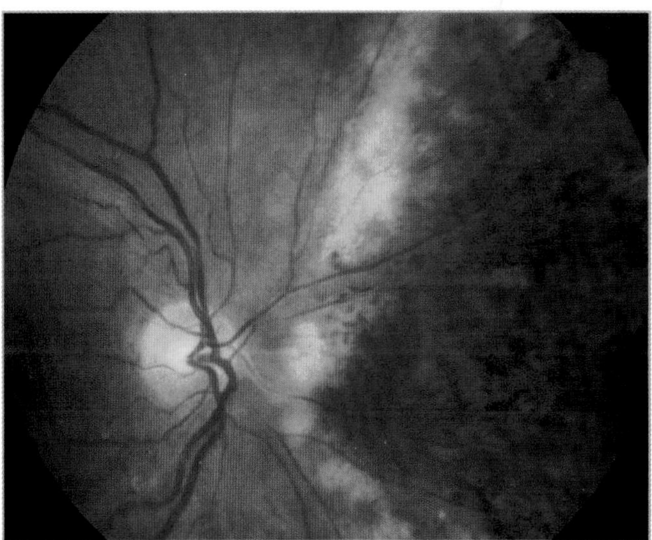

Figure 11.29 As cytomegalovirus retinitis spreads posteriorly its leading edge, showing more pale than its hemorrhagic centre, resembles a 'brush-fire.' (Courtesy of Mr AB Tullo.)

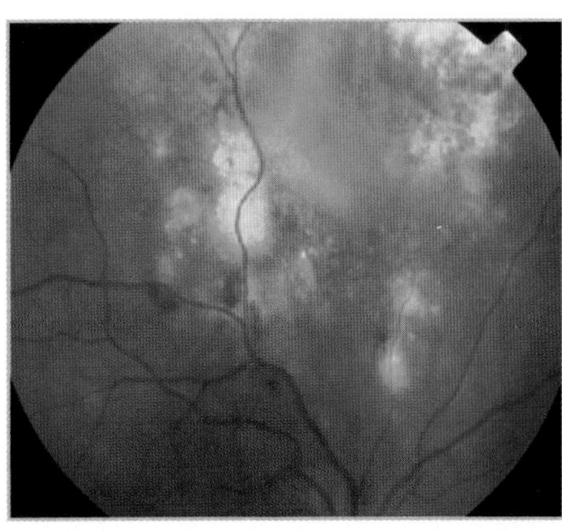

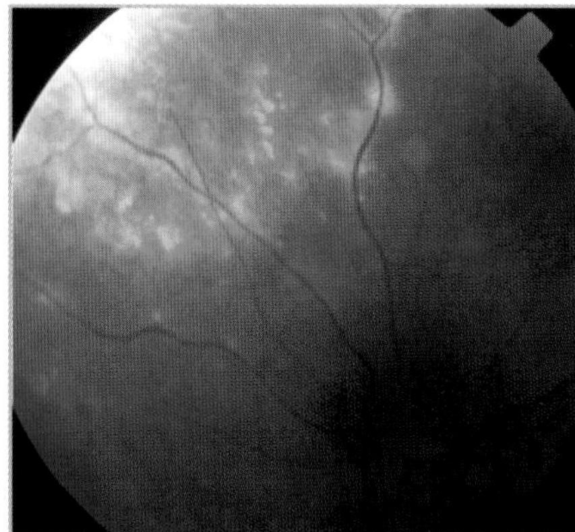

Figure 11.30 Low-grade cytomegalovirus retinitis may appear multifocal. Some areas of inflammation cluster around retinal vessels.

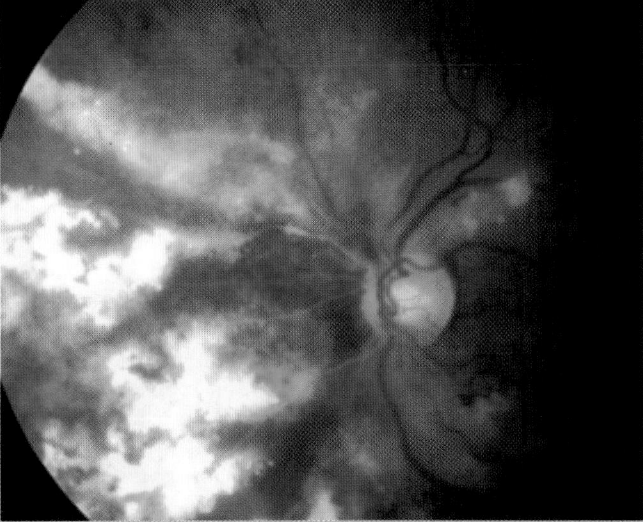

Figure 11.31 Advanced cytomegalovirus retinitis in a patient with AIDS. There is associated occlusive retinal vasculitis with silver-wired vessels.

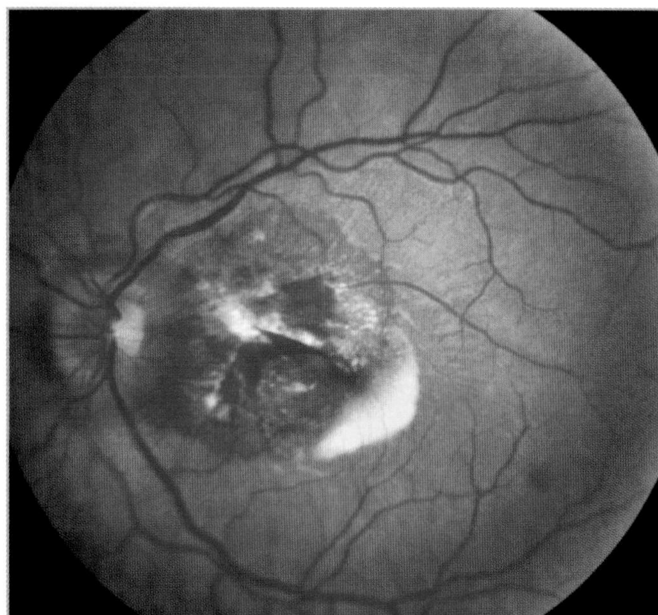

Figure 11.33 Primary macular retinitis in cytomegalovirus. The leading edge has crossed the fovea.

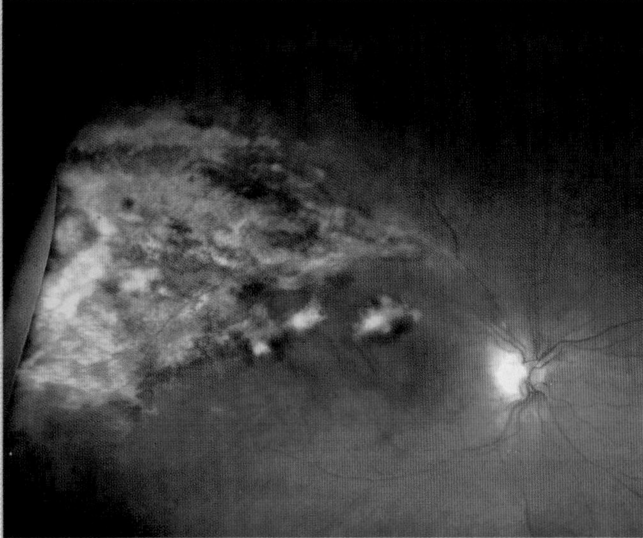

Figure 11.32 Widefield photography of a large sector of cytomegalovirus retinitis at presentation. Inflammation had clearly been present for weeks, but a pericentral scotoma was the reason for seeking consultation.

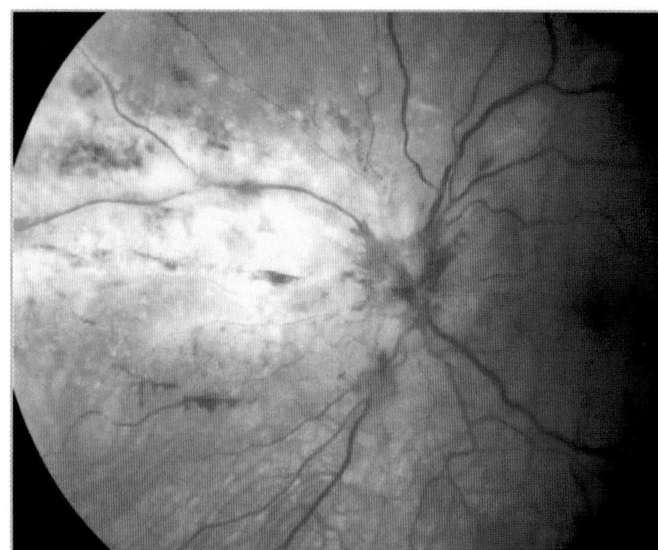

Figure 11.34 A sector of cytomegalovirus retinitis is associated with papillitis, leading to severe and permanent visual loss.

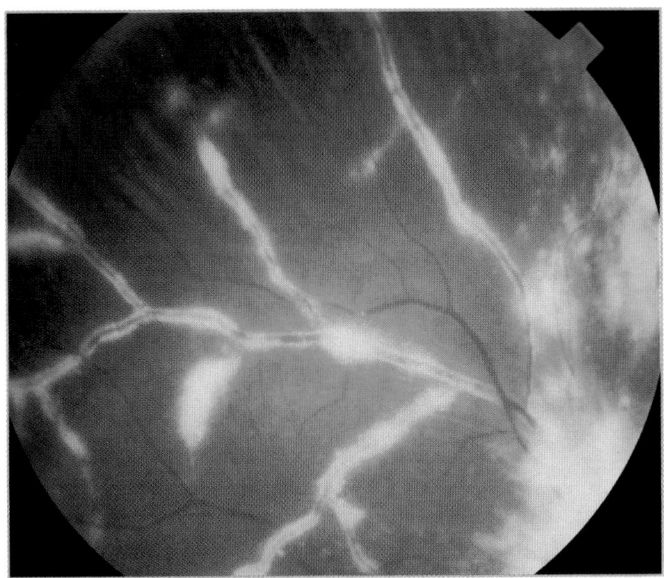

Figure 11.35 Sectoral frosted branch angiitis in association with cytomegalovirus retinitis and papillitis, seen to the right.

corresponding visual field defect. Sometimes progressive expansion of affected retinal areas, documented by fundus photography and visual field assessments, may be encountered without any apparent evidence of reactivation of retinitis. Monitoring should therefore ideally include both visual field assessment and serial retinal photography.

Retinal break formation and consequent rhegmatogenous detachment is very common, affecting about a quarter of eyes within 1 year of CMVR. Such a high incidence is predictable in the presence of such profound retinal atrophy. The likelihood of detachment increases with the area of retina involved and if active retinitis is present. Breaks may be multiple and are frequently very posterior. Early breaks in such thinned retina may be difficult to see against a background of RPE atrophy, but may occur either within or at the edge of the atrophic area.

The most common causes of visual loss in CMVR are direct macular involvement and retinal detachment (Thorne et al. 2006).

CMV anterior uveitis

It has become apparent from aqueous PCR studies that CMV is capable of causing a relapsing or chronic anterior uveitis both in those with intact immune systems and in some eyes with or following retinitis. The uveitis resembles other herpetic anterior uveitis in being commonly associated with a high IOP and causing iris atrophy. There may be corneal endotheliitis and decompensation may result. Myriad fine-pigmented KPs are characteristic (**Fig. 11.38**). Others have described Posner–Schlossman syndrome or Fuchs' heterochromic uveitis in association with CMV atrophy (van Boxtel et al. 2007). Topical steroid alone does not adequately control the inflammation. Systemic valganciclovir or intraocular ganciclovir has been used with short-term success, but recurrence after discontinuation is routine (Chee and Jap 2010) and a long-term solution has not been identified.

Diagnosis

In diagnosing systemic CMV infection, virus can be demonstrated in body fluids using monoclonal antibody tests. Primary infection can be confirmed by the conversion of serum previously tested negative, or by rising titers of both IgG and IgM in those previously untested. Rising IgG titers will also appear in reactivations or reinfections. It may not be possible to distinguish between reactivation of retained virus and reinfection with a new strain. Viral DNA load in peripheral blood is routinely measured in some transplant recipients and AIDS patients by PCR, and some real-time methods can be sensitive to 200 copies/ml. The copy levels normally associated with systemic problems range from 40 000 to several million but pre-emptive treatment is often started in transplant recipients if more than 3000–5000 copies are measured. Occasionally frank CMV retinitis is seen in patients with very low viral load, but this is unusual.

It is presumed that reactivation of latent CMV, rather than primary infection, is responsible for the great majority of cases of CMVR.

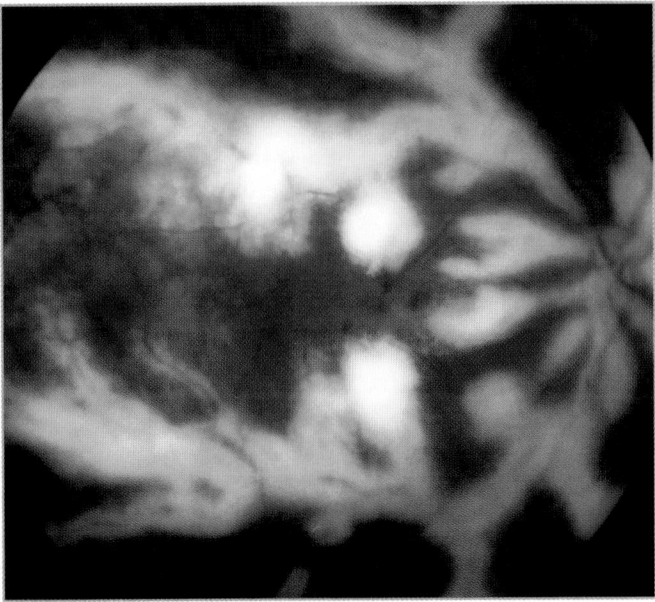

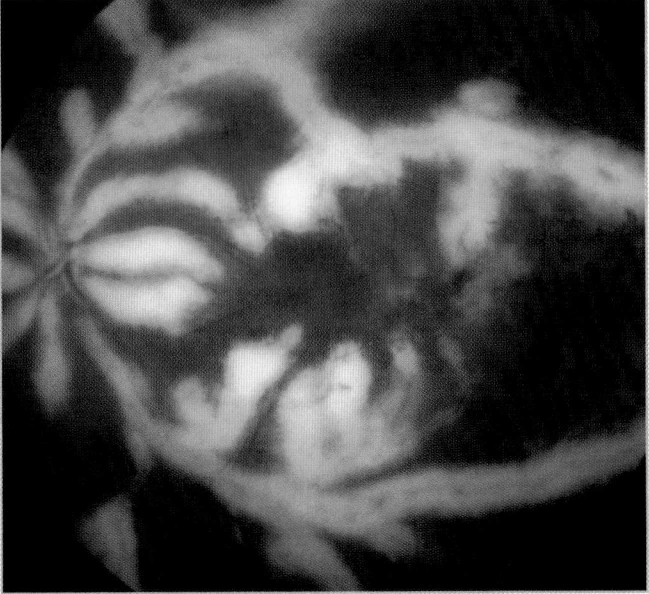

Figure 11.36 Florid bilateral frosted branch angiitis in a young man with ganciclovir-resistant cytomegalovirus retinitis, immunosuppressed after renal transplantation.

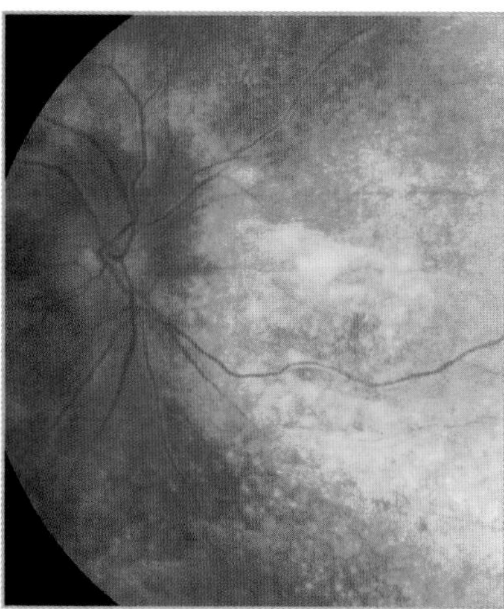
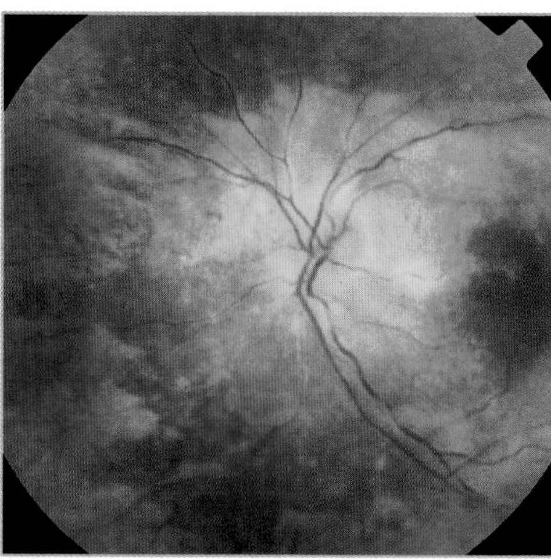

Figure 11.37 Bilateral end-stage cytomegalovirus retinitis in a middle-aged woman undergoing chemotherapy for myelomatosis.

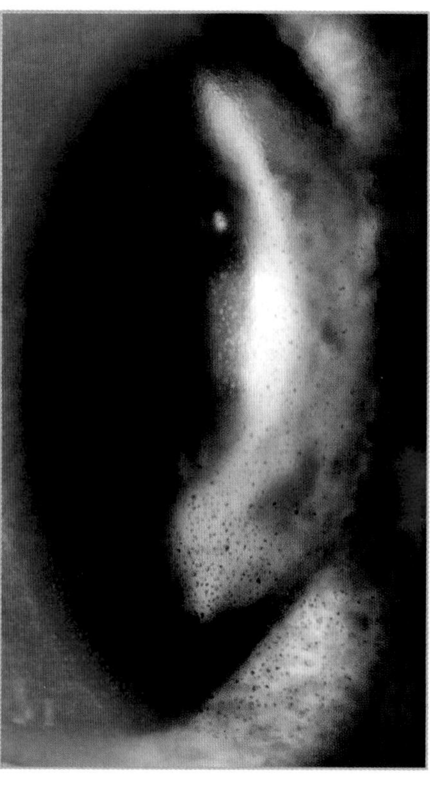

Figure 11.38 Multiple pigmented keratic precipitates in an eye with chronic cytomegalovirus anterior uveitis.

Usually the clinical appearance is typical and may be treated aggressively with confidence. If the signs are unclear, aqueous sampling for PCR studies (usually for all herpesviruses) will differentiate with high sensitivity and specificity.

Management

Systemic antivirals

Ganciclovir and valganciclovir

All drugs available for treatment of CMV disease have a significant toxicity profile and should be managed either by, or in close consultation with, an AIDS physician. All antiviral drugs are virustatic, not virucidal, so, after effective initial induction treatment of acute CMVR, maintenance is required at least for a period. In an attempt to avoid systemic toxicity, intraocular administration is possible, by either frequently repeated injection or (if available) implantation of a slow-release device.

Ganciclovir is a guanine analog that inhibits viral DNA polymerase. It is poorly absorbed orally and for effective induction treatment against active CMVR requires intravenous administration usually at 5 mg/kg twice daily for at least 10–14 days, after which CMVR usually becomes quiescent. It has a substantial toxicity profile including myelosuppression, especially neutropenia and thrombocytopenia, pyrexia, bowel disturbances, cognitive disorders and renal disturbance. Excretion of ganciclovir is renal and doses must be modified in renal disease. Valganciclovir is a valyl ester prodrug of ganciclovir which is well absorbed orally and esterified in the liver to the active drug. Induction treatment against CMVR is usually 900 mg twice daily for 14–21 days. Side effects are similar but induction avoids intravenous access. Resistance to both drugs is fairly common because CMV has the ability, via the proteins pUL97 and pUL54, to inhibit ganciclovir phosphorylation, thus preventing it from incorporating into viral DNA and therefore allowing synthesis to continue unabated. Combining either drug with reverse transcriptase inhibitors can lead to life-threatening myelosuppression, so that AIDS physicians may delay the onset of HAART where CMVR is the defining illness, to permit induction treatment to be completed. Additive toxicity may also occur with pentamidine, flucytosine or other nucleoside derivatives. To some extent neutropenia can be ameliorated by using granulocyte colony-stimulating factor (G-CSF), which may be injected up to three times a week; this elevates neutrophil counts by provoking premature release of immature granulocytes from bone marrow.

Foscarnet

Foscarnet is a pyrophosphate mimic that prevents viral replication by inhibiting DNA polymerase though competitive inhibition of phosphorylate-binding sites. Unlike ganciclovir, it also inhibits reverse transcriptase, so it has some anti-HIV activity. It also has activity against HSV. Induction treatment for acute CMVR requires slow intravenous infusion, preferably via a central venous line, of up to 20 mg/kg three times daily for 2–3 weeks. Foscarnet is substantially nephrotoxic, renal impairment occurring in over 40% of patients. Alternate-day serum creatinine measurements are recommended and dosage adjustments may be required. Electrolyte abnormalities may be seen, including hypocalcemia, hypokalemia and hypomagnesemia. Concentrated drug within the urine may cause genital ulceration. Reduced hemoglobin is seen in a third of patients. Fever is very common, and multiple other side effects have been reported, most commonly nausea and gastrointestinal problems. It is rarely a first-line treatment against CMVR.

Cidofovir

Cidofovir is a nucleoside analog that also inhibits CMV viral DNA polymerase. It is also active against HSV and several other virus groups. It is not susceptible to pUL97 CMV and therefore is not susceptible to resistance by this strain, as are ganciclovir and valganciclovir. However, cross-resistance can develop if ganciclovir-resistant CMV is exposed to that drug for long periods. Cidofovir requires intravenous administration, usually 5 mg/kg once weekly for 2 weeks. It is severely nephrotoxic and probenecid is administered before each infusion. It is ancillary to the above and is rarely a first-line choice of antiviral against CMVR.

Leflunomide

Leflunomide is an immunomodulator that inhibits pyrimidine synthesis. It is used to treat rheumatoid arthritis. However, it also has intrinsic antiviral activity and has been used in CMV disease especially after organ transplantation. Its efficacy is low to moderate so that those with high viremia levels benefit less (Avery et al. 2010), but it has potential in ganciclovir-resistant patients although its use in CMVR has not been formally assessed.

In the 1980s CMVR affected 25–40% of AIDS patients and the median survival time after diagnosis was as low as 9 months. A long-term strategy was not required by the ophthalmologist. In the twenty-first century era of HAART, following induction of quiescence in CMVR, a long-term strategy is most certainly required in the knowledge that the drugs used are not virucidal. If the patient has AIDS and is started on HAART, most will respond with a rise in CD4 count within months, to a level that will not permit CMV disease reactivation. In this circumstance discontinuation of anti-CMV maintenance is safe (Waib et al. 2007). A significant proportion, however, cannot tolerate HAART or do not respond adequately. While awaiting CD4 recovery, it is usual to give oral valganciclovir maintenance, usually at a dose of 900 mg/day. Untreated, recurrence of CMVR is likely after a few weeks. For those patients who are long-term immunodeficient, including post-transplant recipients on oral immunosuppression, or patients after bone marrow transplantation with imperfect leukogenesis, recurrence will be regular and frequent unless a tolerable maintenance treatment can be found. In this group valganciclovir resistance is not uncommon and, as most transplant recipients have imperfect renal function, both foscarnet and cidofovir are a long-term risk. There is potential for intraocular treatment, either alone or as an adjunct to systemic antivirals.

Intraocular treatment

Systemic treatment in appropriate dosage may be unacceptable, usually because of myelosuppression or nephrotoxicity. In this circumstance either ganciclovir or foscarnet may be injected intravitreally. The procedure is performed with topical and subconjunctival anesthesia after IOP reduction by a pressure device for 10 min. Ganciclovir 1–2 mg in 0.1 ml, or foscarnet 1.2–2.4 mg in 0.1 ml, is injected through the pars plana. Weekly or more frequent administration is necessary during induction. Cidofovir cannot be injected intravitreally because it causes severe, often fibrinous uveitis and subsequent hypotony.

There are disadvantages to an intraocular approach. Systemic CMV is not suppressed, and both eyes may require treatment separately. Pars plana injection, repeated perhaps many times in each eye, carries some risks including endophthalmitis, retinal break formation, vitreous hemorrhage, central arterial occlusion and lens damage. The frequent hospital procedures are significant for both the patient and the ophthalmologist.

A slow-release ganciclovir implant was introduced in the 1990s. The rather large device enclosing 4.5 mg is implanted through the pars plana following a localized vitrectomy (**Fig. 11.39**). It is intended to release about 1 μg ganciclovir/h into the posterior segment, but rates may vary. On average the implant is effective for 6–8 months (Muccioli et al. 2000). Consecutive implantation, either after removal of the first, spent implant or at a new pars plana site, has been used with success but in the long term there are potential cumulative problems to consider. A higher-dose implant with longer duration of action has not been commercially introduced after the initial anecdotal success, and the HAART era, in reducing the incidence of CMVR in the AIDS community, has led to the unavailability of the ganciclovir implant. Biodegradable scleral plugs with both ganciclovir and foscarnet are in development but phase II studies have not yet commenced.

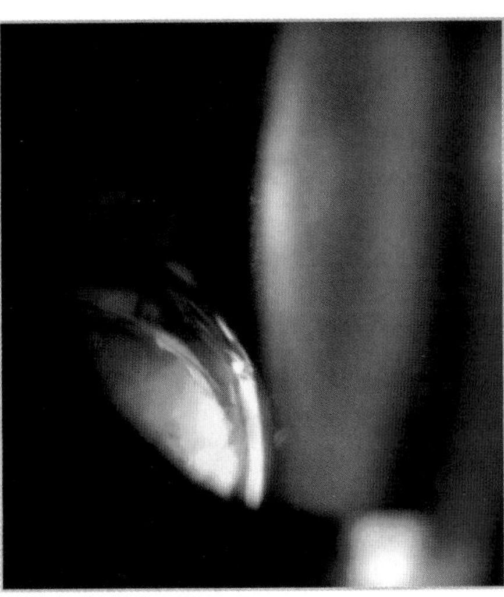

Figure 11.39 A ganciclovir intravitreal implant is seen protruding from the pars plana.

Anti-sense technology uses the knowledge of gene structure within pathogen DNA/RNA to manufacture a nucleotide that has the ability to bind to the pathogen's mRNA and effectively neutralize it. Fomivirsen is a 21-base strand effective against CMV mRNA and is available for intraocular injection. It has been found that it has some efficacy with a reasonable side-effect profile using injections at weeks 0, 2 and 4 for maintenance (Vitravene Study Group 2002) and has therefore been employed where standard treatments have been inadequate.

Intraocular treatment of CMVR has an established place in CMVR management which is likely to increase. The use of intraocular treatment alone for both induction and maintenance has yet to be proven satisfactory.

Laser and surgery in CMV-related retinal detachment

Rhegmatogenous retinal detachment is very common in CMVR, more so when retinal involvement is extensive. Argon laser treatment has been used prophylactically to demarcate quiescent areas of CMVR in an attempt to prevent future detachment of normal retina, as is also practiced for ARN. Such treatment is sometimes successful (Althaus et al. 1998) but is not routinely practiced.

Retinal detachment is characteristically associated with multiple breaks in atrophic retina and requires vitrectomy, substantial endolaser and, usually, the injection of silicone oil. Cataract formation is particularly common in these eyes and rapid posterior capsule opacification is predictable after surgery (Tanna et al. 2003). Silicone oil removal is safely possible only in about half of patients (Morrison et al. 2005) and simultaneous cataract removal increases the risk of re-detachment. Ganciclovir implantation has been proven compatible with silicone oil.

Immune recovery uveitis

Post-CMVR immune recovery uveitis (IRU) is the most important example of the phenomenon of post-infection immune reconstitution inflammatory syndrome (IRIS). In immunodepressed patients who develop opportunistic infection, immune system recovery after, for instance, antiretroviral treatment is then followed by a paradoxical and severe inflammatory reaction at the site of initial infection. The incidence of IRU after CMV retinitis in AIDS patients is about 10% (Kempen et al. 2006) and this is not dependent on the presence or absence of concurrent anti-CMV antivirals. The incidence of IRU is higher if patients are more immunodepressed or have more severe CMVR at presentation. There is some evidence to suggest that delaying HAART onset until after CMVR (or other opportunistic infection) treatment is effective reduces the incidence of IRU. Typically there is a moderate-to-severe non-granulomatous panuveitis, in the absence of retinitis reactivation, but often with macular edema. Typically orbit floor steroid is inadequate to control this but intravitreal triamcinolone appears effective at least in the short term (Morrison et al. 2007), thus far without reports of reactivated CMVR. Oral steroid is sometimes used and can be effective but more severe forms of IRU can be chronic and difficult to treat. The efficacy of anti-CMV antivirals for IRU, if any, is uncertain.

PROGRESSIVE OUTER RETINAL NECROSIS (box 11.6)

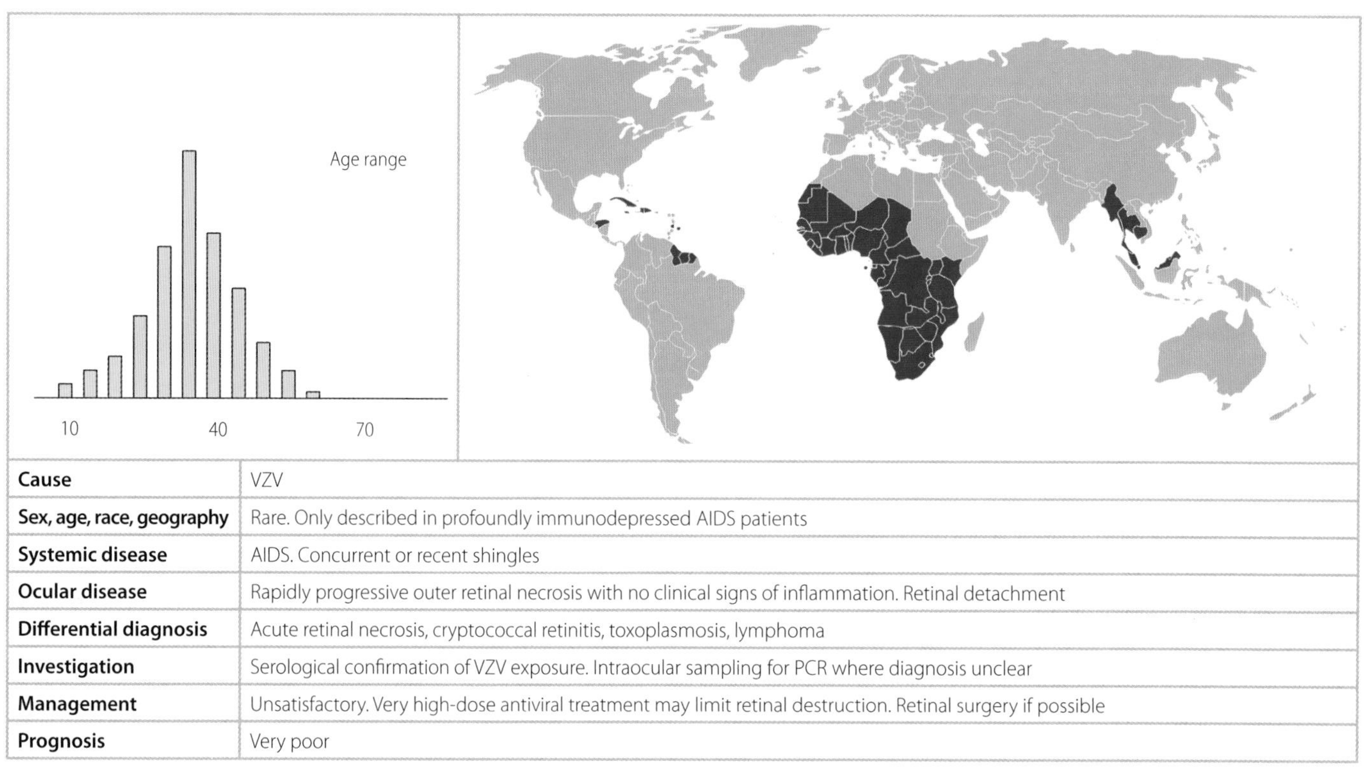

Cause	VZV
Sex, age, race, geography	Rare. Only described in profoundly immunodepressed AIDS patients
Systemic disease	AIDS. Concurrent or recent shingles
Ocular disease	Rapidly progressive outer retinal necrosis with no clinical signs of inflammation. Retinal detachment
Differential diagnosis	Acute retinal necrosis, cryptococcal retinitis, toxoplasmosis, lymphoma
Investigation	Serological confirmation of VZV exposure. Intraocular sampling for PCR where diagnosis unclear
Management	Unsatisfactory. Very high-dose antiviral treatment may limit retinal destruction. Retinal surgery if possible
Prognosis	Very poor

Box 11.6 Progressive outer retinal necrosis

Introduction

Necrotizing retinitis associated with herpesvirus infection in the form known as acute retinal necrosis has been recognized for 40 years. Substantial intraocular inflammation is associated with that condition. Some 20 years later (Forster et al. 1990) a recognizably different form of retinitis was described in AIDS patients, most of whom, it transpires, have concurrent or recent shingles (in any dermatome). The condition affects primarily the outer retina, and has a very poor response to systemic antiviral treatment. The disease, caused by the VZV, is termed PORN. In their classic forms these two extremes of ARN and PORN may be regarded as defining the margins of necrotizing herpetic retinopathies in general with their intermediate forms in between (Guex-Crosier et al. 1997). Many AIDS patients with PORN have CD4 counts <10 – they are incapable of producing a classic inflammatory response (although specimens do show some lymphocytic infiltration) and the ophthalmoscopic appearance represents not primarily an inflammatory condition, but virus proliferating unopposed within a suitable culture medium – the outer retina.

Systemic disease

Almost exclusively PORN is seen in those with advanced AIDS and very low CD4 counts. Some will have defaulted from supervision and HAART treatment. Most have recent or concurrent VZV dermatitis. Any dermatome may be affected and there appears to be no particular association with HZO compared with other dermatomes. Other opportunistic infections may be present.

Ocular disease

Presentation is usually with unilateral symptoms of rapid visual blurring, but bilateral involvement is common on first examination or rapidly thereafter. In contrast to ARN, there is usually very little or no cellular reaction in aqueous or vitreous, giving a very clear retinal view. Again, in contrast to ARN, the post-equatorial retina is usually primarily involved and this may rapidly include the macula. Multifocal, deep retinal (and possibly choroidal), pale areas are seen (**Fig. 11.40**) which rapidly progress within days to coalesce and give widespread retinal edema and whitening (**Fig. 11.41**), affecting both peripheral and central retina. The macula is often primarily involved (**Fig. 11.42**), and edema of this area may give rise to a cherry-red spot. Rapid retinal necrosis ensues and edema subsides, so that, within a week or so, stark white areas are visible (**Figs 11.43** and **11.44**), sometimes sparing perivascular retinal areas so that the retina resembles 'cracked mud.' Optic disk swelling is common. A vasculitic component is not prominent, at least until the late stages of the process (**Fig. 11.45**). Untreated or inadequately treated, retinal fragmentation is the sequel (**Fig. 11.46**), leading to complex and generally inoperable retinal detachment.

Diagnosis

PORN is a new, rare clinical entity, but it has several typical and recognizable features that should allow clinical diagnosis and therefore appropriately urgent treatment. Although also caused by VZV, it has several features that distinguish it from ARN. The differential diagnosis is occasionally challenging. In the early stages, apparent multifocal deep retinal and choroidal involvement may suggest disseminated fungal infection such as cryptococcosis. Toxoplasmosis in immunosuppressed individuals may occupy predominantly the outer retina and may be severe or multifocal. If necessary PCR on intraocular fluid is confirmatory.

Management

Progression of PORN is very unresponsive to conventional antiviral treatment that would normally control ARN. Most affected eyes progress to complete blindness with profound retinal (**Fig. 11.47**) and optic atrophy, the retinal vasculature becoming attenuated. Atrophic retinal break formation and subsequent retinal detachment, in either the acute or the convalescent stages, is virtually

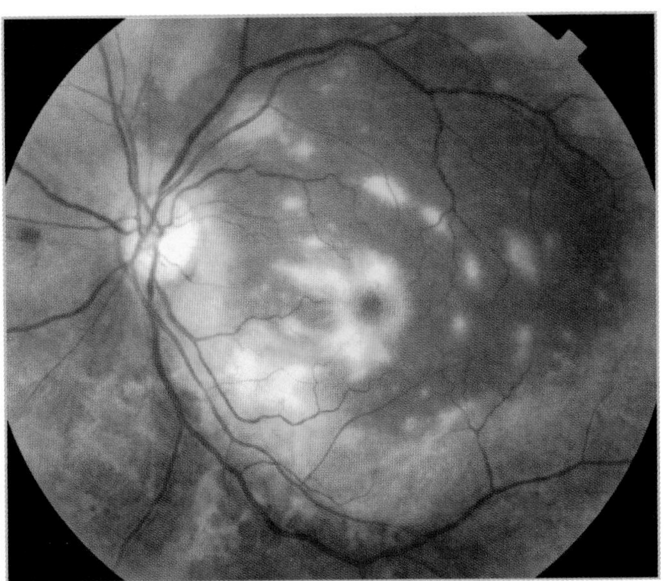

Figure 11.40 Progressive outer retinal necrosis on presentation in a young woman with previously undiagnosed AIDS, newly immigrant to the UK from Africa.

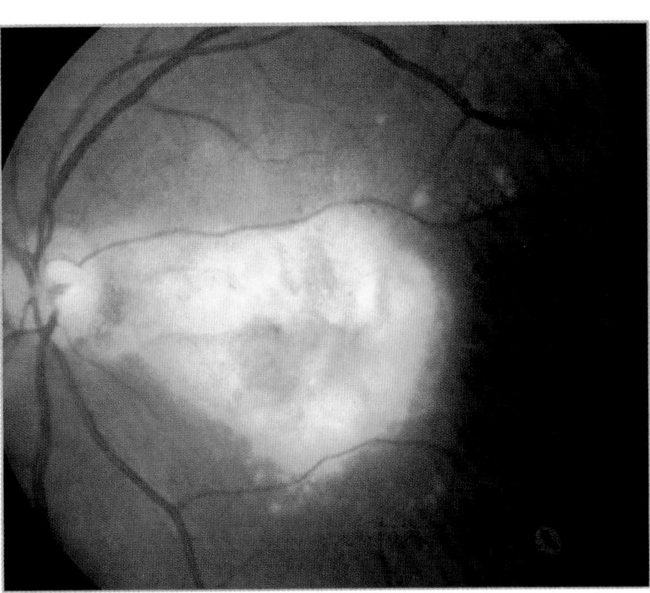

Figure 11.42 Primary macular involvement in progressive outer retinal necrosis on presentation.

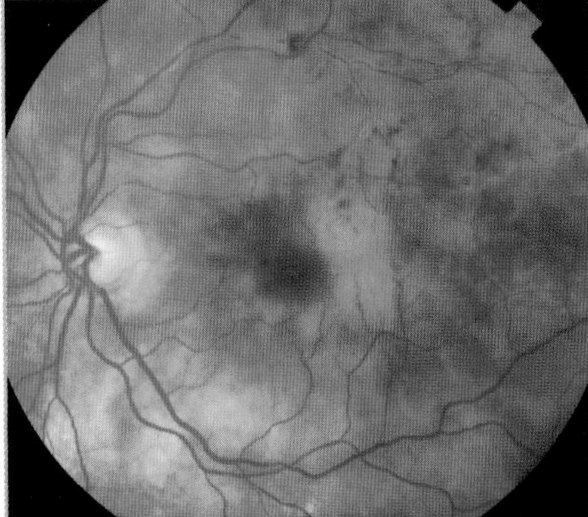

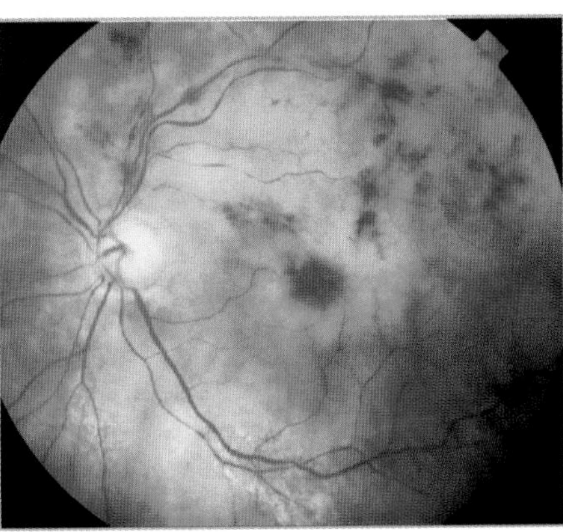

Figure 11.41 Rapidly progressive outer retinal necrosis in a patient with end-stage systemic lupus on immunosuppression.

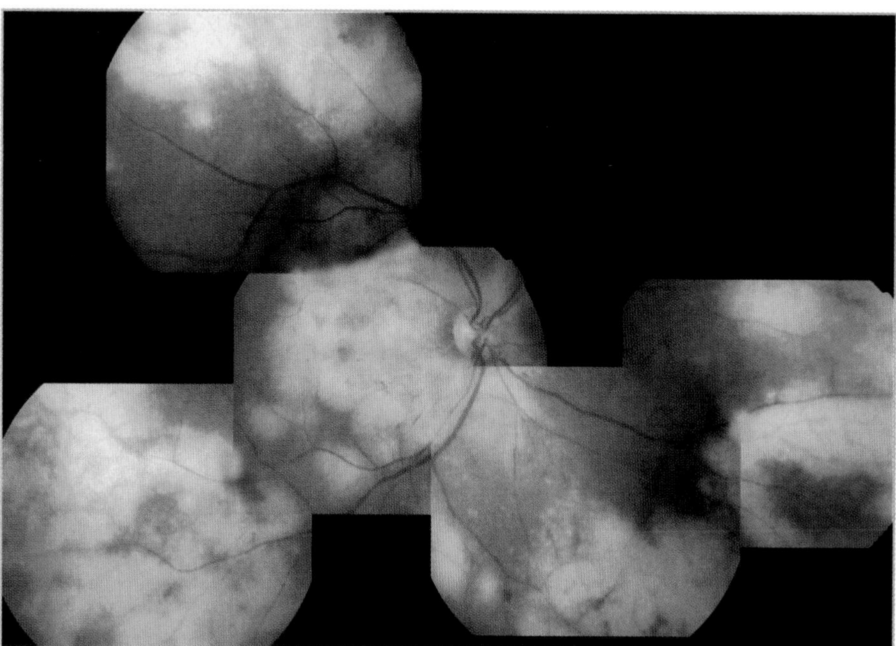

Figure 11.43 Widespread coalescing pale lesions, usually involving the posterior pole, are the hallmark of progressive outer retinal necrosis.

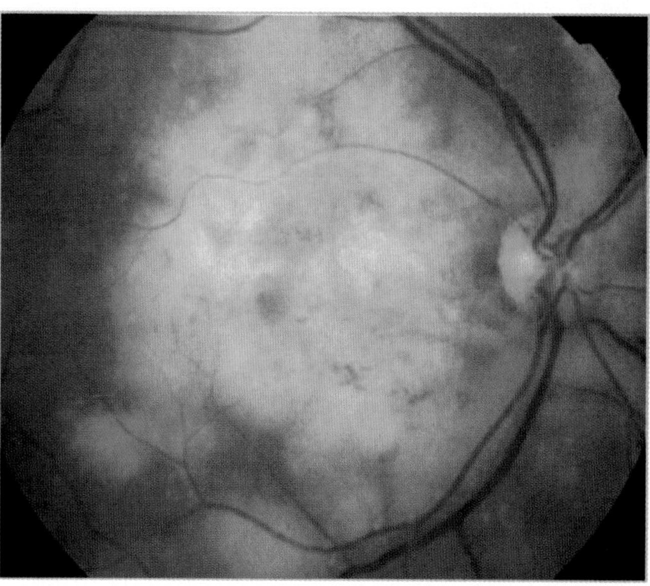

Figure 11.44 Severe macular involvement on presentation. Same patient as Fig. 11.43.

universal. Vitreous organization with tractional effects and PVR, as seen typically in ARN, are not a feature of PORN. This appalling prognosis led to attempts to use very aggressive treatment regimens, usually combining two antivirals from aciclovir, ganciclovir and foscarnet, both in induction doses (Cuilla et al. 1998). To this can be added intraocular ganciclovir or foscarnet, and some have combined intravitreal ganciclovir implantation with regular foscarnet injections. This two-pronged aggressive approach may serve to preserve vision in at least one eye while HAART is instituted, with the hope that CD4 recovery will permit a host immune response to recommence and give intrinsic control. Without this, the visual prognosis remains very poor.

OTHER VIRAL UVEITIS

Chikungunya

Chikungunya, first emerging in the 1950s (Khairallah et al. 2009), is a togavirus that is transmitted by the bites of mosquitoes of the genus *Aedes* and is endemic in parts of Africa and Asia (**Fig. 11.48a**). However, possibly linked to climatic change, a local epidemic in Italy was recently reported, the first in a temperate area. The virus is known to mutate and a further sign of spread is awaited. The illness sustained is very similar to dengue in both symptoms and signs but there tend to be sporadic epidemics of infection. Symptoms rapidly follow an infected bite and usually involve a mild fever lasting 2 or more weeks with musculoskeletal pains. More severe cases develop a bleeding diathesis, prostration and neurological complications including meningoencephalitis or Guillain–Barré syndrome.

Uveitis occurs after, not during, the acute phase and usually affects the anterior segment, and may be granulomatous or non-granulomatous. It may mimic herpetic uveitis. Optic and retrobulbar neuritis are also seen (Lalitha et al. 2007) and in this group visual prognosis is guarded. Retinitis is seen and macular chorioretinitis has been reported (**Fig. 11.49a**). Diagnosis is by qualifying signs in an endemic area, with supportive serology. Aciclovir and prednisolone have been used to treat posterior segment inflammation but no evidence on sensitivity to the aciclovir group is available.

Dengue fever

Dengue virus is a flavivirus that, similar to chikungunya, is transmitted by the bites of Aedes mosquitoes. Infection is most usually asymptomatic but dengue fever is seen in about 5% and is caused by one of four subtypes of the virus; immunity is not common between subtypes. High fever, headache, measles-like rash and severe muscular and arthritic pains begin usually within 2 weeks of infection and last for a week. A small minority develops life-threatening hemorrhagic

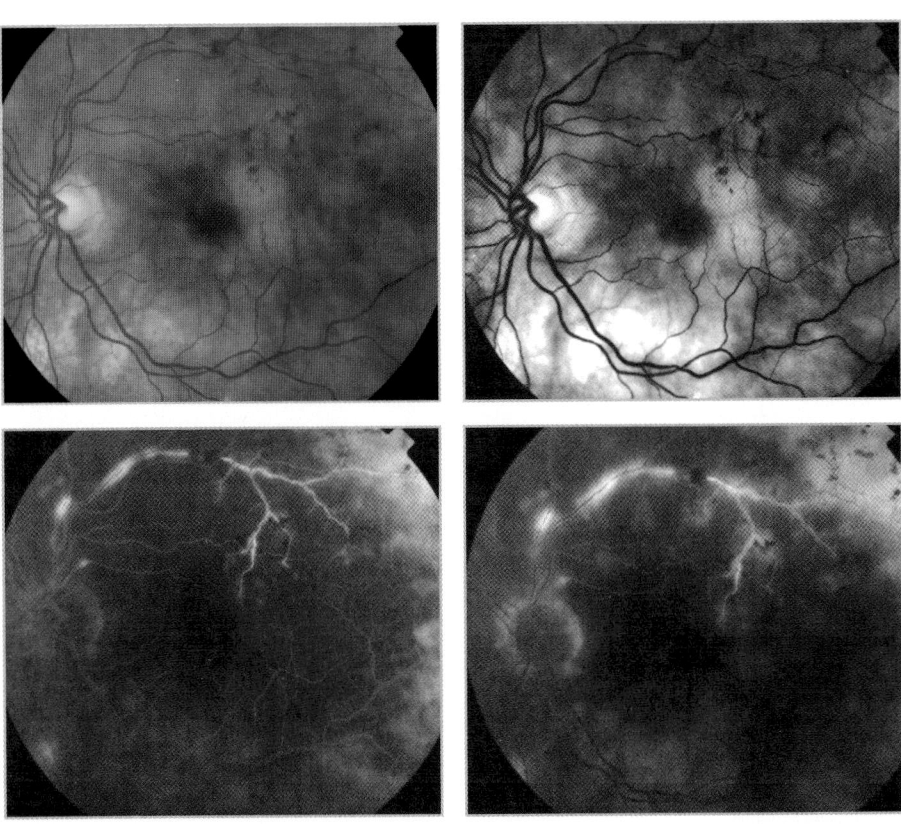

Figure 11.45 Vasculitis and substantial intraretinal leakage in progressive outer retinal necrosis. Same patient as Fig. 11.41.

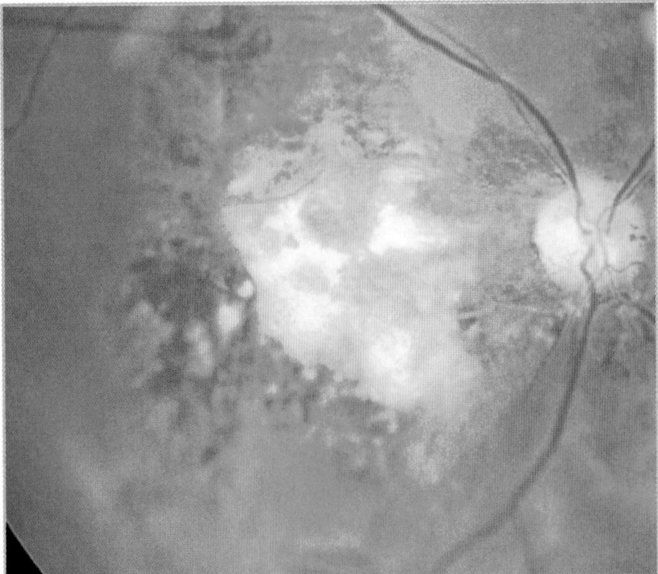

Figure 11.46 Retinal necrosis and fragmentation despite aggressive treatment. Same patient as Figs 11.43 and 11.44. Total inoperable retinal detachment supervened.

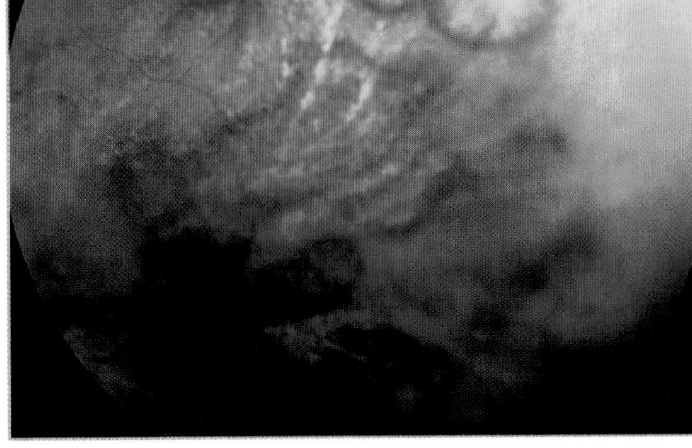

Figure 11.47 Coalescent pale necrotic areas in progressive outer retinal necrosis evolve into atrophic, infarcted retina .

or hypovolemic complications. The disease is substantially more common now than 50 years ago, affecting about 100 million people annually in several world zones (**Fig. 11.48b**).

Uveitis is very uncommon and does not occur in the acute phase but 2–6 months later. There are no pathognomonic features and manifestations are variable. including anterior uveitis (Gupta et al. 2009), vitritis, vasculitis with or without occlusion, multifocal chorioretinitis, and ischemic or hemorrhagic retinopathy. Maculopathy is frequent (Bacsal et al. 2007) comprising clusters of yellow chorioretinal dots, with blot hemorrhages and edema accompanied by substantial retinal and sometimes choroidal vasculitis (**Fig. 11.49b**). A substantial proportion requires oral steroid treatment. Outcomes are variable depending on ischemic change or macular scarring.

Epstein–Barr virus

The Epstein-Barr virus (EBV, HHV-4) is a ubiquitous DNA herpesvirus that is usually transmitted by contact with infected saliva;

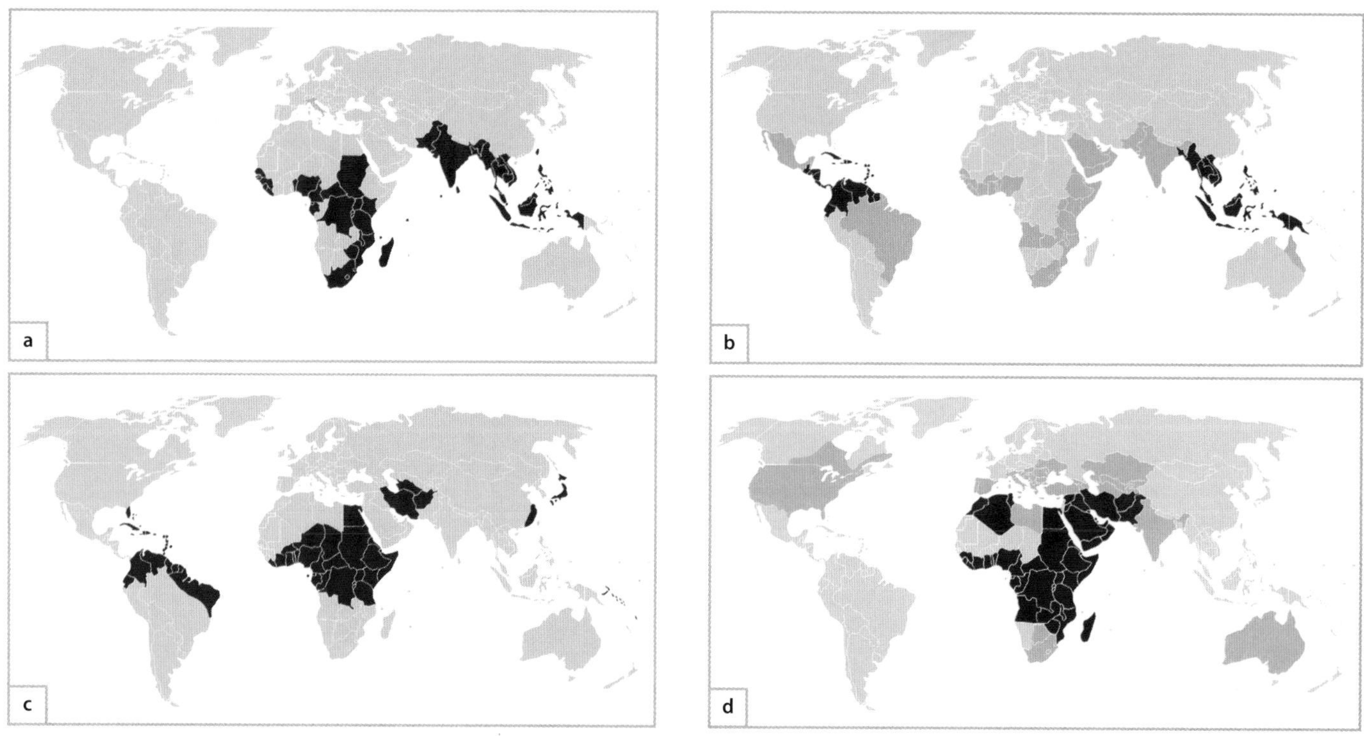

Figure 11.48 World distribution maps for some viral diseases involving uveitis: (a) chikungunya; (b) dengue fever; (c) HTLV-1; (d) West Nile virus.

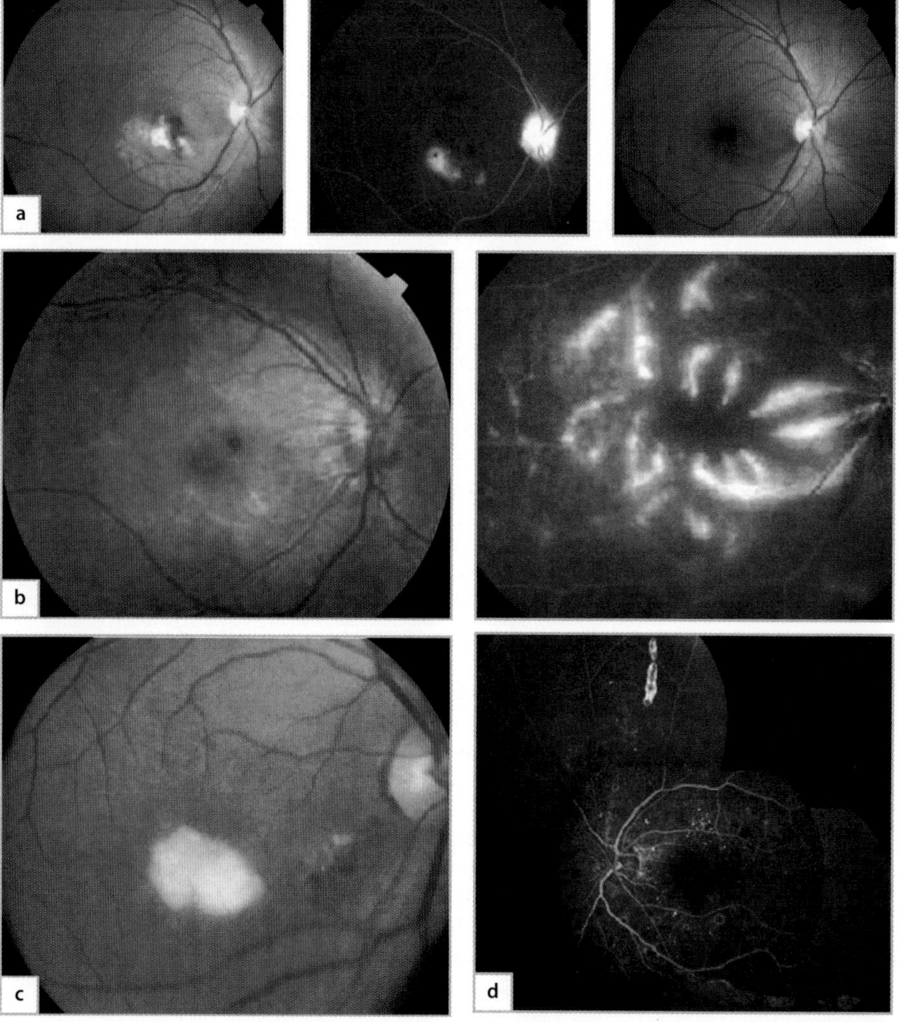

Figure 11.49 Ocular involvement in several viral diseases: a) chikungunya; (b) dengue fever; (c) Rift Valley fever; (d) West Nile virus. (Modified from Khairallah et al. 2009.)

asymptomatic individuals can intermittently shed the virus at any stage after infection. Most acquire the disease in childhood (half are seropositive by 5 years of age) and at this time acquisition is almost always asymptomatic. Most of the rest acquire it by early adulthood (95% seropositive) and from adolescence; about a third develop symptoms and signs of glandular fever. The virus is B-cell lymphotropic, and in some parts of the world infection is also associated with Burkitt's lymphoma.

Both conjunctivitis and superficial keratitis may occur with infectious mononucleosis, the latter resembling the nummular keratitis of adenovirus infection. Uveitis is less common. Although reports of both anterior and posterior uveitis in association with EBV infection are now numerous, an etiological association remains unconfirmed. Higher levels of serum antibodies to EBV have been detected in some patients with uveitis and EBV DNA has been located from intraocular fluid in some. Unifocal retinitis or multifocal outer retinal or choroidal inflammation has also been seen contemporaneously with EBV infection, although not with a convincing etiological connection. Lesions may subside to leave depigmented punctate scars similar to those seen in multifocal choroiditis with panuveitis, or presumed ocular histoplasmosis. Optic disk and macular edema have also been seen. There are interesting anecdotes of tubulointerstitial nephritis with uveitis with EBV infection. Although aciclovir has moderate activity against EBV, the pathogenesis of EBV-associated uveitis is unclear and the use of aciclovir speculative. Evidence of a pathogenic association between EBV and uveitis remains elusive. However, the probable lifelong intralymphocytic infection of affected individuals and the well-known ability of EBV to modify B-cell responses raises the possibility of virus-induced autoimmune inflammation.

Human T-cell lymphotropic virus-I

Human T-lymphotropic virus type I (HTLV-I) is a member of the oncovirus subgroup of retroviruses, which are capable of generating neoplasia, predominantly hematological. HTLV-1 is associated with human T-cell leukemia/lymphoma, and uveitis. Clusters of disease have been reported from Japan and other parts of the Far East, South America, south-eastern USA and the Caribbean, West Africa and the Caucasus (**Fig. 11.48c**). The virus requires venereal or parenteral contact for transmission to occur. A chronic inflammatory myelopathy, probably immune mediated, may occur and was initially named tropical spastic paraparesis. However, the most serious manifestation of HTLV-1 infection is an aggressive adult T-cell leukemia/lymphoma (ATL) with lymphadenopathy, hepatosplenomegaly, bone lesions and skin involvement. The malignancy is resistant to chemotherapy and those with acute presentations or a predominantly lymphomatous process carry a very poor prognosis. Some patients show a chronic course over several years, but the median survival time for ATL is less than 1 year. Diagnosis depends on a high suspicion for the disease in those living within, and traveling to and from, endemic areas where seropositivity may exceed 1%, and is much higher in intravenous drug abusers. An ELISA is available and PCR on blood is also feasible.

Uveitis is not generally seen in those with ATL or myelopathy, but HTLV-1 infection is now definitely associated with uveitis in young adult asymptomatic carriers. Although less than 5% develop uveitis, in some parts of Japan it is the most common cause of uveitis (Miyanaga et al. 2009). Uveitis may be more common in the significant subset of HTLV-1 seropositives that have autoimmune thyroiditis. The inflammation may be unilateral or bilateral, with anterior uveitis a constant feature. Vitritis and retinal vasculitis with retinal exudate and hemorrhage also affect the great majority. Some develop a predominantly intermediate picture but most have relatively benign self-limiting inflammation, which may recur (Nakao et al. 1999). It responds well to topical or, where required, systemic steroid medication. The uveitis appears to respond but has a tendency to recur when treatment is discontinued.

Rift Valley fever

This epidemic viral zoonosis has its reservoir in mammals including livestock and affects predominantly the countries around the Rift Valley, which descends through East Africa. Epidemics have also affected Egypt and parts of the Middle East. The bunyavirus is transmitted mainly by contact with infected animal tissue but also by mosquito bite. Most affected patients have a relatively mild fever, but some develop severe musculoskeletal pains, bleeding diathesis, hepatitis with jaundice or encephalitis. Each epidemic tends to cause hundreds to thousands of human deaths. Diagnosis is by serology, the differential including dengue, West Nile, Ebola, Marburg and Hanta fevers. Treatment is entirely supportive and no specific antiviral is known.

Uveitis affects up to a fifth of patients and almost all develop a macular retinitis (see Fig. 11.49c) with or without retinal vasculitis and papillitis (Al-Hazmi et al. 2005). Permanent visual damage is common and chorioretinal scarring and optic atrophy sometimes remain. There are no data on the effectiveness of either antiviral or steroid treatment.

Rubella and Rubeola viruses

Rubella is caused by airborne transmission of this togavirus, and occurs worldwide. In non-immunized areas infection is very common and normally leads only to a mild and short-lasting febrile illness with upper-body erythematous rash. Acquisition during pregnancy causes major problems to the fetus, hence population immunization, commencing at 1–2 years of age, is widespread. The embryo is affected in over 40% of cases acquired during the first trimester and spontaneous abortion may result. If acquired during the second trimester, over 50% of fetuses develop major organ abnormalities including sensorineural deafness, heart defects including patent ductus, congenital cataract or microphthalmos, learning disabilities, microcephaly, hepatosplenomegaly and thrombocytopenia. The less-severely affected may have developmental delay, learning difficulty and diabetes. Rubella is one of several diseases capable of causing very similar abnormalities if acquired in utero, collectively known as the TORCH complex (**t**oxoplasmosis, **o**ther [including syphilis and VZV], **r**ubella, **c**ytomegalovirus, **h**erpes).

Congenital rubella may cause chorioretinal scarring that is characteristically described as of 'salt and pepper' appearance (**Fig. 11.50**). In the absence of other ocular abnormalities, low vision with macular hypoplasia can be seen, and later macular subretinal neovascular membrane formation is possible. The possibility that active rubella infection can be associated with uveitis is much less well documented. The virus has been suggested as an etiological agent in Fuchs' heterochromic uveitis and this possibility is discussed in Chapter 9. Almost all suggestions of rubella as an etiological agent in uveitis are based on the Goldman–Witmer coefficient rather than RNA isolation through PCR, but there are definite anecdotes of either intermediate or panuveitis during active infection. Anterior uveitis has also followed rubella immunization. Other than these events the evidence for rubella as an etiological agent in uveitis is unconvincing.

Rubeola virus is the paramyxovirus that causes measles. This potentially severe epidemic exanthem is characterized by widespread erythematous rash, moderate pyrexia with pharyngitis, and sometimes hepatitis or encephalitis. Keratitis with ulceration or anterior uveitis has

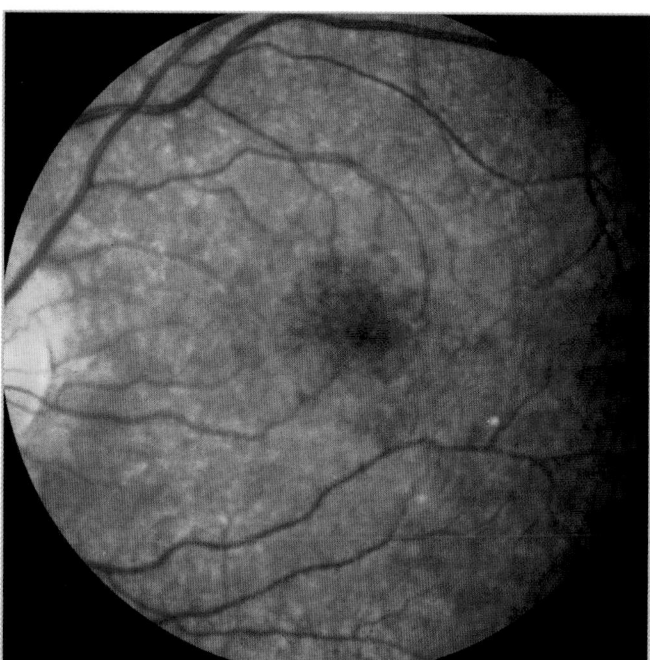

Figure 11.50 Typical mottled salt-and-pepper pigment distribution following congenital rubella infection.

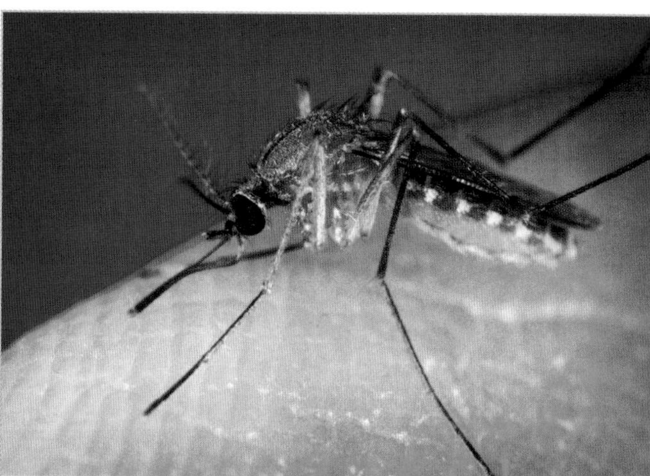

Figure 11.51 A Culex mosquito, the vector of West Nile virus. (Modified from Centers for Disease Control, Public Health Image Library.)

been reported in the acute phase. The disease has a small but significant mortality rate and is subject to population immunization in almost all countries. Subacute sclerosing panencephalitis is a fortunately unusual progressive encephalopathy that is usually fatal, and probably caused by persistent CNS viral infection. Uveitis, particularly chorioretinitis, is not uncommon during this process (Yuksel et al. 2011). Ocular involvement may present before the development of ataxia, epilepsy and personality change. If detected early, lifelong interferon treatment may arrest progression but otherwise the disease is fatal.

West Nile virus

The flavivirus that causes West Nile fever is hosted by wild birds but spread by mosquito bites. Already widespread in most of Africa and the Middle East, it has over the past 20 years caused human infection in North America, southern Europe and the Caucasus (**Fig. 11.48d**). It is spread by Culex mosquitoes (**Fig. 11.51**), some species of which are widespread in temperate climates. The disease is highly likely to continue to widen its range. Most infected humans are asymptomatic, but flu-like fever with headache, muscle aches and pharyngitis, sometimes with rash, is common. A small minority goes on to develop neurological complications including meningoencephalitis with coma, or myelitis. Serology is diagnostic.

Uveitis affects most patients with neurological complications, but not those with mild disease. The resultant multifocal chorioretinitis is virtually pathognomonic of West Nile infection, showing discrete or contiguous lesions distributed in streaks along the line of the nerve fiber layer (see Fig. 11.49d). Active lesions are creamy and scarred, atrophic with RPE loss. For unknown reasons, pre-existing diabetes is a risk factor for chorioretinitis and diabetic retinopathy frequently accompanies images of affected fundi. The management of West Nile infection is supportive only. Ophthalmic disease is treated on its merit and is usually self-limiting. Most do not develop macular scarring.

Immunizations and uveitis

Attacks of uveitis, predominantly bilateral anterior self-limiting uveitis, have been reported anecdotally following shortly after several immunizations against viral diseases. The number of reported cases for hepatitis B vaccine (Frauenfelder et al. 2010) is significant and this requires monitoring. Smaller numbers have been reported after MMR (mumps, measles and rubella), varicella and influenza. Most attacks are mild and require short-term topical steroid treatment.

REFERENCES

Aizman A, Johnson MW, Elner SG. Treatment of acute retinal necrosis syndrome with oral antiviral medications. *Ophthalmology* 2007;**114**:307–12.

Al-Hazmi A, Al-Rajhi AA, Abboud EB, et al. Ocular complications of Rift Valley fever outbreak in Saudi Arabia. *Ophthalmology* 2005;**112**:313–18.

Althaus C, Loeffler KU, Schimkat M, et al. Prophylactic argon laser coagulation for rhegmatogenous retinal detachment in AIDS patients with cytomegalovirus retinitis. *Graefes Arch Clin Exp Ophthalmol* 1998;**236**:359–64.

Avery RK, Mossad SB, Poggio E, et al. Utility of leflunomide in the treatment of complex cytomegalovirus syndromes. *Transplantation* 2010;**90**:419–26.

Bacsal KE, Chee S-P, Cheng C-L, et al. Dengue-associated maculopathy. *Arch Ophthalmol* 2007;**125**:501–10.

Balansard B, Bodaghi B, Cassoux N, et al. Necrotising retinopathies simulating acute retinal necrosis syndrome. *Br J Ophthalmol* 2005;**89**:96–101.

Chee SP, Jap A. Cytomegalovirus anterior uveitis: outcome of treatment. *Br J Ophthalmol* 2010;**94**:1648–52.

Chen N, Yang M, He L, et al. Corticosteroids for preventing postherpetic neuralgia. *Cochrane Database Syst Rev* 2010;**12**:CD005582.

Cuilla TA, Rutledge BK, Morley MG, Duker JS. The progressive outer retinal necrosis syndrome: successful treatment with combination antiviral therapy. *Ophthalmic Surg Lasers* 1998;**29**:198–206 .

de Schryver I, Rozenberg F, Cassoux N, et al. Diagnosis and treatment of cytomegalovirus iridocyclitis without retinal necrosis. *Br J Ophthalmol* 2006;**90**:852–5 .

Dworkin RH, Johnson RW, Breuer J, et al. Recommendations for the management of herpes zoster. *Clin Infect Dis* 2007;**44**:S1–26.

Forster DJ, Dugel PU, Frangieh GT, et al. Rapidly progressive outer retinal necrosis in the acquired immunodeficiency syndrome. *Am J Ophthalmol* 1990;**110**:341–348.

Frauenfelder FW, Suhler EB, Frauenfelder JT. Hepatitis B vaccine and uveitis: an emerging hypothesis suggested by review of 32 case reports. *Cutan Ocul Toxicol* 2010;**29**:26–9.

Guex-Crosier Y, Rochat C, Herbort CP. Necrotising herpetic retinopathies. A spectrum of herpes virus-induced diseases determined by the immune state of the host. *Ocul Immunol Inflamm* 1997;**5**:259–65.

Guo LB, Sun D, Ye JJ, et al. Intravitreal injection of ganciclovir in the treatment of acute retinal necrosis. *Zhonghua Yan Ke Za Zhi* 2007;**43**:631–7.

Gupta A, Srinivasan R, Setia S, et al. Uveitis following Dengue fever. *Eye* 2009;**23**:873–6.

Holland GN. Standard diagnostic criteria for the acute retinal necrosis syndrome. *Am J Ophthalmol* 1994;**117**:663–666.

Ishida T, Sugamoto Y, Sugita S, Mochizuki M. Prophylactic vitrectomy for acute retinal necrosis. *Jpn J Ophthalmol* 2009;**53**:486–9.

Kempen JH, Min YI, Freeman WR, et al. Risk of immune recovery uveitis in patients with AIDS and cytomegalovirus retinitis. *Ophthalmology* 2006;**113**:684–94.

Khairallah M, Jelliti B, Jenzeri S. Emergent infectious uveitis. *Middle East Afr J Ophthalmol* 2009;**16**:225–38.

Kido S, Sugita S, Horie S, et al. Association of varicella zoster virus load in the aqueous humour with clinical manifestations of anterior uveitis in herpes zoster ophthalmicus and zoster sine herpete. *Br J Ophthalmol* 2008;**92**:505–8.

Lalitha P, Rathinam S, Banushree K, et al. Ocular involvement associated with an epidemic outbreak of chikungunya virus infection. *Am J Ophthalmol* 2007;**144**:552–6.

Miserocchi E, Waheed NK, Dios E, et al. Visual outcome in herpes simplex virus and varicella zoster virus uveitis: a clinical evaluation and comparison. *Ophthalmology* 2002;**109**:1532–7.

Morrison VL, Labree LD, Azen SP, et al. Results of silicone oil removal in patients with cytomegalovirus retinitis related retinal detachments. *Am J Ophthalmol* 2005;**140**:786–93.

Morrison VL, Kozak I, LaBree LD, et al. Intravitreal triamcinolone acetonide for the treatment of immune recovery uveitis macular edema. *Ophthalmology* 2007;**114**:334–9 .

Miyanaga M, Shimizu K, Kawaguchi T, et al. A clinical survey of uveitis in HTLV-1 endemic region. *Ocul Immunol Inflamm* 2009;**17**:335–41.

Muccioli C, Belfort R. Treatment of cytomegalovirus retinitis with an intraocular sustained-release ganciclovir implant. *Braz J Med Biol Res* 2000;**33**:779–89.

Nakao K, Ohba N, Nakagawa M, Osame M. Clinical course of HTLV-1 associated uveitis. *Jpn J Ophthalmol* 1999;**43**:404–9.

Nithyanandam S, Stephen J, Joseph M, Dabir S. Factors affecting visual outcome in herpes zoster ophthalmicus: a prospective study. *Clin Exp Ophthalmol* 2010;**38**:845–50.

Tanna AP, Kempen JH, Dunn JP, et al. Incidence and management of cataract after retinal detachment repair with silicone oil in immune compromised patients with cytomegalovirus retinitis. *Am J Ophthalmol* 2003;**136**:1009–15.

Thorne JE, Jabs DA, Kempen JH, et al. Causes of visual acuity loss amongst patients with AIDS and cytomegalovirus retinitis in the era of highly active anti-retroviral therapy. *Ophthalmology* 2006;**113**:1441–5.

Tibbetts MD, Shah CP, Yopung LH, et al. Treatment of acute retinal necrosis. *Ophthalmology* 2010;**117**:818–24.

Urayama A, Yamada N, Sasaki T, et al. Unilateral acute uveitis with retinal periarteritis and detachment. *Jpn J Clin Ophthalmol* 1971;**25**:607–612.

Usui Y, Takeuchi M, Yamauchi Y, et al. Pars plana vitrectomy in patients with acute retinal necrosis syndrome: surgical results in 52 patients. *Nihon Ganka Gakkai Zasshi* 2010;**114**:362–8.

van Boxtel LA, van der Lelij A, van der Meer J, Los LI. Cytomegalovirus as a cause of anterior uveitis in immunocompetent patients. *Ophthalmology* 2007;**114**:1358–62.

van der Lelij A, Ooijman FM, Kijlstra A, Rothova A. Anterior uveitis with sectoral iris atrophy in the absence of keratitis: a distinct clinical entity among *herpetic eye diseases Ophthalmology* 2000;**107**:1164–70.

Vitravene Study Group. Randomized dose-comparison studies of intravitreous fomivirsen for treatment of cytomegalovirus retinitis that has reactivated or is persistently active despite other therapies in patients with AIDS. *Am J Ophthalmol* 2002;**133**:475–83.

Waib LF, Bonon SH, Salles AC, et al. Withdrawal of maintenance therapy for cytomegalovirus retinitis in AIDS patients exhibiting immunological response to HAART. *Rev Inst Med Trop Sao Paulo* 2007;**49**:215–19.

Wong R, Pavesio CE, Laidlaw DA, et al. Acute retinal necrosis: the effects of intravitreal foscarnet and virus type on outcome. *Ophthalmology* 2010;**117**: 556–60.

Yuksel D, Sonmez PA, Yilmaz D, et al. Ocular findings in subacute sclerosing panencephalitis. *Ocul Immunol Inflamm* 2011;**19**:135–8.

Chapter 12 Fungal infection

The true fungi or *Eumycota* are, unlike plants, incapable of synthesizing their own nutrition. They are either saprobes (consuming dead organic matter) or parasites (consuming living organic matter), the latter including the human pathogens. Those classes of medical importance are the Ascomycota (including *Aspergillus, Penicillium, Blastomyces* and *Histoplasma* spp.), the Basidiomycota (including cryptococci) and the Deuteromycota (including *Candida, Sporothrix* and *Coccidioides* spp.). The proper classification of some 'fungal' microorganisms is a regular topic of debate. *Nocardia* sp., once considered a fungus, is now classified with the bacteria. *Coccidioides* sp. has some lifecycle features of a protozoon but is normally considered with the fungi. *Pneumocystis* sp., previously considered a protozoon, is now reclassified as a fungus of the Ascomycota group.

Most fungi have a filamentous hyphal structure, with cell walls made predominantly of chitin. Individual cells are usually incompletely separated by perforated septa. Some fungi are unicellular and known as yeasts. Propagation is by spore formation, either sexual or asexual. Most pathogenic fungi are dimorphic, thriving in a yeast-like phase at 37°C and in a filamentous phase at 25°C, and many are acidophilic. Cellular immunity appears to be of prime importance in human infection. Fungal contact, at least on body surfaces, is universal and frequent, but most human disease is limited to the skin (dermatomycosis) or mucosae. Intravenous inoculation or immunodeficiency, particularly T-lymphocyte disease, is normally required to permit dissemination. In this way hematogenous spread may lead to intraocular infection. This chapter deals with endogenous fungal endophthalmitis, and also with presumed ocular histoplasmosis, a syndrome with an unproven etiology, but with strong evidence linking it to infection with *Histoplasma* spp.

PRESUMED OCULAR HISTOPLASMOSIS SYNDROME (box 12.1)

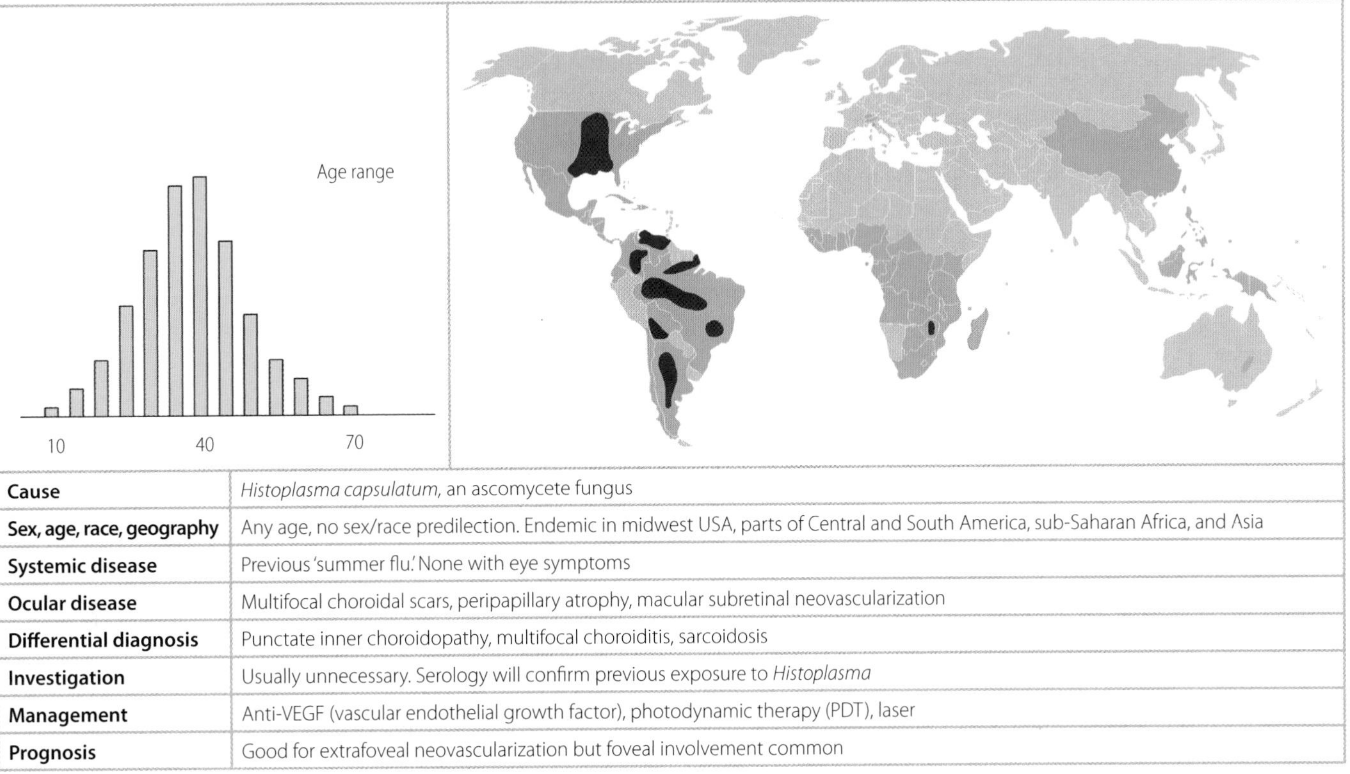

Cause	*Histoplasma capsulatum*, an ascomycete fungus
Sex, age, race, geography	Any age, no sex/race predilection. Endemic in midwest USA, parts of Central and South America, sub-Saharan Africa, and Asia
Systemic disease	Previous 'summer flu.' None with eye symptoms
Ocular disease	Multifocal choroidal scars, peripapillary atrophy, macular subretinal neovascularization
Differential diagnosis	Punctate inner choroidopathy, multifocal choroiditis, sarcoidosis
Investigation	Usually unnecessary. Serology will confirm previous exposure to *Histoplasma*
Management	Anti-VEGF (vascular endothelial growth factor), photodynamic therapy (PDT), laser
Prognosis	Good for extrafoveal neovascularization but foveal involvement common

Box 12.1 Presumed ocular histoplasmosis syndrome

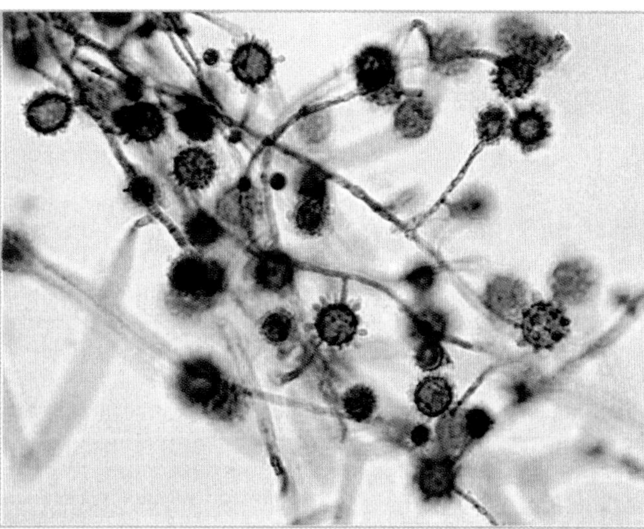

Figure 12.1 The hyphae and macroconidia of *Histoplasma capsulatum*. (Modified from Centers for Disease Control, Public Health Image Library.)

Introduction

Histoplasma capsulatum (**Fig. 12.1**) is a fungus that proliferates on the excreta of bats and birds (including domestic fowl), its highest concentrations being found in the nesting sites of these animals. It is endemic in the midwest USA, particularly in the valleys of the Mississippi and Ohio rivers and their tributaries, being most common in the states of Tennessee, Kentucky and Ohio. It is also commonly found in Central and South America, parts of the West Indies, Indonesia and the Philippines, and isolated pockets exist in Switzerland, Italy and Australasia. The fungus may be inhaled from dry soil or guano, and evidence of previous exposure is found in up to 95% of those tested in US endemic areas. Human disease is uncommon outside the USA.

Acquisition of *H. capsulatum* is usually asymptomatic. In endemic areas, minor exposure is frequent and tolerance develops. Acute symptoms tend to occur only in those who inhale a large inoculum (especially those who venture into bat caves), and who have not previously been exposed. Cavers and spelunkers are a risk group. In this circumstance acute pulmonary histoplasmosis may develop, with pyrexia, pneumonitis, arthralgia and skin rash. In mild form the condition is described as 'summer flu' in the USA. More severe pneumonitis is uncommon but rarely may be fatal. Occasionally pulmonary histoplasmosis can become chronic with lung fibrosis, emphysema and cavitation, not dissimilar to tuberculosis. A small minority, including immunocompromised individuals, may develop disseminated histoplasmosis with weight loss, hepatosplenomegaly, thrombocytopenia, endocarditis, meningitis and other manifestations. More chronic dissemination may present as persistent oral ulcers and chronic laryngitis. Treatment with itraconazole, ketoconazole or amphotericin B is necessary. There are usually no ocular manifestations to disseminated histoplasmosis, but postmortem intraocular involvement has been demonstrated and multifocal chorioretinitis has been reported in a moribund AIDS patient.

In US endemic areas, multifocal chorioretinal scars can be found in up to 13% of the population. It has been postulated that, in those who test positive for previous exposure to *H. capsulatum*, the organism is the cause of the scars. The term 'presumed ocular histoplasmosis syndrome' (POHS) has been used to describe a typical pattern of chorioretinal scarring without vitreous inflammation, often with consequent subretinal neovascularization, in a patient with proven exposure by skin testing or serology. The association between *H. capsulatum* and this syndrome remains conjectural, but, although Koch's postulates for infection have by no means been fulfilled, circumstantial and epidemiological evidence is persuasive. Unfortunately, the term 'POHS' has been mistakenly and confusingly extended to include similar multifocal choroidal syndromes, often with active inflammation, that occur outside known endemic areas. These syndromes are discussed in Chapter 19.

Systemic disease

Patients with POHS do not have active systemic disease. Indeed, as perhaps 99% of those who acquire *H. capsulatum* do so asymptomatically, a previous history of acute infection is rare.

Ocular disease

True POHS is rare outside the midwest USA. Multifocal choroidal scars are typical. The 'histo spots' are small, round and depigmented with some internal pigment clumping. They may be few in number, and are located primarily around the posterior pole (**Fig. 12.2**). In some patients heavily pigmented linear scars are seen, usually more peripherally and usually running parallel to the ora serrata (**Fig. 12.3**). Peripapillary choroidal depigmentation (**Fig. 12.4**) is also characteristic. There are no vitreous cells.

It is the presence or absence of macular histo spots that usually determines the likelihood of visual problems in POHS. Most do not lose vision. Those with macular choroidal scars have a significant incidence of complications. An acute maculopathy, even with central serous detachment, may occur. Recurrences may be frequent and lead to disciform changes (**Fig. 12.5**), typically arising adjacent to old scars, but occasionally subretinal neovascularization may arise anew. Breakthrough of hemorrhage into the vitreous is seen rarely.

Diagnosis

The presence of intraocular inflammation should lead the ophthalmologist to consider similar syndromes such as punctate inner

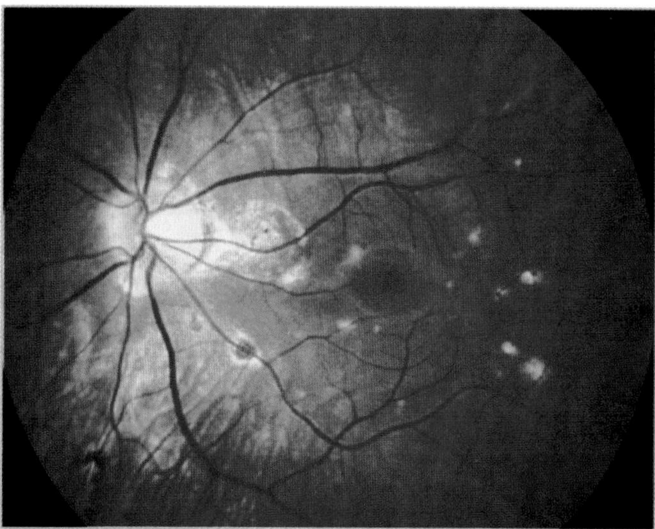

Figure 12.2 Multiple 'histo spots' and peripapillary atrophy in presumed ocular histoplasmosis.

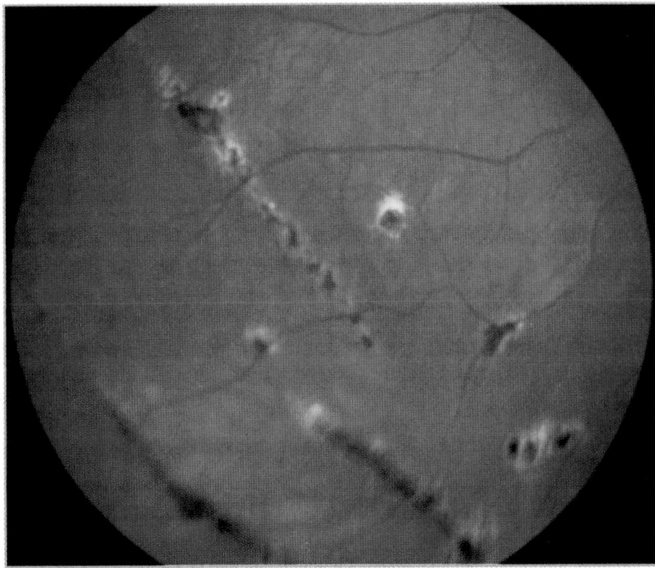

Figure 12.3 Peripheral linear grouped pigmentary scars in a patient with presumed ocular histoplasmosis.

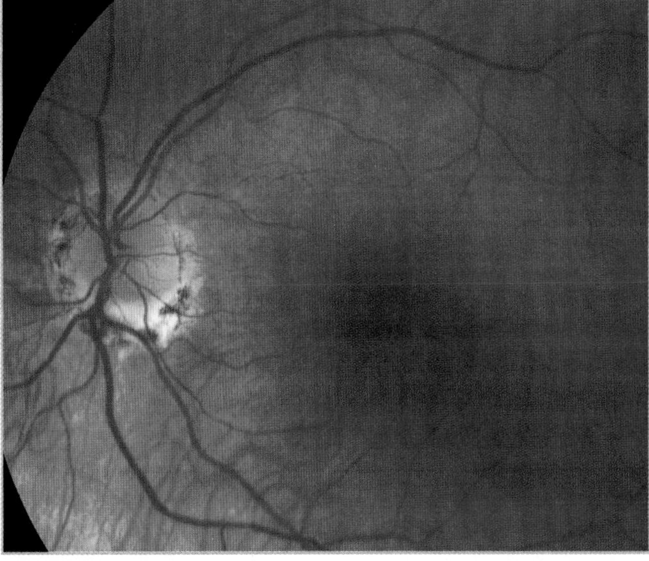

Figure 12.4 Peripapillary atrophy as the only sign indicative of presumed ocular histoplasmosis syndrome in the left eye. The right had developed a macular choroidal neovascular membrane.

choroidopathy (PIC) or multifocal choroiditis with panuveitis, which may, nevertheless, have similar outcomes. Sarcoidosis should also be considered. Early serological assessments by complement fixation were confounded by high rates of cross-reactivity with other fungi but modern ELISA (enzyme-linked immunosorbent assay) methods are superior. The histoplasmin skin test is now rarely used.

Management

The recurrent macular lesions are often steroid responsive in their early stages and oral steroid is better than depot steroid injection (Martidis et al. 1999), but this is not curative and a substantial course may be required. Intravitreal triamcinolone has also been used with good effect. Photodynamic therapy (PDT) has shown considerable promise in several forms of inflammatory choroidal neovascularization including POHS (Lui et al. 2004) but the introduction of anti-VEGF treatments has eclipsed this method of treatment for age-related macular degeneration, which has remained inadequately trialed in POHS and may yet provide a future alternative treatment. Intravitreal anti-vascular endothelial growth factor (VEGF) injections are effective, including both ranibizumab and bevacizumab (Ehrlich et al. 2009, Nielsen et al. 2011) but ongoing treatment is required at an average 4.5 injections in the first year. Combined PDT and anti-VEGF injection has been used in some eyes with weak evidence of additive effect. Persistent membranes, both macular and peripapillary, have been removed surgically with some evidence of efficacy (Almony et al. 2008). In extremis when both maculae are scarred, macular translocation has been used with minor improvement in visual function.

The approaches to, and outcomes of treatment for, choroidal neovascular membranes secondary to POHS and PIC are similar

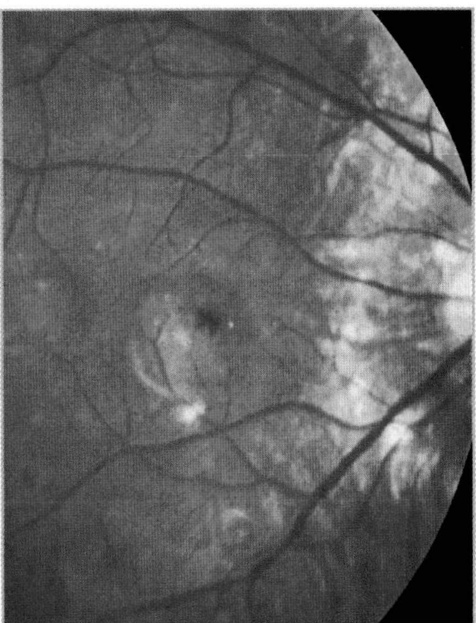

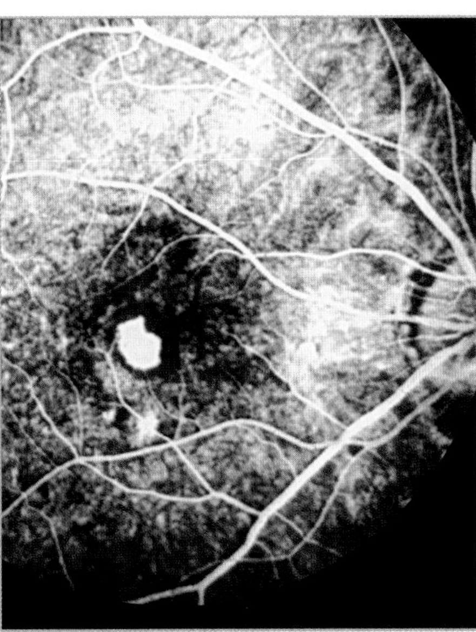

Figure 12.5 Choroidal neovascular membrane formation in presumed ocular histoplasmosis syndrome.

and some would argue, indistinguishable. Our general approach is to initiate high-dose oral steroid therapy and arrange early bevacizumab injection, repeating when necessary after 4–6 weeks and thereafter. There are anecdotal risks of provoking choroidal neovascularization in those with histo spots, including refractive laser surgery and the acquisition of other fungal infection, including dermatomycosis, and some advocate regular Amsler grid self-testing (Trevino and Salvat 2006).

CANDIDIASIS (box 12.2)

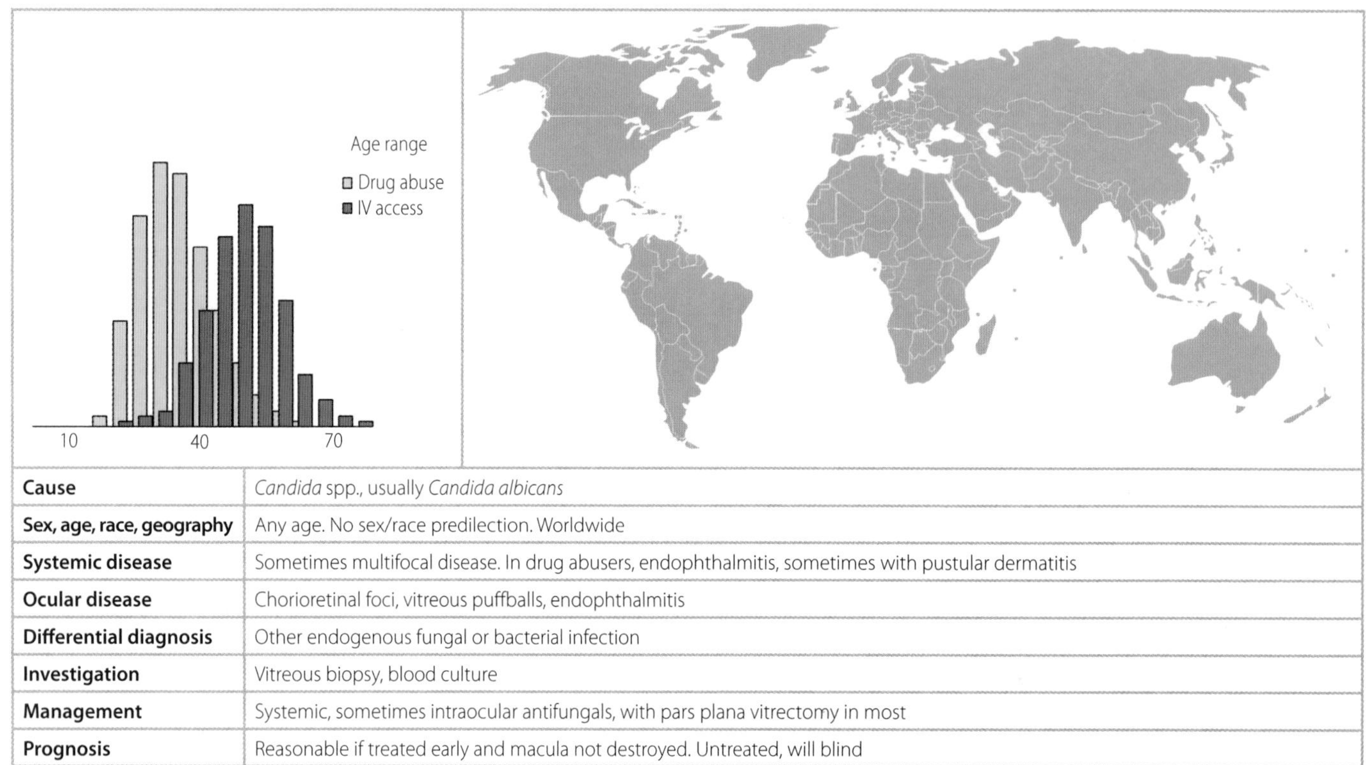

Cause	*Candida* spp., usually *Candida albicans*
Sex, age, race, geography	Any age. No sex/race predilection. Worldwide
Systemic disease	Sometimes multifocal disease. In drug abusers, endophthalmitis, sometimes with pustular dermatitis
Ocular disease	Chorioretinal foci, vitreous puffballs, endophthalmitis
Differential diagnosis	Other endogenous fungal or bacterial infection
Investigation	Vitreous biopsy, blood culture
Management	Systemic, sometimes intraocular antifungals, with pars plana vitrectomy in most
Prognosis	Reasonable if treated early and macula not destroyed. Untreated, will blind

Box 12.2 Candidiasis

Introduction

Members of the genus *Candida* are deuteromycete fungi, several of which are universal skin commensals, and *C. albicans* is a normal inhabitant also of human mucosae including respiratory, gastrointestinal and genital tracts. Of the 80 or so species in the genus, *C. albicans* (**Fig. 12.6**) remains the most frequent human pathogen, but over time the relative proportion of other species has increased, including *C. glabrata, C. tropicalis, C. lusitaniae, C. krusei* and *C. parapsilosis.* Firm identification of species is important because of variable susceptibility to antifungal agents. The organisms are not virulent pathogens, and disseminated candidiasis usually affects only those susceptible, such as during recovery from major surgery and during immunosuppression. There is a 1–2% incidence among organ transplant recipients and generally candidiasis is a risk for patients under intensive care. Intravenous inoculation is usually necessary for intraocular infection to occur.

Candida spp. may access the bloodstream directly via intravenous lines, usually those that have been indwelling for some time. It may be injected as a contaminant of self-administered heroin, a possibility facilitated by the use of lemon juice as a heroin solvent, an ideal culture medium for this acidophilic fungus. Indeed, fungal infection accounts for up to 50% of serious infections in drug abusers, *Candida* and *Aspergillus* spp. being the most commonly involved organisms. *Candida* spp. may also colonize implanted foreign bodies such as artificial heart valves and prosthetic joints. Invasion is facilitated by the use of broad-spectrum antibiotics. Esophagitis, gastrointestinal mucosa damaged by

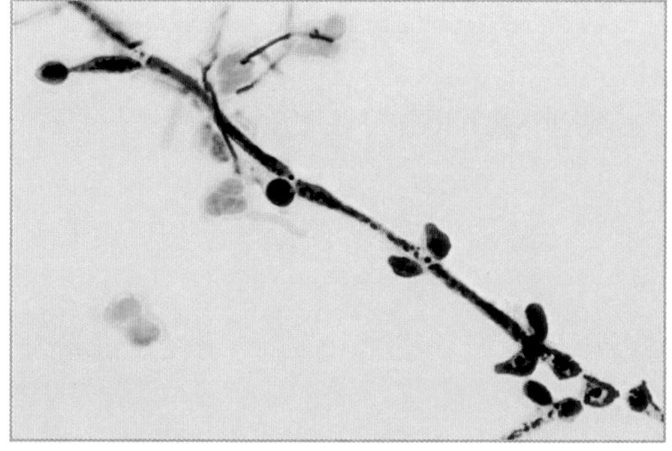

Figure 12.6 *Candida albicans*, showing both pseudohyphae (responsible for spread and tissue invasion) and yeast buds. (Modified from Centers for Disease Control, Public Health Image Library.)

surgery or cytotoxic therapy may provide sites for intravascular access. Immune deficiency, either natural or iatrogenic, malignancy or general debilitation may all provoke dissemination.

Systemic disease

Disseminated candidiasis may present with generalized signs of pyrexia, nodular or pustular skin lesions, failure to respond to antibacterial treatment and organ failure, either acute or chronic. For those with widespread signs, the mortality rate is in excess of 30% and is higher in critically ill individuals. It may also present with focal organ involvement, and it is here that the ophthalmologist is most likely to become involved; most cases of endophthalmitis occur in the absence of other systemic disease.

Ocular disease

Endophthalmitis is seen in a variable but small proportion of those with candidemia, and *C. albicans* is the organism most frequently responsible. Although predisposing factors for dissemination are numerous, cases of endophthalmitis occur overwhelmingly either as a result of intravenous drug abuse or from indwelling intravenous lines.

Progression of intraocular candidiasis is usually slow. Posterior segment infection seems to start in the choriocapillaris, early lesions appearing to be subretinal, but occasionally large (**Fig. 12.7**). Invasion of the retinal pigment epithelium (RPE) may occur, typically causing one or more whitish, elevated retinal lesions to appear at the posterior pole either unilaterally (**Fig. 12.8**) or bilaterally (**Fig. 12.9**). If untreated the retina will be perforated to involve the vitreous (**Fig. 12.10**) and an expanding lesion may form (**Fig. 12.11**). It is characteristic for *Candida* spp. proliferating within the vitreous to form 'puffballs' and these, when linked together, can resemble a 'string of pearls' (**Fig. 12.12**). The infection may progress to become a panophthalmitis with complete vitreous opacification, and patients may present with leukocoria (**Fig. 12.13**). Subsequent traction on sites of posterior hyaloid adhesion may cause retinal detachment, which can progress to become inoperable (**Fig. 12.14**). Successful elimination of the organism will leave atrophic chorioretinal scars.

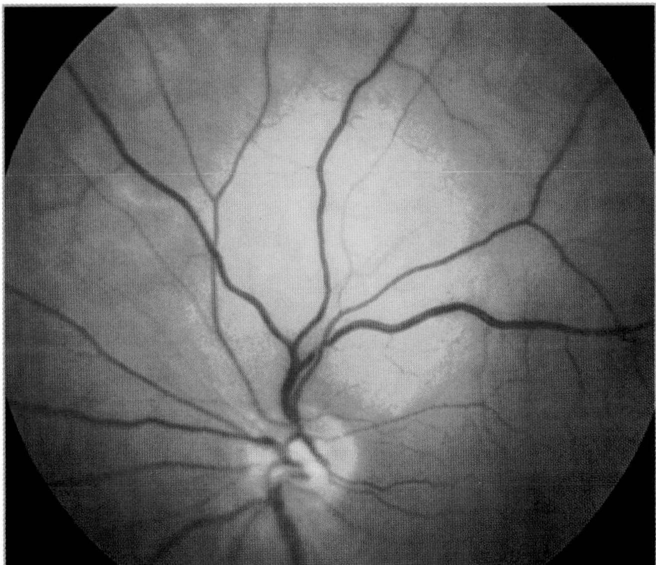

Figure 12.7 A large subretinal focus of endogenous candidiasis. The lesion has yet to invade retina.

Diagnosis

Blood culture is positive in only 50% of those with disseminated candidiasis, but should be repeated if necessary, preferably on 3 consecutive days. In drug abusers blood culture is rarely positive because the condition may have been the result of only one contaminated injection at some previous date. Those with an indwelling intravenous line should have the line removed and the line tip cultured. In those with neutropenia the presence of *Candida* spp. at two or more body sites predicts dissemination in a majority. Pars plana vitrectomy is commonly required, and vitreous microscopy and culture will be confirmatory.

Management

The potential for ocular involvement in those with candidemia is understood and therefore the prospect of ophthalmological screening has been raised. One recent study (Dozier et al. 2011) found that the proportion affected was 1% and that no asymptomatic patients were diagnosed on screening. In contrast, another study (Oude Lashof et al. 2011) identified over 15% affected. These results are inconsistent even accounting for the different populations under study and clearer data are required. However, for those patients unable to express visual symptoms who are found to have candidemia, a single posterior segment examination seems wise.

For those patients who are ill and receiving intravenous therapies, attempts to retain central or peripheral venous catheters in the presence of candidemia lead to a poor outcome; they should be removed and their tips cultured. The treatment of those with intraocular involvement will depend on the layer involved. Those presenting early with small subretinal lesions at the macula (typically intravenous drug abusers) often respond well to oral antifungal treatment without the need for either vitrectomy or intraocular injection. For those whose lesions have broken through into vitreous, this will not suffice and intraocular intervention is also required, sometimes by intraocular injection alone, more often combined with vitrectomy. There has been substantial evolution of systemic antifungals over the past 20 years, such that toxic historical mainstays including amphotericin B and flucytosine are less frequently required. The optimal choice will become apparent if sensitivity in culture can be demonstrated, and intraocular penetration varies substantially between groups.

Azole antifungals

The large group of azoles (predominantly for *Candida* spp., the triazoles, which in general have wider and better antifungal activity than the imidazoles) inhibits the production of fungal ergosterol which is essential for cell membrane metabolism and growth. They are fungistatic, not fungicidal. In general (with the exception of ketoconazole and itraconazole which penetrate poorly) the group produces adequate intravitreal concentrations when administered systemically, particularly **fluconazole** and **voriconazole** (Riddell et al. 2011). Indeed, even topical voriconazole 1% is said to achieve adequate concentration in vitreous (Vemulakonda et al. 2008) and it requires a lower minimum inhibitory concentration (MIC) than fluconazole. Both of the preferred drugs can be administered either orally or intravenously: fluconazole orally at up to 800 mg/day in very severe infection, more usually 400 mg/day for endophthalmitis; voriconazole also at 400 mg/day orally or 4 mg/kg twice daily intravenously. Intraocular penetration from the oral route is good and the advantage of intravenous usage for well patients with candida endophthalmitis is unproven. Each has wide activity against many *Candida* spp. and strains, but *C. glabrata* and *C. krusei* are the fungi most frequently resistant. A large number of

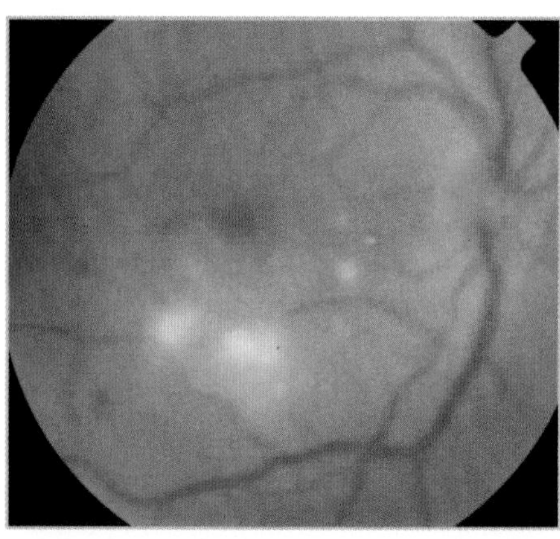
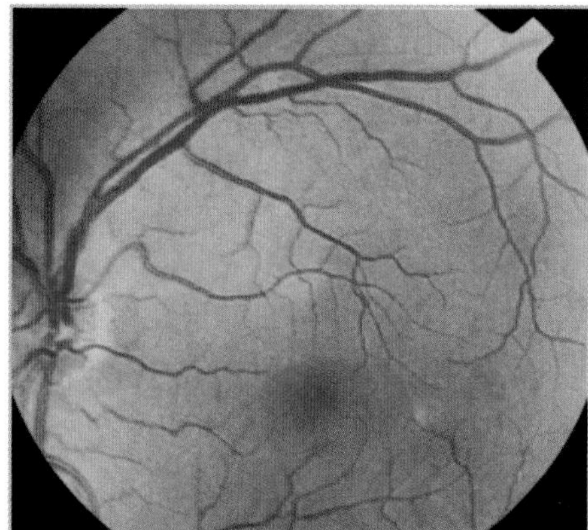

Figure 12.8 Bilateral endogenous candidiasis in an intravenous drug abuser. The left eye shows only a subtle perifoveal choroidal infiltrate, whereas the right has foci that have broken through the retina causing vitritis.

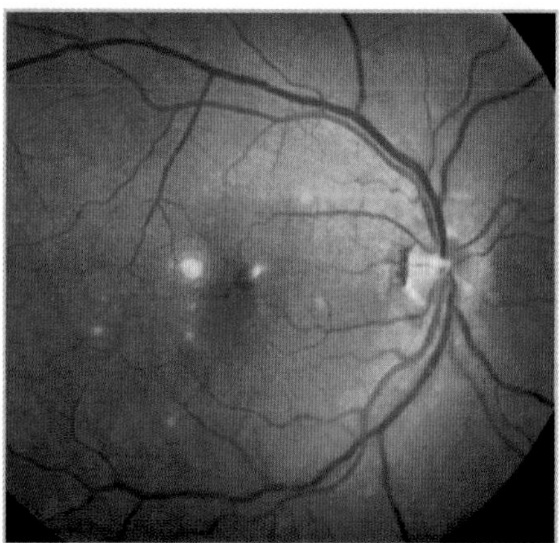
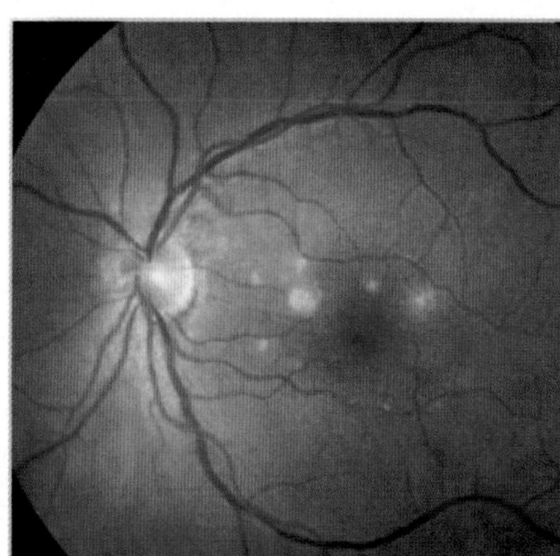

Figure 12.9 Bilateral submacular candida infiltrates without vitreous involvement. The patient had shared the same lemon juice and syringe as the patient in Fig. 12.8 when injecting heroin.

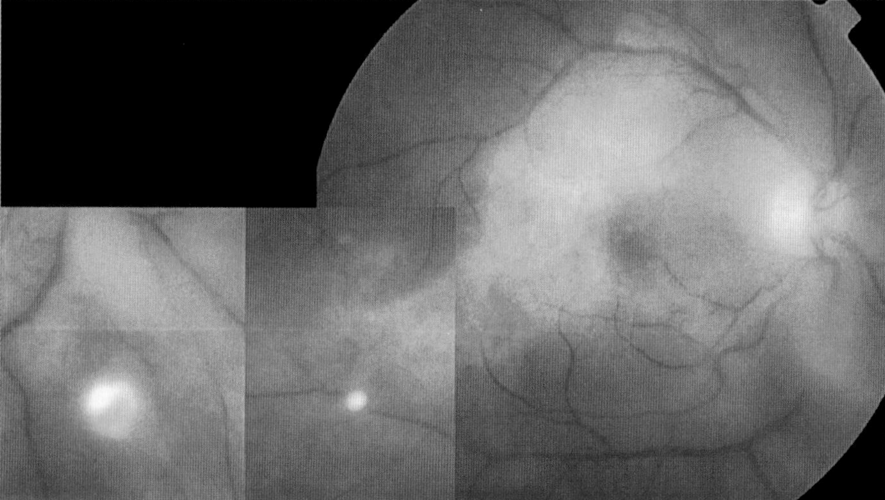

Figure 12.10 Unilateral endogenous candidiasis in a patient with an indwelling central line. Substantial vitritis accompanies two retinal foci (the one at left transposed from inferior fundus).

publications deal with comparative in vitro efficacy of fluconazole and voriconazole, characteristically awarding slight superiority (e.g. 95% vs 90% susceptibility) to voriconazole but, with substantial cross-resistance, only a third of fluconazole-resistant strains being sensitive to voriconazole (Pfaller et al. 2007). Voriconazole has not been demonstrated superior to fluconazole in the prevention of invasive candidiasis (Wingard et al. 2010) or specifically to treat endophthalmitis, but is currently riding a wave of popularity. Clearer evidence is required, preferably from double-blind studies. Another new triazole, **posaconazole**, does not achieve adequate intravitreal MIC from systemic administration but may be useful in exogenous fungal keratitis.

Echinocandin antifungals

This is a relatively new drug class, its members acting by inhibiting synthesis of polysaccharides within the fungal cell wall. They are fungicidal. **Caspofungin** has high efficacy against *Candida* spp. and also against *Aspergillus* spp. It is given intravenously at 50–70 mg daily. It shares a toxicity profile with many antifungals including organ toxicity, leukopenia and anaphylaxis. It is a large molecule

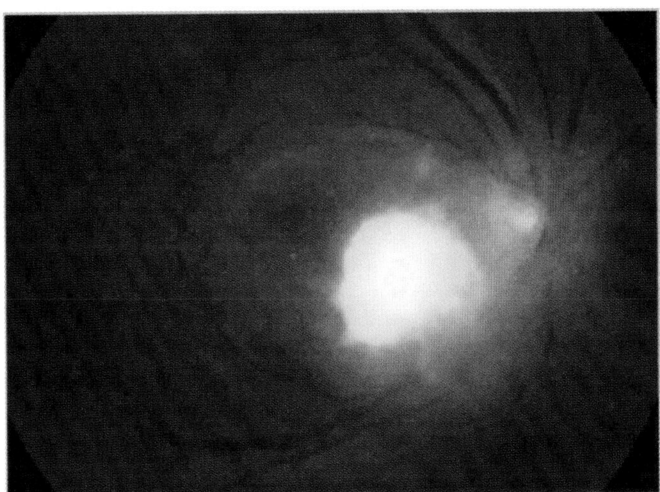

Figure 12.11 An advanced retinal and preretinal candida abscess, probably sustained from a tattoo needle.

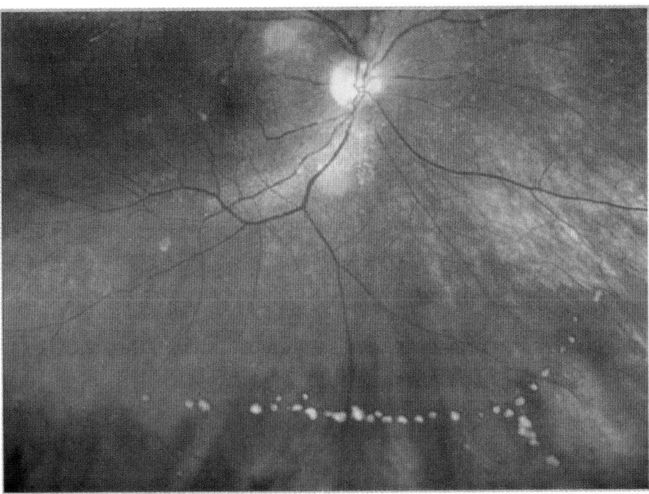

Figure 12.12 Diffuse vitritis and multiple small retinal foci are accompanied by a classic intravitreal 'strong of pearls' in polymerase chain reaction-confirmed intraocular candidiasis.

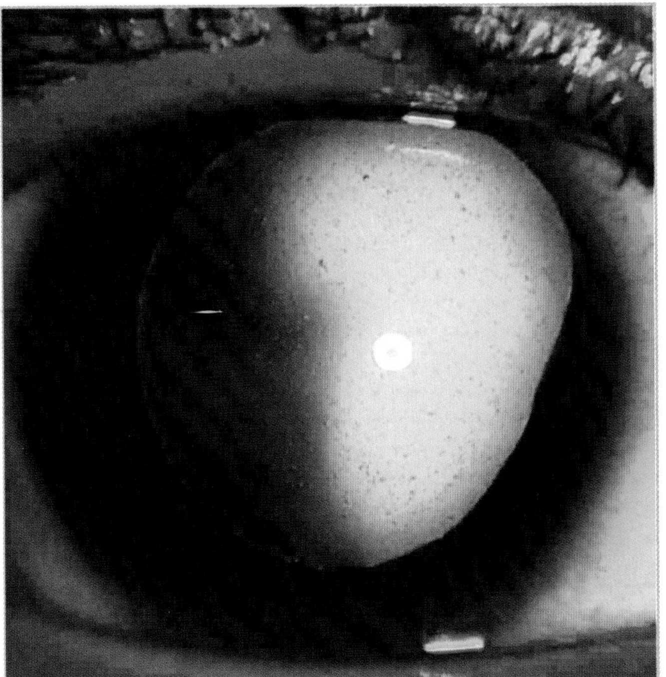

Figure 12.13 Late presentation in candida endophthalmitis (typically in an intravenous drug addict or a comatose patient on an intensive care unit) may exhibit leukocoria. Vision will not be preserved in this eye.

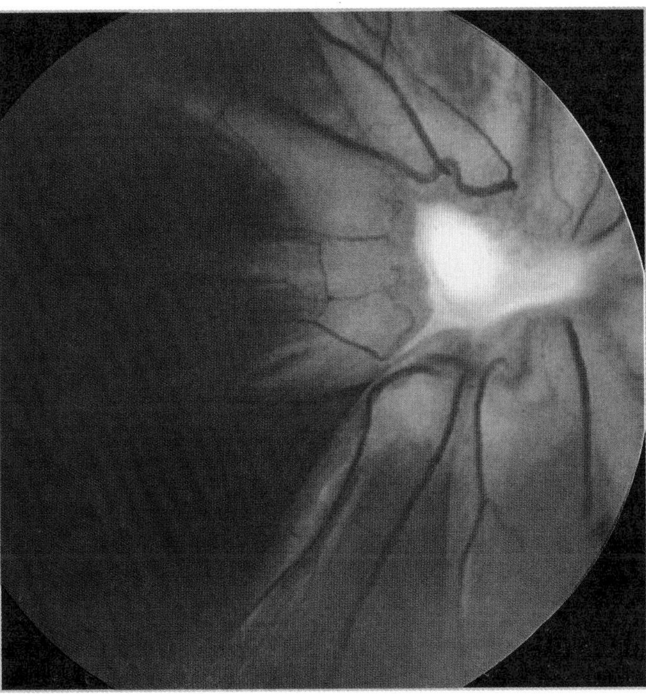

Figure 12.14 Late-presenting candida endophthalmitis with total funnel-shaped retinal detachment and proliferative vitreoretinopathy.

of > 1200 Da and therefore has poor intraocular penetration when administered systemically. There is a paucity of evidence on efficacy in endophthalmitis and the intraocular MIC is not well established. Published anecdotes of success from systemic administration should be viewed with caution. **Micafungin** is the second echinocandin useful in systemic candidiasis. It is given intravenously at 100–200 mg/day for 2 weeks or more. Animal models do not conclusively show enough intravitreal penetration from systemic administration and anecdotes of human usage are also inconclusive. The likely future usage of the echinocandins in human fungal endophthalmitis will be limited to intraocular use if it is demonstrated to be safe, unless similar drugs with molecular weights <500 Da can be manufactured, in which case they are likely to pass the blood-ocular barrier in adequate concentration from intravenous administration.

Polyene antifungals

This group of sterol-based cyclic antifungals works by disrupting cell membrane architecture to cause breaks, allowing cell contents to escape. They are fungicidal. **Amphotericin B** is an old drug, first extracted from streptomyces bacteria in 1955. It is very poorly absorbed orally, and hence can be safely used as lozenges to treat oral thrush. Systemically it requires slow intravenous infusion over 6 hours, in a dose of up to 1 mg/kg per day. Infusion reactions are common and cause pyrexia, rigors and vomiting. Local thrombophlebitis, marrow depression and renal dysfunction are frequent, so regular assessment of organ function is mandatory. Discontinuation of treatment because of intolerance is common. Irreversible renal toxicity may result from administration of a cumulative total dose in excess of 2000 mg. Intraocular penetration is poor from the intravenous route. This drug has now been virtually replaced by liposomal forms (myriad lipid bilayer vesicles containing active drug). These variants retain antifungal activity with reduced toxicity but must still be used with great care systemically. The availability of more effective and less toxic triazoles has removed amphotericins from the systemic armamentarium against candida endophthalmitis. Nystatin is in this group but has not been investigated for intraocular use.

Flucytosine

Flucytosine has been available as an antifungal for over 40 years, being active against some *Candida* spp. and cryptococci. It is a fluorinated pyrimidine that inhibits uracil metabolism and therefore RNA synthesis within fungi. It is available orally in some countries but is normally used intravenously in the management of severe fungal infections at a dose of 100–200 mg/kg per day, divided in four doses and usually for no more than 1 week. Serum concentrations should be monitored with the aim of achieving trough levels of 25–30 mg/l and peak levels of 70–80 mg/l. Care should be taken in renal impairment. Adverse reactions include vomiting, diarrhea, rashes, hepatotoxicity, thrombocytopenia and leukopenia. It is not used alone because of emerging resistance, but this is created through a different mechanism to azole resistance and so cross-resistance is uncommon. It has additive toxicity with amphotericin.

Intravitreal antifungal injection

Amphotericin can be injected intravitreally but is highly toxic and must be diluted appropriately. Normally 5 μg is used, and a maximum of 10 μg. Solutions of the correct dilution should not retain the drug's yellow color. There is no human evidence base for the relative efficacy of liposomal amphotericin intravitreally, but, in rabbit models, retinal toxicity is also reduced allowing the safe usage of 20 μg (40 μg being retinotoxic). In the clinical setting it has been used anecdotally and we have used the same dilution technique as for amphotericin B with good effect.

Voriconazole can be injected intravitreally and in doses up to 25 μg is not retinotoxic. It has been used with success in a variety of cases of fungal endophthalmitis but anecdotal evidence suggests superior efficacy in non-candida cases (which may be less sensitive to systemic triazoles). An intravitreal voriconazole implant is currently undergoing animal studies, its sustained effect likely to enhance efficacy without the need for repeated injection (Yang et al. 2011). Fluconazole is more toxic to retina in animal models but, similar to amphotericin, a liposomal vehicle decreases that toxicity. Studies have not progressed fluconazole as an intraocular formulation and voriconazole is becoming established in that role. Caspofungin is not yet established as a safe drug for human intraocular injection but animal and in vitro studies suggest that it should be well tolerated (Kernt and Kampik 2010) and it is likely to find a very useful place in human endophthalmitis, especially against azole-resistant *Candida* spp.; topically it does not penetrate healthy cornea.

Surgical management

Pars plana vitrectomy will provide a specimen for microscopy, polymerase chain reaction (PCR) and possibly culture with sensitivities. It will remove opaque vitreous to improve funduscopy, can be combined with intravitreal injection of an antifungal agent, and can remove the tractional elements that may lead to retinal detachment. It will also remove a substantial nidus of live fungi. However, areas of firm vitreoretinal adhesion are common and may be traumatized during surgery. Adherent intra- and preretinal accumulations, including typically those around the ora serrata, may not be excisable. Reports on vitrectomy for candida endophthalmitis during the 1980s and 1990s are no longer applicable because of the modern availability of triazoles. However, where diagnosis is in dispute and microbiology is mandatory, and where vitritis is substantial, vitrectomy is difficult to avoid and is generally recommended.

In summary, our own approach to presumed candida intraocular inflammation is to use oral fluconazole alone where lesions are limited to the submacular layer, to add intravitreal antifungal (still most commonly, amphotericin) where there is clear retinal penetration of one or more lesions, generalized vitritis or strings of pearls, and to proceed to vitrectomy with full microbiological investigation where the diagnosis is insecure, vitritis worsens after the above treatment, or multiple or severe vitreous infiltration is seen. A stubborn response is met with repeated intravitreal injection and, sometimes, combined systemic treatment, always based on microbiological advice after culture and sensitivity. Occasionally repeat surgery to remove recurrent peripheral inflammatory foci or to repeat sampling is necessary. Early and aggressive treatment can rescue useful vision in an eye that may otherwise be irreparable within 2–3 weeks.

ASPERGILLOSIS (box 12.3)

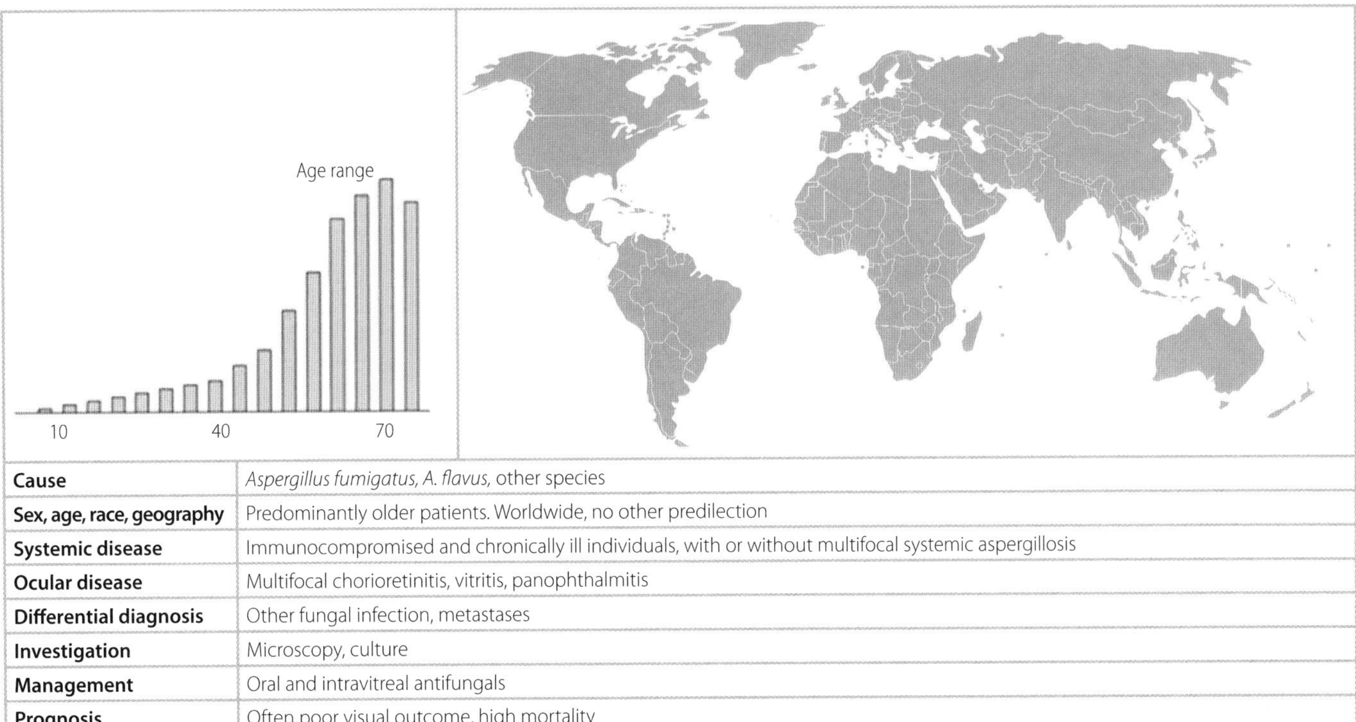

Cause	*Aspergillus fumigatus, A. flavus,* other species
Sex, age, race, geography	Predominantly older patients. Worldwide, no other predilection
Systemic disease	Immunocompromised and chronically ill individuals, with or without multifocal systemic aspergillosis
Ocular disease	Multifocal chorioretinitis, vitritis, panophthalmitis
Differential diagnosis	Other fungal infection, metastases
Investigation	Microscopy, culture
Management	Oral and intravitreal antifungals
Prognosis	Often poor visual outcome, high mortality

Box 12.3 Aspergillosis

Introduction

Aspergillus fungi are widespread aerobic ascomycete fungi that are commonly seen as environmental moulds, but are not human commensals. They are, however, common enough to be inhaled universally and occasionally cause invasive human mycosis. There are several hundred species, but *Aspergillus fumigatus* (**Fig. 12.15**) and *Aspergillus flavus* are the most likely to cause invasive human mycosis. Infection is most likely in immunocompromised individuals, especially in those with profound neutropenia and particularly in those after a heart transplantation or myelodysplasia, but is also seen in intravenous drug abusers, elderly people with diabetes, and those with liver failure or tuberculosis.

Systemic disease

The initial site is usually pulmonary, and a single mass (aspergilloma) may be located asymptomatically on chest radiograph or may cause chronic productive cough or hemoptysis. The rapid development of an area of pulmonary consolidation with cavitation is suspicious. Rapid dissemination with dyspnea and pyrexia may follow. Other primary sites for aspergillosis include facial sinuses, and an invasive paranasal granuloma may invade orbit or brain. In immunodeficient or immunosuppressed individuals, hematogenous dissemination may occur to brain, kidney, liver, skin and eye. Signs will depend on the sites of infection. The mortality from invasive aspergillosis is high, indeed the highest in a series of patients with endogenous endophthalmitis of all types (Schiedler et al. 2004).

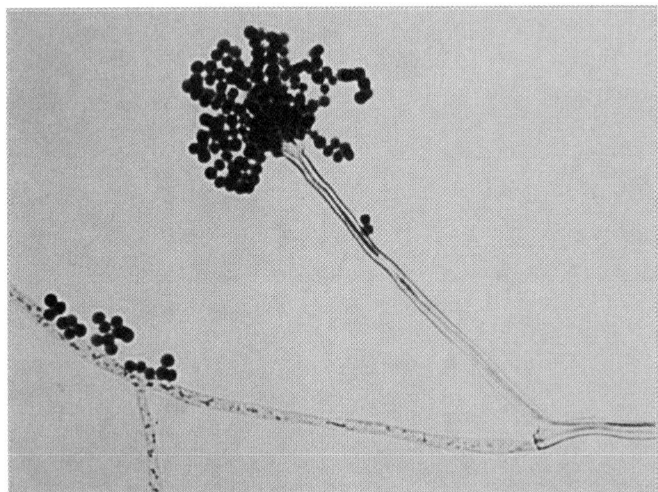

Figure 12.15 *Aspergillus fumigatus,* showing the cluster of microsporidia on a hypha, which were together thought by its discoverer to resemble an aspergillum (a holy water sprinkler). (Modified from Centers for Disease Control, Public Health Image Library.)

Ocular disease

Intraocular involvement in disseminated aspergillus infection may present similarly to intraocular candidiasis, with single or multiple chorioretinal and/or vitreal lesions, usually bilateral, but eyes may be painful and visual loss more acute. There is a tendency in aspergillosis (Rao and Hidayat 2001) to form larger discrete chorioretinal fungal masses (**Fig. 12.16**) that may break through into vitreous to cause severe vitritis (**Fig. 12.17**). We have seen an intravitreal mass resembling a 'dandelion head', spreading centrifugally from a small focus. Intraretinal or vitreous hemorrhage and hypopyon are sometimes seen. Sometimes intraocular involvement is by direct spread from a paranasal sinus and orbital lesion. Panophthalmitis and blindness may ensue.

Diagnosis

Aspergillus endophthalmitis is rare. Those presenting to an ophthalmologist may have the systemic diagnosis already made and, if not, are identified as high risk by a clear history of organ transplantation, neutropenia or immunodeficiency. Blood culture is frequently unrewarding and vitrectomy to confirm diagnosis is necessary for those without systemic confirmation (Weishaar et al. 1998). Galactomannan is a component of the cell wall of *Aspergillus* spp. and is detectable in blood during fungemia. The galactomannan blood test is an ELISA which is therefore useful when microbiology is unavailable.

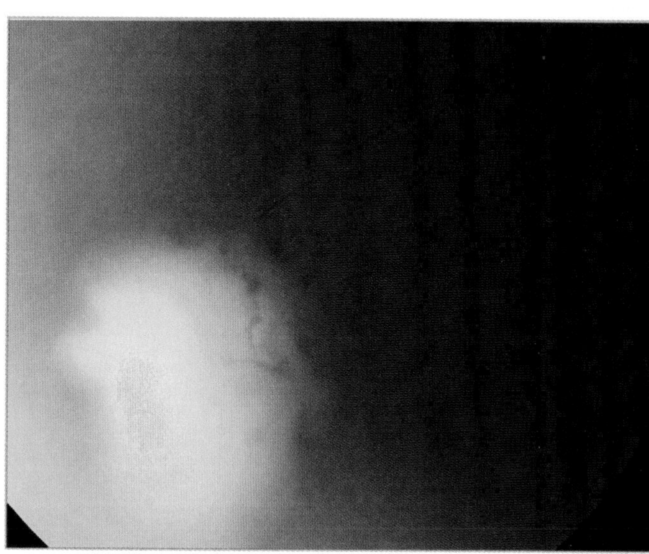

Figure 12.17 Unilateral chorioretinal aspergillosis and vitritis in an immunosuppressed patient after a heart transplantation.

Management

There is a small but significant incidence of aspergillosis in high-risk inpatients so that prophylaxis is used, traditionally, with fluconazole but frequently now with posaconazole. For invasive disease voriconazole is more frequently used (Chai and Hsu 2011) but both these latter drugs have good activity against *Aspergillus spp.*, which are increasingly resistant to other triazoles. Posaconazole does not penetrate the eye adequately to treat endophthalmitis. The antifungals are discussed in detailed in the section on candidiasis above. Intravitreal injection of either voriconazole or amphotericin B has been successful, but systemic treatment is mandatory because systemic foci are likely to develop even in those without signs elsewhere. Voriconazole is preferred to caspofungin or amphotericin now as first-line treatment, although combinations may be required systemically. Despite treatment mortality is high as typically patients have severe combined systemic problems.

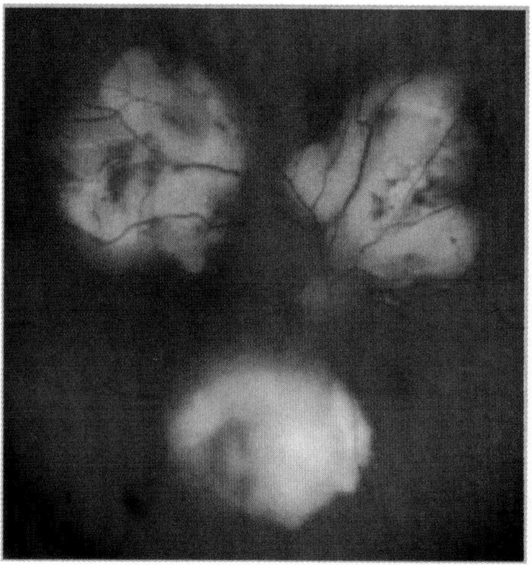

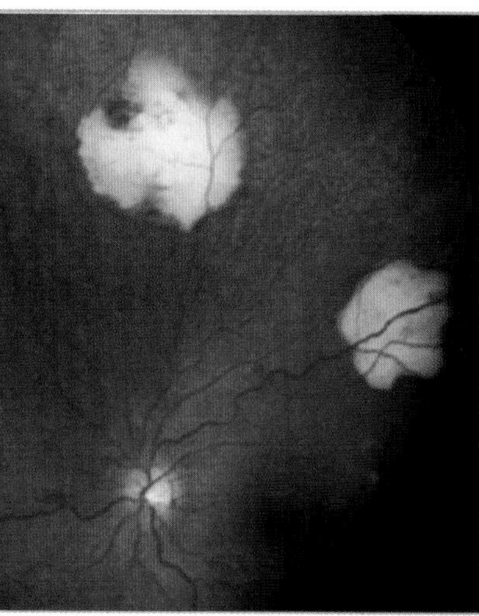

Figure 12.16 Bilateral chorioretinal aspergillosis in a 10-year-old boy with subsequently fatal disseminated disease following heavy immunosuppression. (Courtesy of Mr S Biswas.)

PNEUMOCYSTOSIS (box 12.4)

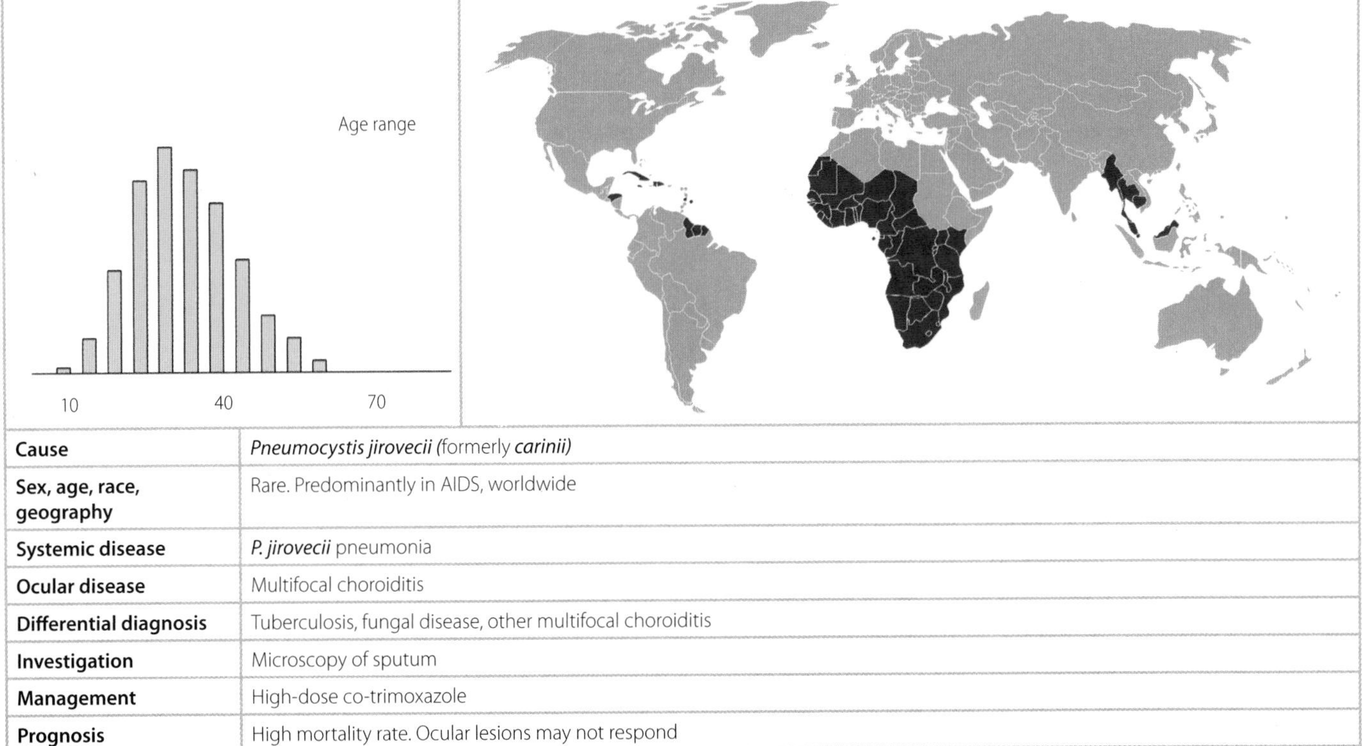

Cause	*Pneumocystis jirovecii* (formerly *carinii)*
Sex, age, race, geography	Rare. Predominantly in AIDS, worldwide
Systemic disease	*P. jirovecii* pneumonia
Ocular disease	Multifocal choroiditis
Differential diagnosis	Tuberculosis, fungal disease, other multifocal choroiditis
Investigation	Microscopy of sputum
Management	High-dose co-trimoxazole
Prognosis	High mortality rate. Ocular lesions may not respond

Box 12.4 Pneumocystosis

Introduction

The organism *Pneumocystis jirovecii* was renamed recently from *P. carinii*. Its precise identification has provided something of a debate; it has morphological and lifecycle features of a protozoon and was previously classified with the subphylum *Sporozoa*. However, RNA sequence studies and other evidence have shown a closer resemblance to the fungi and therefore it is reclassified here (**Fig. 12.18**). The organism is an opportunist but its environmental source is unclear. It may be a commensal. Exposure is virtually universal and most children are seropositive. It is capable of causing invasive disease only in immunodeficient individuals, and characteristically in AIDS patients.

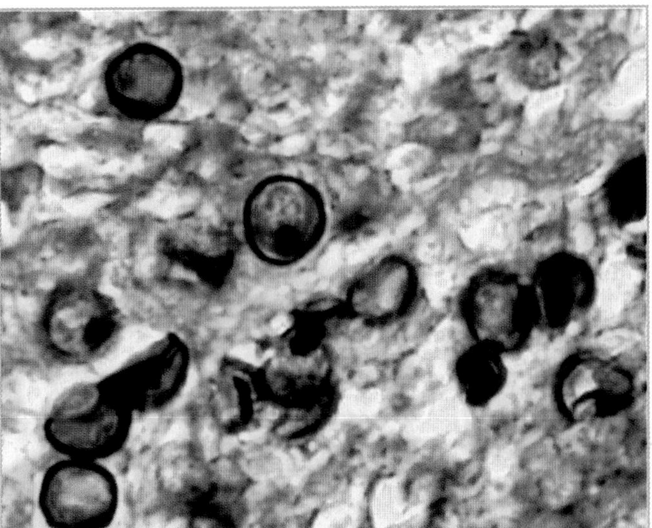

Figure 12.18 Pneumocystis cysts in lung tissue in PCP pneumonia. The spheroid cysts with local thickenings have been likened to 'squashed ping-pong balls.' (Modified from Centers for Disease Control, Public Health Image Library.)

Systemic disease

In the early years of AIDS, *Pneumocystis carinii* pneumonia (as it was then known, and is still known in short as PCP) was the most common AIDS-defining illness and ultimately affected over four-fifths of patients. Pyrexia, malaise, dry cough and dyspnea suggest possible PCP. Diffuse bilateral pulmonary infiltration or hilar node enlargement may be seen on chest radiograph. Respiratory symptoms are usually more severe in those without AIDS, and include tachypnea, cyanosis and respiratory failure. Extrapulmonary infection is rare but may be fatal. Systemic treatment of pneumonia is usually successful but most develop a recurrence within 1 year unless prophylaxis is used. Inhaled pentamidine was the usual prophylactic drug used by AIDS patients with CD4 counts $<0.2 \times 10^9/l$. However, although this protected reasonably against PCP it did not prevent disseminated disease including ocular involvement, and prophylaxis was switched to oral co-trimoxazole in the 1990s, after which the incidence of ocular disease changed from the merely rare to the very rare.

Ocular disease

Pneumocystis sp. may cause a very characteristic choroidal infection (Sha et al. 1992), usually bilateral. There are multiple, pale, well-demarcated, thick, yellowish placoid lesions, usually with no overlying retinal or vitreous inflammation (**Fig. 12.19**), each lesion often being larger than a disk diameter. Patients generally show no signs of other extrapulmonary involvement. This may either indicate a particular predilection of this organism for the choroid, or be an early manifestation of more severe dissemination.

Diagnosis

Pulmonary involvement can be proven by bronchial biopsy but this is rarely justified. The chest radiograph findings are often highly specific. Bronchoalveolar lavage with biopsy has more than a 90% diagnosis rate. However, microscopy of sputum after inhalation of salinified air is often adequate. Ocular tissue is not available for diagnostic purposes; vitreous is usually uninvolved and chorioretinal biopsy should not be necessary in the context of systemic inflammation; the presence of pulmonary organisms together with characteristic fundal lesions is presumptive of the diagnosis.

Management

High-dose co-trimoxazole (trimethoprim 20 mg/kg per day with sulfamethoxazole 100 mg/kg per day, divided into four doses) is given for 2 weeks. The adverse effects of co-trimoxazole, including skin rashes and blood dyscrasias, are more frequent in AIDS patients. Alternatively, dapsone, clindamycin, pentamidine or atovaquone can be used. The mortality rate from PCP in AIDS patients is still around 10%. The responsiveness of choroidal lesions to standard systemic medications is essentially undocumented.

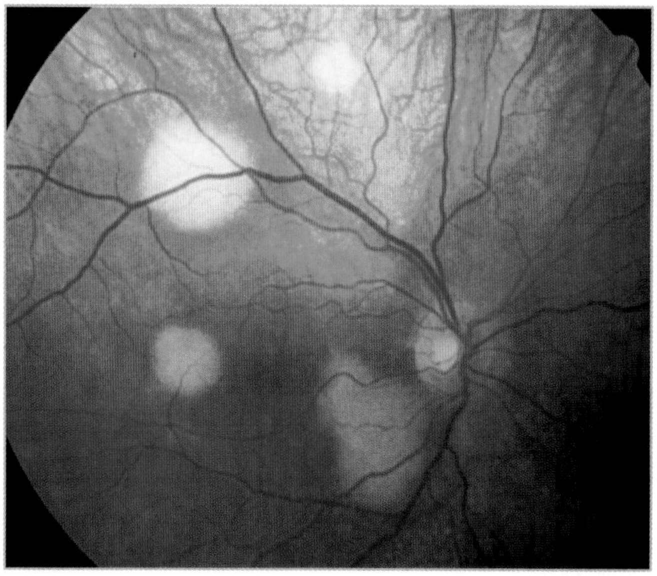

Figure 12.19 Pneumocystis choroiditis in a patient with advanced AIDS from the pre-HAART (highly antiretroviral treatment) era. He succumbed to disseminated infection.

OTHER FUNGAL INFECTIONS

Cryptococcosis

Cryptococcus neoformans is a basidiomycete yeast that thrives in the soil in urban environments and similar to *Histoplasma* sp. has a fondness for guano, particularly that of the pigeon. Infection is by inhalation of dried particles. It is a well-recognized but rare cause of meningitis in immunocompetent individuals, and of disseminated disease (including meningoencephalitis) in immunodeficient individuals, especially in AIDS patients. A third of such patients have ocular or periocular involvement, about a third have papillitis (Kestelyn et al. 1993) but endophthalmitis is rare. Multifocal small choroidal or retinal white lesions progress to apparent retinal nerve fiber infarcts with associated hemorrhage (**Fig. 12.20**). Intravitreal foci may develop, and bilateral anterior uveitis has been seen. Diagnosis requires serology or culture of CSF and urine, with brain imaging. Disseminated cryptococcosis has a high mortality rate and aggressive antifungal treatment, usually with combined flucytosine and amphotericin, may offer the best outcomes. Response to treatment may be followed by IRIS including intraocular inflammation. A subspecies *C. neoformans* var. *gatti* has been causing occasional meningoencephalitis in immunocompetent individuals in some countries. As yet there are no reports of intraocular involvement but this may transpire.

Coccidioidomycosis

Coccidioides immitis is a dimorphic deuteromycete fungus that thrives in arid conditions, particularly in the south-western deserts of the USA and in drier parts of Central and South America. Infection is pulmonary and may be asymptomatic or may cause acute pneumonitis or chronic cavitating infection. Dissemination is uncommon. Intraocular infection is rare in immunocompetent individuals, but may occur with

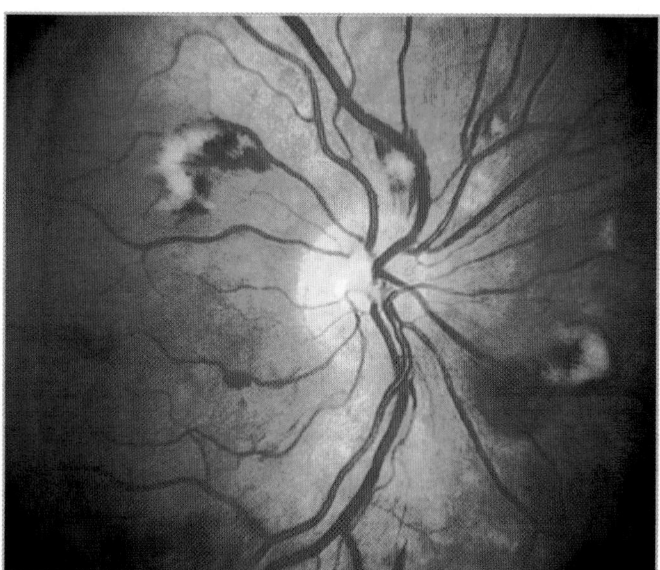

Figure 12.20 Multifocal hemorrhagic nerve fiber layer infarcts in disseminated cryptococcosis. (Courtesy of Dr D Denning.)

or without other manifestations of dissemination, in either anterior or posterior segments but most typically with granulomatous anterior uveitis with iris nodules. Many patients have an associated rash and skin biopsy can be diagnostic. Systemic treatment has been enhanced by the use of fluconazole, but amphotericin is also still used.

Others

Sporothrix schenckii is the causative agent of sporotrichosis, a subcutaneous mycosis that is acquired particularly by nurserymen and gardeners, especially from infected sphagnum moss. It may occasionally disseminate and cause intraocular infection in immunocompetent or immunodeficient individuals. *Blastomyces dermatitidis*, an organism also encountered within the orbit, may rarely cause intraocular involvement in disseminated (North American) blastomycosis, usually a choroiditis. *Penicillium* spp. are rare causes of endophthalmitis after intravenous drug abuse and we have encountered it in an AIDS patient (**Fig. 12.21**). Endophthalmitis has also been described from endogenous infection with *Fusarium, Trichosporon, Pseudallescheria, Monosporium* spp. and others. Naso-orbital mucormycosis, most commonly from *Mucor* or *Rhizopus* spp., may cause intraocular inflammation from direct invasion via the orbit, but this is very rare. Mortality is extremely high.

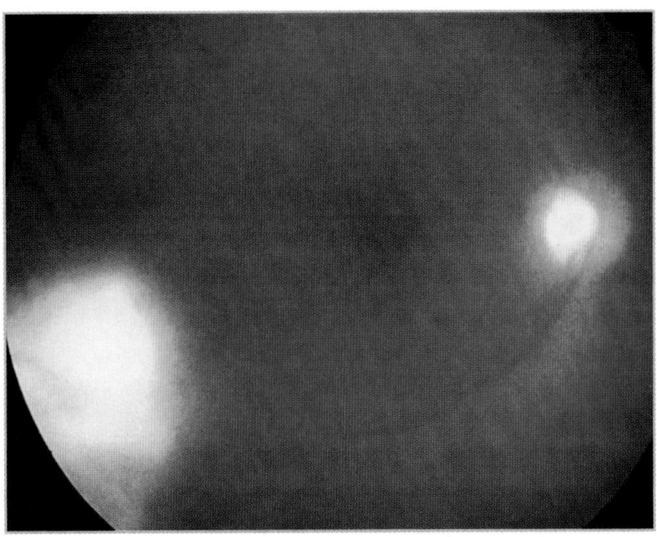

Figure 12.21 Endophthalmitis caused by Penicillium sp. in a patient with AIDS.

REFERENCES

Almony A, Thomas MA, Atebara MH, et al. Long-term follow-up of surgical removal of extensive peripapillary choroidal neovascularisation in presumed ocular histoplasmosis syndrome. *Ophthalmology* 2008;**115**:540–5.

Chai LY, Hsu LY. Recent advances in invasive pulmonary aspergillosis. *Curr Opin Pulmon Med* 2011;**17**:160–6.

Dozier CC, Tarantola RM, Jiramongkolchai K, Donahue SP. Fungal eye disease at a tertiary care center: the utility of routine inpatient consultation. *Ophthalmology* 2011;**118**:1671–6.

Ehrlich R, Cuilla TA, Maturi R, et al. Intravitreal bevacizumab for choroidal neovascularisation secondary to presumed ocular histoplasmosis syndrome. *Retina* 2009;**29**:1418–23.

Kernt M, Kampik A. Intraocular caspofingun: in vitro safety profile for human ocular cells. *Mycoses* 2011;**54**:e110–21.

Kestelyn P, Taelman H, Bogaerts J, et al. Ophthalmic manifestations of infections with *Cryptococcus neoformans* in patients with the acquired immunodeficiency syndrome. *Am J Ophthalmol* 1993;**116**:721–7.

Lui JC, Boldt HC, Folk JC, Gehrs KM. Photodynamic therapy of subfoveal and juxtafoveal choroidal neovascularisation in ocular histoplasmosis: a retrospective case series. *Retina* 2004;**24**:863–70.

Martidis A, Miller DG, Cuilla TA, et al. Corticosteroids as an antiangiogenic agent for histoplasmosis-related subfoveal choroidal neovascularisation. *J Ocul Pharmacol Ther* 1999;**15**:425–8.

Nielsen JS, Fick TA, Saggau DD, Barnes CH. Intravitreal anti-vascular endothelial growth factor therapy for choroidal neovascularisation secondary to ocular histoplasmosis syndrome. *Retina* 2011;Epub.

Oude Lashof AM, Rothova A, Sobel JD, et al. Ocular manifestations of candidaemia. *Clin Infect Dis* 2011;**53**:262–8.

Pfaller MA, Diekema DJ, Gibbs DL, et al. Results from the ARTEMIS DISK global antifungal surveillance study, 1997–2005: an 8.5yr analysis of susceptibilities of *Candida* and other yeast species to fluconazole and voriconazole by CLSI standardised disk diffusion testing. *J Clin Microbiol* 2007;**45**:1735–45.

Rao NA, Hidayat AA. Endogenous mycotic endophthalmitis: variations in clinical and histopathologic changes in candidiasis compared with aspergillosis. *Am J Ophthalmol* 2001;**132**:244–51.

Riddell J, Comer GM, Kauffman CA. Treatment of endogenous fungal endophthalmitis: focus in new antifungal agents. *Clin Infect Dis* 2011;**52**: 648–53.

Schiedler V, Scott IU, Flynn HW, et al. Culture-proven endogenous endophthalmitis: clinical features and visual acuity outcomes. *Am J Ophthalmol* 2004;**137**:725–31.

Sha BE, Benson CA, Deutsch T, et al. *Pneumocystis carinii* choroiditis in patients with AIDS: clinical features, response to therapy, and outcome. *J Acquir Immune Def Syndrome* 1992;**5**:1051–8.

Trevino R, Salvat R. Preventing reactivation of ocular histoplasmosis: guidance for patients at risk. *Optometry* 2006;**77**:10–16.

Vemulakonda GA, Hariprasad SM, Mieler WF, et al. Aqueous and vitreous concentrations following topical administration of 1% voriconazole in humans. *Arch Ophthalmol* 2008;**126**:18–22.

Weishaar PD, Flynn HW, Murray TG, et al. Endogenous aspergillus endophthalmitis. Clinical features and treatment outcomes. *Ophthalmology* 1998;**105**:57–65.

Wingard JR, Carter SL, Walsh TJ. Randomized, double-blind trial of fluconazole versus voriconazole for prevention of invasive fungal infection after allogeneic haemopoietic cell transplantation. *Blood* 2010;**116**:5111–18.

Yang L, Dong X, Wu X, et al. Intravitreally implantable voriconazole delivery system for experimental fungal endophthalmitis. *Retina* 2011:Epub.

Chapter 13 Protozoal infection

The protozoa are unicellular microorganisms with clearly defined nuclei. Of the pathogenic species, some are independent and others are obligate intracellular parasites. The phylum *Protozoa* is subdivided into four subphyla, namely *Sporozoa* (including *Toxoplasma gondii* [and previously *Pneumocystis carinii*, now reclassified as a fungus *Pneumocystis jiroveci*]), *Mastigophora* (including *Giardia lamblia* and *Acanthamoeba* spp.), *Sarcodina* (including *Entamoeba histolytica*) and *Ciliophora*. Only one protozoon, *Toxoplasma gondii*, is a major cause of uveitis, but it is a substantial cause of morbidity especially in the developing world.

TOXOPLASMOSIS (box 13.1)

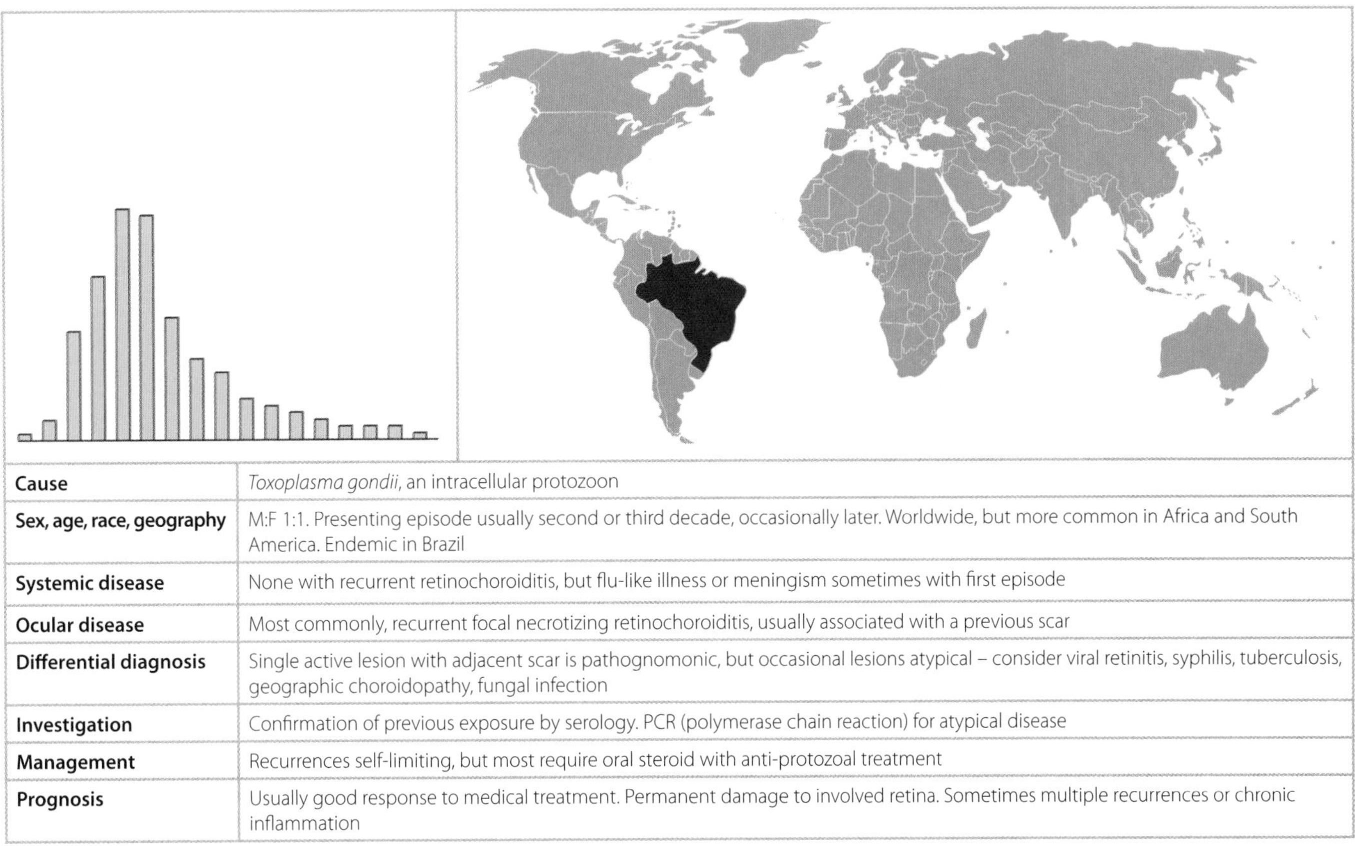

Cause	*Toxoplasma gondii*, an intracellular protozoon
Sex, age, race, geography	M:F 1:1. Presenting episode usually second or third decade, occasionally later. Worldwide, but more common in Africa and South America. Endemic in Brazil
Systemic disease	None with recurrent retinochoroiditis, but flu-like illness or meningism sometimes with first episode
Ocular disease	Most commonly, recurrent focal necrotizing retinochoroiditis, usually associated with a previous scar
Differential diagnosis	Single active lesion with adjacent scar is pathognomonic, but occasional lesions atypical – consider viral retinitis, syphilis, tuberculosis, geographic choroidopathy, fungal infection
Investigation	Confirmation of previous exposure by serology. PCR (polymerase chain reaction) for atypical disease
Management	Recurrences self-limiting, but most require oral steroid with anti-protozoal treatment
Prognosis	Usually good response to medical treatment. Permanent damage to involved retina. Sometimes multiple recurrences or chronic inflammation

Box 13.1 Toxoplasmosis

Introduction

Toxoplasmosis is a zoonotic infection, the causative organism being *Toxoplasma gondii*, a crescentic intracellular protozoon (**Fig. 13.1**) first identified in the Gundi (*Ctenodactylus gundi*, **Fig. 13.2**, a north African rodent) by Nicolle and Manceaux, working in Tunis in 1908. Toxoplasmosis is found almost worldwide but is most common in subtropical areas.

The primary host of *T. gondii* is the cat, which excretes oocysts. These robust bodies can survive in feces for several days, or in water for weeks or more, and are resistant to standard disinfection. They may be ingested by any intermediate host, including humans (**Fig. 13.3**). This direct route of infection may be common in childhood especially in tropical areas, whereas adults in western countries more commonly ingest tissue cysts infecting other intermediate hosts, by eating undercooked meat, especially pork. The disease may also be acquired by drinking unpasteurized goats' milk or cheeses made from it, as is common in some European and many other countries.

The disease is common in humans, but prevalence varies depending on climate, dietary habits and standards of hygiene. Overall prevalence in the USA is approximately 25% whereas, in some parts of France, probably attributable to the ingestion of undercooked meats and unpasteurized cheeses, it is 90%. It is the most common known cause of posterior uveitis in humans.

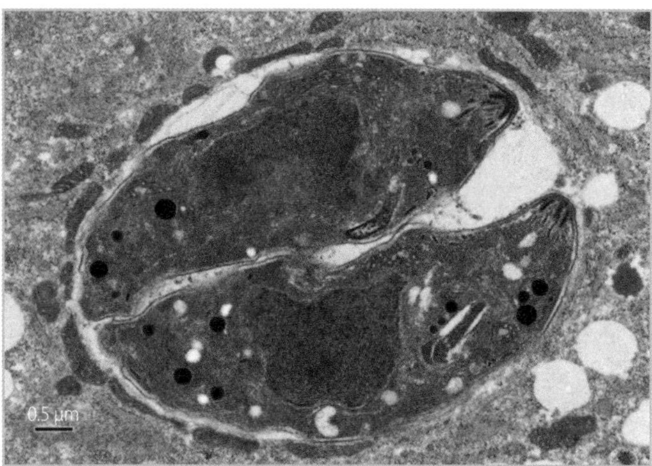

Figure 13.1 A transmission electron micrograph of a pair of toxoplasma trophozoites lying side to side with their apical complexes to the right. (Courtesy of Dr L Pernas.)

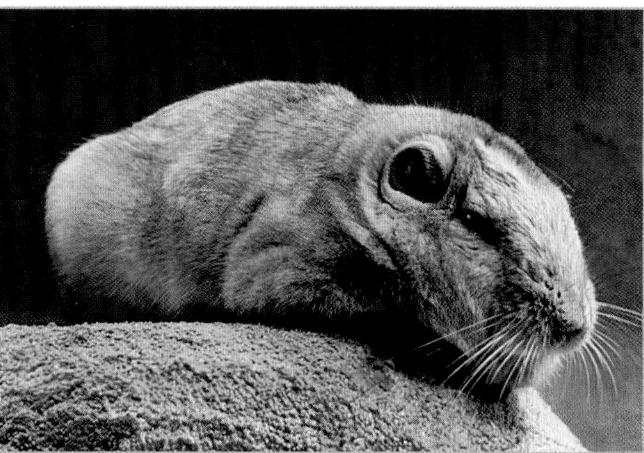

Figure 13.2 The gundi *(Ctenodactylus gundi)*, the North African rodent in which *Toxoplasma gondii* was first isolated.

T. gondii exists in various genotypic strains, types 1, 2 and 3 being found in Europe and North America, of which type 2 is the most common cause of human disease. In South America in contrast, where prevalence, virulence and disease severity all tend to be greater, genetic diversity is far greater and type 1 is common in humans. An excellent review of the development of knowledge of *T. gondii* natural history is available (Ferguson 2009).

In the intermediate host, organisms spread through the lymphatic system. Eventually cystic forms of *T. gondii* may be demonstrated in any tissue but have a particular predilection for heart, muscle, brain and retina. The cyst wall incorporates host elements and is thus immunologically isolated. However, slow multiplication of organisms (bradyzoites) within a cyst (**Fig. 13.4**) may lead to cyst rupture and release of individual free organisms (trophozoites – see Fig. 13.1), which provoke a vigorous inflammatory response. In the immunocompetent host this occasional release of organisms is asymptomatic unless involving the retina, but, in the immunodeficient host, dissemination and fulminating infection may occur.

T. gondii infection is acquired during about 0.5% of pregnancies. It has about a 40% chance of crossing the placenta to infect the fetus, although this chance is greater in the third trimester. As with most transplacental infections the severity of effects on the fetus depend on the phase of pregnancy. Early infection may be lethal, leading to spontaneous abortion. Some 20% of affected liveborn babies have significant systemic effects, including microcephaly, hydrocephalus, microphthalmia, optic neuropathy, deafness, learning disabilities, fits and failure to thrive. Longitudinal studies have shown neurological or ocular involvement in up to 80% of cases (Lower-Steiger et al. 1984), and the result for a UK-born population is a predicted incidence for toxoplasma retinochoroiditis of 0.4/100 000 population per year (Gilbert et al. 1995) compared with 57/100 000 per year for an African-born population.

Received wisdom taught us that all patients presenting with recurrent ocular toxoplasmosis had initially acquired their infection transplacentally. However, there is now evidence that postnatal acquisition can lead to ocular inflammation and reactivation. A survey in the UK (Stanford et al. 2006) found that 50% of children with ocular lesions had acquired their toxoplasmosis postnatally. Accounts of consecutively affected siblings (Glasner et al. 1992) support this view (transplacental transmission presumably occurs only during acute infection, and immunity follows first exposure; subsequent pregnancies should therefore be unaffected). Postnatal acquisition is considered to be most likely in Brazil, where the population prevalence of ocular toxoplasmosis may be as high as 20% despite a very low incidence of ocular lesions in young children.

Systemic disease

The patient presenting to the ophthalmologist with a first episode of symptomatic ocular toxoplasmosis is likely to be a fit young adult, but some patients may be middle-aged or even elderly. The disease is usually reactivated, not newly acquired, and there is therefore no systemic illness. However, ocular involvement may also be seen in newly acquired toxoplasmosis, which may be asymptomatic, but usually causes some systemic upset, often a mild flu-like illness. Sometimes significant lymphadenopathy, particularly affecting the posterior cervical nodes, may occur. Pyrexia, malaise and fatigue, sore throat, maculopapular rash and sometimes hepatosplenomegaly may be seen. A constellation of symptoms sometimes persists to cause a chronic form of glandular fever. More severe effects are rare in immunocompetent individuals, but in immunocompromised individuals meningoencephalitis, pneumonitis, myocarditis and hemolytic anemia may be seen.

Perkins (1973) and others stated that most cases of newly acquired ocular toxoplasmosis were seen in those with severe symptoms of systemic infection, especially where meningoencephalitis was present. However, in this clinic most patients with newly acquired ocular inflammation are systemically well.

Ocular disease

Most patients presenting with ocular toxoplasmosis will describe unilateral subacute painless visual loss with many floaters. However, some will describe pain and redness, and others a more chronic accumulation of floaters. Undoubtedly some minor reactivations of foci outside the arcades will pass without medical presentation. Bilateral symptoms are rare.

The anterior segment

Most but not all patients will have a degree of active anterior uveitis in association with their active posterior segment disease. This may range from a few anterior chamber cells to a very severe uveitis with multiple posterior synechiae. Many but by no means all patients exhibit large

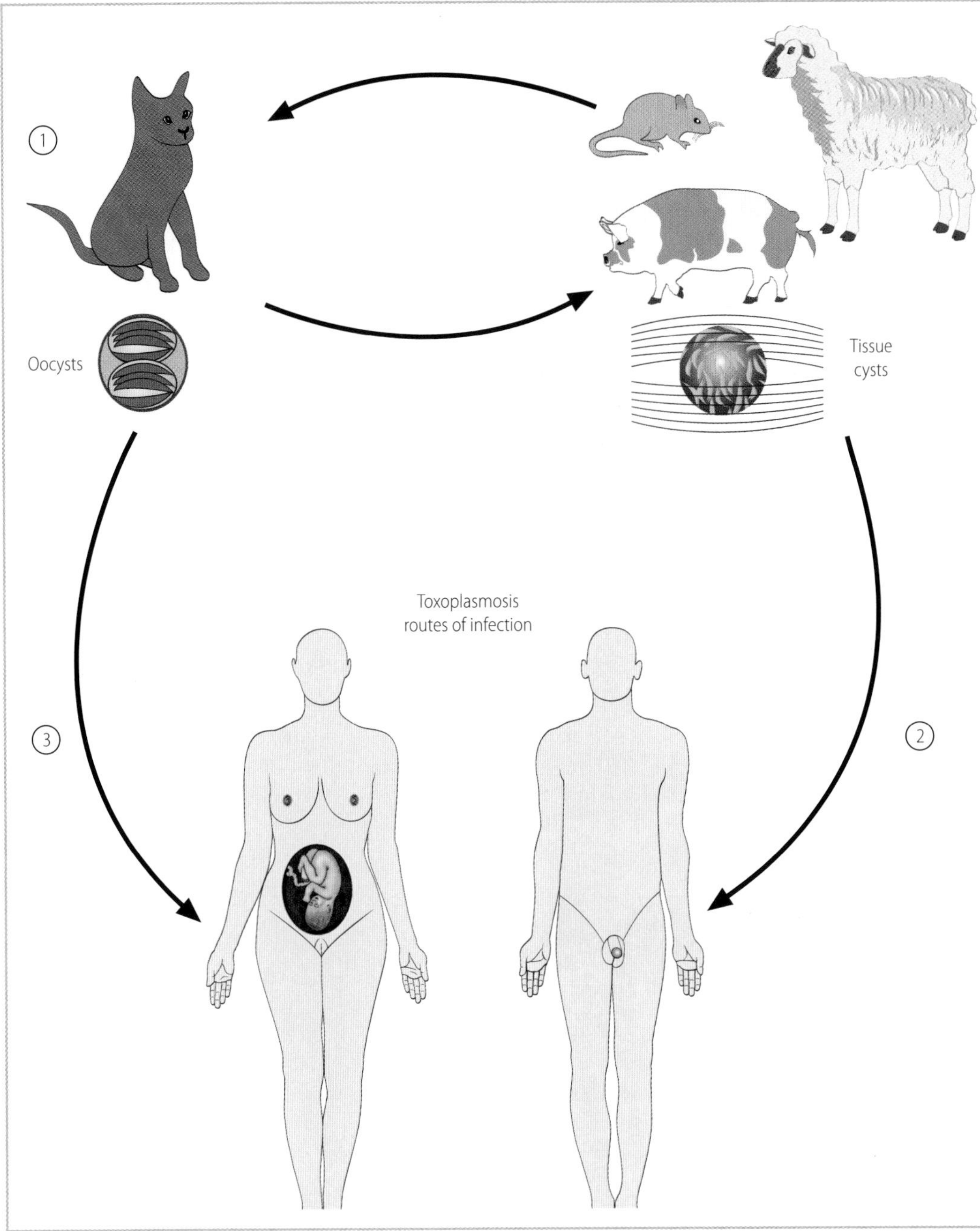

Figure 13.3 The life cycle of *Toxoplasma gondii*. The primary hosts (1) are members of the cat genus, who excrete oocysts in the faces. These are ingested by intermediate animals, through which the life cycle cannot be completed, but within which tissue cysts form. Human infection may occur either through ingestion of undercooked meat containing live cysts (2) or by direct ingestion of oocysts from cat litter (3), which may contaminate water or vegetables or unpasteurized dairy produce. Vertical transmission from mother to fetus may also occur. (Modified from Centers for Disease Control, DPDx Image Library.)

mutton-fat keratic precipitates. The intraocular pressure is raised in 40% of patients (Westfall et al. 2005). In a small proportion of patients, especially in those with recalcitrant or recurrent retinochoroiditis, a chronic non-infective anterior uveitis may persist, as may happen after other posterior segment infections.

The posterior segment

Typical recurrent retinochoroiditis

The characteristic lesions of previous ocular toxoplasmosis are atrophic chorioretinal scars of variable size with pigment clumping, often in a ring around the edge of the lesion (**Fig. 13.5**). It is now thought that most macular colobomas (**Fig. 13.6**) result from congenital ocular toxoplasmosis. Aberrant chorioretinal vascular anastomoses may be present in some scars, and attest to their prenatal development.

Most foci of active retinitis are contiguous with or close to an old scar, but any focal inner retinitis in which the same or the fellow eye has an old chorioretinal scar is compatible with a diagnosis of toxoplasmosis.

Characteristically a new lesion will be oval, white and slightly raised, with poorly demarcated edges. Being centered in the inner retinal layers, small lesions will orient themselves along the nerve fiber layer (**Fig. 13.7**), although such orientation becomes less obvious for larger lesions, which tend to be rounded and dome shaped (**Fig. 13.8**). Occasionally a small pre-existing chorioretinal scar is virtually covered by its adjacent new focus of inflammation causing confusion in diagnosis; a careful search of both fundi for old scars should take place for every new patient with unifocal retinitis.

An associated retinal vasculitis (which may involve both venules and arterioles) is very common and often overlooked. It usually occurs

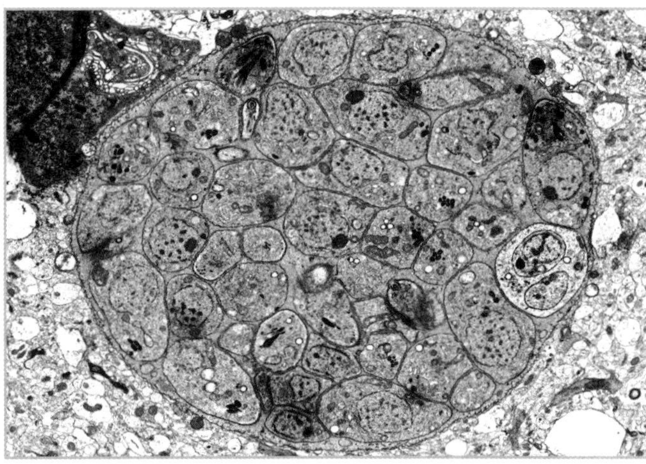

Figure 13.4 A transmission electron micrograph of an intracerebral toxoplasma tissue cyst (strain Me49) containing multiple bradyzoites. At the 3 o'clock periphery is a pair of dividing bradyzoites. (Courtesy of Dr C Caffaro.)

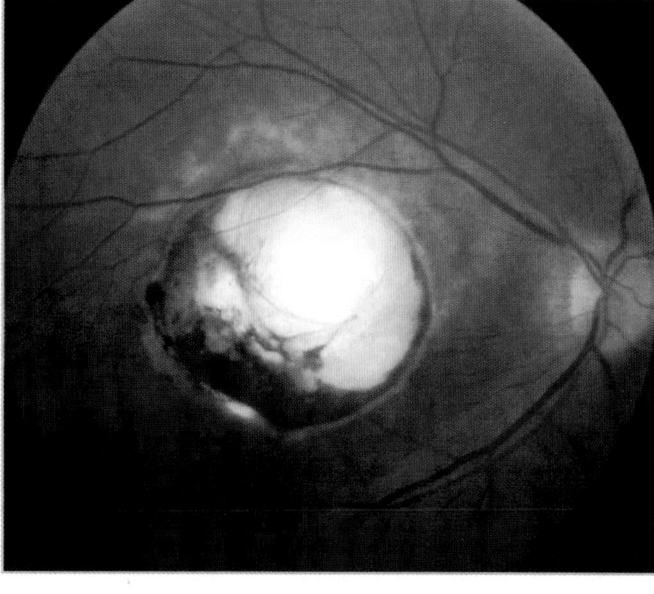

Figure 13.6 A large macular coloboma following congenital toxoplasmosis

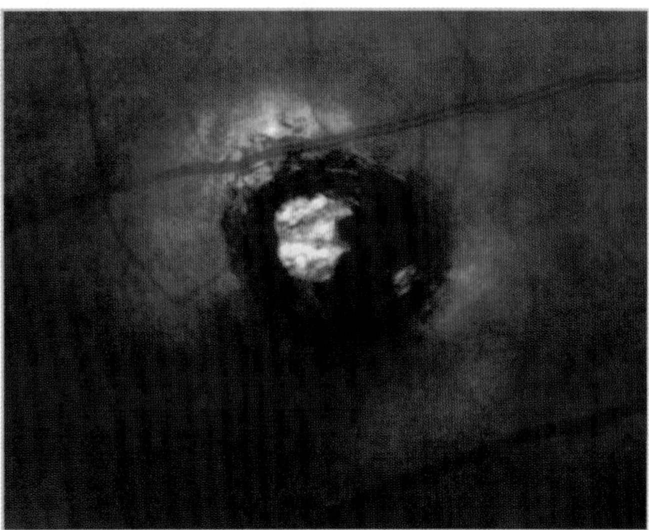

Figure 13.5 A post-inflammatory chorioretinal scar following previously acquired toxoplasmosis.

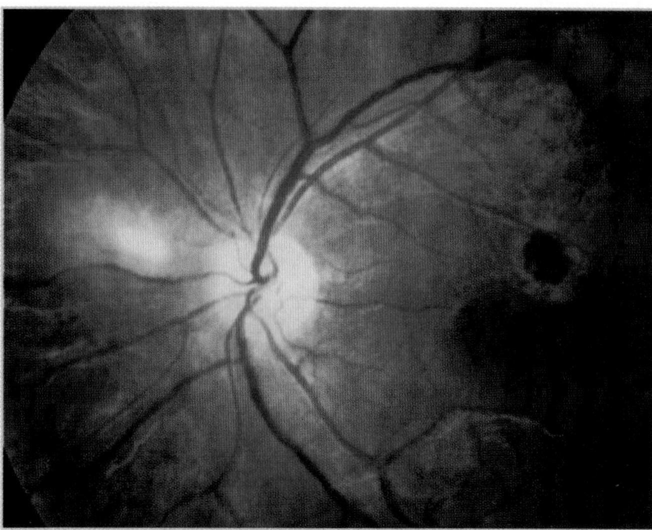

Figure 13.7 A focus of recurrent inflammation has its long axis orientated with the nerve fiber layer, in which it commences.

as patchy perivascular cuffing and may be seen at any position in the affected retina. It is most common near to the active focus (**Fig. 13.9**), may selectively affect a 'feeder' arteriole (**Fig. 13.10**), or arterioles throughout the fundus (**Fig. 13.11**). There may in contrast be widespread phlebitis (**Fig. 13.12**) or, rarely, extremely florid vasculitis with enormous exudation (**Fig. 13.13**). Inflammation straddling a vessel may occlude it (**Fig. 13.14**) and this may be accompanied by intraretinal hemorrhage (**Fig. 13.15**). Uncommonly, neovascularization may supervene, which is responsive to photocoagulation. Posterior pole lesions may cause significant macular edema or star formation (**Fig. 13.16**).

As the episode of inflammation runs its course or responds to treatment, the lesion changes its appearance. The edges 'harden off,' becoming much more distinct and resembling hard exudate, but probably representing necrotic retina (**Fig. 13.17**). The active lesion shrinks slightly, surrounding retinal edema disappears and overlying vitreous opacification subsides (**Fig. 13.18**). In due course the white retinal focus will disappear and chorioretinal scarring and pigmentation will supervene, characteristically occupying an area larger than the active focus. An episode of inflammation usually lasts no more than 8 weeks in immunocompetent patients. However, the residual vitreous opacities will often take several months to clear.

The degree of vitreous opacification overlying an area of active retinitis varies enormously, but all inner retinal foci have at least local overlying inflammatory infiltrate, often appearing fibrinous (**Fig. 13.19**) and some show profound vitreous opacification (**Fig. 13.20**), which may at worst compromise a fundal view with the indirect ophthalmoscope. Even in such cases a pale retinal focus is visible through the semi-opaque vitreous, the so-called 'headlight in the fog' appearance. Rarely multiple vitreous strands appear which may mimic toxocara endophthalmitis (**Fig. 13.21**) After an acute episode vitreous clarity will progressively improve but severe or repeated inflammation is likely to lead to permanent vitreous changes.

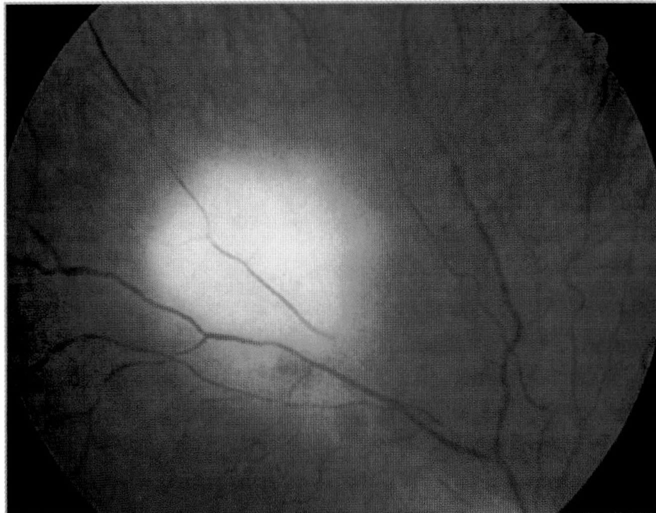

Figure 13.8 A larger focus of reactivation in ocular toxoplasmosis. The lesion is rounded, domed and surrounded by retinal edema. Old chorioretinal scars are just visible adjacent to the new lesion.

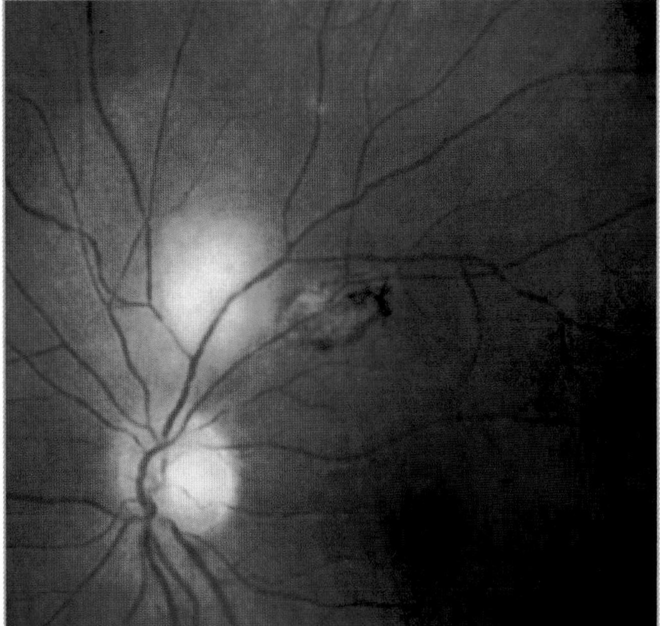

Figure 13.9 A focus of recurrent toxoplasma retinochoroiditis. A white, soft-edged, inflammatory focus with surrounding pale retinal edema is seen together with an old chorioretinal scar. There are scattered patches of retinal vasculitis showing as perivascular cuffing and caliber change.

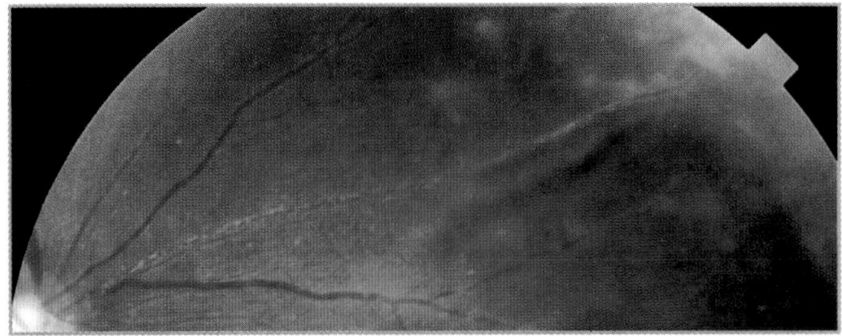

Figure 13.10 An arteriole running directly from disk to active focus shows intermittent cuffing.

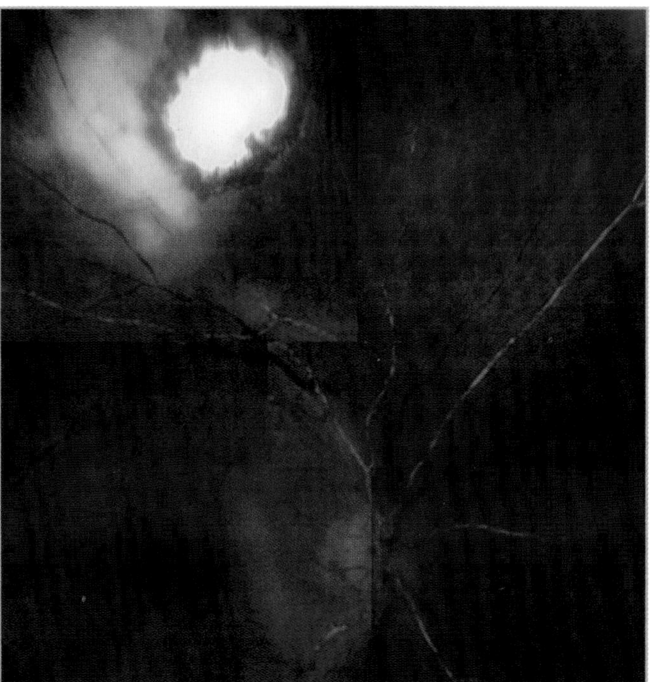

Figure 13.11 A large focus adjacent to an old scar is accompanied by widespread arteriolitis.

The vitreous may become organized into 'veils', and vitreous 'cylinders' (Roizenblatt et al. 1980) (**Fig. 13.22**) have been most commonly associated with toxoplasmosis. Posterior vitreous detachment is usual in those eyes with recurrent attacks, and this event often provokes new symptoms of floaters which will mimic an inflammatory episode. In addition to characteristic recurrent retinochoroiditis as described above, toxoplasmosis may present in the following ways.

Other manifestations

Peripapillary foci, neuroretinitis, papillitis and retrobulbar neuritis

Peripapillary foci of toxoplasmosis are not uncommon. Their proximity to the optic disk augurs poorly for permanent visual field loss (Stanford et al. 2005) and lesions should be aggressively treated (**Figs 13.23** and **13.24**). It is likely that such lesions explained most cases historically diagnosed as 'Jensen's peripapillary choroiditis,' at that time presumed to be tubercular in origin. *T. gondii* is known to be neurophilic and cysts may reside anywhere within the central nervous system. It is therefore likely that reactivations will occasionally involve an intraneural focus of the optic nerve, superficially leading to neuroretinitis or papillitis, and probably further posterior. We have treated a small number of patients with retinal scarring (but without active intraocular inflammation and with a normal optic disk) consistent with toxoplasmosis who have presented with symptoms typical of retrobulbar neuritis and acute sectoral visual field defects (**Fig. 13.25**).

Neuroretinitis usually presents with substantial visual loss, optic nerve head swelling, and peripapillary exudate and a macular star (**Fig. 13.26**). There may be peripapillary splinter hemorrhages. Severe nerve fiber field defects may result. There may be a visible focus of inflammation either contiguous with the optic nerve head or overlying it, and vitreous opacification is usual. The possibility of toxoplasmosis as a cause of neuroretinitis should always be borne in mind, and it is reasonable to accept the presence of a typical chorioretinal scar as

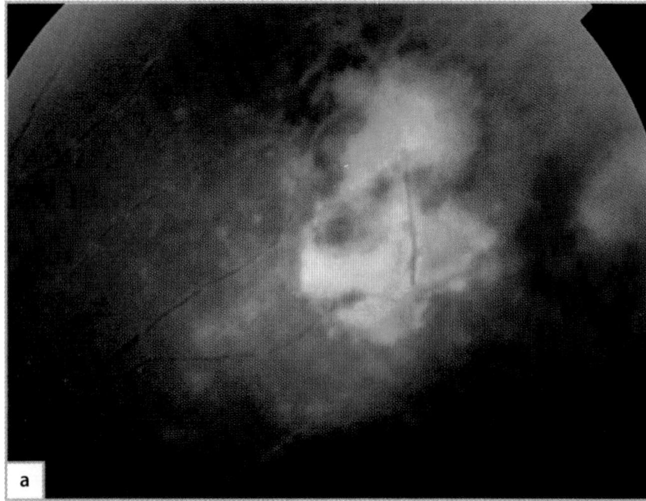

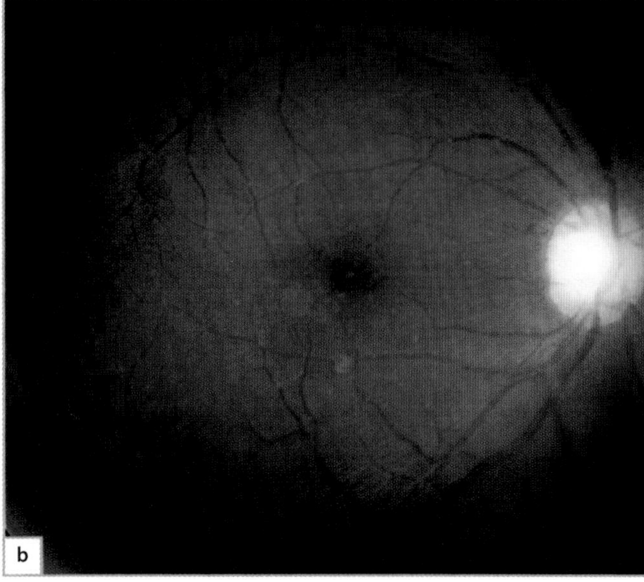

Figure 13.12 A superonasal active focus of toxoplasmosis (a) is associated with widespread vasculitis, mainly affecting venules, which also extends to the posterior pole (b).

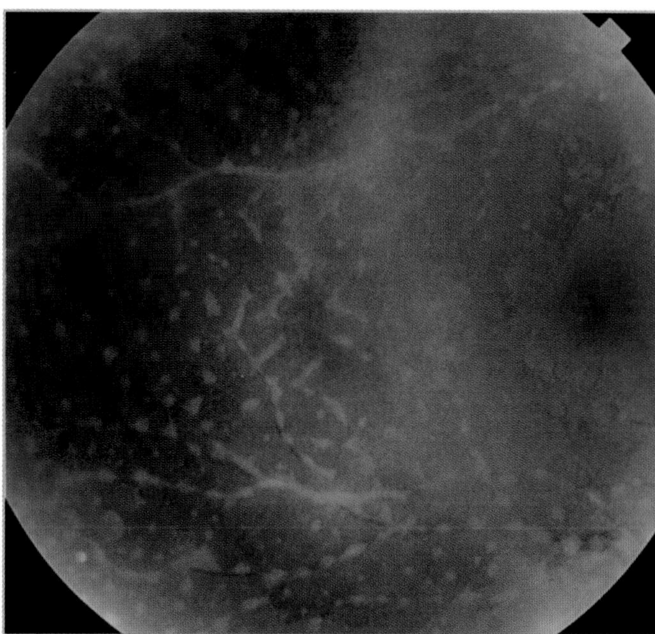

Figure 13.13 Massive perivascular exudation accompanies recurrent peripheral toxoplasmosis

presumptive of the association. However, the differential diagnosis will include sarcoidosis, toxocariasis, bartonellosis, optic neuritis secondary to demyelination, ischemic optic neuropathy or tumors of the optic nerve.

Outer retinal or diffuse retinal toxoplasmosis

Some foci of inflammation may primarily affect the outer retina (Doft and Gass 1985, Matthews and Weiter 1988), in which case deep retinal, sometimes multifocal, gray-white lesions are seen (**Fig. 13.27**), with little or no vitreous reaction. The macula is commonly involved. A more characteristic inner retinal focus may accompany (**Fig. 13.28**) or follow in time (**Fig. 13.29**). The differential diagnosis of outer retinal toxoplasmosis will include acute posterior multifocal placoid pigment epitheliopathy (APMPPE), serpiginous choroidopathy and sarcoid choroiditis. Rarely, large confluent retinal areas may be inflamed (Benson et al. 1992), usually but not necessarily in immunodeficient patients. Diagnosis is challenging; syphilis and herpetic necrotizing retinopathy will be considered in the differential diagnosis.

Acquired toxoplasma retinochoroiditis

Toxoplasmosis may cause retinochoroiditis during the first infection. This circumstance was once thought unusual, occurring in perhaps 2–3% of new infections (Perkins 1973), but is more common in this clinic. The retinal lesion will usually be single and unilateral, but there will be no visible chorioretinal scar indicating previous infection (**Fig. 13.30**). In our experience acquired lesions affect the macula much more often than recurrent foci, are often associated with retinal elevation (**Fig. 13.31**) and often permanently affect central vision.

Multifocal or extended inflammation

Rarely, severe retinochoroiditis may cause panuveitis, and associated scleritis has been reported which in some cases resulted in enucleation. In immunodeficient individuals, a characteristic single focus of reactivation may be seen, but atypical presentations are common. Lesions may be multifocal within one eye (**Fig. 13.32**), although in 18% (Cochereau-Massin et al. 1992) they are bilateral. Lesions may be particularly large or associated with widespread ocular inflammation. Herpetic retinal necrosis may be mimicked (Moshfeghi et al. 2004). Rarely infection may spread to give orbital cellulitis (Moorthy et al. 1993). Sometimes immunodeficient patients may already have suffered intraocular inflammation from other causes, particularly cytomegalovirus (CMV) retinitis, and two active intraocular inflammations may coexist, giving confusing physical signs (**Fig. 13.33**). In the differential diagnosis of toxoplasma retinochoroiditis in immunodeficient, especially AIDS, patients other opportunistic infections must also be considered including various fungi, tuberculosis and herpesviruses. Although the differentiation of toxoplasmosis from CMV retinitis is usually straightforward, the two conditions have sometimes been confused (Elkins et al. 1994).

The atypical features of ocular infection in immunosuppressed individuals may be combined with systemic symptoms and signs (particularly those of encephalitis, including reduced conscious level, and focal signs of brain abscesses), which suggest dissemination. Encephalitis may occur in up to 30% of seropositive AIDS patients at

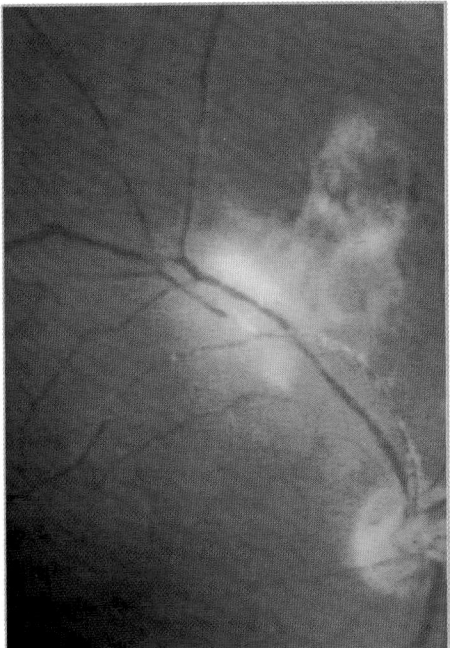

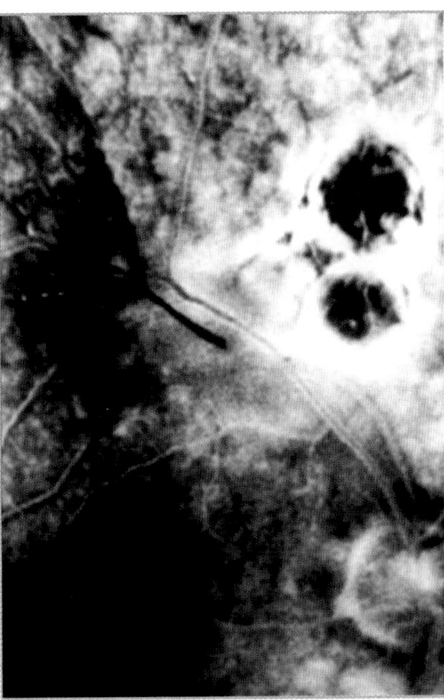

Figure 13.14 An active focus of retinochoroiditis straddles the superotemporal arcade, producing enough vasculitis and/or tissue edema to occlude the superior macular arteriole. Central vision was abruptly and permanently reduced despite the macula being free of inflammation.

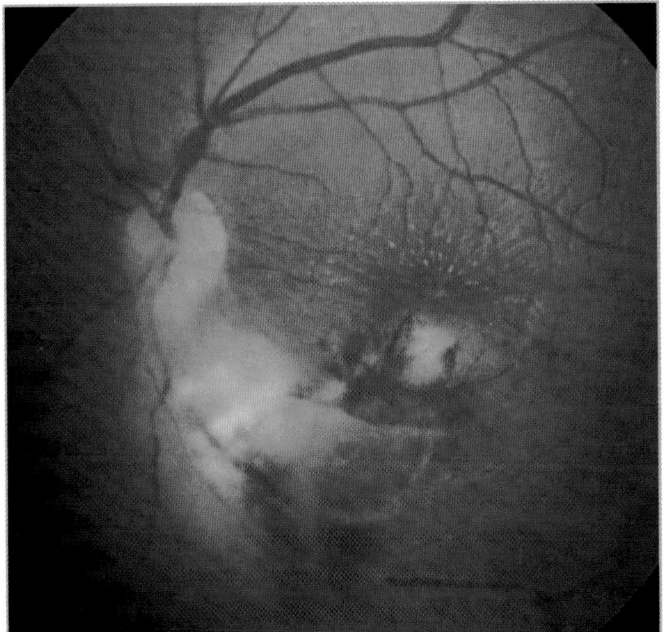

Figure 13.15 A large posterior pole focus is accompanied by occlusive phlebitis with macular hemorrhage and exudate.

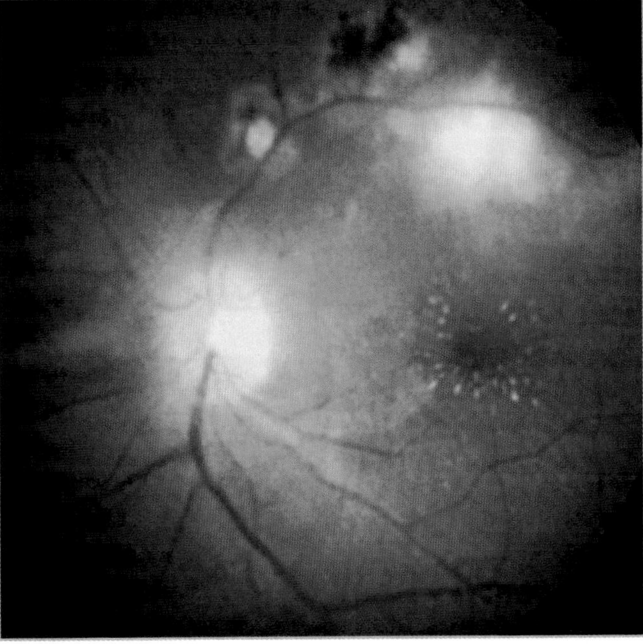

Figure 13.16 Through significant vitritis, a large posterior pole focus is accompanied by macular star exudate.

some time. The diagnosis of atypical intraocular infection in immunosuppressed individuals must always be made in close liaison with the infectious diseases physician.

Large, indolent peripheral foci of inflammation (**Fig. 13.34**), most often in middle-aged or elderly people, probably a result of an age-related decline in cell-mediated immunity (Johnson et al. 1997) can be challenging to treat, often remaining active despite longer courses of antibiotic and steroid treatment. We have sometimes found extremely high toxoplasma IgG titers in such patients. Reactivation has also been described in those taking systemic corticosteroid treatment for other reasons (Morhun et al. 1996).

Non-inflammatory sequelae

As with any inflammatory chorioretinitis, a subretinal neovascular membrane may develop (**Fig. 13.35**), but after toxoplasma retinochoroiditis these are very uncommon. In this clinic they are treated with oral steroid followed by intravitreal bevacizumab injection (with prophylactic co-trimoxazole in addition). Retinal vessel occlusion may lead to substantial ischemia. The resultant neovascularization may later present with vitreous hemorrhage. Rarely post-inflammatory retinal atrophy may lead to break formation and rhegmatogenous detachment. Macular or perimacular lesions may lead to epiretinal membrane formation (**Fig. 13.36**).

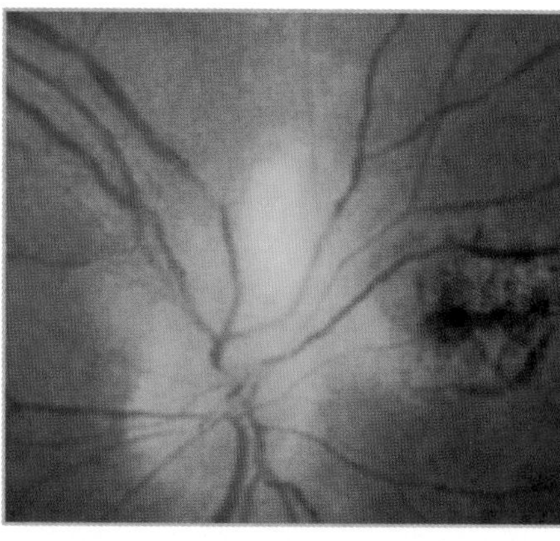
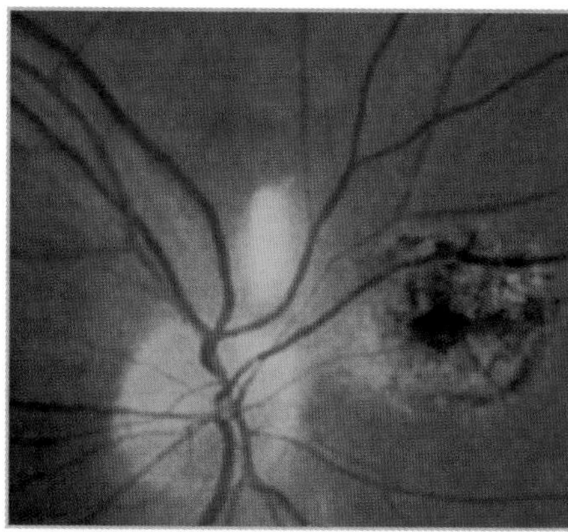

Figure 13.17 An active focus is shown at presentation and after 2 weeks of treatment. The lesion is smaller and better defined, pale retinal edema is subsiding, and the view is clearer as overlying vitreous infiltrate clears.

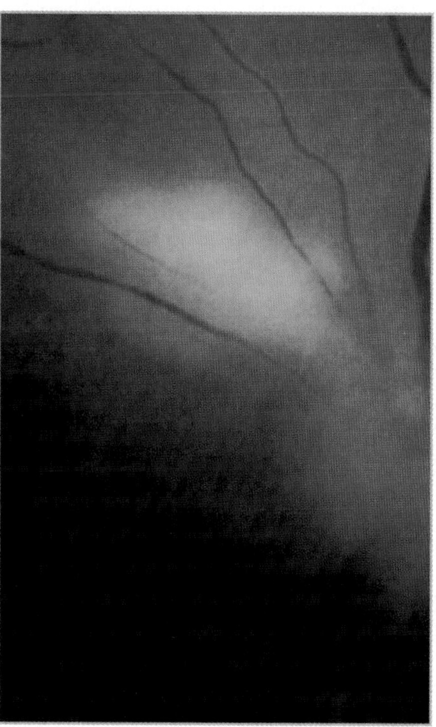
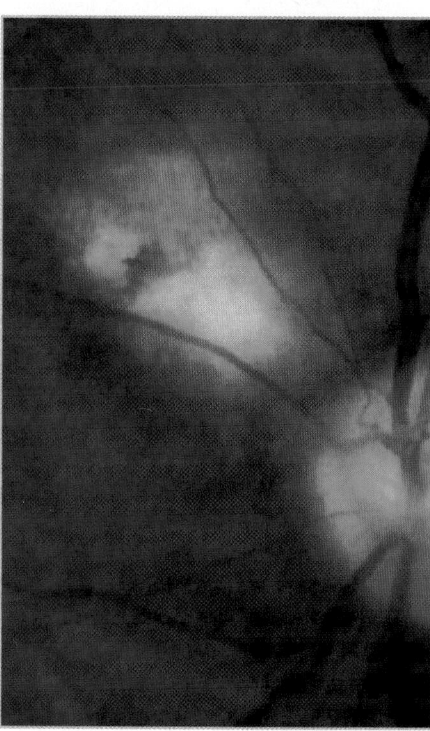

Figure 13.18 An active focus at presentation and after 4 weeks of treatment. Inflammation is virtually settled, leaving a new chorioretinal scar that characteristically is slightly larger than the original focus.

Diagnosis

The features most helpful in diagnosing acute ocular toxoplasmosis are unilateral inflammation, the presence of a single white inner retinal active focus and old chorioretinal scarring (which may also be contralateral). Few other conditions cause unifocal, localized retinitis (as opposed to choroiditis). Where inflammation is atypical or multifocal, herpetic or bacterial infections are possible alternative diagnoses. In the immunodeficient patient other opportunists, particularly fungi, should be considered.

Parasites may readily be identified from tissue specimens but ocular tissue is rarely available for diagnosis. However, organisms have been isolated from vitreous humor in atypical retinitis (Greven and Teot 1994). Although tissue culture of *T. gondii* may provide a diagnosis within 4 days, the technique has not become a practical diagnostic aid. In most patients, the characteristic picture, together with serological confirmation of previous exposure, is adequate to justify the use of anti-toxoplasma medication. Toxoplasma serology should be performed in any patient where the diagnosis is not absolutely clear. Aqueous humor sampling for toxoplasma PCR should be considered; several primers are available, all giving virtually 100% specificity. A comparison of primers against B1, P30 and 18S ribosomal DNA (rDNA) genes found that B1 was the most sensitive (Jones et al. 2000) and this has subsequently been used most commonly. Real-time PCR has advantages, and the addition of more sensitive primers improves sensitivity (Cassaing et al. 2006).

Serological testing

All cases of toxoplasma retinochoroiditis with a pre-existing chorioretinal scar are reactivations of a previously acquired infection. Serological changes indicative of acute infection are therefore not expected and IgM titers are of no relevance. However, after a delay following initial exposure to *Toxoplasma* spp., IgG titers usually remain positive for life. It is possible, using serological testing of adequate sensitivity, to confirm previous exposure to *Toxoplasma* spp.

The population prevalence of toxoplasmosis varies from country to country dependent on standards of hygiene and dietary habits.

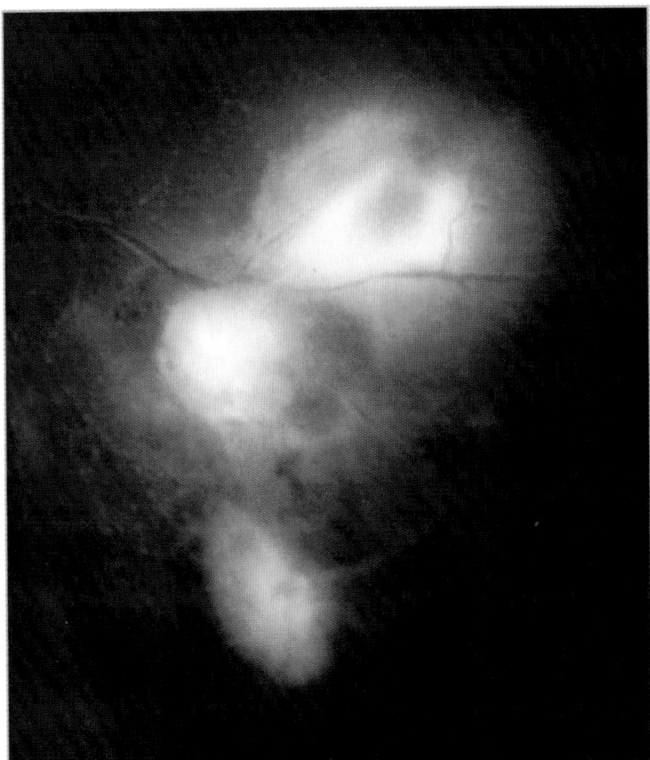

Figure 13.19 Strands of vitreous infiltrate overlying an active focus.

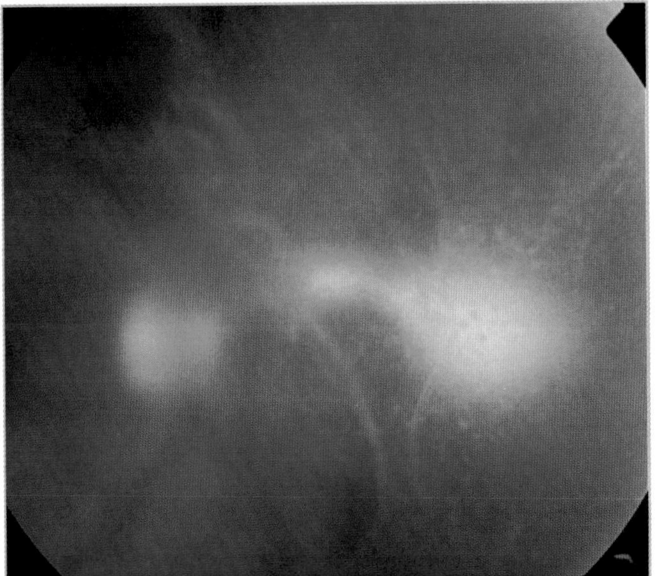

Figure 13.20 Substantial vitreous opacification obscuring an active focus of retinochoroiditis.

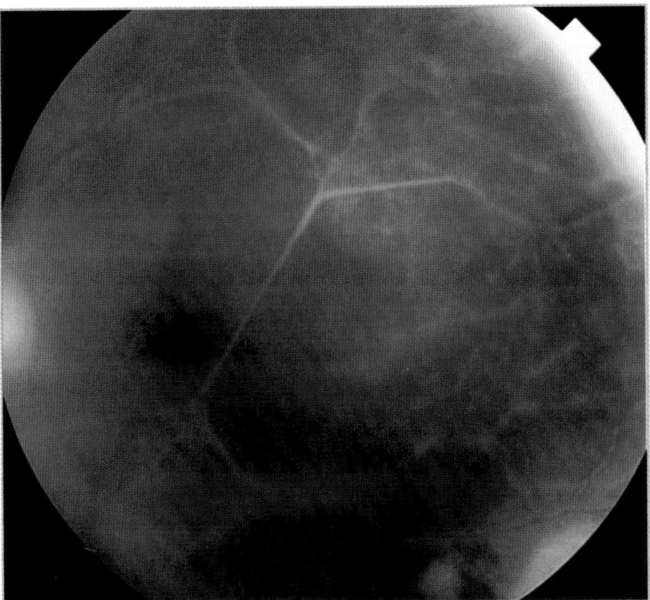

Figure 13.21 An inferotemporal focus of retinochoroiditis is associated with retinal vasculitis and a complex web of vitreous fibrils.

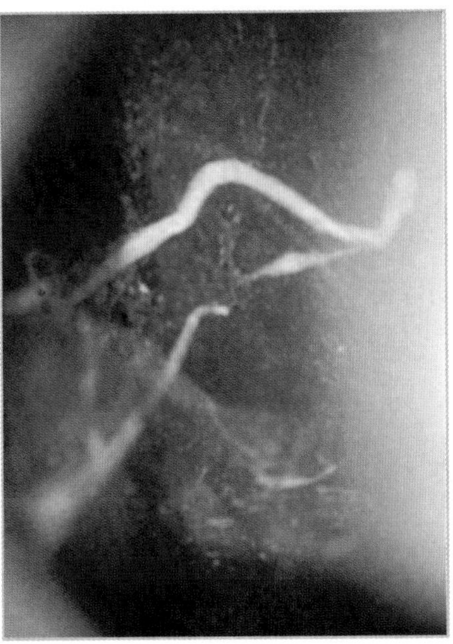

Figure 13.22 Vitreous 'cylinders' after recurrent toxoplasma retinochoroiditis.

Gilbert et al. (1993) showed that, among inhabitants of London tested during pregnancy, white Europeans born in the UK had a 13.3% seropositivity rate, whereas the figure was 12.2% for African-Caribbeans born in the UK, 45.9% for African-Caribbeans born in Africa and 71.4% for white Europeans born in France. Any serological test should be interpreted with local prevalence in mind; positive toxoplasma serology is common and is therefore by no means confirmatory of ocular toxoplasmosis. However, a trustworthy negative test should encourage a diagnostic reappraisal in any patient exhibiting atypical features. Immunodeficient patients, even with disseminated toxoplasmosis, may be unable to generate a detectable serological response and therefore negative serology is less helpful in this group.

The long-standing Sabin–Feldman dye test (the dye test) remains for many the gold standard for serological testing. However, in practice enzyme-linked immunosorbent assay (ELISA) tests have become the standard laboratory test in most centers. Indirect agglutination or fluorescent antibody tests are becoming obsolete. In this clinic, IgG ELISA is primarily used, with IgM ELISA and IgM immunosorbent agglutination assay (ISAGA) if requested, with confirmation by dye test for any ELISA-positive individuals.

If newly acquired acute infection is suspected, serology may confirm this diagnosis with rising titers, first of IgM, then of IgG, usually to very high levels. Two or more blood samples, acute (on presentation) and

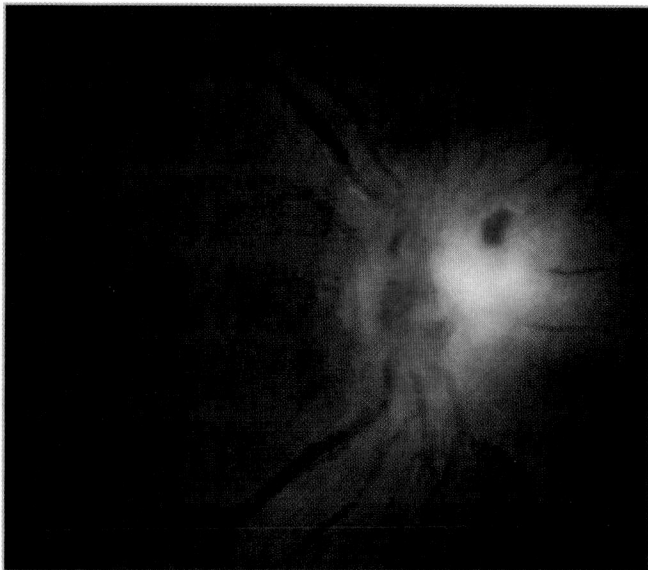

Figure 13.23 Peripapillary toxoplasmosis with associated disc edema and hemorrhage. These lesions can leave large visual field defects.

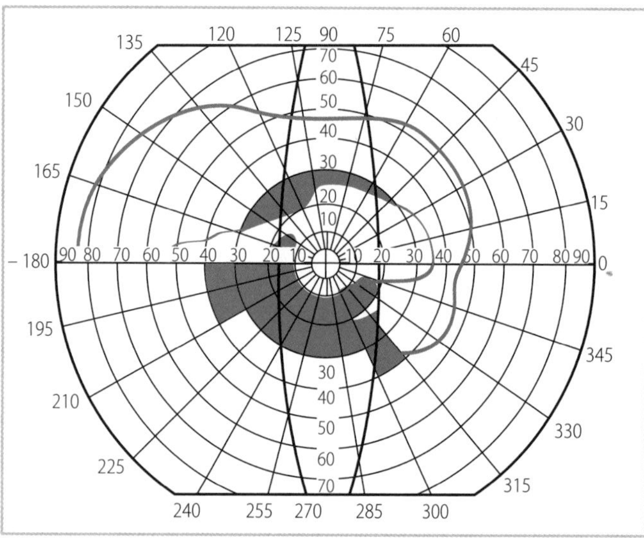

Figure 13.24 Large visual field defects may result from peripapillary foci.

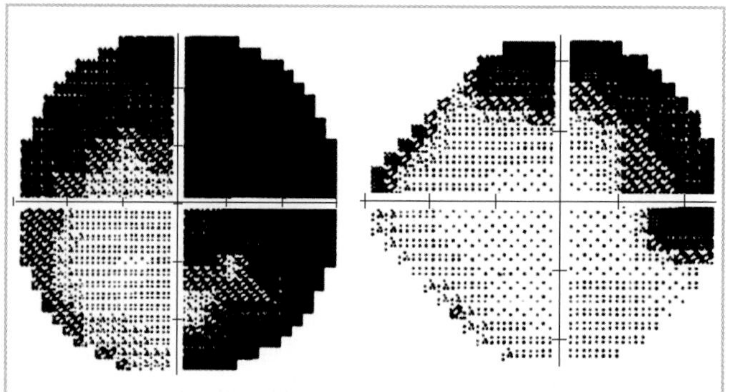

Figure 13.25 Bilateral visual field loss after presumed retrobulbar toxoplasmosis.

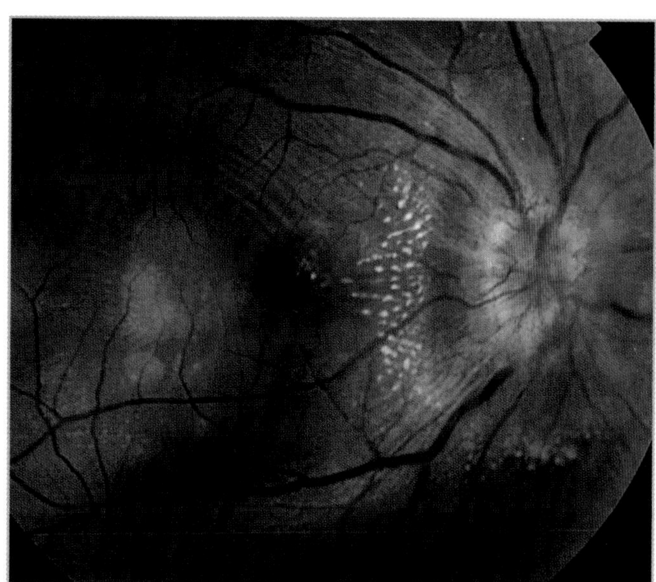

Figure 13.26 Toxoplasma neuroretinitis. The optic disk is swollen and hyperemic with surrounding retinal edema and exudate, forming a macular star and retinal folds. Lateral to the fovea are several patches of outer retinal toxoplasmosis.

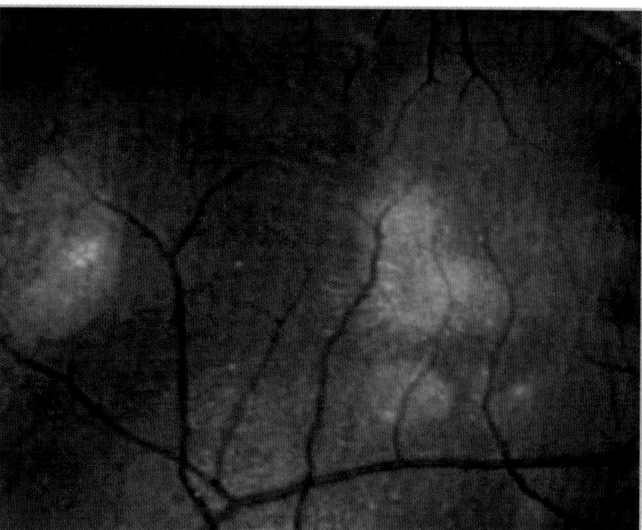

Figure 13.27 A magnified view of the perimacular area of Fig. 13.26, showing several plaques of outer retinal toxoplasmosis. There is a degree of overlying retinal distortion, but little vitreous activity.

convalescent (2–4 weeks later) are ideal but single measurements of high titers of IgM are usually considered sufficient for the diagnosis of acute infection.

ELISA test

For both IgG and IgM detection, most ELISA tests available approach 100% for both specificity and sensitivity, exceeding the performance of the dye test. Diluted patient serum is added to wells pre-coated with *T. gondii* antigen. Specific Ig will bind to the antigen. An enzyme conjugate is added which then, upon incubation, hydrolyses a substrate only if antigen–antibody complexes have formed. The result is read by colorimetry.

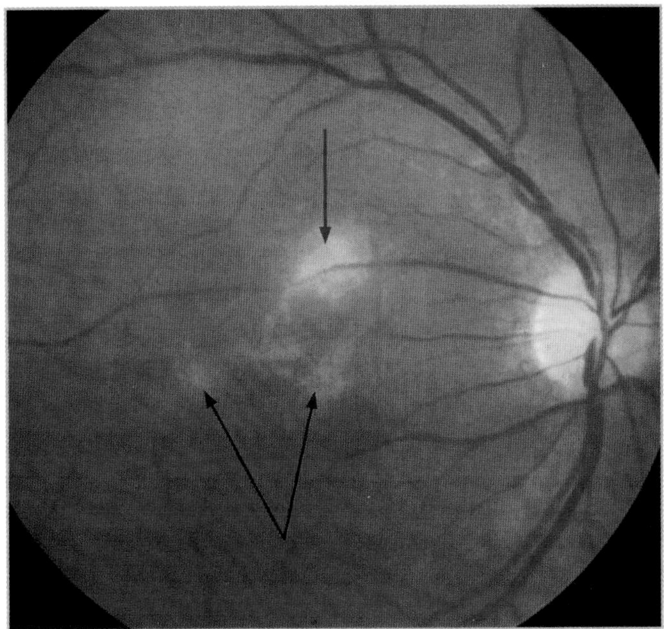

Figure 13.28 Acquired toxoplasmosis manifesting as a combination of inner (red arrow) and outer (black arrow) retinal inflammation.

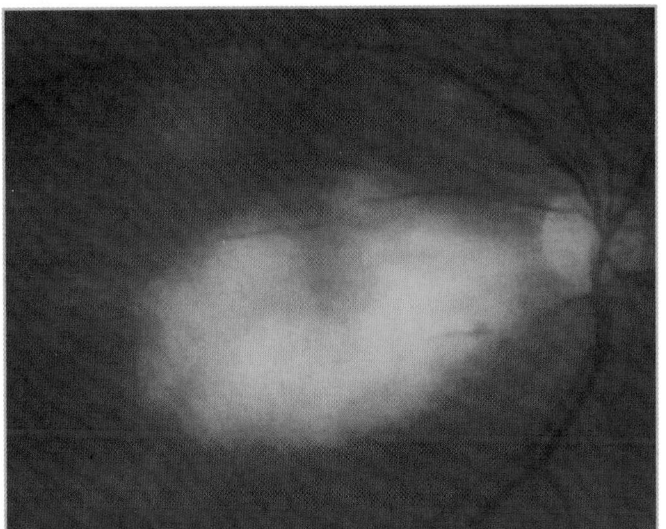

Figure 13.29 Aggressive toxoplasmosis, same eye as Fig. 13.28 despite 1 week of treatment. The patient was immunosuppressed by chemotherapy for myelomatosis.

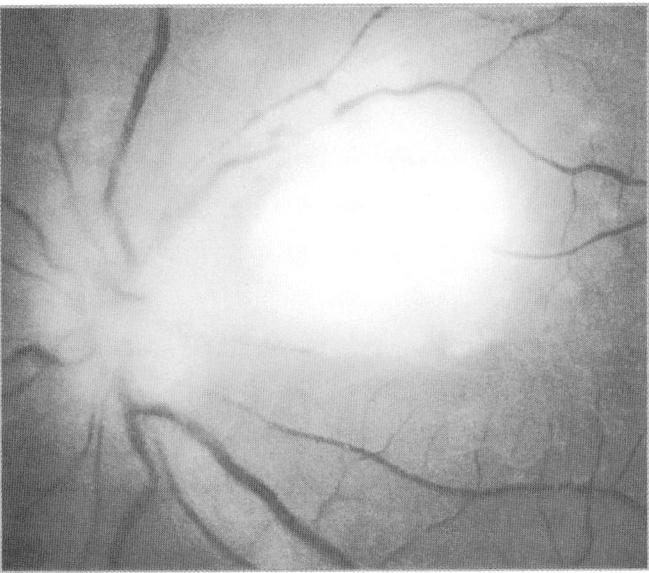

Figure 13.30 Acquired toxoplasmosis in association with pyrexia, lymphadenopathy and meningism. Rising IgM titers confirmed the diagnosis. Central vision was lost.

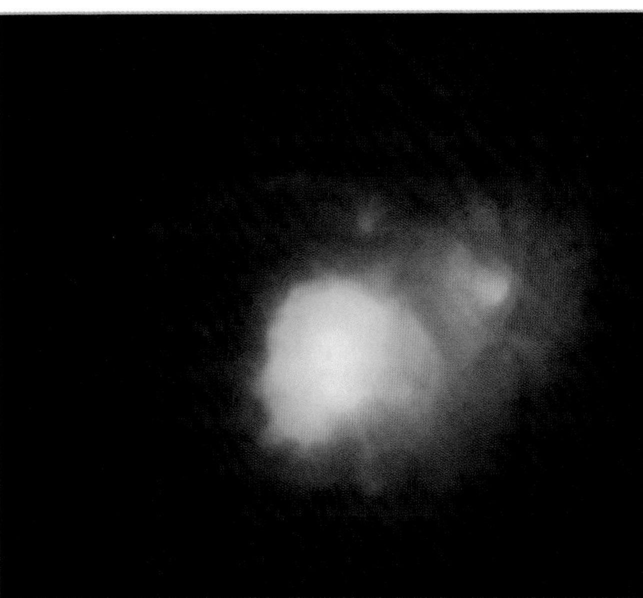

Figure 13.31 Acquired toxoplasmosis in an African–Caribbean patient. A large macular lesion is associated with cystic retinal elevation. Central vision was lost.

Sabin–Feldman dye test

This test depends on the reaction of antibodies from seropositive individuals with live *T. gondii* organisms, to render the latter permeable to the dye methylene blue. In a positive reaction they are thus unstained by the dye, whereas they stain blue if the test is negative. The test takes 2–3 weeks to complete. As a result of the risk to laboratory staff of keeping live cultures of *T. gondii*, this test is confined to reference laboratories. Despite the high performance of ELISA tests, it remains a respected 'confirmatory' test.

Both the indirect fluorescent antibody test and indirect agglutination tests are now largely supplanted by ELISA testing and are virtually obsolete.

Management

Medical treatment

Each episode of active toxoplasma retinochoroiditis is self-limiting. During the period of active inflammation, symptoms will depend on both the location of the lesion and the degree of vitreous opacification. No treatment can prevent necrosis and scarring of the active retinal focus. However, treatment, it is hoped, will limit the size of the resultant scar (and therefore the visual field defect), and limit the intensity and duration of vitreous opacification, limit the duration of symptoms and, perhaps most importantly, kill free intraocular tachyzoites, which (it is assumed) will reduce the number of newly formed bradyzoites, each of which may trigger a further attack.

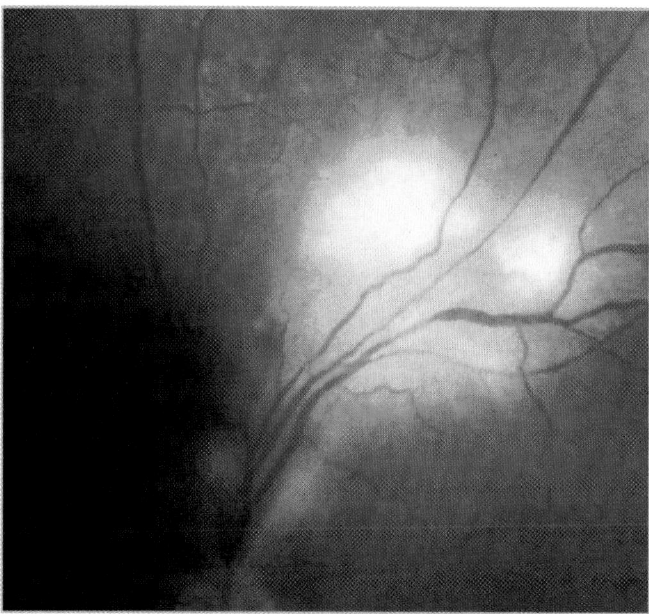

Figure 13.32 Multifocal toxoplasmosis in an HIV-positive patient.

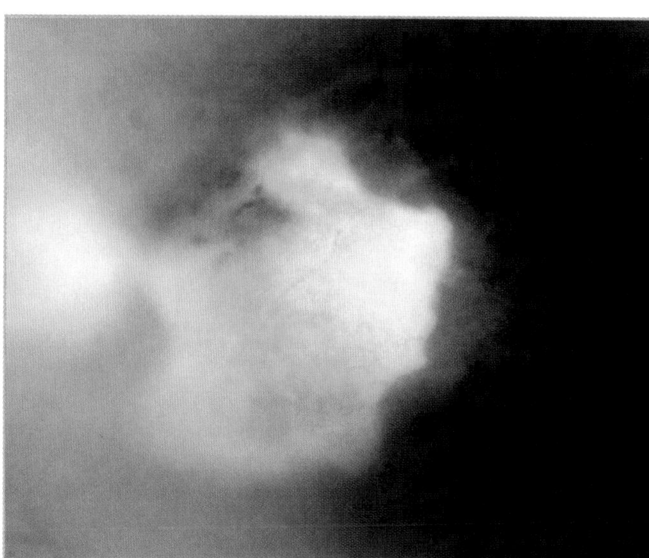

Figure 13.34 A large persistent peripheral lesion in a 65-year-old patient.

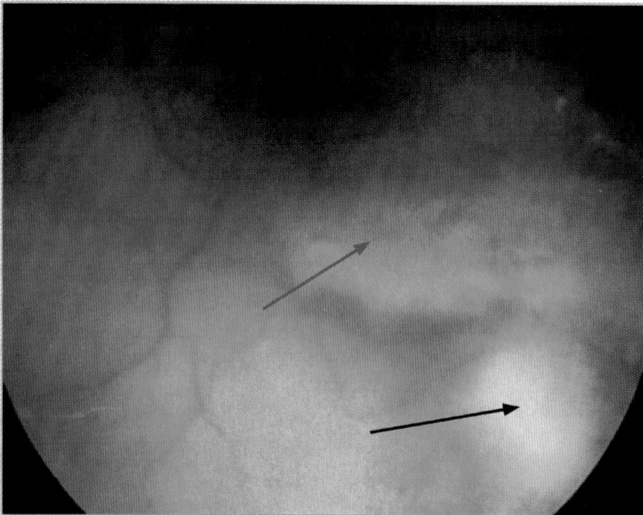

Figure 13.33 Coexistent cytomegalovirus retinitis (red arrow) and toxoplasmosis (black arrow) in the same eye of an HIV-positive patient.

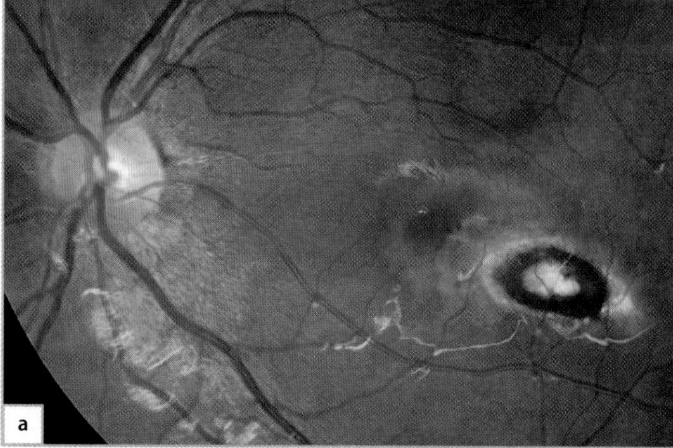

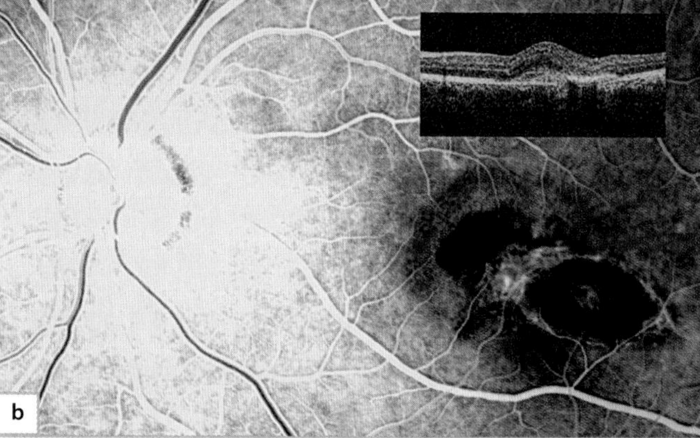

Figure 13.35 A choroidal neovascular membrane with associated subretinal fluid and hemorrhage has formed on the foveal side of an old congenital toxoplasma scar.

However, it is possible that free tachyzoites may form new tissue cysts within only a few days of release (Luder et al. 1999), thus making a prescription of antibiotics at presentation of dubious value for many patients.

The pathogenesis of inflammation in toxoplasma retinochoroiditis is incompletely understood. It is known that active trophozoites are released from a ruptured cyst, and that live organisms are therefore present in the lesion at least for a time. However, it is likely that other mechanisms are involved, such as cytotoxic effects from protozoal components, possibly a hypersensitivity reaction and probably an element of autoimmune damage (Whittle et al. 1998). There is therefore a rational basis for the use of both anti-protozoal therapy and anti-inflammatory medication. However, the evidence in humans for the efficacy of either remains poor (Stanford and Gilbert 2009) and drug-induced side effects may affect 40% of patients (Iaccheri et al. 2008). Pyrimethamine, the longstanding aminoquinolone, needs to have its anti-folate action ameliorated with carefully dosed folinic acid, otherwise hematological problems including thrombocytopenia, are common; sulfas frequently cause allergic reactions

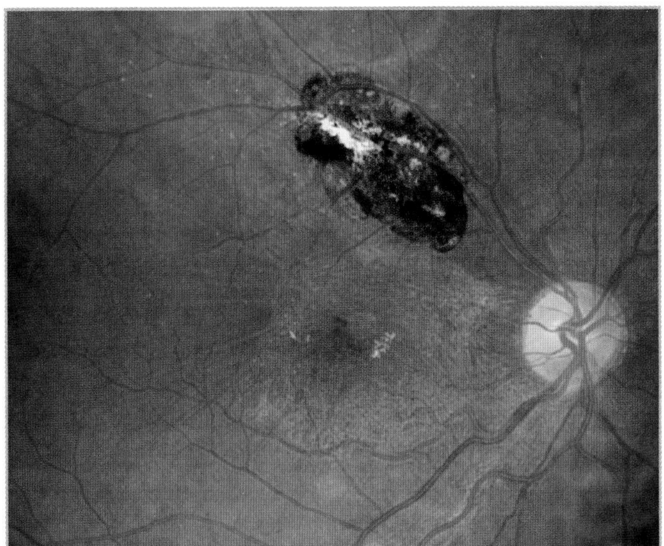

Figure 13.36 Epiretinal membrane with macular pucker following previous toxoplasma retinochoroiditis at the posterior pole.

including erythema multiforme and, occasionally, the Stevens–Johnson syndrome; clindamycin risks severe diarrhea and is expensive. Information on comparative efficacy would therefore be welcome. Anti-protozoal treatments include the following.

Sulfonamides

Sulfonamides suppress folate synthesis, and therefore purine and DNA synthesis. Humans may ingest folate, but microorganisms are obliged to synthesize their own. Sulfonamides act by competitive inhibition, blocking synthesis. For the treatment of toxoplasmosis, either sulfadiazine or sulfadimidine is usually chosen, both being taken orally in a dose of 1 g four times daily. Sulfonamides (including sulfamethoxazole, the sulfa in co-trimoxazole) have a high incidence of skin rashes, occasionally including erythema multiforme or the Stevens–Johnson syndrome. Occasional blood dyscrasias are seen. Sulfas and quinolones act on adjacent components of the folate pathway, thus being complementary when used together.

Quinolones

Pyrimethamine is a 4-aminoquinoline derivative similar to quinine. It inhibits dihydrofolate reductase, which converts folic to folinic acid. The folate pathway exists in both protozoa and humans, but the drug's affinity for this enzyme is far greater in the former. Nevertheless, the folate pathway in the patient may be sufficiently impeded to cause marrow suppression, particularly thrombocytopenia. Hematological monitoring is therefore necessary. Pyrimethamine is given orally at a dose of 25 mg twice daily, usually after a single loading dose of 50 mg. to alleviate marrow toxicity, folinic acid (not folic acid) is given at a dose of 3–5 mg three times per week. A dose smaller than this may not prevent thrombocytopenia, whereas higher doses may compromise the therapeutic effect of the pyrimethamine.

Trimethoprim is similar to pyrimethamine but less potent. Bacterial folate synthesis is exquisitely sensitive to blockage by trimethoprim, the protozoal pathway less so. The pre-prepared combination with sulfamethoxazole (co-trimoxazole 960 mg twice daily) is convenient but the patient is still exposed to the side effects of both drugs.

Macrolides

Clindamycin acts on microbial ribosomes to inhibit protein synthesis. It is taken orally in a dose of 300 mg four times daily. Its most important side effect is the development of *Clostridium difficile* enterocolitis, which may cause severe, occasionally fatal, pseudomembranous enterocolitis (although usually in elderly people). Patients taking clindamycin should therefore be warned to discontinue the drug and contact their physician should significant diarrhea occur. Unfortunately minor diarrhea affects up to 20% of those using clindamycin, so premature curtailment of treatment is not infrequent.

Spiramycin, a macrolide similar to erythromycin, is a second-choice agent in ocular toxoplasmosis, and is not generally available and normally used only in pregnancy (see below). Azithromycin is taken orally in a dose of 500 mg/day for just 3 days. It is therefore a convenient medication, and the toxicity profile of the drug compares favorably with others used to treat toxoplasmosis. It may prove useful for immediate self-administration in patients who have frequent recurrences of ocular disease.

Others

Atovaquone is unrelated to other antibiotics, and inhibits mitochondrial activity in protozoa. It is taken orally at a dose of 750 mg three times daily and has been used mainly for the management of pneumocystis and toxoplasma infections in AIDS patients, with variable results. It is said to have some activity against toxoplasma cysts.

Rothova and others (1993) compared three groups (each receiving oral steroid) treated by pyrimethamine and sulfadiazine, clindamycin and sulfadiazine or trimethoprim/sulfamethoxazole. The evidence for efficacy of any group was poor, but slightly better results were found in the pyrimethamine group, which also caused more side effects. A comparison of trimethoprim with sulfamethoxazole versus pyrimethamine and sulfadiazine (Soheilian et al. 2005) showed comparable efficacy. Another trial exchanged sulfa for azithromycin in combination with pyrimethamine (Bosch-Drierssen et al. 2002), and again found similar results but, predictably, a lower rate of drug-induced side effects. It should also be noted that the use of orbital steroid injections has been found to be deleterious.

Overall, no antibiotic is outstanding. It is clear from the differences in treatment for toxoplasmosis in various centers that no ideal solution has been agreed. There does, however, appear to be a consensus that oral steroid should not be used alone, mainly based on anecdotes of fulminating endophthalmitis in such patients, even when immunocompetent. With our current, incomplete knowledge of the natural history of ocular toxoplasmosis, and understanding the potential risk of treatment side effects, patients in our clinic are treated according to a protocol (see MUC Protocol: Toxoplasmosis on the attached disk). The following lesions are treated (**Fig. 13.37**):

1 Any active focus at the posterior pole that is inside or straddling the temporal vascular arcades (because such lesions are close to fixation, may enlarge to involve the fovea or may cause permanent secondary macular effects)
2 Any peripapillary active focus (within one disk diameter of the disk at its closest) or one involving optic disk swelling (because involvement near or on the optic nerve head tends to leave large visual field defects)
3 Any active focus threatening occlusion of a major retinal vessel (because retinal neovascularization and intraocular hemorrhage are a reported complication, and to avoid large visual field defects)

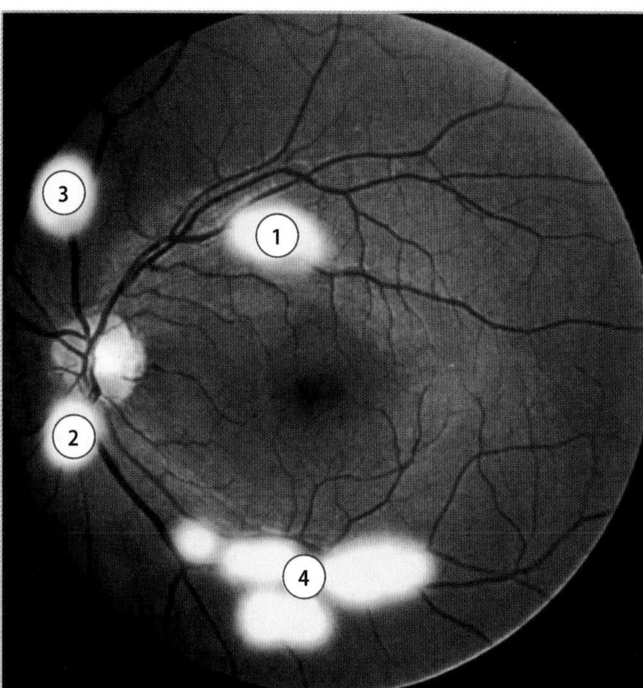

Figure 13.37 A composite diagram of toxoplasma lesions requiring treatment (see text). (1) A lesion within the arcade; (2) a peripapillary lesion; (3) a lesion at risk of occluding a major vessel; (4) multifocal active foci.

4 Multifocal lesions or toxoplasmosis in immunodeficient individuals (because of the risk of fulminating infection).
5 Any active focus with substantial vitreous clouding so that a view of the macula is difficult even with the indirect ophthalmoscope (because macular involvement, direct or indirect, cannot be ruled out)
6 Vitreous whiteout with a confirmed history of recurrent toxoplasmosis (because in the absence of other indicators the etiology is clear, and the degree of inflammation is clearly severe)

Patients with active foci falling outside these criteria may have significant visual loss or floaters due to vitreous opacification, but in these instances the risk–benefit balance is in favor of observation rather than treatment. The episode will be self-limiting and vitreous clarity usually returns to normal.

In this clinic all patients fulfilling the above treatment criteria, with no known contraindications, are treated with prednisolone at a dosage dependent on the degree of intraocular inflammation, but starting at an average 40 mg/day, and not more than 60 mg/day. This dosage is maintained for 2 weeks and then tapered depending on the response. Co-trimoxazole 960 mg twice daily is started simultaneously and continued for 4 weeks.

In the immunodeficient patient, reactivated retinochoroiditis may combine with disseminated toxoplasmosis, particularly encephalitis. In this circumstance vigorous management with antimicrobials is necessary but systemic steroids should not be used. Maintenance treatment, e.g. pyrimethamine 25 mg/day if tolerated, must be continued for life. Even with maintenance treatment a recurrence rate of 20% is reported and when these occur additional agents must be added. Atovaquone has also been used for maintenance in these circumstances, with variable results.

Ocular toxoplasmosis in pregnancy

The development of acute toxoplasma retinochoroiditis during pregnancy is a substantial and complex management challenge (Montoya et al. 2008), the crux questions being: Is it newly acquired or recurrent? Which stage of pregnancy does it present in? Does the focus definitely need treatment?

Newly acquired toxoplasmosis during pregnancy often leads to fetal abnormalities ranging from spontaneous abortion or major abnormality in the first trimester, to a range of abnormalities characterized by the TORCH syndrome. The earlier in pregnancy the infection is sustained, the greater the risk to the fetus. If considered newly acquired through ocular appearance and IgM positivity, the patient's obstetrician should be involved at an early stage to discuss management. If the focus is clearly recurrent (and it seems that recurrent ocular toxoplasmosis may have a predilection for pregnant women), and if the patient is immunocompetent, the risk to the fetus is extremely low. If the disease is newly acquired and the pregnancy is to continue, the risk of placental transmission is high, and both obstetrician and ophthalmologist may prefer to treat. In an immunodeficient woman, there is a fetal risk even if the ocular lesion is recurrent, but this risk is difficult to quantify.

It may be entirely appropriate to observe, but not treat, recurrent lesions that are not high risk for vision. If treatment is considered essential, then, as for other patients, the use of oral steroid without an anti-protozoal is not ideal but may be appropriate in these difficult circumstances. If anti-protozoal treatment is to be used, which drug should we choose? There is no clear consensus, but it is known that pyrimethamine is teratogenic in the first trimester and sulfonamides carry a risk of severe hematological effects when used later in pregnancy. Neither these drugs nor co-trimoxazole is therefore safe. Atovaquone is probably not safe, and azithromycin possibly not. The macrolides clindamycin and spiramycin are both thought to be safe in pregnancy, and spiramycin may reduce the fetal risk. However, the efficacy of oral clindamycin alone in ocular toxoplasmosis is unproven and therefore there is no clear available advice on the preferred regimen. It may be that a future direction for the management of ocular toxoplasmosis during pregnancy is intraocular anti-protozoal injection.

Prophylaxis of recurrent ocular toxoplasmosis

The efficacy of low-dose (co-trimoxazole 960 mg 3–4 times weekly) prophylaxis against *Toxoplasma* encephalitis in AIDS patients (Carr et al. 1992) and against acute systemic reactivation in immunosuppressed heart transplant patients (Baden et al. 2003) is fairly well-established. There is some evidence that similar prophylaxis in the immunocompetent can reduce the incidence of ocular recurrences (Silveira et al. 2002).

Surgical/laser treatment

Where patients are intolerant of medication, in pregnancy, or where medical treatment is unsuccessful, intraocular therapy may be considered. Clindamycin (1 mg in 0.1 ml) has been used with claims of good efficacy either alone (Sobrin et al. 2007) or with dexamethasone (Soheilian et al. 2010). At one time it was felt that peri-scar retinal laser treatment may prevent recurrent disease. If dormant cysts were located only directly around the scar this may have been successful. However, the variable location of new foci, which may develop some distance from the old scar, suggests that laser treatment is unlikely to be successful, and so it has proved.

Vitrectomy has been used during acute inflammation with unhelpful results, including reduced vision and retinal traction. In some patients vitreous organization following repeated inflammation can be permanent. In these circumstances vitrectomy has been used (Adan et al. 2009), although the prophylactic use of anti-protozoal therapy commencing just before surgery, and continuing for some time afterwards, has been recommended. Vitrectomy can be technically challenging in these patients because of the adherent nature of fibrinous scarring.

Choroidal neovascularization secondary to toxoplasmosis is unusual but reported. Both verteporfin photodynamic therapy (PDT) (Wirthlin et al. 2006) and intravitreal anti-VEGF (vascular endothelial growth factor) injection (Benvenuto et al. 2008) have been successful in treatment.

As for any zoonosis with a single-genus primary host, eradication of disease can be a target. Currently the hyperendemic nature of toxoplasmosis in some parts of the world makes this a daunting task. No new anti-protozoal drugs are close to availability. Much work has been done on the development of *T. gondii* vaccines and these are routinely used in some domestic animal groups including sheep (Silveira et al. 2009). However, human trials are not in development. It is likely that the junior ophthalmologist will continue to see and treat ocular toxoplasmosis through his career.

OTHER PROTOZOAL INFECTIONS

Acanthamoeba keratouveitis

Acanthamoeba spp. are well recognized as a cause of progressive keratitis in contact lens wearers. Associated uveitis may be seen and misdiagnosis as herpes simplex keratouveitis is a common but avoidable error (Moore et al. 1985). The contact lens and its case should be obtained for microscopy and culture. Where corneal epithelial defects are present, corneal scrape should be performed. In refractory cases corneal biopsy may be necessary. The medical treatment of keratitis has proved difficult. Propamidine, neomycin, miconazole, clotrimazole, chlorhexidine and metronidazole have been used with variable effect. Corneal transplantation may be necessary, accompanied by a substantial rate of both rejection and recurrence.

Entamoeba uveitis

Entamoeba histolytica is an intestinal parasite and may infect the large bowel of humans and some other large mammals. The worldwide prevalence of infection is estimated at 10%, rising to 50% in Asia. Transmission is usually by contaminated water or food, although infection is also more common in homosexuals. Ulcerative bowel disease with dysentery may result. Occasionally extraintestinal infection occurs, including hepatitis with abscess formation, but pulmonary or brain abscesses may also be seen.

Uveitis, including intermediate uveitis, has been reported in patients with amoebic dysentery. *E. histolytica*, or its subspecies *E. hartmanni*, has also been thought to cause focal serous or exudative chorioretinitis, in the form of a cystic macular lesion with surrounding subretinal hemorrhage and apparent hyperplasia of the retinal pigment epithelium. Small yellowish granular retinal lesions are also seen and the vitreous is usually clear. Histological confirmation has not been possible. Diagnosis is by fecal microscopy or serology. For chronic extraintestinal disease including uveitis, metronidazole and diiodohydroxyquin may be sequentially combined with chloroquine or dehydroemetine.

Giardia uveitis

Giardia lamblia may be ingested with contaminated water or food, and similar to *Entamoeba* sp. is more common in homosexuals. It is worldwide in distribution. Some infections are asymptomatic, but diarrhea, malaise, fatigue, colic and vomiting are usual. Chronic infection may lead to malabsorption and weight loss. Iridocyclitis, chorioretinitis and hemorrhagic retinopathy have been seen, as has retinal arteritis (Knox and King 1982). No histological confirmation has been possible, but resolution of the ocular inflammation followed systemic treatment. Examination of feces or duodenal fluid for cysts is diagnostic. If necessary, jejunal biopsy may be performed. ELISA or indirect immunofluorescence tests may detect serum antibodies. Metronidazole, furazolidone and quinacrine have all been successfully used to treat giardiasis in adults.

Cryptosporidium and Plasmodium spp.

Uveitis has been reported as a rare complication of both cryptosporidiosis and malaria. The former can also be responsible for provoking reactive arthritis syndrome.

REFERENCES

Adan A, Giralt J, Alvarez G, et al. Pars plana vitrectomy for vitreoretinal complications of ocular toxoplasmosis. *Eur J Ophthalmol* 2009;**19**: 1039–43.

Baden LR, Katz JT, Franck L. Successful toxoplasmosis prophylaxis after orthotopic cardiac transplantation with trimethoprim-sulfamethoxazole. *Clin Transplant* 2003;**75**:339–43.

Benson MT, Parsons MA, Talbot JF, et al. Aggressive toxoplasma retinitis. *Acta Ophthalmol* 1992;**70**:795–800.

Benevento JD, Jager RD, Noble AG, et al. Toxoplasmosis-associated neovascular lesions treated successfully with ranibizumab and antiparasitic therapy. *Arch Ophthalmol* 2008;**126**:1152–6.

Bosch-Driessen LH, Verbraak FD, Suttorp-Schulten MA, et al. A prospective randomised trial of pyrimethamine and azithromycin vs pyrimethamine and sulfadiazine for the treatment of ocular toxoplasmosis. *Am J Ophthalmol* 2002;**134**:34–40.

Carr A, Tindall B, Brew BJ, et al. Low-dose trimethoprim–sulfamethoxazole prophylaxis for toxoplasmic encephalitis in patients with AIDS. *Ann Internal Med* 1992;**117**:106–11.

Cassaing S, Bessieres MH, Berry A, et al. Comparison between two amplification sets for molecular diagnosis of toxoplasmosis by real-time PCR. *J Clin Microbiol* 2006;**44**:720–4.

Cochereau-Massin I, LeHoang P, Lautier-Frau M, et al. Ocular toxoplasmosis in human immunodeficiency virus-infected patients. *Am J Ophthalmol* 1992;**114**:130–5.

Doft BH, Gass JDM. Punctate outer retinal toxoplasmosis. *Arch Ophthalmol* 1985;**103**:1332–6.

Elkins BS, Holland GN, Opremcak EM, et al. Ocular toxoplasmosis misdiagnosed as cytomegalovirus retinopathy in immunocompromised patients. *Ophthalmology* 1994;**101**:499–507.

Ferguson DJ. *Toxoplasma gondii*: 1908–2008, homage to Nicolle, Manceaux and Splendore. *Mem Inst Oswaldo Cruz* 2009;**104**:2.

Gilbert RE, Tookey PA, Ades AE, et al. Prevalence of toxoplasma IgG among pregnant women in west London according to country of birth and ethnic group. *BMJ* 1993;**306**:185.

Gilbert RE, Stanford MR, Sanders MD, et al. Incidence of acute symptomatic toxoplasma retinochoroiditis in south London according to country of birth. *BMJ* 1995;**310**:1037–40.

Glasner PD, Silveira C, Kruszon-Moran D, et al. An unusually high prevalence of ocular toxoplasmosis in southern Brazil. *Am J Ophthalmol* 1992:**114**:136–44.
Greven CM, Teot LA. Cytologic identification of Toxoplasma gondii from vitreous fluid. *Arch Ophthalmol* 1994;**112**:1086–8.
Iaccheri B, Fiore T, Papadaki T, et al. Adverse drug reactions to treatments for ocular toxoplasmosis: a retrospective chart review. *Clin Ther* 2008;**30**:2069–74.
Johnson MW, Greven CM, Jaffe GJ, et al. Atypical, severe toxoplasmic retinochoroiditis in elderly patients. *Ophthalmology* 1997;**104**:48–57.
Jones CD, Okhravi N, Adamson P, et al. Comparison of PCR detection methods for B1, P30 and 18S rDNA genes of T. *gondii* in aqueous humour. *Invest Ophth Vis Sci* 2000;**41**:634–44.
Knox DL, King J. Retinal arteritis, iridocyclitis and giardiasis. *Ophthalmology* 1982;**89**:1303–8.
Lower-Sieger DH, Rothova A, Koppe JG, et al. Congenital Toxoplasmosis: a prospective study based on 1821 pregnant women. In: Saari KM (ed.), *Uveitis Update*. Amsterdam: Elsevier 1984: 203–7.
Luder CG, Giraldo-Velasquez M, Sendtner M, et al. *Toxoplasma gondii* in primary rat CNS cells: differential contribution of neurones, astrocytes and microglial cells for the intracerebral development and stage differentiation. *Exp Parasitol* 1999;**93**:23–32.
Matthews JD, Weiter JJ. Outer retinal toxoplasmosis. *Ophthalmology* 1988;**95**:941–6.
Montoya JG, Remington JS. Management of *Toxoplasma gondii* infection during pregnancy. *Clin Infect Dis* 2008;**47**:554–66.
Moore MB, McCulley JP, Luckenbach M, et al. Acanthamoeba keratitis associated with soft contact lens wear. *Am J Ophthalmol* 1985;**100**:396.
Moorthy RS, Smith RE, Rao NA. Progressive ocular toxoplasmosis in patients with acquired immunodeficiency syndrome. *Am J Ophthalmol* 1993;**115**:742–7.
Morhun PJ, Weisz JM, Elias SJ, et al. Recurrent ocular toxoplasmosis in patients treated with systemic corticosteroids. *Retina* 1996;**16**:383–7.
Moshfeghi DM, Dodds EM, Couto CA, et al. Diagnostic approaches to severe, atypical toxoplasmosis mimicking acute retinal necrosis. *Ophthalmology* 2004;**111**:716–25.
Perkins ES. Ocular toxoplasmosis. *Br J Ophthalmol* 1973;**57**:1–17.
Roizenblatt J, Grant S, Foos R. Vitreous cylinders. *Arch Ophthalmol* 1980;**98**: 734–39.
Rothova A, Meenken C, Buitenhuis HJ, et al. Therapy for ocular toxoplasmosis. *Am J Ophthalmol* 1993;**115**:517–23.
Silveira C, Belfort R Jnr, Muccioli C, et al. The effect of long-term intermittent trimethoprim/sulfamethoxazole treatment on recurrences of toxoplasmic retinochoroiditis. *Am J Ophthalmol* 2002;**134**:41–6.
Silveira C, Gargano N, Kijlstra A, et al. Toxoplasma vaccines: appropriate end points and sample size in future human clinical trials. *Expert Rev Anti Infect Ther* 2009;7:**905**–8.
Sobrin L, Kump L, Foster CS. Intravitreal clindamycin for toxoplasmic retinochoroiditis. *Retina* 2007;**27**:952–7.
Soheilian M, Sadoughi M-M, Ghajarnia M, et al. Prospective randomised trial of trimethoprim/sulfamethoxazole versus pyrimethamine and sulfadiazine in the treatment of ocular toxoplasmosis. *Ophsource* 2005;**112**:1876–82.
Soheilian M, Ramezani A, Azimzadeh Z, et al. Randomised trial of intravitreal clindamycin and dexamethasone versus pyrimethamine, sulfadiazine and prednisolone in treatment of ocular toxoplasmosis. *Ophthalmology* 2010;epub.
Stanford MR, Gilbert RE. Treating ocular toxoplasmosis – current evidence. *Mem Inst Oswaldo Cruz* 2009;**104**:2.
Stanford MR, Tomlin EA, Comyn O, et al. The visual field in toxoplasmic retinochoroiditis. *Br J Ophthalmol* 2005;**89**:812–14.
Stanford MR, Tan HK, Gilbert RE. Toxoplasmic retinochoroiditis presenting in childhood: clinical findings in a UK survey. *Br J Ophthalmol* 2006;**90**:1464–7.
Westfall AC, Lauer AK, Suhler EB, Rosenbaum JT. Toxoplasmosis retinochoroiditis and elevated intraocular pressure: a retrospective study. *J Glaucoma* 2005;**14**:3–10.
Whittle RM, Wallace GR, Whiston RA, et al. Human antiretinal antibodies in toxoplasma retinochoroiditis. *Br J Ophthalmol* 1998;**82**:1017–21.
Wirthlin R, Song A, Dong J, et al. Verteporfin photodynamic therapy of choroidal neovascularisation secondary to ocular toxoplasmosis. *Arch Ophthalmol* 2006;**124**:741–3.

Chapter 14 Parasite infestations and toxic uveitis

In medical parasitology, a vast array of organisms is capable of infesting humans. The eye may be involved in several of these, most of which are rare in the developed world. Those infestations that may cause, or masquerade as, uveitis are included here, although several others are capable of involving the cornea, conjunctiva and adnexae. The most important parasites are the helminths, or worms.

The roundworms, a subgroup of the phylum *Aschelminthes*, are also known as *Nematoda* or *Nemathelminthes*. Members of this group causing uveitis include *Toxocara canis*, *Onchocerca volvulus* and probably *Baylisascaris procyonis*. The flatworms, or phylum *Platyhelminthes*, have three classes. Members of two of these may cause uveitis. The tapeworms, or *Cestoda*, include *Taenia saginata* (the cow tapeworm) and *Taenia solium* (the pig tapeworm), both of which may cause intraocular inflammation. The flukes, or *Trematoda*, include *Schistosoma* spp. and *Paragonimus westermani*, both of which may cause uveitis.

Various *Arthropoda* may induce intraocular inflammation, either by the entry of larvae, especially of botflies, or by the ocular penetration of body parts, e.g. caterpillar setae. Various animal or vegetable toxins may also cause intraocular inflammation after direct contact, and these are also discussed here.

TOXOCARIASIS (box 14.1)

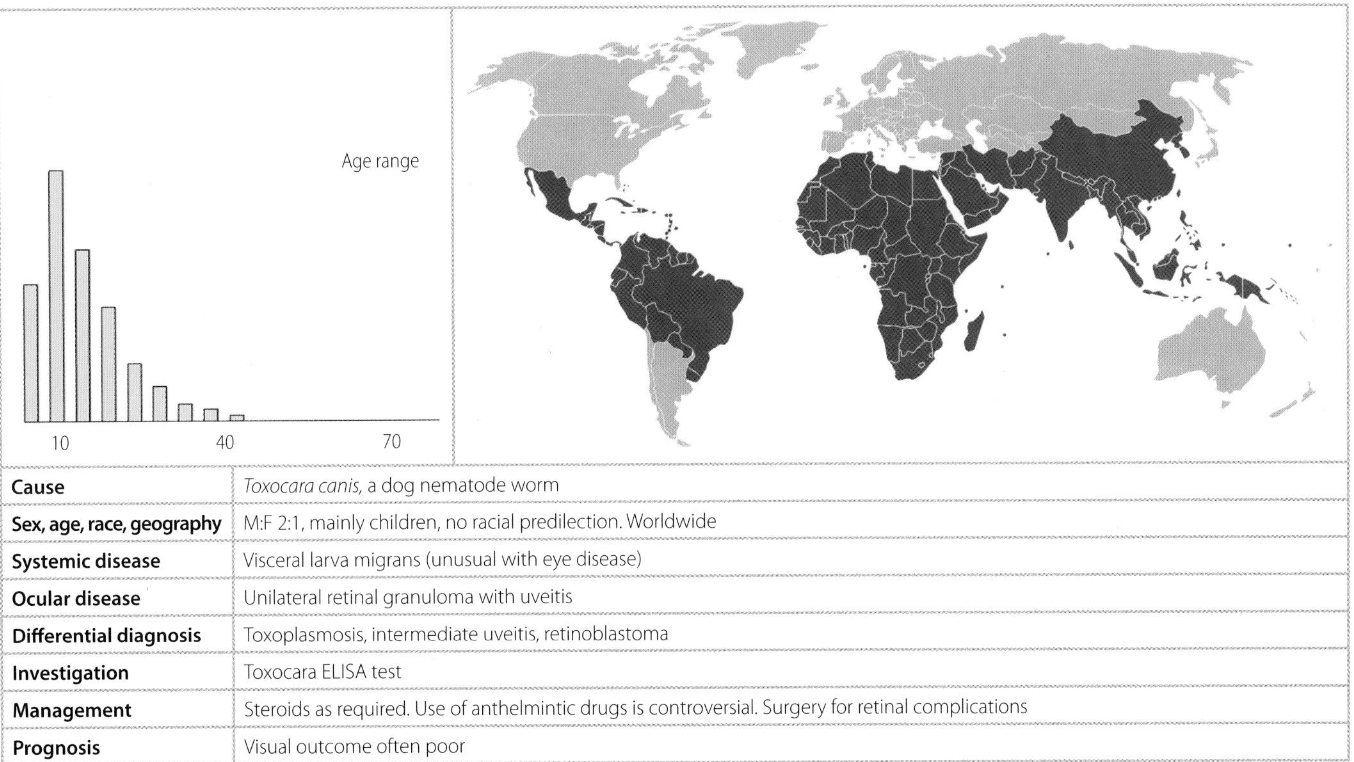

Cause	*Toxocara canis*, a dog nematode worm
Sex, age, race, geography	M:F 2:1, mainly children, no racial predilection. Worldwide
Systemic disease	Visceral larva migrans (unusual with eye disease)
Ocular disease	Unilateral retinal granuloma with uveitis
Differential diagnosis	Toxoplasmosis, intermediate uveitis, retinoblastoma
Investigation	Toxocara ELISA test
Management	Steroids as required. Use of anthelmintic drugs is controversial. Surgery for retinal complications
Prognosis	Visual outcome often poor

Box 14.1 Toxocariasis

Introduction

Toxocara canis is a nematode (**Fig. 14.1**) with primary hosts that are members of the dog family, both wild and domesticated. Up to 80% of domesticated puppies may be infested. The disease may be acquired transplacentally or by mouth, from maternal milk, by direct ingestion of ova from contaminated feces, by eating the meat of intermediate hosts containing tissue cysts or by drinking contaminated water. The lifecycle (**Fig. 14.2**) resembles that of other parasitic nematodes, the larvae maturing within the intestine before invading the lymphatics and migrating widely within the body. Pulmonary larvae may be coughed and swallowed, and the larvae mature into adults in the large intestine, constantly producing eggs which are excreted. Soil contamination by ova is therefore common in areas populated by domestic dogs. Embryonated eggs may be viable for years and are highly resistant to disinfection. The similar helminth *Toxocara cati* infests cats as primary host. The importance of *T. cati* in human disease is unknown (because diagnostic antigens are shared) but probably under-estimated.

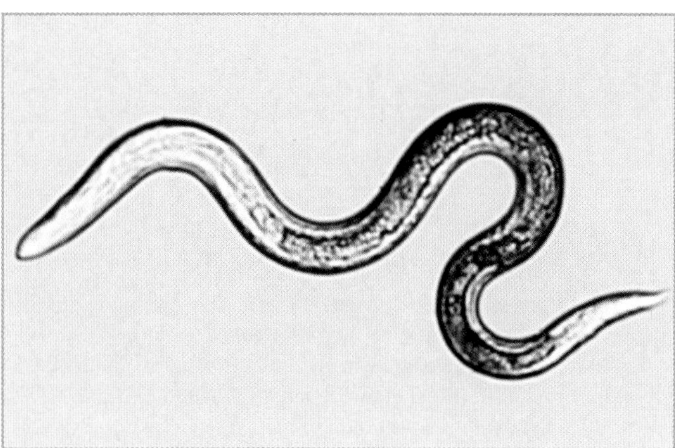

Figure 14.1 The larval stage of *Toxocara canis*. (Modified from Centers for Disease Control, DPDx Image Library.)

Human acquisition is by ingestion of ova from contaminated soil, fomites or direct contact with infested animals. Seropositivity is more common in dog breeders but acquisition is most common in early childhood. In the USA, in certain population groups the seropositivity rate was as high as 14% (Won et al. 2008). The eating of soil is reported by some parents of affected children. The human is an intermediate host within which the nematode cannot mature. Larvae migrate from the small intestine into the portal circulation and thence are widely distributed, most notably to the liver, lung, brain and eye. The larvae, in an arrested state of development, may continue to migrate for extended periods, or become immobile and produce a markedly eosinophilic granulomatous inflammation, within which the larva may survive for long periods.

The tissue reaction to helminth parasites including *T. canis* follows predictable stages. Initially a marked eosinophil abscess surrounds the larva, followed by a vigorous granulomatous reaction, adding lymphocytes, epithelioid cells and some foreign body-type giant cells (**Fig. 14.3**). Occasionally a marked eosinophilic deposit of amorphous material, possibly representing an in vivo immune complex precipitate, is seen, although the phenomenon is not unique to *T. canis* granulomas. Older lesions predominantly consist of epithelioid cells with pronounced fibrosis. The larva itself may disintegrate and become unrecognizable.

Systemic disease

Acquisition of toxocariasis is usually asymptomatic, but some develop a constellation of symptoms and signs known as visceral larva migrans (VLM). VLM may also follow infestation with *T. cati* and other nematodes. Although urticarial skin rash is often a feature, the condition should be distinguished from cutaneous larva migrans, which follows hookworm infestation and causes migratory serpiginous itchy papules. In VLM, pyrexia, muscular pains, urticarial rash, coughing, tiredness, pallor and weight loss are accompanied by hepatosplenomegaly, lymphadenopathy and eosinophilia, which may be dramatic, both relative (up to 90%) and absolute (up to 90×10^9/l). Recovery is usual within 3 weeks without treatment, but occasionally symptoms may linger for months. The usefulness and safety of systemic anthelmintic drugs remain debatable. Infrequently, systemic steroids are required where pulmonary, cerebral or myocardial involvement is severe. Deaths occur rarely, usually from myocarditis or encephalitis.

Ocular disease

Intraocular larvae were first located (Wilder 1950) after scrupulous histological examination of eyes enucleated for suspected retinoblastoma, and later identified (Nichols 1956) as *T. canis*. The proportion of those infested with *T. canis* who develop ocular involvement is unknown, but in the UK 2.6% are seropositive for previous exposure yet ocular involvement is much less common. Even in high-risk groups such as New Zealand hydatid control officers, with a seropositivity rate of 28% (Clemett et al. 1987), ocular involvement is rare. Presumably, as reproduction of the nematode does not occur in the human, the likelihood of ocular involvement will increase with the number of larvae ingested.

Acquisition of *T. canis* usually causes no systemic symptoms, so only a minority of those who develop ocular involvement have a history of VLM. Nevertheless a history of VLM should be sought, and if found will strongly support the diagnosis. Simultaneous visceral and ocular disease is occasionally reported (Paul et al. 2009)

Most patients with ocular toxocariasis are children, more commonly boys (Gillespie et al. 1993), but presentation may be in adulthood. Involvement is unilateral in the vast majority but bilateral cases are well recognized and in a series from the USA affected 2 of 22 patients (Stewart et al. 2005). Ocular toxocariasis has traditionally been described in three main forms: peripheral retinochoroiditis, posterior pole retinochoroiditis and endophthalmitis. However, in practice the clinical spectrum of involvement is wide and includes milder cases that would not normally be reported. Features within each traditional category may be mixed. The signs will depend upon, first, the location of the larva and its developing granuloma and, second, the degree of intraocular inflammation associated with it.

The larval granuloma

Toxocaral granulomas have long been recognized to show a predilection for the retinal periphery, to a lesser extent the posterior pole and occasionally the optic nerve head. It has been suggested, quite logically, that this distribution is explained by the relative diameters of the larva and the arteriolar vessel within which it is disseminated. The second-stage *T. canis* larva has a diameter of 18–20 μm, whereas the retinal capillary bed narrows to 15 μm in places. The larva may impact where such narrowing occurs, having bypassed deeper side branches.

Most patients present with a peripheral retinal granuloma (**Fig. 14.4**). The lesion may be clearly visible with indirect ophthalmoscopy or require careful indentation, if necessary under general anesthesia in young children. The early lesion will be white and ill-defined, later developing pigmented chorioretinal scarring. Characteristically vitreoretinal traction develops (**Fig. 14.5**) which may be progressive. Macular heterotopia may follow (**Fig. 14.6**), the retinal vascular pattern may shift and, in severe cases, retinal folding will result. Massive tractional bands (**Fig. 14.7**) may cause tractional or rhegmatogenous retinal detachment. Organized preretinal and vitreous bands branching around the posterior hemisphere are common (**Fig. 14.8**) and on occasion, particularly if episodes of inflammation are repeated, they may form a lattice crossing most of the vitreous cavity (**Fig. 14.9**).

The macula is a less frequent site for granuloma formation but seems to present more commonly in older children and adults. Early on the lesion is raised, white and poorly defined. As inflammation settles, the lesion will become more sharply defined and white, characteristically drawing in the retina and causing tractional folds (**Fig. 14.10**). In time funnel detachment may occur (**Fig. 14.11**).

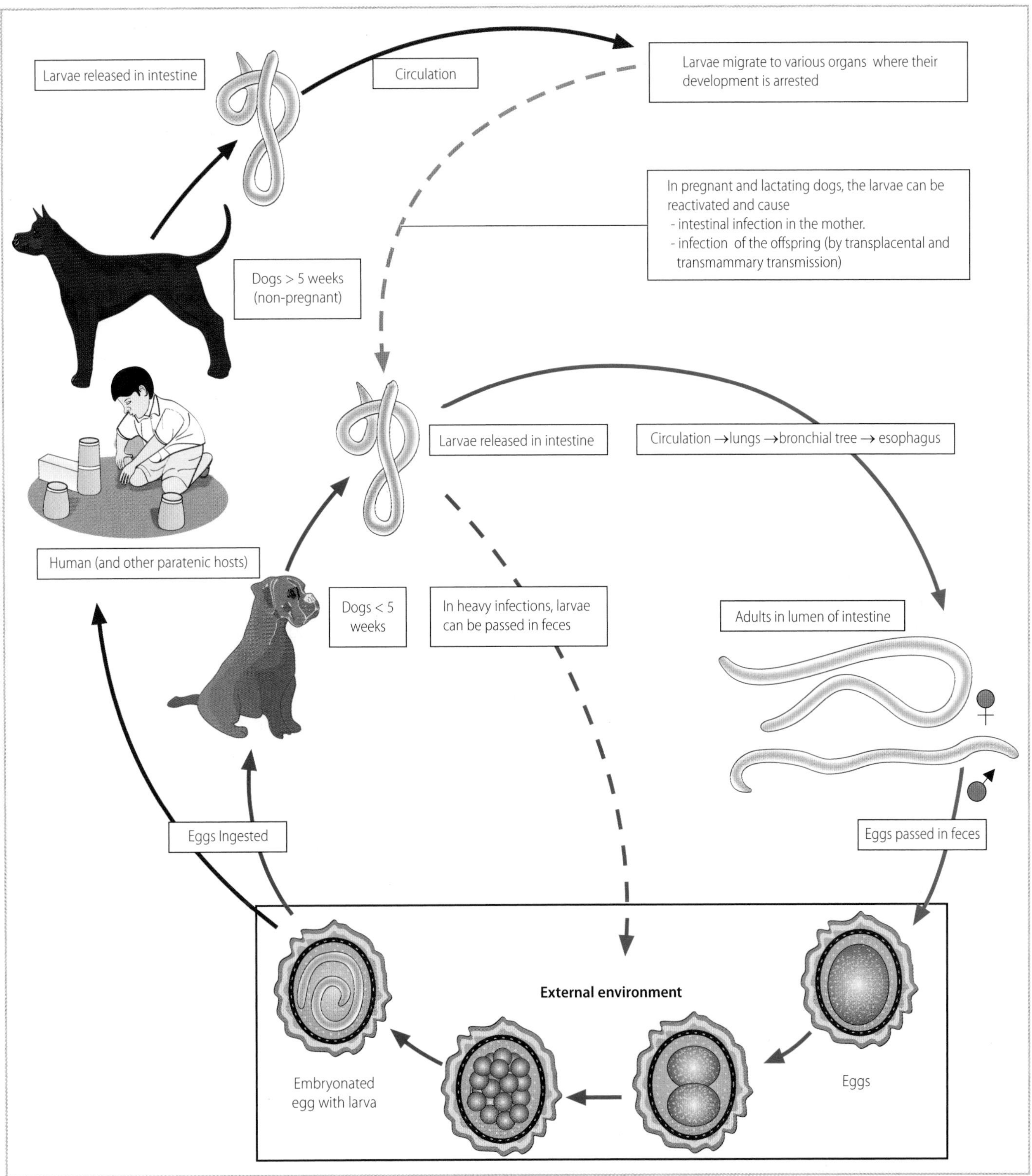

Figure 14.2 The life cycle of *Toxocara canis*. The primary hosts are members of the dog genus, which harbor adult worms in their intestine, the eggs of which are excreted in feces. Human infection occurs most commonly by ingestion of eggs from contaminated soil. Vertical transmission from mother to fetus may also occur. (Modified from Centers for Disease Control, DPDx Image Library.)

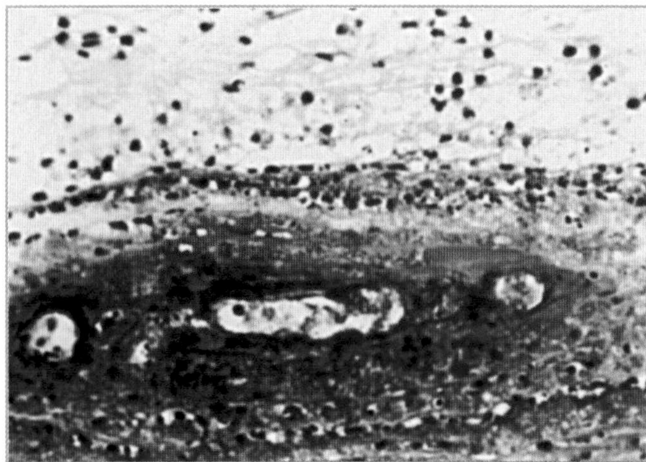

Figure 14.3 A histological preparation showing an intraocular *Toxocara canis* larva. The coiled larva is sectioned three times and fragments of the eosinophilic cuticle are visible to the right. There is a prominent granulomatous cell infiltrate. (Courtesy of Dr R Bonshek.)

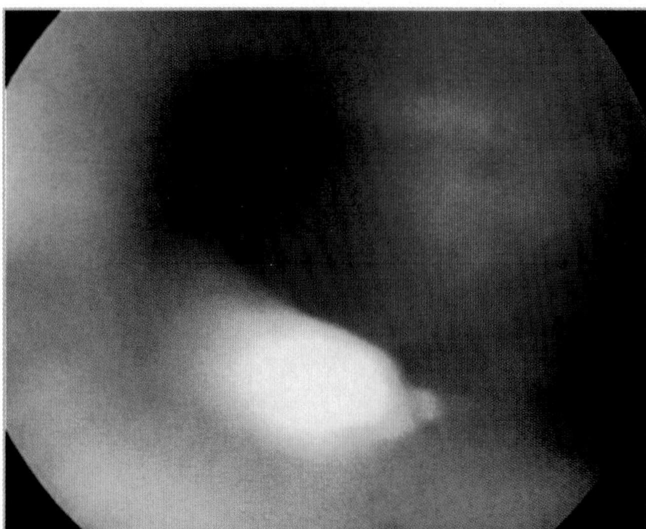

Figure 14.4 A raised white peripheral retinal toxocara granuloma.

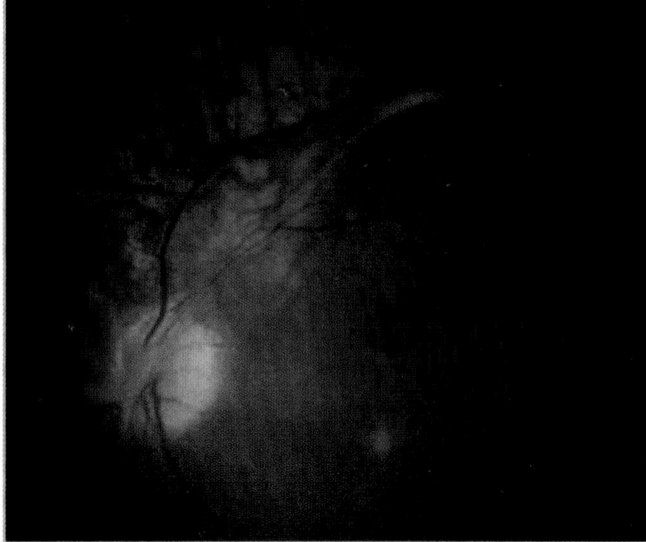

Figure 14.5 A toxocara granuloma in the superotemporal periphery exerts traction via fibroglial tissue towards the optic disk.

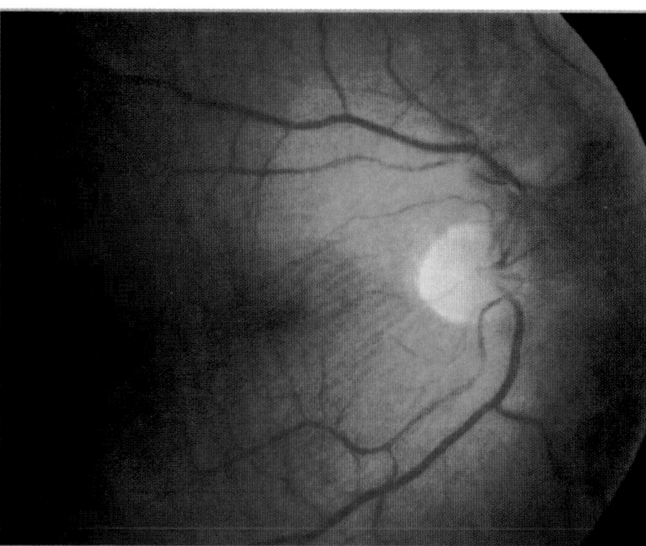

Figure 14.6 A granuloma in the nasal periphery distorts the main vascular arcades and causes macular retinal folding with heterotopia.

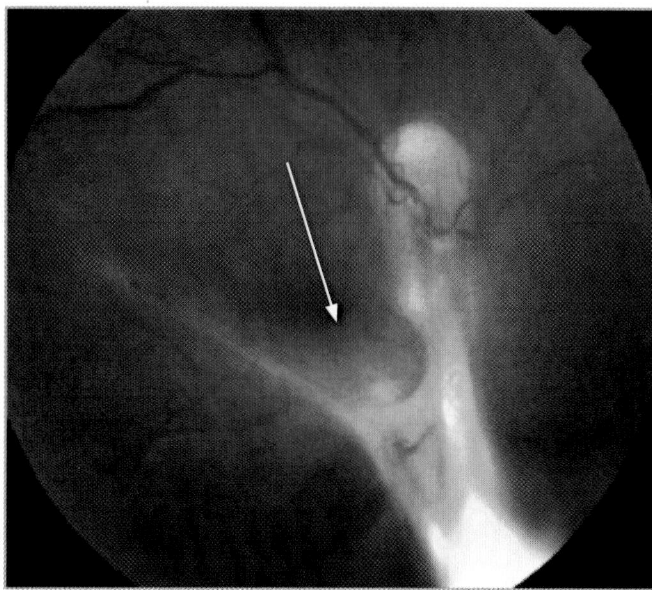

Figure 14.7 Massive fibroglial traction to an inferior peripheral granuloma incorporates major retinal vessels and induces tractional retinal detachment. The fovea (arrow) is drawn inferonasally.

The optic nerve head is rarely a site for inflammation. Substantial swelling may occur, with altered overlying blood vessels. Occasionally inflammation is severe enough to cause central vessel occlusion. Inflammation will subside to leave a degree of peripapillary fibrosis. Wherever the primary granuloma, extensive fibrosis in young children may lead to a presentation with leukocoria.

Intraocular inflammation

Whatever the location of the larval granuloma, the degree of associated intraocular inflammation can vary markedly. In some, the granuloma may form without any apparent cellular infiltrate into the vitreous humor, although tractional retinal effects may ensue. More commonly a granuloma may have overlying vitreous opacification, which may be quite localized. Generalized vitreous opacification affects some and may be severe enough to prevent an

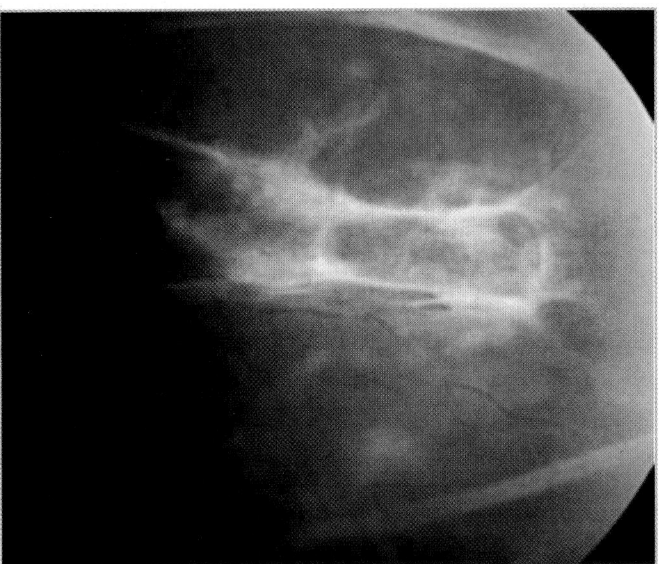

Figure 14.8 Multiple fibroglial preretinal vitreous bands are seen, after episodes of uveitis induced by a toxocara granuloma.

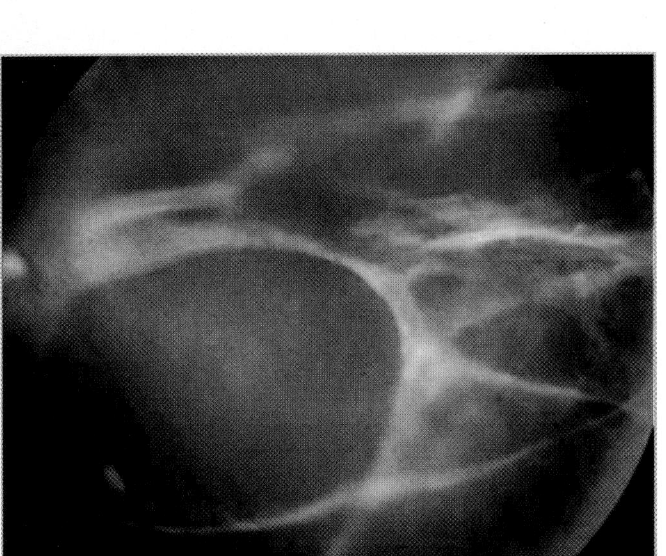

Figure 14.9 Fibrotic strands extensively criss-cross the vitreous cavity after repeated inflammation.

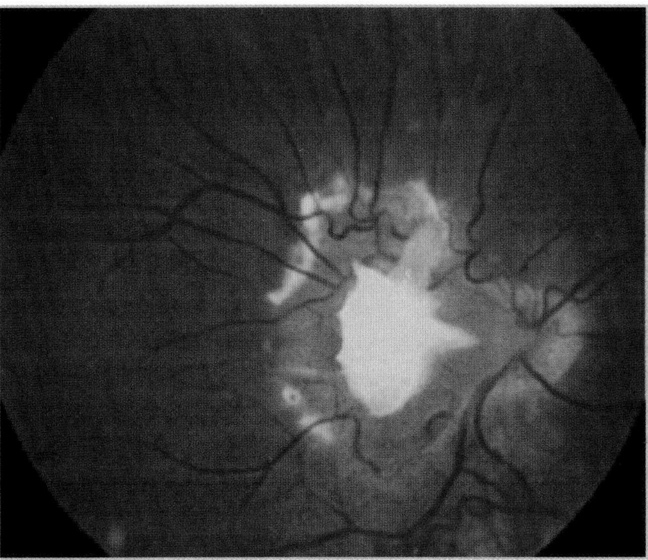

Figure 14.10 A quiescent toxocara granuloma at the macula with resultant severe tractional change, the vascular arcades being indrawn. There is a ring of retinal exudate.

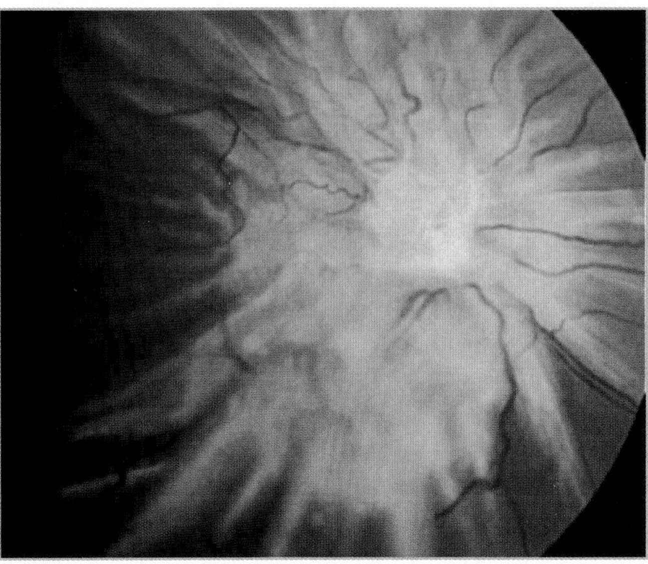

Figure 14.11 A funnel-shaped retinal detachment has resulted from the tractional effects of a toxocara granuloma.

adequate view of the fundus. Even so the location of the granuloma can usually be seen.

A significant minority of patients presents with very vigorous intraocular inflammation. Pain and photophobia are not common but severe anterior chamber inflammation may be present, with keratic precipitates that may be confluent, and there may even be a hypopyon. If inflammation is very severe, serous retinal detachment may occur, and later cyclitic membrane, cataract and leukocoria may appear. At worst the eye may become phthisical.

Motile nematode larvae

Motile nematode larvae have been seen in the human retina and have been destroyed by laser. Measurements of some of these larvae were compatible with *T. canis*. Larvae may break free from granulomas and migrate after a period of quiescence, explaining multifocal scars in toxocariasis. It may be that *T. canis* larvae are one cause of diffuse unilateral subacute neuroretinitis.

Diagnosis

Differential diagnosis

Toxocariasis in its typical forms, with a readily identifiable granuloma, associated inflammation and vitreous bands or tractional retinal changes, is not a challenging diagnosis. However, the spectrum of presentation does vary and the differential diagnosis for the individual patient may be wide.

Peripheral toxocara retinochoroiditis may resemble intermediate uveitis. However, intermediate uveitis is usually bilateral and tends to present in older children or young adults. Pars plana exudate may be seen in intermediate uveitis, but this is usually widespread or multifocal and is not generally concentrated into a single focus that resembles a larval granuloma. Also, vitreous opacification is usually in the form of large 'snowballs' rather than the diffuse cellular inflammation and subsequent bands seen in toxocariasis. Nevertheless toxocara serology should be performed in cases of unilateral intermediate uveitis. Retinal traction is a common feature of toxocariasis, but may also be seen in retinopathy of prematurity (where it is directed towards the temporal quadrant) or familial exudative retinopathy (where findings are usually bilateral and familial), or it may be idiopathic and congenital. Inferior tractional retinal elevation is also well recognized in intermediate uveitis in young people (Jalil et al. 2010).

Retinoblastoma is an important diagnosis to consider in some cases. Indeed, enucleation specimens with this proposed diagnosis have regularly provided histological evidence of nematode larvae. Retinoblastoma usually presents earlier than toxocariasis, there may be a family history, and cataract, cyclitic membrane or vitreous bands are not seen. In those presenting late with the sequelae of inflammation, persistent hyperplastic primary vitreous may be considered. In this case, the eye is often microphthalmic and may have a pupillary membrane or a visible persistent hyaloid arterial system.

Where the vitreous humor is very hazy and an inflammatory lesion is seen indistinctly through it, toxoplasmosis is a possibility. In this condition, the presence of pigmented chorioretinal scarring, often adjacent to the lesion, makes the differential diagnosis easier, and presentation is most common in adulthood. Serological testing will be helpful, but initiation of treatment must often precede the results and should be made on the basis of the clinical appearance. In a few patients both toxocara and toxoplasma titers may be high in a patient with ocular toxocariasis. Coinfection is well described (Jones et al. 2008), explained in part by common means of infection in patients living in environments populated by unwormed dogs and cats. In addition, *Toxoplasma gondii* has been isolated from the gut of *Toxocara canis*, leading to speculation that the nematode can act as a vector for toxoplasmosis.

ELISA

Current ELISA (enzyme-linked immunosorbent assay) methods use toxocara excretory/secretory exoantigens and assess total IgG response. The test has several problems: first there is cross-reactivity with other helminth exoantigens, reducing specificity in countries with high rates of infestation; second, sensitivity is known to be substantially less for those with ocular disease compared with those with VLM, probably reflecting both the smaller antigenic load, and possibly its immune sequestration within the eye; and third, not all IgG subclasses may be involved in the immune reaction. Various recombinant antigens may enhance specificity (Mohamad et al. 2009), probably selecting IgG4 as target. Thus sensitivity and specificity may be enhanced from 78–92% to 93–96%, respectively (for systemic disease). Western blotting is more sensitive, and enhanced specificity may be achieved by the supplementary use of an immunoelectrotransfer blot (Roldan and Espinoza 2009) for seropositive patients. Nevertheless there is a tendency for seropositivity to wane over time.

Serology can also be performed on intraocular fluid (Felberg et al. 1981). A titer positive at a dilution of 1:8 is usually considered positive. The test is alternatively expressed as an optical density reading, those > 0.25 usually being considered positive. Proven ocular toxocariasis is described with negative blood serology (Sharkey et al. 1993) as may be expected. Aqueous humor sampling may therefore be justified in certain cases.

Although overall population prevalence (in samples from blood donors) is as low as 2.6%, some populations of children may have seropositivity rates approaching 90% (in the Caribbean, for instance) and the relevance of positive serology in the individual patient should be considered with local population prevalence in mind. Positive serology is not proof of ocular toxocariasis, but in the context of clinically suggestive signs is very supportive. In contrast the presumptive diagnosis is frequently made in the setting of typical clinical features, even with negative serology.

Ocular ultrasonography

In those in whom the lesion cannot be visualized, especially in those with late presentation and cataract, ultrasonography can be useful. The highly reflective granulomas can be identified, as can vitreous bands and retinal detachment or traction (Wan et al. 1991). Appearances in general are different from those of retinoblastoma, although the signs are not pathognomonic. Ultrasonography appears to be at least as good as magnetic resonance imaging (MRI) or computed tomography (CT) in assisting the diagnosis of ocular toxocariasis.

Non-specific tests

If intraocular fluid is taken for an ELISA test, the presence of eosinophils will support the diagnosis of parasite infestation. Blood eosinophilia, although a constant feature of VLM, is usually absent in ocular toxocariasis because the systemic effects, if any, have usually settled before presentation. Occasionally a relative eosinophilia may still be detected, although, in those unusual instances of recent or simultaneous VLM, absolute eosinophilia is likely.

Management

Presentation varies widely in ocular toxocariasis and the need for treatment will depend first on the degree of intraocular inflammation and its consequent effects, and second on the degree of traction resulting from progressive granuloma formation, and the sequelae of this. Our experience is that, in young children, progressive macular distortion and heterotopia may affect visual acuity only moderately, but fusional capacity is often lost with resultant amblyopia. Early treatment to prevent progression if possible is therefore desirable.

Medical treatment

Discussion of the appropriate management of ocular toxocariasis has for decades generated heat, but not light. Anthelmintic drugs are available but their efficacy for ocular (as opposed to systemic) disease is unimpressive and they carry significant toxicity. Fears are often expressed (based on well-described events after treatment for other infestations including with *Echinococcus* sp.) that the disruption of a larva may provoke more inflammation and scarring, and that allowing gradual encapsulation by local granulomatous reaction may be preferable. It is known that most of the vigorous eosinophilic response is directed not against the larval contents but against the excretory/secretory antigens that it exudes. Objections to treatment on these grounds therefore remain speculative and should probably concentrate instead on the known side effects of anthelmintic drugs.

Benzimidazoles and other anthelmintics

This group of antifungal, anthelmintic drugs acts against nematodal fumarate reductase or other enzyme systems. Thiabendazole substantially inhibits larval migration but does not appear to be larvicidal. Although albendazole is larvicidal in ascariasis and trichuriasis, that effect has not been observed in toxocariasis. Fenbendazole is larvicidal in the gut but poorly absorbed and toxic. Levamisole is now reserved for veterinary use. Diethylcarbamazine is effective in filariasis and has been used anecdotally in toxocariasis without evidence of effect. Ivermectin may be larvicidal for *Toxocara* spp. but does not cross the blood–brain barrier in tolerable doses. Data on intraocular penetration of any of these drugs are non-existent. No adequate studies on efficacy in human ocular disease are available. The rationale for anthelmintic treatment is thus weak, especially where sequestration of a single larva within an intraocular granuloma has already occurred. Intolerance of benzimidazoles is not uncommon. Hypersensitivity reactions, hepatotoxicity and erythema multiforme have been reported. Side effects include anorexia, vomiting, dizziness, headache, drowsiness, blurred vision and xanthopsia (yellow vision). Overall there is inadequate evidence to risk anthelmintic drugs as a primary treatment in ocular toxocariasis.

Anti-inflammatory and immunosuppressive treatment

Associated anterior uveitis will be treated with topical steroids and mydriasis as required. Some lesions may be controlled with the use of periocular steroid, but, where intraocular inflammation is severe, systemic steroids are appropriate and effective. If not, some sources consider the use of systemic anthelmintics appropriate (Magnaval and Glickman 2006). In rare instances with inflammation inadequately responsive to oral steroid, immunosuppression has been used (Mora et al. 2006).

Surgical treatment

Where vitreous bands develop, or where macular heterotopia, retinal folding or detachment occurs, surgery has been used (**Fig. 14.12**) with both anatomical and visual success (Amin et al. 2000). As tractional effects are often progressive, early surgery has been advocated (Rodriguez 1986).

Ocular toxocariasis is rare but worldwide systemic infection regarded as a major health issue, with *Toxocara* spp. regarded as a possible etiological factor in disease ranging from atopy and chronic asthma to epilepsy and other neurological disorders. Attempts to control disease by worming pets and limiting fecal dissemination will not be successful in the developing world. No significant developments are being made in immunization or in the creation of new effective anthelmintics. The ophthalmologist will continue to see ocular involvement in young people into the future.

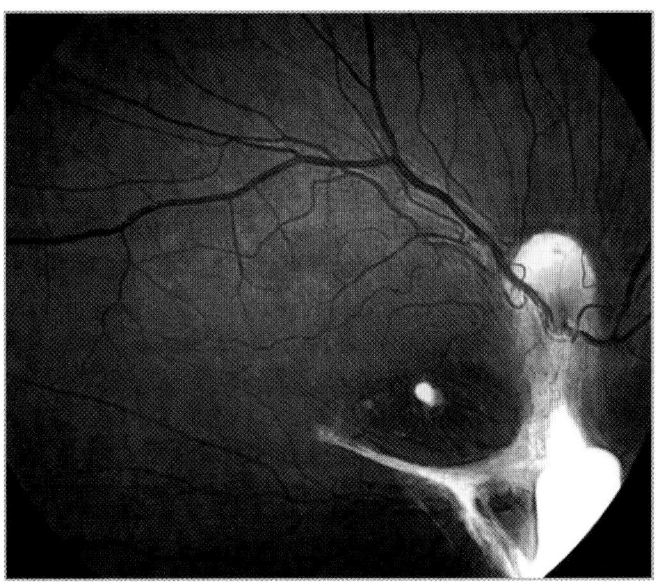

Figure 14.12 Same patient as Fig. 14.7 after oral steroid treatment and vitrectomy with division of vitreoretinal traction band. Complete retinal flattening proved impossible and, although retinal exudate temporarily formed, macular traction was partially relieved with stabilization of visual acuity.

DIFFUSE UNILATERAL SUBACUTE NEURORETINITIS (box 14.2)

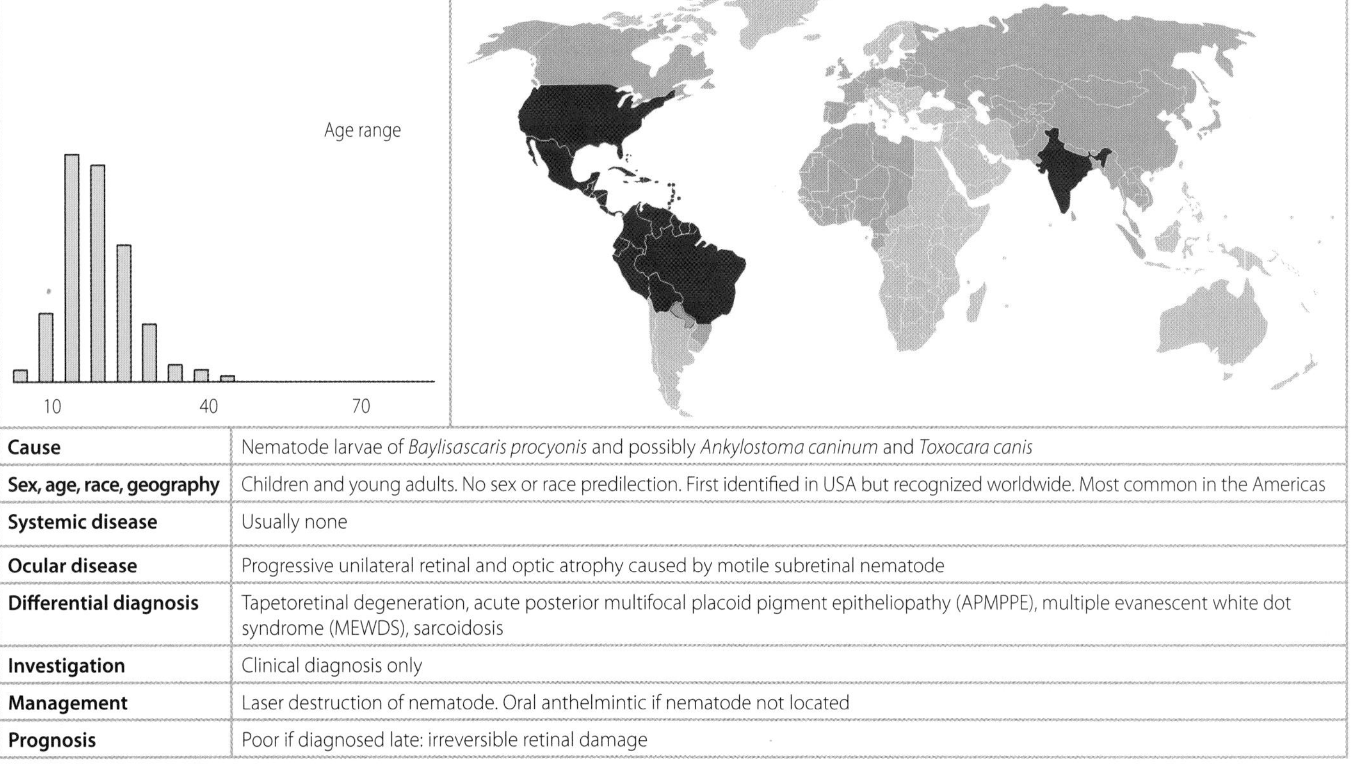

Cause	Nematode larvae of *Baylisascaris procyonis* and possibly *Ankylostoma caninum* and *Toxocara canis*
Sex, age, race, geography	Children and young adults. No sex or race predilection. First identified in USA but recognized worldwide. Most common in the Americas
Systemic disease	Usually none
Ocular disease	Progressive unilateral retinal and optic atrophy caused by motile subretinal nematode
Differential diagnosis	Tapetoretinal degeneration, acute posterior multifocal placoid pigment epitheliopathy (APMPPE), multiple evanescent white dot syndrome (MEWDS), sarcoidosis
Investigation	Clinical diagnosis only
Management	Laser destruction of nematode. Oral anthelmintic if nematode not located
Prognosis	Poor if diagnosed late: irreversible retinal damage

Box 14.2 Neuroretinitis

Introduction

A disorder, characterized by unilateral progressive retinal destruction and optic atrophy with retinal vessel attenuation and retinal pigment epithelium (RPE) damage, was first described by Gass in 1977 and then renamed (Gass and Scelfo 1978) diffuse unilateral subacute neuroretinitis (DUSN). In due course patients with DUSN were seen to have a motile subretinal worm in the affected eye (Gass and Braunstein 1983) and nematode worm larvae of a range of sizes have subsequently been observed from 0.4 mm to 2.0 mm in length and from 0.02 mm to 0.10 mm in diameter. Observations fall broadly into two types: the smaller and the larger. It has been suggested that either several nematodes may cause DUSN or a single species may be observed at different stages of development. Although DUSN is increasingly well reported (Cortez et al. 2005), no histological specimen has yet confirmed the species involved. The smaller larva may be *Toxocara canis* or *Ankylostoma caninum*, the dog hookworm (although it is unclear how *T. canis* larvae could cause two strikingly different forms of intraocular pathology). The larger worm was soon suggested (Kazakos et al. 1985) to be *Baylisascaris procyonis*, the raccoon roundworm, and accumulated circumstantial evidence (Goldberg et al. 1993) makes this association virtually certain.

The raccoon, *Procyon lotor*, is indigenous to temperate North America but increasing urbanization has led to its proximity to human garbage in large numbers, and in some American states it is a major pest (**Fig. 14.13**). Exported to zoos around the world, escapees have also colonized large areas elsewhere, particularly eastern Europe, the Caucasus and Japan. It is the natural host of *B. procyonis* (**Fig. 14.14**) and its excreta contain myriad ova which if ingested cause sometimes fatal visceral or neural larva migrans in many (> 90 identified to date) mammalian paratenic hosts, including humans (**Fig. 14.15**). Dogs, however, can harbor larvae and shed ova and become an alternative primary host in areas of the world where the raccoon is not indigenous. Ova are long-lived in soil and are resistant to disinfection and bleach (Sorvillo et al. 2002). Human infestation leads to extraintestinal migration and resultant eosinophilia. Complications include encephalitis or myocarditis, which may be fatal, and *B. procyonis* has been identified in some cases *post mortem*. Animal models have proven the ability of *B. procyonis* to cause ocular DUSN after oral ingestion. About 5% of ingested larvae migrate to the central nervous system (CNS) (Shafir et al. 2006).

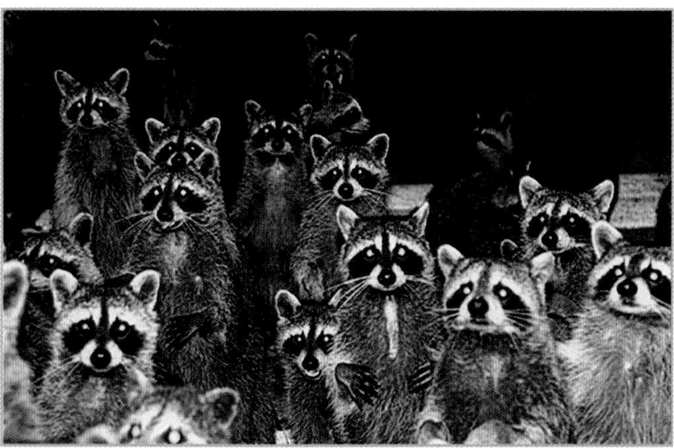

Figure 14.13 A group of suburbanized raccoons wait for garbage disposal in the USA.

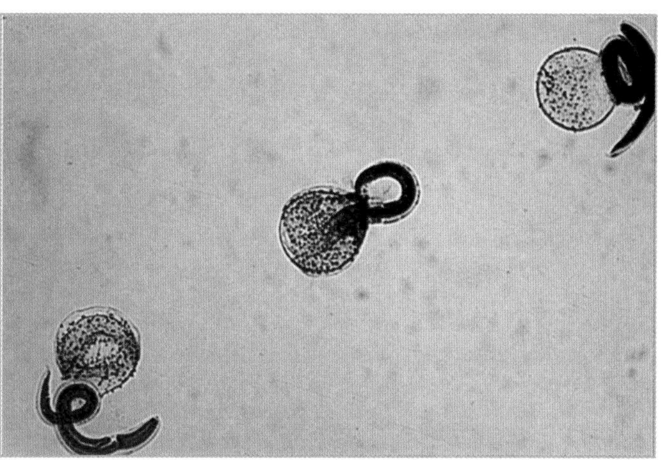

Figure 14.14 Larvae of *Baylisascaris procyonis* hatching from ova. (Modified from Centers for Disease Control, DPDx Image Library.)

Systemic disease

Patients with DUSN typically have no systemic symptoms or signs. It has not been associated with VLM. However, coexisting DUSN and neural larva migrans confirmed by cerebrospinal fluid (CSF) serology have been reported (Mets et al. 2003).

Ocular disease

In the early stages poorly defined, grouped, yellow-white, deep retinal lesions occur apparently in crops, each subsiding within days (**Fig. 14.16**). Visual acuity is decreased, with vitreous inflammation and, in some cases, optic papillitis. A careful (and if necessary repeated) retinal search may reveal the nematode larva (**Fig. 14.17**), most often near to active retinal lesions, its movement being provoked by light. Occasionally the passage of the worm seems to leave visible retinal tracks. In time (possibly years rather than months) progressive optic atrophy with retinal arteriolar attenuation and sheathing combines with diffuse and focal scarring of the RPE. Non-specific visual field loss and abnormal electroretinogram (ERG) responses are seen, superficially resembling a unilateral tapetoretinal degeneration. Retinal damage in DUSN is irreversible and severe visual acuity loss is seen in the majority, reflecting that presentation is often late and diagnosis sometimes later despite increasing familiarity with the disease.

Diagnosis

Diagnosis is essentially clinical, the ophthalmoscopic search for the nematode being sometimes prolonged and, if necessary, repeated. However, the clinical pattern of grouped evanescent retinitis is typical and treatment is often instituted without locating the larva. Both ELISA and western blot analysis for excretory/secretory exoantigens of *B. procyonis* have been developed, but neither is widely available.

Management

The motile larva can be destroyed by laser coagulation without inducing a vigorous inflammation. If achieved in the early stage of disease, this is effective in arresting inflammation and may improve visual acuity (Garcia et al. 2004). In typical cases where no larva is located, it has become accepted practice to administer the anthelmintic albendazole in high dose (400 mg daily for 30 days in adults). There is clear evidence of success for this mode of treatment (Souza et al. 2005).

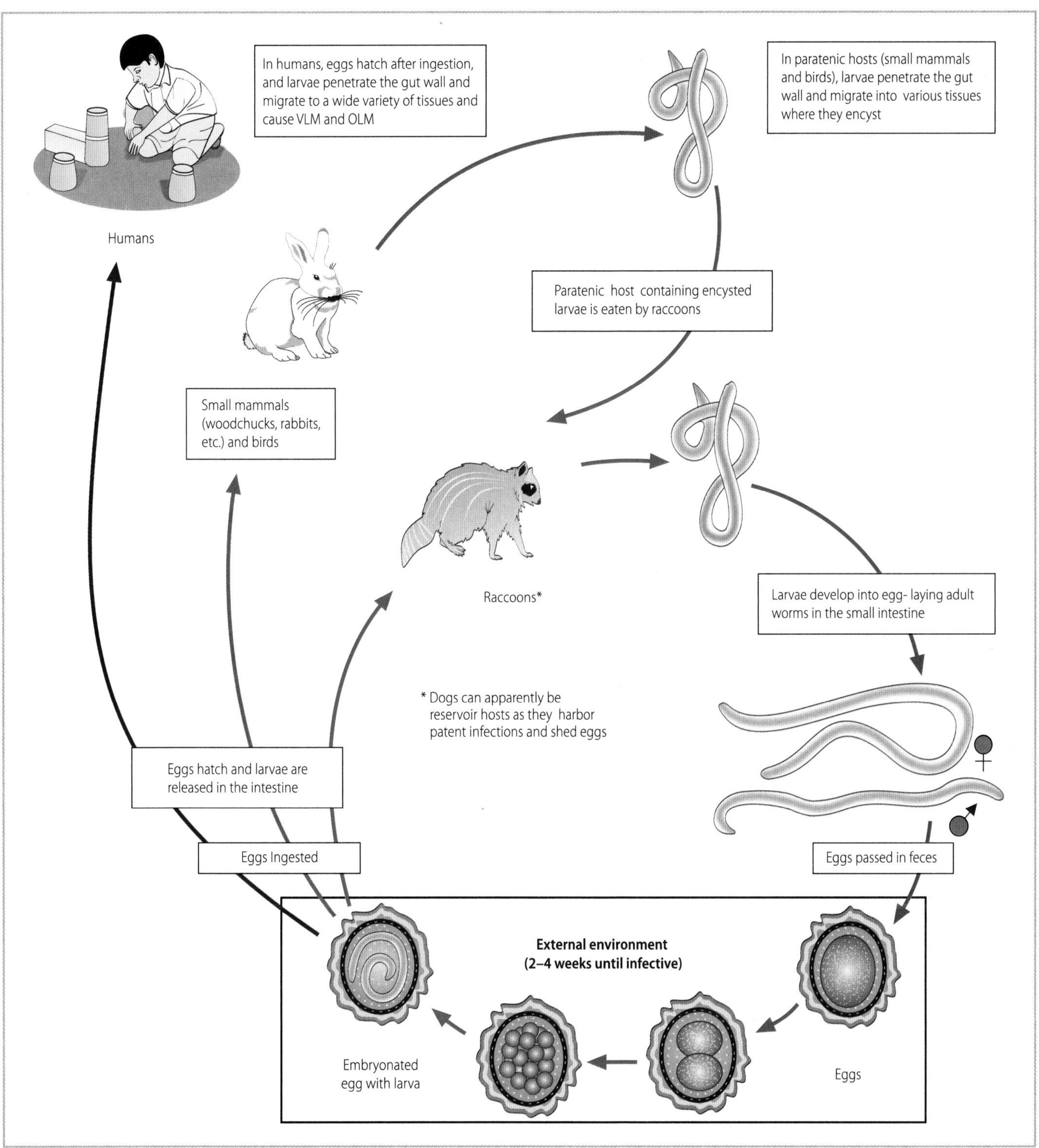

Figure 14.15 The life cycle of *Baylisascaris procyonis*. (Modified from Centers for Disease Control, DPDx Image Library.)

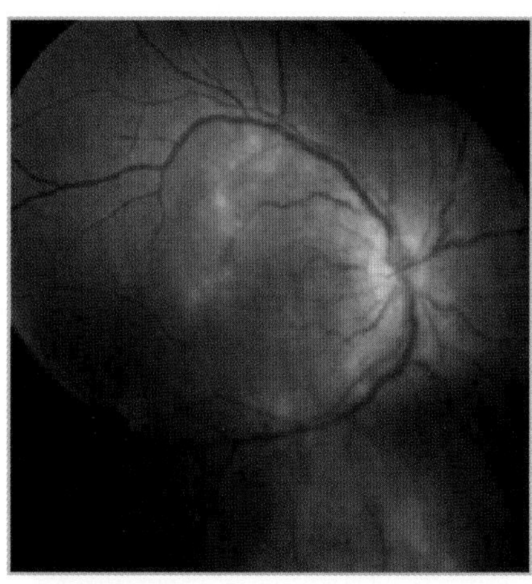

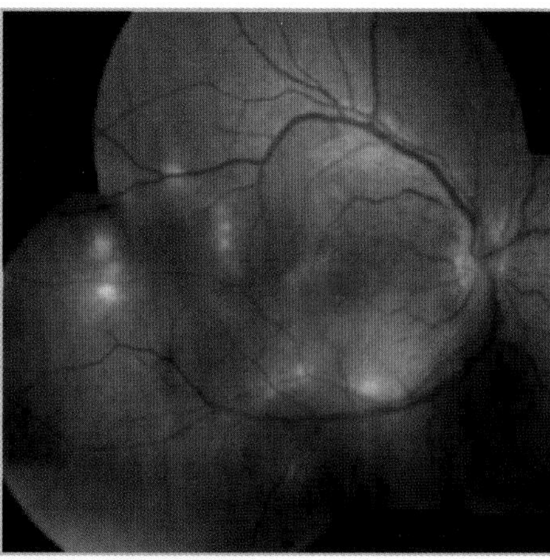

Figure 14.16 The early appearances of diffuse unilateral subacute neuroretinitis. Two retinal montages taken 1 week apart showing evanescent grouped retinal lesions. (Courtesy of Dr A Curi.)

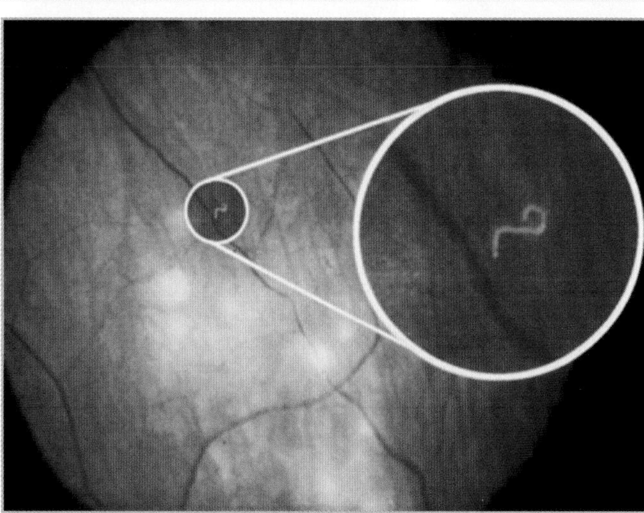

Figure 14.17 Deep retinal grouped cream-colored lesions are the hallmark of early diffuse unilateral subacute neuroretinitis. Adjacent is a nematode larva, also shown magnified, (Courtesy of the late Dr JDM Gass.)

ONCHOCERCIASIS (box 14.3)

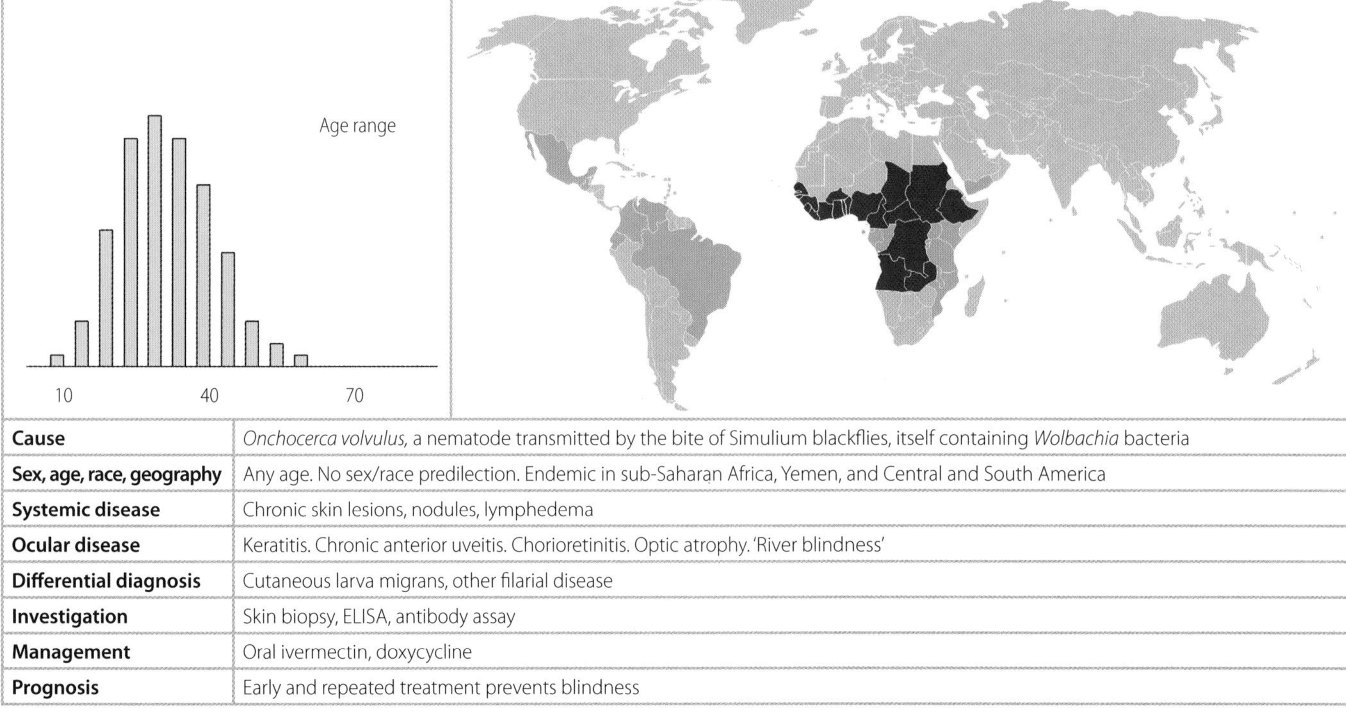

Cause	*Onchocerca volvulus*, a nematode transmitted by the bite of Simulium blackflies, itself containing *Wolbachia* bacteria
Sex, age, race, geography	Any age. No sex/race predilection. Endemic in sub-Saharan Africa, Yemen, and Central and South America
Systemic disease	Chronic skin lesions, nodules, lymphedema
Ocular disease	Keratitis. Chronic anterior uveitis. Chorioretinitis. Optic atrophy. 'River blindness'
Differential diagnosis	Cutaneous larva migrans, other filarial disease
Investigation	Skin biopsy, ELISA, antibody assay
Management	Oral ivermectin, doxycycline
Prognosis	Early and repeated treatment prevents blindness

Box 14.3 Onchocerciasis

Introduction

Onchocerciasis probably affects more than 20 million people, and its possible sequel, river blindness, affects more than a million of these, placing it high on the list of major causes of world blindness. It is endemic in sub-Saharan Africa, with lesser-affected areas in Yemen and Saudi Arabia, and Central and South America. The pathogenesis of ocular disease has been clarified in recent years, and involves blackflies of the *Simulium* genus, the parasitic nematode *Onchocerca volvulus* and, now realized to be of great importance, the symbiotic bacterium *Wolbachia pipientis*. Female blackflies (which require running water in which to lay eggs) are biting flies, and its many species are worldwide pests. It is required on both afferent and efferent loops of the *O. volvulus* lifecycle (**Fig. 14.18**) for which humans are the primary host. Adult worms live in the dermis and subcutaneous tissues, the coiled females (up to 5 cm long) each producing thousands of microfilarial larvae daily (**Fig. 14.19**), which migrate widely and are aspirated into the blood meal of the next blackfly bite. A phase of the lifecycle is passed within *Simulium* sp. and microfilariae are then transmitted back to other humans during subsequent bites, maintaining the cycle.

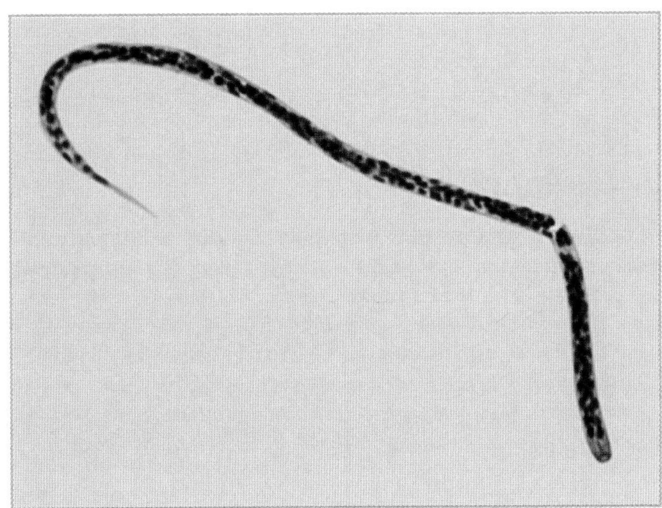

Figure 14.19 The larval (microfilarial) stage of O. volvulus. The head end is at lower right. (Modified from Centers for Disease Control, DPDx Image Library.)

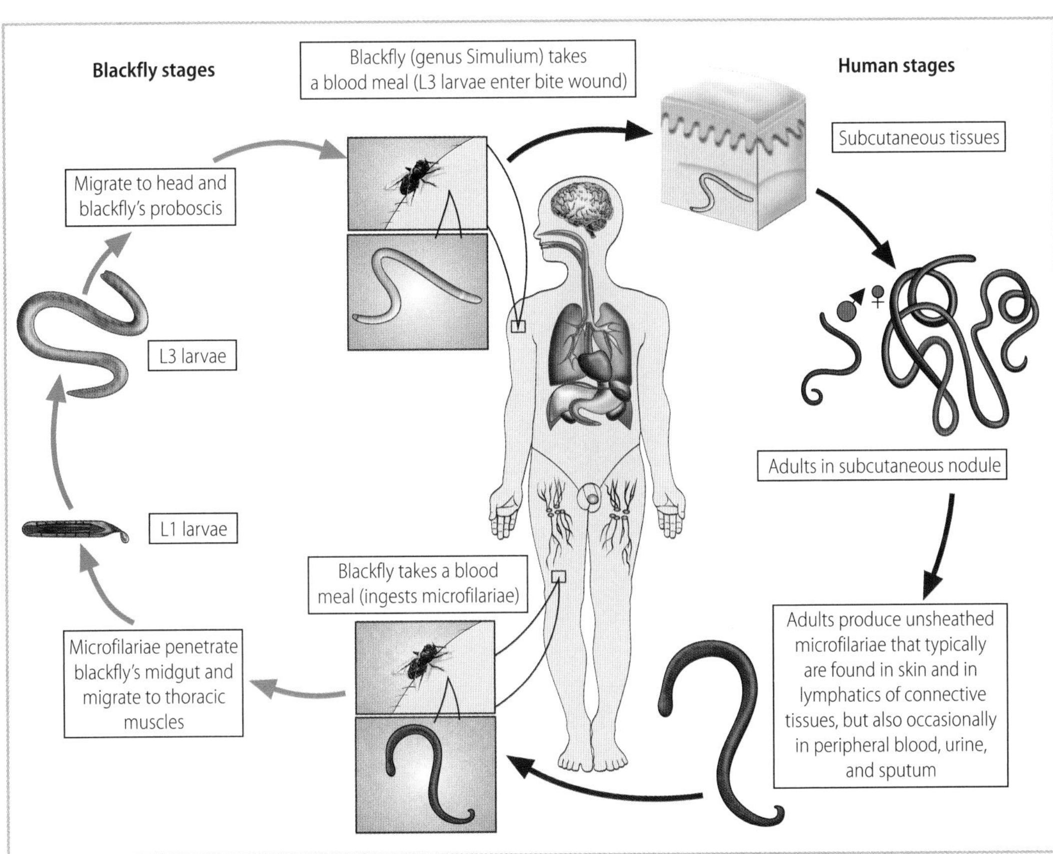

Figure 14.18 The lifecycle of *Onchocerca volvulus*. (Modified from Centers for Disease Control, DPDx Image Library.)

Although both adult and larval forms generate a degree of eosinophilic response as do other nematodes, live microfilariae do not generate an intraocular inflammatory reaction. It is now known that the endosymbiont bacterium *Wolbachia pipientis*, which resides within a very high proportion of arthropod and other invertebrate species (including *O. volvulus*) and which are released upon the death of the larvae, are responsible for the resultant keratitis and uveitis.

Systemic disease

Manifestations of onchocerciasis differ according to geographical area, but all show cutaneous involvement, with papular pruritic dermatitis, subcutaneous nodules and sclerosing lymphadenitis. Coiled adult worms may become enclosed in fibrotic capsules, and these palpable nodules (onchocercomas) are especially found in the scalp or over bony prominences. Lymphadenitis may become obstructive, causing lymphedema and elephantiasis, especially in the groin. Intense pruritus leads to excoriation and secondary infection. Microfilariae may also involve deep tissues and, although glomerulonephritis, pulmonary abscesses and hepatitis may be found, they are rarely symptomatic.

Ocular disease

Microfilariae migrate to the eye and have been found in all layers and compartments. They may die within the cornea, especially in the periphery, and the surrounding inflammatory reaction causes punctate 'snowflake' opacities. In severe cases, sclerosing keratitis is seen (**Fig. 14.20**). Microfilariae may be seen in the anterior chamber (**Fig. 14.21**), but in doubtful cases more will appear after a period in the dark. Iridocyclitis may ensue, including fibrinous exudate and synechia formation, and subsequently secondary glaucoma and cataract may occur. The inflammation is non-granulomatous and chronic. Bilateral chorioretinitis is common and manifests as focal RPE scarring, in some cases becoming generalized and severe (**Fig. 14.22**) with loss of the choriocapillaris. Although profound visual loss can result, it is optic atrophy, secondary to optic neuritis rather than to chorioretinitis, that is responsible for most cases of blindness. Visitors to endemic areas who acquire onchocerciasis and then return home typically develop dermatitis but do not develop ocular involvement (McCarthy et al. 1994).

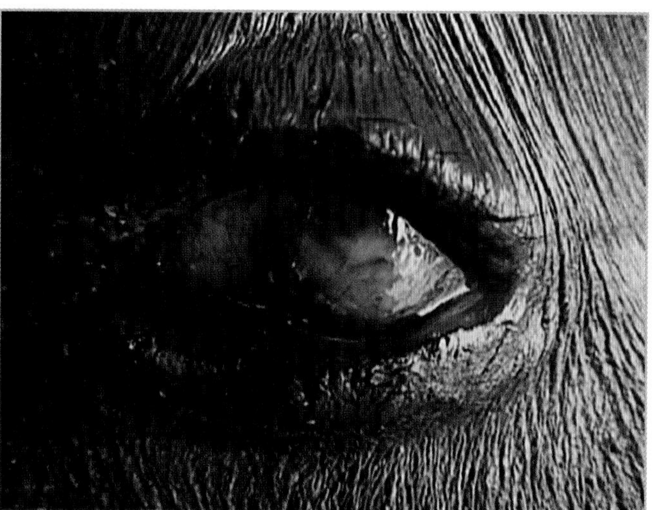

Figure 14.20 Corneal opacification in onchocerciasis.

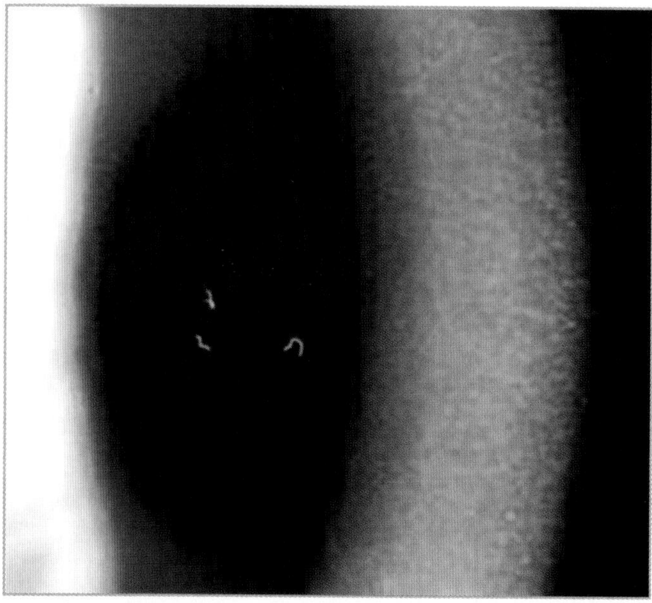

Figure 14.21 Diagrammatic microfilariae to scale in the anterior chamber. A created image.

Diagnosis

A skin-snip biopsy is examined microscopically for microfilariae after allowing it to soak in saline. The anterior chamber may also demonstrate larvae. If none is found the suspect can receive a single dose of diethylcarbamazine (DEC) 50 mg (the Mazzotti test), in which case a pruritic rash usually develops within 2–4 hours, reflecting the intradermal death of the larvae. However, occasional severe reactions may ensue, so a DEC patch test is now available that induces a local rather than a systemic reaction. An ELISA is available (although not readily in endemic countries) which has > 95% specificity but cannot differentiate active from old disease. A recent alternative is a rapid-format antibody test to Ov16 antigen (Weil et al. 2000), which shows promising reliability and can be rapidly administered in the field using patient serum. A polymerase chain reaction (PCR) has been developed that has adequate sensitivity to detect microfilarial debris within skin scrapes, but the costs limit the availability of this technique. Perhaps the most promising recent development is the Oncho-dipstick antibody assay (Ayong et al. 2005), which can detect the Oncho-C27 protein in urine or tears with sensitivity/specificity of 100%/100% and 92%/100% respectively. Finally, definitive identification of adult worms is achieved by excision of onchocercomas, which also reduces antigenic load.

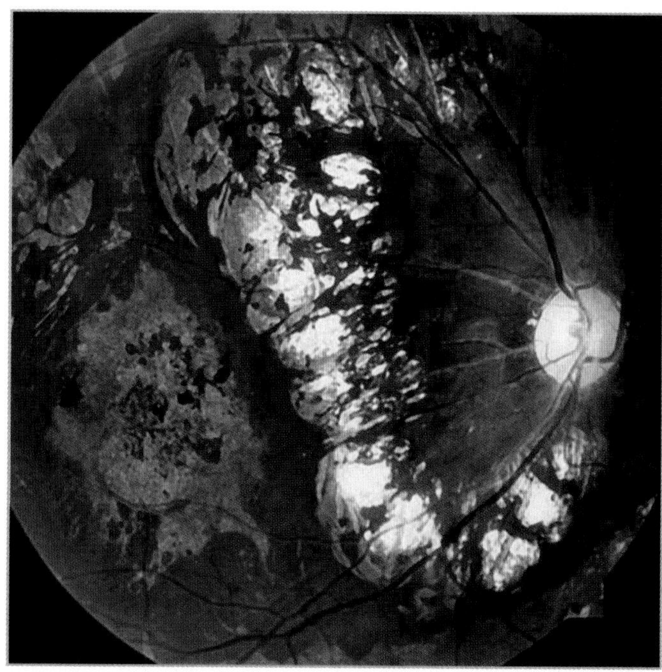

Figure 14.22 Widespread and severe pigmentary chorioretinal scarring following onchocerciasis.

Management

Eradication programs

As humans are the primary host for *O. volvulus*, the disease can theoretically be eradicated. This realization has led to several such programs in affected areas, beginning in Africa with the Onchocerciasis Control Programme (OCP) in 1974, which concentrated initially on blackfly control using larvicides in affected rivers, followed by the use of ivermectin treatment. The OCP was extended by the African Programme for Onchocerciasis control (APOC) in 1995 which, using ivermectin donated by Merck, treated over 40 million people in 30 African countries. *Simulium* elimination is demonstrably successful (Garms et al. 2009). There are similar initiatives outside Africa and their combined result is a substantial decline in morbidity. However, ivermectin is larvicidal but does not kill adult worms (which have a lifespan of up to 15 years within their human subcutaneous nodules). Control remains imperfect and the APOC concluded in 2010. It is, however, estimated (Hopkins 2005) that a further 20 years of treatment involving up to 90 million people would be necessary to achieve elimination. Matters are further complicated by developing resistance to ivermectin (Osei-Atweneboama et al. 2007). Eradication remains an elusive goal.

The patient

Historically onchocerciasis was treated for 3 weeks with oral DEC, but this did not kill adult worms, which required surgical removal. The Mazzotti reaction, a violent cutaneous and systemic reaction to the death of microfilariae, was common and worsening of ocular inflammation was reported. Relapse of the disease within a few months was universal (because of reinfection by further fly bites), and re-treatment was poorly tolerated. Suramin killed adult worms but required intravenous administration and was extremely toxic. Neither of these drugs is now considered useful.

The later introduction of ivermectin proved extremely important. This broad-spectrum parasiticide was derived initially from *Streptomyces* spp. and is neurotoxic to a variety of worms and some arthropods. The effect of a single oral dose of 150 μg/kg may be sustained for 2–3 years. However, more frequent dosage is necessary to control posterior segment ocular inflammation and, in adults, the dose is usually repeated every 6–12 months. Allergic skin rashes are less problematic than with DEC.

It is known that the death of microfilariae, either by natural attrition or after anthelmintic treatment, releases *Wolbachia* bacteria which induce vigorous inflammation. These bacteria are sensitive to doxycycline which induces long-lasting sterility in adult worms (Hoerauf et al. 2003). Preceding ivermectin treatment with 4–6 weeks of doxycycline 200 mg/day has been shown to kill adult worms (Hoerauf et al. 2008) and the drug is clearly a useful adjunct to ivermectin.

CYSTICERCOSIS (box 14.4)

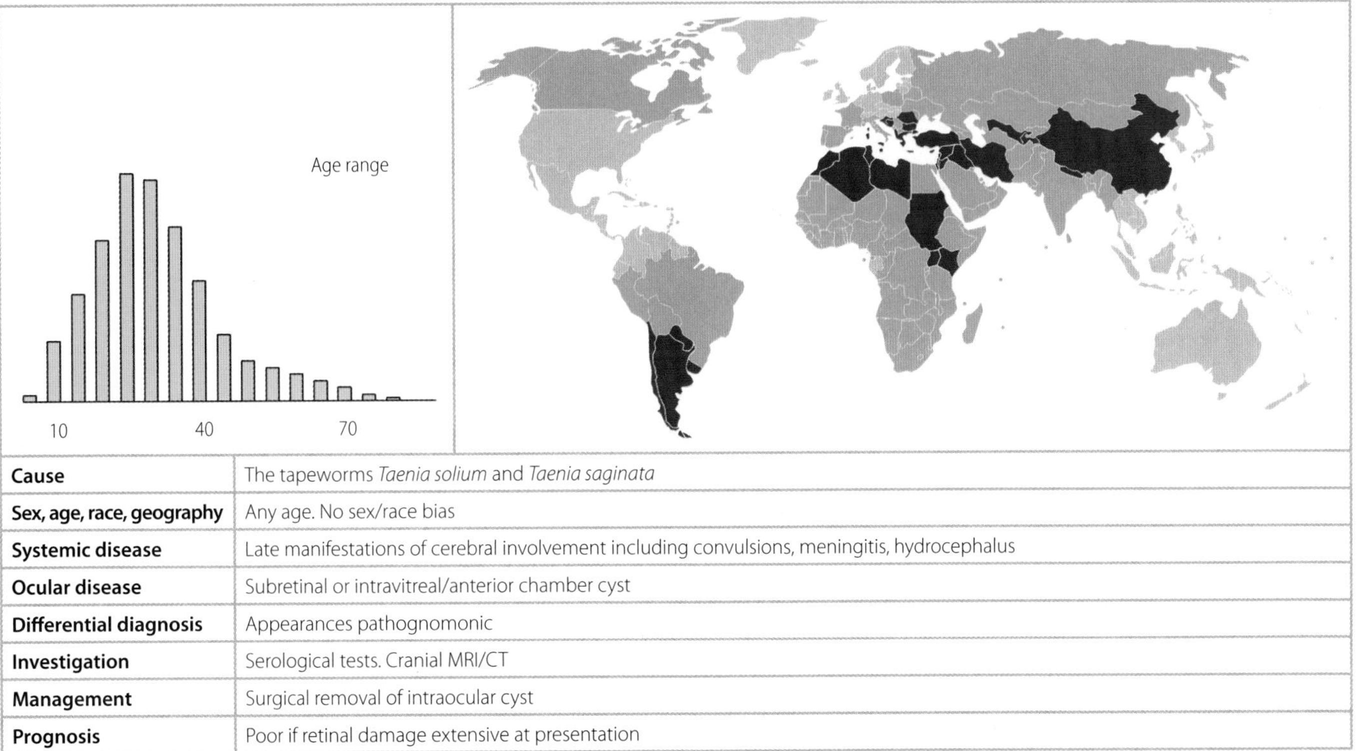

Cause	The tapeworms *Taenia solium* and *Taenia saginata*
Sex, age, race, geography	Any age. No sex/race bias
Systemic disease	Late manifestations of cerebral involvement including convulsions, meningitis, hydrocephalus
Ocular disease	Subretinal or intravitreal/anterior chamber cyst
Differential diagnosis	Appearances pathognomonic
Investigation	Serological tests. Cranial MRI/CT
Management	Surgical removal of intraocular cyst
Prognosis	Poor if retinal damage extensive at presentation

Box 14.4 Cysticercosis

Introduction

The pig tapeworm *Taenia solium* primarily infests humans. The adult worm, usually single, inhabits the small intestine, its head being firmly attached to intestinal epithelium via the scolex. Tail segments (proglottids) containing eggs are regularly shed and defecated. Eggs are ingested by the intermediate host (the pig), hatch in the small intestine and migrate via the lymphatics or portal system, the embryos becoming encysted as cysticerci within skeletal muscle and various organs including the eye. The human ingests cysticerci via inadequately cooked pork, and the developing cestode attaches to the small intestine (**Fig. 14.23**). Human infestation by an adult *T. solium* (taeniasis) does not lead to cysticercosis in the host.

However, confusingly humans may also act as an intermediate host, by directly ingesting eggs from contaminated food or water, in which case cysticercosis may occur. In some cases this happens in the individual who is host to an adult worm because of feco-oral self-contamination. The ingested larvae then penetrate into human tissue as occurs in the usual intermediate host, the pig. In this way ocular involvement is possible. The lifecycle of *T. saginata* is similar, but the intermediate host is the cow. It is a less common cause of human cysticercosis. The diseases are common in areas with inadequate food hygiene.

Systemic disease

Most patients are children and young adults. The location of the cysticerci determines the symptomatology of human cysticercosis. Cerebral involvement is common but symptoms from cysts, some of which are more than 1 cm in diameter, may not arise for several years. It is the death of a cyst that causes osmotic cyst swelling and pressure effects, sometimes with focalizing signs, and the leakage of cyst contents generates an inflammatory reaction. Convulsions, focal neurological deficits, hemiparesis, meningitis or hydrocephalus may result. In children, acute encephalitis may occur.

Ocular disease

Intraocular or periocular cysticerci are found (Madigubba et al. 2007) in about a quarter of infested patients, the posterior segment being more commonly involved, especially the subretinal space. Presentation is often with symptoms of retinal displacement or serous detachment, with photopsia and visual loss, although a free intraocular cysticercus, having perforated the retina, may be seen as a floater. On examination the intracameral (**Fig. 14.24**) or intravitreal (**Fig. 14.25**) translucent cyst may pulsate or spontaneously evaginate its scolex, immediately withdrawing it on response to light, or may be observed in the subretinal space. Irreversible damage occurs due to macular involvement, retinal detachment or transretinal migration. Leakage from a cyst will cause inflammatory signs.

Diagnosis

The intraocular detection of a cysticercus is usually pathognomonic, but cerebral involvement (which should always be searched for by MRI

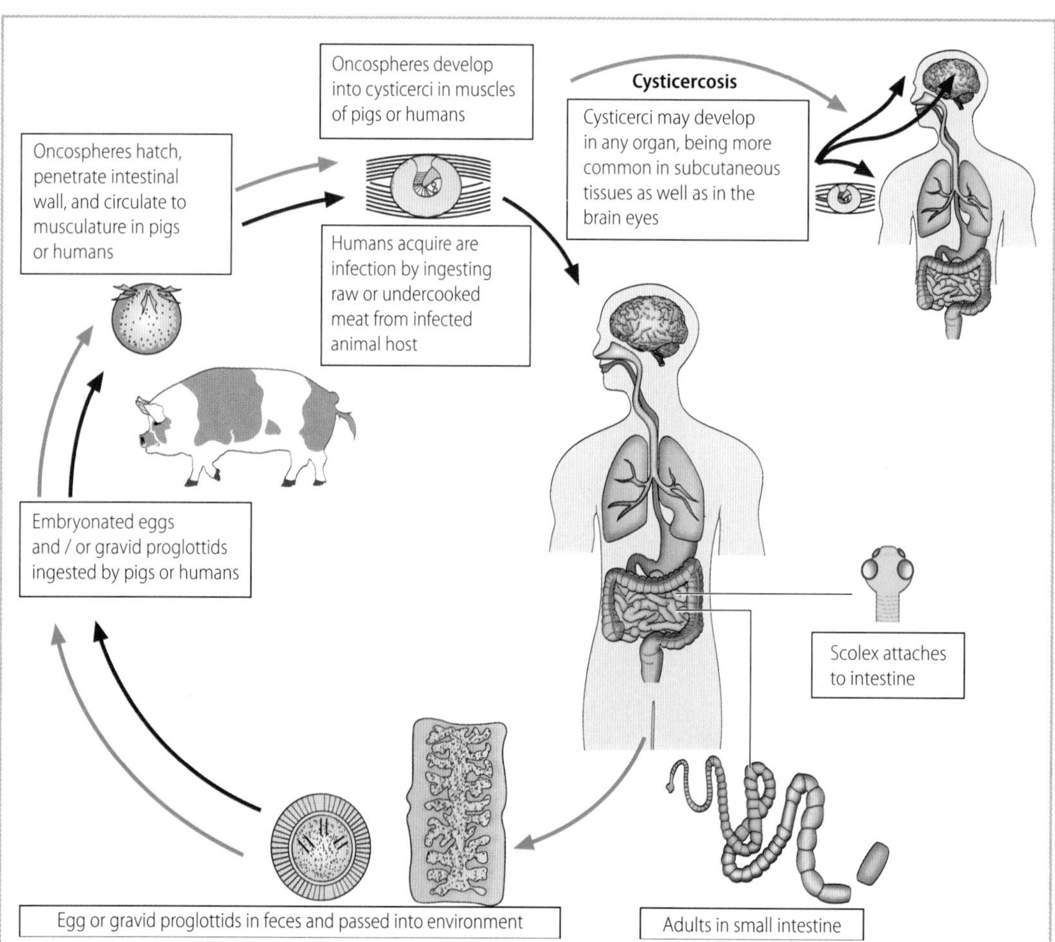

Figure 14.23 The life cycle of *Taenia solium*. (Modified from Centers for Disease Control, DPDx Image Library.)

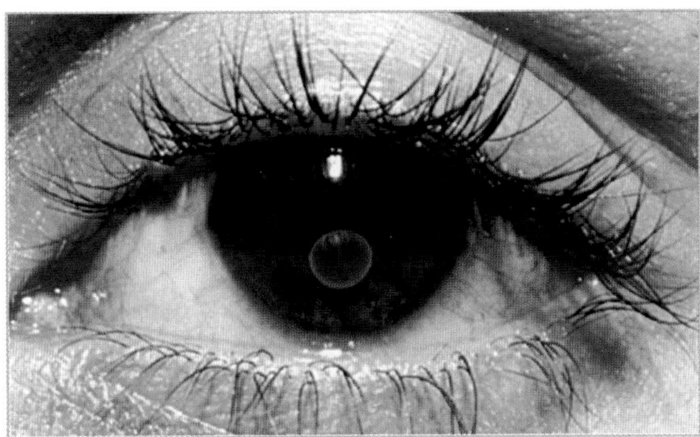

Figure 14.24 A cysticerca of *Taenia solium* in the anterior chamber. The invaginated scolex can be seen pointing upwards. (Courtesy of Professor F Orefice.)

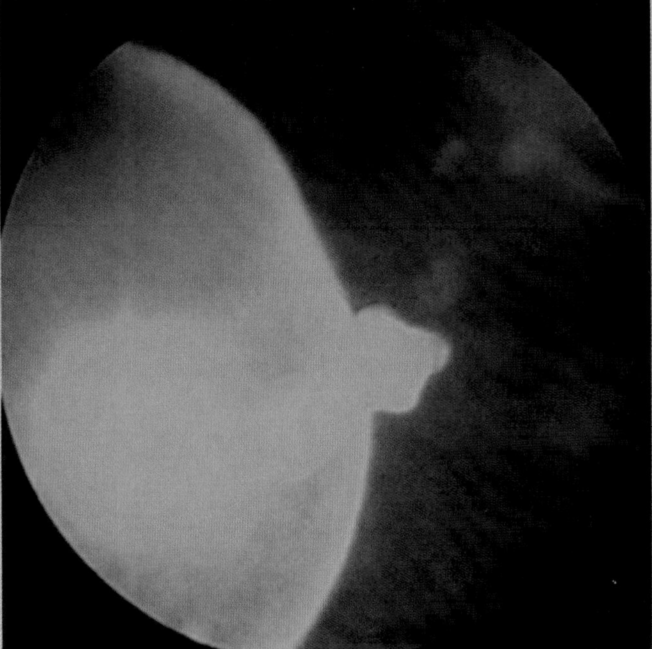

Figure 14.25 A cysticerca in the vitreous, with the scolex evaginated to the right. (Courtesy of Professor F Orefice.)

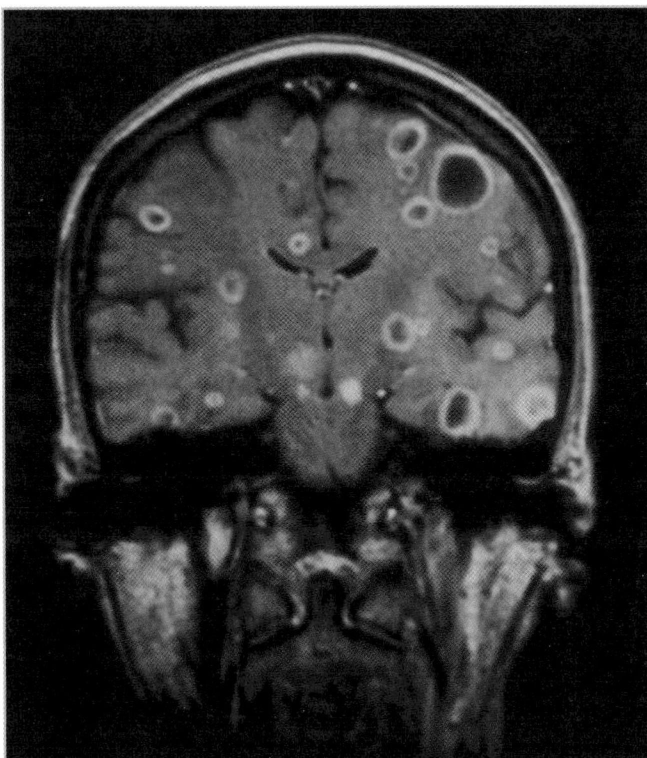

Figure 14.26 Multiple ring-enhancing intracranial cysticerci shown on a post-contrast coronal MR scan. (Courtesy of Dr K Cumming.)

or CT when an intraocular cyst is located) will demonstrate gadolinium ring-enhancing intracranial cysts (**Fig. 14.26**). Both an ELISA test and immunoblot assay are useful, but any serological assessment may be negative where only a single cyst is present. In some cases brain biopsy is necessary. Histology of any cyst will confirm the species involved, and patients with multiple cysticerci may have at least one readily accessible to biopsy, e.g. in a mucous membrane.

Management

Optimal anthelmintic treatment for neurocysticercosis remains unclear. Both praziquantel and albendazole have been used and it is clear that both have some effect (Del Brutto et al. 2006), but it is equally clear that active cysts remain after a standard single treatment of albendazole 400 mg twice daily for 8 days (Carpio et al. 2008). Concomitant oral steroid treatment is required. Medical treatment alone is inadequate for an intraocular organism, because retained cysticerci usually lead to irreversible damage, dead or alive. Removal from aqueous or vitreous humor may be straightforward, but subretinal organisms are a surgical challenge. Pre-surgical treatment with albendazole may be helpful (Yadav et al. 2009). Intraocular disruption of a cyst will cause vigorous inflammation, so perioperative steroid cover is recommended.

OTHER NEMATODE AND TREMATODE INFESTATIONS

The remaining parasitic nematode infestations (loiasis, dirofilariasis and bancroftian filariasis) are most commonly associated with periocular adult worms, but uveitis has been reported in each (Kean et al. 1991). Intraocular penetration has been reported in gnathostomiasis and angiostrongyliasis. Uveitis can also occur in the trematodal diseases schistosomiasis and paragonimiasis.

Ophthalmomyiasis

The first-instar larvae of certain parasitic flies develop within host tissue and are rarely capable of ocular penetration. Intraocular larvae, often subretinal, may therefore be seen occasionally, especially in farm workers. The genera involved include *Cuterebra* (rodent botfly), *Hypoderma* (cattle grub), *Gasterophilus* (horse bot) and *Chrysomyia bezziana* (screw-worm fly), although the intraocular larvae are indistinguishable. Presentation may be acute, with pain and visual loss. Typically the larva moves to and fro beneath the retina, leaving behind it visible criss-cross tracks of retinal damage (**Fig. 14.27**). The larva can be destroyed by argon laser photocoagulation, apparently without inducing inflammation, but others have elected to remove it surgically.

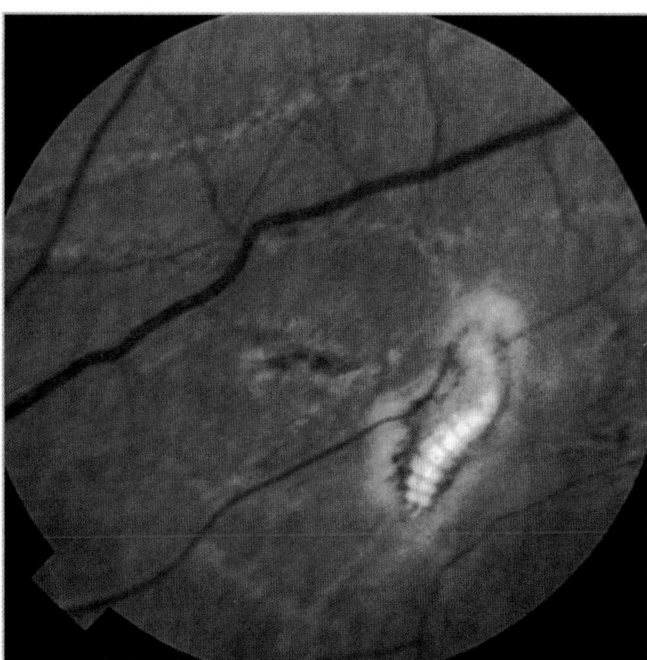

Figure 14.27 Ophthalmomyiasis. The subretinal larva, killed by argon laser photocoagulation, lies among its old subretinal tracks. (Reprinted with permission from Forman et al. 1984.)

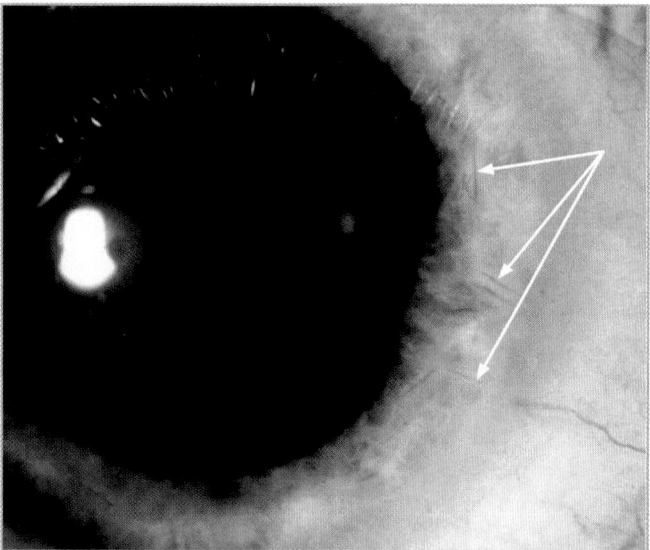

Figure 14.28 Caterpillar setae embedded within the iris (arrowed), with adjacent pale swelling and posterior synechiae.

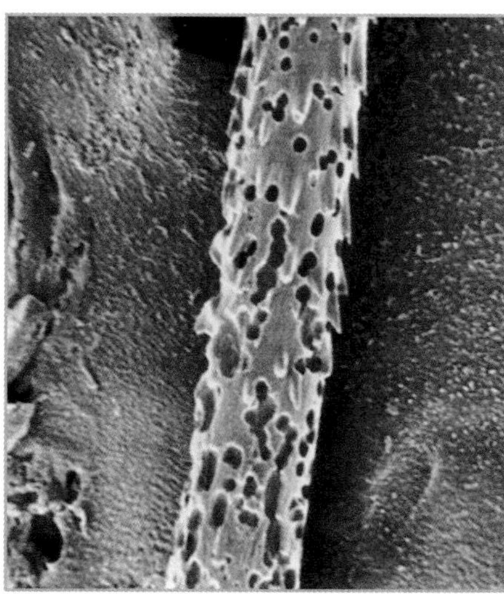

Figure 14.29 A scanning electron microscope image of a caterpillar seta extracted from the eye in Fig. 14.27. The barbs facilitate progressive penetration and make surgical removal difficult.

Toxic uveitis

Spiders, stings, setae, snakes and spurge

Toxic effects may result from ocular penetration of fragments from insects or spiders. The severe keratitis resulting from bee stings is well reported and there may be associated toxic uveitis with hypopyon. Certain beetles can emit powerful vesicant chemicals and ocular surface contact may lead to corneal necrosis and severe uveitis. The hairs of spiders, in addition to causing ophthalmia nodosa, have caused chorioretinal lesions. However, most reports of ocular penetration involve caterpillar setae (hairs). These can easily penetrate the ocular surface and the hooked barbs tend to migrate internally. A violent keratoconjunctivitis occurs which may become chronic. Intraocular penetration is heralded by acute uveitis which may include iris nodules (**Fig. 14.28**). Intravitreal or chorioretinal penetration is reported, sometimes with papillitis. Chorioretinal tracks tend to be pigmented, with a white, inflamed leading edge. Removal of setae may be more traumatic than allowing them to remain, but placing a laser barrage in front of the leading edge of the track to prevent progression has been suggested. Setae have been removed from both the anterior chamber (**Fig. 14.29**) and vitreous.

Spitting cobras achieve their aim of disablement by spraying venom at the eyes, and accidental ocular exposure to other snake venoms is occasionally seen. The resultant ophthalmia has been reported in humans (Chu et al. 2010). Severe keratoconjunctivitis is usually accompanied by severe anterior uveitis, which requires aggressive anti-inflammatory treatment but may lead to necrotic change. Rarely uveitis is reported as a consequence of a snake bite itself and, ironically, also as a consequence of the administration of anti-snake venom.

Lovers of the typical English herbaceous border will appreciate the characteristic display of various euphorbias (spurges) but gardeners are well aware that they should be pruned with care. The milky sap contains alkaline terpene esters that cause intense pain to mucosae, reportedly worse than capsaicin, and if reaching the eye can induce severe keratouveitis. After irrigation with buffered saline, support is non-specific with topical steroid and mydriasis.

REFERENCES

Amin HI, McDonald HR, Han DP, et al. Citrectomy update for macular traction in ocular toxocariasis. *Retina* 2000;**20**:80–5.

Ayong LS, Tume CB, Wembe FE, et al. Development and evaluation of an antigen detection dipstick assay for the diagnosis of human onchocerciasis. *Trop Med Int Health* 2005;**10**:228–33.

Carpio A, Kelvin EA, Bagiella E, et al. Effects of albendazole treatment on neurocysticercosis: a randomised controlled trial. *J Neurol Neurosurg Psychiatry* 2008;**79**:1050–5.

Chu ER, Weinstein SA, White J, Warrell DA. Venom ophthalmia caused by venoms of spitting elapid and other snakes: report of ten cases with review of epidemiology, clinical features, pathophysiology and management. *Toxicon* 2010;**6**:259–72.

Clemett RS, Williamson HJ, Hidajat RR, et al. Ocular Toxocara canis infections: diagnosis by enzyme immunoassay. *Aust NZ J Ophthalmol* 1987;**15**:145–150.

Cortez R, Denny JP, Muci-Mendoza R, et al. Diffuse unilateral subacute neuroretinitis in Venezuela. *Ophthalmology* 2005;**112**:2110–14.

Del Brutto OH, Roos KL, Coffey CS, Garcia HH. Meta-analysis: cysticidal drugs for neurocysticercosis: albendazole and praziquantel. *Ann Intern Med* 2006;**145**:43–51.

Felberg NT, Shields JA, Federman JL. Antibody to *Toxocara canis* in the aqueous humor. *Arch Ophthalmol* 1981;**99**:1563–64.

Foreman AR, Cruess AF, Benson WE. Ophthalmomyiasis treated by argon-laser photocoagulation. *Retina* 1984;**4**:163–65.

Garcia CA, Gomes AH, Garcia Filho CA, Vianna RN. Early stage diffuse unilateral subacute neuroretinitis: improvement of vision after photocoagulation of the worm. *Eye* 2004;**18**:624–27.

Garms R, Lakwo TL, Ndyomugyenyi R, et al. The elimination of the vector *Simulium neavei* from the Itwara onchocerciasis focus in Uganda by ground larviciding. *Acta Tropica* 2009;**111**:203–10.

Gass JDM, Braunstein RA. Further observations concerning the diffuse unilateral subacute neuroretinitis syndrome. *Arch Ophthalmol* 1983;**101**:1689–97.

Gass JDM, Scelfo R. Diffuse unilateral subacute neuroretinitis. *J R Soc Med* 1978;**71**:95–111.

Gillespie SH, Dinning WJ, Voller A, et al. The spectrum of ocular toxocariasis. *Eye* 1993;**7**:415–18.

Goldberg MA, Kazacos KR, Boyce WM, et al. Diffuse unilateral subacute neuroretinitis. Morphometric, serologic, and epidemiologic support for Baylisascaris as a causative agent. *Ophthalmology* 1993;**100**:1695–701.

Hoerauf A, Mand S, Volkmann L, et al. Doxycycline in the treatment of human onchocerciasis: kinetics of *Wolbachia* endobacteria reduction and of inhibition of embryogenesis in female *Onchocerca worms*. *Microbes Infect* 2003;**5**:261–73.

Hoerauf A, Specht S, Buttner M, et al. *Wolbachia* endobacteria depletion by doxycycline as antifilarial therapy has macrofilaricidal activity in onchocerciasis: a randomised placebo-controlled study. *Med Microbiol Immunol* 2008;**197**:295–311.

Hopkins AD. Ivermectin and onchocerciasis: is it all solved? *Eye* 2005;**19**: 1057–66.

Jalil A, Dhawahir-Scala F, Jones NP. Non-progressive tractional inferior retinal elevations in intermediate uveitis. *Ocul Immunol Inflamm* 2010;**18**:60–3.

Jones JL, Kruszon-Moran D, Won K, et al. *Toxoplasma gondii* and *Toxocara* spp. co-infection. *Am J Trop Med Hyg* 2008;**78**:35–9.

Kazacos KR, Raymond LA, Kazacos EA, et al. The raccoon ascarid. A probable cause of human ocular larva migrans. *Ophthalmology* 1985;**92**:1735–44.

Kean BH, Sun T, Ellsworth RM. Diseases caused by nematodes. In: *Ophthalmic Parasitology*. New York: Igaku-Shoin, 1991.

McCarthy JS, Ottensen EA, Nutman TB. Onchocerciasis in endemic and nonendemic populations: differences in clinical presentation and immunologic findings. *J Infect Dis* 1994;**170**:736–41.

Madigubba S, Vishwanath K, Reddy GB, Vemuganti GK. Changing trends in ocular cysticercosis over two decades: an analysis of 118 surgically excised cysts. *Int J Med Microbiol* 2007;**25**:214–19.

Magnaval JF, Glickman LT. Management and treatment options for human toxocariasis. In: Holland C, Smith HV (eds), *Toxocara: The enigmatic parasite*. Wallingford: CAB 2006: 113–22.

Mets MB, Noble AG, Basti S, et al. Eye findings of diffuse unilateral subacute neuroretinitis and multiple choroidal infiltrates associated with neural larva migrans due to *Baylisascaris procyonis*. *Am J Ophthalmol* 2003;135:888–90.

Mohamad S, Azmi RC, Noordin R. Development and evaluation of a sensitive and specific assay for diagnosis of human toxocariasis by use of three recombinant antigens (TES-26, TES-30USM, and TES-120). *J Clin Microbiol* 2009;**47**:1712–17.

Mora P, Vecchi M, Barbera L, et al. Use of systemic cyclosporin A in a case of severe toxocara uveitis. *J Infect* 2006;**52**:159–61.

Nichols RL. The aetiology of visceral larva migrans I diagnostic morphology of infective second stage toxocara larvae. *J Parasitol* 1956;**42**:349–62.

Osei-Atweneboama MY, Eng JK, Boakye DA, et al. Prevalence and intensity of *Onchocerca volvulus* infection and efficacy of ivermectin in endemic communities in Ghana: a two-phase epidemiological study. *Lancet* 2007;**369**:2021–9.

Paul M, Stefaniak J, Twardosz-Paulik H, Pecold K. The co-occurrence of Toxocara ocular and visceral larva migrans syndrome: a case series. *Cases J* 2009;**2**:6881.

Rodriguez A. Early pars plana vitrectomy in chronic endophthalmitis of toxocariasis. *Graefes Arch Clin Exp Ophthalmol* 1986;**224**:218–20.

Roldan WH, Espinoza YA. Evaluation of an enzyme-linked immunoelectrotransfer blot test for the confirmatory serodiagnosis of human toxocariasis. *Mem Inst Oswaldo Cruz* 2009;**104**:3.

Shafir SC, Wise ME, Sorvillo SJ, Ash LR. Central nervous system and eye manifestations of infection with Baylisascaris procyonis. *Curr Infect Dis Reports* 2006;8:307–13.

Sharkey JA, McKay PS. Ocular toxocariasis in a patient with repeatedly negative ELISA titre to Toxocara canis. *Br J Ophthalmol* 1993;**77**:253–254.

Sorvillo F, Ash LR, Berlin OG, et al. *Baylisascaris procyonis:* an emerging helminthic zoonosis. *Emerg Infect Dis* 2002;**4**:355–9.

Souza EC, Casella AM, Nakashima Y, Monteiro LR. Clinical features and outcomes of patients with diffuse unilateral subacute neuroretinitis treated with oral albendazole. *Am J Ophthalmol* 2005;**140**:437–9.

Stewart JM, Cubillan LD, Cunningham ET. Prevalence, clinical features and causes of vision loss among patients with ocular toxocariasis. *Retina* 2005;**25**:1005–13.

Wan WL, Cano MR, Pince KJ, et al. Echographic characteristics of ocular toxocariasis. *Ophthalmology* 1991;**98**:28–32.

Weil GJ, Steel C, Liftis F, et al. A rapid-format antibody card test for diagnosis of onchocerciasis. *J Infect Dis* 2000;**182**:1796–9.

Wilder HC. Nematode endophthalmitis. Trans *Am Acad Ophthalmol Otolaryngol* 1950;**55**:99–109.

Won KY, Kruszon-Moran D, Schantz PM, Jones JL. National seroprevalence and risk factors for zoonotic Toxocara spp. infection. *Am J Trop Med Hyg* 2008;**79**:552–7.

Yadav SK, Winter I, Singh SK. Management of intra-vitreal cysticercosis. *Nep J Ophthal* 2009;**1**:143–5.

Chapter 15 Intermediate uveitis and idiopathic chronic vitritis

The terms 'intermediate uveitis' and 'idiopathic chronic vitritis' describe two forms of intraocular inflammation both of which tend to be very long term. The former characteristically affects younger adults, the latter elderly people. Although some patients with intermediate uveitis have underlying systemic inflammation, most cases of both diseases remain idiopathic. They are dealt with together here for convenience, but there is no suggestion of a shared aetiology.

INTERMEDIATE UVEITIS (box 15.1)

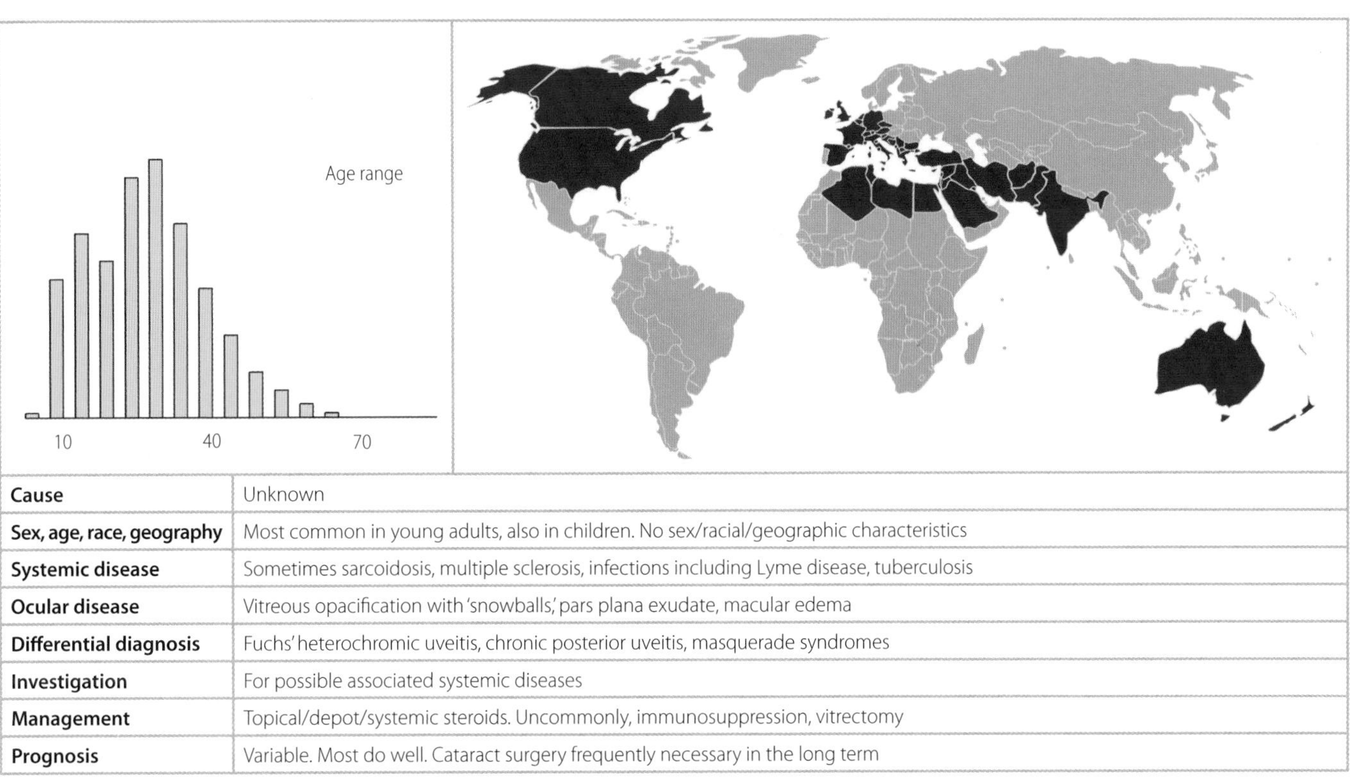

Cause	Unknown
Sex, age, race, geography	Most common in young adults, also in children. No sex/racial/geographic characteristics
Systemic disease	Sometimes sarcoidosis, multiple sclerosis, infections including Lyme disease, tuberculosis
Ocular disease	Vitreous opacification with 'snowballs,' pars plana exudate, macular edema
Differential diagnosis	Fuchs' heterochromic uveitis, chronic posterior uveitis, masquerade syndromes
Investigation	For possible associated systemic diseases
Management	Topical/depot/systemic steroids. Uncommonly, immunosuppression, vitrectomy
Prognosis	Variable. Most do well. Cataract surgery frequently necessary in the long term

Box 15.1 Intermediate uveitis

Introduction

The term 'intermediate uveitis' is an attempt by the International Uveitis Study Group to generate a term acceptable to the ophthalmological community, to describe the condition first described as 'cyclitis' by Ernst Fuchs in 1906, and then variously as 'peripheral uveitis,' 'peripheral cyclitis,' 'pars planitis' and 'chronic cyclitis.' Despite the now widespread use of the preferred term, 'pars planitis' is still used confusingly, in two different ways: first (and, if at all, preferably) to describe a subset of about 10% of patients with substantial snowbanking over the pars plana, and second (and unhelpfully) as a historic, alternative term for intermediate uveitis generally. 'Intermediate uveitis' is a descriptive, not a diagnostic, term, and in most cases no underlying cause is found. However, its presence implies that the ophthalmologist should be considering a variety of possible etiologies, some of which require modified or specific treatment.

Intermediate uveitis is a common diagnosis in a specialist uveitis clinic. Epidemiological studies from such sources find that, with some geographical variation, it accounts for between 3% and 15% of uveitis. However, the population of specialist clinics is clearly subject to referral bias, and in a general ophthalmological practice a figure as low as 1.4% is quoted in comparison to a figure of 12% for a referral centre in the same area (McCannel et al. 1996). The proportion is, however, much higher in childhood uveitis, where it may account for as many as 25% of all cases (Althaus and Sundmacher 1992).

Intermediate uveitis is bilateral in the vast majority of patients, although asymmetrical involvement is common. Familial cases are intermittently reported but are actually scarce. Evidence of an association with HLA-DR2 (an antigen also associated with optic neuritis and demyelinating disease in addition to some other posterior segment inflammatory disorders) was initially inconclusive, but the identification of its allelic subtype HLA-DR15 has provided more support for an inherited predisposition (Raja et al. 1999, Oruc et al. 2001). Some have suggested that the condition is less common in black than in white individuals in the USA, and rare in Chinese and Japanese individuals, but epidemiology at present is speculative. The disease predominantly affects young people. There may be two major groups of patients: the first present in childhood between the ages of 5 and 15, and the second between 20 and 40 years, although the validity of this bimodal distribution has been questioned because of the greater incidence of underlying systemic disease (including sarcoidosis) in the older age group. Only very uncommonly do patients present over the age of 40. Many patients present with a longstanding history of symptoms and therefore the true onset age is likely to be significantly earlier than the age at presentation to an ophthalmologist.

The pathogenesis of intermediate uveitis is unknown. Rare histological studies, while demonstrating peripheral retinal phlebitis and epiretinal changes, have not in general demonstrated substantial uveal inflammation. An immune-mediated response has been assumed, but hypotheses of autoimmunity have been speculative. Demonstrations of large populations of B-cell infiltrates into the vitreous, with few T-cells, have led to the suggestion that T-cell immunoregulation of B-cell function may be impeded, at least during the chronic phase of the disease. The occurrence of intermediate uveitis or very similar processes in connection with diverse diseases such as sarcoidosis, multiple sclerosis and Lyme disease, suggest the possibility of a converging pathogenetic pathway, probably immune-mediated, perhaps provoked by a number of different antigens.

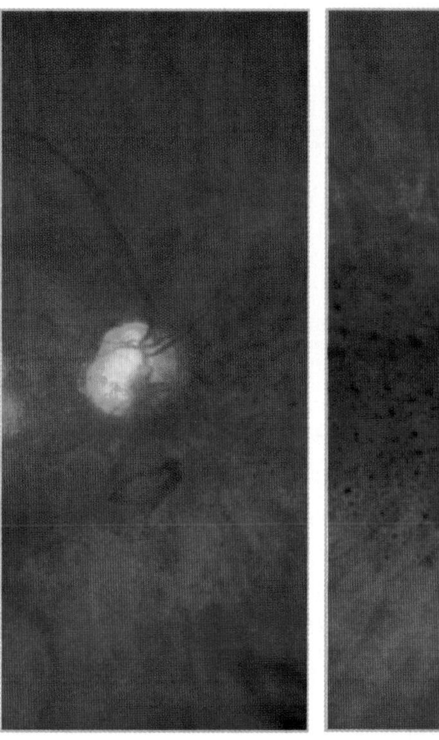
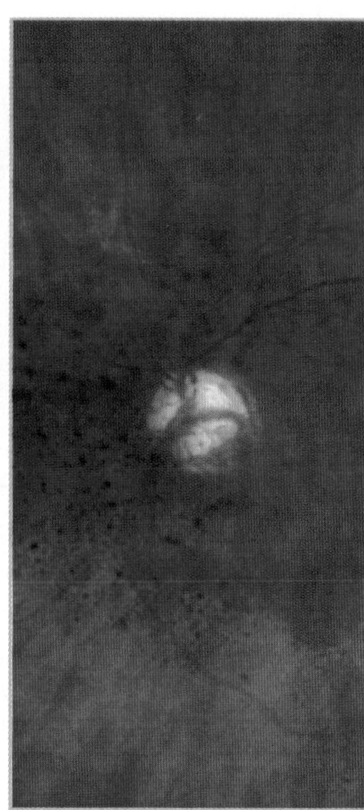

Figure 15.1 Incipient posterior vitreous detachment in intermediate uveitis, as imaged on widefield photography. The right Weiss ring is detached from the disk, the left nearly so. There are a large number of cell deposits on the posterior hyaloid, seen as silhouettes.

Systemic disease

Most patients with intermediate uveitis have no associated systemic disease and the condition is idiopathic. However, associated disease may be found in a substantial minority, possibly up to 31% (Boskovitch et al 1993). An association with sarcoidosis is well recognized (Jones 2002), as is a link with multiple sclerosis (Wagemans et al. 1992), which affects possibly more than 15% of cases and up to 30% of women. An intermediate uveitis-like picture may occur in tuberculosis, syphilis, Behçet's disease and Lyme disease. A form of intermediate uveitis has also been described in Japanese patients infected with human T-lymphotropic virus type I. In our clinic, following a comprehensive general history, all patients presenting with intermediate uveitis are investigated for sarcoidosis and syphilis. Lyme serology and tuberculin testing would not be requested without further evidence of disease or a history of exposure, although that approach would differ in an endemic area.

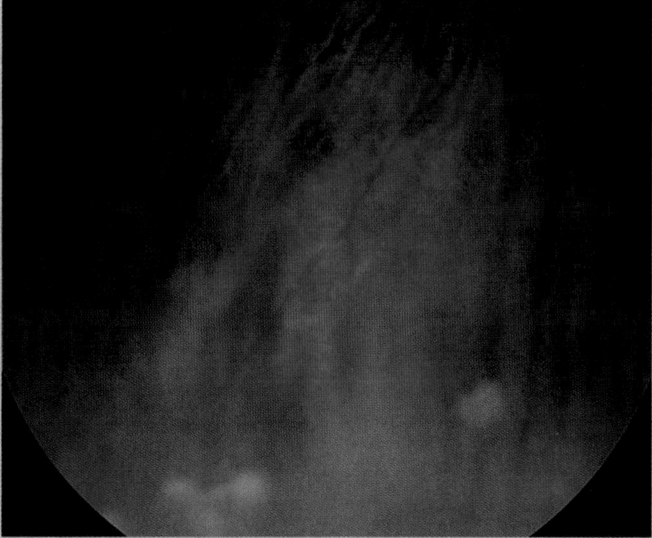

Figure 15.2 Inferior preretinal snowballs in intermediate uveitis.

Ocular disease

Symptoms and signs

The primary site of inflammation in intermediate uveitis is unknown, but the spectrum of signs is quite narrow. Typically there will be some vitreous opacification, and it is these visible floaters, often unilateral, that most commonly bring the patient to an ophthalmologist. Not uncommonly presentation is provoked by the worsened floaters of posterior vitreous detachment, often an early phenomenon in intermediate uveitis (**Fig. 15.1**). The greatest concentration of such opacities is invariably inferior, and severity varies from mild (**Fig. 15.2**) to very severe (**Fig. 15.3**). Careful examination of the fellow eye is mandatory because it is common to find inflammatory signs, sometimes very subtle, in the other eye of a patient who has presented with uniocular symptoms. The vitreous opacities are often conglomerated into suspended 'snowballs' (**Fig. 15.4**), which appear to be composed of active and degenerate macrophages. Snowballs may hover in small numbers over the inferior peripheral retina, or may encroach substantially into central vision (**Fig. 15.5**), especially in children. Vitreous cellular activity is variable but may be severe. Flare is not usually a major component.

Involvement of the anterior segment in intermediate uveitis is variable, but significant anterior chamber (AC) activity requiring

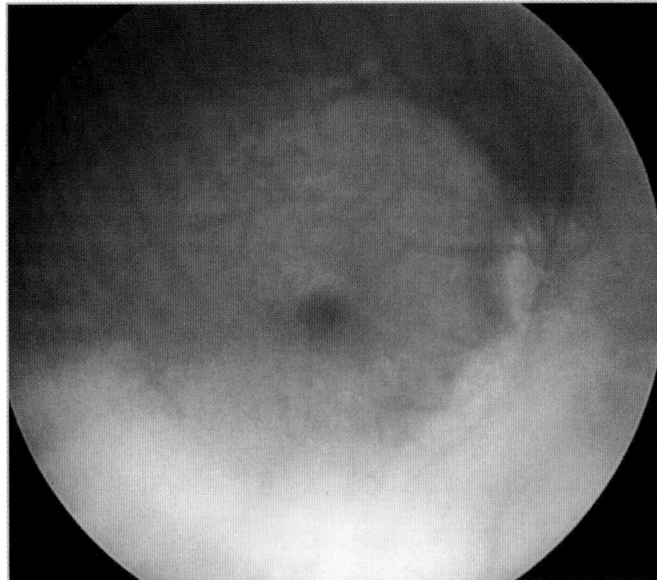

Figure 15.3 Severe vitreous opacification especially inferiorly, adjacent to pars plana exudate in the right eye of a 14 year old with intermediate uveitis.

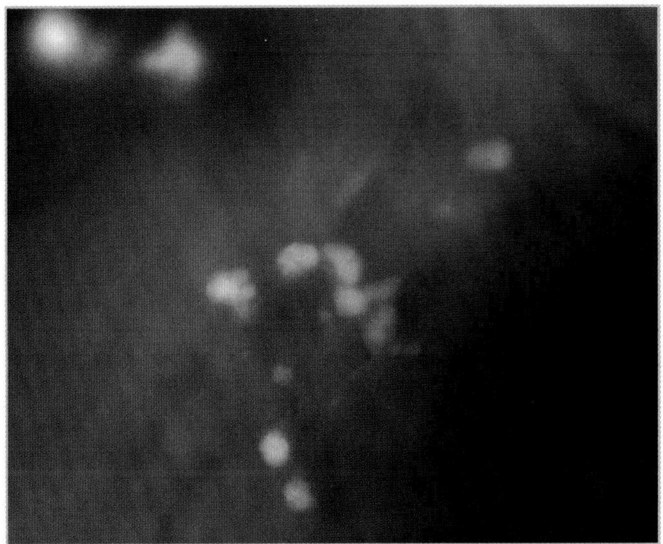

Figure 15.4 Vitreous snowballs overlying the inferior retina in intermediate uveitis.

topical steroids is not uncommon, and some patients need long-term treatment. On occasion patients will present for the first time with substantial anterior uveitis, discomfort, ciliary injection and sometimes posterior synechiae. Some patients probably pass through an acute phase before settling into the more recognizable, chronic form of the disease. Patients may have intermittent flare-ups of AC activity but severe inflammation is uncommon and most patients will have a few AC cells at most. It is most unusual for large confluent keratic precipitates (KPs) to be present in intermediate uveitis and, if seen, sarcoidosis in particular should be considered.

It should be mentioned that patients with Fuchs' heterochromic uveitis, a condition presenting in approximately the same age group with similar symptoms of floaters, sometimes have very significant vitreous involvement (Jones 1991) and on occasion inferior snowballs may be seen. Peripheral retinal vessel sheathing may also be seen,

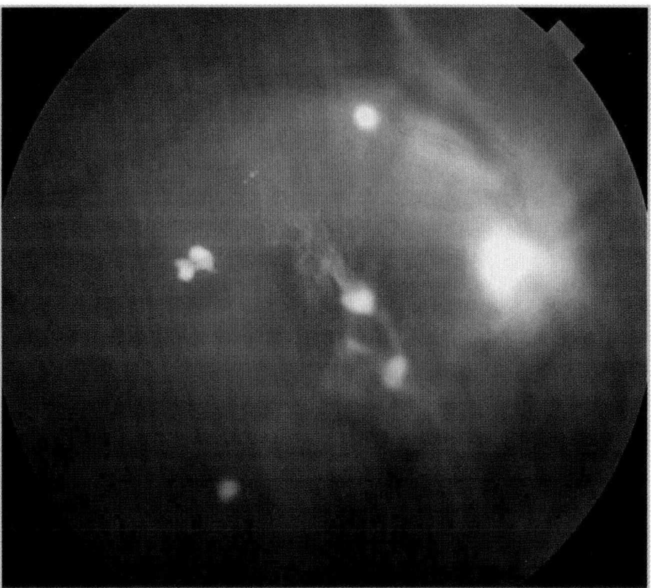

Figure 15.5 Vitreous snowballs and sheet-like opacities in the central vitreous in chronic intermediate uveitis.

although less commonly than in intermediate uveitis. The very occasional mild heterochromia seen in intermediate uveitis may also confuse the issue. However, the differential diagnosis is aided by the fact that Fuchs' disease is usually unilateral, anterior segment signs, with stellate KPs involving most of the corneal endothelium, are usually distinct, glaucoma is a much more common complication, and macular edema is most uncommon, if indeed it occurs at all (Jones 1993).

A careful examination of peripheral retina and pars plana is important in a patient with intermediate uveitis. Exudation, described as 'snowbanking,' over pars plana and peripheral retina may be patchy and is usually concentrated inferiorly, but in severe instances may occupy 360° of the peripheral fundus. Fibrotic changes in these areas may persist, and histology in this situation has shown fibrous tissue with moderate lymphocytic infiltration. Subtle sheathing of peripheral retinal venules (**Fig. 15.6**) is a common feature of intermediate uveitis and its presence enhances the association with optic neuritis and demyelinating disease (Malinowski et al. 1993). Peripheral retinal, pars plana and disc neovascularization are occasionally seen.

Vitreous opacification may cause many floaters but visual acuity measurements are often surprisingly well preserved; only in very severe cases do the floaters become intolerable. The hallmark of intermediate uveitis and the most important visual threat is macular edema, which is very common (**Fig. 15.7**). This, if allowed to persist for months or more, may lead to permanent retinal damage or epiretinal membrane formation and irremediable visual loss. It is the need to suppress macular edema that usually sets the therapeutic level in individual patients.

Course, complications and prognosis

The behavior of intermediate uveitis over time varies enormously between patients and prognostication can be difficult. One thing is certain; intermediate uveitis is a very chronic disease. A new patient may expect to have inflammatory signs for years to come, and some observers have doubted that intermediate uveitis ever 'burns out,' at least for adult-onset disease. However, broadly speaking the severity

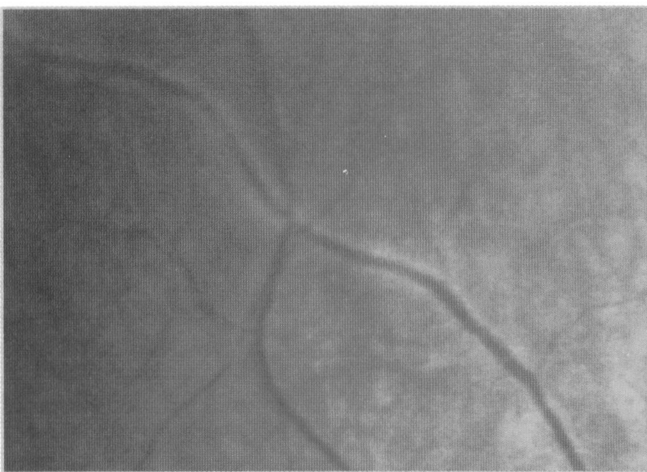

Figure 15.6 Sheathing of peripheral retinal venules in intermediate uveitis.

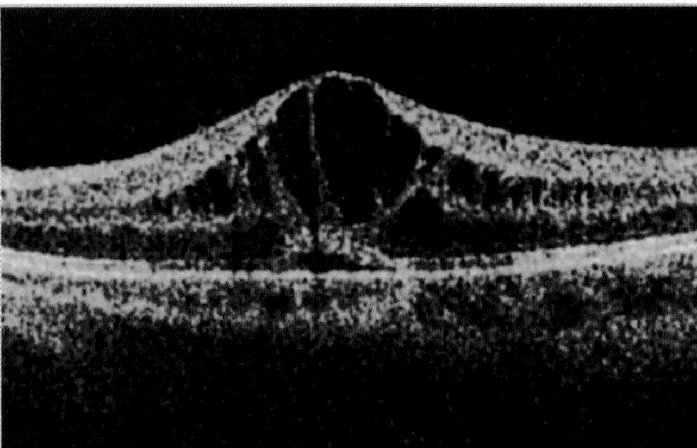

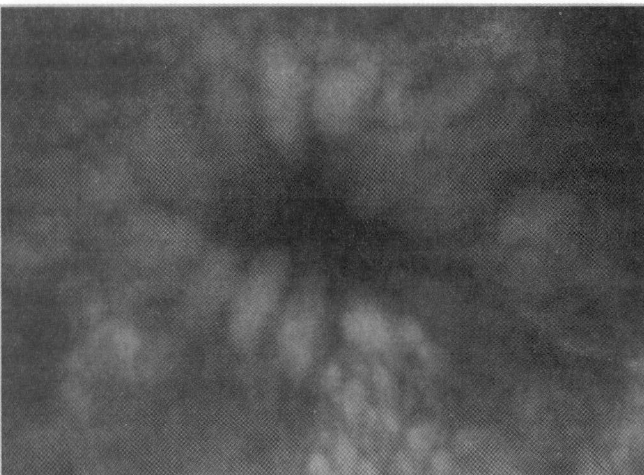

Figure 15.7 Severe cystoid macular edema, shown on ocular coherence tomography and fluorescein angiography, in intermediate uveitis.

of signs at onset is a reasonable marker for future decrease in visual acuity. Observations of the natural pattern of behavior of the condition are modified by the need to treat, and surveys showing a greater rate of improvement for moderate and severe forms will be compromised by this bias. However, some have divided intermediate uveitis into three broad groups of severity: first, a benign group with only low-grade activity and a tendency to intermittent remissions (comprising perhaps 10% of the total); second, a chronic insidious group (the majority); and third a progressive chronic group (about a third of the total) with a tendency to recurrent episodes and worsening vision. Individuals will notice fluctuations in symptoms over periods of months rather than days or weeks.

Cataract formation is common in intermediate uveitis, eventually affecting almost half the eyes. Undoubtedly systemic steroids contribute to this complication. However, macular edema and its resultant damage remain the predominant cause of visual loss in about three-quarters of eyes. Smoking increases the risk of macular edema (Thorne et al. 2008). Its management is discussed in detail in Chapter 7. Glaucoma is not a frequent complication of intermediate uveitis, a fact that probably reflects the absence of substantial anterior segment inflammation in most eyes, with few resultant anterior synechiae. However, a significant minority of patients will develop glaucoma after steroid therapy.

Inferior pars plana exudate and gliosis creates tractional effects and retinal elevations are not infrequently observed, especially in younger patients (Jalil et al 2010). Distinguishing between tractional retinal detachment and retinoschisis can be difficult, but our observation is that, in the absence of coincident macular traction, progression to rhegmatogenous detachment is very unusual. Preretinal tractional effects can occasionally lead to retinal vessel dragging (**Fig. 15.8**) and macular heterotopia. Rhegmatogenous detachment may also follow vitreous organization and traction, but historically also after cryotherapy. Occasionally neovascularization, usually of peripheral retina, less commonly at the disk or posterior pole, may cause vitreous hemorrhage. The pathogenesis of such new vessels is uncertain, because retinal ischemia is generally not a feature of intermediate uveitis.

Retinal vasoproliferative tumor

A wide variety of terms has been used to describe the phenomenon of non-malignant masses within or under the retina, usually peripherally, consisting predominantly of vascular fibroglial tissue.

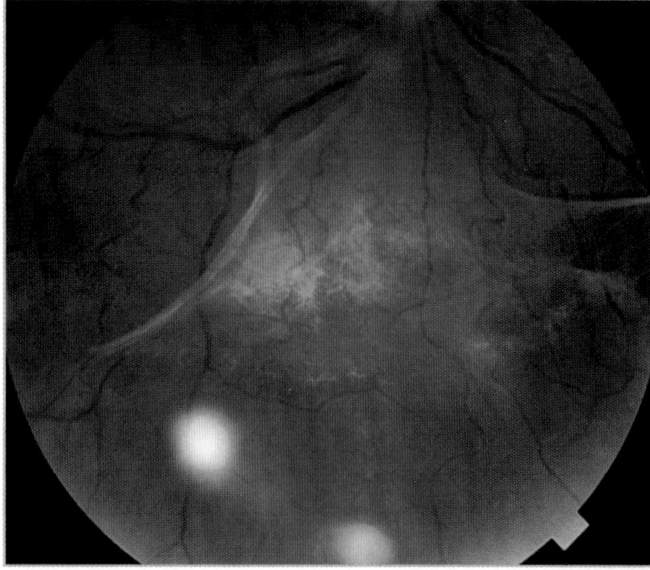

Figure 15.8 Vitreoretinal adhesion of fibroglial sheets in intermediate uveitis causes retinal traction as evidenced by vessel distortions. Tractional elevation and secondary rhegmatogenous detachment follow in a minority.

In addition to the above, the terms **peripheral nodular telangiectasis** and **reactive retinal glioangiosis** have been used, among others. The phenomenon occurs secondary to a wide variety of predisposing intraocular pathology including retinopathy of prematurity, retinitis pigmentosa, retinal detachment, and forms of uveitis including toxoplasmosis, toxocariasis and tuberculosis. However, it is included here because, in a very large series of vasoproliferative tumors, intermediate uveitis was the most frequently identified underlying cause, being associated with 28% of the secondary lesions (Sheilds et al. 1995).

Most tumors are inferotemporal and vary from slightly raised telangiectatic areas simulating Coats' disease, to large nodules suggesting malignant tumor. The lesions are usually single and red/yellow, with minimal dilation of feeder vessels, in contrast to the retinal hemangiomas of von Hippel–Lindau syndrome. There is usually a considerable exudative reaction (**Fig. 15.9**). Management is dependent on visual effect (and by no means all require treatment) but, if severe, cryotherapy, laser, photodynamic therapy and proton beam therapy have all been applied, with mixed results. Ruthenium plaque therapy has been found to be safe and effective for a large group (Anastassiou et al. 2006) with cataract and epiretinal gliosis being the most frequent sequelae. Intraocular anti-VEGF (vascular endothelial growth factor) monoclonal antibody injection has been used anecdotally with unproven effect. If in doubt on the etiology of such a lesion the management of these tumors is the preserve of the ocular oncologist.

Diagnosis

The diagnosis of intermediate uveitis is entirely clinical. Typically cases will demonstrate minimal anterior segment activity, vitreous cells and snowballs, pars plana exudate, macular edema and sometimes subtle peripheral retinal vessel sheathing. The coexistence of other signs such as granulomatous anterior uveitis, frank retinal vasculitis or focal retinal or choroidal lesions should suggest another entity. The possibility of sarcoidosis should always be investigated. On occasion, focal peripheral inflammation including toxoplasmosis and toxocariasis may mimic intermediate uveitis, as may intraocular large-cell lymphoma. Fluorescein angiography will identify subclinical vasculitis and this or ocular coherence tomography (OCT) will clarify the extent of macular edema; it is this that will modify management.

Management

The treatment of intermediate uveitis has two aims in mind: first, the improvement of vision and, second, the avoidance of postinflammatory sequelae such as glaucoma, macular damage and vitreous traction, which will complicate management and may cause permanent visual loss.

A significant minority of patients have mild intermediate uveitis with only a few vitreous floaters, and even these may be experienced for periods only of a few months at a time. No treatment is required and it is our practice, after perhaps a year of observation, to discharge and to invite re-attendance if new symptoms are experienced. In those who develop persistent macular edema, permanent macular damage may occur and treatment is necessary. Many patients with intermediate uveitis have very asymmetrical disease, and often only one eye requires treatment. This circumstance is not an indication for systemic steroids. For unilateral treatment, or where bilateral treatment is necessary but systemic steroids are to be avoided, a deep periocular depot of methylprednisolone or triamcinolone is preferred, using general anesthesia for children. One injection often leads to significant improvement, which may persist, but if unsuccessful we would now progress to intraocular triamcinolone injection.

For bilateral macular edema, or after failed periocular treatment, systemic steroid treatment is usually successful. For adults, a starting dose of about 40 mg/day prednisolone is sustained for 2–4 weeks until a response is achieved, and dose reduction to 15 mg/day is then usually possible over a further 6–8 weeks. Further dose reduction is then in smaller increments. It is often possible to discontinue steroid treatment without a recurrence of edema, and this quiescence may be prolonged. In others, edema will recur readily. The future course of management will then depend on the tolerance of the required maintenance dose, which varies substantially between patients. Intermittent depot methylprednisolone may be used to supplement maintenance oral steroids and, in a small minority of cases, oral immunosuppression may be required. The evidence base for macular edema treatment is dealt with more fully in Chapter 7.

Where vitritis and vitreous debris are persistent, or asymmetrical intermediate uveitis is inadequately responsive to medical treatment, vitrectomy may be considered. It is doubtless effective in improving visual acuity in most and has been found often to be successful in improving macular edema (Wiechens et al. 2001) and to reduce the need for systemic medication (Giuliari et al. 2010). Whether longer-term inflammatory response is reduced is a more contentious issue. A meta-analysis of vitrectomy in uveitis generally, but with more than half of patients having intermediate uveitis, found only equivocal evidence of success (Becker and Davis 2005). It has become our practice frequently to combine vitrectomy where used, with intravitreal triamcinolone injection. There is probably an additive short-term effect but, as for injection alone, not sustained (Gutfleisch et al. 2007).

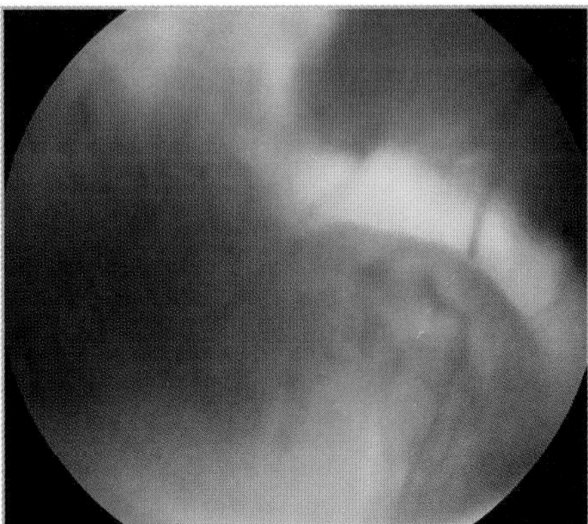

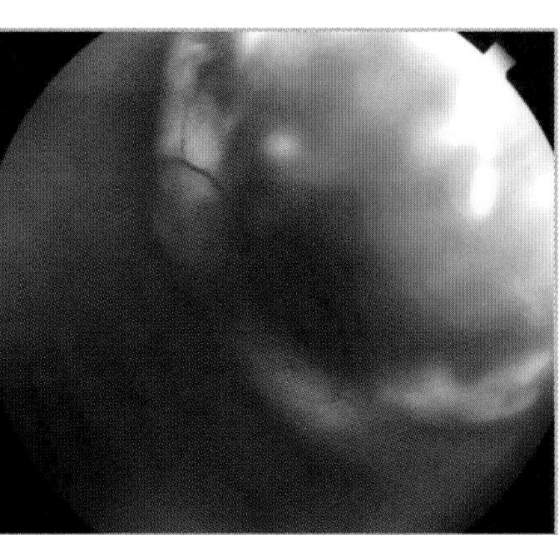

Figure 15.9 Peripheral nodular telangiectasis with substantial surrounding exudative reaction, in two patients with intermediate uveitis.

Cataract is a not uncommon complication of intermediate uveitis and its treatment. With careful preoperative control of inflammation, results of extraction with intraocular lens implantation are generally reliable. Indeed, intermediate uveitis is a form of intraocular inflammation that causes less concern than many when considering cataract surgery (Rahman and Jones 2005). In those with secondary glaucoma requiring surgery, enhancement is required and we would use a similar peroperative steroid regimen for this, and for vitrectomy in those few for whom it is required.

Neovascularization of the pars plana and peripheral retina, or more rarely at the optic disk or posterior pole, may lead to recurrent vitreous hemorrhage. Inflammatory neovascularization may be steroid responsive, but, if not, indirect peripheral laser ablation may be effective. Cryotherapy is no longer used. For non-clearing hemorrhage, where residual vitreous opacification is severe or tractional changes are found, vitrectomy may be required and combined with internal search and peripheral laser photocoagulation. Although complications may be encountered in those with active neovascularization, outcomes have been largely satisfactory and long-term benefit may be seen (Potter et al. 2001). Retinal detachment is an important complication following vitrectomy in these eyes.

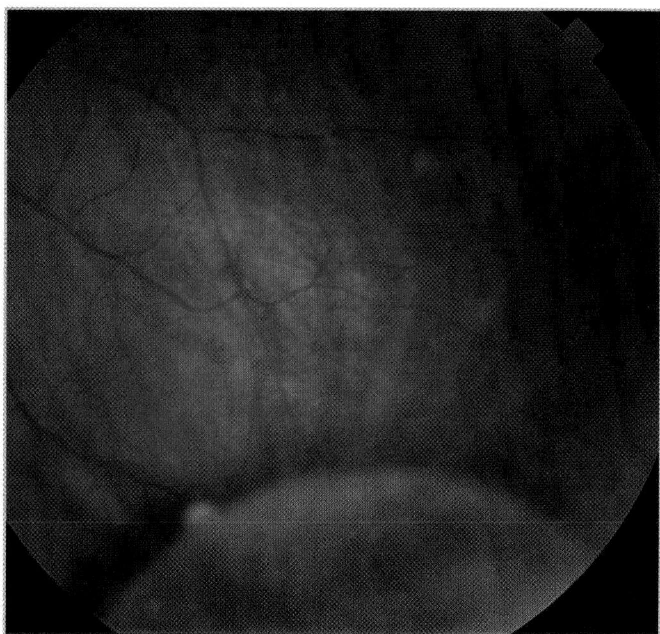

Figure 15.11 Inferior retinal elevation in a boy with intermediate uveitis. No progression was observed over a period of several years.

INTERMEDIATE UVEITIS IN CHILDREN

Intermediate uveitis may present in childhood, only rarely (1 in 54 aged <16 years in our experience) under the age of 5. It has certain characteristics that are distinct from adult-onset disease. Children are more likely to present with worse vision and severe vitreous opacification (**Fig. 15.10**), quite often present with vitreous hemorrhage (Lauer et al. 2002), and with disease that is very asymmetrical. They often have florid pars plana exudate and are more likely to develop inferior retinal elevations (**Fig. 15.11**) (Jalil et al. 2010). In contrast to adults with intermediate uveitis, children do not often develop macular edema, but instead they very often develop associated optic nerve head swelling (**Fig. 15.12**), its severity varying in tandem with inflammation control.

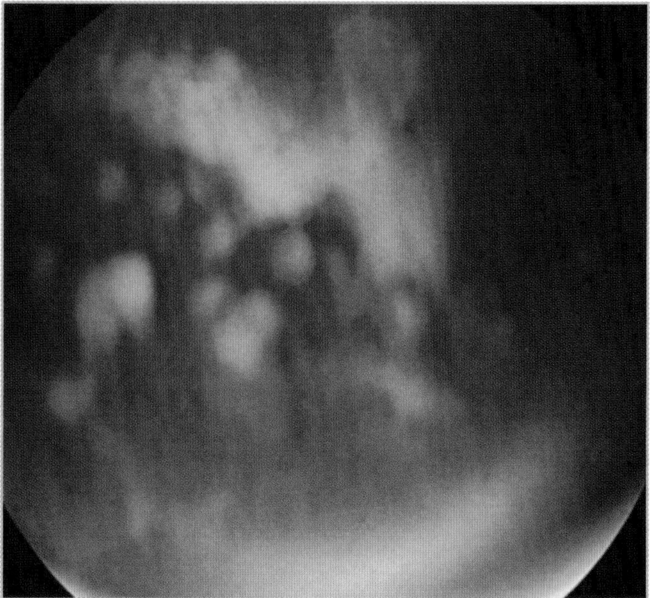

Figure 15.10 Severe vitreous opacification in a boy with intermediate uveitis.

This papillitis is rarely severe, and in our experience has not been associated with disk hemorrhage, vascular occlusion, visual obscuration or nerve fiber bundle defects. In the absence of focal neurological signs (which should of course always be excluded), and with the confidence that this type of papillitis is uveitis related and entirely an intraocular feature, we no longer arrange neurological referral or brain imaging in these children.

We have not made a diagnosis of multiple sclerosis in childhood-onset intermediate uveitis, in contrast to adults. Unilateral intermediate uveitis (usually somewhat atypical) may be related to toxocariasis in children. Sarcoidosis seems to occur with approximately the same incidence as in adults (12% in our cohort). Others have found that early onset is a marker for a higher risk of poor outcome and a complicated course (Ayuso et al. 2010), but we have found that children are more likely to remit after some time compared with adults, a finding shared by others (de Boer et al. 2006). Most children require orbital depot steroid injection and/or systemic steroid treatment, but, in contrast to some other forms of childhood uveitis, the need for oral immunosuppression to treat juvenile-onset intermediate uveitis is quite uncommon (Schatz et al. 2007).

IDIOPATHIC CHRONIC VITRITIS

This well-recognized but poorly reported chronic intraocular inflammation particularly affects middle-aged or elderly people, usually women. Vitritis may be profound, but usually with diffuse cellular activity rather than clumping as seen in intermediate uveitis. Pars plana exudation is not seen, but peripheral retinal pigment epithelium (RPE) scarring and depigmentation is common. Cystoid macular edema is frequently seen and may be troublesome to manage. Although predominantly a vitritis, there is often evidence of anterior segment inflammation and some develop chronic panuveitis which is difficult to treat. Anterior segment sequelae including cataract, synechiae and glaucoma may occur. It is important to consider and exclude sarcoidosis and intraocular lymphoma. In view of the last, primary vitrectomy is a valid approach to initial management especially where vitreous cellular activity is profound.

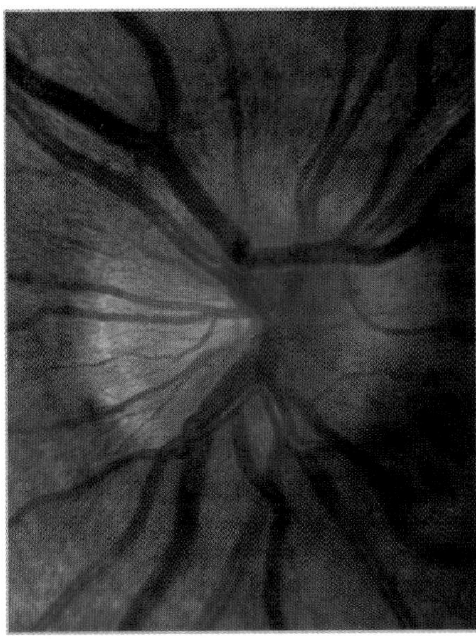
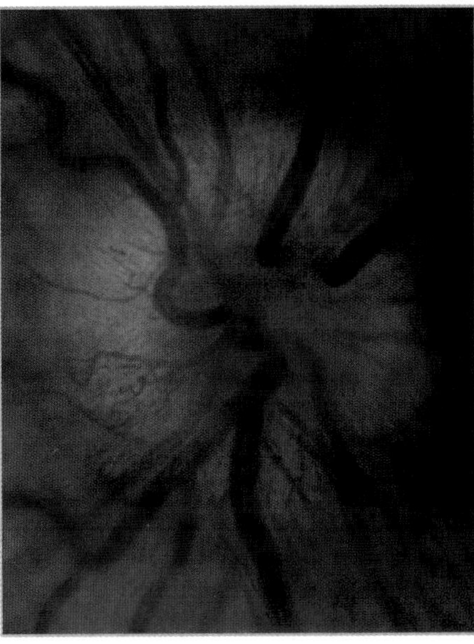

Figure 15.12 Bilateral optic nerve head hyperemia and swelling in a girl with intermediate uveitis. There were no associated neurological signs and a CT of the brain was normal. The swelling resolved on treatment of the uveitis.

REFERENCES

Althaus C, Sundmacher R. Intermediate uveitis: Epidemiology, age and sex distribution. *Intermediate uveitis. Dev Ophthalmol* 1992:**23**:9–14.

Anastassiou G, Bornfeld N, Schueler AO, et al. Ruthrnium-106 plaque brachytherapy for symptomatic vasoproliferative tumours of the retina. *Br J Ophthalmol* 2006;**90**:447–50.

Ayuso VK, ten Kate HA, van der Does P, et al. Young age as a risk factor for complicated course and visual outcome in intermediate uveitis in children. *Br J Ophthalmol* 2010;**184**:267 [online].

Becker M, Davis J. Vitrectomy in the treatment of uveitis. *Am J Ophthalmol* 2005;**140**:1096–105.

de Boer J, Berendschot TT, van der Does P, Rothova A. Long-term follow-up of intermediate uveitis in children. *Am J Ophthalmol* 2006;**141**:616–21.

Boskovich SA, Lowder CY, Meisler DM, et al. Systemic diseases associated with intermediate uveitis. *Cleve Clin J Med* 1993;**60**:460–465.

Giuliari GP, Chang PY, Thakuria P, et al. Pars plana vitrectomy in the management of paediatric uveitis: the Massachusetts eye research and surgery institution experience. *Eye* 2010;**24**:7–13.

Gutfleisch M, Spital G, Mingels A, et al. Pars plana vitrectomy with intravitreal triamcinolone: effect on uveitis cystoid macular oedema and treatment limitations. *Br J Ophthalmol* 2007;**91**:345–8.

Jalil A, Dhawahir-Scala F, Jones NP. Non-progressive tractional inferior retinal elevations in intermediate uveitis. *Ocul Immunol Inflamm* 2010;**18**: 60–63.

Jones NP. Fuchs' heterochromic uveitis: a reappraisal of the clinical spectrum. *Eye* 1991;**5**:649–661.

Jones NP. Major Review: Fuchs' heterochromic uveitis. *Surv Ophthalmol* 1993;**37**:253–272.

Jones NP. Sarcoidosis and uveitis. *Ophthalmol Clin N Am* 2002;**15**:319–26.

Lauer AK, Smith JR, Robertson JE, Rosenbaum JT. Vitreous hemorrhage is a common complication of pediatric pars planitis. *Ophthalmology* 2002;**109**:95–8.

Malinowski SM, Pulido JS, Folk JC. Long-term visual outcome and complications associated with pars planitis. *Ophthalmology* 1993;**100**:818–824.

McCannel CA, Holland GN, Helm CJ, et al. Causes of uveitis in the general practice of ophthalmology. *Am J Ophthalmol* 1996;**121**:35–46.

Oruc S, Duffy BF, Mohanakumar T, Kaplan HJ. The association of HLA class II with pars planitis. *Am J Ophthalmol* 2001;**131**:657–9.

Potter MJ, Myckatyn SO, Maberley AL, Lee AS. Vitrectomy for pars planitis complicated by vitreous hemorrhage: visual outcome and long-term follow-up. *Am J Ophthalmol* 2001;**131**:514–15.

Rahman I, Jones NP. Long-term follow-up of cataract extraction with intraocular lens implantation in patients with uveitis. *Eye* 2005;**19**:191–7.

Raja SC, Jabs DA, Dunn JP, et al. Pars planitis: clinical features and class II HLA associations. *Ophthalmology* 1999;106:594–9.

Schatz CS, Uzel JL, Leininger L, et al. Immunosuppressants used in a steroid-sparing strategy for childhood uveitis. *J Pediatr Ophthalmol Strabismus* 2007;**44**:28–34.

Shields CL, Shields JA, Barrett J, et al. Vasoproliferative tumors of the ocular fundus. *Arch Ophthalmol* 1995;**113**:615–23.

Thorne JE, Daniel E, Jabs DA, et al. Smoking as a risk factor for cystoid macular edema complicating intermediate uveitis. *Am J Ophthalmol* 2008;**145**:841–6.

Wagemans MA, Breebart AC. Association between intermediate uveitis and multiple sclerosis. In: Böke WRF, Manthey KF, Nussenblatt RB (eds). Intermediate Uveitis. Dev Ophthalmol Basel: *Karger* 1992;**23**:99–105.

Wiechens B, Nolle B, Reichelt JA. Pars-plana vitrectomy in cystoid macular edema associated with intermediate uveitis. *Graefes Arch Clin Exp Ophthalmol* 2001;**239**:474–81.

Chapter 16 Sarcoidosis and granulomatous diseases

Many different diseases form granulomatous foci of inflammation and many give intraocular appearances that suggest an underlying granulomatous process, but the paradigm of both is sarcoidosis. In its common and varied forms it is a disease of older children and adults, but a specific early onset form of sarcoidosis has markedly different characteristics and an identified genetic mutation which, if giving rise to familial cases, is known as Blau syndrome. These and other rarer forms of chronic granulomatous inflammation are discussed here.

SARCOIDOSIS (box 16.1)

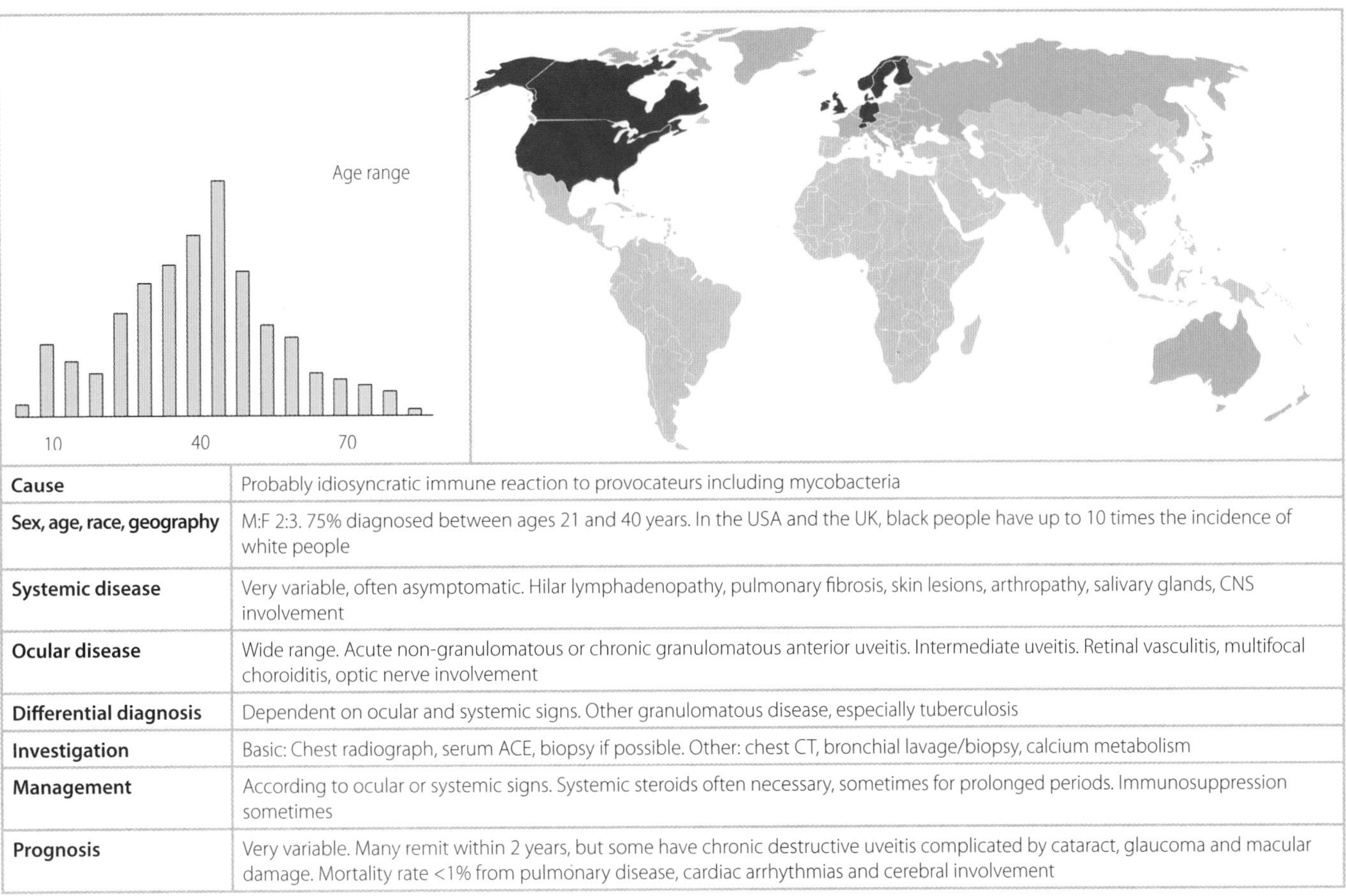

Cause	Probably idiosyncratic immune reaction to provocateurs including mycobacteria
Sex, age, race, geography	M:F 2:3. 75% diagnosed between ages 21 and 40 years. In the USA and the UK, black people have up to 10 times the incidence of white people
Systemic disease	Very variable, often asymptomatic. Hilar lymphadenopathy, pulmonary fibrosis, skin lesions, arthropathy, salivary glands, CNS involvement
Ocular disease	Wide range. Acute non-granulomatous or chronic granulomatous anterior uveitis. Intermediate uveitis. Retinal vasculitis, multifocal choroiditis, optic nerve involvement
Differential diagnosis	Dependent on ocular and systemic signs. Other granulomatous disease, especially tuberculosis
Investigation	Basic: Chest radiograph, serum ACE, biopsy if possible. Other: chest CT, bronchial lavage/biopsy, calcium metabolism
Management	According to ocular or systemic signs. Systemic steroids often necessary, sometimes for prolonged periods. Immunosuppression sometimes
Prognosis	Very variable. Many remit within 2 years, but some have chronic destructive uveitis complicated by cataract, glaucoma and macular damage. Mortality rate <1% from pulmonary disease, cardiac arrhythmias and cerebral involvement

Box 16.1 Sarcoidosis

Introduction

Sarcoidosis is an inflammatory disease causing multifocal granulomas. Its precise cause remains unknown. However, current theories suppose a genetic predisposition activated by one of a variety of different triggers. Studies on large populations have suggested certain environmental factors, possibly seasonal, including exposure to vegetable dust, high humidity (or microorganisms associated with such an environment), metal working in general and titanium in particular, and others as abstruse as inkjet printer toner. An association with infection by *Propionibacterium* spp. has long been suggested, and the finding of *P. acnes* and *P. granulosum* DNA from vitreous samples is intriguing (Yasuhara et al. 2005). Antigens from *Mycobacterium tuberculosis* have been found in 55% of sarcoid tissue samples (Song et al. 2005) and are potent inducers of interferon-γ which normally act to control the microorganism but which may, via an idiosyncratic route, lead to sarcoidosis. Interferon-α, used therapeutically either in hepatitis C or melanoma patients, is well described as a cause of sarcoidosis (Heinzerling et al. 2010) and this has included ocular disease (Doycheva et al. 2009). The well-described role of interferons in provoking sarcoidosis has led to the interesting recent hypothesis that sarcoidosis may be mediated by STAT-1, a transcription factor responsible for upregulating interferon-stimulated genes, in response to stimulation by interferons (Rosenbaum et al. 2009).

The prevalence, racial predilection, familial, geographic, climatic and occupational clustering of sarcoidosis have been extensively studied (Sharma 2008). However, some results are inconsistent, and sarcoidosis produces a varied clinical presentation in different parts of the world, making this a confusing field. There are also changes over time, sarcoidosis apparently evolving from an anecdotal dermatological problem (Boeck's sarcoid) in the nineteenth century to a very common multisystem disorder, in parallel with a decline in tuberculosis. Sarcoidosis is now the most common cause of interstitial lung disease in the west (Demedts et al. 2001). However, striking differences in disease prevalence between countries are seen, varying from 3.7:100 000 in Japan to 28.2:100 000 in Finland (Pietinalho et al. 1995); women are apparently affected in a minority in India or a majority in Greece, African-Caribbean individuals in 0% in Sweden or 66% in the USA, 96% of patients in the UK present between 20 and 40 years of age, but only 18% do so in Greece. Löfgren's syndrome affects 28% of patients in the UK but is almost unknown in Japan. In contrast, up to 70% of Japanese patients have uveitis, but as few as 5% in Denmark. It was initially believed that sarcoidosis increased in prevalence with distance from the equator, but further studies have not confirmed this and population comparisons are inevitably confounded by the greater impact of racial clustering.

Large cohort research programs including the ACCESS study (emanating from 10 specialist centers across the USA [Newman et al. 2004]) have clarified some of these disparities; women do appear slightly more likely to be affected, and there were also sex differences in clinical manifestations; women tended more to ocular and neurological involvement, whereas men had a higher risk of hypercalcemia. African-Caribbean individuals were more likely to have uveitis, skin and liver disease. In the USA the lifetime risk of sarcoidosis for those of African-Caribbean origin (2.4%) is nearly three times that for white people (0.85%). Most studies find that the peak incidence for men with sarcoidosis is about 40 years, whereas that for women is later at about 55 years. The latter phenomenon appears to be becoming more well defined with the use of chest CT in the diagnosis of later-onset sarcoidosis (Jones 2002a). Some, including our group, have also found a smaller peak of incidence in children at 8–14 years.

Clustering of sarcoidosis in families has been well reported: 5.9% of patients in the UK have an affected relative (McGrath et al. 2000) and in the USA the relative risk of sarcoidosis for family members of affected patients is 4.7, siblings being at highest risk (5.8). Such risks are, for unknown reasons, far higher for white than for black families. However, most familial cases involve only parent–child pairs or sibling pairs, more complex pedigrees being rare. This does not suggest a single causative gene mutation but, rather, a summation of several more minor genetic influences.

Definitive diagnosis is by biopsy. A sarcoid lesion is characteristically a well-defined granuloma with epithelioid cells arranged concentrically around multinucleate Langhans-type giant cells, which may contain inclusion bodies (**Fig. 16.1**). There may be frequent plasma cells around the periphery of the lesion and, if longstanding, peripheral fibroblastic activity may also be seen. Central necrosis of the lesion may occur, but caseation does not; its presence implies tuberculosis (TB). Healed granulomas leave a residual hyaline scar.

Sarcoidosis is a truly protean disease, being acute or chronic in presentation, widespread or localized, self-limiting or prolonged, trivial or lethal. However, there appears to be a reasonably well-defined subgroup of patients, usually young adults, presenting with subacute symptoms of erythema nodosum, hilar lymphadenopathy, arthropathy and sometimes acute uveitis (Löfgren's syndrome), who often have a self-limiting form of the disease that remits spontaneously within 2 years. Those middle-aged patients with a more insidious onset, including granulomatous uveitis, skin plaques, nerve palsies and pulmonary parenchymal involvement, often have a more chronic and destructive course. Resolution is less likely with widespread extrapulmonary disease. Overall some two-thirds of white patients spontaneously remit, but only a third of black patients. A minority are permanently handicapped by the resultant tissue damage and the disease is ultimately fatal in up to 1% of cases.

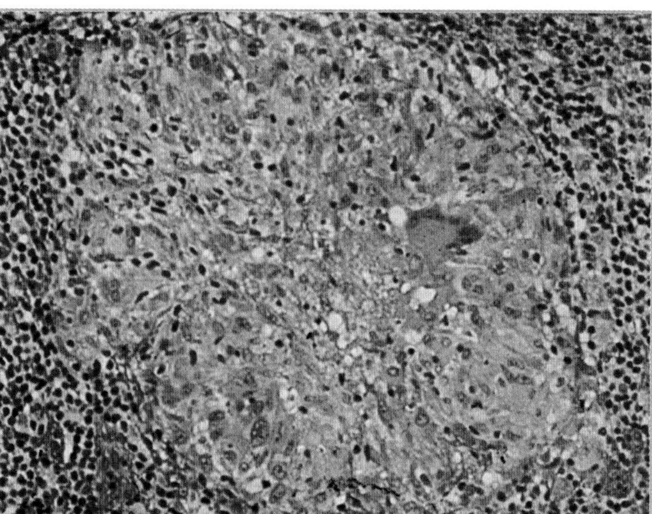

Figure 16.1 A sarcoid granuloma within a lymph node, comprising epithelioid cells and multinucleate giant cells. There is no caseation. (Courtesy of Dr R Bonshek.)

Systemic disease

There are doubtless a large number who go through an episode of sarcoidosis without symptoms, and undiagnosed. Of those who are symptomatic, many experience involvement in only one or two organ systems but a few develop profound and widespread disease. General constitutional symptoms are common, particularly at presentation; these include fatigue, malaise, weight loss and fever with night sweats (Mihailovic-Vucinic and Jovanivic 2008). However, the most commonly involved region is the chest.

The chest

Up to 95% have radiological chest involvement (Baughman et al. 2001) but far fewer, perhaps half the patients have chest symptoms, predominantly dyspnea, dry cough or wheeze (Lynch et al. 2007). Radiologically, pulmonary sarcoidosis may be staged. In early disease (stage 1) there is usually bilateral hilar lymphadenopathy without lung involvement (**Fig. 16.2**). Unilateral node enlargement is much less common and should suggest investigation for TB, lymphoma or fungal pneumonitis. Stage 2 implies parenchymal involvement (**Fig. 16.3**) and resolution of lymphadenopathy with continuing lung inflammation is denoted stage 3. End-stage pulmonary fibrosis is stage 4. The prognosis is substantially affected by the radiological stage: up to 97% of stage 1 patients become asymptomatic in due course, but, in stages 2 and 3, these figures fall to 58% and 25%, respectively. Lung function tests may be normal in early stages, but progressive impairment reflects diminished compliance and reduced forced vital capacity, although the forced expiratory volume in 1 s/forced

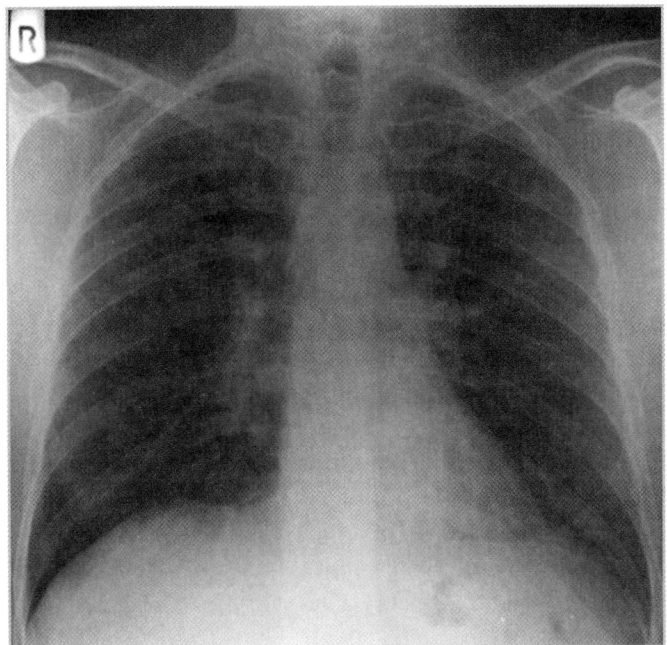

Figure 16.2 A chest radiograph of stage 1 pulmonary sarcoidosis showing bilateral hilar lymphadenopathy but no evidence of lung parenchymal involvement.

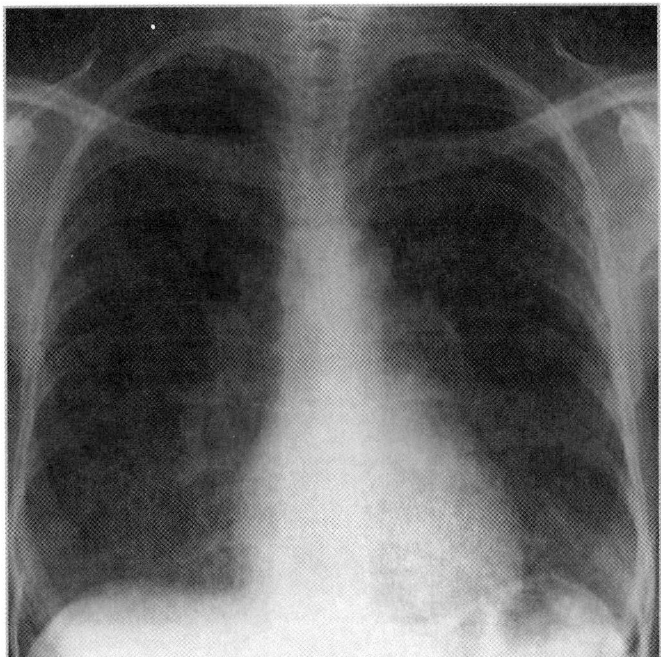

Figure 16.3 Stage 2 pulmonary sarcoidosis with hilar lymphadenopathy and parenchymal involvement manifesting as micronodular shadowing.

vital capacity (FEV_1:FVC) ratio usually remains normal. Advanced fibrosis causes hypoxemia and cyanosis, and lung involvement may ultimately be fatal in a few cases. The overall mortality rate in sarcoidosis is now low, but lung fibrosis remains the most common cause of death and, in those clinics providing specialist care to those with severe lung disease, the mortality rate may be as high as 4.8% (Reich 2002).

In patients with clinical suspicion of sarcoidosis but a normal chest radiograph, high-resolution computed tomography (HRCT) can be very helpful. The technique is particularly useful in older patients with punched-out chorioretinal lesions and posterior synechiae (Clement et al. 2010). Typical features include strings of bronchovascular or perilymphatic micronodules, subpleural micronodules and ground-glass parenchymal involvement (Lynch 2003) with or without fibrosis (**Fig. 16.4**). Occasionally honeycomb cysts or miliary opacities are seen. Importantly, patterns of parenchymal involvement can be both obvious and virtually pathognomonic, in the absence of abnormal plain radiological findings.

Pulmonary involvement may indirectly cause cardiac changes through cor pulmonale and sometimes direct myocardial involvement will be manifested in conduction defects, tachycardias or heart failure. Sudden death from undiagnosed myocardial sarcoidosis is occasionally reported.

The skin

Erythema nodosum (**Fig. 16.5**) is a well-recognized feature of sarcoidosis, especially in association with polyarthropathy and hilar lymphadenopathy. Sarcoidosis is its most common cause, although by no means the only one; it may also be a response to streptococcal infection, following the administration of drugs, especially sulfonamides, penicillin and salicylates; it may accompany inflammatory bowel disease; and rarely it is seen after fungal infection, leprosy or TB, and sometimes as an isolated idiopathic disorder, in which case it may be recurrent. The lesions may involve any part of the body but classically are pretibial and initially raised, purple and tender, then flattening and becoming violaceous before fading within a few weeks. Histology shows deep dermal inflammation and panniculitis with perivascular mixed-cell infiltrate, giant cell formation, and vascular occlusion with some extravasation of blood. Occasionally sarcoid-like granulomas are seen in erythema nodosum biopsy specimens, but in general biopsy is not considered appropriate because in most cases histology does not identify the underlying diagnosis.

Cutaneous sarcoid may have widely differing appearances, but the most recognizable is lupus pernio, a chronic progressive raised cyanotic plaque, most often affecting the face and ears (**Fig. 16.6**). Boeck's sarcoids are papular or nodular lesions, sometimes clustered and especially occurring on the face and arms. They often have a brown tint and may be intradermal or subcutaneous. Other lesions may be multifocal or singular, nodular or placoid, pigmented or vitiliginous, sessile or necrotic and ulcerated (**Fig. 16.7**). If in doubt, biopsy is imperative if tissue diagnosis has not been made elsewhere. Lesions are sometimes periocular and may involve eyelid margins (**Fig. 16.8**).

Bone, joint and muscle

Polyarthropathy, especially of the larger joints, is a frequent presenting feature of sarcoidosis, often with erythema nodosum, and is often self-limiting without permanent change. Enthesitis, tenosynovitis and dactylitis may occur. In chronic sarcoidosis, destructive joint changes are seen, usually in a small number of joints. The phalanges of the hands and feet may be involved (**Fig. 16.9**) and phalangeal cysts may be seen. In severe acute sarcoidosis myalgia may be a feature. Occasionally polymyositis will become chronic.

Abdominal organs

Liver biopsy reveals granulomas in 60% of cases but palpable hepatomegaly is uncommon and cirrhotic changes or liver failure is rare. However, splenomegaly affects 10% or more of patients and occasionally the spleen is large enough to warrant splenectomy. Renal granulomas

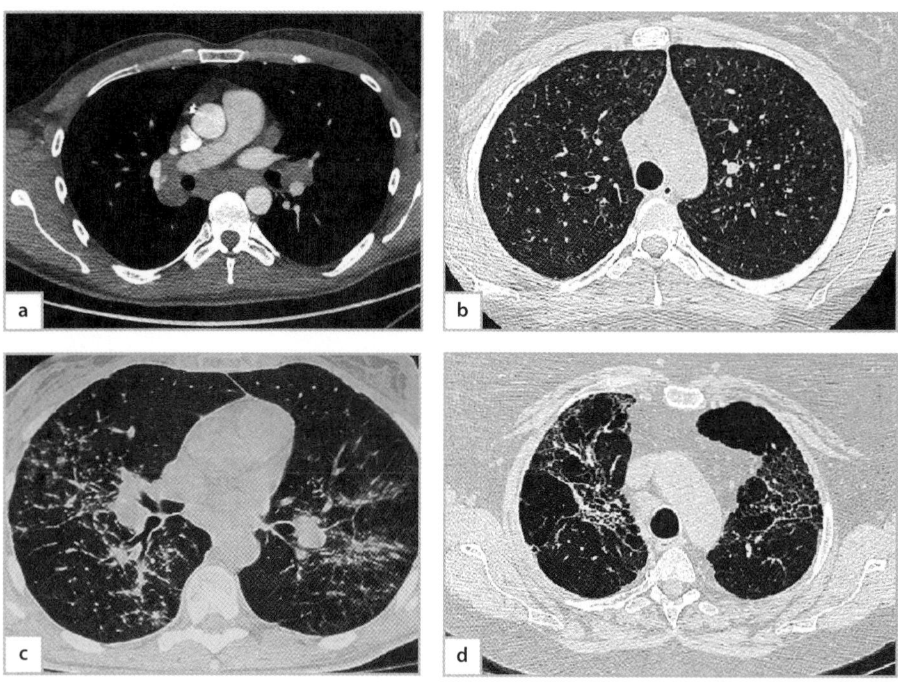

Figure 16.4 Chest CT characteristics of sarcoidosis: (a) massive hilar and mediastinal lymphadenopathy; (b) multiple micronodular opacities in active parenchymal disease; (c) peribronchial beading; and (d) end-stage upper-lobe pulmonary fibrosis. (Courtesy of Dr P Taylor.)

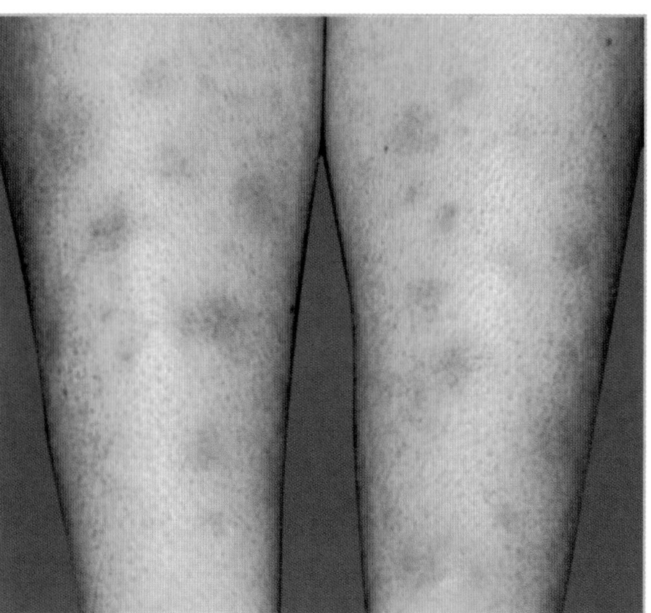

Figure 16.5 Bilateral pretibial erythema nodosum in a patient with sarcoidosis. The lesions are tender.

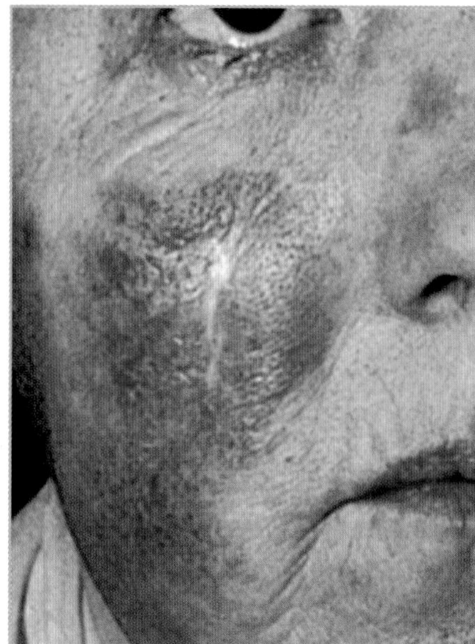

Figure 16.6 Lupus pernio affecting the cheek. The lesion has previously been biopsied.

are usually sparse and insignificant, deterioration in renal function probably affecting less than 1% of sarcoid patients. Hypercalcemia affects more than a third of patients with renal involvement, and damage from nephrocalcinosis may be more common than direct inflammation or fibrosis.

Salivary and lacrimal glands

Involvement of these glands may provide distinct changes on gallium-67 scintigraphy (see below). Clinical enlargement is unusual, but may be dramatic. Mikulicz's syndrome comprises the diffuse swelling of most or all lacrimal and salivary glands, and usually results from sarcoidosis but may also be caused by leukemias and lymphomas.

Heerfordt's syndrome (uveoparotid fever) is a well-recognized but uncommon presentation of sarcoidosis comprising parotid and submaxillary gland enlargement, uveitis and facial nerve palsy. Lacrimal gland involvement does not always cause enlargement, but may lead to dry eye. On occasion salivary and lacrimal gland enlargement is accompanied by transient mild orchitis and may be misdiagnosed as mumps.

The nervous system

Neurosarcoidosis probably affects 5–10% of those with sarcoid but this proportion is said to rise to over a third for those with fundal inflammation; indeed the pathology of the periphlebitis in retina

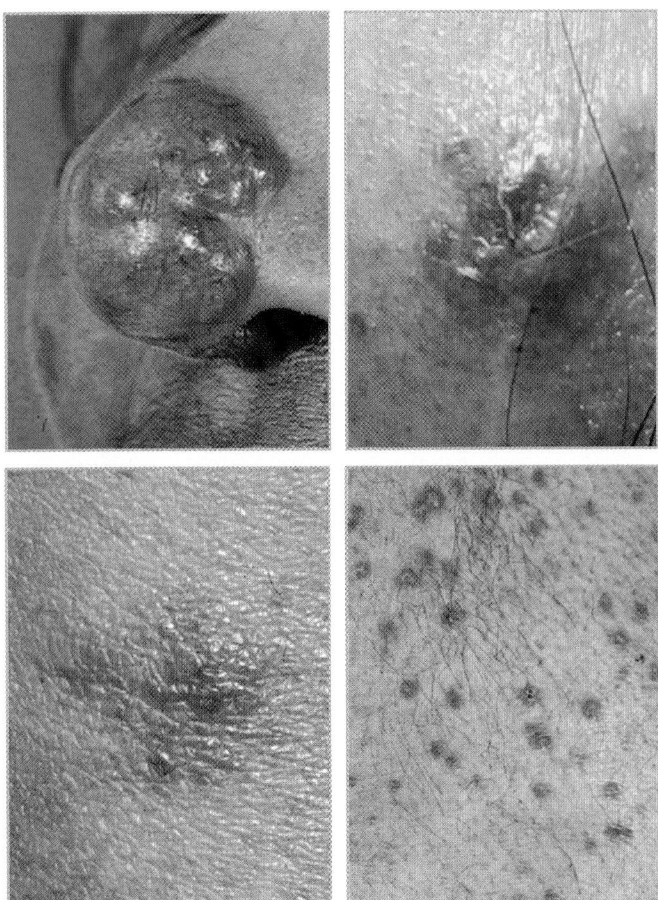

Figure 16.7 A collection of skin lesions in sarcoidosis. Boeck's sarcoid often involves the face (top left) and arms (bottom left). Other lesions may be multifocal and pigmented (bottom right) and, less commonly, necrotic or ulcerated (top right).

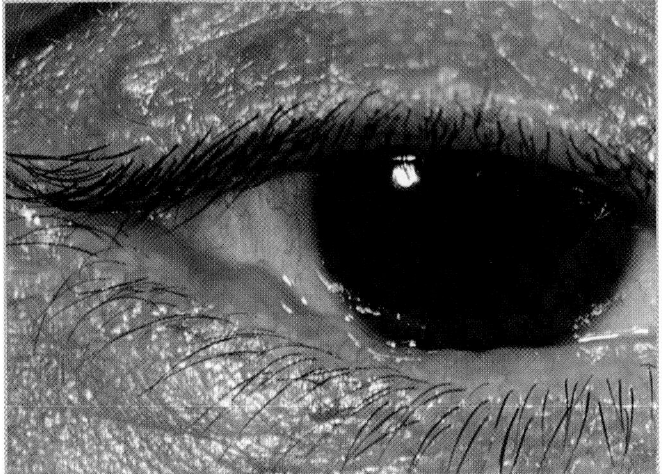

Figure 16.8 Sarcoid skin lesions involving the lateral upper lid and lateral bottom lid margin, where small nodular swellings can be seen.

and meninges appears to be similar. Cranial neuropathy affects up to 80% of patients (Joseph and Scolding 2009) and 50% may present with a cranial nerve palsy, most commonly facial. Myelopathy and peripheral polyneuropathy may also occur, the former tending towards a poor prognosis. Usually clear evidence of systemic sarcoidosis accompanies such lesions. Involvement of the central nervous system (CNS) is, however, notorious for its diagnostic difficulty and signs will depend on the sites of granuloma formation. Presentation may mimic a well-localized tumor or, as a result of its patchy and intermittent symptomatology, impersonate demyelinating disease. The hypothalamus or pituitary may be involved, as may the roots of cranial nerves. Leptomeningeal involvement with thickening is supportive of the diagnosis (**Fig. 16.10**), and involvement of basal meninges may result in hydrocephalus. Findings on MRI may be confusing but are aided by gadolinium enhancement. The ophthalmologist may be asked to help with diagnosis. In these circumstances he or she will be particularly considering sarcoidosis, multiple sclerosis and CNS/ocular lymphoma in the differential diagnosis, and occasionally ocular signs or intraocular sampling will help to make this distinction. Chronic intracranial sarcoidosis may be resistant to both systemic steroid and oral immunosuppression, but the introduction of anti-tumor necrosis factor α TNF-α monoclonal antibody treatment has improved the prognosis (Santos et al. 2010).

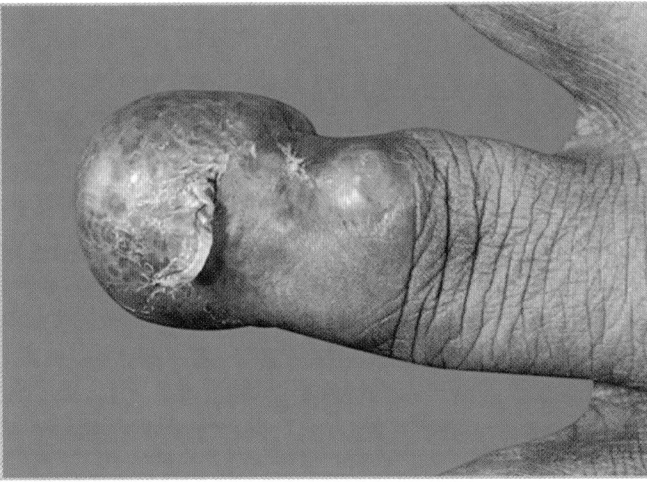

Figure 16.9 Destruction of the terminal phalanx in sarcoid dactylitis.

Ocular disease

Sarcoidosis causes some 5–15% of all cases of uveitis. On average the eyes are involved in a third of patients with sarcoidosis. Although uveitis in sarcoidosis is commonly perceived as being typically 'granulomatous', in fact the spectrum of inflammation is wide. Uveitis may be acute and non-granulomatous or chronic and granulomatous, and the posterior segment may be involved in various ways. The visual outcome of sarcoid uveitis therefore varies depending especially on duration, posterior segment inflammation and the development of macular edema or glaucoma. Up to 5% of patients have a visual acuity worse than 6/60 in both eyes (Edelston et al. 1999). The salient ocular signs have recently been summarized (Jones et al. 2010).

Acute non-granulomatous anterior uveitis

Many patients with classic Löfgren's syndrome will develop, in the early stages, an acute or subacute non-granulomatous uveitis, which is usually bilateral and symmetrical. Keratic precipitates (KPs) are fine and not confluent. The inflammation is usually rapidly responsive to

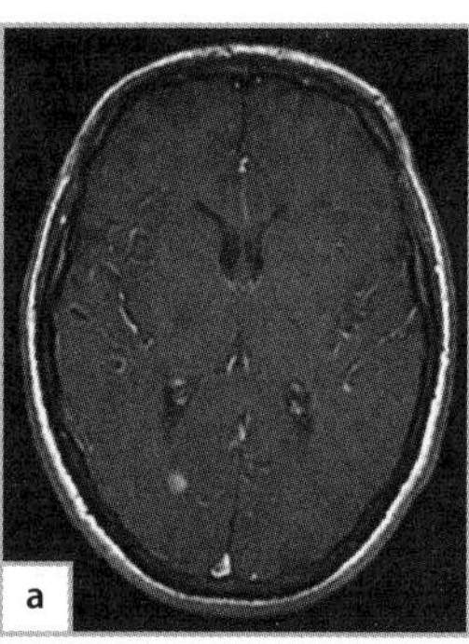

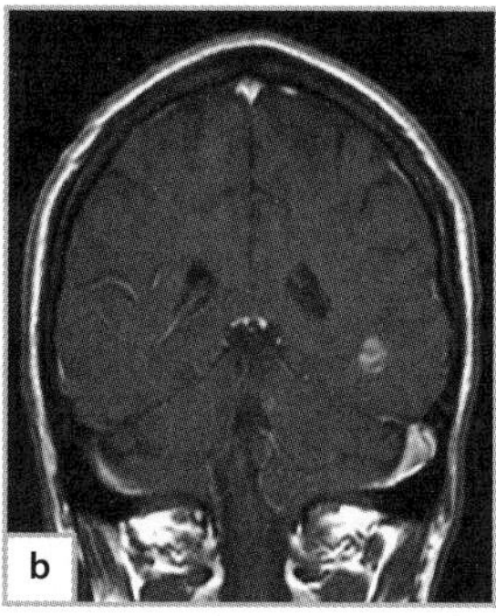

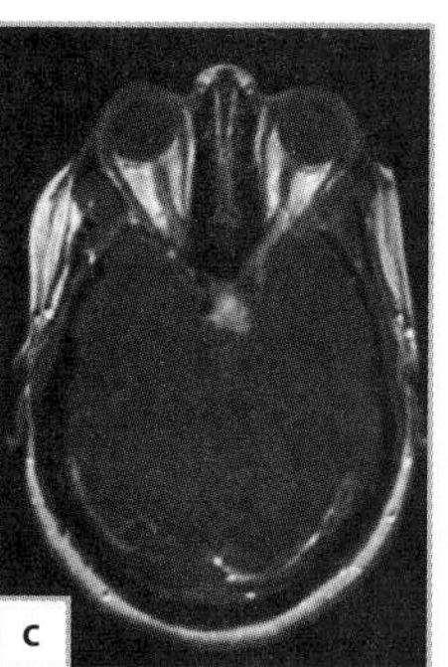

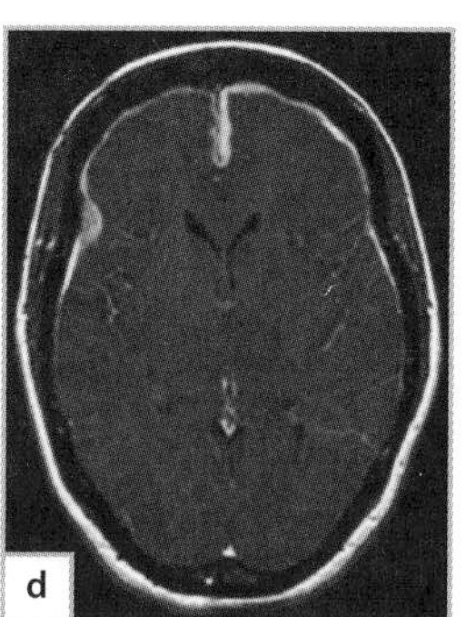

Figure 16.10 Four patients with neurosarcoidosis; focal parenchymal lesions are seen in (a) and (b), hypothalamic involvement in (c) and leptomeningeal thickening in (d).

topical steroid treatment. The episode may last only for a few weeks or months and often does not recur, reflecting the self-limiting nature of this form of sarcoidosis. In general our experience is that this form of uveitis with subacute sarcoidosis has an excellent prognosis.

Chronic granulomatous anterior uveitis

Tending to affect older patients, this form of inflammation is characteristically associated with chronic pulmonary involvement and affects more than 50% of those with sarcoid uveitis. Bilateral involvement is usual, although very asymmetrical disease is not uncommon. Visual loss rather than discomfort is the usual reason for presentation to an ophthalmologist and many patients will have impressive collections of 'mutton-fat' KPs at presentation (**Fig. 16.11**), often in a fairly white eye. Posterior synechiae are the rule and may be well advanced (**Fig. 16.12**). Peripheral anterior synechiae (PAS) may also be formed at presentation and this form of uveitis is commonly accompanied by glaucoma. Some authors feel that tent-shaped PAS are particularly associated with sarcoid uveitis (Kawaguchi et al. 2007). Although iris nodules are sometimes considered a typical part of this form of uveitis, they are actually very uncommon. Even when present, they are often quite small (**Fig. 16.13**). Only rarely is florid nodulation of the iris seen (**Fig. 16.14**), and then usually in association with severe multisystem sarcoidosis. The nodules may become vascularized. This form of uveitis requires vigorous topical treatment and complications may require medical or surgical intervention. Mutton-fat KPs may take weeks to clear. Examination of the fundus, although often difficult in such eyes, is important because granulomatous anterior uveitis is commonly associated with chorioretinal changes.

Intermediate uveitis

Inferior vitreous snowballs, pars plana exudate and often peripheral retinal vascular sheathing are common manifestations of sarcoidosis, being the presenting type of uveitis in 10–20% of sarcoid patients. The perceived incidence of sarcoidosis as a cause of intermediate uveitis varies widely around the world, from about 2% to 20% or more, and of course such discrepancies reflect well-recognized regional variations in the prevalence of sarcoidosis in general. Evidence of focal posterior segment inflammation may also be present but often sarcoid-related intermediate uveitis is clinically indistinguishable from idiopathic types. It is therefore important that all patients presenting with intermediate uveitis are investigated for sarcoidosis.

Retinal vasculitis

Sarcoidosis predominantly affects retinal venules, much less commonly arterioles. Patchy retinal periphlebitis is seen usually in the subacute, rather than the chronic, form of sarcoidosis and is one of the hallmarks

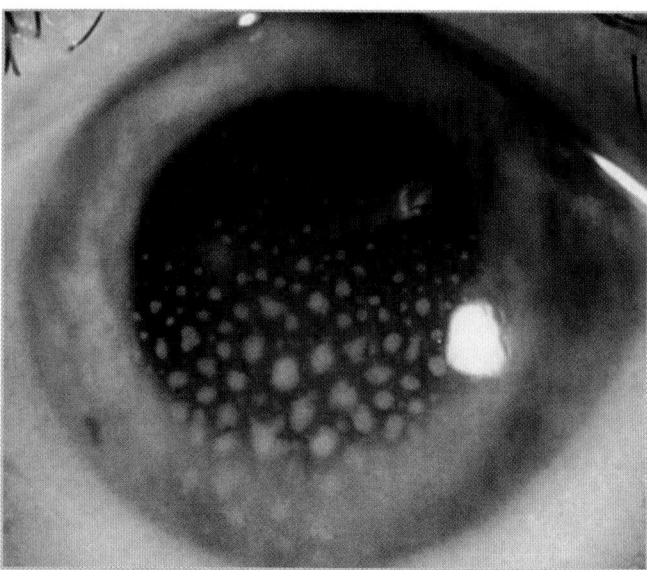

Figure 16.11 Multiple large 'mutton-fat' keratic precipitates in a patient presenting with sarcoidosis.

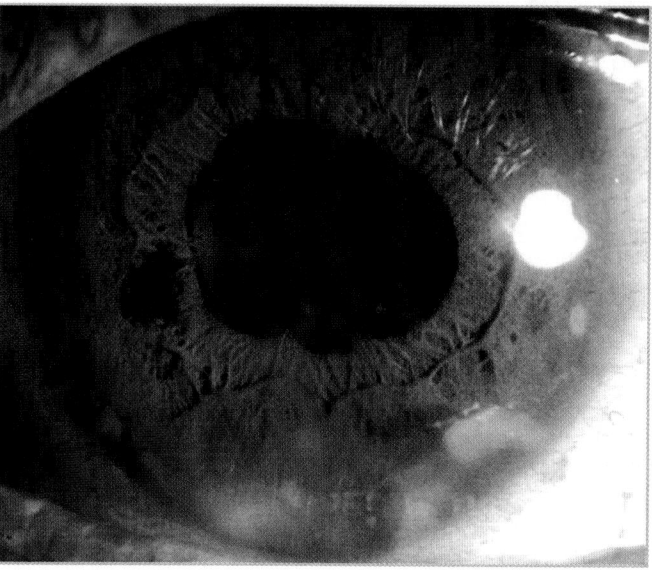

Figure 16.12 Extensive posterior synechiae and large confluent keratic precipitates in a patients with sarcoid uveitis.

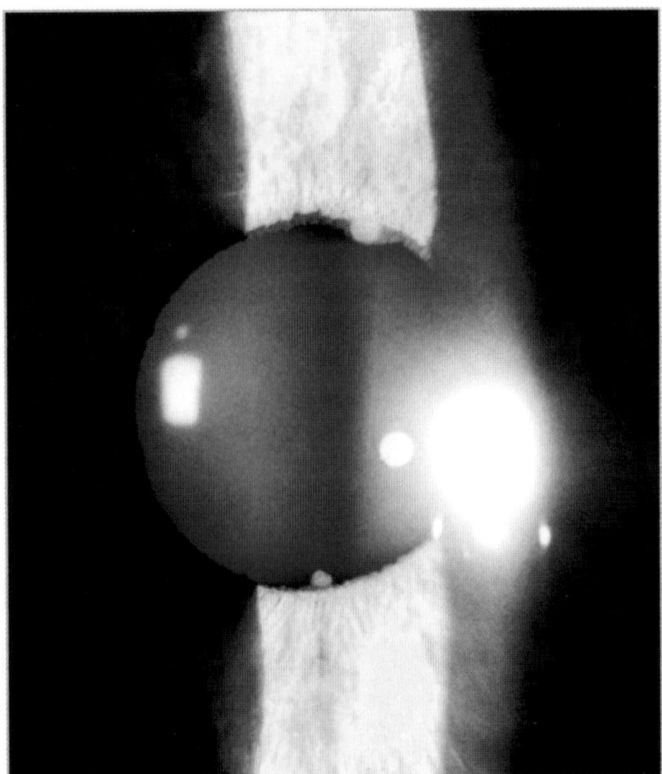

Figure 16.13 Two nodules at the pupil margin in a patient with sarcoid uveitis.

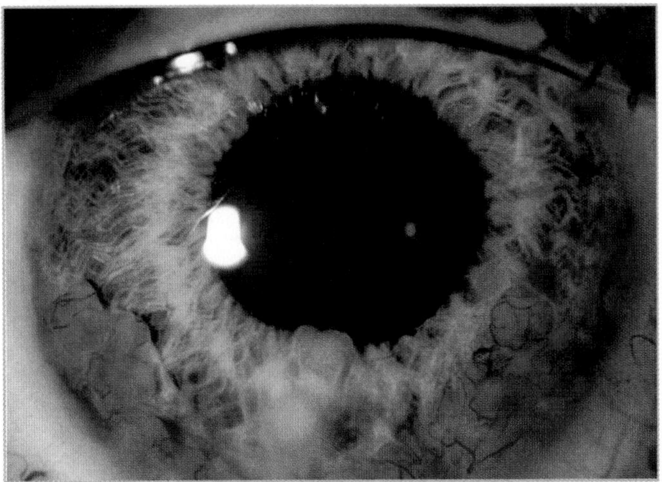

Figure 16.14 Florid confluent and vascularized iris nodules in a young man with severe multisystem sarcoidosis and bilateral granulomatous uveitis.

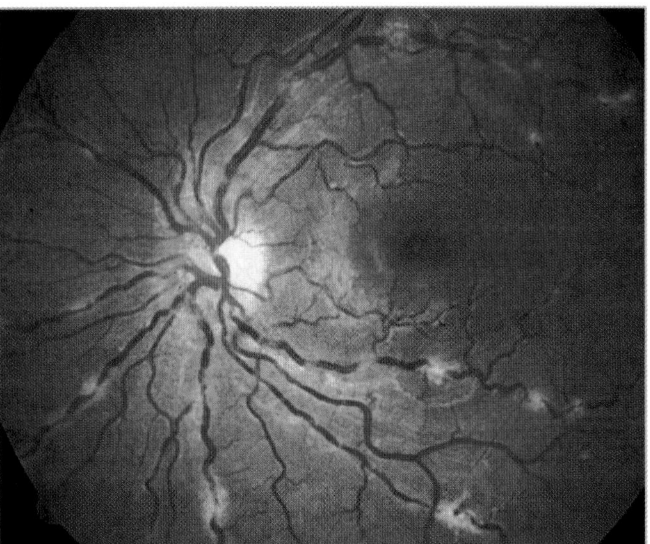

Figure 16.15 Widespread retinal periphlebitis in a 19-year-old young woman with acute sarcoidosis presenting with fever, night sweats, dyspnea and hepatosplenomegaly. The retinal veins are engorged and tortuous and there are patches of perivenous exudate corresponding to areas of vascular leakage.

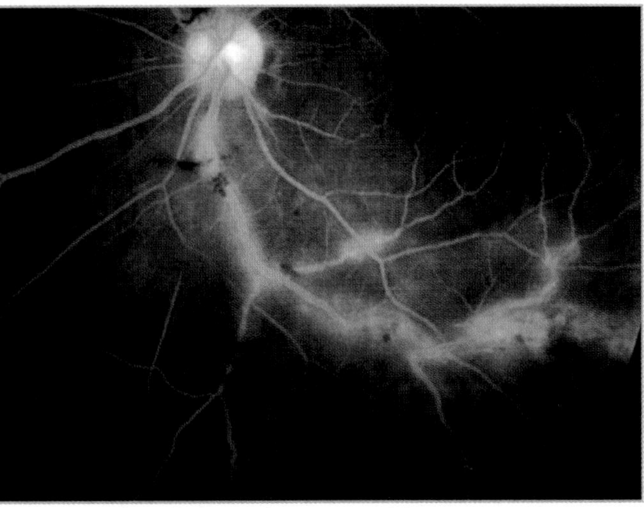

Figure 16.16 Widespread vein wall staining and leakage in a patient with severe sarcoid panuveitis.

of the disease. The veins may be somewhat engorged and tortuous and will be intermittently obscured or surrounded by fluffy white plasma protein exudate (**Fig. 16.15**) from areas of leaky vessel wall. These areas show well on fluorescein angiography (**Fig. 16.16**), which usually shows intermittent vessel wall staining and leakage, but venous occlusion is actually very uncommon in sarcoidosis and is rarely acute.

Although retinal periphlebitis is the characteristic vascular change in retinal sarcoidosis, arteries are clearly affected in some patients. Insidious peripheral vascular shutdown (**Fig. 16.17**) and neovascularization may occur (**Fig. 16.18**). Acute ischemic vasculitis is rare but has been reported (Suresh and Jones 1999). There is a tendency to arterial ectasia formation, sometimes with frank macroaneurysm (**Fig. 16.19**), especially in older women (Rothova and Lardenove 1998), particularly those with associated multifocal choroiditis. Further studies have shown that sarcoidosis is very strongly associated with this finding, and the phenomenon has recently been included in the list of suggestive diagnostic features of the disease (Herbort et al. 2009).

Choroidal involvement

Multifocal choroiditis is the second hallmark of posterior segment sarcoidosis. Lesions are likely to be in various stages of evolution, actively inflamed foci being pale, creamy-yellow and indistinct, often with slightly oval shapes (**Fig. 16.20**), healed areas showing pigmentary scarring. For unknown reasons, the inferior and nasal choroid are particularly likely to be affected, although in some cases circumferential

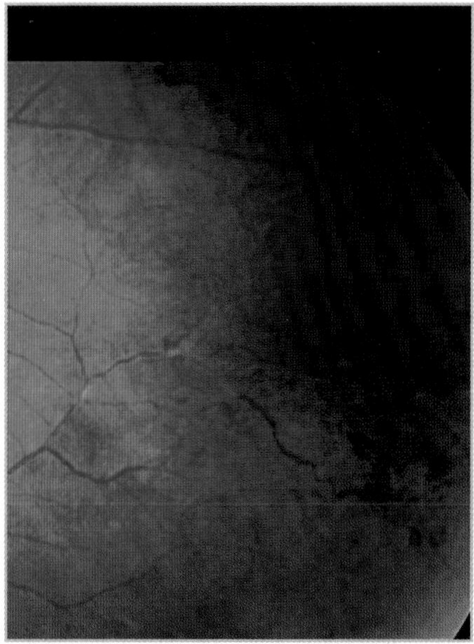

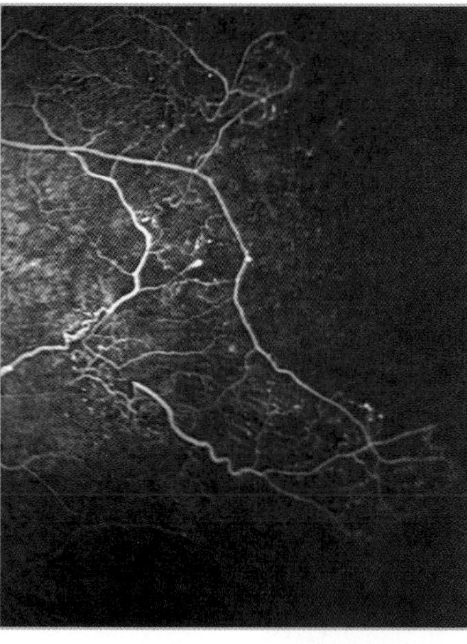

Figure 16.17 Peripheral vascular occlusion in a patient with sarcoidosis. In addition to venous caliber changes, beading and shunting there is arteriolar silver-wiring.

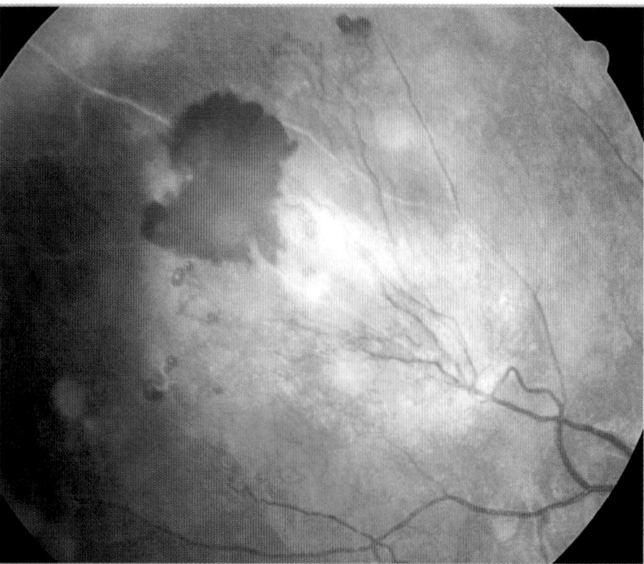

Figure 16.18 Peripheral vascular occlusion with neovascularization and preretinal hemorrhage in sarcoidosis. There is marked telangiectasia and silver-wiring.

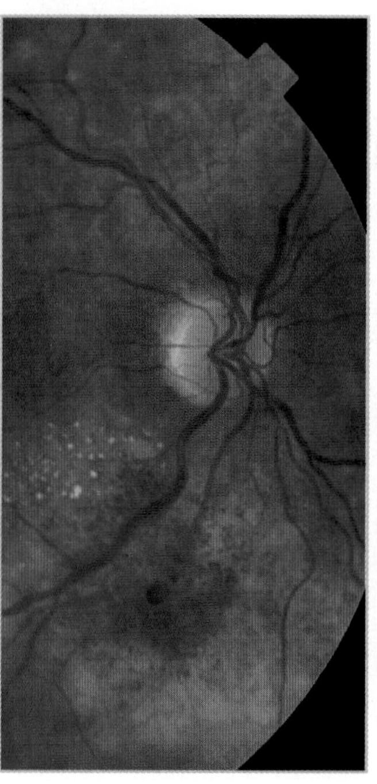

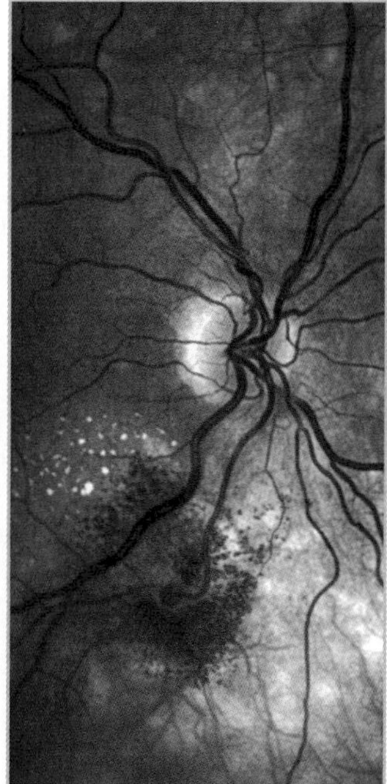

Figure 16.19 An arterial macroaneurysm in a patient with multifocal choroiditis (seen better on red free) in sarcoidosis.

involvement can be extensive. Larger lesions are unusual, but if present may raise the retina (**Fig. 16.21**) and even be associated with subretinal fluid. In such cases the differential diagnosis includes tuberculoma or metastatic carcinoma.

Sarcoidosis is a great mimic and in some circumstances is associated with atypical fundal appearances. Conjunctival biopsies indicative of sarcoidosis have been reported in a group of patients with punctate inner choroidopathy, suggesting an etiological role for sarcoidosis in at least some of these patients (Hershey et al. 1994). Acute posterior multifocal placoid pigment epitheliopathy has been anecdotally described in association with sarcoidosis (Prokosch et al. 2010) and sarcoidosis may certainly mimic birdshot retinochoroidopathy (Read et al. 2000).

Optic nerve involvement

Very unusually a granuloma will directly affect the optic nerve head (**Fig. 16.22**), being typically near the disk margin and yellowish in color. Larger lesions can be visually destructive (**Fig. 16.23**), by causing either nerve fiber bundle field defects or vascular occlusion. The optic nerve may also be involved in neurosarcoidosis and this may manifest as nerve head edema (sometimes with opticociliary shunt formation or vascular occlusion) or progressive optic atrophy. On rare occasions a fundus presents a picture so strongly suggestive of sarcoidosis that it is itself virtually pathognomonic (**Fig. 16.24**).

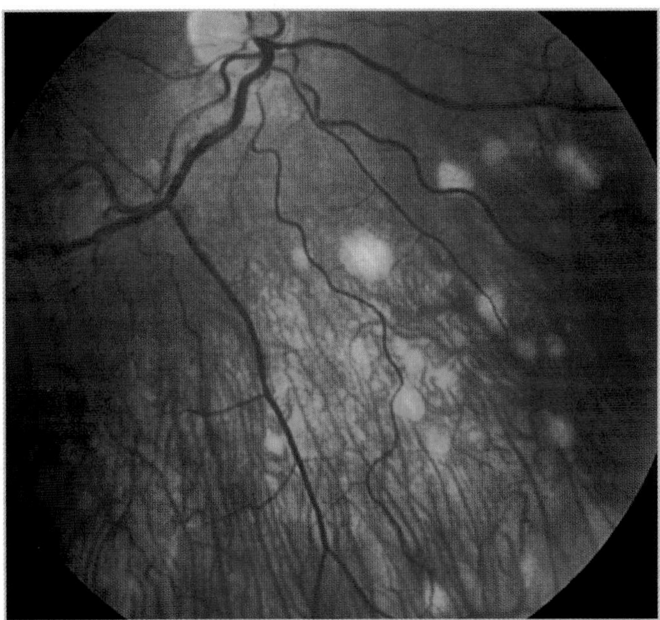

Figure 16.20 Multifocal choroiditis especially affecting the inferonasal retina. The active lesions are smallish, creamy and with slightly indistinct edges.

Sequelae of inflammation

As with any chronic insidious anterior uveitis, posterior synechiae may lead to pupil block, and PAS may lead to glaucoma that is likely to need enhanced drainage surgery. Chronic inflammation, together with the use of systemic steroids, may lead to cataract formation. Both cataract and glaucoma are common in sarcoid uveitis, and the latter is definitely a marker for severe disease (Asukata et al. 2006) and poorer prognosis. Retinal or optic disk neovascularization may respond to systemic steroid therapy. Subretinal neovascular membranes are extremely uncommon in sarcoidosis (Perentes et al. 2005) and are managed as for other uveitic membranes (see Chapter 7).

Diagnosis

Histological or cytological diagnosis

By definition a confirmed diagnosis of sarcoidosis requires histology. However, biopsy is invasive and there are many circumstances where a panel of circumstantial evidence will combine to make the presumptive diagnosis of sarcoidosis acceptable. However, where the differential diagnosis is difficult, and definitive diagnosis would change patient management, histological diagnosis assumes a greater importance. Any straightforward opportunity to obtain histological confirmation should be pursued. For many years the Kveim–Siltzbach test (in which a suspension of human-derived sarcoid lymph node or splenic material was injected intradermally, then biopsied 6 weeks later to identify new granulomas) was used as a proxy for lesional biopsy. In the UK, the test was abandoned over a decade ago as material became unavailable and the concern over prion diseases mounted. It should now be regarded as historical.

Bronchoscopic cytology

Bronchoalveolar lavage requires the use of a fiberoptic bronchoscope under sedation. The scope is inserted into a distal bronchus and 100 ml of buffered saline is injected and then reaspirated. The aspirate is spun down and cytologically analyzed. In sarcoidosis there are usually increased lymphocyte counts, particularly activated CD4 cells. A proportion of lymphocytes > 15% is alone highly suggestive of sarcoidosis (sensitivity 90%). A specificity of 94% is obtained if the CD4:CD8 ratio is > 3.5 (Judson 2008). Macrophages are also common but neutrophils and eosinophils are few. Similar cell profiles may be seen in pulmonary TB, allergic alveolitis and other conditions, therefore cytology alone can never be diagnostic.

Transbronchial, endobronchial or mediastinal biopsy

Transbronchial lung biopsy (TLB) may be diagnostic, especially if the recommended four to five sites are sampled. It can provide a histological diagnosis of sarcoidosis in 40–90% of those with compatible

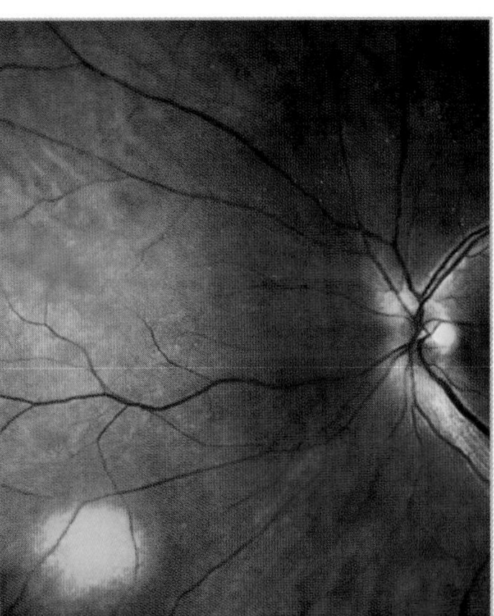

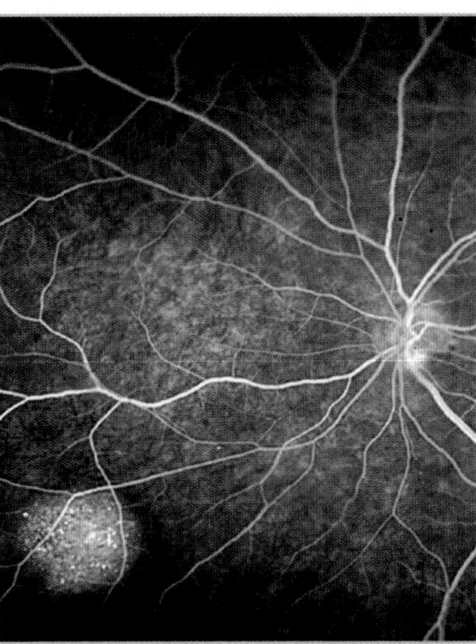

Figure 16.21 A large choroidal granuloma in a man with sarcoidosis, lifting overlying retina, in color and fluorescein angiography.

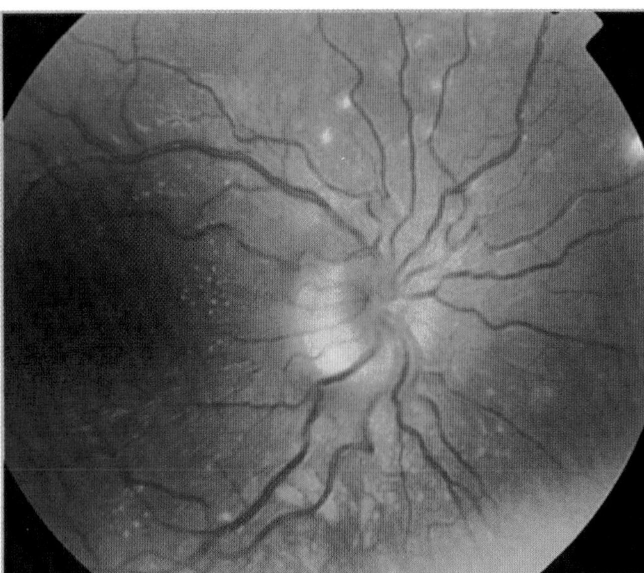

Figure 16.22 Direct optic nerve head involvement in sarcoidosis, with multifocal choroiditis and macular exudate.

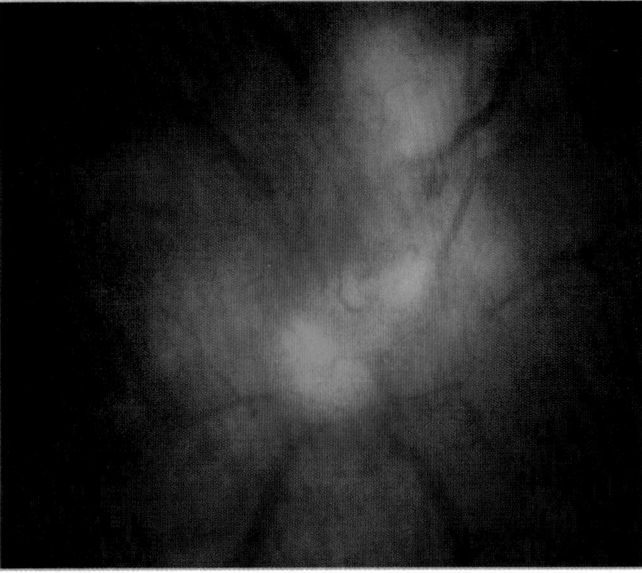

Figure 16.23 A large optic nerve head and peripapillary granuloma seen through dense vitritis in a young man with sarcoidosis.

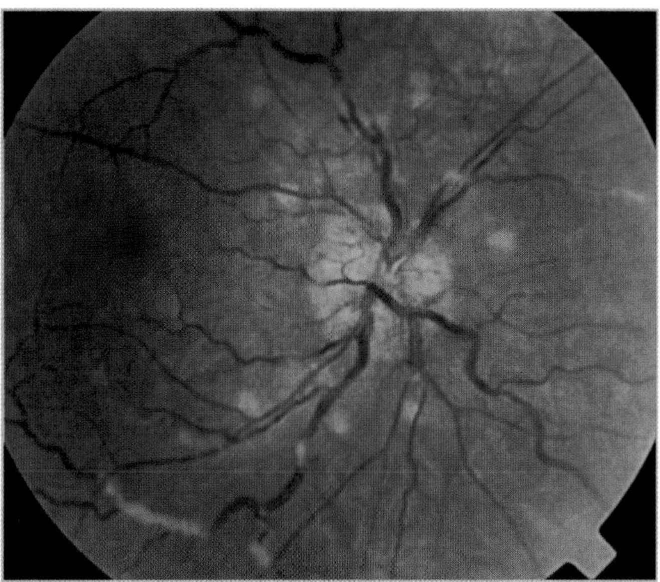

Figure 16.24 A paradigm for sarcoidosis: multifocal choroiditis, patchy periphlebitis and papillitis.

ocular lesions, even when no other evidence of pulmonary or systemic involvement was present (although as expected the pick-up rate is higher where parenchymal disease is present on chest radiograph), and where the hila appeared radiologically normal. Although other granulomatous diseases such as histoplasmosis and brucellosis may cause pulmonary non-caseating granulomas, the ocular signs are unlikely to cause confusion in the differential diagnosis. Transbronchial lung biopsy is an invasive procedure that carries a small morbidity, including the risk of pneumothorax and hemothorax. It will therefore be used with circumspection by most chest physicians in the absence of pulmonary symptoms or radiological signs. Endobronchial biopsy has a lower diagnostic rate of 40–60% but if performed together with TLB the combined diagnostic rate is higher than for TLB alone. Transthoracoscopic peripheral lung biopsy or mediastinoscopy with node biopsy may be used if considered justified. However, these are major invasive procedures. More recently, ultrasound-guided, endobronchial, fine-needle biopsy has produced high diagnostic rates with low morbidity (Tremblay et al. 2009) and is likely to replace the mediastinal approach biopsy in the great majority of cases.

Conjunctival and lacrimal gland biopsy

The conjunctiva is readily accessible for biopsy and the procedure has less morbidity than for many other sites. The use of blind biopsy (where no lesions are visible) in patients with possible sarcoidosis has generated much heat in discussion, the pick-up rate being unimpressive and certainly not justifying the procedure as a first-line biopsy site for possible sarcoid patients as some have suggested. However, in examining the patient with suspected sarcoidosis, the ophthalmologist should always take the opportunity to look for conjunctival granulomas, especially in the inferior fornix. Biopsy of visible lesions may be highly productive, and the procedure is associated with low morbidity and discomfort. Although 20% of lacrimal gland biopsies provide diagnostic histology in suspected sarcoidosis, the procedure has significant potential for damage to lacrimal ducts with consequent dry eye. As the disease may itself reduce lacrimal gland function, biopsy is not recommended unless the lacrimal gland is enlarged and diagnosis has not yet been established.

Biopsy of skin and other sites

Cutaneous sarcoidosis is extremely heterogeneous (Marchell and Judson 2007) but biopsy of a suspicious skin lesion, if accessible and cosmetically acceptable, is highly likely to be productive and may avoid more invasive biopsy. Biopsy of skin nodules in acute sarcoidosis is less productive, and, although some instances of non-caseating granulomas have been reported in classic erythema nodosum, biopsy of these lesions is often unhelpful and therefore unjustified in most instances. Palpable lymph nodes may also be productive. Modern fine-needle aspiration biopsy of the liver is associated with low morbidity, but its use may be justifiable only in the presence of abnormal liver function. Positive histology has been found in 70% of those with active proven sarcoidosis elsewhere. Other biopsy choices are driven by symptomatic organ involvement.

Immune changes

Sarcoidosis appears to depress delayed-type hypersensitivity reactions, and patients with the disease react poorly to antigens (anergy). Atopy is also probably suppressed. The causes of this phenomenon remain under investigation. It is known that dendritic cells malfunction, and an imbalance in regulatory T-cell function has been proposed (Miyara et al. 2006). In practice a tuberculin test may prove negative after documented prior positivity. The test is not particularly useful except in those instances where tuberculosis is high on the differential diagnosis list. A positive reaction to a 1-unit PPD (purified protein derivative) test makes a diagnosis of sarcoidosis unlikely, whereas a negative reaction to a 100-U PPD test supports, although does not prove, the diagnosis. Some centers use an extended anergy panel, where a range of allergens and antigens is applied by skin prick, in an attempt to identify a wide anergic response. The method has not gained widespread acceptance as a diagnostic test.

Hematological changes

In widespread active disease, mild normochromic anemia is common, as is a raised erythrocyte sedimentation rate (ESR). Eosinophilia may be seen. Where splenomegaly is present, thrombocytopenia or hemolytic anemia may be present.

Serum angiotensin-converting enzyme

Angiotensin-converting enzyme (ACE) is normally present throughout the human body but especially in endothelial cells of the lung and kidney and in seminal fluid. It is responsible for the conversion of angiotensin I to angiotensin II (a potent vasopressor), and degrades bradykinin (a potent vasodilator), thereby contributing to the control of blood pressure. The enzyme may be synthesized by macrophages under certain conditions, and has been found in epithelioid cells and macrophages in sarcoid granulomas. In sarcoidosis, therefore, and in some other diseases, raised serum ACE levels may be found.

The normal range for serum ACE differs between laboratories depending on the method of assay, but, in general, for adults a normal level is 32.1 ± 8.5 IU/l, with an upper level of normal usually given as 50 or 55 IU/l. Fit children aged > 4 years have higher ACE levels than adults, increasing until puberty when levels may be raised to 40% above normal adult levels. From puberty, levels decline during adolescence (Bénéteau-Burnat et al. 1990). Higher levels are maintained for a longer time in boys (until about age 18) than in girls (until about age 14). The reasons for these changes are unknown, but the greater relative mass of active lymphoid tissue, which degrades in adolescence, may play a part. In our clinic we will accept levels of up to 70 IU/l as normal in children when considering juvenile sarcoidosis.

ACE levels may also be raised in conditions that are part of the differential diagnosis of sarcoid, including pulmonary (4% of patients) or miliary TB (90%), atypical mycobacterial infection, systemic fungal infection, leprosy (40%), Hodgkin's disease, allergic alveolitis, or fibrosing lung disease including silicosis (30%), asbestosis (17%), berylliosis and lung carcinoma. Raised levels are also seen in almost all patients with Gaucher's disease, most with hyperthyroidism, and in pneumocystosis, alcoholic liver disease, diabetes mellitus and systemic lupus erythematosus. However, where uveitis is the starting point for ACE estimation, the likelihood of sarcoidosis is obviously greater than several others on this list. It is also said that only sarcoidosis is capable of generating very high levels of ACE. Some would argue that, if the level is > 100 IU/l, the specificity for sarcoidosis approaches 100%.

Sarcoidosis is by far the most common cause of raised ACE levels. The sensitivity of the test is about 80%, but opinions on specificity differ widely, ranging between 60% and 95%. In sarcoidosis, levels are thought to represent the total body mass of secreting granulomas, so very high ACE levels tend to occur in those with clinically obvious disease, whereas, in those with limited organ involvement, levels may not be raised. In some forms of sarcoidosis, particularly neurosarcoid, ACE levels are often normal. However, in the presence of uveitis within the accepted spectrum of sarcoidosis, a raised ACE level is highly significant but normal ACE levels cannot rule out the disease. It is now known that the individual's capability of secreting ACE is altered by the possibility of insertions or deletions at the ACE gene (Kruit et al. 2007), and therefore it has been suggested that a correcting factor be inserted after testing. The use of ACE inhibitors (increasingly common as first-line treatments for systemic hypertension) is known to reduce ACE levels, often very substantially, but their effect on levels in patients with sarcoidosis has not been well quantified. Our practice, when requesting ACE levels in patients suspected of sarcoidosis, is to note when the patient is taking an ACE inhibitor and to apply an informal upward 'correction,' while being aware that the investigation is much less valuable.

For an ACE level raised to > 50 IU/l, a predictive value approaching 50% has been found (ie the patient has almost a 50% chance of having sarcoidosis based on this result alone). Further interpretation should then depend on ocular and other signs. In the absence of other diseases on the above list, and in the absence of any other evidence of a different disease, we would accept, for a patient exhibiting ocular disease 'typical' of sarcoidosis, any raised ACE level as being presumptive of the disease, even in the absence of other symptoms and signs. Others agree (Stavrou et al. 1997). Systemic steroid treatment rapidly lowers ACE levels in those with sarcoidosis, so serum samples for diagnosis must be taken first. Physicians often use ACE levels as a marker for disease activity, but the ophthalmologist rarely has to call upon indirect methods in the context of treated uveitis.

Serum lysozyme

Lysozyme is an enzyme capable of breaking down bacterial cell walls. It is a normal component of tears, saliva and serum, but is thought to be secreted by granuloma cells and levels are raised in granulomatous disease, including sarcoidosis. Levels are considered raised if 8 mg/l or above. This level, with a predictive value for sarcoidosis of a mere 12%, means that the test has much lower specificity for sarcoidosis than serum ACE estimation. For this reason many laboratories, including our own, have withdrawn serum lysozyme estimation. However, the increasingly common use of ACE inhibitors may give the test a 'second wind'; the old but neglected finding (Baarsma et al. 1987), that using a combination of results > 40 IU/l for ACE and 10 mg/l for lysozyme, the predictive value rises to 83%, may lead to a reintroduction of lysozyme testing.

Calcium metabolism

Sarcoidosis can cause changes in calcium metabolism but only 2% are symptomatic due to hypercalcemia. Biochemical changes will resemble hypervitaminosis D, including hypercalcemia (sometimes as high as 4 mmol/l), normal serum phosphate, serum phosphatase either normal or slightly raised, and elevated urine calcium (usually 10–20 mmol/l in 24 h). A raised plasma urea may also be found. We do not routinely use detailed investigation of calcium metabolism for diagnosis, but a 24-h urine calcium estimation is sometimes used, and is the test most likely to be abnormal.

Chest radiography

A posteroanterior chest radiograph should be requested for any non-pregnant patient suspected of having sarcoidosis, whether or not pulmonary symptoms are present. About a third of diagnoses are initially suggested by an abnormal chest radiograph and eventual involvement of lung parenchyma or hilar lymph nodes may occur in over 90% of all patients affected by the disease. If a plain film gives equivocal results, or is reported normal in any patient with ocular signs highly suggestive of sarcoidosis, it is now our practice to request chest HRCT which can be virtually diagnostic (see above).

Gallium-67 scintigraphy

Gallium-67 can become localized at sites of active inflammation in a variety of diseases. This is presumed to be a function of macrophages and possibly of activated lymphocytes. Gallium-67 citrate is injected intravenously and 2 or 3 days later sites of active isotope uptake are demonstrated by imaging with a gamma camera. Whole body imaging is preferable because of the protean nature of sarcoidosis, which may be localized to one or two extrapulmonary sites. The imaging process is sometimes used to identify likely sites for biopsy. Uptake is not specific to sarcoidosis but certain uptake patterns are quite typical of it. Combined lacrimal and salivary gland uptake is known as the 'panda' sign (**Fig. 16.25**), whereas uptake into the right paratracheal and bilateral hilar nodes is known as the 'lambda' sign. This sign is virtually pathognomonic of sarcoidosis. Orbital uptake may be a function not only of lacrimal gland and lymphoid foci of the conjunctiva, but also of the uvea itself, and is typical of acute, rather than chronic, sarcoidosis. Gallium-67 uptake into lacrimal and salivary glands may also be seen in Sjögren's disease, TB and after radiation treatment. In both pulmonary and extrapulmonary sites, both inflammatory and neoplastic disease may cause ^{67}Ga uptake. The test is therefore sensitive for sarcoidosis but not particularly specific. The use of both ^{67}Ga scanning and serum ACE level together, it is claimed (Neves et al. 1994), produces specificity approaching 100% for sarcoidosis. However, in practice scanning is expensive and only rarely used as part of a diagnostic system.

A diagnostic protocol for sarcoidosis

The individual ophthalmologist, being aware of the characteristics of sarcoidosis in his or her region, will usefully devise an appropriate protocol for diagnosis (Jones 2002b). In this clinic, any patient exhibiting signs of sarcoid-related uveitis (including all patients with intermediate uveitis of unproven etiology) and in whom a diagnosis of sarcoidosis has not already been made, will undergo plain chest radiograph, serum ACE estimation and liver/renal function tests. Visible conjunctival or skin lesions will be biopsied and those exhibiting pulmonary symptoms or demonstrating radiological parenchymal involvement are referred to our colleague chest physician who runs a specialist sarcoidosis clinic. This is important because, even for asymptomatic patients, baseline lung function should be performed. We request chest HRCT if findings are equivocal. Bronchopulmonary lavage or biopsy is less frequently performed as pick-up rates from CT increase. Calcium metabolism, organ screens or more invasive investigations are reserved for those with severe disease where the differential diagnosis is confusing. Some authors argue that tissue diagnosis should always be pursued to confirm diagnosis. However, in managing over 200 patients with presumed sarcoid uveitis, we have used a pragmatic presumption of the disease on many occasions and only in rare instances has a changed diagnosis been necessary.

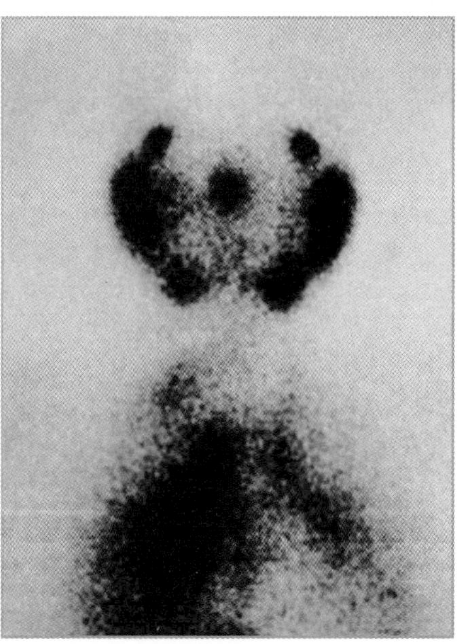

Figure 16.25 A gallium-67 scan of upper torso of a patient with active sarcoidosis, showing uptake into salivary and lacrimal glands, mediastinum and lung parenchyma. (Courtesy of Dr HJ Testa.)

Management

Anterior uveitis is adequately managed with topical steroids. Sometimes periocular steroids are required. A minority of patients will require treatment with systemic steroids, some for long periods, accompanied by the usual precautions. It is our experience that, in most patients with widespread sarcoidosis including uveitis, it is the ophthalmologist who most often requires the highest dose of steroids to control his or her component of the disease. Physicians may use serial serum ACE levels to determine the level of disease activity in those on steroid treatment, but this is not necessary for the ocular component, which can be judged adequately on the basis of symptoms and signs. Where systemic steroid leads to complications, supplementation with deep peribulbar injections may assist.

Immunosuppression for sarcoid uveitis is not well studied. A variety of small case series exist. Methotrexate is the most commonly used immunosuppressive, with generally good results (Baughman 2008). There is little evidence that azathioprine is helpful. Ciclosporin is not considered useful for pulmonary sarcoidosis but may be helpful in some with neurosarcoid. Mycophenolate has been used with some promise in refractory sarcoid in the eye and elsewhere, and more recently, together with infliximab, is considered a potentially very useful treatment for difficult neurosarcoid (Moravan and Segal 2009). There is increasing interest in the use of anti-TNF-α therapy for both pulmonary and extrapulmonary disease. Etanercept does not appear helpful but infliximab shows promise (Baughman et al. 2010). Information on adalimumab is as yet only anecdotal.

Cataract is common in eyes with chronic sarcoid uveitis. Surgery is likely to be straightforward if the usual precautions are followed. Secondary glaucoma is also common. The extensive PAS that can form may occlude the angle internally, but examination of trabeculectomy specimens suggests that, where the angle is open, infiltration and fibrosis of Schlemm's canal may be of substantial importance (Hamanaka et al. 2002). Those requiring surgery benefit from both steroid cover and antimetabolite enhancement.

SARCOIDOSIS IN CHILDREN

Sarcoidosis in children is unusual, but the ophthalmologist has an important role to play in diagnosis. Two clear subsets of children appear to be identified: older children (with disease onset age 5 years or over) almost invariably have lung involvement, with eye, liver, skin and spleen also commonly affected; the much rarer, early onset patients typically develop uveitis, arthropathy and skin rash, only a minority having lung disease. Patients from this subset, although sporadic rather than familial, are likely to demonstrate the same CARD15 mutation as for Blau syndrome (see below).

In the child with uveitis and arthropathy, juvenile chronic arthritis is the prime differential diagnosis. Other seronegative arthropathies should be considered including psoriatic arthritis and juvenile ankylosing spondylitis; Behçet's disease is even less common and Muckle-Wells or chronic infantile neurological cutaneous and articular (CINCA) syndrome is rare. Older children with sarcoidosis are likely to have elevated levels of ACE, but the test cannot be relied on in those under 5, because, even in those with an established diagnosis, levels are usually normal. Enlarged lymph nodes, affected skin or conjunctiva is a therefore site for consideration of biopsy.

The long-term prognosis and the outcome after management of the disease and its complications have not been well reported. Cataract and glaucoma may occur and surgery for either will require special precautions. For glaucoma drainage surgery, the coexistence of two (childhood and uveitis), and possibly a third (racial) risk factors deleterious to the success of drainage surgery, will be challenging.

BLAU SYNDROME AND OTHER GRANULOMATOUS DISEASES

A rare syndrome comprising multisystem granulomatous inflammation closely resembling juvenile sarcoidosis was first described in two American families by Blau (1985) and is otherwise known as **familial juvenile systemic granulomatosis.** It presents in childhood with anterior or posterior uveitis, sometimes including multifocal choroiditis (Latkany et al. 2002), granulomatous skin lesions, arthropathy with periarticular synovial cysts and cranial neuropathies. The disease is autosomal dominant with high penetrance and is virtually identical to, or at least considerably overlaps the clinical spectrum of, infantile sporadic sarcoidosis. At least 30 families and 150 patients worldwide have now been described. Affected patients consistently express a CARD15 (NOD2) mutation (Miceli-Richard et al. 2001), the locus being on chromosome 16. The mutation appears to provoke granulomatous inflammation when triggered, and is also seen in Crohn's disease. It should be considered in the differential diagnosis of childhood sarcoidosis where a family history is identified. Lesions tend to respond to low-dose steroid treatment.

A possibly new disease of infantile-onset panniculitis with uveitis and systemic granulomatosis (Wouters et al. 2007) has recently been described. It does not appear to be associated with *CARD15* mutations. Uveitis has also been associated with granuloma annulare (Oz et al. 2003) and systemic elastolytic granulomatosis (Kurose et al. 1992). The chronic granulomatous disease spectrum is a group of similar disorders characterized by a failure of phagocytosis, with recurrent infections leading to granulomatous change. They are usually X-linked, present in infancy and can include recurrent or chronic uveitis (Al-Muhsen et al. 2009).

REFERENCES

Al-Muhsen S, Al-Hemidan A, Al-Shehri A, et al. Ocular manifestations in chronic granulomatous disease in Saudi Arabia. *J Am Assoc Pediatr Ophthalmol Strabismus* 2009;**13**:396–9.

Asukata Y, Ishihara M, Hasumi Y, et al. Ocular conditions associated with severe or intractable ocular sarcoidosis. *Nippon Ganka Kiyo* 2006;**57**:877–80.

Baarsma GS, La Hey E, Glasius E, et al. The predictive value of serum angiotensin converting enzyme and lysozyme levels in the diagnosis of ocular sarcoidosis. *Am J Ophthalmol* 1987;**104**:211–17.

Baughman RP, Teirstein AS, Judson MA, et al. Clinical characteristics of patients in a case control study of sarcoidosis. *Am J Respir Crit Care Med* 2001;**164**:1885–9.

Baughman RP, Costabel U, duBois RM. Treatment of sarcoidosis. *Clin Chest Med* 2008;**29**:533–48.

Baughman RP, Lower EE, Kaufman AH. Ocular sarcoidosis. *Semin Respir Crit Care Med* 2010;**31**:452–62.

Bénéteau-Burnat B, Baudin B, Morgant G, et al. Serum angiotensin-converting enzyme in healthy and sarcoidotic children: comparison with the reference interval for adults. *Clin Chem* 1990;**36**:344–6.

Blau EB. Familial granulomatous arthritis, iritis, and rash. *J Pediatr* 1985;**107**:689–93.

Clement DS, Postma G, Rothova A, et al. Intraocular sarcoidosis: association of clinical characteristics of uveitis with positive chest high-resolution computed tomography findings. *Br J Ophthalmol* 2010;**94**:219–22.

Demedts M, Wells AU, Anto JM, et al. Interstitial lung disease: an epidemiological overview. *Eur Respir J* 2001;32(suppl):2S–16S.

Doycheva D, Deuter C, Stuebiger N, Zierhut M. Interferon-alpha-associated presumed ocular sarcoidosis. *Graefes Arch Clin Exp Ophthalmol* 2009;**247**:675–80.

Edelston C, Pearson A, Joynes E, et al. The ocular and systemic prognosis of patients presenting with sarcoid uveitis. *Eye* 1999;**13**:748–53.

Hamanaka T, Takei A, Takemura T, Oritsu M. Pathological study of cases with secondary open-angle glaucoma due to sarcoidosis. *Am J Ophthalmol* 2002;**134**:17–26.

Heinzerling LM, Anliker MD, Muller J, et al. Sarcoidosis induced by interferon-alpha in melanoma patients: incidence, clinical manifestations and management strategies. *J Immunother* 2010;**33**:834–9.

Herbort CP, Rao NA, Mochizuki M, et al. International criteria for the diagnosis of ocular sarcoidosis: results of the first international workshop on ocular sarcoidosis. *Ocul Immunol Inflamm* 2009;**17**:160–9.

Hershey JM, Pulido JS, Folberg R, et al. Non-caseating conjunctival granuloma in patients with multifocal choroiditis and panuveitis. *Ophthalmology* 1994:**101**:596–601.

Jones NP. Sarcoidosis. *Curr Opin Ophthalmol* 2002a;**13**:393–6.

Jones NP. Sarcoidosis and uveitis. *Ophthalmol Clin N Am* 2002b;**15**:319–26.

Jones NP, Mochizuki M. Sarcoidosis: Epidemiology and clinical features. *Ocul Immunol Inflamm* 2010;**18**:72–9.

Joseph FG, Scolding NJ. Neurosarcoidosis: a study of 30 new cases. *J Neurol Neurosurg Psychiatry* 2009;**80**:297–304.

Judson MA. The diagnosis of sarcoidosis. *Clin Chest Med* 2008;**29**:415–27.

Kawaguchi T, Hanada A, Horie S, et al. Evaluation of characteristic ocular signs and systemic investigations in ocular sarcoidosis patients. *Jpn J Ophthalmol* 2007;**51**:121–6.

Kruit A, Grutters JC, Gerritson WB, et al. ACE I/D-corrected Z scores to identify normal and elevated ACE activity in sarcoidosis. *Respir Med* 2007;**101**:510–15.

Kurose N, Nakagawa H, Iozumi K, et al. Systemic elastolytic granulomatosis with cutaneous, ocular, lymph nodal and intestinal involvement. Spectrum of annular elastolytic giant cell granuloma and sarcoidosis. *J Am Acad Dermatol* 1992;**26**:359–63.

Latkany PA, Jabs DA, Smith JR, et al. Multifocal choroiditis in patients with familial juvenile systemic granulomatosis. *Am J Ophthalmol* 2002;**134**:897–904.

Lynch JP III. Computed tomography scanning in sarcoidosis. *Semin Respir Crit Care Med* 2003;**24**:393–418.

Lynch JP III, Ma YL, Koss MN, et al. Pulmonary sarcoidosis. *Semin Respir Crit Care* Med 2007;**28**:53–74.

Marchell RM, Judson MA. Chronic cutaneous lesions of sarcoidosis. *Clin Dermatol* 2007;**25**:295–302.

McGrath DS, Daniil Z, Foley P, et al. Epidemiology of familial sarcoidosis in the UK. *Thorax* 2000;**55**:751–4.

Miceli-Richard C, Lesage S, Rybojad M, et al. *CARD15* mutations in Blau syndrome. *Nat Genet* 2001;**29**:19–20.

Mihailovic-Vucinic V, Jovanivic D. Pulmonary sarcoidosis. *Clin Chest Med* 2008;**29**:459–73.

Miyara M, Amoura Z, Parizot C, et al. The immune paradox of sarcoidosis and regulatory T cells. *J Exp Med* 2006;**203**:359–70.

Moravan M, Segal BM. Treatment of CNS sarcoidosis with infliximab and mycophenolate mofetil. *Neurology* 2009;**72**:337–40.

Neves RA, Rodrigues A, Power WJ, et al. The value of combined serum angiotensin converting enzyme and gallium scan in the diagnosis of ocular sarcoidosis. In: Nussenblatt RB, Whitcup SM, Caspi RR, Gery I (eds), Advances in Ocular Immunology. *Amsterdam*: Elsevier, 1994:353–356.

Newman L, Rose C, Bresnitz R, et al. A case control etiologic study of sarcoidosis: environmental and occupational risk factors. *Am J Respir Crit Care Med* 2004;**170**:1324–30.

Oz O, Tursen U, Yildirim O, et al. Uveitis associated with granuloma annulare. *Eur J Ophthalmol* 2003;**13**:93–5.

Perentes Y, Tran VT, Sickenberg M, Herbort CP. Subretinal neovascular membranes complicating uveitis: frequency, treatments and visual outcome. *Ocul Immunol Inflamm* 2005;**13**:219–24.

Pietinalho A, Hiraga Y, Hosoda Y, Lofroos AB, Yamaguchi M, Selroos O. The frequency of sarcoidosis in Finland and Hokkaido, Japan. A comparative epidemiological study. *Sarcoidosis* 1995;**12**:61–7.

Prokosch V, Becker H, Thanos S, Stupp T. acute posterior multifocal placoid pigment epitheliopathy with concurrent cerebral vasculitis and sarcoidosis. *Graefes Arch Clin Exp Ophthalmol* 2010;**248**:151–2.

Read RW, Rao NA, Sharma OP. Sarcoid choroiditis initially diagnosed as birdshot choroidopathy. *Sarcoidosis Vasc Diffuse Lung Dis* 2000;**17**:85–6.

Reich JM. Mortality of intrathoracic sarcoidosis in referral vs population-based settings: influence of stage, ethnicity, and corticosteroid therapy. *Chest* 2002;**121**:32–9.

Rosenbaum JT, Pasadhika S, Crouser ED, et al. Hypothesis: sarcoidosis is a STAT1-mediated disease. *Clin Immunol* 2009;**132**:174–83.

Rothova A, Lardenove C. Arterial macroaneurysms in peripheral multifocal choroiditis associated with sarcoidosis. *Ophthalmology* 1998;**105**:1393–7.

Santos E, Shaunak S, Renowden S, Scolding NJ. Treatment of refractory neurosarcoidosis with infliximab. *J Neurol Neurosurg Psychiatry* 2010;**81**:241–6.

Sharma OP. Sarcoidosis around the world. *Clin Chest Med* 2008;**29**:357–363.

Song Z, Marzilli L, Greenlee BL, et al. Mycobacterial catalase-peroxidase is a tissue antigen and target of the adaptive immune response in systemic sarcoidosis. *J Exp Med* 2005;**201**:755–67.

Stavrou P, Linton S, Young DW, et al. Clinical Diagnosis of ocular sarcoidosis. *Eye* 1997;**11**:365–70.

Suresh P, Jones NP. Ischaemic retinal vasculitis in biopsy-proven sarcoidosis. *Eye* 1999;**13**:800–1.

Tremblay A, Stather DR, MacEachern P, et al. A randomised controlled trial of standard vs endobronchial ultrasonography-guided transbronchial needle aspiration in patients with suspected sarcoidosis. *Chest* 2009;**136**:340–6.

Wouters CH, Martin TM, Stichweh D, et al. Infantile onset panniculitis with uveitis and systemic granulomatosis: a new clinicopathological entity. *J Pediatr* 2007;**151**:707–9.

Yasuhara T, Tada R, Nakano Y, et al. The presence of *Propionobacterium* spp. in the vitreous fluid of patients with sarcoidosis. *Acta Ophthalmol* 2005;**83**:364–9.

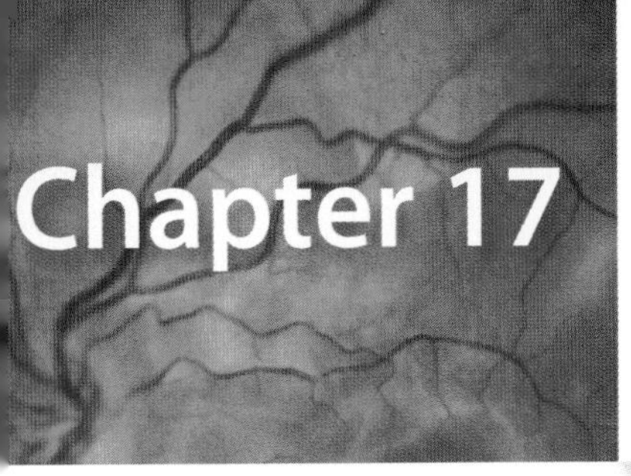

Sympathetic uveitis and Vogt–Koyanagi–Harada syndrome

Sympathetic uveitis and the Vogt–Koyanagi–Harada (VKH) syndrome are probably distinct and separate entities, but they have several close similarities, both clinical and histological. Both are bilateral granulomatous uveitides, usually including widespread choroidal inflammation, of presumed autoimmune etiology. Ocular features, both anterior and posterior, may be strikingly similar, and on occasion certain systemic findings may be common to both conditions. They are considered here together.

SYMPATHETIC UVEITIS (box 17.1)

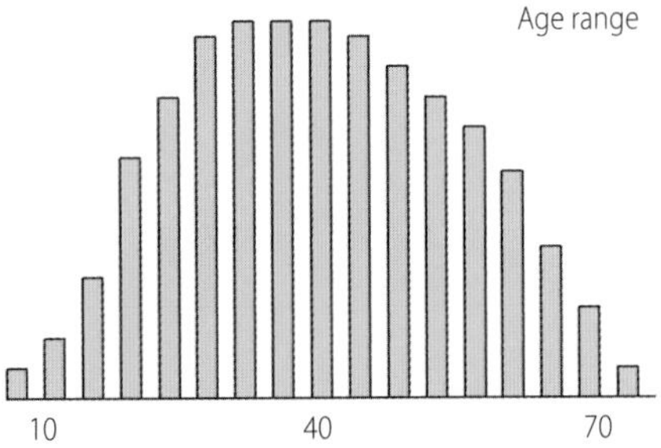

Age range

10 40 70

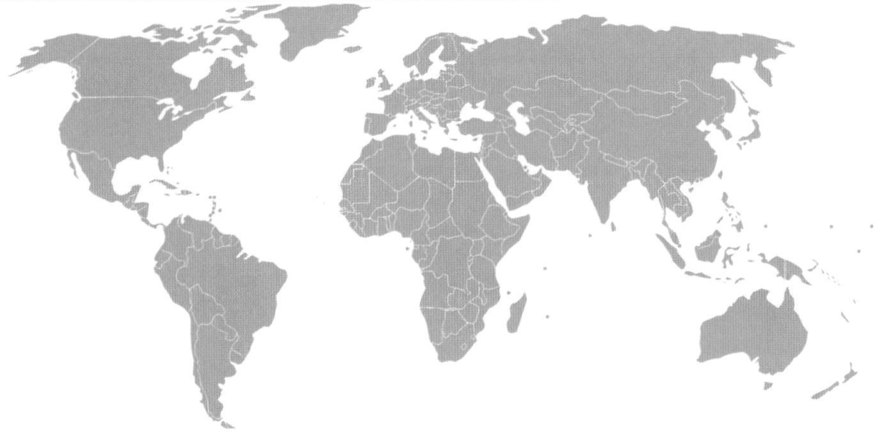

Cause	Presumed autoimmune uveitis after exposure of intraocular antigens, probably photoreceptor components, by ocular penetration, increasingly following elective retinal surgery
Sex, age, race, geography	More young males affected by trauma, but both sexes affected after surgery later in life. No racial characteristics. Worldwide
Systemic disease	Usually none
Ocular disease	Bilateral granulomatous panuveitis with diffuse choroidal involvement, often Dalen–Fuchs nodules and optic nerve inflammation, sometimes retinal vasculitis
Differential diagnosis	VKH syndrome, multifocal choroiditis, phakoanaphylactic uveitis, sarcoidosis
Investigation	Unnecessary. Histological proof if exciting eye enucleated
Management	Prophylactic enucleation of injured eyes. Systemic steroid therapy, often with additional immunosuppression
Prognosis	Reasonable or good with early diagnosis and aggressive management, otherwise blinding

Box 17.1 Sympathetic uveitis

Introduction

Sympathetic uveitis (SU), or sympathetic ophthalmia as it was named by MacKenzie in 1830, is a rare bilateral granulomatous uveitis that characteristically follows penetrating injury or surgery involving uveal tissue. Loss of the fellow eye after penetrating injury had been recognized and feared well before MacKenzie's formal description; the eighteenth-century English oculist Benjamin Duddell wrote of a penetrating injury:

> ... the uvea digested came through the wound in the cornea. The eye that is not hurt must always be drest for fear of a flux of humours upon it: I have seen several that have lost both eyes, though only one has been hurt at first ...

The pathogenesis of SU remains unconfirmed, but it is now generally accepted that the disease is an autoimmune response to intraocular (probably retinal) antigens which gain access by penetrating injury or surgery to conjunctival lymphatics, exposing them to cell-mediated responses. The possibility that an infective agent may also be necessary to provoke SU is speculative, but would help to explain the rarity of the disease following trauma or surgery (during which the extraocular release of small quantities of intraocular antigen must be quite common). The responsible intraocular antigen(s) remains unknown; retinal components including S-antigen and inter-photoreceptor retinoid-binding protein are known to be highly antigenic and are used to induce experimental uveitis in animal models, and are possible suspects; uveal components appear to be less likely candidates.

In at least some patients, SU is associated with HLA-DRB1*04 and HLA-DQA1*03, which appear to be markers for both susceptibility and severity (Kilmartin et al. 2001). Polymorphisms in cytokine genes can also identify likelihood of severity and recurrence, e.g. the interleukin IL-10 –1082 single nucleotide polymorphism (Atan et al. 2005).

No controlled study has been undertaken or could ethically be designed to give the true incidence of SU, and previous estimates are fundamentally flawed by the therapeutic necessity of enucleation in some cases of trauma. Calculations of 0.19% after penetrating injury, and of 0.007% after ocular surgery, have historically been made, although other estimates have differed widely. The disease, it is said, used to be much more common, but claims of increasing rarity must be interpreted in the context of incomparable retrospective studies of dubious epidemiological significance, and against a background of changing methods of management and differing attitudes to early enucleation. A prospective 15-month study in the UK (Kilmartin et al. 2000) identified a minimum incidence of 0.03/100 000 population per year, but not the incidence following trauma or surgery, which remains unknown. However, it can be said with confidence that SU is rare after elective ocular surgery but becomes less rare with consecutive procedures, especially involving the posterior segment. In the west the disease is now probably more common after surgery than trauma, but this ratio probably remains reversed for most of the world. The recent introduction of small-incision, sutureless, vitrectomy techniques has led to some concern that uveal exposure and the risk of SU may be increased, a concern not ameliorated by a few anecdotes of 23-gauge vitrectomy-induced SU. The incidence of post-traumatic SU is substantially reduced when it is the practice to enucleate at-risk blind eyes early (as evidenced by US military records during the Second World War and Korean war, where SU was not recorded).

There is no evidence of a sex bias in SU. The historically higher incidence in males was almost certainly explained by their greater tendency to suffer penetrating injury; in postsurgical sympathetic uveitis the incidence is equal between the sexes. The disease may occur at any age and in any racial group, although it was observed that, despite a high incidence of penetrating injury, the condition is particularly rare in Australasia and the south-west Pacific. This may be a fruitful area for genetic research.

Whatever the true incidence, the risk of SU impinges heavily (and probably disproportionately) on the thoughts of the ophthalmologist dealing with penetrating injury, and has occurred not only after elective posterior segment surgery, but also after glaucoma surgery, cataract surgery and non-penetrating cyclodestructive procedures, particularly using the Nd:YAG (neodymium:yttrium–aluminium–garnet) laser. It has been said that this carries the greatest risk for SU of any ophthalmic surgical procedure. It has also occurred with uveal melanoma (and specifically after ruthenium plaque brachytherapy).

Systemic disease

Typical SU has no systemic features. However, a small minority have symptoms and signs normally associated with the VKH syndrome and sometimes seen in acute posterior multifocal placoid pigment epitheliopathy (APMPPE), namely vitiligo, poliosis, alopecia, hearing disturbance including tinnitus, vertigo and cerebrospinal fluid (CSF) pleocytosis.

Ocular disease

Sympathetic uveitis has been known to start as early as 5 days or as late as 66 years after trauma, but the majority start between 1 and 12 months after the initiating event. In a study of 32 patients (Chan et al. 1995) it was found that, in two cases (6%), the inflammation had started within 2 weeks, 37% within 3 months, 56% within 1 year and 69% within 3 years.

In its typical bilateral granulomatous form, in the context of a clear history of penetrating injury or surgery, SU is not a diagnostic challenge. Symptoms of discomfort or visual loss are usually subacute. Severe anterior chamber inflammation with confluent keratic precipitates (KPs) is often seen. Vitreous opacification is variable but may be so severe that indirect funduscopy is compromised. Choroidal involvement may at its most severe be diffuse and widespread, or multifocal. Papillitis may be seen but peripapillary edema is common (**Fig. 17.1**) and may leave substantial peripapillary atrophy. The archetypal small yellow lesions (Dalen–Fuchs nodules) at the level of Bruch's membrane are seen especially pre-equatorially (**Fig. 17.2**), but may occur anywhere including the posterior pole, and gradually fade into

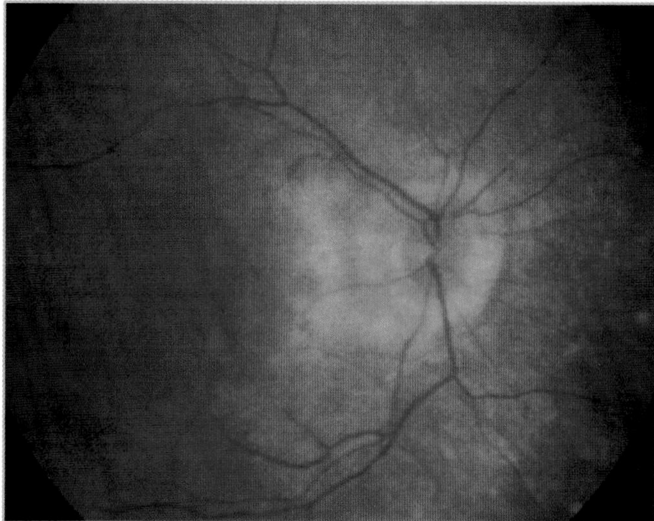

Figure 17.1 Acute sympathetic uveitis demonstrating multifocal choroidal infiltrates and peripapillary pallor representing choroiditis and edema.

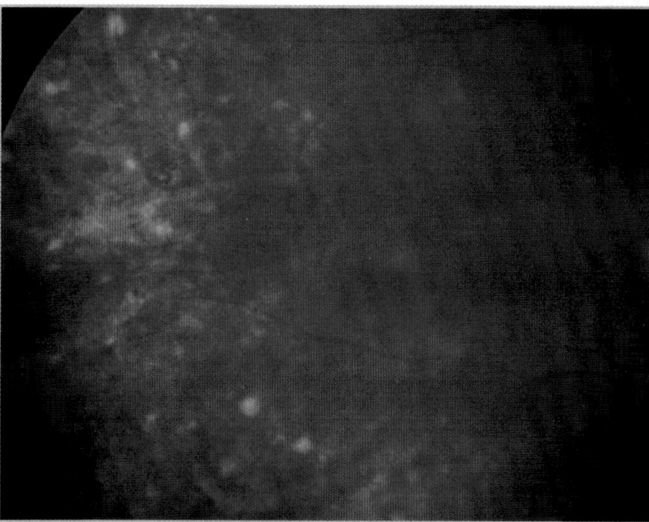

Figure 17.2 Multifocal Dalen–Fuchs nodules scattered on Bruch's membrane, together with more widespread choroidal infiltration, in the retinal periphery in acute sympathetic uveitis.

depigmented scars (**Fig. 17.3**). Exudative retinal detachment may occur, and rarely retinal vasculitis may be seen (**Fig. 17.4**). Anterior segment complications include rapid synechia formation, glaucoma and cataract, and ultimately, in some eyes, severe disorganization (**Fig. 17.5**). In the long term, progressive optic nerve damage may occur, and this may be insidious despite apparent good control of intraocular inflammation. Monitoring with serial visual fields is useful. Despite this constellation of possible complications, if appropriately managed good vision can be maintained in a majority (Galor et al. 2009).

Although historically portrayed as a catastrophic disease, SU actually has a wide spectrum of severity and, for those less severe and less characteristic, diagnosis may be difficult. Often the exciting eye is severely disorganized after its injury, and intraocular inflammation may be difficult to detect and the posterior segment impossible to examine. Inflammation may be non-granulomatous, mild (initially at least) or virtually confined to the anterior segment.

The first histopathological study of SU was written by one of the giants of ophthalmology (Fuchs 1905) and several specimens, mainly of the exciting rather than the sympathizing eye, have been described. Histologically, the whole uveal tract may be thickened by a cellular infiltrate comprising epithelioid and giant cells (which phagocytose choroidal and retinal pigment epithelium [RPE] pigment) and T lymphocytes (**Fig. 17.6**), which sometimes, together with depigmented RPE cells, form the aggregations known as Dalen–Fuchs nodules on the retinal aspect of Bruch's membrane (**Fig. 17.7**). These do not occur in all cases of SU and are not pathognomonic for the disease (also being a feature of VKH syndrome, for example). The cellular infiltrate also sometimes aggregates around posterior ciliary and retinal arterioles and vortex veins. The choriocapillaris is usually spared.

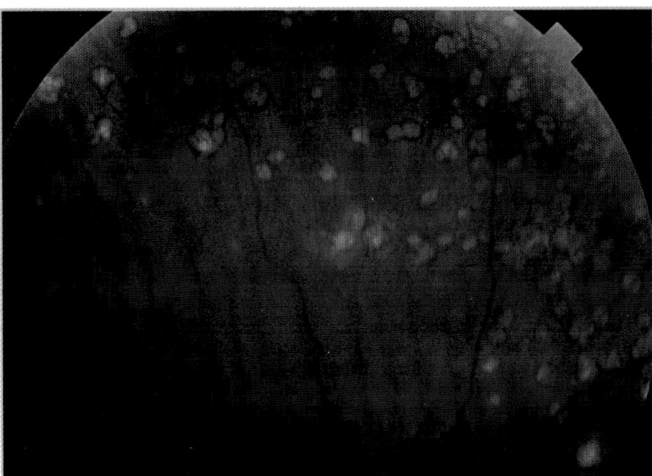

Figure 17.3 Peripheral multifocal chorioretinal atrophy representing the loci of previous Dalen–Fuchs nodules.

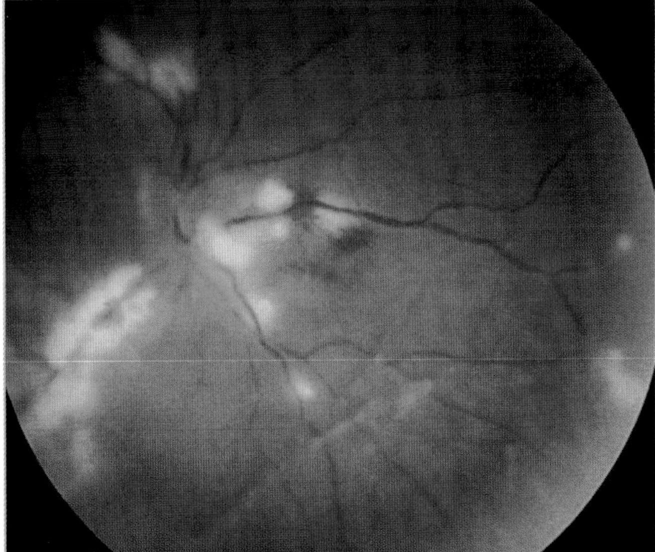

Figure 17.4 Acute retinal vasculitis in sympathetic uveitis, showing perivascular exudate and substantial caliber change.

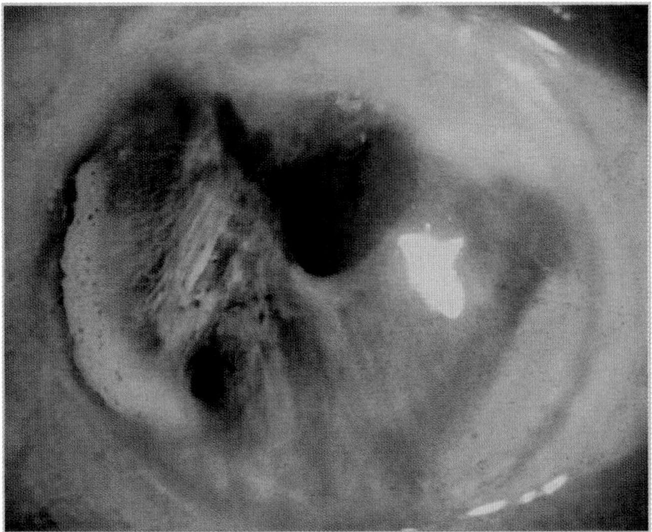

Figure 17.5 The anterior segment sequelae of sympathetic uveitis from the era before systemic immunosuppression: band keratopathy, aphakia, iris atrophy with corectopia and glaucoma.

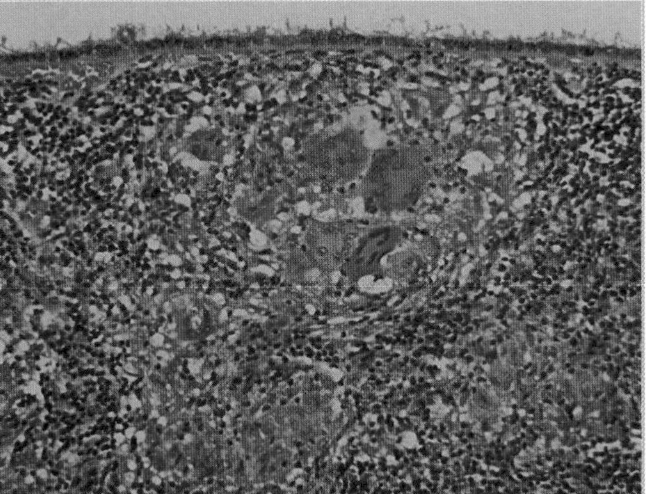

Figure 17.6 Massive granulomatous inflammatory infiltration of the choroid in sympathetic uveitis, comprising especially lymphocytes and epithelioid cells, the latter often agglomerated into multinucleate giant cells as here. The retinal pigment epithelium is at the top. (Courtesy of Dr R Bonshek.)

Diagnosis

Diagnosis is essentially clinical. Fluorescein angiography may be helpful in milder cases and will show early hypo- or hyperfluorescent RPE lesions with late-phase leakage (**Fig. 17.8**), the latter also affecting the optic disk (**Fig. 17.9**). When quiescent, multiple RPE window defects are seen corresponding to visible depigmented scars (**Fig. 17.10**). In general fluorescein angiography is similar to the findings in the VKH syndrome, but with substantially less tendency to serous retinal detachment. In the context of a clear clinical picture the test is not of diagnostic significance.

The clinical diagnosis of sympathetic uveitis is often straightforward, but substantial diagnostic delay sometimes occurs and this has been associated with a worse outcome. On occasion the condition can closely resemble the VKH syndrome, the intraocular appearances sometimes being identical. VKH syndrome is much more common in certain racial groups and a history of penetrating trauma is almost always detectable for SU. The appropriate management for both conditions is in any case similar: early and aggressive.

The differential diagnosis of SU will include other forms of granulomatous uveitis, including sarcoid, which can present with granulomatous anterior uveitis and multifocal fundal lesions (although not usually with a subacute presentation); multifocal choroiditis from other causes should also be considered. In one case of SU, placoid lesions resembling APMPPE have been described. When in doubt, the history of penetrating trauma is crucial.

SU is not the only form of intraocular inflammation capable of affecting the uninjured eye after a penetrating trauma. Phakoanaphylactic uveitis is well described and is usually caused by traumatic disruption of the lens capsule. It may also follow elective extracapsular cataract surgery. Typically a localized nidus of inflammation is centered around

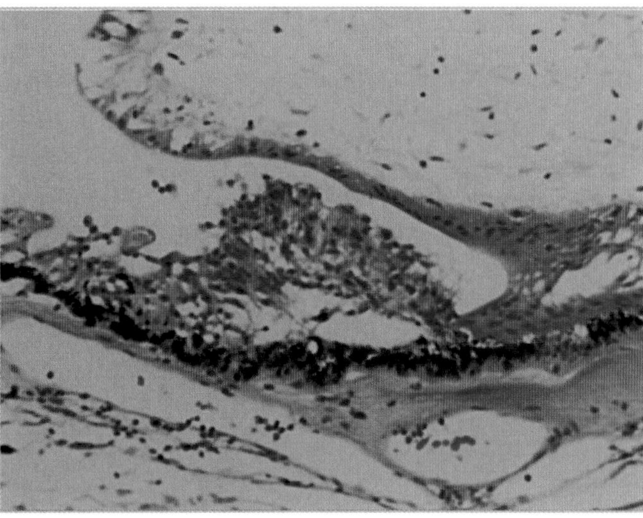

Figure 17.7 A Dalen–Fuchs nodule sits atop a disordered retinal pigment epithelium in acute sympathetic uveitis. (Courtesy of Dr R Bonshek.)

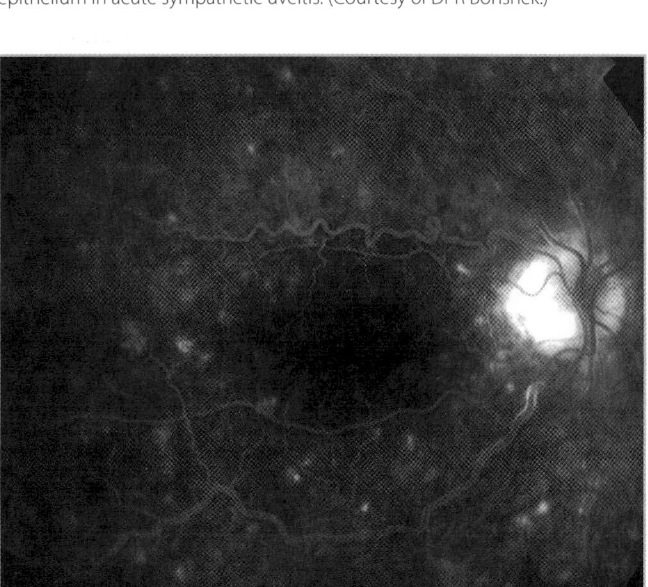

Figure 17.8 Fluorescein angiography in early sympathetic uveitis showing multifocal pinpoint leaks. There is also peripapillary vessel wall staining indicating active retinal vasculitis.

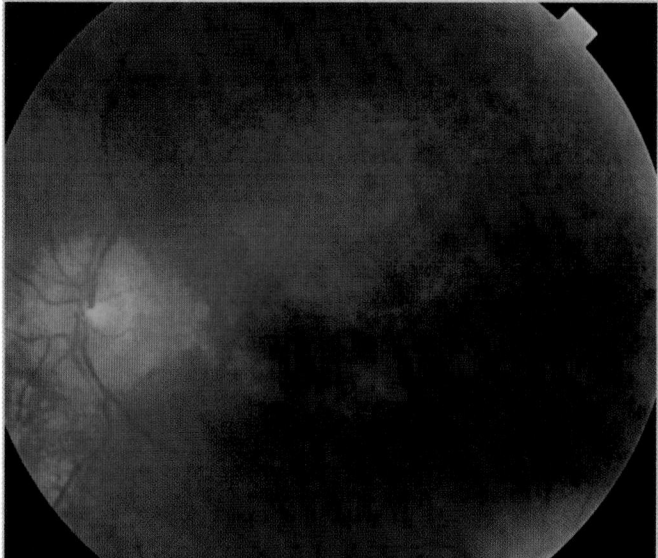

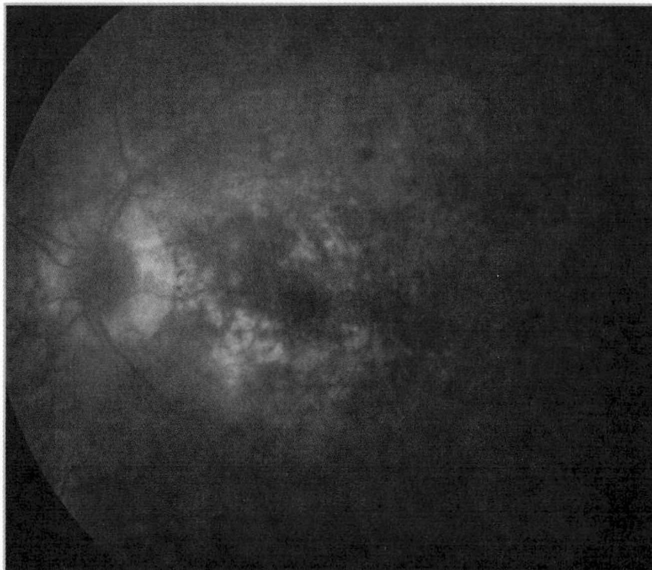

Figure 17.9 Active sympathetic uveitis with substantial vitritis showing widespread pale choroidal involvement and substantial peripapillary atrophy. There is also scattered intraretinal hemorrhage.

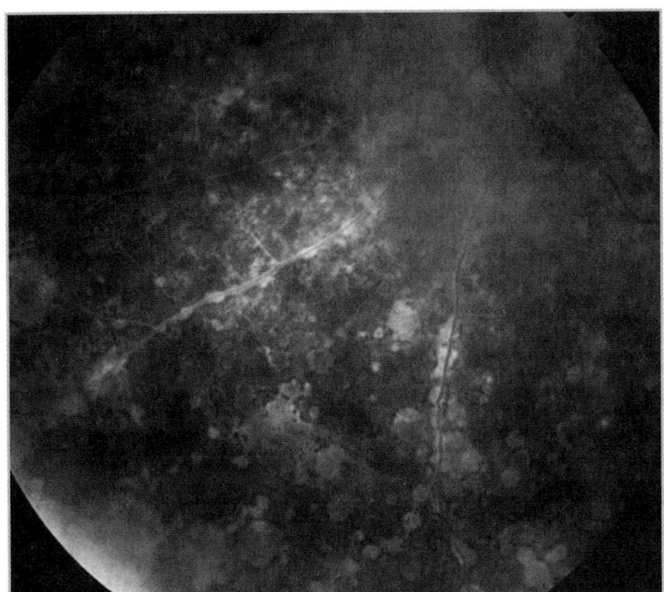

Figure 17.10 Late-phase fluorescein angiography in sympathetic uveitis showing multiple wide areas of choroidal involvement, some of which have a distinctly perivascular pattern. There is also patchy retinal vasculitis.

retained lens matter, at which stage an infective process may be suspected. However, in phakoanaphylactic uveitis the histological appearances are typical. In a minority of instances, the other eye may develop uveitis, although usually after inflammation in the first has subsided. The vitreous may be hazy, but posterior segment lesions are not seen. Sympathetic uveitis and phakoanaphylaxis can coexist; histologically, an element of phakoanaphylactic uveitis has been detected in a high proportion of cases of SU. Recalcitrant phakoanaphylaxis may respond poorly to steroid treatment and removal of the offending lens matter is likely to be necessary.

A condition designated 'sympathetic irritation' has been described, which may comprise anterior segment inflammation with ciliary injection and photophobia, in the uninjured eye after trauma to the other. It tends to be self-limiting. Whether this represents a mild form of sympathetic uveitis or a distinct entity is unknown.

Progressive subretinal fibrosis and uveitis (see later) is a chronic vitritis associated with progressive subretinal lesions which slowly formed a subretinal sheet. Recently the histological examination of an affected eye and the demonstration of autoantibodies against photoreceptor and RPE led to the suggestion that this may be a variant of sympathetic ophthalmia (Wang et al. 2002), hence its mention here. It is, however, dealt with more fully in Chapter 19.

Management

Prevention of Injury

Intraocular penetration, whether traumatic or iatrogenic, is the prerequisite for almost all instances of sympathetic uveitis. Despite national legislature and an increasing awareness of the risks of eye injury, the incidence of ocular trauma, both blunt and penetrating, is capable of further substantial reduction. Ophthalmologists, in regularly treating those who have been injured, some of whom are habitually at increased risk of injury, should not underestimate their preventive and educational role. The expertise of ophthalmologists is essential in the development of safety protocols, especially occupational and sporting, and the enthusiastic participation of a few has contributed substantially to enhanced eye safety. Nevertheless more could be done.

Prophylactic enucleation

Following penetrating trauma, enucleation is the only sure prophylaxis against SU. The ophthalmologist encountering a perforated globe is required, in the knowledge that SU is a risk, to make a judgment with some speed on the future of the injured eye. Although SU has been recorded as early as 5 days after injury, this is exceptional. It is generally agreed that the ophthalmologist has up to 2 weeks in which to assess the potential usefulness of the injured eye, and the safety of allowing it to remain. Fortunately many penetrated globes have reparable damage and, after primary and often secondary surgical intervention, clearly have the potential for substantial vision. There is no question of enucleation in these circumstances. For those eyes that are badly injured and have little visual prognosis, there are several factors that will impinge on the decision whether or not to enucleate.

First, the eye may be perceived to be at greater or lesser risk of SU. In fact there is little evidence that penetrating injuries of different anatomical types carry different risks of SU, but uveal incarceration, either anterior or posterior, has been found to be a consistent factor. Second, the degree of discomfort in, and the cosmetic appearance of, the injured eye will be taken into account. Older enucleation methods often resulted in cosmetic and other problems, including orbit volume deficit, ptosis, socket contracture, implant extrusion and orbital infection. However, current techniques using baseball or hydroxyapatite implants have significantly improved the cosmetic results of enucleation. Nevertheless the modern trend is to consider evisceration rather than enucleation after globe injuries. Concerns have been raised about the risk of SU because of inadvertently retained uveoretinal fragments and anecdotes of SU have been reported. However, no cases were identified in a large retrospective study (du Toit et al. 2008) and the risk may be exaggerated.

Clearly no decision about enucleation can be made without a comprehensive examination of the fellow eye. Any pre-existing problems such as amblyopia, risk factors for retinal detachment or any visual deficit may modify the decision to enucleate the injured eye.

Therapeutic enucleation

The effectiveness of enucleating the exciting eye once bilateral inflammation has started has been the subject of debate. It is difficult to conceive of pathogenic reasons why this procedure should help, because by this stage the autoimmune priming and clonal lymphocytic expansion process is well under way. Nevertheless, it has been suggested that the outcome in the sympathizing eye can be improved in this way. Although this advantage is unproven, it is our practice to discuss it with the patient, and to offer enucleation of the exciting eye if it is blind and cosmetically poor. We would not, however, enucleate an eye with any useful vision.

Medical and surgical treatment

It is now clear that both early recognition and aggressive management contribute to a satisfactory outcome in SU. Most patients will require systemic steroid treatment. Oral prednisolone starting at a dose of 80 mg/day or more is usual. Anterior segment involvement is managed by the use of topical steroids and mydriasis as usual. Often intensive treatment is required at first. Inflammation usually responds well to the initiation of treatment and, after a satisfactory response, the steroid dosage is reduced slowly and progressively. At some stage reactivation of the process is likely, usually in the posterior segment, where fresh Dalen–Fuchs nodules may occur. We have found that peripapillary edema is a sensitive sign of reactivation. If this occurs, once more the process of initiation and reduction must be repeated, but this time with a greater knowledge of the likely maintenance dosage. Occasionally periocular steroids are helpful as adjunctive treatment, but are inadequate if used alone for posterior segment involvement.

The level of systemic treatment required to maintain quiescence varies considerably between patients, but is usually life-long. Our practice is to establish the steroid dose required to suppress active inflammation and to decide whether this is tolerable to the patient in the long term. For the majority in whom it is not (the dose in these cases often exceeding 20 mg/day) we add immunosuppressive treatment. A substantial steroid dose reduction is usually possible in those on combined treatment, and for some patients with chronic uveitis such dose reduction becomes an imperative. In this, as in other forms of very chronic severe uveitis, intraocular steroid implantation clearly has a place for some patients (Mahajan et al. 2009).

Using adequate immunosuppression, SU can be suppressed in the long term and useful, sometimes excellent vision can be maintained in what is usually the patient's only functioning eye. Nevertheless complications may ensue; cataract is a common sequel to long-term steroid treatment, and glaucoma may result from anterior segment damage. The surgical management of these conditions needs care, and the necessary precautions are discussed in Chapter 7.

VOGT–KOYANAGI–HARADA SYNDROME (box 17.2)

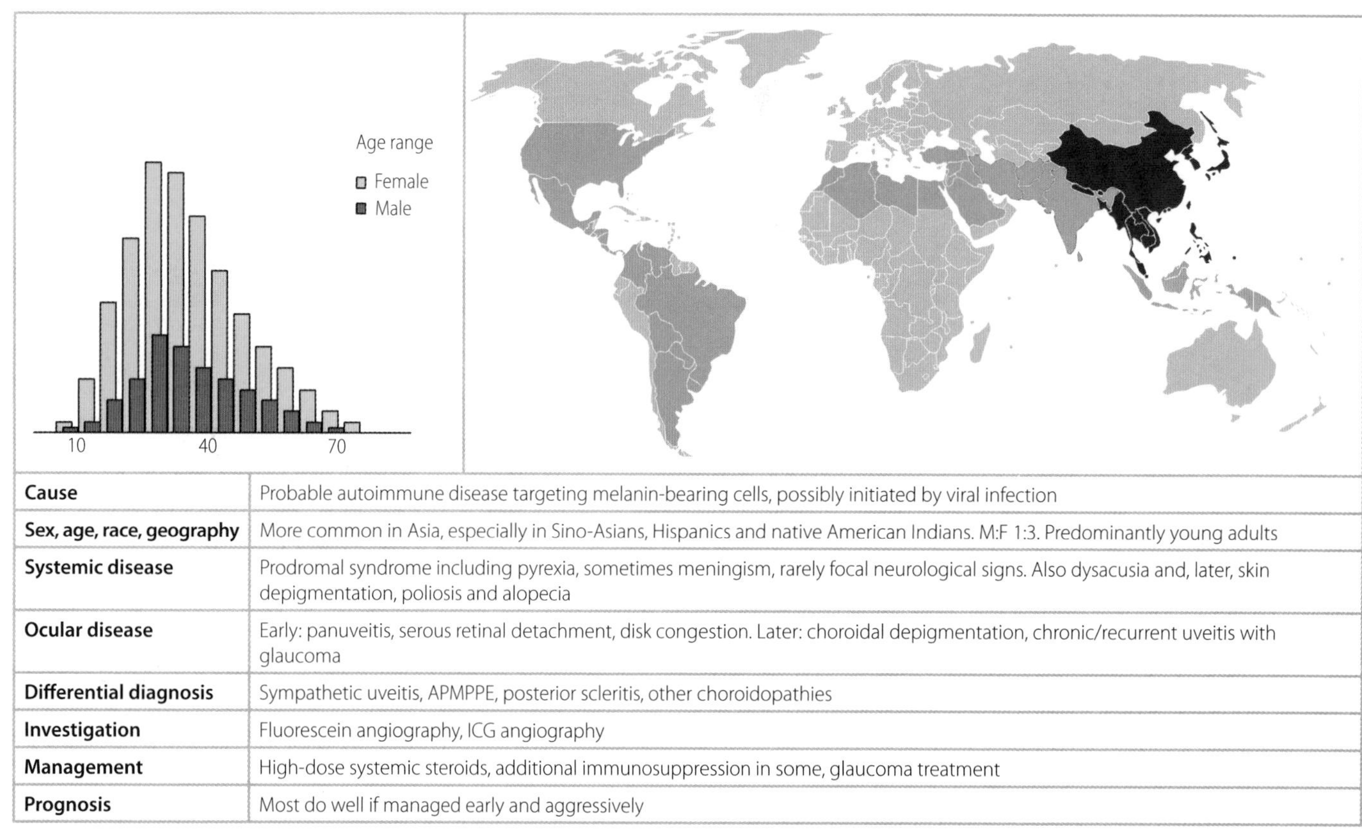

Cause	Probable autoimmune disease targeting melanin-bearing cells, possibly initiated by viral infection
Sex, age, race, geography	More common in Asia, especially in Sino-Asians, Hispanics and native American Indians. M:F 1:3. Predominantly young adults
Systemic disease	Prodromal syndrome including pyrexia, sometimes meningism, rarely focal neurological signs. Also dysacusia and, later, skin depigmentation, poliosis and alopecia
Ocular disease	Early: panuveitis, serous retinal detachment, disk congestion. Later: choroidal depigmentation, chronic/recurrent uveitis with glaucoma
Differential diagnosis	Sympathetic uveitis, APMPPE, posterior scleritis, other choroidopathies
Investigation	Fluorescein angiography, ICG angiography
Management	High-dose systemic steroids, additional immunosuppression in some, glaucoma treatment
Prognosis	Most do well if managed early and aggressively

Box 17.2 Vogt–Koyanagi–Harada syndrome

Introduction

The coexistence of depigmentation and inflamed eyes was noted in the Middle East over 1000 years ago. Although seen previously by others, Vogt first reported poliosis and uveitis (Vogt 1906); later Koyanagi reported the coexistence of vitiligo and alopecia with uveitis (Koyanagi 1929) and Harada described serous retinal detachment in association with cerebrospinal fluid (CSF) abnormalities (Harada 1926). Soon afterwards these signs were grouped together as components of a single entity, henceforth described as the VKH syndrome.

The syndrome is common in Japan (accounting for perhaps 8% of all cases of uveitis) and in China and the Far East. It has a significant frequency throughout Asia, the Middle East, and South and Central America. It is uncommon in North America and rare in Europe. These differences in incidence are probably explained by racial predilection. The syndrome is extremely rare in white people but is much more common in Asian, Hispanic and in indigenous native American individuals. There is a significant association of VKH with HLA-DR4 and HLA-DRB1 (various alleles in different ethnic groups, but most commonly HLA-DRB1*0405) (Goldberg et al. 1998). The alleles DQA*0301 and DQB*0401 may also be associated, at least in Chinese patients (Liu et al. 1999).

Patients as young as 7 can present with VKH syndrome, but most are in early to middle adulthood, the most common age at presentation being 30–35 years. Women are affected at least twice as often as men in most countries, the apparent exception being Japan; here, where the disease is most common, there does not appear to be a sex bias.

The cause of VKH syndrome is unproven but the prodrome that frequently occurs suggests a viral trigger for a disease that has all the characteristics of an autoimmune process against melanin-containing cells. Such cells are present not only within the eye and skin, where the major manifestations of the disease are seen, but also within the stria vascularis of the cochlea, in the leptomeninges and in the pineal gland. Inflammation directed against pigment-bearing cells in these latter areas probably explains dysacusia and meningism, respectively. Support for a T-cell-mediated autoimmune pathogenesis comes from lymphocyte studies, immunohistochemistry and electron microscopy. Histologically, VKH syndrome is a granulomatous panuveitis with diffuse infiltration of epithelioid cells, giant cells and lymphocytes similar to sympathetic uveitis. Dalen-Fuchs nodules may be present. The epithelioid cells may contain melanin pigment. As for SU, the choriocapillaris and RPE are largely spared. It has been suggested that this sparing might be the result of transforming growth factor β (TGF-β) or RPE-protective protein (suppressing phagocyte superoxide production), both secreted by the RPE (Rao 1997).

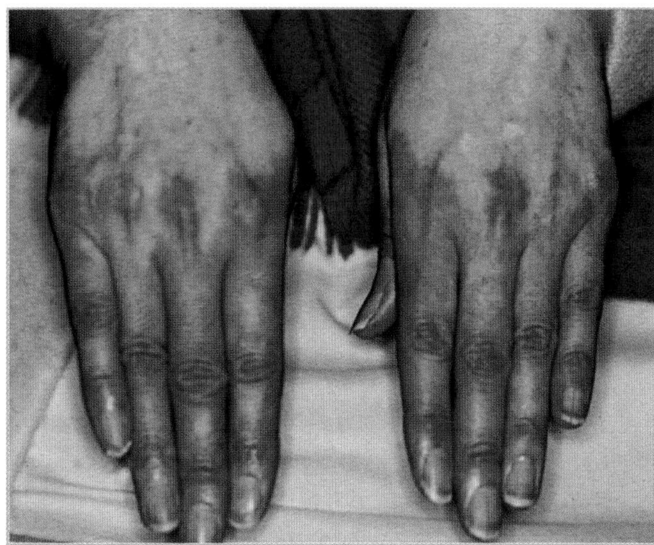

Figure 17.11 Severe symmetrical vitiligo in an Indian woman with VKH syndrome. The face was similarly affected and ultimately all racial pigmentation was lost.

Systemic disease

The syndrome varies substantially from patient to patient, but, where systemic involvement occurs, there is a distinct phasic progression. Most patients present later with ocular problems, but a prodrome may be recalled that resembled a viral illness with malaise, pyrexia, headache, and sometimes dizziness or meningism. Rarely, focal neurological signs may occur at this stage, even including dysphasia, cranial nerve palsy or hemiparesis. In those who undergo central nervous system (CNS) investigation, CSF pleocytosis is usually found. Also starting at this stage or soon afterwards, tinnitus in about 40% and symmetrical high-frequency hearing loss in about 50% are experienced, which usually improves spontaneously within weeks. Labyrinthine inflammation may occur (Oku and Ishikawa 1994) but vertigo is less common, affecting less than 20% (Al Dousary 2010). Altered sensation with hypersensitivity to touch may also be reported as a prodromal symptom.

In the convalescent phase, which usually follows many weeks after the onset and rarely any earlier, signs of damage to cutaneous melanocytes may develop, with vitiligo (**Fig. 17.11**), alopecia or poliosis (**Fig. 17.12**) occurring in up to 60% of patients. These manifestations may be progressive and severe and treatment has been unsatisfactory. The signs are often markedly symmetrical. In those dark-skinned patients who have perilimbal conjunctival pigmentation, its disappearance (Sigiura's sign) tends to occur early in the convalescent phase.

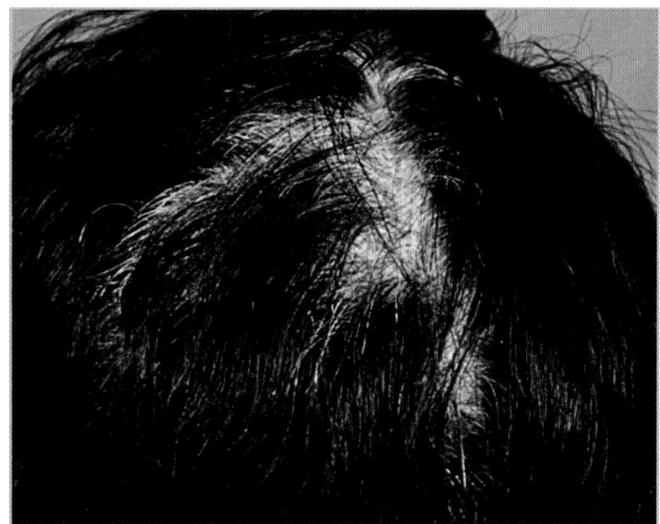

Figure 17.12 Patchy alopecia with marginal poliosis, developing some 3 months after presentation with uveitis, in a young Malaysian with VKH syndrome

As a presumed autoimmune disease, VKH syndrome has been reported in association with thyroiditis, inflammatory bowel disease and diabetes.

Ocular disease

The uveitic phase may be preceded by a prodrome or may be the initial manifestation. The uveitis is always bilateral. There is usually a symmetrical onset, but sequential involvement of the second eye may be delayed by a week or so. Diffuse choroiditis is usual, with papillary edema or, in particular, hyperemia (**Fig. 17.13**). Peripapillary retinal edema is frequent. Multifocal lesions may be seen both in the periphery and further posteriorly (**Fig. 17.14**), indistinguishable from Dalen–Fuchs nodules in SU. Where there is substantial breakdown of the RPE, serous elevations of the retina may occur (**Fig. 17.15**) and may become confluent; this is the Harada form of the disease. At the posterior pole, pale areas of choroidal inflammation are often visible, even through elevated retina. These may be multifocal or aggregated.

Anterior uveitis is usual, but may not be present at onset. Large KPs and iris nodules may be seen but are not essential for diagnosis. A substantial rise in intraocular pressure is common, the associated anterior chamber shallowing indicating forward displacement of the iris/lens diaphragm caused by ciliary body swelling. Annular choroidal detachment has been reported. Acute angle closure may occur, but this is rare.

Active uveitis usually persists for 2–3 months at least, and during this time foci of posterior segment inflammation develop RPE scars in the midperiphery, indistinguishable from SU (**Fig. 17.16**). In those dark-skinned patients with heavy choroidal pigmentation, generalized pigment loss over a period of months leads to a gradual color change

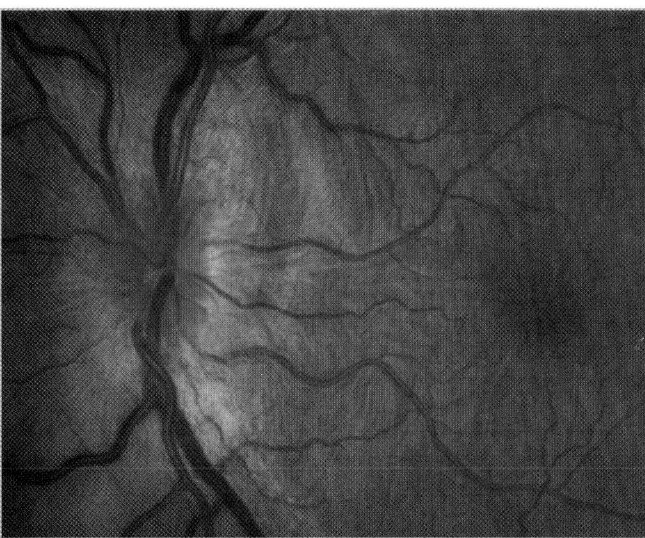

Figure 17.13 Optic disk blurring and hyperemia, together with peripapillary and retinal edema with folding, in acute VKH syndrome.

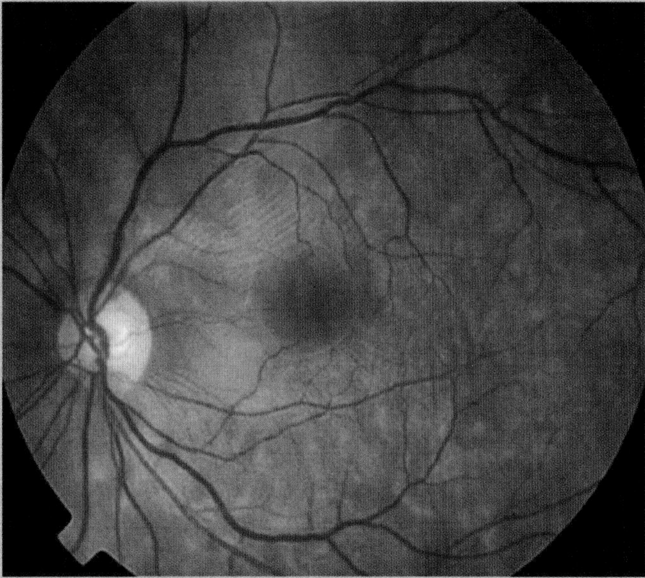

Figure 17.14 Multifocal choroidal infiltration in acute Vogt–Koyanagi–Harada syndrome, with associated serous retinal elevation affecting the macula.

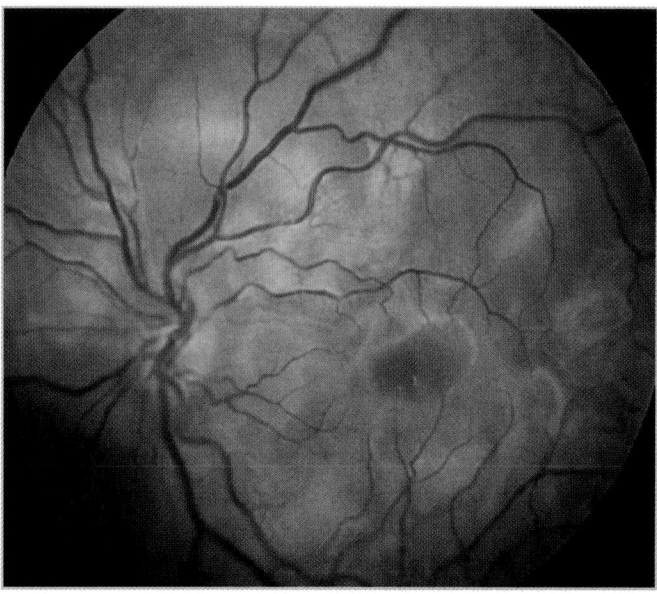

Figure 17.15 Multifocal serous retinal detachment, becoming confluent in acute Vogt–Koyanagi–Harada syndrome. Areas of pale choroidal inflammation are visible through the edematous retina.

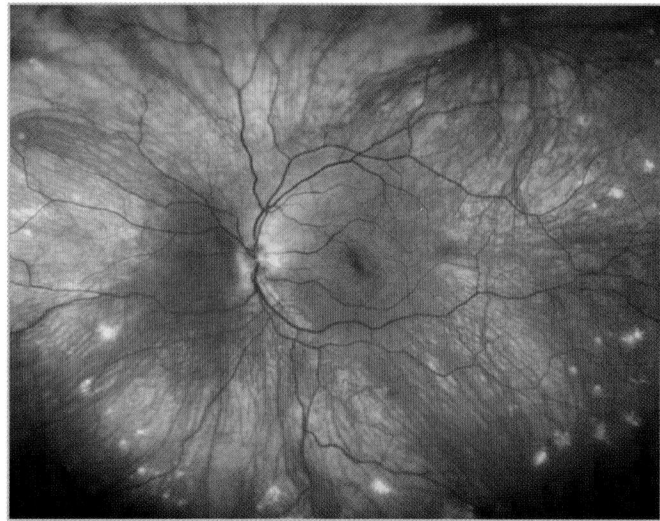

Figure 17.16 Multifocal depigmented chorioretinal scars in late-phase Vogt–Koyanagi–Harada syndrome, representing the sites of old Dalen–Fuchs nodules.

in the fundus, typically a light reddish-orange that has been likened to a 'sunset glow' sky (**Fig. 17.17**). The rarely affected fundus in white people will also depigment, but less dramatically because there is less choroidal pigment to lose. Peripapillary atrophy is common.

Typically the syndrome now enters a chronic, relapsing or recurrent phase with exacerbations of uveitis, sometimes granulomatous, affecting mainly the anterior segment and subsiding to an underlying mild chronic panuveitis. At this stage, in contrast to the uveitis at presentation, mutton-fat KPs and iris nodules are quite frequent. Posterior segment recurrences are seen much less frequently (in less than 10%) but are usually bilateral and require treatment as for the acute phase (Sachdev et al. 2008). Consecutive exacerbations of uveitis frequently lead to complications including glaucoma and cataract. As with any inflammatory choroidopathy, subretinal neovascular membranes may develop late in the course of the disease. In VKH syndrome up to 10% of patients develop this complication and the membranes have a predilection for the peripapillary and macular areas.

Diagnosis

There is no diagnostic test for VKH syndrome; the diagnosis is entirely clinical. For this reason a variety of diagnostic criteria has been discussed in recent decades. Sigiura's original criteria, although clinically useful, regarded CSF analysis as essential for complete diagnosis but current practice regards this as unnecessarily invasive. An international group met to formulate modified diagnostic criteria in 2001 (Read et al. 2001) and these are shown in slightly modified form in **Table 17.1**. Notably, the disease can be classified as probable, incomplete or complete depending on how many criteria are met.

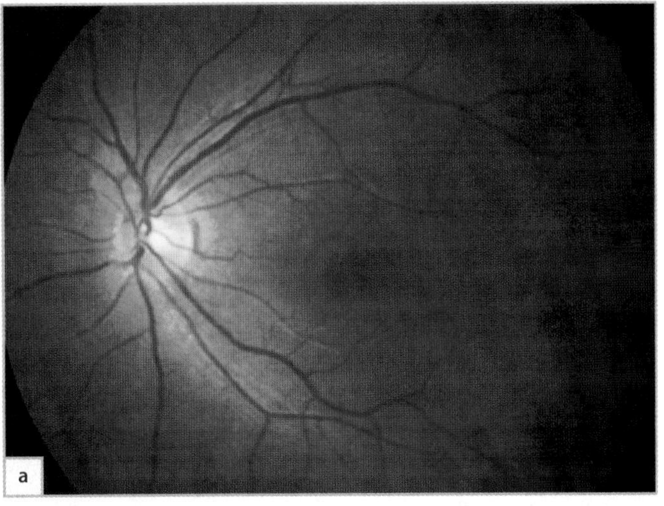

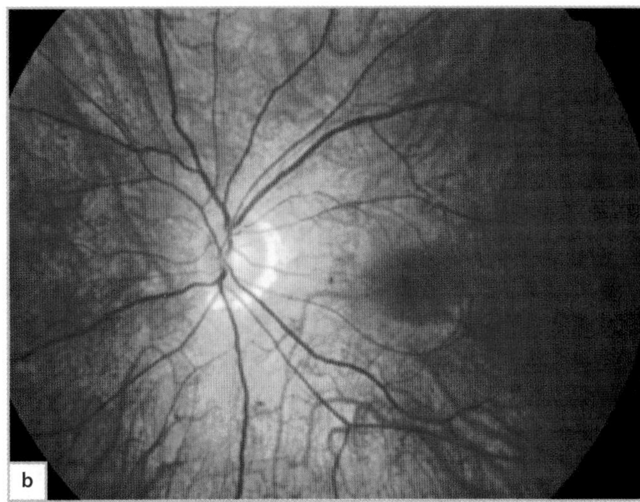

Figure 17.17 The left fundus of a young Malaysian woman shortly after the onset of Vogt–Koyanagi–Harada syndrome (a). The retinal pigment epithelium (RPE) and choroid are deeply pigmented as expected in one of her racial origin. Eighteen months later (b) there is substantial choroidal and RPE depigmentation, giving a 'sunset glow' to the fundus. There is also a peripapillary white atrophic crescent.

Table 17.1 Revised International Diagnostic Criteria for Vogt–Koyanagi–Harada (VKH) syndrome, 2001

1. There should be no history of ocular trauma or surgery	
2. There should be no clinical or laboratory evidence of other ocular disease entities	
3. The uveitis must be bilateral, exhibiting either A or B below: A. (Early disease): i. Diffuse choroiditis with either focal or bullous subretinal fluid ii. If fundal appearances are equivocal, must have: a. Focal choroidal perfusion delay, pinpoint leakage, placoid fluorescence and optic nerve staining on fluorescein angiography and b. Diffuse choroidal thickening, but no scleritis B. (Late disease): i. A suggestive history of 3A and either ii or iii: ii. Depigmentation; either sunset glow or Sigiura's sign iii. Nummular chorioretinal scars with retinal pigment epithelium clumping and migration and recurrent or chronic anterior uveitis	
4. Active or history of any one of: meningism, tinnitus, cerebrospinal fluid pleocytosis	
5. Any one of: alopecia, poliosis, vitiligo	
Complete VKH syndrome	Requires all of 1–5 criteria
Incomplete	Requires 1–3 and either 4 or 5
Probable	Requires 1–3

Adapted from Read et al. (2001).

Fluorescein angiography may be helpful, typically showing early multifocal punctate hyperfluorescence, these patches enlarging and coalescing through the sequence (**Fig. 17.18**). In those with focal serous retinal detachment, fluorescein will pool in these spaces to give a dramatic appearance (**Figs 17.19** and **17.20**). Disk leakage is frequent. Indocyanine green (ICG) angiography may show active choroidal lesions not visible clinically or on fluorescein angiography (Bouchenaki et al. 2000) and this may indicate subclinical recurrence. Characteristic features are hypofluorescent dark dots and diffuse late choroidal hyperfluorescence.

The coexistence of focal neurological signs with uveitis is justification for lumbar puncture. Whether meningism without focal signs justifies the procedure is more contentious; where ocular involvement is characteristic, this is not our practice. CSF lymphocyte pleocytosis, although typical of VKH syndrome. is by no means pathognomonic of the disease; it may be present in several different causes of uveitis with neurological signs, and may be seen with APMPPE, which may share several common features with VKH syndrome. Abnormal electroencephalography is another indicator of neurological involvement, although again changes are variable and non-specific.

In its paradigm, the diagnosis of VKH syndrome is unequivocal. However, its formes frustes may confuse. Sympathetic uveitis may present with a pattern of intraocular involvement that is strikingly similar to VKH syndrome, and a history of penetrating trauma (including a suspicion of occult penetration) or of ocular surgery, including cyclodestructive procedures, should be sought. The 2001 criteria do not allow the diagnosis of VKH syndrome if such findings are positive. Whether the exclusion of any and all intraocular surgery is sensible is a matter of opinion. APMPPE may closely resemble VKH syndrome, first because ocular involvement may include multifocal serous reti-

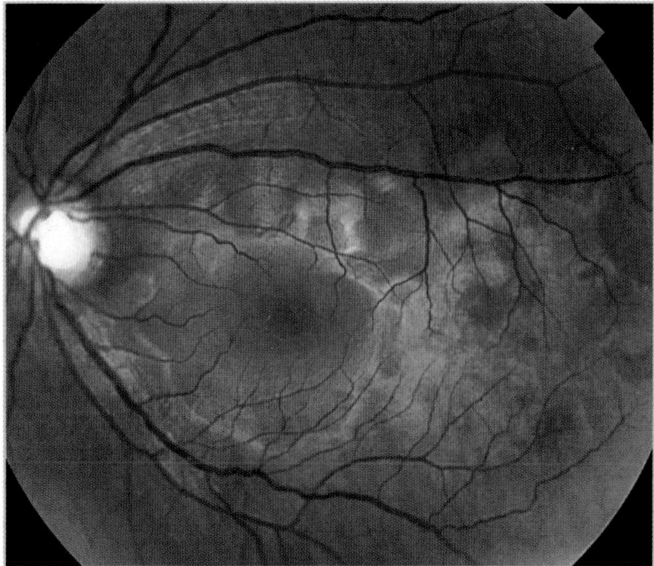

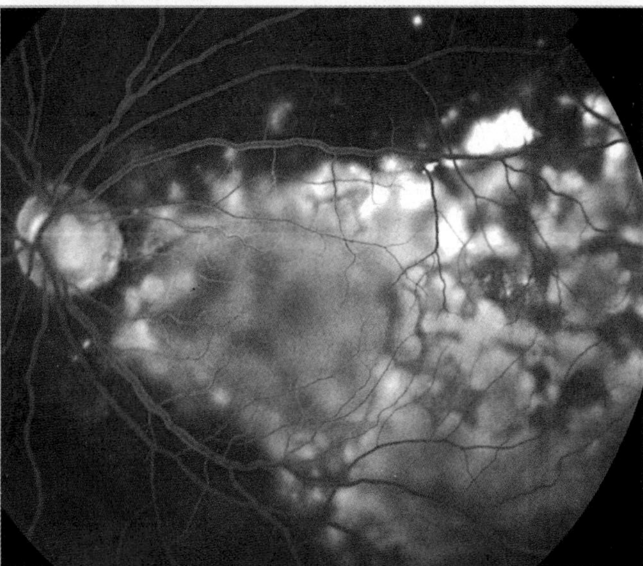

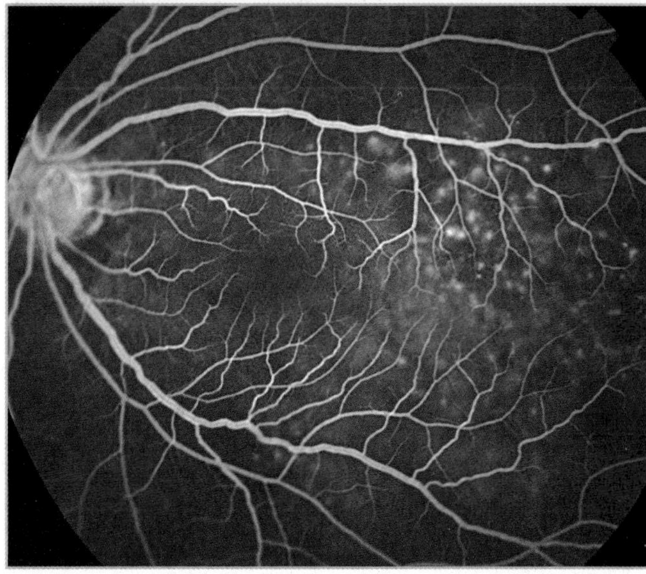

Figure 17.18 The fundus in acute Vogt–Koyanagi–Harada syndrome with arterial and late-phase fluorescein angiography. Early multifocal punctate leakage is followed by pooling of fluorescein within subretinal fluid.

nal detachment, and second because systemic accompaniments to APMPPE may include a viral prodrome, dysacusia and sometimes encephalomeningeal symptoms, in the most severe cases reflecting cerebral vasculitis. However, lesions in APMPPE are typically only at the posterior pole, or at least posterior to the equator, and there are distinct differences on fluorescein angiography reflecting choriocapillaris ischemia: placoid lesions show early blockage and late staining, rather than the multifocal punctate leakage of VKH syndrome. There is characteristically little vitreous, and no anterior chamber cellular infiltrate in APMPPE, in contrast to the significant uveitis of VKH syndrome.

Sarcoidosis may occasionally provide diagnostic difficulty, but posterior segment changes are usually distinct. Multifocal choroiditis is predominantly inferior, diffuse choroidal involvement is unusual and retinal periphlebitis may be marked, whereas it is unusual in VKH syndrome. Both granulomatous and non-granulomatous uveitis may occur in sarcoidosis, but glaucoma is less common compared with VKH syndrome. Standard tests for sarcoidosis should be performed if doubt exists.

Serous retinal detachment or generalized choroidal thickening with pallor is a feature of posterior scleritis, the uveal effusion syndrome or choroidal necrosis in systemic lupus erythematosus. Systemic signs of the latter are usually clear, this severe form of ocular involvement usually being associated with a significant worsening of the disease, often with severe renal involvement. The uveal effusion syndrome may mimic VKH syndrome in its early stages, although the degree of intraocular inflammation is at worst mild, and its serous detachments are predominantly peripheral, but accompanying glaucoma is frequent. In time, the spontaneous reduction of the detachments will leave the characteristic 'thrush-breast' RPE pigmentation, which is distinctly different from late-stage appearances in VKH syndrome. Posterior scleritis frequently generates a severe and radiating aching pain, and there is often a clear history of predisposing illness such as rheumatoid arthritis. Choroidal folds may be present (although these are also occasionally seen in VKH syndrome) but ultrasonography, in demonstrating marked scleral thickening, can distinguish the condition from VKH syndrome. Other conditions that may occasionally mimic VKH syndrome include masquerade syndromes, the multiple evanescent white dot syndrome (MEWDS) and Lyme disease, although diagnostic confusion would be unusual for all of these conditions.

Management

As for SU, early recognition and aggressive management of VKH syndrome is likely to improve the outcome. High-dose systemic steroid treatment is necessary for the early panuveitis. Some would use 100 mg/day or more orally; an alternative is to start therapy with intravenous methylprednisolone; treatment may be tapered once control is established. Not only may such management halt the process before it enters the chronic recurrent phase, but it may also reduce the likelihood of vitiligo and alopecia. Inflammation may reactivate if steroids are tapered too quickly; such episodes are felt to increase the risk of steroid-resistant disease in the future. Some authors feel that at least 6 months of initial oral steroid treatment is preferable (Lai et al. 2009).

Unfortunately recurrences of inflammation may not respond to steroid treatment, even in high dose. The addition of adjunctive therapy is then necessary. The results of low-dose ciclosporin treatment have been favorable (Moorthy 1995) and the drug may act by downregulating Th1 and Th17 lymphocytes (Lui et al. 2009). Azathioprine has also been used successfully as a steroid-sparing agent in both acute and

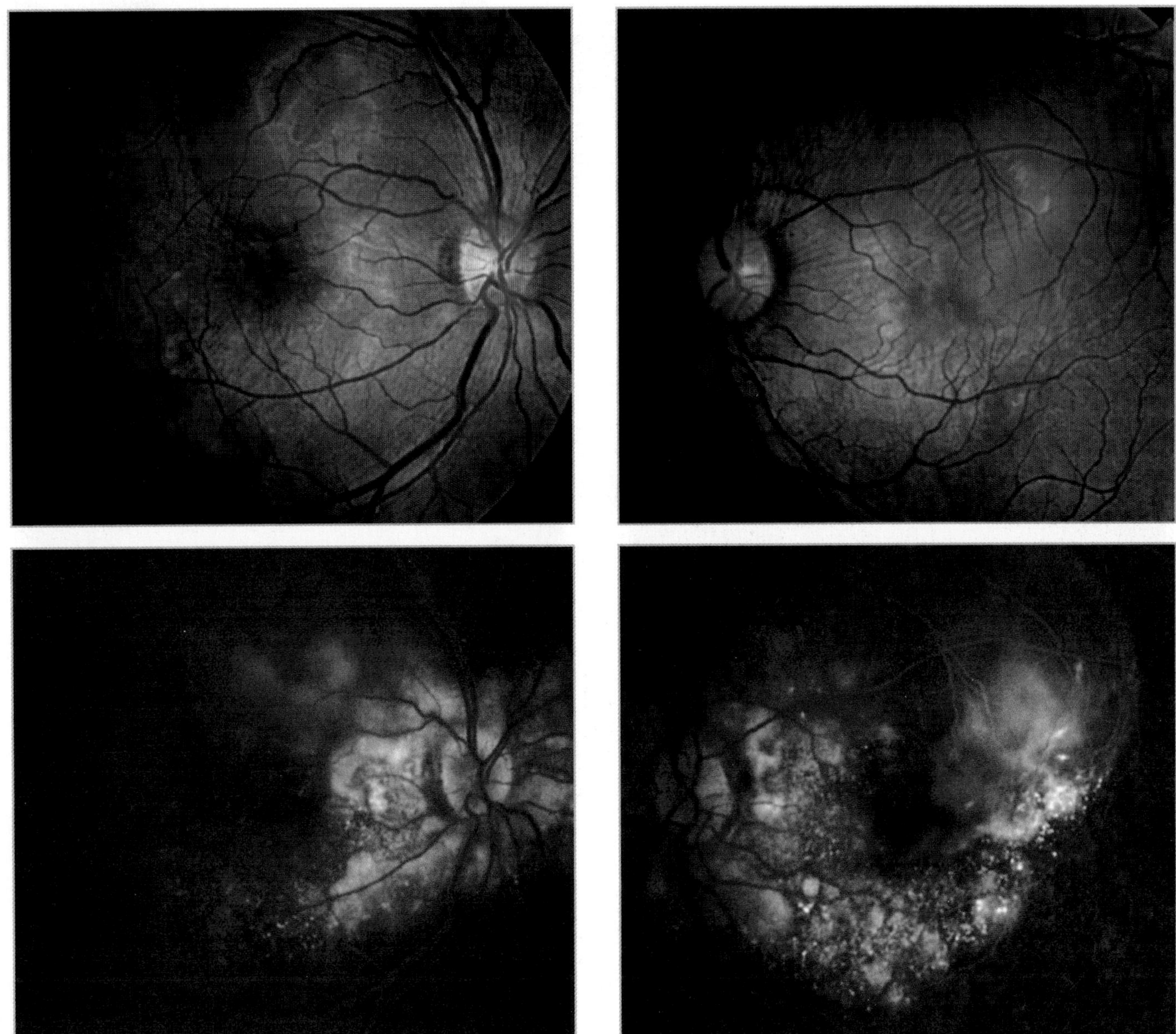

Figure 17.19 Acute Vogt–Koyanagi–Harada syndrome with disc hyperemia and serous retinal elevation showing as dramatic subretinal pooling of fluorescein.

chronic disease (Kim and Hu 2007). For those with treatment-resistant disease, infliximab has been used successfully in a small number of patients (Wang et al. 2008).

Aggressive early management with systemic steroids, and if necessary additional immunosuppression, is accepted to be necessary in VKH syndrome and has favorably affected outcomes, but the prognosis for eventual visual function must remain guarded; a few patients may still progress to substantial visual loss. In general, half to two-thirds of patients retain visual acuities of 6/9 or better, and severe visual loss affects fewer than 10%.

Eventual cataract formation is common in VKH syndrome. As for other forms of uveitis, performing surgery during a period free of inflammation maximizes the likelihood of successful outcome, but in general surgery is not troublesome. Glaucoma may occur early in VKH syndrome due to anterior movement of the iris base secondary to cyclitis. Rarely this may be severe enough to cause acute angle closure. The use of laser iridotomy to relieve pupillary block may fail in this circumstance and surgical iridectomy will then be required. Later, anterior synechia formation or response to steroid treatment may also raise intraocular pressure, but secondary open-angle glaucoma is anyway common in chronic phase VKH syndrome. Overall more than half the patients are affected at some stage, and it is prolonged in two-thirds of these (Forster et al. 1993). A high proportion of patients require surgical intervention. Formal drainage procedures require enhancement, as for all uveitic glaucomas. Some will need drainage tube implantation.

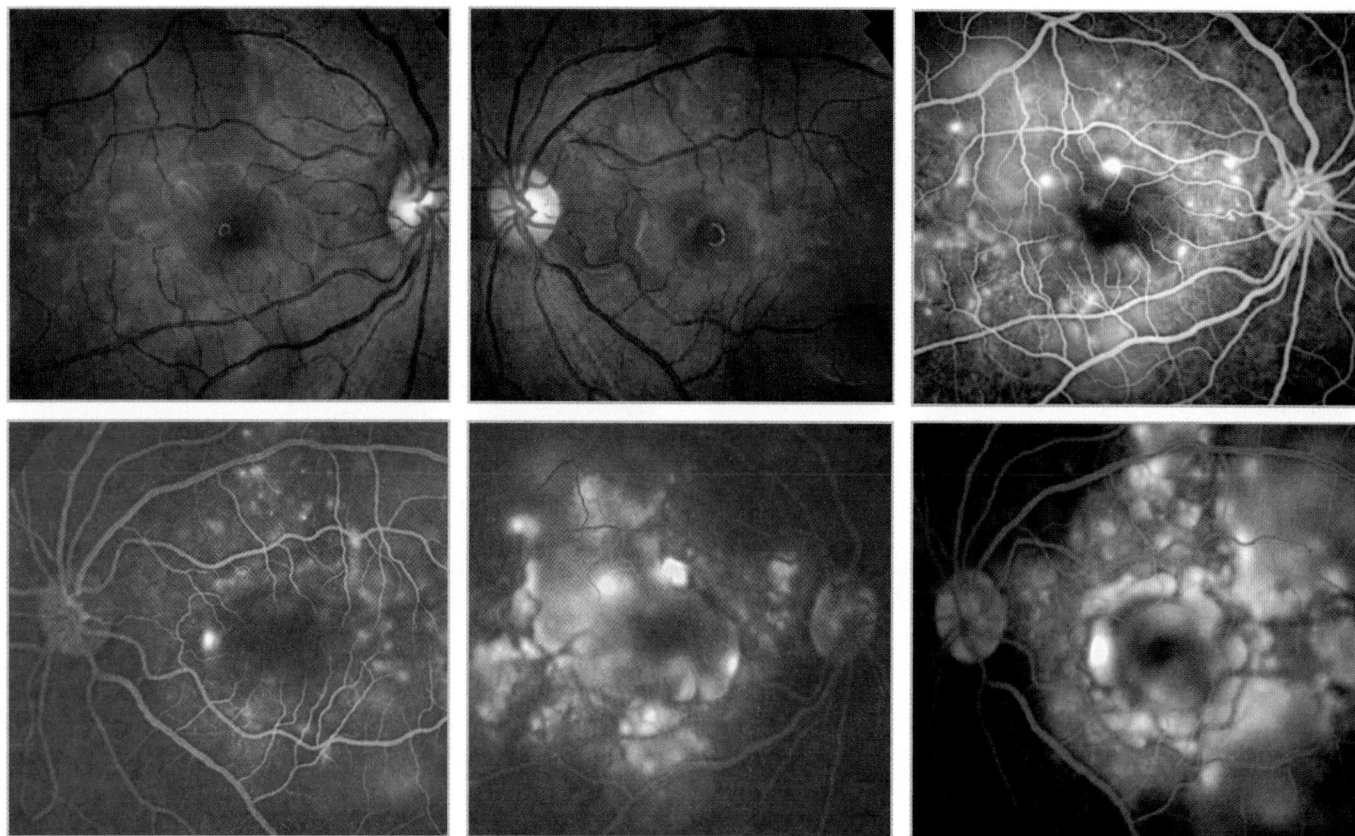

Figure 17.20 Acute Vogt–Koyanagi–Harada syndrome with multifocal punctate fluorescein leakage coalescing into subretinal pooling.

REFERENCES

Al Dousary S. Auditory and vestibular manifestations of Vogt–Koyanagi–Harada disease. *J Laryngol Otol* 2010;**30**:1–4.

Atan D, Turner SJ, Kilmartin DJ, et al. Cytokine gene polymorphism in sympathetic ophthalmia. *Invest Ophthalmol Vis Sci* 2005;**46**:4245–50.

Bouchenaki N, Morisod L, Herbort CP. Vogt–Koyanagi–Harada syndrome: importance of rapid diagnosis and therapeutic intervention. *Klin Monatsbl Augenheilkd* 2000;**216**:290–4.

Chan CC, Roberge FG, Whitcup SM, et al. 32 cases of sympathetic ophthalmia. *Arch Ophthalmol* 1995;**113**:597–600.

Forster DJ, Rao NA, Hill RA, et al. Incidence and management of glaucoma in Vogt–Koyanagi–Harada syndrome. *Ophthalmology* 1993;**100**:613–18.

Fuchs E. Uber sympathisierende Entzundung (Zuerst Bermerkunen uber serose traumatische Iritis). *Graefes Arch Clin Exp Ophthalmol* 1905;**61**:365.

Galor A, Davis JL, Flynn HW, et al. Sympathetic ophthalmia: incidence of ocular complications and vision loss in the sympathizing eye. *Am J Ophthalmol* 2009;**148**:704–10.

Goldberg AC, Yamamoto JH, Chiarella JM, et al. HLA-DRB*0405 is the predominant allele in Brazilian patients with Vogt-Koyanagi-Harada disease. *Hum Immunol* 1998;**59**:183–8.

Harada E. Beitrag zur klinischen Kenntnis von Michteitriger Choroiditis (choroiditis diffusa acta). *Acta Soc Ophthalmol Jpn* 1926:**30**:356–78.

Kilmartin DJ, Dick AD, Forrester JV. Prospective surveillance of sympathetic ophthalmia in the UK and Republic of Ireland. *Br J Ophthalmol* 2000;**84**:259–63.

Kilmartin D, Wilson D, Liversedge J, et al. Immunogenetics and clinical phenotype of sympathetic ophthalmia in British and Irish patients. *Br J Ophthalmol* 2001;**85**:281–6.

Kim SJ, Yu HG. The use of low-dose azathioprine in patients with Vogt-Koyanagi-Harada disease. *Ocul Immunol Inflamm* 2007;**15**:381–7.

Koyanagi Y. Dysakusis, Alopecia und Poliosis bei schwerer Uveitis nicht traumatischen Ursprungs. *Klin Monatsbl Augenheilkd* 1929;**82**:1 94–211.

Lai TY, Chan RP, Chan CK, Lam DS. Effects of the duration of initial oral corticosteroid treatment on the recurrence of inflammation in Vogt-Koyanagi-Harada disease. *Eye* 2009;**23**:543–8.

Liu Q, Zhang M, Qiu C, Hu T. Association of HLA-DQA1 and DQB1 alleles with Vogt–Koyanagi–Harada syndrome in Han Chinese population. *Zhongua Yan Ke Za Zhi* 1999;**35**:210–15.

Liu X, Yang P, Lin X, et al. Inhibitory effect of cyclosporin A and corticosteroids on the production of IFN-gamma and IL-17 by T cells in Vogt–Koyanagi–Harada syndrome. *Clin Immunol* 2009;**131**:333–42.

Mahajan VB, Gehrs KM, Goldstein DA, et al. Management of sympathetic ophthalmia with the fluocinolone acetonide implant. Ophthalmology 2009;116:552–7.

Moorthy RS, Inomata H, Rao NA. Vogt–Koyanagi–Harada syndrome. *Surv Ophthalmol* 1995;**39**:265–92.

Oku H, Ishikawa S. Vestibulo-ocular reflex abnormality in Vogt–Koyanagi–Harada syndrome. *Br J Ophthalmol* 1994;**78**:912–16.

Rao N. Mechanisms of inflammatory response in sympathetic ophthalmia and VKH syndrome. *Eye* 1997;**11**:213–16.

Read RW, Holland GN, Rao NA, et al. Revised criteria for Vogt–Koyanagi–Harada disease: report of an international committee on nomenclature. *Am J Ophthalmol* 2001;**131**:647–52.

Sachdev N, Gupta V, Gupta A, Singh R. Posterior segment recurrences in Vogt–Koyanagi–Harada disease. *Int Ophthalmol* 2008;**28**:339–45.

du Toit N, Motala MI, Richards J, et al. The risk of sympathetic ophthalmia following evisceration for penetrating eye injuries at Groote Schuur hospital. *Br J Ophthalmol* 2008;**92**:61–3.

Vogt A. Frühzeitiges Ergrauen der Zilien und Bemerkungen über den sogenannten plötlzichen Eintritt dieser Veränderung. *Klin Monatsbl Augenheilkd* 1906;**4**:228–42.

Wang RC, Zamir E, Dugel PU, et al. Progressive subretinal fibrosis and blindness associated with multifocal granulomatous chorioretinitis: a variant of sympathetic ophthalmia. *Ophthalmology* 2002;**109**:1527–31.

Wang Y, Gaudio PA. Infliximab therapy for 2 patients with Vogt–Koyanagi–Harada syndrome. *Ocul Immunol Inflamm* 2008;**16**:167–71.

Chapter 18 Vasculitis

Vasculitis is a common manifestation of both systemic and intraocular inflammatory disease. The inflammation may simultaneously involve several systems as in Behçet's disease, or may be confined to a single site as in cutaneous or primary retinal vasculitis. Some connective tissue inflammatory diseases such as systemic lupus erythematosus and rheumatoid disease may have a significant vasculitic element. The group of diseases now classified as the systemic vasculitides may have significant ophthalmic involvement including uveitis or, much less commonly, intraocular vasculitis. Perivascular inflammation is a significant component of multiple sclerosis.

Retinal vasculitis may be a component of many different forms of intraocular inflammation. It is characteristic of Behçet's disease. It may also be prominent in a variety of inflammatory disorders discussed elsewhere, including sarcoidosis, birdshot retinochoroidopathy, viral retinitis and others. This chapter discusses those diseases in which systemic vasculitis is associated with intraocular inflammation, or where retinal vasculitis is the predominant form of intraocular inflammation. Behçet's disease is discussed first, followed by the systemic vasculitides and their relationship to intraocular inflammation. The various forms of primary retinal vasculitis unassociated with systemic disease are then discussed. Systemic lupus erythematosus and multiple sclerosis are included here for convenience because both may include a vasculitic process. The implications of thrombophilia in association with retinal vasculitis draw the chapter to a close.

BEHÇET'S DISEASE (box 18.1)

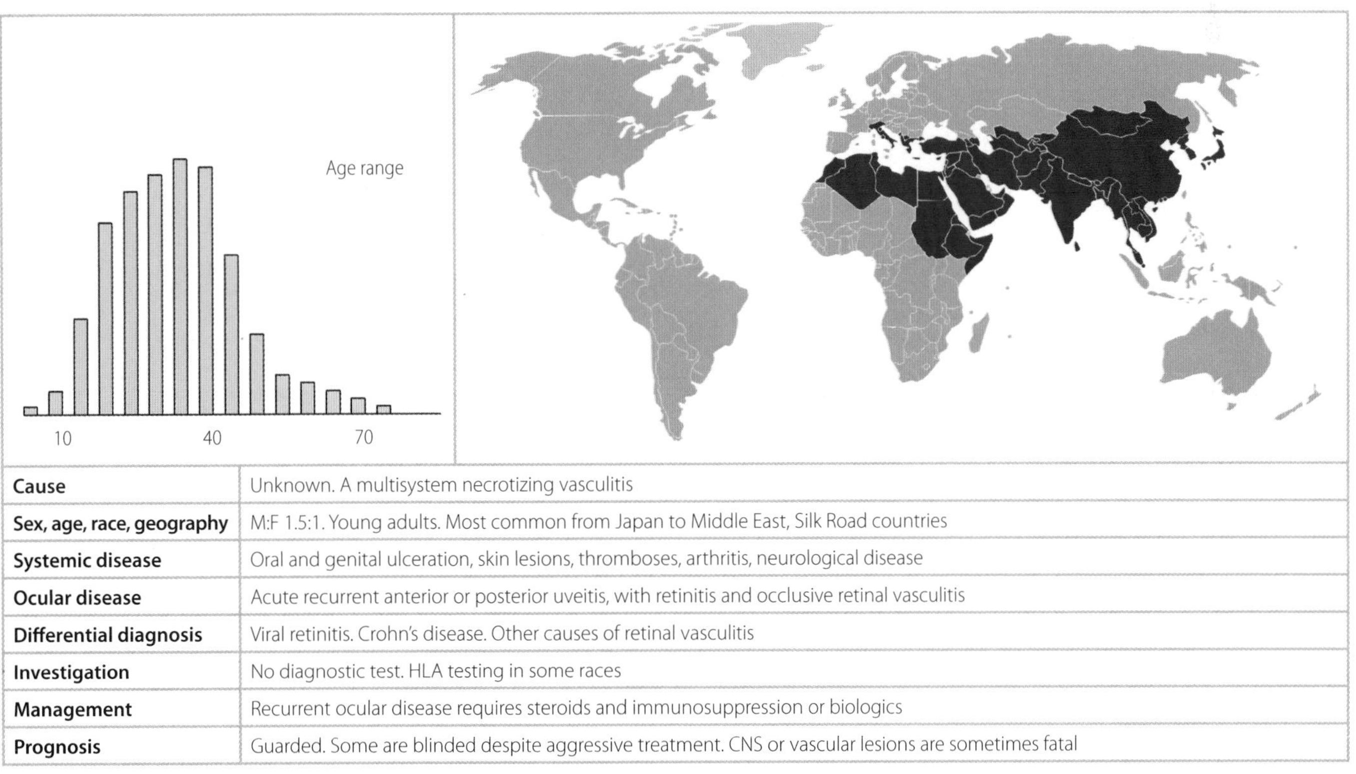

Cause	Unknown. A multisystem necrotizing vasculitis
Sex, age, race, geography	M:F 1.5:1. Young adults. Most common from Japan to Middle East, Silk Road countries
Systemic disease	Oral and genital ulceration, skin lesions, thromboses, arthritis, neurological disease
Ocular disease	Acute recurrent anterior or posterior uveitis, with retinitis and occlusive retinal vasculitis
Differential diagnosis	Viral retinitis. Crohn's disease. Other causes of retinal vasculitis
Investigation	No diagnostic test. HLA testing in some races
Management	Recurrent ocular disease requires steroids and immunosuppression or biologics
Prognosis	Guarded. Some are blinded despite aggressive treatment. CNS or vascular lesions are sometimes fatal

Box 18.1 Behçet's disease

Introduction

In 1937 Hulusi Behçet, a Turkish dermatologist (Behçet 1937), described the association between intraocular inflammation and oral ulceration that continues almost exclusively to bear his name. The disease had in fact been described in 1931 by Benedict Adamantiades in Greece, and the Graeco-Ottoman dispute over the eponym lingers even now. In fact by far the earliest, albeit brief, description (about 400 BC) emanated from the *Epidemics Book III* of Hippocrates of Kos (a Greek island, although geographically closer to Turkey) in which he refers to 'Many had aphthae and sores in the mouth. Fluxes about the genitals were frequent ... watery ophthalmia, chronic and painful.' Although physicians in Greece and some other European countries remain loyal to 'Adamantiades' disease', the term 'Behçet's disease' is deeply embedded in medical history and is used here.

In addition to the classic triad of uveitis, oral and genital ulceration, other manifestations are now known to be protean. Any body system may become involved and, although most patients develop signs in two or more locations simultaneously, in some the various manifestations may be separated in time so that diagnosis is delayed by years.

Behçet's disease typically affects young adults, and its onset is very uncommon over the age of 50 years. There is a clear geographic distribution; it is particularly common in Japan where the prevalence is as high as 13.5/100 000, and the disease accounts for 20% of patients in some uveitis clinics. It is also very common in the Middle East, the eastern Mediterranean and North Africa, and much less common in northern Europe and the USA. In the UK, for instance, there is a prevalence of a mere 0.6/100 000. It has long been noted that the greatest concentration of the disease occurs in the countries of the Silk Roads, those ancient interweaving trade routes running from the great eastern Mediterranean ports of Tyre and Antioch, past the Caucasus and Himalaya, through Samarkand and Kashgar, skirting the Gobi into China and beyond. Over centuries many thousands of travelers and locals indubitably shared both their microbes and their genes, leading to the well-recognized geographical distribution of today, even though, frustratingly, the etiology of the disease still eludes us.

A male predominance is well recognized but varies from as few as 1.5:1 to as high as 9:1 in some Middle Eastern countries, the latter possibly in part representing access to medical services. There are many reports of familial cases and there is a significant association with HLA-B51, at least in Japanese and Middle Eastern patients, which has also been found to predict a greater likelihood of both uveitis and neurological involvement. Further analysis indicates that the allele HLA-B*5101 (which is far more common in males) is linked to disease and may at least in part explain male predominance. The introduction of genome-wide association studies has permitted non-targeted comparisons between affected and unaffected individuals with various diseases, and Behçet's disease is one inflammation that has been so studied (Remmers et al. 2010). In addition to confirming the association with HLA-B*51, variants at interleukins IL-10 and IL-23R–IL-12RB2 have been identified.

The manifestations of Behçet's disease are known to be caused by a necrotizing vasculitis, but the underlying cause is unknown. A viral etiology (especially implicating herpes simplex virus) or a bacterial etiology (especially implicating streptococci) has been suggested. The typical inflammatory foci commence with lymphocytic infiltration, followed by polymorph migration and fibrinoid necrosis in blood vessels. Massive polymorph extravasation is a typical feature, although there is substantial evidence that the disease is T-cell driven, and this notion is strongly supported by the effectiveness of ciclosporin.

Systemic disease

Oral ulceration

This is the most common sign of Behçet's disease, affecting more than 97% of patients (International Study Group for Behçet's Disease or ISGBD 1992). Indeed, in some diagnostic systems it is used as a prerequisite for diagnosis (ISGBD 1990). As a diagnostic sign, oral ulceration has low specificity because the symptom is so common in those who do not have Behçet's disease. However, there do appear to be features of the oral aphthous ulceration in Behçet's disease that distinguish them from other causes. Recurrences of ulcers may be frequent, or in severe cases virtually continuous. Although most ulcers are small, some may be large and particularly painful. They may occur in crops, and adjacent ulcers may form an irregular confluent lesion. Involvement of areas of the mouth where aphthous ulceration is unusual, such as the lips (**Fig. 18.1**), tongue, palate (**Fig. 18.2**), fauces and pharynx, is suspicious of Behçet's disease.

Most oral ulcers in Behçet's disease heal without scarring, but particularly large and deep lesions may leave a puckered scar visible on the surface of the mucosa and this may be useful in diagnosis. Less commonly, oropharyngeal ulceration can be widespread and severe, with dysphagia even preventing the intake of oral fluids and necessitating parenteral administration (see Fig. 18.2). In such circumstances, herpetic or bacterial tonsillopharyngitis is sometimes misdiagnosed.

Other inflammatory conditions may cause oral ulceration, including the Stevens–Johnson syndrome (which is not usually a problem in differential diagnosis), lupus, Crohn's disease or reactive arthritis with uveitis (both of the last two may be a challenge to diagnosis, but tend to be associated with a different form of uveitis).

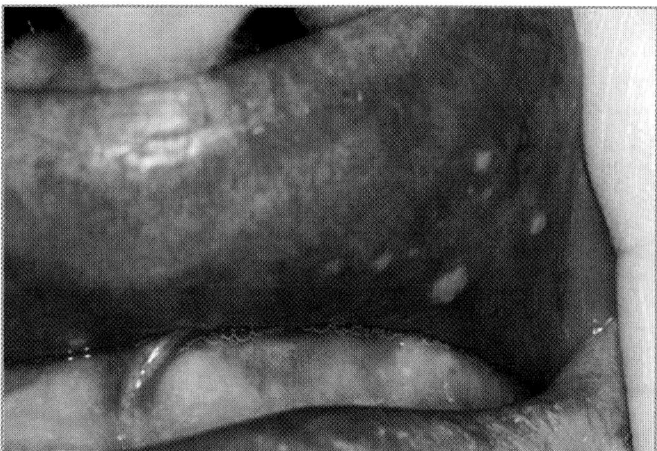

Figure 18.1 A crop of new aphthous ulcers on the buccal surface of the upper lip in Behçet's disease.

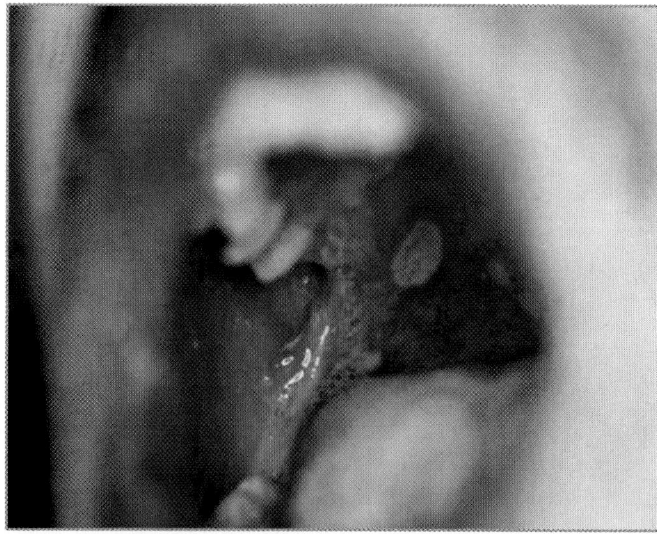

Figure 18.2 A large palatal ulcer, also with fauceal and pharyngeal ulcers, in a young man with Behçet's disease. Before diagnosis and high-dose steroid therapy, persistent dysphagia was severe enough to warrant parenteral feeding.

Genital ulceration

In men, ulcers on the penis or more commonly on the anterior scrotum are usually clearly evident. However, lesions on the posterior scrotum (**Fig. 18.3**) or perineum may also occur and, although they may cause discomfort, their presence may not be volunteered by the patient to an ophthalmologist; a direct enquiry should therefore be made and, if necessary, a search for both active lesions and scars. Not all ulcers leave scars - larger ulcers tend to do so but overall about 60% of genital ulcers result in scarring, in both men and women (Cem Mat et al. 2006). In women, uncommonly intravaginal lesions may occur alone but more frequently the vulva is involved and such lesions may be widespread and extremely painful. Perianal ulceration is less common, and if present Crohn's disease should be considered in the differential diagnosis.

Skin lesions

Erythema nodosum is a non-specific panniculitis/dermatitis that may occur in a variety of inflammatory diseases associated with uveitis. However, in Behçet's disease, the red-purple, tender discoid lesions have a particular tendency to occur not only in the pretibial area, but also on the arms, chest, head and neck. Other lesions suggestive of cutaneous vasculitis may be seen, and superficial or deep thrombophlebitis, usually of the lower legs, is an occasional feature. Erythema multiforme is much less common. Folliculitis, papulopustular eruption or acneiform nodules are all seen in Behçet's disease; in comparison to acne (whether or not steroid induced), the lesions may be atypical in distribution (e.g. involving the forearms, **Fig. 18.4**) and dramatic. The pustular lesions are sterile.

Neuro-Behçet's disease

Neurological complications of Behçet's disease occur in perhaps 10% of most cohorts and can be life threatening. Patients tend to be aged 25–40 at presentation. Many will present with a subacute meningoencephalitis, often involving the brain stem. Some develop cranial nerve palsies or the manifestations of focal lesions involving the spinal cord, brain stem, basal ganglia and thalamus, but the cerebellum or cerebrum may also be involved. Presentations can include ataxia, oculomotor disturbance, sensorineural deafness, bulbar palsy, hemiparesis (**Fig. 18.5**), confusional state or transverse myelitis (Kidd et al. 1999) but, for focal lesions, preceding meningism is common. Lesions may be transient or permanent. Thrombosis of the dural sinus or cerebral veins may occur but is much less common. Cerebrospinal fluid (CSF) analysis usually shows leukocytosis and increased protein. Magnetic resonance imaging (MRI) studies

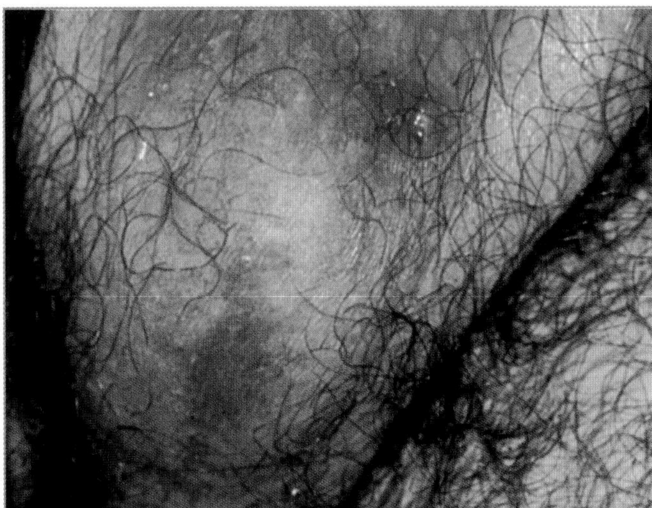

Figure 18.3 An active posterior scrotal ulcer in Behçet's disease, and a healed one below it. The patient was only aware of mild discomfort, not of ulceration.

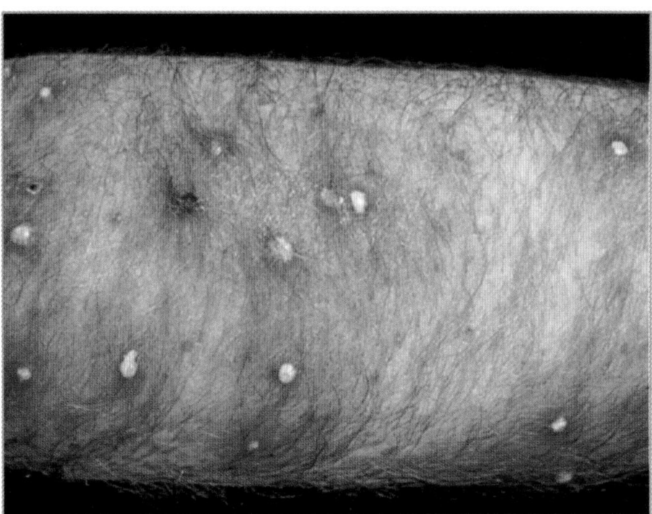

Figure 18.4 Pustular folliculitis of the forearm in Behçet's disease; the sterile lesions were widespread over the trunk, arms and thighs.

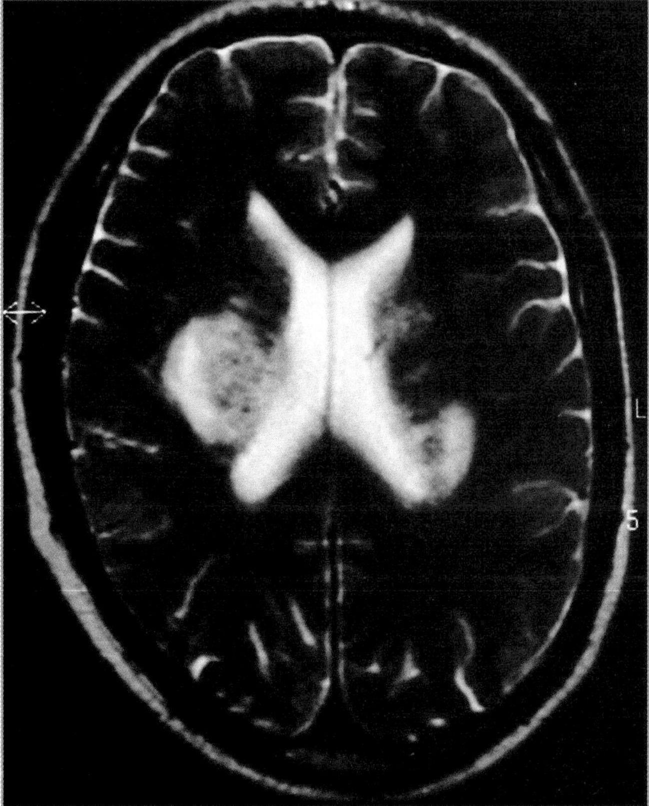

Figure 18.5 Horizontal T2-weighted MRI in a patient with Behçet's disease presenting with meningitis, hemiparesis and dysarthria, showing bilateral periventricular foci of inflammation. Full recovery followed intravenous methylprednisolone and cyclophosphamide.

show a predilection for the mesodiencephalic junction and the pontobulbar region (Koçer et al. 1999) and, in general, it is thought that parenchymal involvement supports the likely pathogenesis of small-vessel vasculitis. FLAIR sequence imaging may be particularly helpful in delineating periventricular lesions. The distribution and appearance of lesions will help to differentiate demyelination and other vasculitides.

Optic neuropathy is an uncommon and poorly described manifestation of Behçet's disease but it may be less uncommon in white patients (Joseph et al. 2007). Acute optic neuritis and ischemic neuropathy have been reported. Chronic optic neuropathy with progressive visual loss in the absence of retinal ischemia is also seen and is difficult to manage.

Other manifestations

About half the patients will develop joint involvement, usually a polysynovitis, especially in the ankles and knees. The severity varies from a mild arthralgia to a severe arthritis with effusion, but erosive damage is uncommon. Onset is usually subacute but occasionally sudden and severe, mimicking septic arthritis. Epididymitis or epididymo-orchitis is not infrequent. A variety of gastrointestinal manifestations has been reported in over 10% of patients, but the lower esophagus and ileocaecal regions are most commonly affected. Anorexia, abdominal distension and discomfort are frequent. Ulceration and bleeding, enteritis, diarrhea, perforation (occasionally multiple or sequential) and perianal fistula are all recorded.

Major thrombotic episodes occur in a few patients with Behçet's disease, sometimes involving the superior or inferior venae cavae; intraventricular thrombosis is also a risk, as is mesenteric thrombosis which may present with acute abdomen. Peripheral superficial or deep thrombophlebitis is common. Large-vessel arteritis (including aortitis) may occur, and this may lead to obstruction. Arterial aneurysms (at any location) are an uncommon but serious occurrence, although they are most likely to be problematic in the pulmonary circulation, where ruptured aneurysms may lead to hemoptysis, or in the mesenteric circulation, where rupture has caused massive internal bleeding. Renal involvement is uncommon and usually mild; proteinuria or microscopic hematuria is detected in some and a few have developed glomerulonephritis. Pneumonitis is seen occasionally. Most patients with Behçet's disease are generally well but intermittently symptomatic because of the focal problems described above. However, some experience an acute onset of the disease, with malaise, fever and weight loss in addition to characteristic manifestations.

Behçet's disease has a significant mortality rate. In a 20-year outcome survey, a 10% mortality rate was demonstrated (Yazici and Esen 2008). The most common causes of death were major vessel disease (40% of deaths, including ruptured pulmonary artery aneurysm, which was seen almost exclusively in men), followed by heart and central nervous system (CNS) disease (12% each). Surprisingly there does not appear to be an increased risk of coronary disease.

Ocular disease

Intraocular inflammation occurs in about 80% of patients with Behçet's disease, but is more common in men than in women. Men are also more likely to develop posterior segment involvement and macular lesions. Uveitis is not usually the first manifestation of the disease, but may arise soon after the onset. Those who develop the disease aged <25 years have a higher incidence of eye inflammation. In those with Behçet's disease who have failed to develop ocular inflammation after several years, the likelihood of such development is low, but nevertheless we have seen patients presenting with uveitis many years after the first onset of mucocutaneous symptoms.

The uveitis in Behçet's disease is typically recurrent, with extremely rapid exacerbations. Attacks are symptomatic and may involve the anterior or posterior segment, or both. The disease is almost always eventually bilateral but individual attacks are usually unilateral or asymmetrical. Sequential involvement of the second eye may be delayed for years; we have seen patients, who were blind in one eye after many recurrences of occlusive retinal vasculitis, developing involvement of the second eye for the first time more than a decade later. It is the progressive damage caused by recurrent posterior uveitis that leads to the high incidence of visual loss in this disease. In some patients, inflammation may occur only in the anterior segment, although this is by no means benign.

Anterior uveitis is common. It is symptomatic, with pain and photophobia. Hypopyon is frequently seen (**Fig. 18.6**) but is usually small and sometimes visible only on gonioscopy of the inferior angle. A fibrinous reaction is not usually seen in Behçet's disease, and this lack of intracameral fibrinogen means that the hypopyon is sometimes slowly mobile if the patient's head is tilted. Presumably this is a manifestation of the rapid migration and extravasation of leukocytes in Behçet's disease, in contrast to the vascular protein 'leakage' seen in HLA-B27-associated uveitis. Nevertheless, posterior synechiae may occur in Behçet's disease. Glaucoma and cataract may complicate the picture.

The posterior segment lesions are usually characteristic. An attack is often accompanied by rapid-onset vitreous opacification, the 'smoky' appearance being caused by myriads of free-floating inflammatory cells, which tend not to coagulate into large opacities. Through this hazy medium, areas of fluffy white focal retinitis may be punctate, often multifocal (**Fig. 18.7**) or larger and accompanied by retinal edema and flame-shaped hemorrhages (**Fig. 18.8**). Small retinal branch arteriole or vein occlusions may also be seen. The macula is frequently affected and vision therefore often profoundly reduced (**Fig. 18.9**). Although

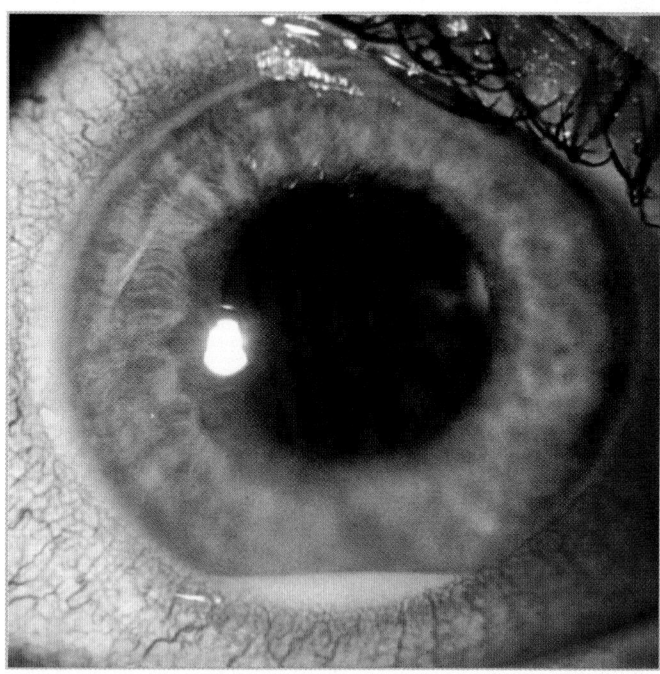

Figure 18.6 Hypopyon anterior uveitis during an acute flare-up of Behçet's disease.

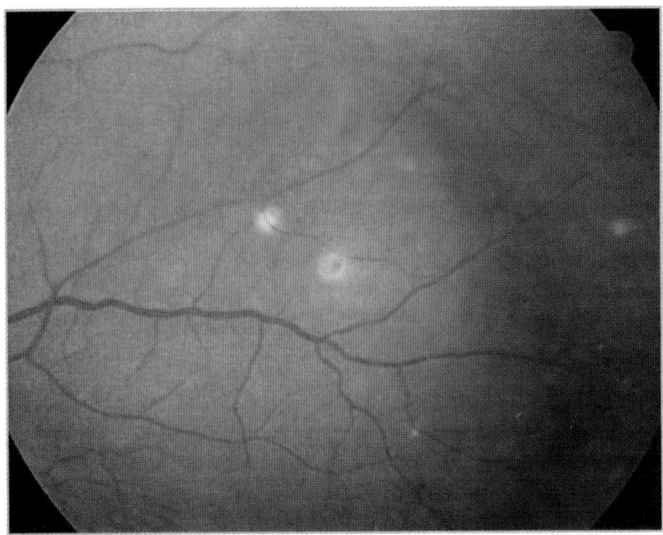

Figure 18.7 Acute multifocal punctate retinitis in a retinal recurrence, seen through slightly hazy vitreous.

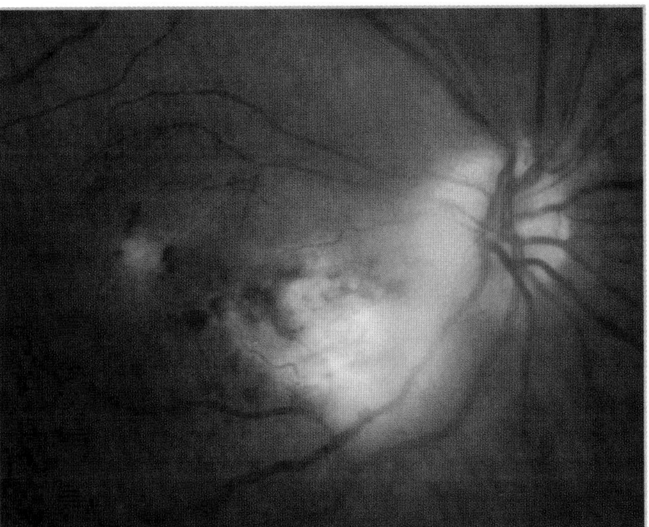

Figure 18.9 Acute macular retinitis in Behçet's disease.

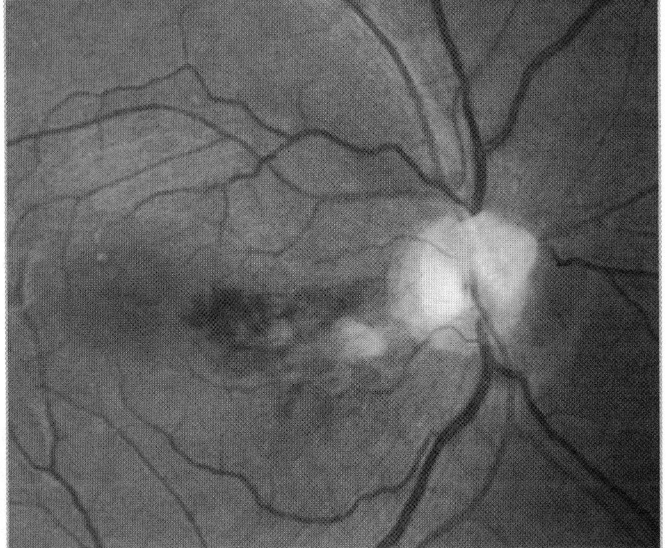

Figure 18.8 An active retinal focus in the papillomacular bundle with associated flame hemorrhages, together with an active disk lesion.

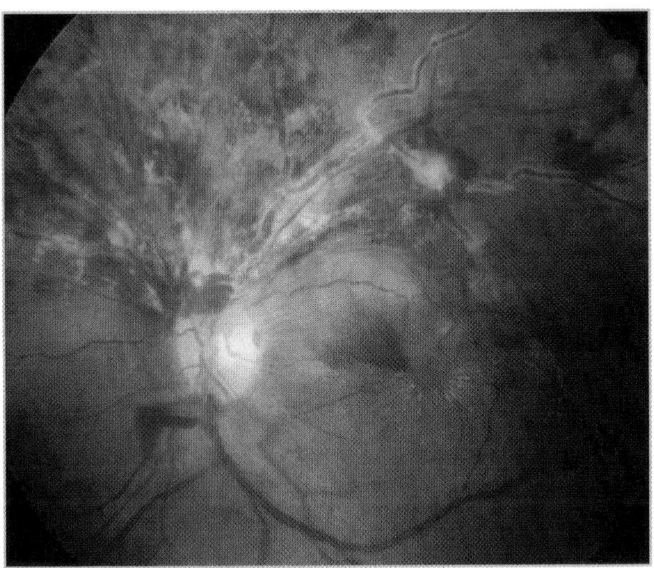

Figure 18.10 Hemispheric vein occlusion with substantial perivenous frosting, associated with a macular star; the presenting sign in a young woman with simultaneous-onset severe orogenital ulceration. She did not recover central vision.

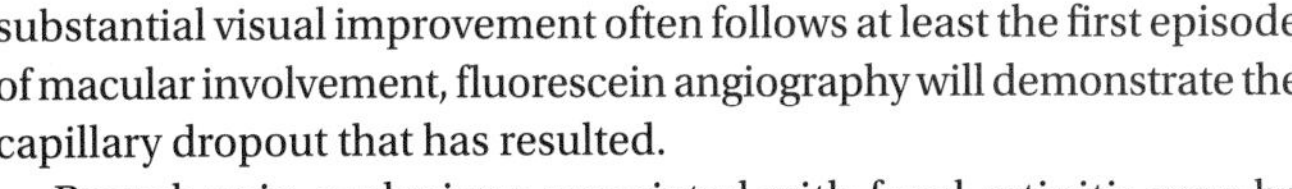

substantial visual improvement often follows at least the first episode of macular involvement, fluorescein angiography will demonstrate the capillary dropout that has resulted.

Branch vein occlusions associated with focal retinitis may be limited to small areas, but sometimes hemisphere (**Fig. 18.10**) or central vein occlusions are seen. It is common in such circumstances to see clear 'frosting' of affected veins, and Behçet's disease should be on the differential diagnosis list for secondary frosted branch angiitis. Widespread capillaritis manifesting as diffuse capillary bed leakage (**Fig. 18.11**) is considered by some to be characteristic of Behçet's disease but in fact is seen in primary retinal vasculitis and some other conditions. Sequential episodes of retinitis or occlusive vasculitis will lead to frank arterial occlusion and silver-wiring (**Fig. 18.12**). Although Behçet's disease is characteristically recurrent and acute, sometimes indolent chronic vitritis or intermediate-like uveitis is seen, and in these cases fibrotic epiretinal reactions may occur, leading to substantial tractional effects (**Fig. 18.13**). In some eyes, an inexorable decline into overlapping reactivations and gross retinal ischemia, often one hemisphere before the other (**Fig. 18.14**), leads eventually to profound optic atrophy, empty or attenuated retinal vessels and blindness (**Fig. 18.15**). Historically, untreated patients almost inevitably suffered this fate. Modern interventions make this outcome much less common.

The optic nerve may be involved in several ways: papilledema, as a sign of intracranial hypertension secondary to cerebral vein or dural sinus thrombosis, has been reported. Patients with disk swelling therefore require appropriate investigation, including brain imaging; acute or chronic optic neuropathy is recognized and slow stepwise field deterioration can be seen (**Fig. 18.16**); retinal or disk

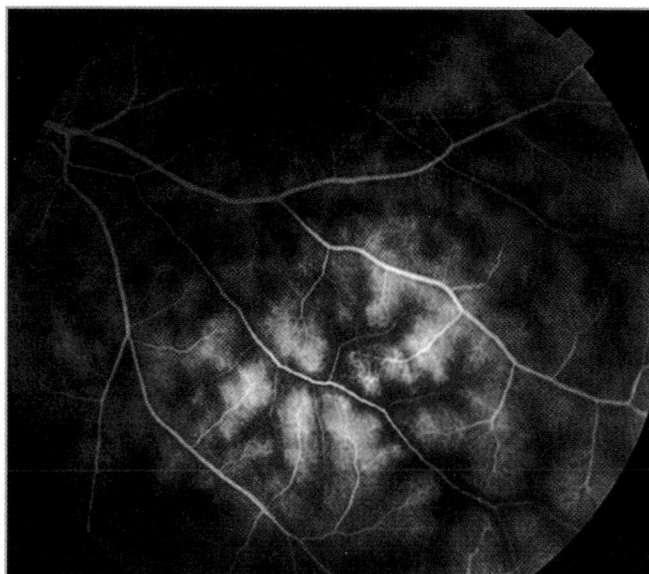

Figure 18.11 The characteristic feathery pattern of retinal capillary bed leakage secondary to capillaritis, in a patient with Behçet's disease.

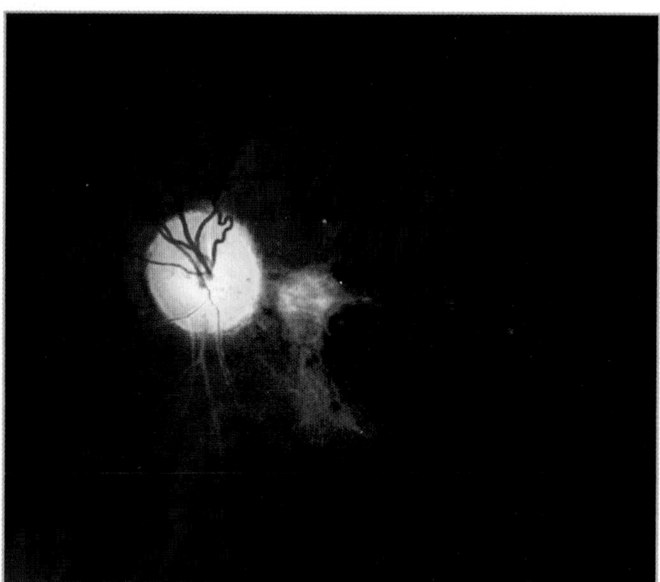

Figure 18.12 Later-stage retinal disease showing inferior hemisphere ischemia with arterial silver-wiring, together with optic atrophy, retinal pigment epithelium clumping and epiretinal membrane.

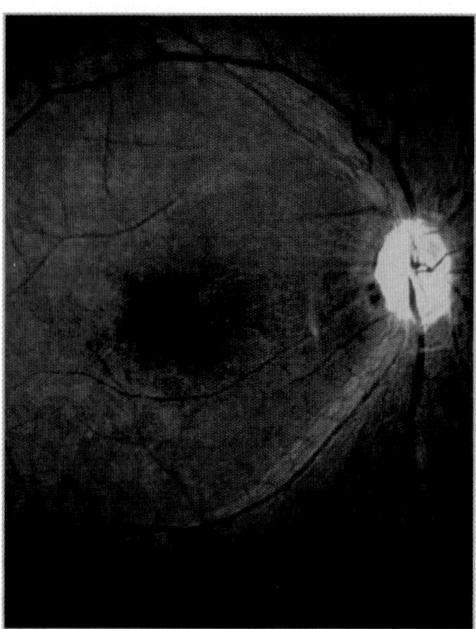

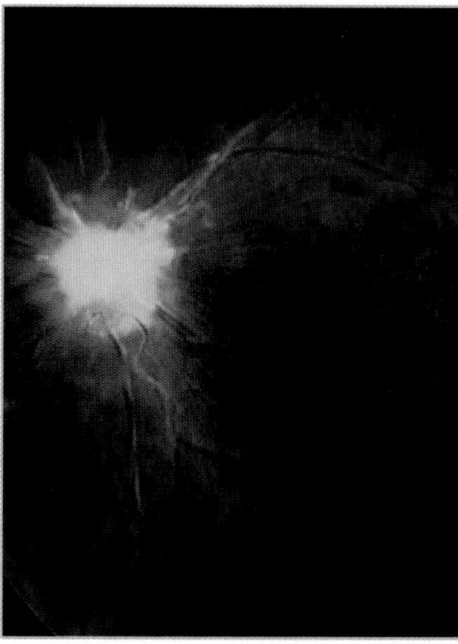

Figure 18.13 Preretinal and optic nerve head gliosis with substantial retinal traction is associated with widespread vascular sheathing and retinal atrophy in a patient with chronic vitritis in Behçet's disease.

neovascularization is not common in Behçet's disease, occurring in perhaps 5% of those with retinal involvement (Atmaca et al. 1996) but when present causes recurrent vitreous hemorrhage and requires laser photocoagulation.

The outlook for vision in Behçet's disease must remain guarded despite progressive improvements in treatment. In 2004 a large series from Turkey describing 880 patients followed during the 1980s and 1990s demonstrated a 30% blindness rate for males with the disease (Tugal-Tutkun et al. 2004).

Diagnosis

Behçet's disease is a disorder with protean manifestations that may present to any one of several specialists, sometimes sequentially over several years, and that may be a diagnostic challenge. Some consider that the disease falls into four broad subtypes: mucocutaneous, with predominant oral and genital ulceration, sometimes with skin lesions; arthritic, with joint involvement prominent in addition to mucocutaneous disease; neurological; and ocular, the last two including any or all of the other manifestations. It is possible that such groups represent the predominant experience of different specialists, rather than the existence of discrete subtypes, but evidence is accumulating of predispositions to certain manifestations because of gene mutations. In those patients with uveitis and arthritis with or without oral ulceration, reactive arthritis and uveitis enter the differential diagnosis; those with severe gastrointestinal involvement with or without oral or perianal ulceration are difficult to distinguish from patients with Crohn's disease; some vascular manifestations can mimic Takayasu's disease; neurological manifestations may suggest herpetic encephalitis or sarcoidosis; retinitis or retinal vasculitis may appear to be viral.

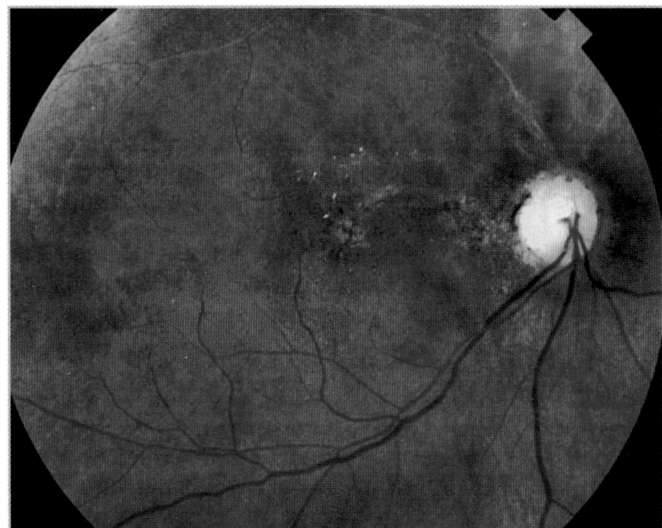

Figure 18.14 The lower hemisphere of this eye is relatively intact, but in contrast the upper is blind, with complete retinal infarction and resultant atrophy, together with optic hemiatrophy and macular scarring.

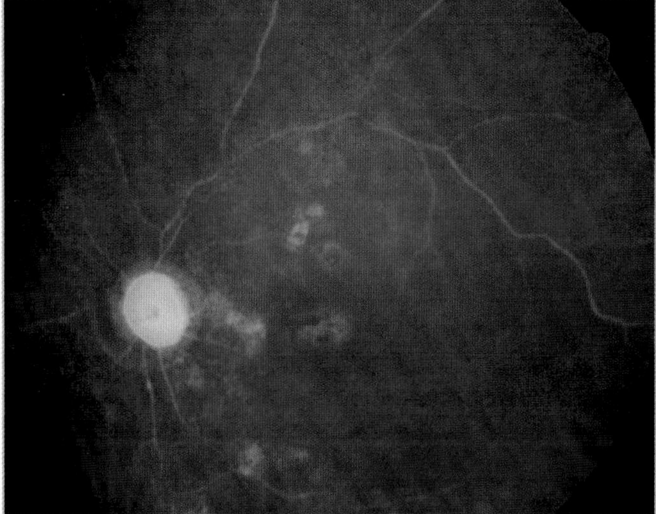

Figure 18.15 Terminal optic atrophy and vascular wipeout with widespread retinal atrophy and pigmentary scarring in a blind eye.

Such diagnostic difficulties are frequent, especially in the west where 'complete' Behçet's disease presenting as a combined entity, is rare.

The diagnosis of Behçet's disease is entirely clinical. However, in such a variable disease the diagnosis may be in dispute and those with possible Behçet's disease may be labeled 'incomplete' or 'suspect.' At least seven diagnostic systems have been proposed since the initial Mason and Barnes system in 1969 (Dervis et al. 2005), which are broadly similar although each may be more clinically useful within different specialty areas. It is usually accepted that the 'minor' diagnostic criteria, although often highly significant for the patient, do not add to the reliability of a diagnostic system, which should therefore be based on the 'major' criteria only. The diagnostic criteria of the ISGBD (1990), based on multicenter studies in seven countries, are given in **Table 18.1** and the minor criteria in **Table 18.2**.

Table 18.1 ISG Diagnostic criteria for Behçet's disease

Patients must have:
1. Aphthous or herpetiform oral ulceration recurring at least three times per year and any two of:
2. Active ulcers or evidence (by examination or history) of scars from previous ulcers, on penis, scrotum, vulva, vagina, perineal or perianal
3. Anterior or posterior uveitis including retinal vasculitis
4. Relevant skin lesions: a. Erythema nodosum b. Folliculitis including papulopustular lesions or acneiform nodules (not related to corticosteroid treatment)
5. A positive pathergy test
Adapted from International Study Group for Behçet's Disease (1990).

Table 18.2 Minor criteria of Behçet's disease – not used for diagnosis

Gastrointestinal ulceration, abdominal pain, diarrhea
Polyarthritis or arthralgia, especially of large joints
Venous thrombosis, aneurysms
Pneumonitis, hemoptysis
Epididymo-orchitis
Erythema multiforme
Meningitis, encephalitis, confusional states, brain-stem disease
Proteinuria and hematuria

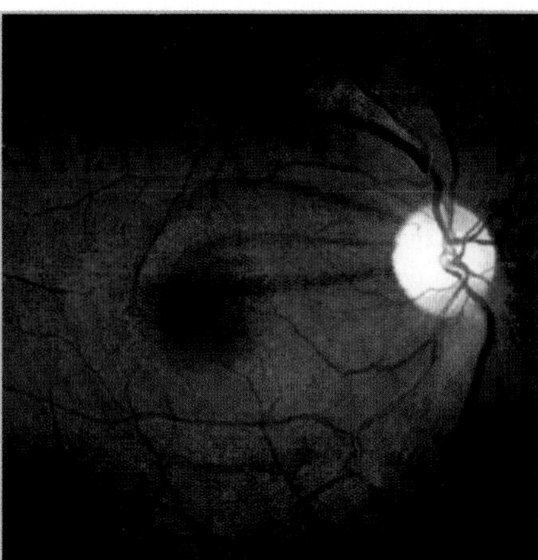

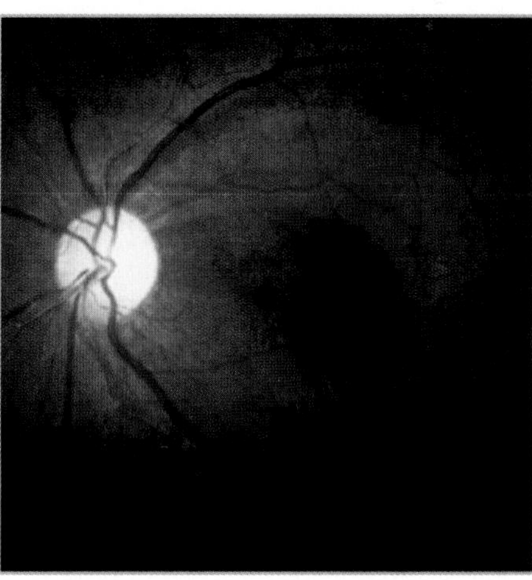

Figure 18.16 An enhanced-contrast fundus photograph showing multiple nerve fiber bundle defects in a patient with Behçet's chronic optic neuropathy. There is accompanying temporal optic atrophy.

This diagnostic system requires the presence of aphthous ulceration in all patients. This, and the exclusion of minor criteria from the diagnostic process, creates a rigid system. Such systems are helpful in the comparison of patient groups and imperative for multicenter studies of treatment, but are perhaps less helpful in the diagnosis of the individual patient, who may be considered by the ophthalmologist to have ocular features characteristic of the disease but may not adequately fulfill the diagnostic criteria. In this clinic we would consider the existence of two minor criteria to 'substitute' for one major criterion if necessary, and manifestations widely separated in time; over a period of years the diagnosis may become more clear by the progressive involvement of systems. Despite this less stringent approach to the diagnosis of an individual patient, there will still remain some whose ocular manifestations are quite typical of Behçet's disease, but who are otherwise well. In practice it seems highly likely that some patients do have Behçet's disease, but in incomplete or localized forms. The term 'ocular Behçet's disease' has been used in these circumstances. This is a useful label, because these eyes tend to behave in a way characteristic of those in patients with typical Behçet's disease and similar treatment options can be considered.

Pathergy test

A significant proportion of patients with Behçet's disease (although probably more patients in the Middle East than elsewhere) develop a sterile pustule at the site of skin trauma. The phenomenon is known as 'pathergy.' This reaction forms the basis of the pathergy test; a subcutaneous puncture may provoke such a pustule within a day or two. A positive pathergy test is used as a major criterion for diagnosis in some diagnostic systems (see Table 18.1). However, there is some evidence that its incidence is decreasing, to perhaps as few as a third of patients with Behçet's disease (Davatchi et al. 2007). It has always been considered of limited use for diagnosis in white people and has not been used in this clinic.

Blood tests

Circulating immune complexes are found in about half the patients and acute-phase proteins are increased. Complement C9 level is a sensitive marker for disease activity and has been used to monitor treatment efficacy. Serum IgA may be increased. General markers of autoimmune disease such as antinuclear antibodies (ANAs), anti-thyroid antibody and antibodies to gastric parietal cells are not found. Patients with arthritis are rheumatoid factor negative. Those with clinical evidence of deep venous thrombosis or arterial occlusion should be investigated for thrombophilic factors which are often abnormal, including anti-phospholipid antibodies and deficiency of protein C or S (Caramaschi et al. 2010) and possibly factor V Leiden (Batioglu et al. 2003). HLA-B51 testing may be of some use depending on the relative risk for specific populations but is not diagnostically useful in a UK population.

Management

The patient with Behçet's disease may develop severe manifestations within the areas of expertise of several specialists and, as for other multisystem diseases, close liaisons are required to optimize treatment. In some centers this is best achieved by combined clinics. For the majority who develop sight-threatening uveitis, it usually falls to the ophthalmologist to be the main arbiter of treatment because it is the eyes that usually require the most potent anti-inflammatory or immunosuppressive therapy.

Anterior uveitis in Behçet's disease is often hyperacute and requires intensive topical steroid therapy, sometimes combined with subconjunctival administration. Acute posterior uveitis or retinitis usually requires high-dose systemic steroids and, with particularly severe involvement, intravenous methylprednisolone. Long-term maintenance with systemic steroids alone is highly unsatisfactory at preventing recurrences, associated with substantial side effects and, in the long term, ineffective. Immunosuppressives are therefore usually required.

Historically, chlorambucil was the immunosuppressive of choice. However, the considerable side effects of this drug, especially in young people, led to the search for alternatives. Azathioprine is widely used with early demonstration of success by controlled trial (Yazici et al. 1990), being followed by several confirmatory reports (Saadoun et al. 2010). Colchicine is frequently used to treat other manifestations of Behçet's disease, particularly the arthropathy and mucocutaneous manifestations, but it is not considered useful in the management of uveitis. Cyclophosphamide is still used in some patients (Davatchi et al. 2004), usually for severe episodes in patients already immunosuppressed. The efficacy of ciclosporin especially for the uveitis element of the disease is well accepted, and long-term low-dose therapy may be both well tolerated and effective (Özdal et al. 2002). However, reports of a higher incidence of neurological involvement in ciclosporin-treated patients are a substantial concern (Kötter et al. 2006), which has modified our approach to treatment. Opinion on the efficacy of mycophenolate mofetil is conflicting; it is not considered particularly useful for mucocutaneous manifestations but it has been used successfully for the uveitis and in our clinic it has been a useful addition to the armamentarium.

The varying manifestations of Behçet's disease dictate the approach to treatment. Anterior uveitis may be managed by topical steroid alone. Unilateral focal retinitis outside the macula may respond to orbital floor depot steroid. Inflammatory or vaso-occlusive macular involvement mandates the use of high-dose (and sometimes, preferably, intravenous) steroid. The latter approach remains the most effective and rapidly acting treatment of an acute recurrence. However, maintenance treatment should aim to reduce or if possible prevent recurrent disease, both intraocularly and systemically, without the use of systemic steroids. For patients with multisystem disease close cooperation with their rheumatologist or dermatologist will be necessary.

Previously in our clinic there was a definite preference for ciclosporin as the first-line immunosuppressive where disease warranted. The emerging evidence on neurological involvement in ciclosporin-treated patients and the availability of mycophenolate have tailored our approach depending on patient age, sex and system involvement. Whichever immunosuppressive is chosen, a steroid taper follows at the appropriate time with an intention to discontinue if possible. Recurrent disease is followed either by immunosuppressive dose increase or by the addition of a second agent. We do not use colchicine but our rheumatological colleagues do – it must be used with caution if combined with ciclosporin (as of course should non-steroidal anti-inflammatory drugs – NSAIDs). One year disease free will lead to a slow taper of immunosuppressive dosage. A few patients maintain quiescence for years after cessation of treatment, but many recur. Each recurrence is treated with steroid as required, followed by adjustment of immunosuppression maintenance and a further steroid taper. We have found that ciclosporin, in particular, has the ability in some patients to suppress recurrence even in very low doses (e.g. 1 mg/kg per day) that are undetectable on measurement of serum trough levels; after a false reassurance of disease burn-out, we have discontinued such doses only to encounter immediate recurrences. Tacrolimus is an alternative to ciclosporin (Sakane et al. 1995) but the effects if any on neuro-Behçet's disease have not been well described. Some authors consider the efficacy/toxicity profile to be somewhat better overall for tacrolimus. We have not found methotrexate to be of adequate potency to suppress this form of recurrent uveitis.

It is our policy to treat unilateral sight-threatening uveitis in Behçet's disease as we would bilateral disease; sequential involvement is common and therefore to be anticipated, and the risk of immunosuppression is justified in this circumstance.

Using this approach most patients can be maintained uveitis free without oral steroid treatment. A few have chronic vitritis or intermediate uveitis, which does require low-dose steroids. Many who are uveitis free on immunosuppression continue to suffer mucocutaneous symptoms. In these circumstances, if local treatment, such as steroid lozenges, nicotine patches or gum, is unsuccessful, some will respond to colchicine. Others do well on thalidomide (Franks et al. 2004) but this is of no relevance to uveitis and the control of this drug (which should normally remain with the rheumatologist) is rightly very stringent.

Our approach to surgery, if required in patients with uveitis, follows basic principles: stringent and stable control of intraocular inflammation and careful postoperative follow-up. Postoperative disease flares are unusual and intraocular lenses are well tolerated if such methods are followed. Postoperative visual results are mainly a factor of macular status.

Interferon

Interferon-α (IFNα, specifically IFN-α2a), in addition to being an antiviral and anti-cancer drug, has immunosuppressive properties and has been used in Behçet's disease. Its action is not fully understood. It is effective in the majority (Stübinger et al. 2001) and, importantly, some consider that it may lead to long-term remission of disease (Deuter et al. 2010); others disagree (Gendron et al. 2003). Unfortunately it is unpleasant to use; it is pyrogenic and flu-like symptoms are universal, other side effects including injection site reactions also being common. Adverse effects may be temporary or may persist. Pegylation prolongs the efficacy of a single dose but has not yet been evaluated in Behçet's disease. There is clearly a place for IFN-α2a in some patients with immunosuppression-resistant uveitis, but that place is difficult to confirm in the context of developing enthusiasm for monoclonal antibody therapy:

Monoclonal antibody therapy

There is great enthusiasm currently for the use of anti-TNF-α (tumor necrosis factor α) monoclonal antibody treatment in both combined immunosuppression-resistant Behçet's disease and some other forms of severe uveitis. Infliximab in particular has been widely but anecdotally used but no controlled trial has been published. Its efficacy is well described (Tugal-Tutkun et al. 2005), usually in an infusion dosage of 5 mg/kg at weeks 0, 2, (4), (6), 8 initially, and notably its speed of effect can be impressive. Using an intensive regimen, a degree of remission has been claimed (Tabbara et al. 2008). Where antibodies have developed, anecdotes of a switch to adalimumab have been largely positive. Neither the indications nor the optimal regimen for anti-TNF-α monoclonal antibody treatment have yet been clarified and, for such expensive drugs, a controlled trial is sorely needed.

B-cell suppression with rituximab (anti-CD20 monoclonal antibody) is gaining ground in the management of several rheumatic diseases and forms of systemic vasculitis. Initial reports of its use in difficult uveitis in Behçet's disease (Davatchi et al. 2010) suggest its superiority to cyclophosphamide, but more studies are required. Anakinra (IL-1R antagonist) has been used only anecdotally and no firm conclusions have been drawn. Tocilizumab (IL-6R antagonist) has a theoretical basis for use but no data currently exist. Further possibilities will doubtless arise.

Sweet syndrome

Sweet's or Sweet syndrome (acute febrile neutrophilic dermatosis) is a rare sudden-onset inflammatory disorder comprising fever, neutrophilia and multifocal tender skin papules with a characteristic leukocytic and histiocytic histology. It may also cause arthritis, aphthous ulceration and uveitis (usually iridocyclitis) and, more rarely, widespread systemic inflammation. It is usually seen in association with underlying autoimmune inflammations such as inflammatory bowel disease or rheumatoid arthritis, or with leukemia or other malignancies. It may also be drug induced.

It is included here first because Behçet's disease may be on the differential diagnostic list for a patient presenting with combinations of the above symptoms and signs and second because, confusingly, Sweet syndrome has anecdotally been reported as a complication of Behçet's disease itself. All manifestations are normally steroid responsive but occasionally require additional treatment including immunosuppression or dapsone.

PRIMARY SYSTEMIC VASCULITIS AND UVEITIS (box 18.2)

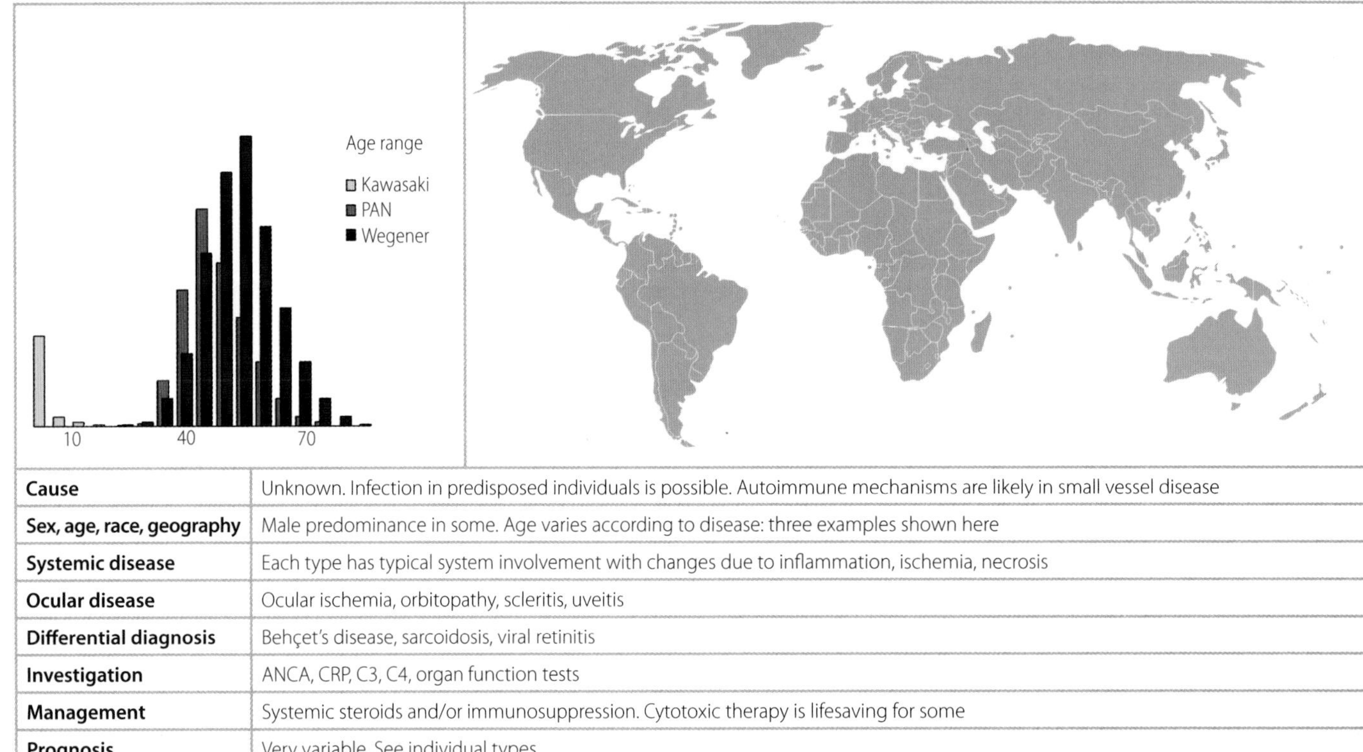

Cause	Unknown. Infection in predisposed individuals is possible. Autoimmune mechanisms are likely in small vessel disease
Sex, age, race, geography	Male predominance in some. Age varies according to disease: three examples shown here
Systemic disease	Each type has typical system involvement with changes due to inflammation, ischemia, necrosis
Ocular disease	Ocular ischemia, orbitopathy, scleritis, uveitis
Differential diagnosis	Behçet's disease, sarcoidosis, viral retinitis
Investigation	ANCA, CRP, C3, C4, organ function tests
Management	Systemic steroids and/or immunosuppression. Cytotoxic therapy is lifesaving for some
Prognosis	Very variable. See individual types

Box 18.2 Primary systemic vasculitis and uveitis

Introduction

Necrotizing inflammation of blood vessels is the primary abnormality in the systemic vasculitides. Vasculitis may also be a prominent component of several other diseases, but in these, blood vessel inflammation is secondary and they are discussed elsewhere. Primary systemic necrotizing vasculitis may take many forms and differential diagnosis and classification had been confusing until the Chapel Hill Consensus Conference was held in North Carolina in 1994, establishing a simple classification that is the most commonly used today. It is based first on the size of blood vessel primarily involved by the inflammation (large, medium or small) and second by the presence or absence of granulomas. The Chapel Hill system is shown in **Table 18.3**. It is not a comprehensive system for vasculitis, excluding secondary causes and some 'unclassifiable' forms.

It is a strange but undeniable feature of the primary systemic vasculitides that retinal vasculitis is so uncommon. The most common cause of ocular or visual involvement by these diseases is ischemia secondary to extraocular vasculitis (predominantly, ischemic optic neuropathy) or granulomatous orbital or scleral inflammation. Uveitis is very uncommon, but only intraocular inflammation is discussed here.

Table 18.3 Chapel Hill classification of the systemic vasculitides

Vessel size	With granulomas	Without granulomas
Large	Giant cell arteritis	Takayasu's disease
Medium	Churg–Strauss syndrome	Polyarteritis nodosa Kawasaki's disease
Small	Wegener's granulomatosis	Microscopic polyarteritis Henoch–Schönlein purpura

Giant cell arteritis

Acute posterior segment ischemia in the form of central retinal artery occlusion or, more commonly, ischemic optic neuropathy is the characteristic ocular lesion in giant cell arteritis. A few rare cases of primary intraocular inflammation have been reported, and chronic ocular ischemia may occur that may mimic uveitis. This is discussed in Chapter 9.

Churg–Strauss syndrome

Churg-Strauss syndrome (allergic granulomatosis) was first recognized as an entity separate from polyarteritis nodosa in 1951 (Churg and Strauss 1951) because of the association of asthma and eosinophilia with vasculitis. It is very rare. The disease affects young adults and often presents with severe allergic rhinitis with polyp formation. Vasculitis starts later and may be widespread. This phase usually lasts only a few months, and if survived settles to leave severe chronic asthma and vasculitic damage to other systems. Ocular involvement in is uncommon but usually consists of the neuro-ophthalmic complications of intracranial involvement or of ischemic optic neuropathy similar to that seen in giant cell arteritis. A tiny number of anecdotes of uveitis, usually with papilledema or neurological complications, have been reported.

Wegener's granulomatosis

This is a granulomatous necrotizing vasculitis of small vessels which especially affects the respiratory tract and kidneys, but which may also become more generalized. Some patients present with a non-specific illness including malaise and weight loss before proceeding with variable speed to a vasculitis, which had a mortality rate approaching 100% before the introduction of cytotoxic immunosuppression.

Classic Wegener's granulomatosis predominantly affects the upper respiratory tract, the mucosal necrosis causing a foul bloody rhinorrhea with intranasal crusting, ulceration and septal perforation. Sinusitis, glue ear and hoarseness reflect spreading involvement. Stridor, cough, dyspnea, pleurisy or hemoptysis indicates lower respiratory tract involvement. Chest radiograph typically shows cavitating pulmonary nodules. Glomerulonephritis or necrotizing cutaneous vasculitis may be seen.

In its widespread and aggressive form, Wegener's granulomatosis is a sinister diagnosis even with the cytotoxic immunosuppressives now available. However, milder or anatomically limited forms are known to exist, and the orbital region is one well-recognized area for limited disease. Such variants may be initially less aggressive, but may at any time convert into more aggressive and widespread disease, and caution in both management and prognostication should always be maintained.

There is ophthalmic involvement in about half the patients but orbital inflammation, scleritis and/or keratitis predominates (Tarabishy et al. 2010). Uveitis if present is usually secondary to sclerokeratitis but may be seen in isolation (Watkins et al. 2009). Retinal vasculitis is uncommon but may be occlusive. Choroidal involvement may present as a placoid-like segmental ischemia, granulomatous choroiditis or massive choroidal vasculitis with infarction and serous retinal detachment, as is seen in some patients with lupus.

Takayasu's arteritis

Takayasu's disease is a rare vasculitis affecting large arteries including the aorta and its major branches. It is most common in women in Japan and the Orient. The eyes are involved in many patients, predominantly by vascular occlusion, either ischemic neuropathy or ocular ischemic syndrome (Jayanthi et al. 2010), but anecdotal reports of intraocular inflammation have appeared.

Polyarteritis nodosa

After the initial descriptions of systemic vasculitis in the nineteenth century by Kussmaul and Maier and others, the term 'polyarteritis nodosa' was used very broadly to encompass several vasculitides that are now separately recognized. The use of the term has gradually narrowed and has more recently been used to describe one subset of these patients.

Polyarteritis nodosa (PAN) is a rare vasculitis of medium-sized arteries leading to end-organ infarction. Presentations include acute abdomen from perforation of mucosal ulcers, mesenteric infarction or pancreatitis, myocardial infarction, purpuric skin rashes or subcutaneous thrombosis. Pea-sized aneurysmal nodules may follow the course of superficial arteries and are a hallmark of the disease. Neurological involvement is uncommon; CNS lesions may lead to stroke and peripheral neuropathies occur. The eyes are involved in 10–20% of patients with PAN (Akova et al. 1993). Necrotizing scleritis, peripheral ulcerative keratitis, anterior uveitis (with or without scleritis), and retinal or choroidal vasculitis with ischemia are all possible features. Aggressive immunosuppression is life saving.

Kawasaki's disease

Kawasaki's disease (the mucocutaneous lymph node syndrome) is an idiopathic vasculitis of moderate-sized arteries with pathological features very similar to polyarteritis nodosa, occurring most commonly in children of Asian origin. It presents most commonly in infants and young children (but rarely up to late adolescence) with persistent high pyrexia, lymphadenopathy, mucosal inflammation involving the mouth, lips and conjunctiva, and a variable skin rash that may include vesicles. Severe redness of palms and soles is later followed by progressive desquamation of the extremities. Involvement of any major system may occur, but coronary aneurysms are characteristic. Kawasaki's disease is now the leading cause of acquired heart disease in children, and the mortality rate is about 3%.

Conjunctivitis is almost universal. Bilateral anterior uveitis is not uncommon (Perrin et al. 2009) but is usually mild and short-lived. However, posterior segment inflammation with visual loss has been reported.

Other systemic vasculitides

Uveitis or retinal vascular involvement is a rare feature of microscopic polyangiitis (Mihara et al. 2005), leukocytoclastic vasculitis, urticarial vasculitis and Henoch–Schönlein purpura. Anterior uveitis is rarely seen in histiocytic necrotizing lymphadenitis (Kikuchi–Fujimoto disease). Other systemic inflammations may exhibit a retinal vasculitic element. These are discussed either below or in the appropriate chapter.

Diagnosis

Most patients presenting to an ophthalmologist with a systemic vasculitis have been diagnosed elsewhere and are already immunosuppressed. Uncommonly, but most often in limited forms of Wegener's granulomatosis, the presenting symptoms may be ophthalmic. In these situations the ophthalmologist will play a crucial role. In suspected cases, thorough investigation is necessary. Where systemic vasculitis is obvious the urgent involvement of a physician is essential. Otherwise, systemic examination followed by an organ screen is important. Full blood count (FBC), erythrocyte sedimentation rate (ESR), acute-phase proteins, urea and electrolytes, and renal and liver functions are required. Many immunology laboratories will now offer a 'vasculitis screen' for such suspects, which may include anti-neutrophil cytoplasmic antibodies (ANCA), C-reactive protein (CRP), complement C3 and C4 and ANAs. Where connective tissue diseases are also possible, rheumatoid factor and ANA subtypes including extractable nuclear antigen (ENA) antibody and anti-DNA antibody, should be sought.

Anti-neutrophil cytoplasmic antibodies

A group of predominantly IgG-circulating autoantibodies known as ANCAs are found in many patients with systemic vasculitis and seem to indicate small vessel involvement in the inflammatory process. Serum from an affected patient is added to immobilized normal human polymorph leukocytes. Originally an indirect immunofluorescent technique was used to highlight the resultant complexes. In positive tests, the resultant fluorescence falls into three patterns, which are usually distinct, but may have some overlap in appearance. A granular cytoplasmic pattern (**Fig. 18.17**) is defined as c-ANCA,

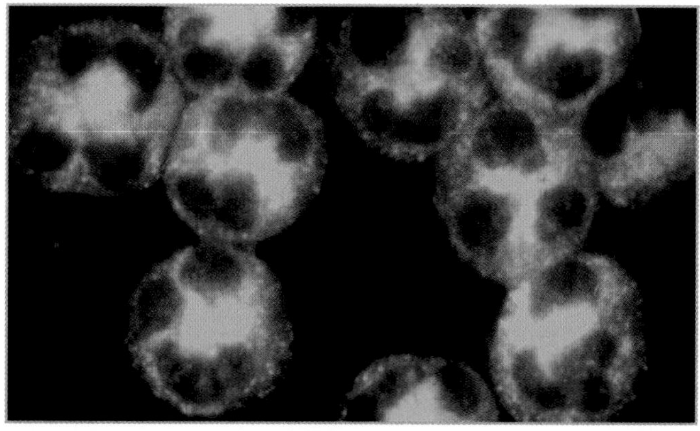

Figure 18.17 Neutrophils demonstrating c-ANCA under indirect immunofluorescence. The stain occupies the whole cytoplasm, in contrast to p-ANCA.

a predominantly perinuclear pattern is denoted p-ANCA and an atypical 'snowdrift' pattern is called x-ANCA. It is now known that the only target molecule for c-ANCA is proteinase 3, whereas the p-ANCA response is less specific, antigens including myeloperoxidase, lysozyme, lactoferrin and elastase. Enzyme-linked immunosorbent assay (ELISA) methods are now available specifically to detect anti-proteinase 3 antibody and anti-myeloperoxidase antibody.

A c-ANCA pattern is supportive of a diagnosis of Wegener's granulomatosis, but is not specific for this disease. However, p-ANCA, as might be suggested from its reaction with several antigens, is much less specific. In a study of 38 patients with a confirmed underlying diagnosis who had anti-proteinase 3 antibody (Geffriaud-Ricouard et al. 1993), 19 had Wegener's granulomatosis, 15 microscopic polyangiitis, 2 crescentic glomerulonephritis and 2 relapsing polychondritis. In the same study, of 45 patients with anti-myeloperoxidase antibody with a confirmed underlying diagnosis, 26 had microscopic polyangiitis, 8 crescentic glomerulonephritis, 5 Wegener's granulomatosis, 3 PAN, 2 systemic lupus erythematosus (SLE) and 1 Churg–Strauss syndrome. Known associations with the three ANCA types are noted in **Table 18.4**.

False-negative ANCA results may occur during intercurrent infection and there is some cross-reactivity with antinuclear antigens, which may in part explain positivity in SLE. Using ELISA testing for proteinase 3 and myeloperoxidase, specificity is enhanced and quantification is possible. Positive ANCA at low titers may not be significant for diagnostic purposes, but ANCA levels seem to be a good indicator of disease activity after diagnosis and more specific than acute phase proteins.

In patients with uveitis but without systemic indicators, ANCA testing is not a useful diagnostic procedure. Either c-ANCA or more commonly p-ANCA may be weakly positive in more than 10% but this does not lead to formal diagnosis. In one study (Chan et al. 1996), 10 of 64 patients (16%) with mixed uveitides were c-ANCA positive, of whom only two had underlying connective tissue disease. Importantly, the test was no more specific for those with retinal vasculitis.

It may be that ANCAs are a sensitive indicator of small vessel vasculitis even in single locations. However, in the absence of systemic symptoms or signs it does not appear to aid ophthalmological diagnosis. Its diagnostic use should be reserved for those in whom there are clear suggestions of the underlying diseases in Table 18.4, in which context ANCA positivity is significant.

Management

In their classic and widespread forms, the systemic vasculitides are life threatening. In small-vessel vasculitis, the use of high-dose systemic steroids alone is inadequate and cytotoxic immunosuppression is required. A variety of regimens has been devised for this purpose, but, most commonly, pulsed intravenous cyclophosphamide and methylprednisolone are used to initiate treatment, followed by oral maintenance treatment, usually with azathioprine but occasionally with methotrexate. Such cytotoxic regimens have led to substantial increases in survival rates. Complete remission can be achieved in over 75% of patients, although later relapse is not uncommon. Information on the efficacy of plasma exchange and ciclosporin is conflicting, but mycophenolate has its adherents for maintenance therapy. Infliximab treatment has been used, but currently greater interest centers on the use of rituximab (Stone et al. 2010), which may prove superior for relapsing disease.

Table 18.4 Associations with anti-neutrophil cytoplasmic antibodies (ANCAs)

ANCA type	Associated conditions
c-ANCA	Wegener's granulomatosis
	Microscopic polyarteritis
	Churg–Strauss syndrome
	Idiopathic crescentic glomerulonephritis
p-ANCA	Microscopic polyarteritis
	Polyarteritis nodosa
	Wegener's granulomatosis
	Churg–Strauss syndrome
	Idiopathic crescentic glomerulonephritis
	Systemic lupus erythematosus
	Rheumatoid arthritis
x-ANCA	Ulcerative colitis, Crohn's disease
	Autoimmune hepatitis, sclerosing cholangitis
	Primary biliary cirrhosis
	Systemic lupus erythematosus
	Rheumatoid arthritis

c-, cytoplasmic/classic; p-, perinuclear; x-, atypical/snowdrift.

PRIMARY RETINAL VASCULITIS (box 18.3)

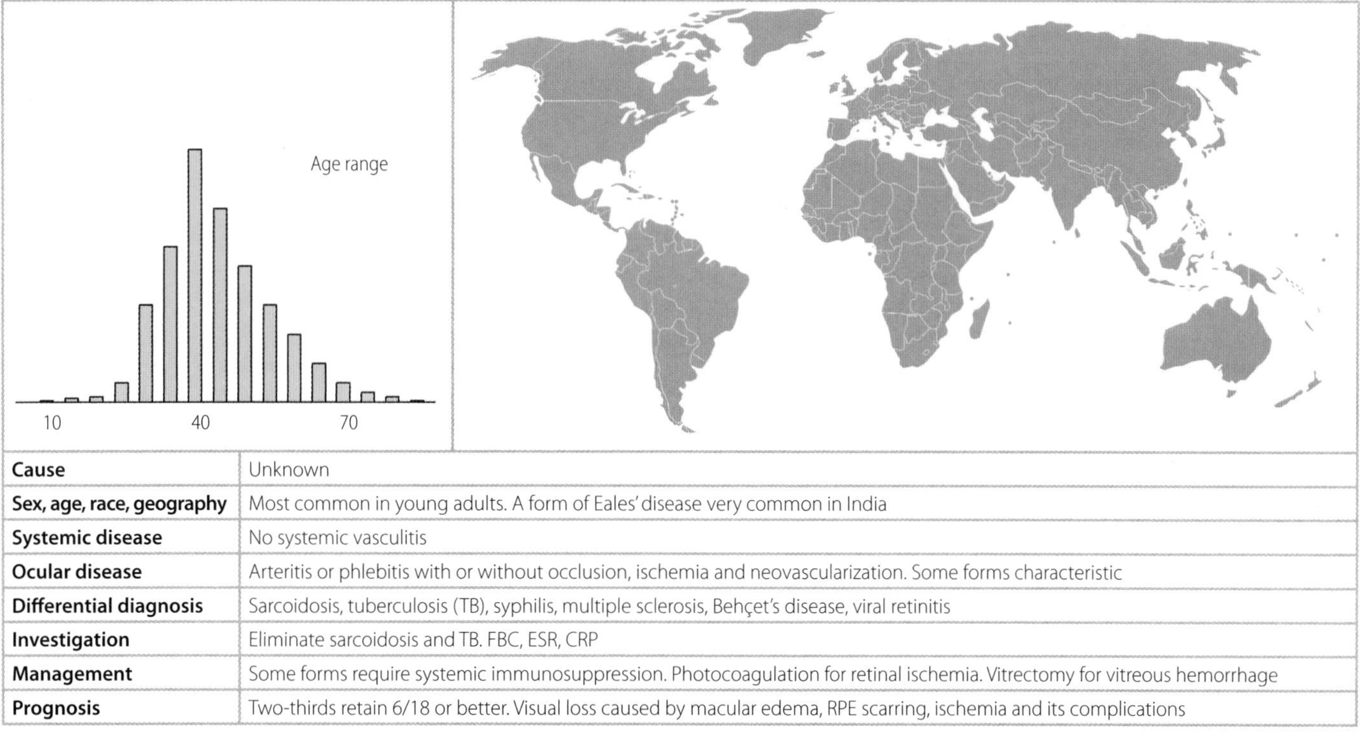

Cause	Unknown
Sex, age, race, geography	Most common in young adults. A form of Eales' disease very common in India
Systemic disease	No systemic vasculitis
Ocular disease	Arteritis or phlebitis with or without occlusion, ischemia and neovascularization. Some forms characteristic
Differential diagnosis	Sarcoidosis, tuberculosis (TB), syphilis, multiple sclerosis, Behçet's disease, viral retinitis
Investigation	Eliminate sarcoidosis and TB. FBC, ESR, CRP
Management	Some forms require systemic immunosuppression. Photocoagulation for retinal ischemia. Vitrectomy for vitreous hemorrhage
Prognosis	Two-thirds retain 6/18 or better. Visual loss caused by macular edema, RPE scarring, ischemia and its complications

Box 18.3 Primary retinal vasculitis

Introduction

Primary (idiopathic) retinal vasculitis (PRV) is by definition not associated with systemic vasculitis or systemic inflammation, and intraocular infection is presumed to be absent. It is much less common than secondary retinal vasculitis, which can occur in sarcoidosis, TB, Behçet's disease, birdshot retinochoroidopathy, viral retinitis and others. It is most commonly seen in young adults, in women rather more often than in men (Graham et al. 1989).

The taxonomy of primary retinal vasculitis has always been confusing; some of this difficulty centers around the varying definitions of 'Eales' disease,' and attempts to categorize different forms of PRV based on appearance alone. In the cases of both primary frosted branch angiitis and idiopathic retinal vasculitis with aneurysms and neuroretinitis (see below), the strikingly individual appearances and behavior render the terms useful for diagnosis and management. However, the umbrella term 'primary retinal vasculitis' has been for some years in use as a generic term for all in this group of retinal vascular inflammations, apparently unassociated with inflammations elsewhere.

Systemic disease

The reader will immediately be confused by the insertion of a paragraph that, as described above, has no place here. Although it is reassuring that, after the initial exclusion of concurrent systemic inflammation, systemic disease does not tend to develop (George et al. 1996), it should nevertheless be noted that patients with ischemic PRV have a significantly raised coronary morbidity (Palmer et al. 1995a) and thrombophilic factors have been found significantly more common in these patients (Palmer et al. 1995b). The impact of smoking on both visual and coronary morbidity is clear and patients should be strongly encouraged to desist. Indeed, even in the absence of firm data, this advice should reasonably be extended to any patient with retinal vasculitis showing a tendency to occlusion.

Ocular disease

Retinal vasculitis most often affects the venous side of the circulation, but arteritis or mixed vasculitis may also occur. Inflammation usually causes perivascular 'sheathing' (**Fig. 18.18**), which occurs in most patients during active inflammation. This phenomenon presumably represents either extravasated or actively migrated perivascular inflammatory cell infiltrate, with or without plasma protein exudate, and when active the sheathing tends to be irregular and fuzzy in outline, often accompanied by changes in vessel caliber (either real or apparent because of obscuration of part of the vessel) and tortuosity. Diffuse capillary leakage (**Fig. 18.19**) and macular edema are also common features of active disease. There is variable vitritis or sometimes anterior uveitis. In some circumstances telangiectasis, or more rarely retinal aneurysms, accompany the inflammation. Following active vessel wall inflammation 'sheathing' may be retained, with a clearer, smoother outline representing perivascular scarring (**Fig. 18.20**). Atrophic retinal pigment epithelium (RPE) scarring may also be seen.

Vessel caliber change showing as patchy attenuation is frequent but only a minority develops vessel shutdown and ischemia. This may be acute and affect major retinal vessels (usually on the venous side), or insidious and progressive. Ischemia obviously gives a worse outlook (**Fig. 18.21**); retinal and disk neovascularization (**Fig. 18.22**), recurrent

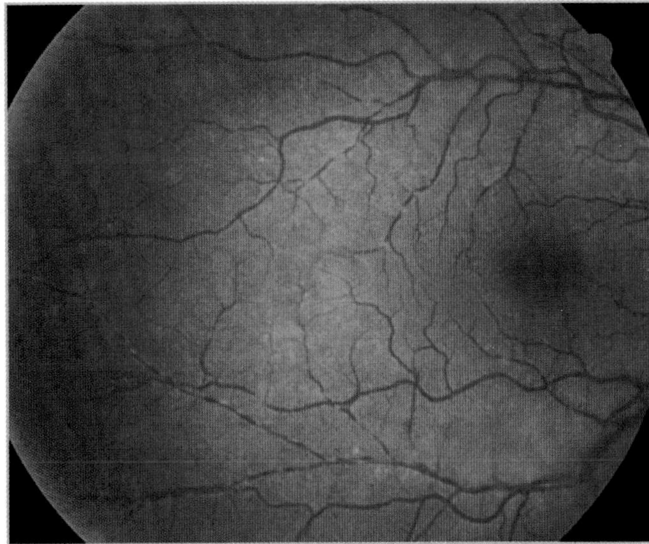

Figure 18.18 Primary retinal vasculitis with widespread perivenous cuffing and caliber changes. In this case the arterial tree is unaffected.

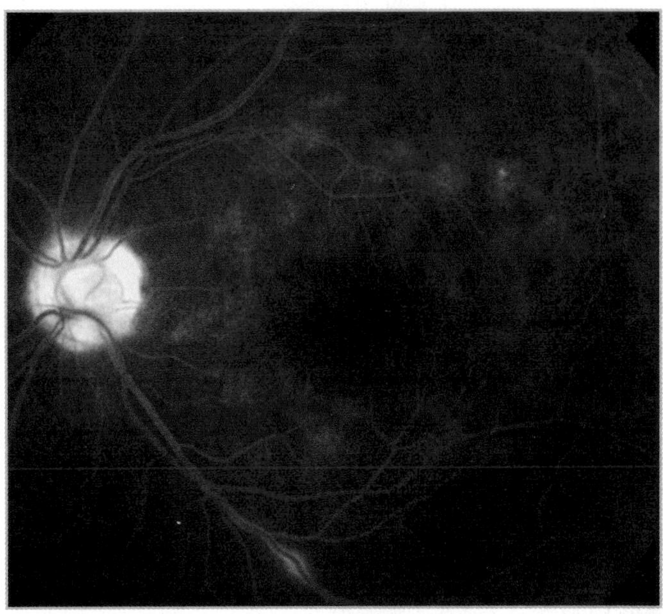

Figure 18.19 Multifocal areas of retinal capillary leakage in primary retinal vasculitis. Such areas will amalgamate to cause cystoid edema. Inferiorly there is also marked venule wall staining and fluorescein leakage indicating focal phlebitis.

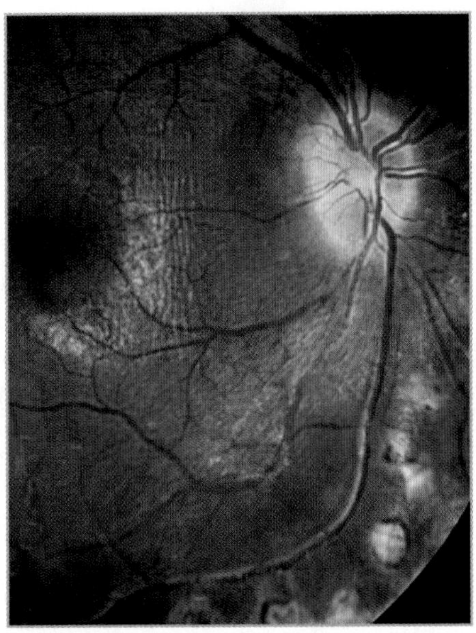

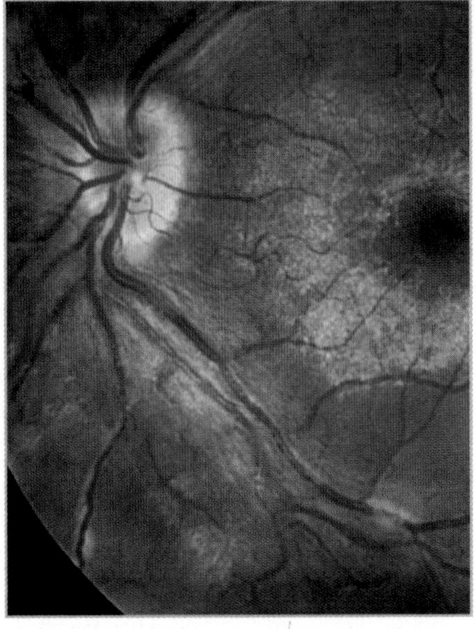

Figure 18.20 Consecutive stages of retinal phlebitis in eyes with ischemic primary retinal vasculitis: in the left eye are two patches of 'fluffy' active vasculitis; in the right, after panretinal laser treatment the inferotemporal vein shows old perivascular scarring.

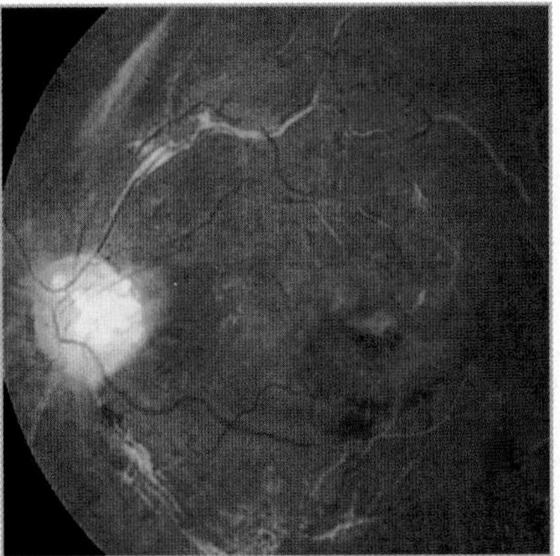

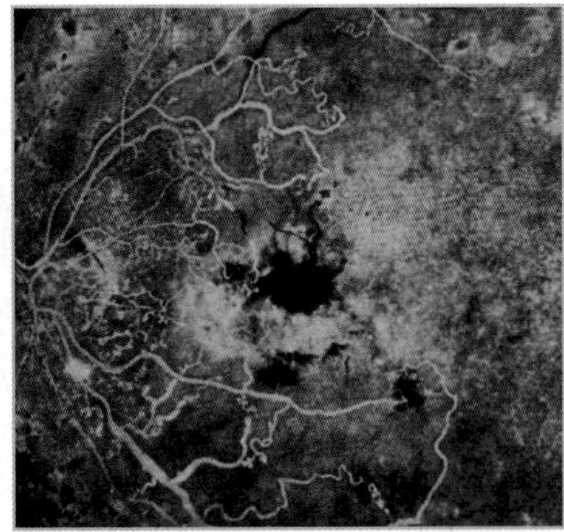

Figure 18.21 Widespread vascular shutdown in primary retinal vasculitis exhibiting as silver-wiring with associated optic atrophy and macular scar. The full extent of the ischemia is, as ever, shown only on fluorescein angiography.

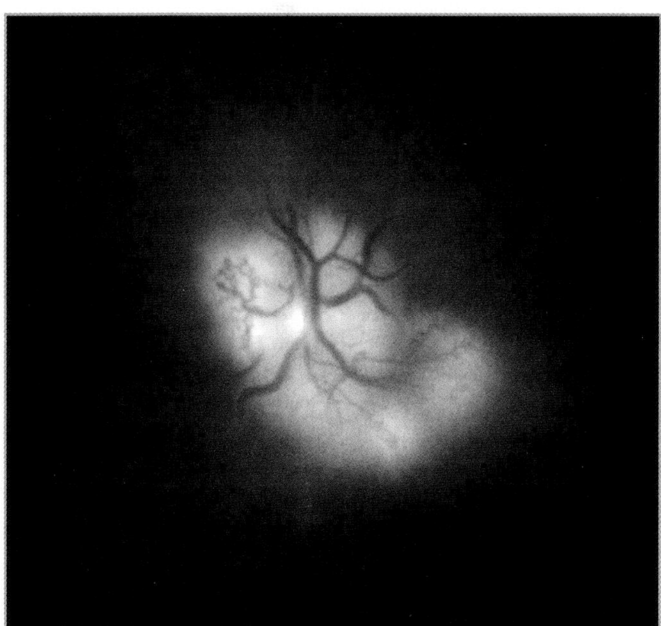

Figure 18.22 Optic disk neovascularization with extensive fluorescein leakage in a young woman with primary retinal vasculitis.

vitreous hemorrhage and neovascular glaucoma are frequent complications. Fluorescein angiography is an essential component of both diagnosis and monitoring and widefield angiography has enhanced the ability to monitor and treat accurately. Patchy areas of vasculitis with staining of vessel walls or fluorescein leakage are often more obvious than on clinical examination, and occult vessel shutdown is clearly shown.

Diagnosis

In patients who present with retinal vasculitis and have, after thorough history-taking and examination, no sign of an accompanying systemic disease, extensive investigation is unlikely to be helpful. However, fluorescein angiography is essential. A chest radiograph and angiotensin-converting enzyme (ACE) level, FBC and ESR or CRP (which are likely to be abnormal in any significant underlying vasculitis) should be included. The relevance of positive ANCA, raised complement C3 or C4, or antinuclear factor in primary retinal vasculitis is dubious; it is rare for a patient later to develop overt manifestations of lupus or systemic vasculitis. Those patients with a family history of multiple sclerosis may be found to have demyelination on MRI (Gass et al. 1995). In the light of increasing evidence on the involvement of TB in patients with retinal vasculitis, especially with vascular occlusion, it is now our practice to submit all patients with apparent PRV to TB testing.

Management

In the experience of most authors the visual outcome of PRV is largely dependent on whether or not it causes vascular occlusion. If it does, it requires vigorous immunosuppression. Acute occlusive PRV usually responds well to high-dose oral or intravenous steroids, but clearly their use is suboptimal for long-term treatment of insidious disease. The early identification of retinal ischemia allows the institution of oral immunosuppression and laser photocoagulation if necessary. The latter does not usually need to be dense or aggressive as for proliferative diabetic retinopathy. Where treatment fails, neovascularization will lead to vitreous hemorrhage. Single events are usually self-clearing, allowing a reappraisal with angiography. However, recurrent hemorrhage is not uncommon and, if this prevents adequate reappraisal between events, matters may spiral out of control. In one large series of patients with ischemic PRV, recurrent vitreous hemorrhage was the most common indication for vitrectomy (Shukla et al. 2008). In our experience, when vitrectomy is provoked, internal search, good endolaser cover (and if necessary epiretinal membrane [ERM] peel) is usually effective. Several anecdotes have been published suggesting the effectiveness of intravitreal injection of anti-VEGF (vascular endothelial growth factor) monoclonal antibody in the management of both macular edema and retinal neovascularization in PRV.

For most patients who show no evidence of retinal ischemia on careful monitoring, decisions on management may be difficult. These patients may show mild chronic vitritis which in itself does not justify treatment; nevertheless after months or years, ERM formation is very common and this, together with untreated mild chronic macular edema, often leads to slightly reduced visual acuity. A careful discussion of risks versus benefits of oral immunosuppression is therefore necessary with each patient.

The preferred choice of immunosuppressive in PRV is unclear. There is some experience of azathioprine (Greenwood et al. 1998) that appears effective and is currently our favored drug in this group; other reports are anecdotal and the area is sorely in need of comparative studies.

Specific subtypes of PRV

Eales' disease

Retinal and vitreous hemorrhage with epistaxis and constipation were the original signs described in a small group of young men by Henry Eales, a Birmingham ophthalmologist in the late nineteenth century (Eales 1880). Subsequently the eponym has been used, confusingly, in several different ways; some have used it mistakenly as an umbrella term for all cases of PRV, others as a synonym for 'idiopathic retinal periphlebitis'; in the west, the term is usually confined to an occlusive retinal periphlebitis starting in the pre-equatorial area with ischemia and neovascularization, often presenting with vitreous hemorrhage (**Fig. 18.23**); in India it frequently describes a florid exudative periphlebitis (**Fig. 18.24**), often in patients who have a clear history of TB or of exposure to that disease; some now require tuberculin hypersensitivity as a prerequisite for diagnosis.

Evidence of a tuberculous etiology for a large number of patients with Eales' disease, at least in countries where the disease is common, is increasing (Therese et al. 2007). The retinal vasculitis in such cases should of course be redefined and ceases to be PRV. The term 'Eales' disease' itself is becoming increasingly unhelpful and, in the opinion of this author, the understanding of retinal vasculitis would be enhanced if it were abandoned.

Frosted branch angiitis

In 1976 Ito and co-workers described a dramatic fundal picture in a child, comprising massive perivenous exudation over substantial lengths of retinal vein. Substantial but patchy perivenous exudation had long been recognized in sarcoidosis and other disorders, but huge and confluent *translucent* exudation affecting retinal veins over a wide area seemed to be a new finding. The appearance of affected vessels was likened to a tree branch covered in heavy frost, and the term 'frosted branch angiitis' (FBA) was coined. The disease is clearly rare and probably new; most patients have been Japanese, and boys and young adults are predominantly affected (Walker et al. 2004). A variable degree of intraocular inflammation accompanies

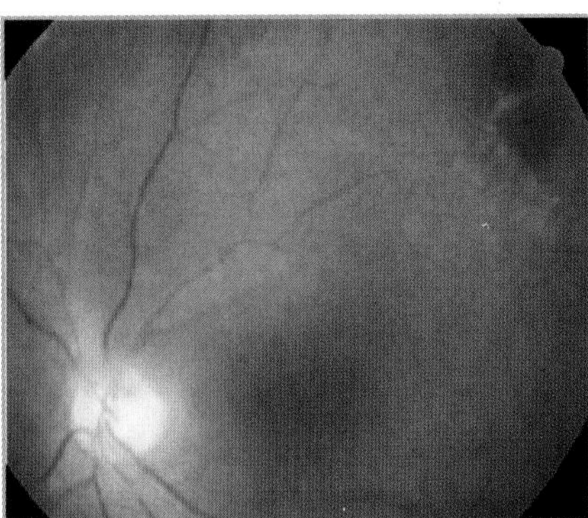

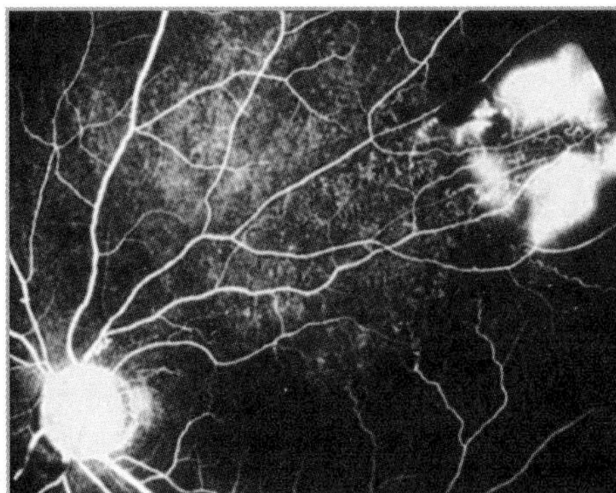

Figure 18.23 The 'western' type of Eales' disease: a young man presented with retinal and vitreous hemorrhage secondary to a frond of retinal neovascularization adjacent to peripheral ischemic phlebitis.

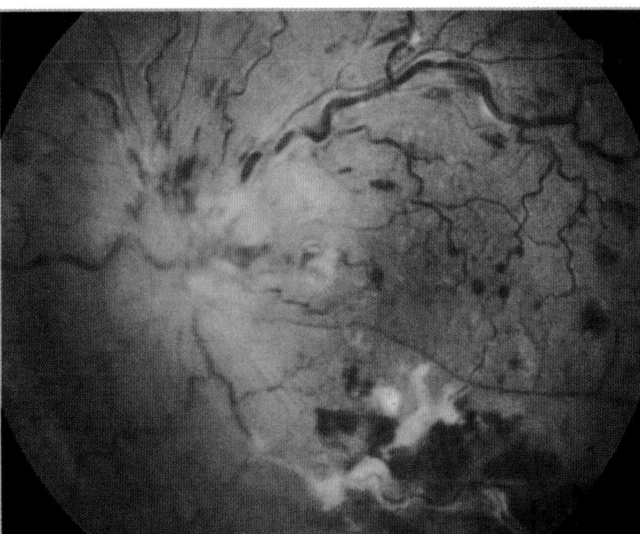

Figure 18.24 Florid exudative periphlebitis with tortuosity, hemorrhage and papillitis in a young Indian man whose wife was on treatment for pulmonary tuberculosis.

the picture, affecting both anterior and posterior segments, but this is rarely severe. Bilateral involvement is more common (**Fig. 18.25**). Systemic steroid treatment has been used, usually with good results. Reports of resolution with only periocular or topical steroid treatment have been made.

Retinal vasculitis of frosted branch type may also occur in association with pre-existing intraocular inflammation caused by cytomegalovirus (see Fig. 11.35), herpes simplex, toxoplasmosis or Behçet's disease (see Fig. 18.10), and has been seen in patients with SLE, leukemia, lymphoma and Crohn's disease (Jones 2012). These are often unilateral and localized. These latter forms of FBA should more properly be regarded as 'secondary,' the term 'primary (idiopathic) FBA' being reserved for bilateral widespread vasculitis as shown in **Fig. 18.25**, with no evidence of other intraocular disease.

The cause of primary FBA is unknown. Occurring often after a prodromal illness, a hypersensitivity reaction may be responsible, possibly including perivascular immune complex deposition. However, there is no histological evidence base. Fluorescein angiography shows florid late vascular leakage from affected vessels, but occlusion is very unusual. The widespread outer retinal and sometimes optic nerve dysfunction has been shown in reduced amplitudes of

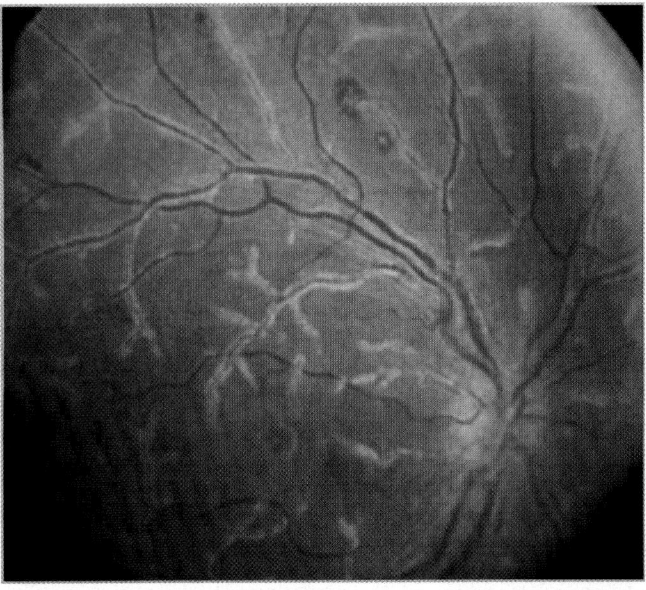

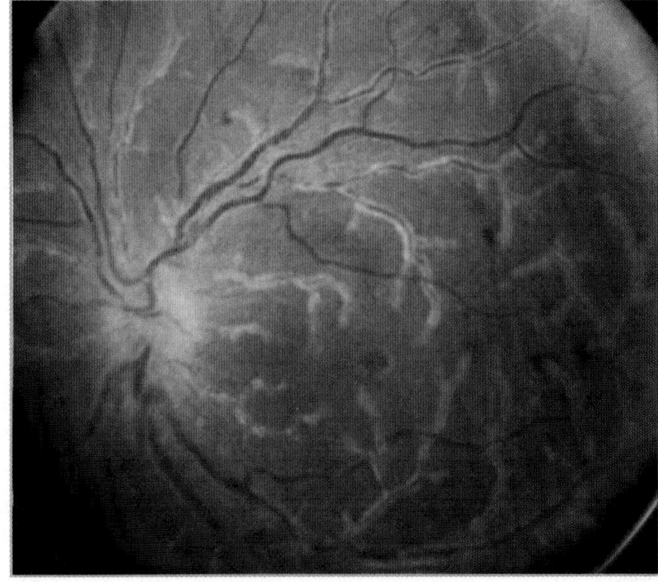

Figure 18.25 Bilateral primary frosted branch uveitis in a 7-year-old boy, showing widespread translucent frosting, disk and macular edema and scattered intraretinal hemorrhage. Vision at this stage was R 6/60, L 2/36, improving to 6/6 in both after oral steroid treatment. (Reproduced from Walker et al. 2004.)

electroretinogram, electro-oculogram and visual evoked potentials. The visual fields may be constricted or may exhibit relative central defects that tend to resolve. The prognosis is generally good with most achieving a return to normal visual acuity. However, recovery may be limited by post-edematous macular scarring or ERM formation, occlusive vasculitis, retinal fibrosis, vitreous hemorrhage or optic atrophy.

Idiopathic retinal vasculitis with aneurysms and neuroretinitis

A small number of patients have been reported to develop a bilateral retinal vasculitis (predominantly an arteriolitis) comprising intermittent sheathing, multifocal vessel distortions including aneurysms (**Fig. 18.26**), vascular leakage with exudate and ischemia (**Fig. 18.27**), leading to neovascularization and hemorrhage. Untreated, the disease tends to progress stepwise over a number of years to a poor visual outcome from exudative maculopathy or retinal ischemia. It has been postulated that focal inflammatory destruction of periarteriolar smooth muscle could cause ectasias and aneurysm formation. The condition has no associated systemic disease, although sarcoidosis should be excluded, because this form of retinal vasculitis is also sometimes associated with aneurysm formation.

A staging system of Idiopathic retinal vasculitis with aneurysms and neuroretinitis (IRVAN) has been proposed (Samuel et al. 2007) which is likely to aid management decision-making. The treatment has been very frustrating; there is no convincing evidence that either systemic steroid (Chang et al. 1995) or immunosuppression is effective; early laser photocoagulation for widespread ischemia has been recommended, and several anecdotal reports of the use of bevacizumab or ranibizumab have suggested short-term success in the management of both macular edema and retinal neovascularization. However, neither of these interventions will prevent the complications of renewed vasculitis, and the prognosis must remain extremely guarded for patients with this intriguing form of retinal vasculitis.

Vasculitis of the eye, ear and CNS

The triad of conditions below are not known to be pathogenically related but share a predilection for the eye, ear and brain. All are rare but the ophthalmologist dealing with inflammatory disease should be aware of them and consider them in the differential diagnosis of uveitis with hearing loss and/or CNS signs.

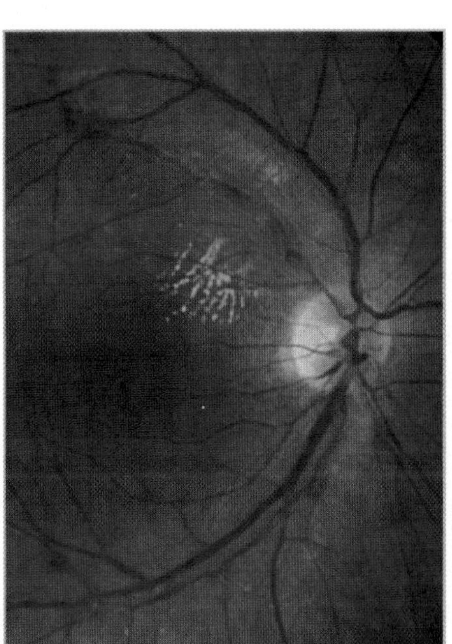

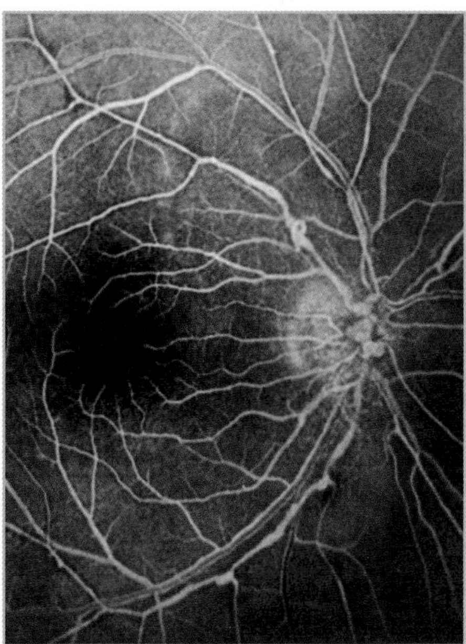

Figure 18.26 The characteristic changes of IRVAN syndrome: multifocal arterial ectasias including both fusiform and saccular aneurysms, associated intraretinal hemorrhage and a partial macular star.

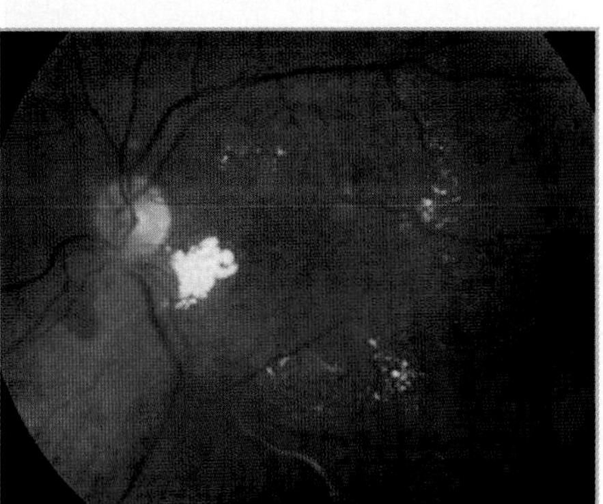

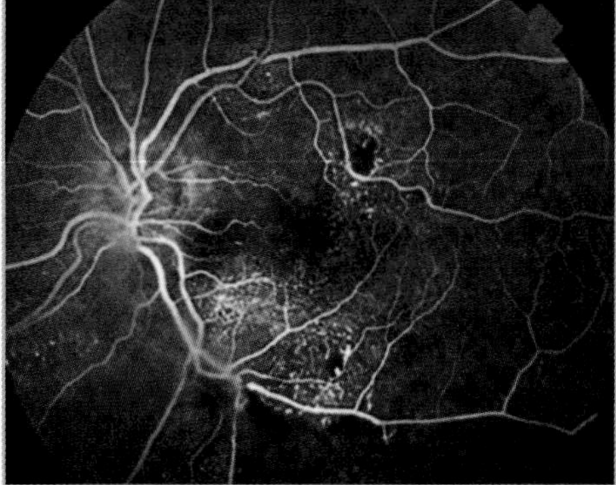

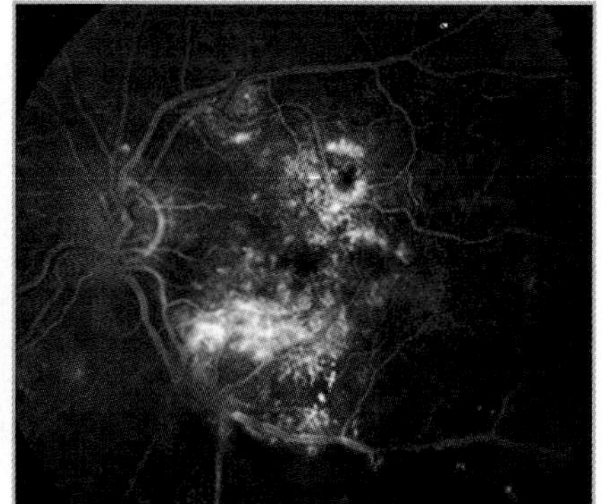

Figure 18.27 More advanced IRVAN showing arterial occlusion with silver-wiring and extensive non-perfusion; substantial macular exudate, an enlarged foveal avascular zone and diffuse macular edema.

Cogan's syndrome

Cogan's syndrome (Cogan 1945) is a rare presumed autoimmune vasculitis predominantly affecting the eye and ear, with systemic vasculitis in some. It may occur at any age, including childhood with acute hearing loss or Ménière-like syndrome accompanied by headache and sometimes fever and arthralgia. A majority later (usually within 1 year) develop the typical ocular manifestation of bilateral interstitial keratitis (Grasland et al. 2004) (**Fig. 18.28**) and/or anterior uveitis, but some develop atypical ocular involvement including episcleritis/scleritis or retinal vasculitis. Patients typically develop progressive sensorineural deafness and half become totally deaf (Gluth et al. 2006) although cochlear implantation has proved successful. Systemic vasculitis may ensue, most prominently carotiditis and aortitis complicated by dissection or aneurysm formation, and commonly severe aortic valve incompetence requiring replacement. Involvement of the kidney and CNS has have been reported.

Diagnosis of this rare disease is often delayed, especially in those with atypical presentations. If identified during the acute phase, high-dose systemic corticosteroids are recommended, usually enhanced with immunosuppression including cyclophosphamide, although some patients may progress despite this. Anecdotes of the use of both infliximab and rituximab are as yet inconclusive. Topical ciclosporin for corneal involvement has been claimed to be useful. Severe visual loss affects perhaps 5% of patients.

Susac's syndrome

Susac's syndrome (Susac et al. 1979) consists of a triad of encephalopathy, multiple branch retinal arteriolar occlusions and hearing loss, presumed to be an autoimmune endotheliopathy affecting precapillary arterioles of the brain, retina and inner ear. Despite the multitude of infarctions resulting from vascular occlusion, no coagulopathy has been found. The disease particularly affects young women and has been associated with pregnancy or oral contraceptive usage. A prodromal flu-like illness may occur. Headache, either constant or migrainous, is common, and the encephalopathy is notorious for its psychiatric symptoms of confusion, amnesia, cognitive failure, paranoia and sometimes, ultimately, dementia. Brain imaging characteristically shows multifocal microinfarcts of the corpus callosum and internal capsules. Vestibulocochlear involvement may lead to a combination of vertigo, tinnitus and fluctuant hearing loss (Roeser et al. 2009), which may progress to severe deafness. Multifocal retinal arteriolar occlusion, usually bilateral, is accompanied by vessel wall staining, particularly discrete plaques, on fluorescein angiography (**Fig. 18.29**), supporting a vasculitic etiology. Uveitis has not been reported and, probably of etiological importance, in contrast to the precapillary arteriolar involvement of placoid pigment epitheliopathy for example, the choroid is unaffected.

Similar to Cogan's syndrome, Susac's syndrome is under-recognized and temporal separation of symptoms will delay diagnosis. Many patients do not present the full diagnostic triad. Management requires high-dose systemic steroid and immunosuppression. Anti-platelet therapy is useful. The optimal regimen is undecided.

Primary CNS angiitis

This rare vasculitis, confined to the CNS, causes multifocal granulomatous inflammation of media and adventitia of small parenchymal and leptomeningeal arteries and veins. It characteristically affects middle-aged men but may affect children or elderly people. It may present with protean neurological deficits and diagnosis is characteristically one of exclusion, with differential diagnoses of thrombotic stroke, lymphoma, reversible cerebral vasoconstriction syndromes and infectious encephalitis. Brain biopsy is necessary for

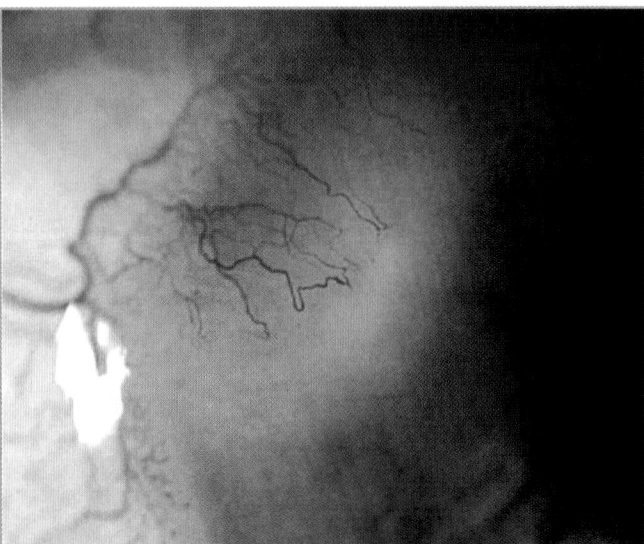

Figure 18.28 Active interstitial keratitis showing both superficial and deep neovascularization with stromal infiltration. There was associated mild anterior uveitis.

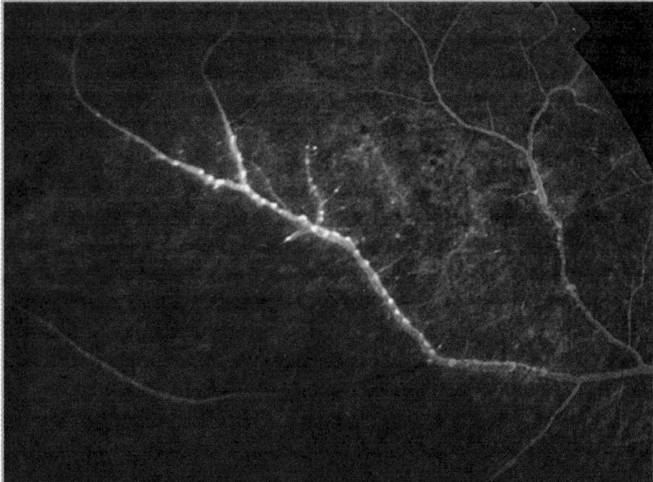

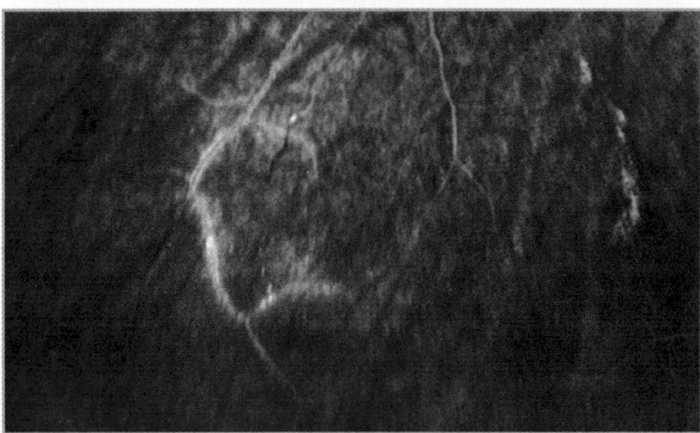

Figure 18.29 Fluorescein angiography in a young woman with Susac's syndrome showing several areas of arteriolar shutdown associated with vessel wall staining.

confirmation. The condition is rarely associated with either anterior uveitis or panuveitis (Rosenbaum et al. 1998).

Systemic lupus erythematosus

Systemic lupus erythematosus is an uncommon chronic autoimmune inflammatory disease of connective tissue. There is a vasculitic element and the underlying mechanism includes immune complex deposition. It is predominantly a disease of young adults with a ratio of nine affected females to every male, and is more common in African-Caribbean and Asian individuals than in white people. The disease has multisystem effects and an immensely variable course with fluctuations and relapses, and as a result diagnostic criteria have been established by the American College of Rheumatology, revised in 1997: for firm diagnosis, a patient should exhibit, either simultaneously or consecutively on no more than two occasions, 4 or more of 11 cardinal features, which include malar or discoid rash, oral ulceration, hemolytic anemia, pericarditis, proteinuria, arthritis and others. Patients may present with malaise, weight loss, pyrexia and lymphadenopathy. The typical malar 'butterfly' rash occupies the cheeks and nasal bridge. Organ-specific inflammation in the kidney, CNS, heart or lungs is a severe complication. A cutaneous vasculitis and Raynaud's phenomenon may occur. An SLE-like disease can follow the administration of drugs including hydralazine, isoniazid and methyldopa.

Some patients require multidisciplinary care. Those with mild disease may require no treatment. Mild inflammation including arthritis may be controlled by NSAIDs, but, if not, hydroxychloroquine may be successful. If these drugs prove inadequate, corticosteroids are added. Azathioprine is frequently used as a steroid-sparing agent where necessary but does not always prevent flares, and mycophenolate may be only marginally better (Houssiau et al. 2010). Cyclophosphamide is usually reserved for severe organ involvement, e.g. nephritis with renal failure, where it is given intravenously. With such immunosuppressive regimens the 10-year mortality rate has been reduced to under 10%. Deaths are usually the result of renal failure, cerebral lupus, intercurrent infection or coronary thrombosis.

Anterior uveitis may be seen in patients with SLE. Retinal involvement may comprise intraretinal hemorrhage, cotton-wool spots, microvascular and arteriolar occlusions (Nag and Wadhwa 2006). The retinal signs of severe and labile systemic/renal hypertension with intermittent hypoperfusion and resultant ischemia are also an occasional feature. Retinal vascular involvement (**Fig. 18.30**) is characteristic of severe SLE and usually occurs in those patients with severe renal or cerebral involvement. With occasional obvious exceptions, it is not clear whether a retinal vasculitis is involved, but, in contrast, the less common inflammation in the choroidal vasculature may be intense, in some cases leading to choroidal necrosis and serous retinal detachment (**Fig. 18.31**). This lupus choroidopathy (Nguyen et al. 2000) usually occurs during a severe systemic flare and is a poor prognostic indicator. Ischemic optic neuropathy or optic neuritis may also occur.

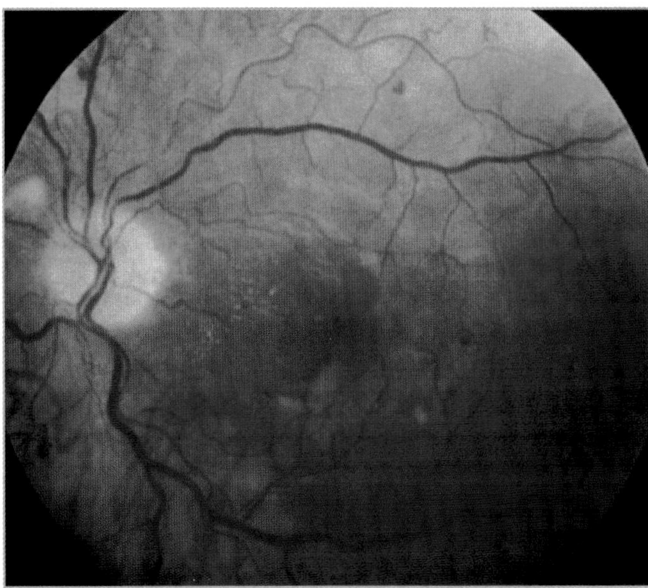

Figure 18.30 Arterial tortuosity and attenuation, retinal ischemia with hemorrhages and cotton-wool spots in systemic lupus erythematosus.

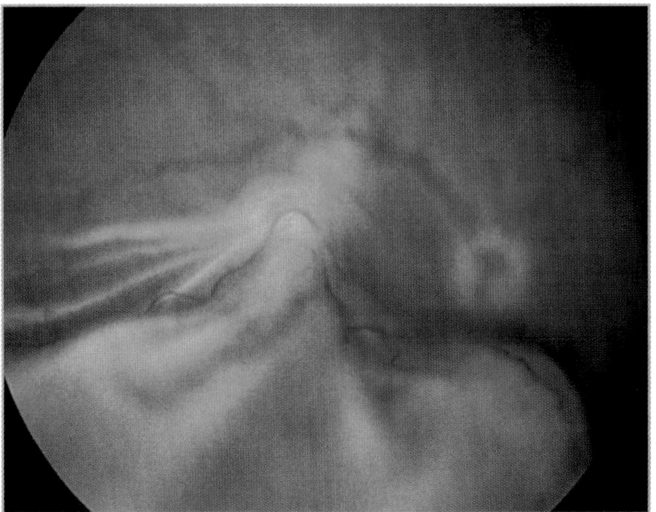

Figure 18.31 Serous retinal detachment in systemic lupus erythematosus resulting from lupus choroidopathy; severe choroidal vasculitis with ischemia and necrosis.

Antinuclear antibodies and other immunological tests

In nearly all patients with SLE and in a high proportion of those with some other connective tissue diseases, ANAs can be demonstrated in serum using immunofluorescent techniques. Antibodies to nuclear components can be formed by all Ig classes and it is clear that ANAs are a heterogeneous group, reacting to several different nuclear antigens. The ANA subtype anti-double-stranded DNA antibody (anti-dsDNA Ab) is specifically associated with SLE and anti-histone Ab is linked to drug-induced lupus. The anti-ENA antibodies (anti-ENA Abs) are of several distinct subtypes, the anti-Sm ENA being specifically associated with SLE (whereas the anti-Ro and anti-La ENAs are associated with Sjögren's syndrome).

Other diseases associated with ANA positivity include mixed connective tissue disease, chronic active hepatitis, biliary cirrhosis, leukemias and Hashimoto's disease, and false positivity in apparently healthy people is occasionally seen. In patients with intraocular inflammation, ANAs have very low specificity for SLE; less than 1% of those with uveitis and positive ANAs actually have SLE (Rosenbaum et al. 1990), so the test has no screening value in adults without symptoms or signs indicative of SLE. However, ANAs are of importance in the diagnosis of juvenile chronic arthritis and uveitis (see Chapter 8).

In SLE and several other connective tissue inflammatory disorders, a high degree of 'immunological noise' may be seen, indicating a heightened response with autoimmune features. Apart from ANAs and anti-DNA Ab, antibodies to RNA, red blood cells and platelets, rheumatoid factor and organ-specific antibodies may be seen and false-positive RPR rapid plasmin reagin) or VDRL (Venereal Disease Reference Laboratory) tests may be found.

Multiple sclerosis

Multiple sclerosis (MS) is a demyelinating disease of the CNS characterized by recurrent subacute focal dysfunction affecting two or more sites. Perivascular inflammation is the initial abnormality and these areas of inflammation evolve into plaques of demyelinated axons. The disease is most common in white people, particularly in northern Europe. Optic neuritis is the manifestation of MS most often seen by the ophthalmologist and almost half the MS patients have optic nerve damage *post mortem*. Intraocular inflammation is also associated with the disease, although there are striking differences of opinion on its incidence, ranging from 0.6% to 18% of MS patients. Opinions differ as to the effect, if any, of the presence of retinal periphlebitis or uveitis on MS severity and behavior. The uveitis precedes the diagnosis of MS in about half the patients (Zein et al. 2004), often by several years. The ophthalmologist will therefore be sensitive to the possibility in the patient with recurrent neurological symptoms. The great majority of affected patients are female.

Peripheral retinal venous sheathing (**Fig. 18.32**) occurs in 10% or more patients. There is an inflammatory infiltrate of the vein wall and perivascular area. Leakage may be seen on fluorescein angiography where periphlebitis is not clinically visible, so occult retinal periphlebitis may affect rather more MS patients than are suspected clinically. Rarely, more significant and extensive retinal periphlebitis is seen, sometimes with occlusion, neovascularization and hemorrhage (Ronzani et al. 1995). In patients with retinal vasculitis with a family history of MS, cranial MRI may identify lesions typical of demyelination (Gass et al. 1995); whether this investigation should be performed in these circumstances is quite another matter.

Intermediate uveitis may affect some 2% of patients with MS (and in long-term follow-up studies, MS is diagnosed in up to 50% of those with intermediate uveitis – Prieto et al. 2001). This particular percentage should be carefully remembered if ever considering the use of anti-TNF-α monoclonal antibodies in those rare patients with intermediate uveitis who are immunosuppression resistant; acute demyelination has followed such treatment. Anterior uveitis affects some 5% and many of these are granulomatous. Bilaterality seems to be the rule, and severe inflammation with mutton-fat keratic precipitates (KPs), posterior synechiae, cataract and macular edema can occur. In those with granulomatous anterior uveitis and neurological signs, sarcoidosis with neurological involvement is the main differential diagnosis, although exclusion of TB and syphilis is also wise.

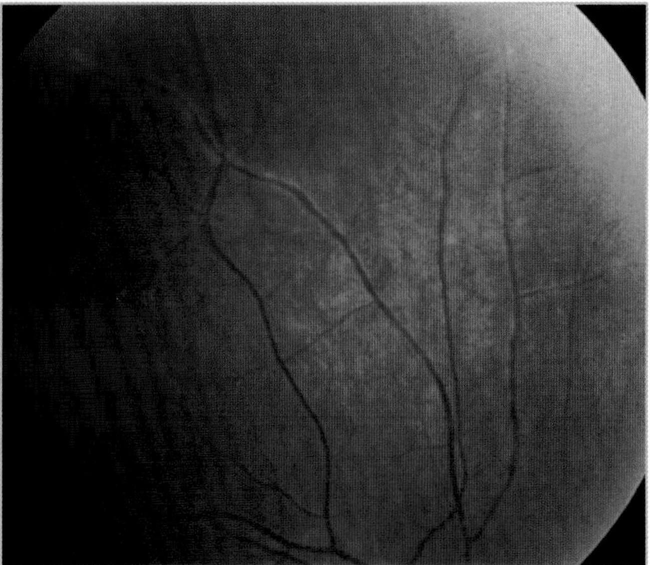

Figure 18.32 Peripheral venous sheathing in multiple sclerosis.

The management of MS is outside the scope of this short account, and associated uveitis is rarely severe enough to justify immunosuppression. However, the ophthalmologist should be aware that interferons, of both α (used to treat viral hepatitis etc) and β (used to treat MS) type, have been associated with an ischemic retinopathy comprising circumpapillary cotton-wool spots and intraretinal hemorrhage, which, if compromising retinal circulation on angiography, will mandate discontinuation.

Thrombophilia and retinal vasculitis

A common thread in the diseases discussed above is the greater severity imposed by vascular occlusion. In a situation where vascular wall integrity, luminal caliber, probable endothelial irregularity and therefore laminar flow are all probably compromised by active vasculitis, it seems obvious that any further rheological difficulty imposed by hypercoagulability will make intravascular thrombosis more likely (Rocca et al. 1994). It is therefore incumbent on the ophthalmologist to be aware of the basics of thrombophilic abnormalities, to investigate appropriately for their presence and to liaise with physicians over treatment where anticoagulation becomes desirable. In the context of vasculitic disease, more information is available on Behçet's disease and lupus than for the other diseases above, but some common factors are likely. However, extrapolation of management advice to other causes of retinal vasculitis, although superficially reasonable, is as yet presumptive. Possible relevant factors include the following.

Anti-phospholipid antibodies

The autoimmune generation of antibodies against the phospholipid components of cell membranes causes spontaneous thrombosis. The primary culprits are anti-cardiolipin Ab and anti-β_2 glycoprotein Ab. The anti-phospholipid antibody (a-PL Ab) syndrome (Hughes' syndrome) comprises repeated venous and arterial thrombosis (with spontaneous abortions or other severe pregnancy complications in affected women). The condition can be secondary to other autoimmune diseases, predominantly lupus. Via a slightly different pathway, another a-PL Ab, lupus anticoagulant (La-C, confusingly named because, first, it is actually prothrombotic in vivo and, second, it is not usually associated with lupus [although SLE patients are more likely to be La-C positive]) causes platelet aggregation by interference with platelet membrane integrity.

Genetic thrombophilia

Certain forms of genetic abnormality leading to hypercoagulability are not uncommon. Factor V Leiden (FVL) is a variant of clotting factor V that acts as a procoagulant. Heterozygosity for this variant is present in about 5% of the population. Prothrombin mutation G20210A or raised homocysteine levels are less common but similarly increase the risk of thrombosis. Much less common are the deficiencies of coagulation inhibitors. Protein C inhibits clotting factors V and VIII and is deficient in up to 0.5%. Protein S is a cofactor to protein C and may also be deficient. There are several other potential genetic abnormalities with complex potential effects on the coagulation cascade.

Sickle cell disease

Sickle genes are most common in malarial regions, which of course have substantial overlap with some diseases causing retinal vasculitis, particularly Behçet's disease. The potential complicating effect of either sickle disease or sickle trait in eyes with coexisting vasculitis has not been formally studied, but anecdotally those dealing with uveitis feel that occlusive tendencies are worsened.

Some uveitis practitioners assert the importance of thrombophilia testing for all patients with retinal vasculitis. However, placing into perspective the not infrequent finding of apparently minor abnormalities, where the influence of such findings on any vaso-occlusive tendency is at best poorly understood and at worst entirely speculative, is difficult. However, the easy availability of anti-platelet treatment, and also if necessary formal anticoagulation, implies that thrombophilia testing should at least be performed on those patients with evidence of either retinal vascular occlusion or thromboembolism elsewhere. Some trends at least are apparent.

Occlusive retinal vasculitis is known to be substantially more common in men with Behçet's disease. It is also thought that thrombotic events in that disease are associated with a diverse variety of thrombophilic factors (Caramaschi et al. 2010), including reduced activated protein C levels (Navarro et al. 2004). FVL, however, although well known to be associated with retinal vein thrombosis generally in the under-60s, is not so clearly associated with retinal thrombosis in Behçet's disease. In contrast FVL is associated with a doubling of thrombosis risk in SLE patients, with or without a-PL Ab (Kaiser et al. 2009). The latter patients are known independently to have increased risk of severity of lupus retinopathy. Indeed, combined central retinal artery and vein occlusion, with or without associated SLE, is almost pathognomonic of a-PL Ab positivity.

By no means all those with a-PL Ab develop recurrent thrombosis and the need for low-dose aspirin is not agreed for a-PL Ab positives without a history of thrombosis. However, there is evidence of a significant reduction in thrombotic episodes for those who are a-PL Ab positive with underlying lupus (Hereng et al. 2008). Similarly, low-dose aspirin is thought useful in Susac's syndrome. There is currently no consensus on the need for aspirin in patients with Behçet's disease and thrombotic episodes, but it is agreed that control of inflammation by immunosuppression is paramount (Mehta et al. 2010). Where severe thrombosis has occurred, anticoagulation has been used, but the risk of bleeding from associated pulmonary or coronary aneurysms should be considered and, for those started on anticoagulation, decisions on duration are problematic.

In summary, the effects of vasculitis together with thrombophilia, particularly two or more varieties of the latter, may worsen the risk of thrombotic episodes both in the retina and elsewhere. However, the precise effects of the various thrombophilic factors are poorly understood and indications for the use of antiplatelet or anticoagulant drugs remain unclear. Currently it is our practice to perform a thrombophilia screen on any patient with recurrent or progressive retinal vascular occlusion in association with retinal vasculitis and, if there are no contraindications, to use low-dose aspirin in the presence of any abnormality.

REFERENCES

Akova YA, Jabbur NS, Foster CS. Ocular presentation of polyarteritis nodosa. Clinical course and management with steroid and cytotoxic therapy. *Ophthalmology* 1993;**100**:1775–81.

Atmaca LS, Batioglu F, Idil A. Retinal and disc neovascularisation in Behçet's disease and efficacy of laser photocoagulation. *Graefe's Arch Clin Exp Ophthalmol* 1996;**234**:94–9.

Batioglu F, Atmaca LS, Karabulut HG, Beyza SD. Factor V Leiden and prothrombin gene G20210A mutations in ocular Behcet disease. *Acta Ophthalmol Scand* 2003;**81**:283–5.

Behçet H. Über rezideivierende, aphthöse, durch ein Virus verursachte Geschwüre am Mund, am Auge und an den Genitalien. *Dermatol Wochenschr* 1937;**46**:414–19.

Caramaschi P, Poli G, Bonora A, et al. A study on thrombophilic factors in Italian Behçet's patients. *Joint Bone Spine* 2010;**77**:330–4.

Cem Mat M, Goksugur N, Engin B, et al. The frequency of scarring after genital ulcers in Behçet's syndrome: a prospective study. *Int J Dermatol* 2006;**45**: 554–6.

Chan TK, Dick AD, Forrester JV, et al. Antineutrophil cytoplasmic antibodies in chronic idiopathic intraocular inflammatory disease. *Ocul Immunol Inflamm* 1996;**4**:83–90.

Chang TS, Aylward GW, Davis JL, et al. Idiopathic retinal vasculitis, aneurysms, and neuro-retinitis. Retinal Vasculitis Study. *Ophthalmology* 1995;**102**:1089–97.

Churg J, Strauss L. Allergic granulomatosis, allergic angiitis and periarteritis nodosa. *Am J Pathol* 1951;**27**:277–301.

Cogan DG. Syndrome of nonsyphilitic interstitial keratitis and vestibuloauditory symptoms. *Arch Ophthalmol* 1945;**33**:144–9.

Davatchi F, Shahram F, Chams H, Akbarian M. Pulse cyclophosphamide in ocular manifestations of Behçet's disease: a double-blind crossover study. *Arch Iranian Med* 2004;**7**:201–5.

Davatchi F, Chams-Davatchi C, Shahram F, et al. Pathergy test in Behçet's disease: change in incidence over the time. *APLAR J Rheumatol* 2007;**10**: 333–5.

Davatchi F, Shams H, Rezaipoor M, et al. Rituximab in intractable ocular lesions of Behçet's disease; randomized single-blind control study (pilot study). *Int J Rheum Dis* 2010;**13**:246–52.

Dervis E, Geyik N. Sensitivity and specificity of different diagnostic criteria f or Behçet's disease in a group of Turkish patients. *J Dermatol* 2005;**32**: 266–72.

Deuter CM, Zierhut M, Möhle A, et al. Long-term remission after cessation of interferon-alpha treatment in patients with severe uveitis due to Behçet's disease. *Arthrit Rheum* 2010;**62**:2796–805.

Eales H. Cases of retinal haemorrhage associated with epistaxis and constipation. *Birmingham Med Rev* 1880;**9**:262–73.

Franks M, MacPherson G, Figg W. Thalidomide. Lancet 2004;363:1802–11.

Gass A, Graham E, Moseley IF, et al. Cranial MRI in idiopathic retinal vasculitis. *J Neurol* 1995;**242**:174–7.

Geffriaud-Ricouard C, Noel LH, Chauveau D, et al. Anti-neutrophil cytoplasm antibodies: diversity and clinical applications. *Clin Nephrol* 1993;**39**:125–36.

Gendron G, Bodaghi B, Wechsler B, et al. Efficacy and safety of interferon alfa-2a in intractable Behçet's disease-associated uveitis. *Invest Ophthalmol Vis Sci* 2003;**44**:E-abstract 2404.

George RK, Walton C, Whitcup SM et al. Primary retinal vasculitis Systemic associations and diagnostic evaluation. *Ophthalmology* 1996;**103**:384–89.

Gluth MB, Baratz KH, Matteson EL, Driscoll CL. Cogan syndrome: a retrospective review of 60 patients throughout a half century. *Mayo Clin Proc* 2006;**81**: 483–88.

Graham EM, Stanford MR, Sanders MD, et al. A point prevalence study of 150 patients with idiopathic retinal vasculitis: 1. Diagnostic value of ophthalmological features. *Br J Ophthalmol* 1989;**73**:714–21.

Grasland A, Pouchot J, Hachulla E, et al. Typical and atypical Cogan's syndrome: 32 cases and review of the literature. *Rheumatology* 2004;**43**:1007–15.

Greenwood AJ, Stanford MR, Graham EM. The role of azathioprine in the management of retinal vasculitis. *Eye* 1998;**12**:783–88.

Hereng T, Lambert M, Hachulla E, et al. Influence of aspirin on the clinical outcomes of 103 anti-phospholipid antibodies-positive patients. *Lupus* 2008;**17**:11–15.

Houssiau FA, D'Cruz D, Sangle S, et al. Azathioprine versus mycophenolate mofetil for long-term immunosuppression in lupus nephritis: results from the MAINTAIN nephritis trial. *Ann Rheum Dis* 2010;13199 5epub.

International Study Group for Behçet's disease. Criteria for diagnosis of Behçet's disease. *Lancet* 1990;**335**:1078–80.

International Study Group for Behçet's disease: Evaluation of diagnostic ('classification') criteria in Behçet's disease – towards internationally agreed criteria. *Br J Rheumatol* 1992;**31**:299–308.

Ito Y, Nakano M, Kyu N, Takeuchi M. Frosted branch angiitis in a child. *Rinsho Ganka (Jpn J Clin Ophthalmol)* 1976;**30**:797–803.

Jayanthi P, Sarada D, George J, et al. Hypoperfusive and hypertensive ocular manifestations in Takayasu arteritis. *Clin Ophthalmol* 2010;**4**:1173–6.

Jones NP. Frosted branch angiitis. In: Zierhut M, Ohno S, Orefice F et al (eds). Intraocular inflammation. New York: *Springer* 2012:**6**.7 (in press).

Joseph FG, Scolding NJ. Neuro-Behçet's disease in Caucasians: a study of 22 patients. *Eur J Neurol* 2007;**14**:174–80.

Kaiser R, Barton JL, Chang M, et al. Factor V Leiden and thrombosis in patients with systemic lupus erythematosus: a meta-analysis. *Genes Immun* 2009;**10**:495–502.

Kidd D, Steuer A, Denman AM, Rudge P. Neurological complications in Behçet's syndrome. *Brain* 1999;**122**:2183–94.

Koçer N, Islak C, Siva A, et al. CNS involvement in neuro-Behçet syndrome: an MR study. *Am J Neuroradiol* 1999;**20**:1015–24.

Kötter I, Günaydin I, Batra M, et al. CNS involvement occurs more frequently in patients with Behçet's disease under cyclosporin A than under other medications – results of a retrospective analysis of 117 cases. *Clin Rheumatol* 2006;**25**:482–6.

Mehta P, Laffan M, Haskard DO. Thrombosis and Behçet's syndrome in non-endemic regions. *Rheumatology* 2010;**49**:2003–4.

Mihara M, Hayasaka S, Watanabe K, et al. Ocular manifestations in patients with microscopic polyangiitis. *Eur J Ophthalmol* 2005;**15**:138–42.

Nag TC, Wadhwa S. Vascular changes of the retina and choroid in systemic lupus erythematosus: pathology and pathogenesis. *Curr Neurovasc Res* 2006;**3**:159–68.

Navarro S, Ricart JM, Medina P, et al. Activated protein C levels in Behçet's disease and risk of venous thrombosis. *Br J Haematol* 2004;**126**:550–6.

Nguyen QD, Uy HS, Akpek EK, et al. Choroidopathy of systemic lupus erythematosus. *Lupus* 2000;**9**:288–98.

Özdal PC, Ortaç S, Taskintuna I, Firat E. Long-term therapy with low-dose cyclosporin-A in ocular Behçet's disease. *Doc Ophthalmol* 2002;**105**:301–12.

Palmer HE, Zaman AG, Edelston CE, et al. Systemic morbidity in patients with isolated idiopathic retinal vasculitis. *Lancet* 1995a;**346**:505–6.

Palmer HE, Jurd KM, Hunt BJ, et al. Thrombophilic factors in ischaemic and non-ischaemic retinal vasculitis. *Eye* 1995b;**9**:507–12.

Perrin L, Letierce A, Guitton C, et al. Comparative study of complete versus incomplete Kawasaki disease in 59 pediatric patients. *Joint Bone Spine* 2009;**76**:481–5.

Prieto JF, Dios E, Gutierrez JM, et al. Pars planitis: epidemiology, treatment, and association with multiple sclerosis. *Ocul Immunol Inflamm* 2001;**9**:93–102.

Remmers EF, Cosan F, Kirino Y, et al. Genome-wide association study identifies variants in the MHC class I, IL-10, and IL-23R-IL-12RB2 regions associated with Behçet's disease. *Nat Genet* 2010;**42**:698–702.

Rocca PV, Siegel LB, Cupps TR. The concomitant expression of vasculitis and coagulopathy: synergy for marked tissue ischaemia. *J Rheumatol* 1994;**21**:556–60.

Roeser MM, Driscoll CL, Shallop JK, et al. Susac syndrome – a report of cochlear implantation and review of otological manifestations in twenty-three patients. *Otol Neuro-otol* 2009;**30**:34–40.

Ronzani M, Lang GE, Wagner P, et al. Severe occlusive retinal periphlebitis with vitreous hemorrhage in multiple sclerosis. *Ger J Ophthalmol* 1995;**4**:328–31.

Rosenbaum JT, Wernick R. The utility of routine screening of patients with uveitis for systemic lupus erythematosus or tuberculosis. A Bayesian analysis. *Arch Ophthalmol* 1990;**108**:1291–3.

Rosenbaum JT, Roman-Goldstein S, Lindquist GR, Rosenbaum RB. Uveitis and central nervous system vasculitis. *J Rheumatol* 1998;**25**:593–7.

Saadoun D, Wechsler B, Terrada C, et al. Azathioprine in severe uveitis of Behçet's disease. *Arthrit Care Res* 2010;**62**:1733–8.

Sakane T, Mochizuki M, Inaba G, Masuda K. A phase II study of FK506 (tacrolimus) on refractory uveitis associated with Behçet's disease and associated conditions. *Ryumachi* 1995;**35**:802–13.

Samuel MA, Equi RA, Chang TS, et al. Idiopathic retinitis, vasculitis, aneurysms, and neuroretinitis (IRVAN): new observations and a proposed staging system. *Ophthalmology* 2007;**114**:1526–9.

Shukla D, Kanungo S, Prasad NM, Kim R. Surgical outcomes for vitrectomy in Eales' disease. *Eye* 2008;**22**:900–4.

Stone JH, Merkel PA, Spiera R, et al. Rituximab versus cyclophosphamide for ANCA-associated vasculitis. *N Eng J Med* 2010;**363**:221–32.

Stübinger N, Kötter I, Deuter C, Zierhut M. Behçet's disease: uveitis-therapy with interferon alpha2a – prospective clinical study in 33 patients. *Klin Monatsbl Augenheilkd* 2001;**218**:768–73.

Susac JO, Hardman JM, Selhorst JB. Microangiopathy of the brain and retina. *Neurology* 1979;**29**:313–6.

Tabbara KF, Al-Hemidan AI. Infliximab effects compared to conventional therapy in the management of retinal vasculitis in Behçet disease. *Am J Ophthalmol* 2008;**146**:845–50 .

Tarabishy AB, Schulte M, Papaliodis GN, Hoffman GS. Wegener's granulomatosis: clinical manifestations, differential diagnosis, and management of ocular and systemic disease. *Surv Ophthalmol* 2010;**55**: 429–44.

Therese KL, Deepa P, Therese J, et al. Association of mycobacteria with Eales' disease. *Indian J Med Res* 2007;**126**:56–62.

Tugal-Tutkun I, Onal S, Altan-Yaycioglu R, et al. Uveitis in Behçet disease: an analysis of 880 patients. *Am J Ophthalmol* 2004;**138**:373–80.

Tugal-Tutkun I, Mudun A, Urgancioglu M, et al. Efficacy of infliximab in the treatment of uveitis that is resistant to treatment with the combination of azathioprine, cyclosporine and corticosteroids in Behçet's disease: an open-label trial. *Arthrit Rheum* 2005;**52**:2478–84.

Walker S, Iguchi A, Jones NP. Frosted branch angiitis: a review. *Eye* 2004;**18**:527–33.

Watkins AS, Kempen JH, Choi D, et al. Ocular disease in patients with ANCA-positive vasculitis. *J Ocul Biol Dis Infor* 2009;**3**:12–19.

Yazici H, Esen F. Mortality in Behçet's syndrome. *Clin Exp Rheumatol* 2008;**26**:S138–40.

Yazici H, Pazarli H, Barnes CG, et al. A controlled trial of azathioprine in Behçet's syndrome. *N Engl J Med* 1990;**322**:281–285.

Zein G, Berta A, Foster CS. Multiple sclerosis-associated uveitis. *Ocul Immunol Inflamm* 2004;**12**:137–42.

Chapter 19 Multifocal or zonal retinochoroiditis

A perusal of Sir Stewart Duke-Elder's *System of Ophthalmology* from 1965 will show that only one of the following conditions is included, and that, helicoid chorioretinal atrophy, was not considered to be inflammatory. A considerable array of multifocal or zonal syndromes affecting outer retina or inner choroid has since been described. Some of these seem to be genuinely new diseases. Others may be newly recognized, having previously been considered under the broad umbrella of 'multifocal choroiditis.' The first three of these syndromes appear to be well defined and discrete; the remainder have many features in common, and probably a considerable degree of overlap in their spectra. Each syndrome is individually described. After this, the similarities and distinctions between the syndromes are discussed and summarized.

At this point I would like to pay tribute to the late J Donald M Gass MD, whose research is liberally referred to within this book. An ophthalmologist of rare skill in observation and interpretation, he was responsible for the first descriptions of more diseases in this chapter than any other, and it is fitting that he is mentioned here as one of the great taxonomists of retinal inflammation.

ACUTE POSTERIOR MULTIFOCAL PLACOID PIGMENT EPITHELIOPATHY (box 19.1)

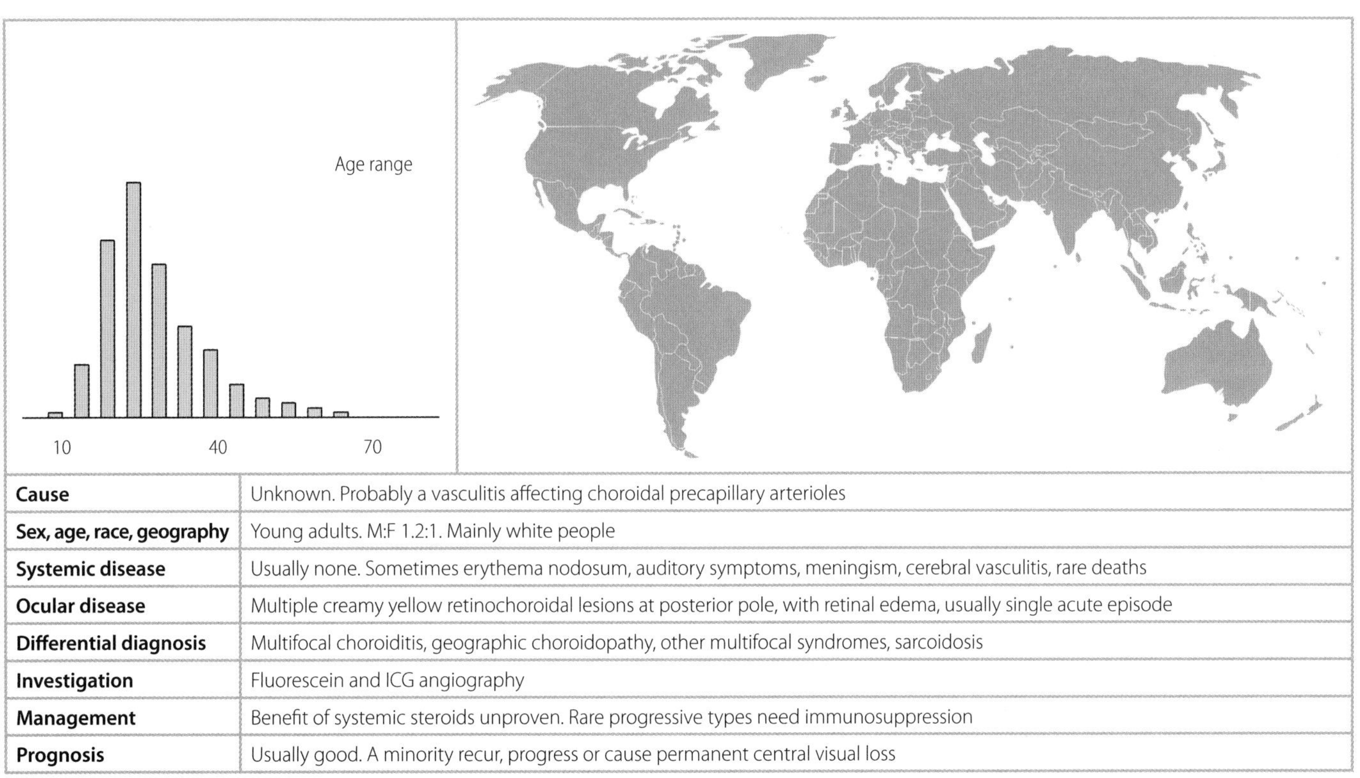

Cause	Unknown. Probably a vasculitis affecting choroidal precapillary arterioles
Sex, age, race, geography	Young adults. M:F 1.2:1. Mainly white people
Systemic disease	Usually none. Sometimes erythema nodosum, auditory symptoms, meningism, cerebral vasculitis, rare deaths
Ocular disease	Multiple creamy yellow retinochoroidal lesions at posterior pole, with retinal edema, usually single acute episode
Differential diagnosis	Multifocal choroiditis, geographic choroidopathy, other multifocal syndromes, sarcoidosis
Investigation	Fluorescein and ICG angiography
Management	Benefit of systemic steroids unproven. Rare progressive types need immunosuppression
Prognosis	Usually good. A minority recur, progress or cause permanent central visual loss

Box 19.1 Acute posterior multifocal placoid pigment epitheliopathy

Introduction

In 1968 Donald Gass described three young women with painless visual loss who developed multiple cream-colored lesions at the posterior pole, apparently deep within the retina. In time the lesions cleared to leave a degree of retinal pigment epithelium (RPE) scarring, but vision returned almost to normal. The condition was named **acute posterior multifocal placoid pigment epitheliopathy** (APMPPE). It is not clear whether APMPPE was genuinely a new disease, or whether the condition was previously considered to be a form of 'multifocal choroiditis.' It may affect children and elderly people but the disease is strikingly more common in young adults, with a mean age at onset of 26 years (Jones 1995). Slightly more males than females are affected. The great majority of reported cases have been in white people, but whether this is a genuine racial predilection or a reporting bias, is unknown.

Systemic disease

Most patients with APMPPE are systemically well and show no signs of underlying disease. However, in about a third other symptoms will be experienced. A prodromal illness suggesting viral infection is quite common, and erythema nodosum, bowel disturbance, upper respiratory tract infection and lymphadenopathy are sometimes seen. There is, however, only anecdotal serological evidence of viral infection, although APMPPE has been associated with mumps, adenovirus, streptococci and *Borrelia* spp. In some, recent immunization (including hepatitis B, influenza, varicella, meningococci and others) or antibiotic prescriptions have been documented. A few patients with APMPPE experience symptoms that may also occur in the Vogt–Koyanagi–Harada (VKH) syndrome, including symptoms of meningeal irritation with headache, stiff neck and dizziness, and vestibuloauditory symptoms including hearing disturbance, tinnitus and vertigo.

In some patients there is direct or indirect evidence of a systemic vasculitis. This may affect the skin (causing erythema nodosum), kidneys or cerebrum or, in rare cases, has been widespread and necrotizing. In a small number of patients a frank cerebral vasculitis or meningoencephalitis has been demonstrated both angiographically and histologically; the multifocal granulomatous arteritis resembles the pathological findings in temporal arteritis. Cavernous or other large cerebral sinus thrombosis has also been reported in association. Significant neurological lesions (O'Halloran et al. 2001) including stroke are reported (Comu et al. 1996) and rare deaths have occurred. It has been speculated that symptoms of meningism seen in some patients may imply a mild cerebral vasculitis or meningitis.

Ocular disease

The typical patient with APMPPE is a young adult with a few days' history of visual loss which is often unilateral or asymmetrical, but usually involves the second eye within 2 weeks. Visual acuity may be substantially reduced. On examination there is usually no anterior segment inflammation and vitreous cells are not usual. Characteristically there are several 'placoid' (meaning plate like, and implying roundish and with a slight thickness like an upside-down plate) creamy-yellow lesions centered in and around the posterior pole, not usually contiguous with the optic disk, varying from very few (**Fig. 19.1**) to very many (**Fig. 19.2**). These lesions usually have slightly blurred outlines and some may be confluent. They appear to be deep within the retina. A degree of surrounding retinal edema is common and the foveal reflex is often abnormal. A serous retinal elevation may develop over one or more placoid lesions (**Fig. 19.3**). In this situation the VKH syndrome will be part of the differential diagnosis, but it is very uncommon for serous detachments to coalesce in APMPPE and angiographically the two conditions are usually very different. A few patients have shown evidence of a concurrent retinal vasculitis, and a few with papillitis.

Most active lesions appear simultaneously, but over the succeeding days and weeks a few more lesions may arise as the first start to settle. This process of resolution will take weeks; the lesions will develop much clearer margins and become flatter, any overlying serous fluid or retinal edema resolving spontaneously (**Fig. 19.4**). Over the succeeding months RPE scarring and pigment accumulation will follow, its extent demonstrating the severity of initial involvement (**Fig. 19.5**) and the degree of pigment clumping and dispersion often being greater in fundi of non-white patients (**Fig. 19.6**). Despite the extent of scarring, central visual acuity is often preserved at or near pre-inflammation levels. However, critical examination of vision will usually reveal significant loss of contrast sensitivity and relative visual field defects, both of which are permanent changes. Foveal involvement at onset is associated with a poorer prognosis.

A minority of patients has a unilateral attack. The prognosis in these cases is guarded and sequential involvement of the second eye at some future date is not unusual. A single episode is the rule for each eye but recurrent disease is well described and may be more visually destructive. It is therefore difficult to reassure completely those who have recovered from a single attack.

Diagnosis

The cause of APMPPE is unknown and there is no diagnostic test. Typical lesions are unlikely to be confused with most other multifocal posterior segment inflammations. The lesions are quite large, unlike many similar syndromes, and subsequent scarring, although severely involving the RPE, tends not to involve the outer choroid. An associated retinal vasculitis is unusual and the vitreous is usually

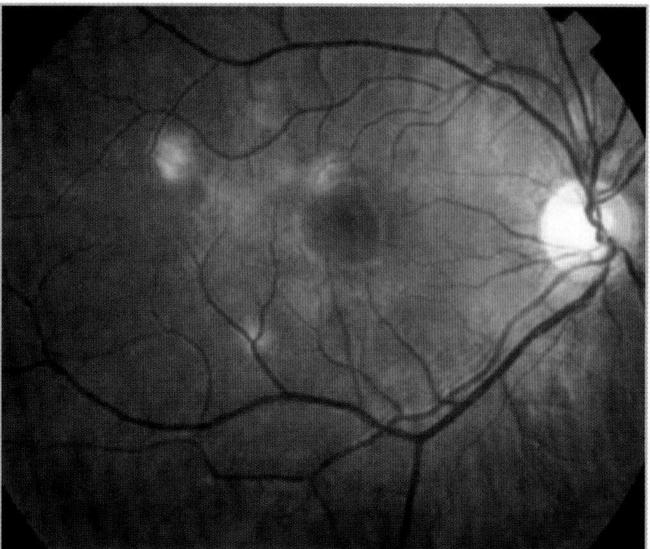

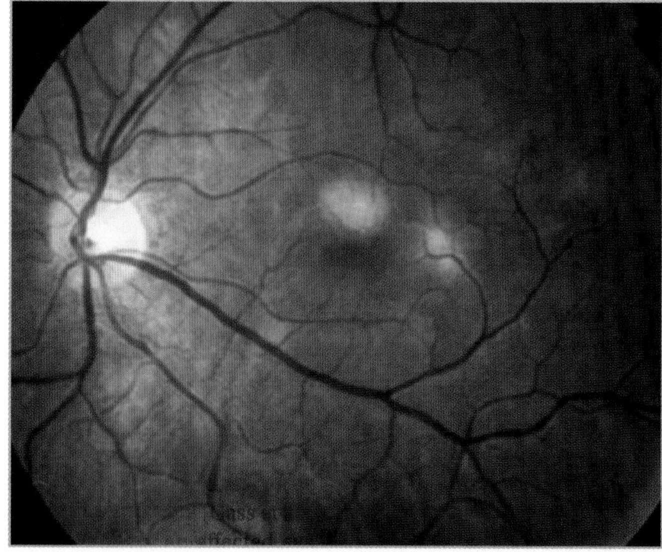

Figure 19.1 A few lesions of varying size in both maculae in a young patient with acute posterior multifocal placoid pigment epitheliopathy.

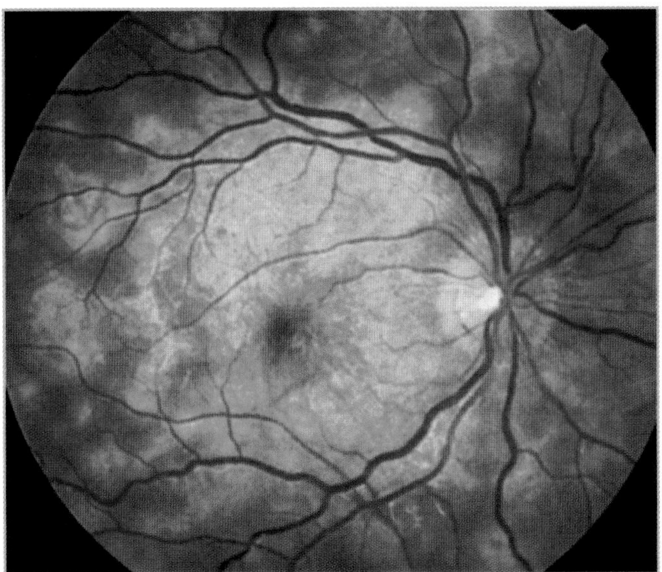

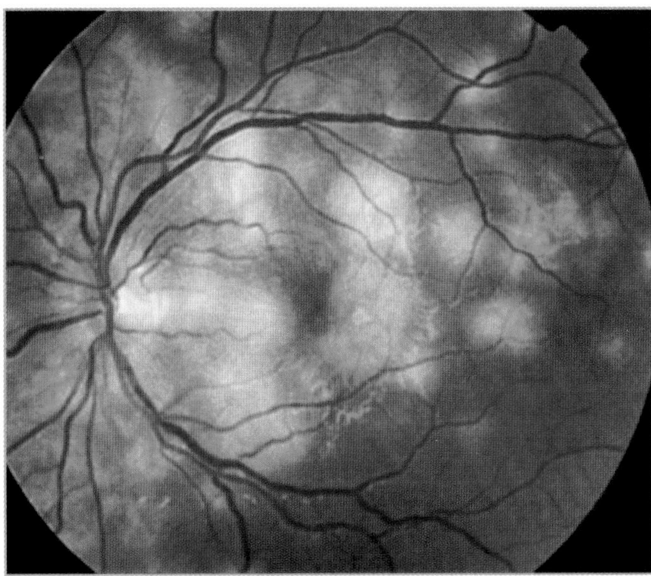

Figure 19.2 Large clusters of acute macular lesions in a patient with acute posterior multifocal placoid pigment epitheliopathy.

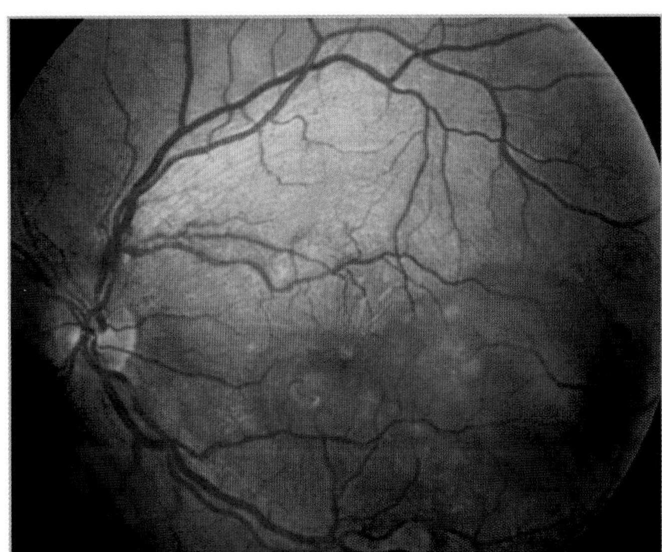

Figure 19.3 Two confluent domes of serous detachment overlie foci of inflammation in acute posterior multifocal placoid pigment epitheliopathy. (Reproduced with permission from BMJ Publishing Group Ltd, from Jones 1995.)

clear. Geographic choroidopathy may show several foci of inflammation and involve the macula while sparing the peripapillary area, and APMPPE may occasionally be peripapillary. On occasion these two conditions are difficult to differentiate, but the subsequent recurrent and progressive behavior of geographic choroidopathy and deeper scarring is diagnostic. Significant serous subretinal fluid accumulations, or the concurrence of meningeal or auditory symptoms, may suggest the VKH syndrome, but APMPPE is not associated with significant anterior or posterior uveitis, and carries none of the later depigmentary stigmata of the VKH syndrome.

Fluorescein angiography is useful and, although there are no signs pathognomonic of APMPPE, a sequence showing early zonal absence of choroidal fluorescence (indicating absence of lobular perfusion presumably caused by occlusion of precapillary arterioles) underlying approximately the areas of swollen and opaque retina, which later become stained but do not leak (**Fig. 19.7**). In contrast fluorescein angiography in VKH syndrome typically shows multifocal punctate leakage (see Fig. 17.19) which is very different from the angiographic appearance of APMPPE. Multifocal choroiditis in granulomatous disease such as sarcoidosis and tuberculosis may cause similar lesions, but usually smaller, with more solid retinal elevation, and more widespread.

Management

APMPPE is usually a self-limiting condition with a reasonably favorable outcome, but a few patients will permanently lose central visual acuity and a tiny minority will develop permanent neurological deficit or die. A recent large follow-up series (Fiore et al. 2009) showed that final acuity was 6/12 or less in a quarter of eyes. However, the three-quarters of patients with 6/9 or better acuity will often report a rather greater subjective handicap, as is common to many patients with widespread macular scarring, despite a reasonable high-contrast acuity measurement. The effect, if any, of oral steroid treatment during the acute phase is unproven, but patients are offered and usually choose this treatment in our clinic. Patients with severe headache or focal neurological symptoms require urgent and full neurological investigation. Those with stroke have been successfully treated with cyclophosphamide. Subretinal neovascularization is occasionally reported after resolution of inflammation, but surprisingly infrequently in comparison with some other forms of inflammation affecting the chorioretinal junction.

During the last decade or so, reports of APMPPE have included more patients with difficult, atypical or progressive disease, and neurological involvement. This may indicate a reporting bias or a change in the pattern of behavior of the disease, if it is a single entity. However, our own clinical experience reflects these trends and the progress of future patients will be observed with interest.

Atypical APMPPE or placoid-like disease

In its typical form few ocular inflammatory syndromes are so straightforward to diagnose as APMPPE. However, variations are common and the clinician is led to question the supposition of APMPPE not

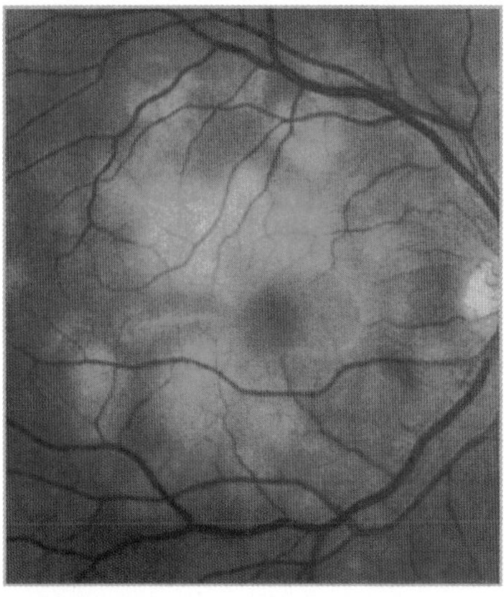
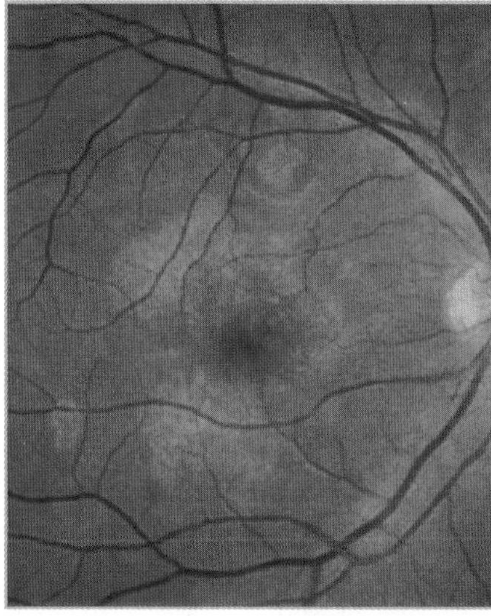

Figure 19.4 Acute-phase acute posterior multifocal placoid pigment epitheliopathy is shown on the left. Two weeks later (on the right), during which time the patient used high-dose oral steroid treatment, the retinal swelling and opacity has subsided and the retinal pigment epithelium has begun to atrophy.

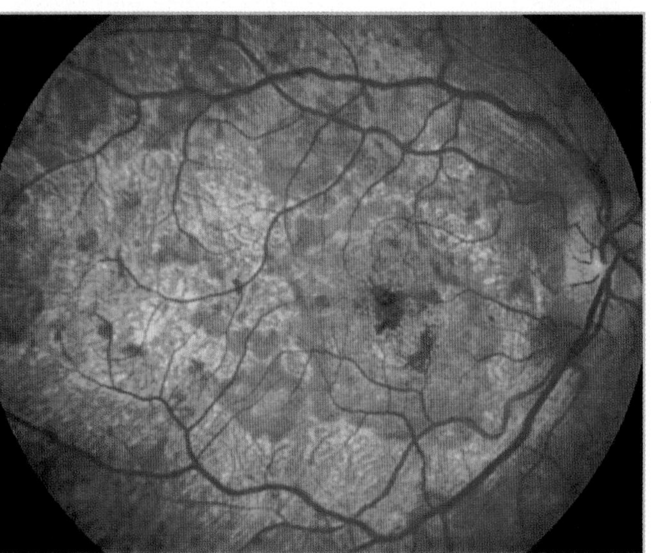

Figure 19.5 An eye some months after an attack of acute posterior multifocal placoid pigment epitheliopathy showing widespread retinal pigment epithelium and inner choroidal atrophy with some pigment clumping. Nevertheless the final visual acuity was 6/9.

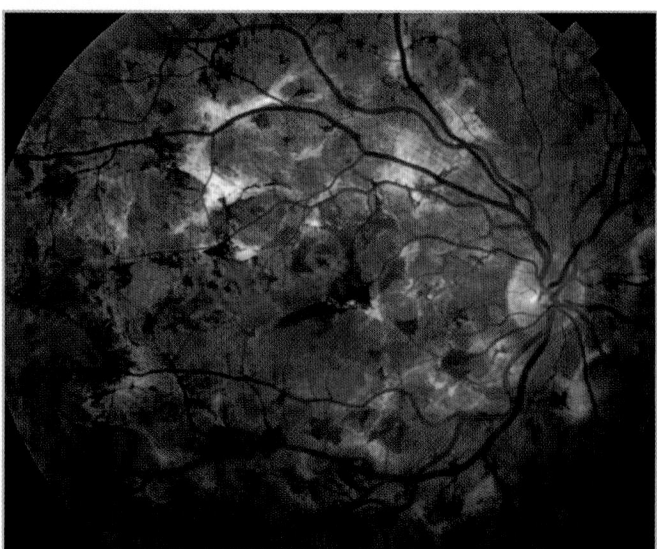

Figure 19.6 Extensive and severe retinal pigment epithelium and inner choroidal scarring in an eye of a non-white patient after acute posterior multifocal placoid pigment epitheliopathy. Visual acuity 6/6.

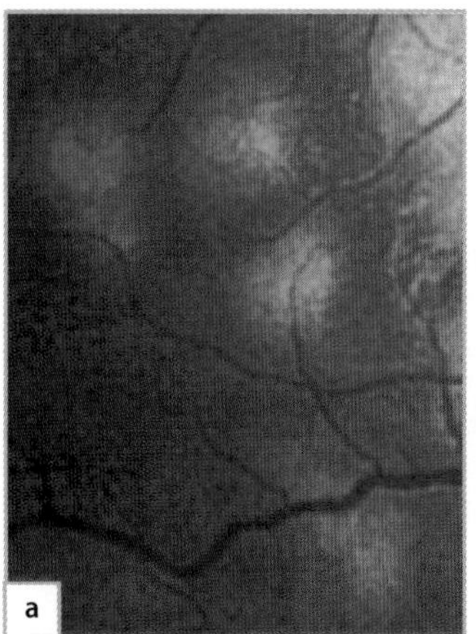

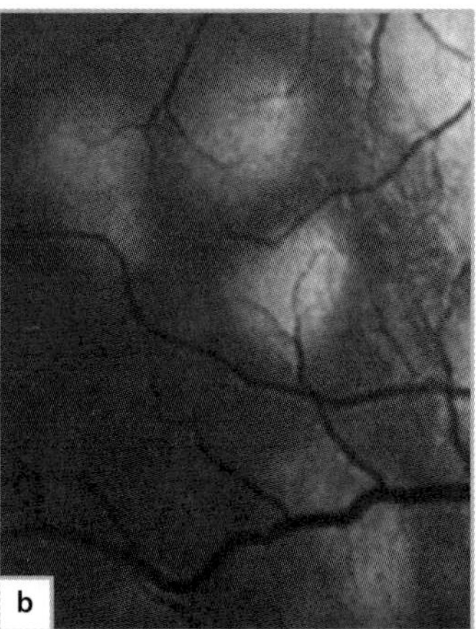

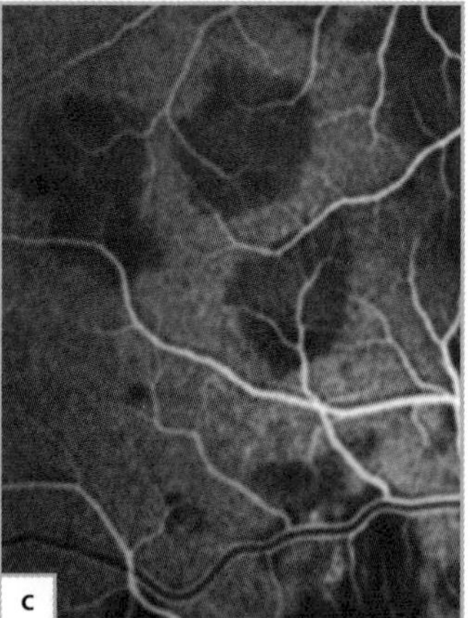

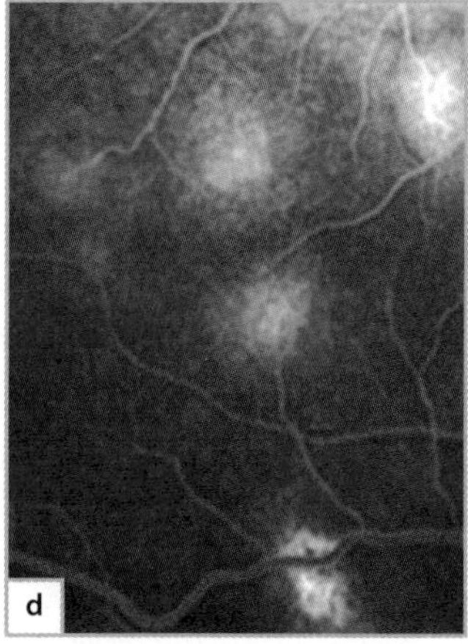

Figure 19.7 Typical acute posterior multifocal placoid pigment epitheliopathy showing retinal swelling and opacity in color (a) and red-free (b) images. The early venous phase fluorescein angiogram (c) shows choroidal hypofluorescence clearly underlying the affected retina. Later in the sequence (d) the retinal lesions stain but do not leak.

infrequently because of initial appearance or subsequent behavior. Unilateral disease may become sequential; monophasic inflammation may recur; lesions may not be placoid in shape but very irregular and numerous (**Fig. 19.8**); lesions may be far more widespread in the fundus and even pre-equatorial; continuing progressive disease may simultaneously show new, resolving and scarred foci; and some may fail to respond to oral steroid and require immunosuppression. Some atypical patients led Nussenblatt and colleagues (1996) to suggest the term **ampiginous choroiditis** to describe patients with features of both APMPPE and serpiginous choroiditis: multifocal acute lesions from the former; recurrence, coalescence and progression from the latter. In 2000, BE Jones and colleagues described a small group of patients with a similar type of placoid-like disease but with widespread lesions progressively appearing over time and they called it **relentless placoid chorioretinitis**. Oral immunosuppression was required in some. Subsequently further case reports have appeared. The authors speculated that this may be a variant of serpiginous choroiditis, but in fact the lesions, being widespread and usually discrete and multifocal rather than contiguous and expansive, seem more to suggest placoid-like disease. We have also encountered similar patients (**Fig. 19.8**) but it is not clear whether either of these stated syndromes (which seem to be one and the same thing) represent a distinct subset of either APMPPE or serpiginous choroiditis (see below) or whether a spectrum of severity of APMPPE exists, which seems more likely. The suggestion by some that there is a continuum between APMPPE and serpiginous choroiditis seems currently an over-statement; the paradigms of these conditions are very different and diagnostic conundrums posed by atypical cases do not necessitate a common etiology.

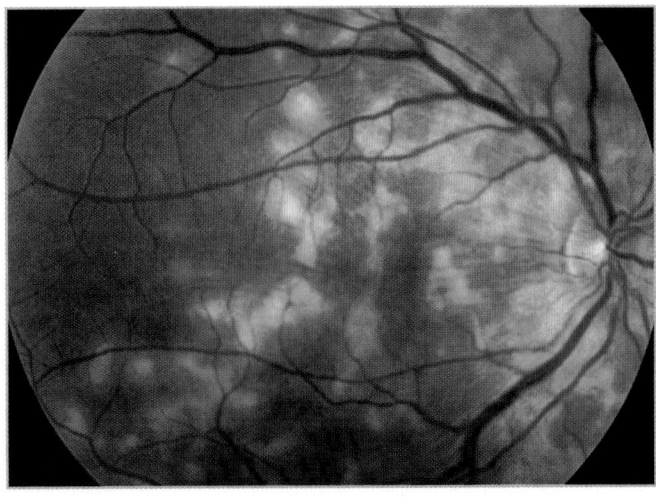

Figure 19.8 An atypical acute posterior multifocal placoid pigment epitheliopathy-like inflammation in a 17-year-old boy with unusual irregular-shaped lesions which continued to progressively appear over a wide area of the fundus. Oral immunosuppression was used.

Arguments over the taxonomy of these descriptive terms will doubtless continue, but in the absence of a suggested etiology are largely semantic. However, one important diagnosis must not be overlooked in any patients with an atypical outer retinopathy/inner choroidopathy, and that is tuberculosis (TB): wherever atypical or steroid-unresponsive APMPPE or geographic choroidopathy is encountered, it has become clear that TB testing is mandatory.

SERPIGINOUS CHOROIDITIS (box 19.2)

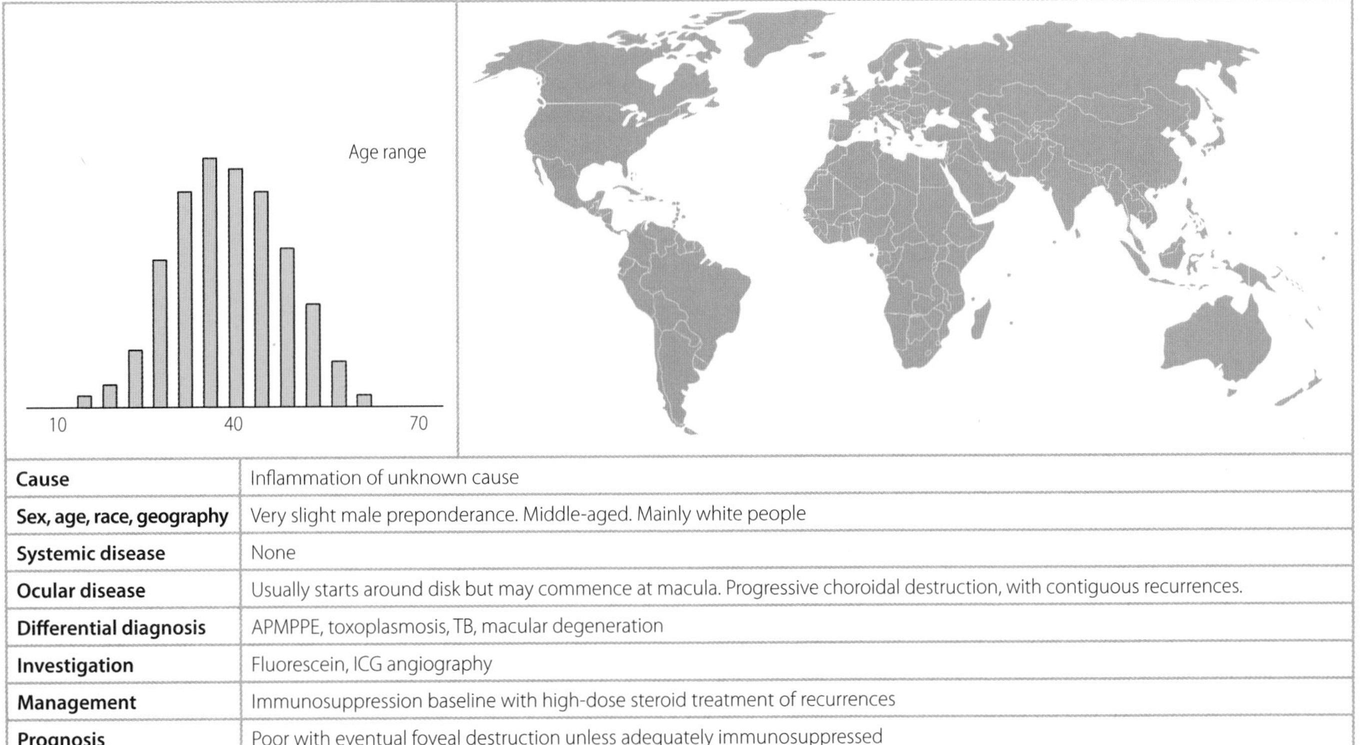

Cause	Inflammation of unknown cause
Sex, age, race, geography	Very slight male preponderance. Middle-aged. Mainly white people
Systemic disease	None
Ocular disease	Usually starts around disk but may commence at macula. Progressive choroidal destruction, with contiguous recurrences.
Differential diagnosis	APMPPE, toxoplasmosis, TB, macular degeneration
Investigation	Fluorescein, ICG angiography
Management	Immunosuppression baseline with high-dose steroid treatment of recurrences
Prognosis	Poor with eventual foveal destruction unless adequately immunosuppressed

Box 19.2 Serpiginous choroiditis

Introduction

This rare disease is a progressive chorioretinal disorder of presumed inflammatory origin. It has borne several descriptive names, including: helicoid choroidopathy, a term now rarely used but describing the tendency of new lesions to expand like blades of a propeller from the optic disk; geographic choroidopathy (the term previously preferred here), describing the irregular map-like configuration of most resultant chorioretinal scars; and **serpiginous choroiditis** (SC), because some lesions seem to snake around the fundus. A brief count of publications on the subject makes it clear that the last term is the clear victor, and this author admits defeat by now using that term. The condition was originally described as atrophic or degenerative, under various historical names. Suggestions of both autoimmune and infectious disease have been proposed, with indirect evidence of the latter for a number of different organisms including varicella-zoster and herpes simplex viruses.

Systemic disease

There is no evidence that SC is linked to a systemic disease. Anecdotes of associations with dystonia, celiac disease and hypoglycemia have been reported but no consistent associations have been found.

Ocular disease

Patients may present with recurrent acute lesions adjacent to the scars of asymptomatic previous attacks, or with the first lesion if it involves the macula. Blurred central vision or paracentral field loss is usually the presenting symptom. New lesions are deep in the fundus and are very poorly defined, cream or gray-colored, and of variable size and shape. There is usually no cellular infiltration into either anterior or posterior compartments, but a few patients have posterior vitreous cells visible. The acute lesions are visible for weeks or months and then subside to leave substantial chorioretinal scarring with overlying loss of function (**Fig. 19.9**). Early lesions have a particular predilection for the peripapillary area, but new lesions may arise anywhere in the posterior pole and occasionally are multiple.

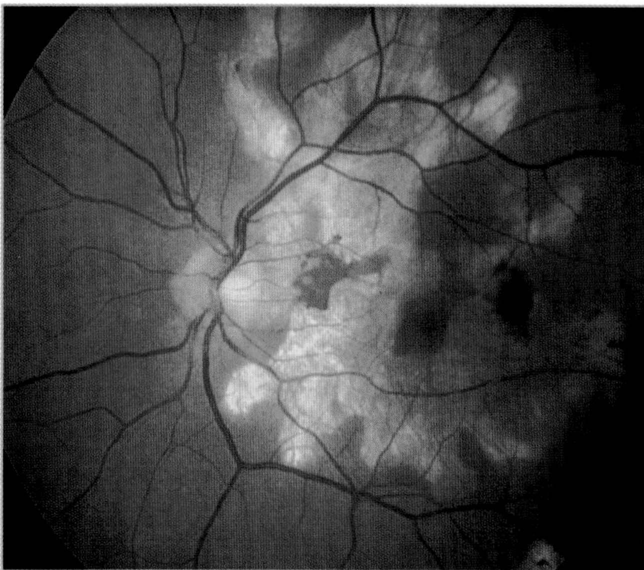

Figure 19.9 Widespread contiguous chorioretinal scarring in serpiginous choroiditis. The fovea is tantalizingly preserved, awaiting destruction by the next recurrence.

SC is a disease that progresses by multiple recurrences, and new lesions tend to arise at intervals varying from months to years, at the edge of an old scar so that, over a period of years, the area of fundal damage enlarges in an irregular and unpredictable way (**Fig. 19.10**), sometimes by multiple serpiginous projections. Involvement of the fovea, which is ultimately likely (although often late in the process), leads to permanent central visual loss. There is depigmentation of the RPE and loss of the choriocapillaris, possibly with involvement of deeper choroidal vessels. The disease may initially be unilateral, but if so almost always consecutively involves the fellow eye leaving bilateral scarring (**Fig. 19.11**).

A variant of SC begins in and expands within the macula without involving the peripapillary area and thus may present with visual loss, which may be permanent. Behavior is as for classic SC except for the location (**Fig. 19.12**). Subretinal neovascularization may occur in up to a quarter of patients with SC and may compound central visual problems. Retinal vasculitis has occasionally been observed and there are reports of branch vessel occlusions. Mild anterior uveitis during recurrences is unusual.

Diagnosis

Fluorescein angiography shows early hypofluorescence corresponding to old scars, presumably reflecting choroidal infarction. Later, mottled fluorescence appears within the area (**Fig. 19.13**) over areas that still retain some choroidal perfusion – the remainder stays dark. Indocyanine green (ICG) angiography confirms persistent hypoperfusion. During an acute reactivation the affected edge shows an extending tongue of subtle retinal opacification (**Fig. 19.14**), which characteristically in late fluorescein angiography has a staining centre but a dark advancing edge.

The differential diagnosis of SC includes APMPPE where the former involves only the macula or the latter has lesions also around the disk, and especially where APMPPE lesions are confluent. In general, APMPPE tends to occur in a significantly earlier age group, the active lesions resolve more quickly and subtotal visual recovery is the rule, the final profound RPE scarring having only subtle effects on central vision in comparison to those of SC. Scar edge reactivation is also a feature of recurrent toxoplasma retinochoroiditis, but the deeply pigmented scar edge and vitritis accompanying toxoplasmosis normally make the diagnosis clear. As for APMPPE, any lesion resembling SC but showing atypical features including multifocal or widespread lesions should provoke a search for TB, which has been increasingly recognized recently (Gupta et al. 2003) as causing atypical serpiginous-like disease.

Management

As recurrent disease may be delayed for long periods and as visual symptoms can be detected earlier with critical self-testing, the regular use of Amsler grids by known patients has been recommended. Acute recurrences have responded to either intravenous methylprednisolone or intravitreal triamcinolone injection, but study numbers are small. Attempts to prevent recurrences have also been made. The usefulness of ciclosporin has been disputed, but claims for the usefulness of azathioprine with prednisolone (Vianna et al. 2006) and interferon-α2a (Sobaci et al. 2005) have been made. In general the efficacy of immunosuppression has been claimed (Christmas et al. 2002) but where inadequately effective, the use of cyclophosphamide has been

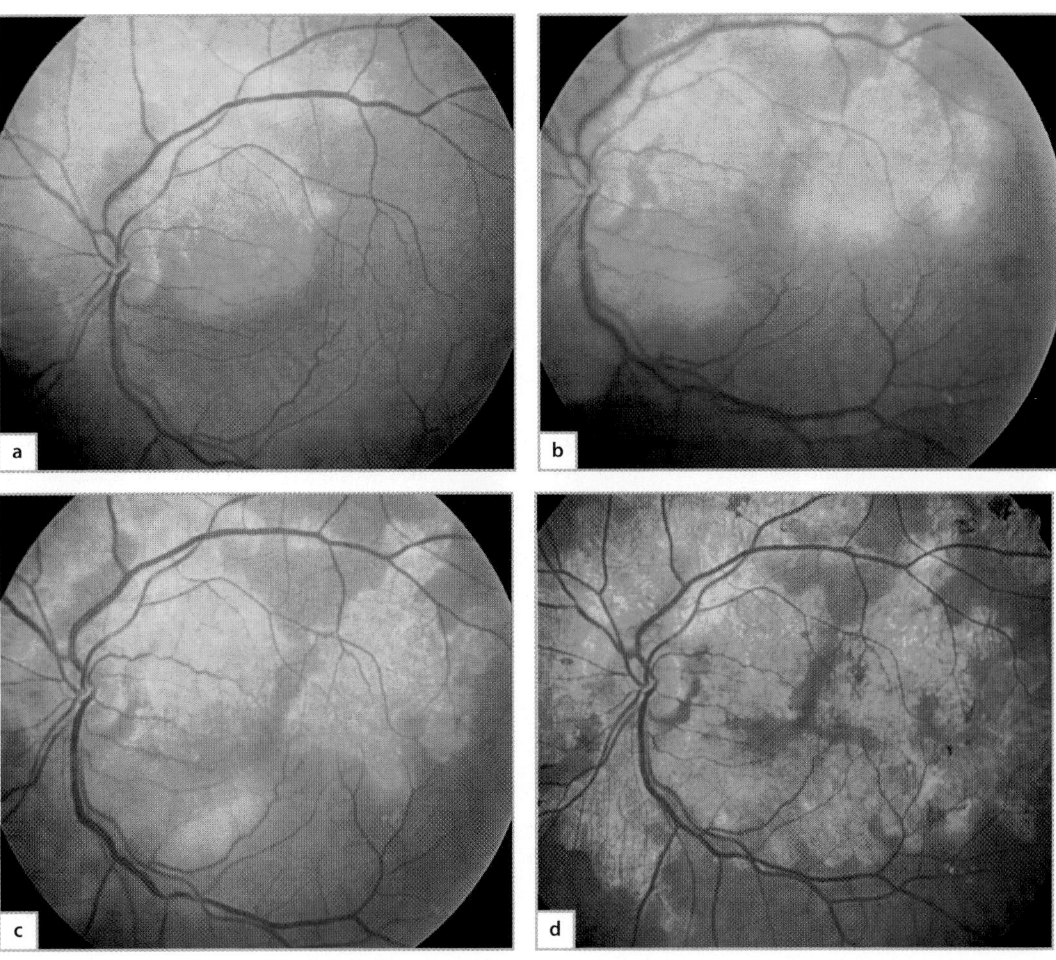

Figure 19.10 Consecutive photos of serpiginous choroiditis in a 58-year-old woman (a) at presentation; (b) 4 months later showing edge reactivation; (c) a further 3 months later and (d) 1 year later showing widespread scarring. Nevertheless the fovea was preserved.

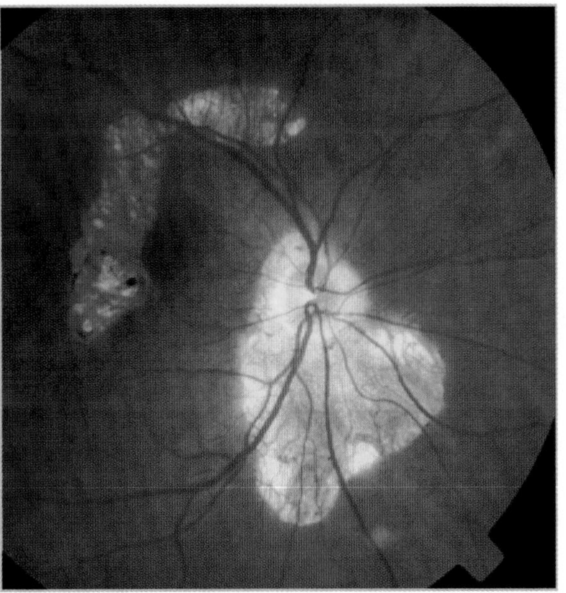

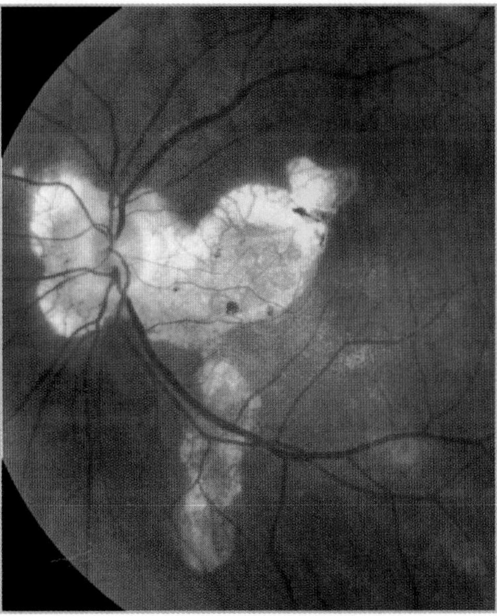

Figure 19.11 Bilateral chorioretinal scarring in serpiginous choroiditis; the right fovea has been lost, the left is threatened.

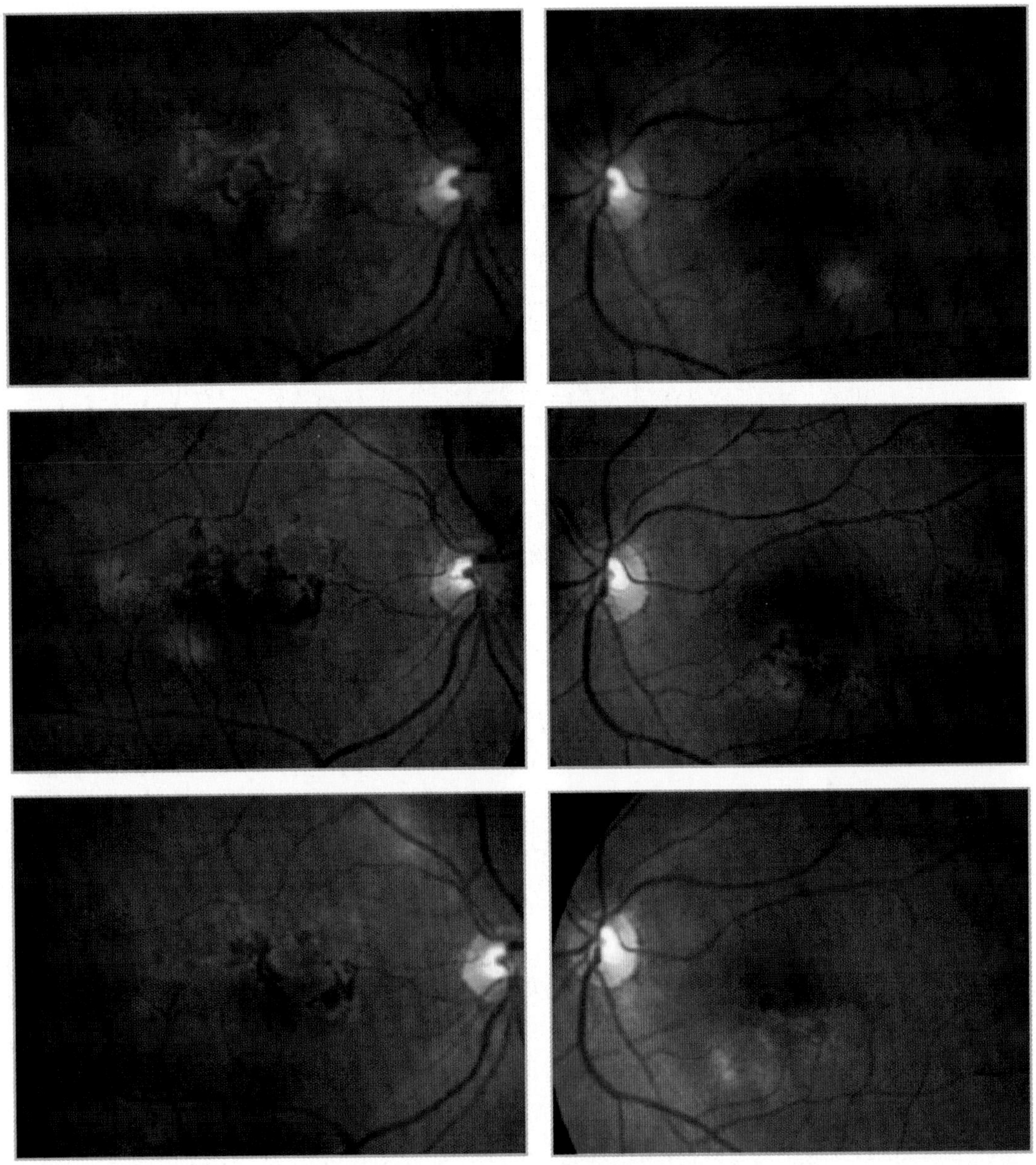

Figure 19.12 Macular serpiginous choroiditis presenting with acute right visual loss in a 45-year-old woman (top) and progressing (middle and bottom) through recurrences to more extensive macular scarring.

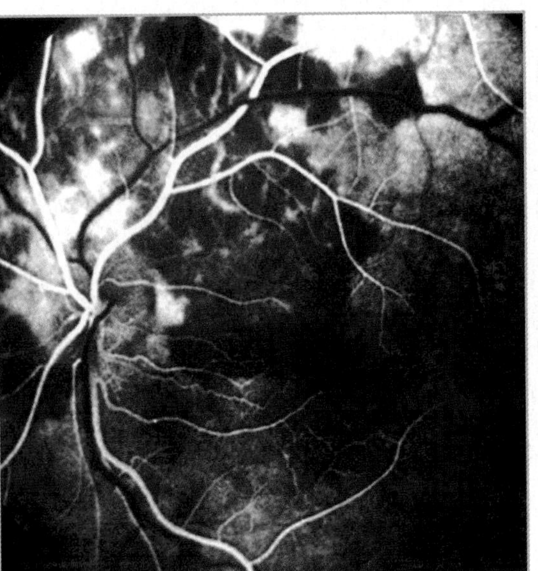

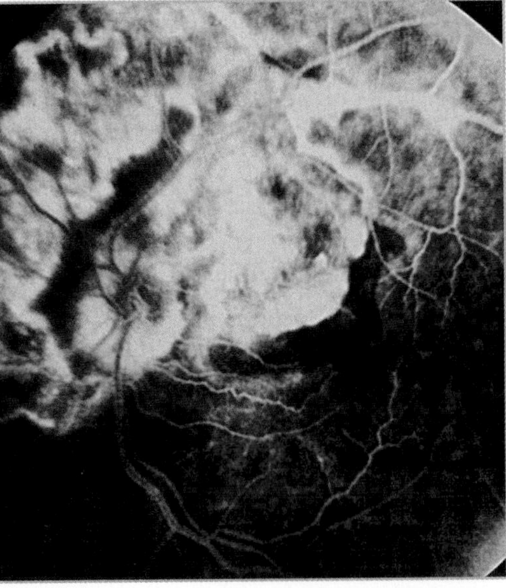

Figure 19.13 Early venous fluorescein angiography shows choroidal infarction, and affected areas stain later in the sequence.

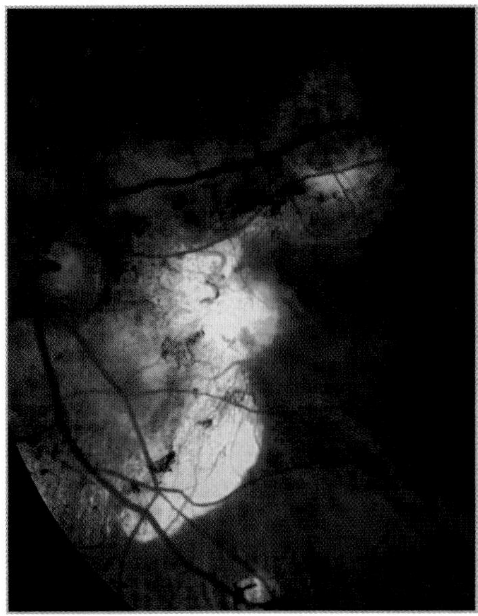

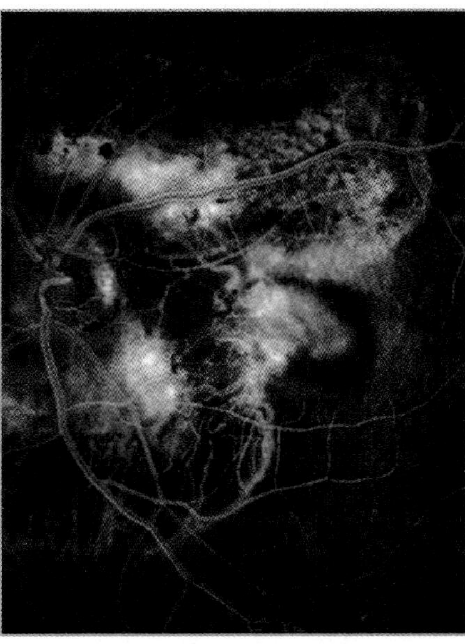

Figure 19.14 An acute reactivation of serpiginous choroiditis showing a tongue of affected chorioretina endangering the fovea. The late fluorescein angiogram shows the active area with a dark edge but a staining centre.

supported (Akpek et al. 2002). Historically, SC has been perceived as a disease that requires high levels of immunosuppression to achieve true remission, and claims for success must be interpreted with the fickle stop-start nature of recurrences in mind. Ultimately the preservation of central vision rests on the ability to prevent progression across the fovea.

Recently a distinctive form of inflammation has been described (Golchet et al. 2006) resembling macular serpiginous choroiditis, but with prolonged choroidal hypoperfusion despite fading of pale retinal lesions over years, and relatively well-preserved acuity until the frequent late development of subretinal neovascularization. The condition was termed **persistent placoid maculopathy (Fig. 19.15)**. The authors considered that, although its appearance and behavior justified its definition as a new entity, it resembled SC rather than placoid epitheliopathy and is thus placed here. It tends to occur in middle-aged or older patients. Anecdotes of successful immunosuppression and the use of intravitreal bevacizumab after subretinal neovascularization have not yet been joined by more concrete information on management.

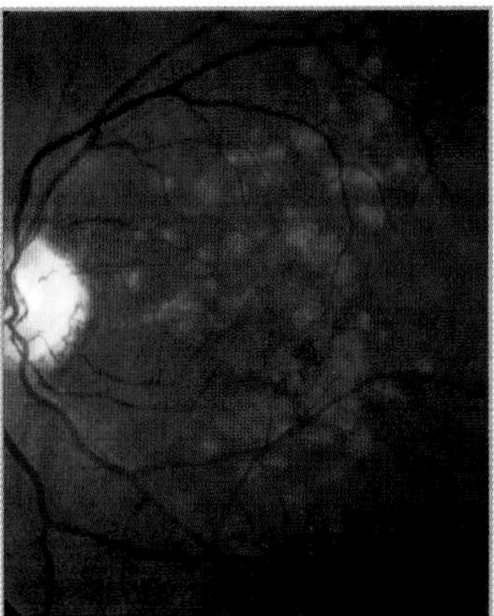

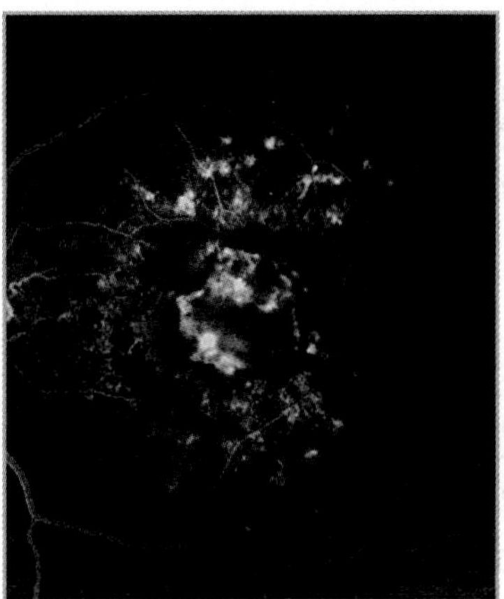

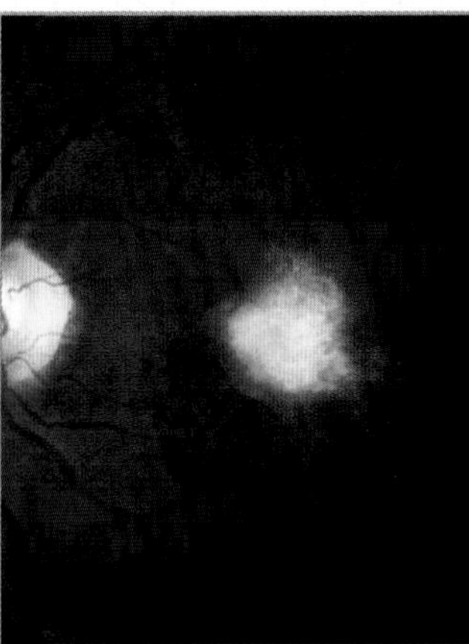

Figure 19.15 A middle-aged woman with persistent placoid maculopathy presents at first with clustered multifocal macular lesions which fade, followed by a large central neovascular membrane, treated with intraocular bevacizumab. A dense macular scar results. Similar changes affected the right eye.

BIRDSHOT RETINOCHOROIDOPATHY (box 19.3)

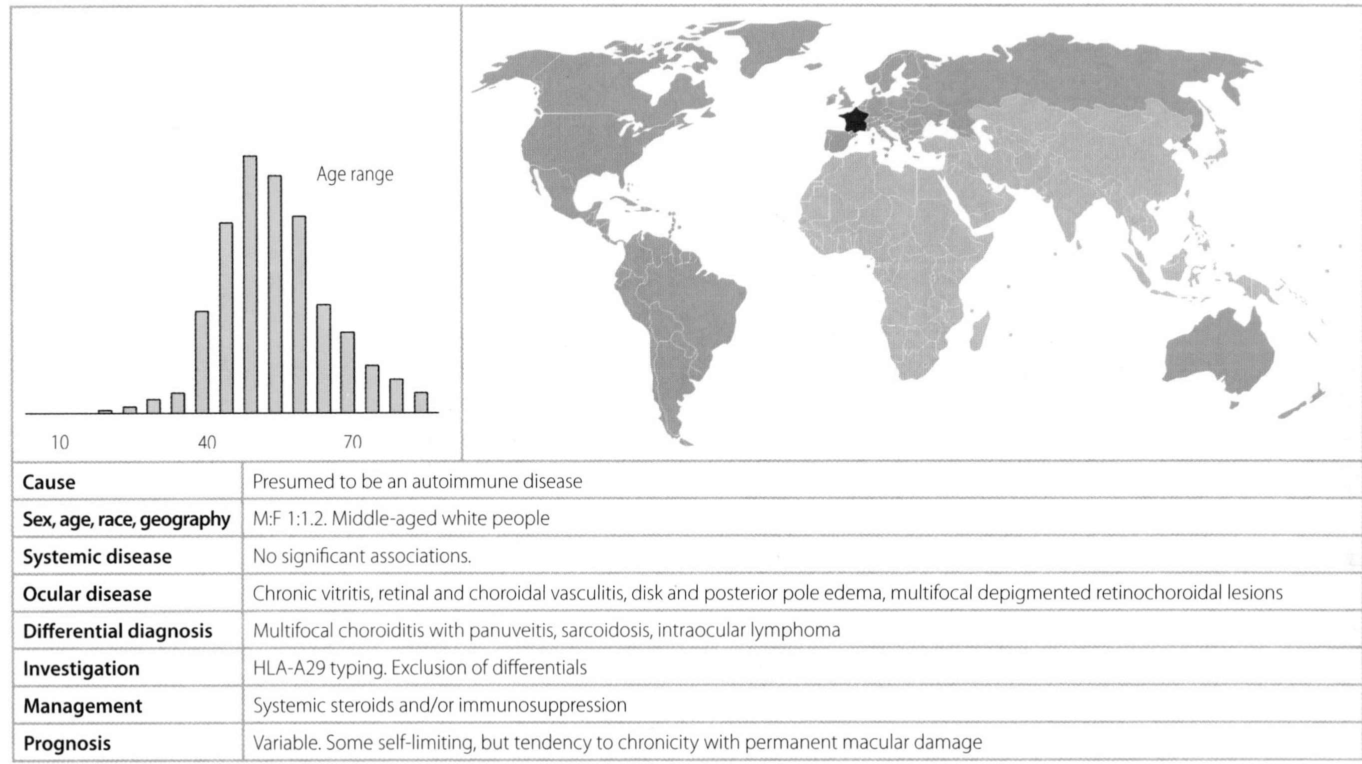

Cause	Presumed to be an autoimmune disease
Sex, age, race, geography	M:F 1:1.2. Middle-aged white people
Systemic disease	No significant associations.
Ocular disease	Chronic vitritis, retinal and choroidal vasculitis, disk and posterior pole edema, multifocal depigmented retinochoroidal lesions
Differential diagnosis	Multifocal choroiditis with panuveitis, sarcoidosis, intraocular lymphoma
Investigation	HLA-A29 typing. Exclusion of differentials
Management	Systemic steroids and/or immunosuppression
Prognosis	Variable. Some self-limiting, but tendency to chronicity with permanent macular damage

Box 19.3 Birdshot retinochoroidopathy

Introduction

Ryan and Maumenee in 1980 and, shortly afterwards, Gass (1981) described a total of 24 patients with common features suggestive of a new type of intraocular inflammation. The first authors coined the term 'birdshot' retinochoroidopathy (BR) to describe the pattern of distribution of the fundal lesions, recalling the wide distribution of pellets from a shotgun loaded with birdshot (buckshot pellets being larger and less dispersed). The second used the term 'vitiliginous' to describe not only the progressive multifocal depigmentation of the fundus lesions, but also the association with cutaneous vitiligo in a minority of patients. This association has not been confirmed with time, and the former term is now used. In 1982 (Nussenblatt et al. 1982) a very strong association with HLA-A29 was established which has subsequently proved to carry a very high relative risk of about 224, currently the highest for any HLA disease association. Further studies initially suggested that the association was uniquely with HLA-A2902 but it now appears that A2901 is occasionally encountered, although probably not any of HLA-A2903–HLA-A2906. About 90% of HLA-A29 positives have the A2902 allele anyway, so the statistical significance of the association remains somewhat unclear. There is some evidence of retinal autoimmunity, especially to retinal S-antigen. Initially considered a rare disease, reports of fairly large cohorts have progressively appeared, but none competes with the group of 225 studied in Paris (Trinh et al. 2009), France apparently being a genuine focus of disease. In contrast the condition is very rare in the Middle East, Africa and Japan and indeed BR is almost exclusive to white people. The prevalence of HLA-A2902 itself (see Fig. 3.2), which is so common in parts of Africa, does not parallel reports of BR from around the world, reflecting on the unknown further trigger(s) required to initiate the disease.

Systemic disease

No concurrent or preceding illness is identified in the great majority of patients with BR. The original claimed association with vitiligo has not been confirmed. Positive serology for *Borrelia burgdorferi* has been found in some patients with BR, but a definite link with Lyme disease has not been established, and the current limitations of such serology are discussed in Chapter 10.

Ocular disease

Patients are almost always white, and middle-aged or older with a mean onset in the fifth decade. There is a slight majority of women, but this is not as pronounced as in some multifocal syndromes. Presentation is usually with floaters and blurred vision, but there may also be subjective visual field constriction, night blindness, metamorphopsia or defective color vision. Photophobia is occasionally a problem.

Affected eyes are white and pain free, and show no evidence of significant anterior chamber (AC) inflammation, but occasional AC cells may be observed. There is vitritis of varying degree, with diffuse cellular activity but without peripheral clumping of opacities as seen in intermediate uveitis. Retinal edema is frequent and may be subclinical (seen only on fluorescein angiography) or lead to chronic cystoid macular edema, or in some cases disk edema.

The hallmark lesions of BR are multifocal and occupy the deep retina and superficial choroid. The lesions vary in number, size and prominence. Most patients have several, some have very many, and in time numbers will increase. The lesions are typically pale, without substance but not excavated, often oval (the long meridian pointing to the posterior pole) and of moderate size (usually quarter to half a disc diameter). They are usually most concentrated at the posterior pole and vary in prominence depending on number, state of progression and underlying fundal pigmentation. The early appearance may be quite subtle (**Fig. 19.16**) or profound (**Fig. 19.17**), the lesions involving most of the post-equatorial fundus, decreasing in frequency with distance from the macula. As for any lesions affecting outer retina or inner choroid, they are more obvious on red-free illumination (**Fig. 19.18**). In some patients these lesions only develop late, sometimes years after the onset of other inflammatory signs. In longstanding disease, widespread coalescent RPE depigmentation has been observed.

Patients with BR may demonstrate a good high-contrast acuity but symptomatically are often unhappy, and this can be highlighted by contrast sensitivity testing (Kappel et al. 2009) or with microperimetry (Giuliari et al. 2010). Widespread macular edema, not necessarily but

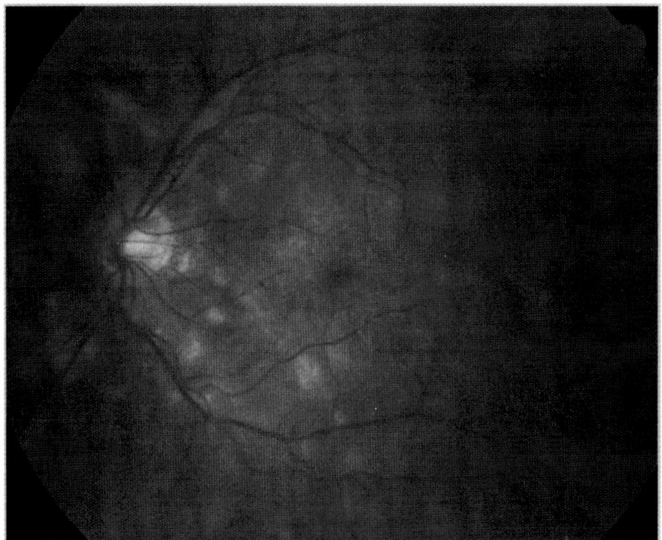

Figure 19.16 Subtle pale lesions in birdshot retinochoroidopathy may be difficult to visualize against a tessellated fundus.

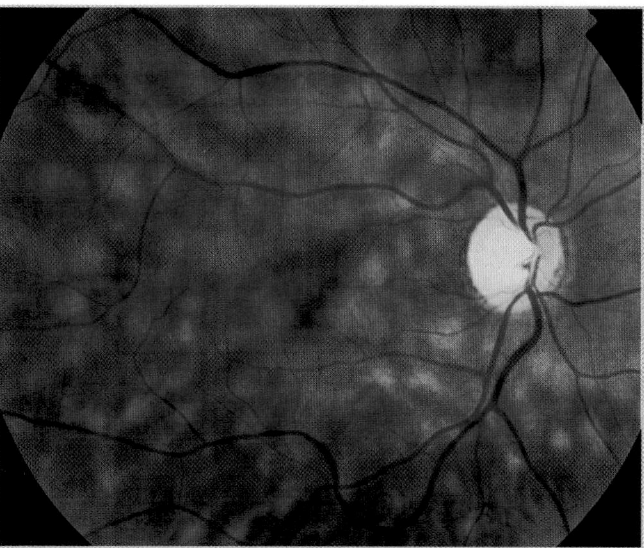

Figure 19.17 Widespread prominent birdshot lesions are almost coalescent in their density especially at the posterior pole. This patient had also developed associated optic neuropathy.

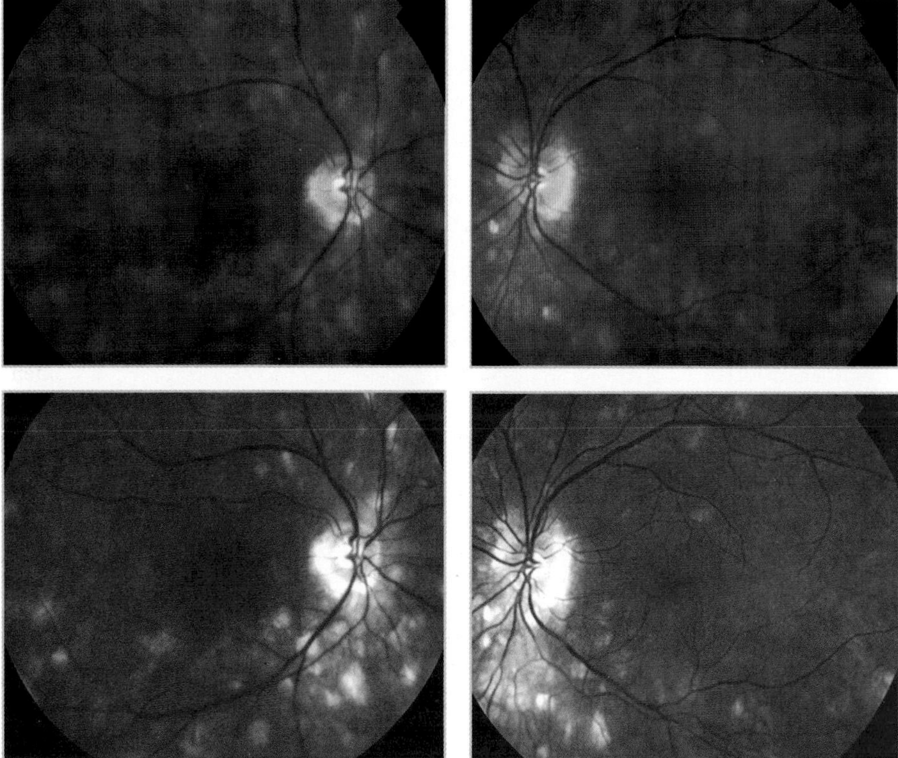

Figure 19.18 Birdshot lesions are more clearly visible under red-free illumination and this may aid examination especially in light-colored fundi.

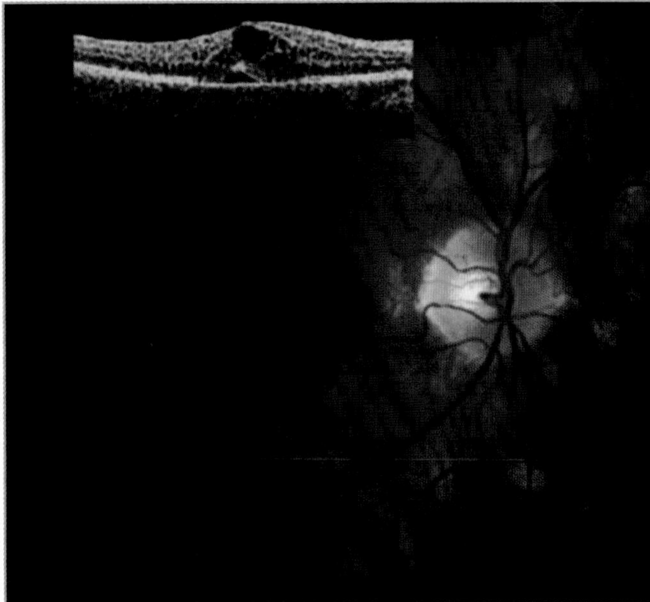

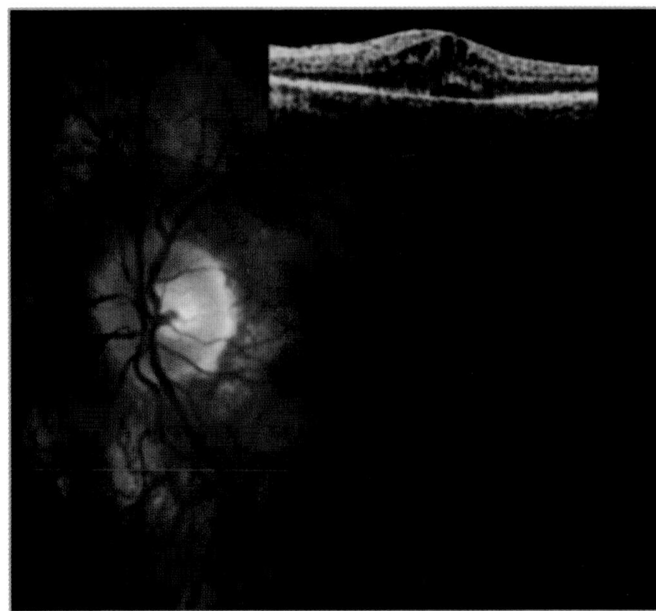

Figure 19.19 Bilateral cystoid macular edema in chronic birdshot retinochoroidopathy as demonstrated by the superimposed ocular coherence tomography images of each fovea.

often including cystoid change (**Fig. 19.19**), often in association with leaking retinal vasculitis, is the predominant cause. Slowly progressive loss of central vision is the natural course for untreated patients, often accompanied by loss of visual field (Thorne et al. 2008). A few patients also develop associated optic neuropathy which can devastate visual function.

Diagnosis

Fluorescein angiography can highlight the vascular leakage, macular edema and disk edema which are important components of BR. Vascular leakage and late perivascular staining, together with leakage from the disk (**Fig. 19.20**), is characteristic. The multifocal lesions themselves are usually not be seen at all on fluorescein angiography but are clearly visible dark spots on ICG angiography. There is sometimes clinical and angiographic evidence of choroidal vasculitis. Retinal function studies have been performed, and the combination of abnormal dark adaptation, dyschromatopsia of the yellow–blue type, a reduced-amplitude electroretinogram (ERG) with increased b-wave latency and abnormal electro-oculogram (EOG), has been interpreted as a predominantly inner retinal abnormality, which is perhaps surprising in view of the ophthalmoscopic signs.

The typical clinical appearance of BR is pathognomonic, but we ask for HLA-A29 testing as routine and revisit the diagnosis if negative. The differential diagnosis of vitritis with multifocal fundal lesions includes multifocal choroiditis with panuveitis, sarcoidosis and lymphoma; any chronic vitritis with fundal lesions in middle-aged patients should raise suspicion of the last. The characteristic distribution of lesions, symptomatology, supportive fluorescein angiography, and most significantly HLA testing, will usually establish the diagnosis of BR.

Management

There is no consensus on the optimum treatment of BR. Although a few patients have self-limiting disease, it tends to be very chronic and over a period of years may lead to permanent visual loss, especially as a result of macular damage. There is a clear correlation between visual acuity on presentation and the visual outcome (Rothova et al. 2004), and poor outcome is also unsurprisingly associated with long duration of symptoms at presentation. The long-term use of systemic steroid treatment is undesirable and of limited use. A variety of oral immunosuppressives has been used, the initial enthusiasm being for ciclosporin (Vitale et al. 1994) but, in general, adequately immunosuppressed patients have a better outcome with sustained visual acuity (Kiss et al. 2005). For those few refractory cases, daclizumab has been helpful in some cases (Sobrin et al. 2008) and further developments are awaited.

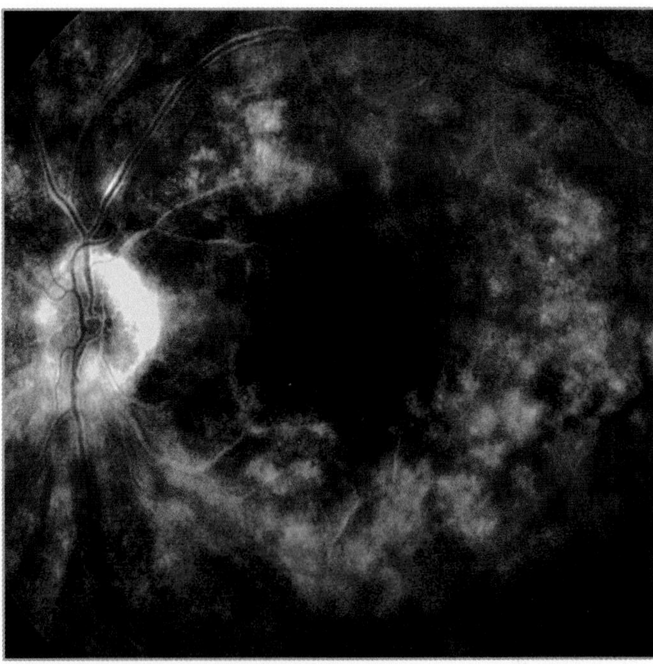

Figure 19.20 A late-phase fluorescein angiogram shows optic disk staining and leakage; multifocal retinal vasculitis with wall staining and widespread intraretinal edema including the macula.

ACUTE ZONAL OCCULT OUTER RETINOPATHY (box 19.4)

Age range
Female
Male
10 40 70

Cause	Unknown, possibly infective
Sex, age, race, geography	Predominantly young women, mostly white
Systemic disease	Occasional transverse myelitis or multiple sclerosis
Ocular disease	Acute visual field loss with shimmering photopsia, late retinal atrophic signs
Differential diagnosis	Anterior visual pathway lesions, retinal dystrophy, syphilis, Diffuse unilateral subacute neuroretinitis (DUSN), paraneoplastic retinopathy
Investigation	Electrophysiology, visual field testing, CNS imaging if necessary
Management	Unknown. Immunosuppression ineffective
Prognosis	Untreated most cases arrest leaving reasonable vision; a few are blinded

Box 19.4 Acute zonal occult outer retinopathy

Introduction

In 1993 Gass described 13 patients, mostly young women, with photopsia, extensive visual field defects and abnormal ERGs, and named this syndrome **acute zonal occult outer retinopathy** (AZOOR). He immediately suggested that the condition may be associated with other white dot syndromes included below. In the succeeding 18 years about 130 cases of AZOOR have been published (Monson et al. 2011), mostly involving white people in the western world, with a few reports from Asia. The disease remains rare but is perhaps increasingly well recognized. Women outnumber men 3.2:1 with an average age at presentation of 37 years. The condition may be unilateral or bilateral. No effective treatment has been proven. A significant proportion of affected patients have previously or simultaneously developed multifocal chorioretinal inflammation including multiple evanescent white dot syndrome (MEWDS) and it is increasingly accepted that AZOOR is either a common end-point or a frequent complication of a group of white dot syndromes, possibly with a common etiology.

Systemic disease

Most patients with AZOOR have no systemic disease, but we and others have seen patients with both transverse myelitis and multiple sclerosis in association. The former condition can be seen as a post-infective phenomenon and suggestions, as yet unconfirmed, of a possible fungal or viral etiology for AZOOR are intriguing.

Ocular disease

The photopsiae are often quite a characteristic symptom; in contrast to the periodic glints or flashes that can occur in vitreoretinal traction, the symptoms of AZOOR are often described as an intrusive shimmering which is frequently present and visually very distracting. If bilateral, asymmetry is typical. The associated visual field defects, which tend to be acute in onset and then slowly progressive for months, are almost always extensions of the blind spot of great variability in size and shape. They are not nerve fiber bundle defects. Afferent pupil defects are inconstant and often temporary. At presentation AZOOR is genuinely 'occult' in that neither the retina nor the optic nerve looks abnormal. Field loss is usually permanent and may progress to severe visual loss. In time widespread retinal atrophy with fine RPE depigmentation and outer retinal sheen, occasionally with bone spicule formation and retinal vessel attenuation, may develop (**Fig. 19.21**), which stains but does not leak on fluorescein angiography (**Fig. 19.22**).

Diagnosis

In the absence of visible intraocular problems, anterior visual pathway disease is the primary differential diagnosis of AZOOR. The coexistence of any sign of active or previous focal retinal inflammation should suggest the diagnosis in the presence of characteristic symptoms and visual field assessment should of course be performed. Electrophysiology tends to show not only photoreceptor abnormality but also inner retinal disease as demonstrated by delayed 30-Hz flicker

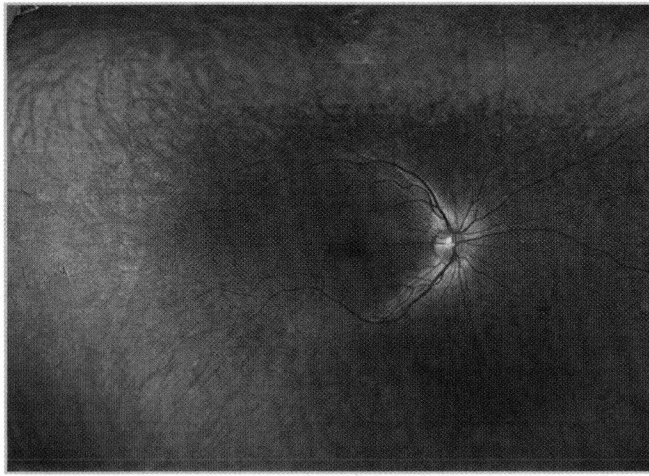

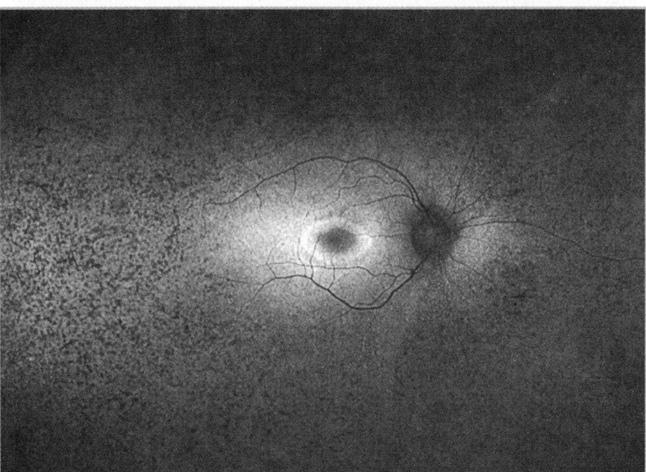

Figure 19.21 Late-stage acute zonal occult outer retinopathy showing subtle outer retinal atrophy and some bone spicule pigmentation. Autofluorescence shows multiple dark punctate areas. Very constricted visual field; VA 6/6.

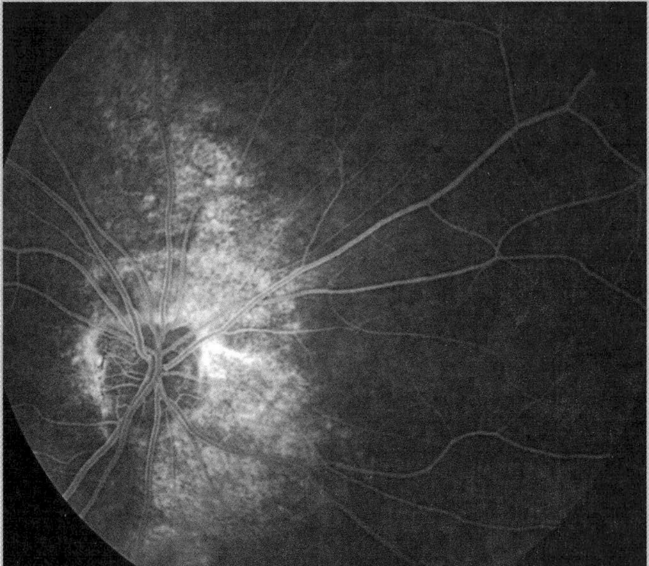

Figure 19.22 Concentric fluorescein staining in late-stage acute zonal occult outer retinopathy.

ERG and reduced EOG light rise (Francis et al. 2005). Both fluorescein and ICG angiography at presentation are normal. If symptoms are atypical it will be difficult to avoid brain imaging which will be normal unless there are association signs of demyelination. For those presenting late, retinal changes may be visible, thus suggesting a differential diagnosis including asymmetrical tapetoretinal degenerations or receptor dystrophies, syphilitic retinitis and (if unilateral) diffuse unilateral subacute neuroretinitis. Long-term follow-up shows that, although most patients retain good visual acuity albeit with significant visual field defects, a proportion is blinded (Gass et al. 2002). In patients presenting with shimmering photopsia, scotomas and absent retinal signs, paraneoplastic retinopathy should always be considered.

Management

Many patients have been treated with either systemic steroid or immunosuppression, and there is a wide consensus that such treatment is unhelpful. Such clear resistance to potent anti-inflammatory or immunosuppressive treatment mitigates against an autoimmune cause and suggests an infective etiology. It is therefore interesting to note the suggestion that infection (past or present) with a *Candida* subspecies has been consistently identified in affected patients (Pisa et al. 2008), although these results have so far been found by only one group. Of equal interest is the report of the cure of three patients with AZOOR-like disease by valaciclovir treatment (Mahajan and Stone 2010). It will be noted with interest that herpetic infection is a well-recognized precursor of transverse myelitis which has been reported in association with AZOOR. Further developments are awaited with interest.

Acute idiopathic blind spot enlargement

In 1988 Fletcher and others described 7 patients with ages ranging from 25 to 39, 5 of whom were women, who presented with acute unilateral visual disturbance, including negative or positive scotomas in the temporal field, associated in most with photopsia or bright haloes in the affected field. They called the syndrome **acute idiopathic blind spot enlargement** (AIBSE). The optic disks were not swollen (in contrast to the previously reported 'big blind spot syndrome'), but blind spot enlargement was documented on perimetry, usually with well-defined irregular borders. Afferent pupil defects are seen in a majority (Singh et al. 1991), which is reminiscent of MEWDS. Only a minority had evidence of peripapillary atrophy, and this did not explain the extent of the field defect. Symptoms and signs resolve spontaneously within months, but bilateral involvement and recurrences are sometimes seen. The occurrence of blind spot enlargement as a common accompaniment to MEWDS suggests a possible etiological connection, but some (Volpe et al. 2001) feel that the conditions are distinct.

The similarities between AIBSE and AZOOR are clear, strongly suggesting that the former is perhaps a more limited type of the latter, albeit with a more reliable afferent pupil defect.

Acute annular outer retinopathy

A young man with a striking and apparently new form of intraocular inflammation was described in 1995 by Gass and Stern, who called it acute annular outer retinopathy (AAOR) and immediately suggested that it may be a form of AZOOR. The condition is by no means occult, but, clearly, similarly involves the outer retina and, in the absence to date of a proven etiology (for either disease), AAOR is presented here as a subset of AZOOR. A small number of further cases of this rare, usually unilateral inflammation have been reported (Fekrat et al. 2000), predominantly in young adults, and we have encountered two. Patients tend to present either with visual distortion or with a scotoma and are found on presentation to have a semi-opaque irregular ring of deep retinal inflammation concentric with the disk, which enlarges progressively over a period of weeks, leaving behind it an atrophic and damaged RPE, often with pigment clumping (**Fig. 19.23**). The severity of inflammation (**Fig. 19.24**) and resultant visual acuity are clearly variable. An autoimmune mechanism for the condition has been hypothesized and, when comparing its appearance with immune ring formation in corneal disease, for example, the idea is attractive. However, its 'brush-fire expansion' behavior is also very reminiscent of cytomegalovirus (CMV) retinitis and further searches for etiology are awaited, although currently there is no evidence of a viral etiology. Our patients seemed unresponsive to oral steroid treatment and no firm conclusions on optimal management have been drawn.

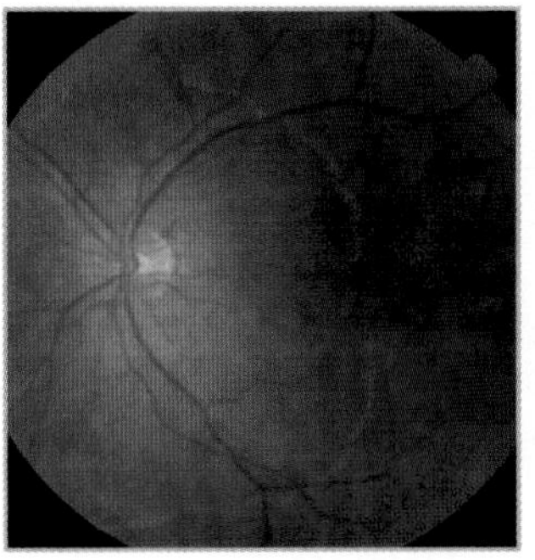
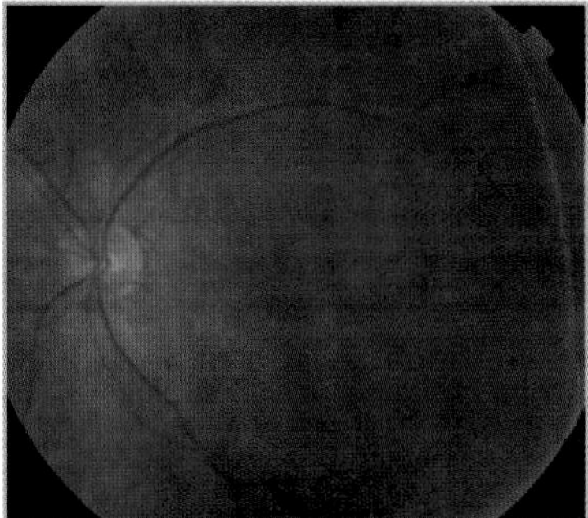
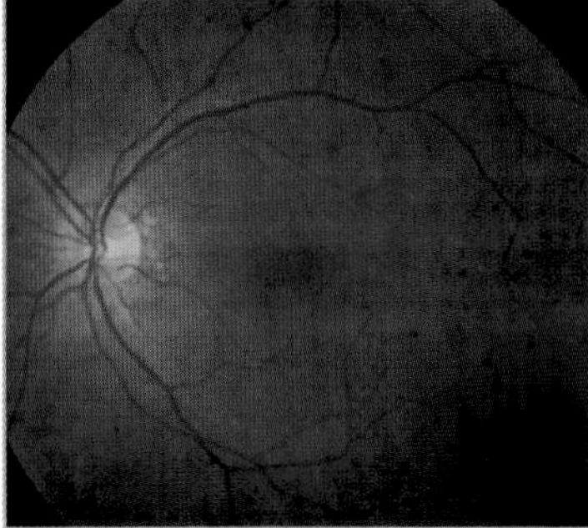

Figure 19.23 Consecutive fundal photographs in acute annular outer retinopathy: at presentation (left) with visual distortion there is an irregular, pale, deep retinal ring concentric with the disc. Six weeks later (middle) the ring has expanded to encompass the posterior pole. Some 3 months later (right) the ring has disappeared to leave retinal pigment epithelium atrophy and widespread pigment clumping with acuity of 6/12.

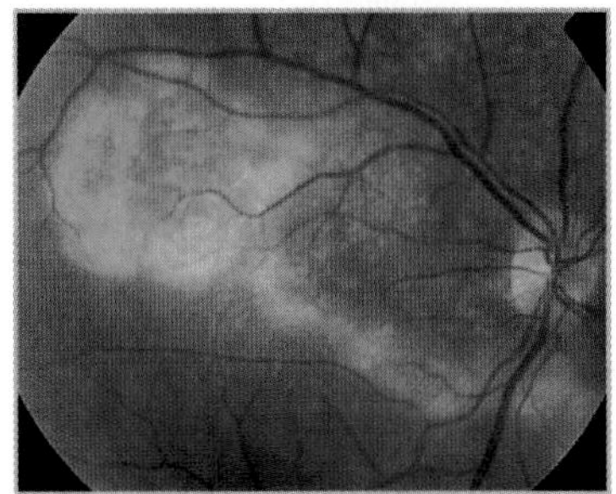
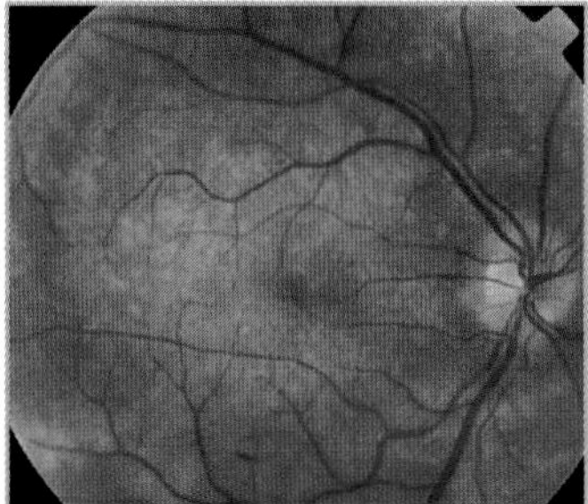
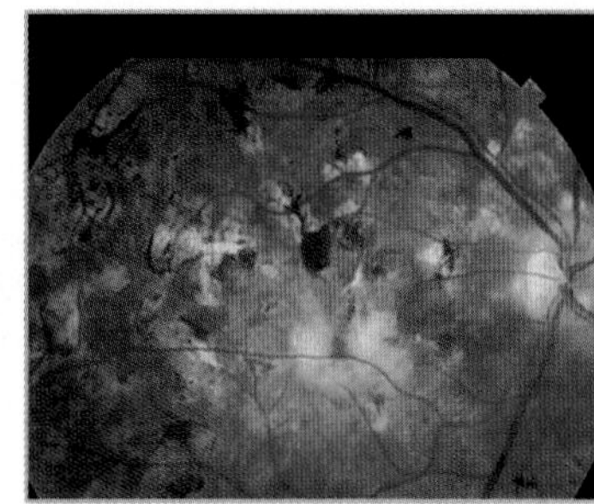

Figure 19.24 A more severe case of acute annular outer retinopathy showing progressive change (despite high-dose oral steroid) leading to severe retinal pigment epithelium scarring and pigmentation with acuity of count fingers only.

MULTIPLE EVANESCENT WHITE DOT SYNDROME (box 19.5)

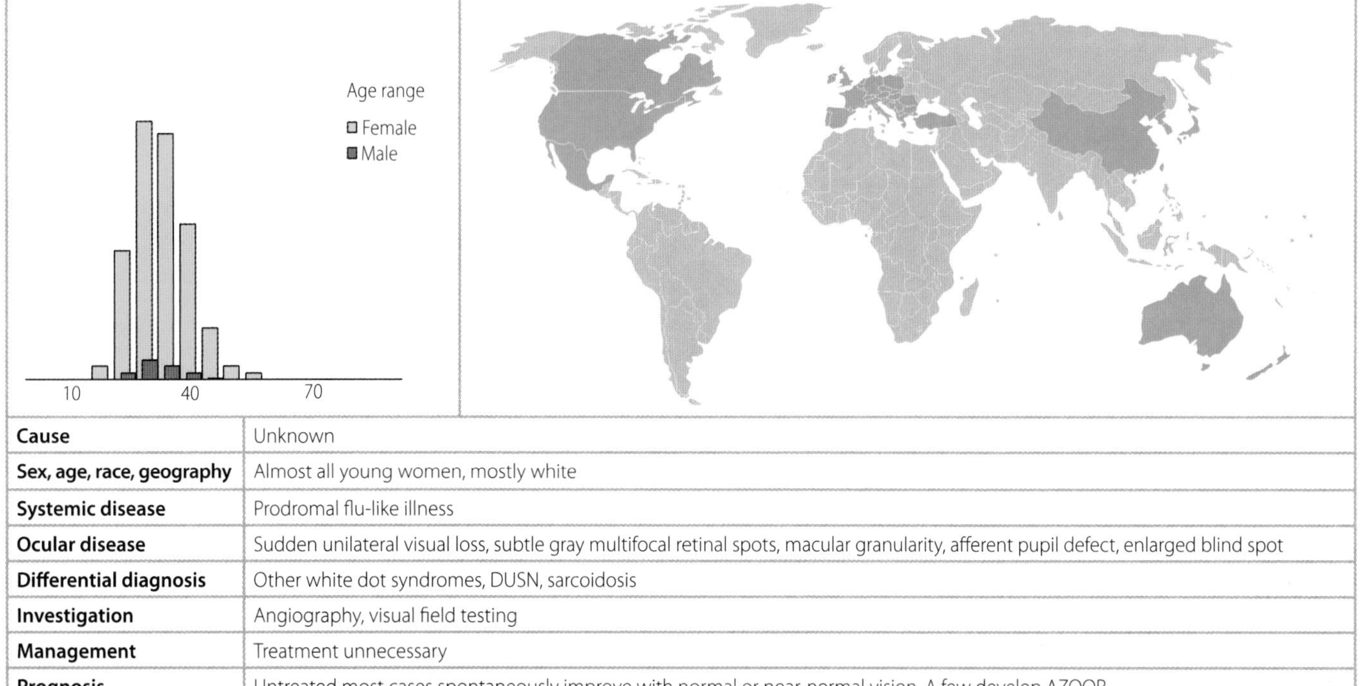

Cause	Unknown
Sex, age, race, geography	Almost all young women, mostly white
Systemic disease	Prodromal flu-like illness
Ocular disease	Sudden unilateral visual loss, subtle gray multifocal retinal spots, macular granularity, afferent pupil defect, enlarged blind spot
Differential diagnosis	Other white dot syndromes, DUSN, sarcoidosis
Investigation	Angiography, visual field testing
Management	Treatment unnecessary
Prognosis	Untreated most cases spontaneously improve with normal or near-normal vision. A few develop AZOOR

Box 19.5 Multiple evanescent white dot syndrome

Introduction

The multiple evanescent white dot syndrome was first described in 11 patients in the USA (10 of whom were women with an average age of 28) by Jampol and co-workers (1984). Early reports emanated from North America but the disease is widespread, mainly in white people. Painless unilateral visual loss or paracentral scotomas of rapid onset, often with photopsia, in a young adult, almost always female, is typical. A recent flu-like illness is common. Multifocal subtle deep retinal lesions around the posterior pole are accompanied by an afferent pupil defect and a low visual acuity out of keeping with the mild retinal observations. Spontaneous recovery is the rule without chorioretinal scarring.

Systemic disease

Patients developing MEWDS characteristically have a flu-like illness preceding the onset of visual symptoms, and a few have followed immunization for hepatitis, but otherwise no significant systemic associations are seen.

Ocular disease

Patients are overwhelmingly young women with unilateral acute symptoms, comprising loss of acuity, photopsia or paracentral scotomas. On examination there is often an afferent pupil defect. There is no anterior segment inflammation, and vitreous cells, although usually seen, are few and posterior. Two significant findings are seen in the fundus: first subtle, grayish, moderate-sized (about 100 μm) deep retinal lesions are seen around the posterior pole (**Fig. 19.25**), most dense within and around the vascular arcades and disk, but tending to spare the perifoveal area. Second, a characteristic dark granular appearance is seen over the macula itself, on closer examination caused by myriads of tiny punctate yellowish or orange spots, and the foveal reflex is abnormal. Occasionally, evidence of mild retinal periphlebitis is seen, and mild optic disk swelling is also possible. Enlargement of the blind spot is common (**Fig. 19.25**) and there is a clear overlap with the findings of AIBSE. This enlargement may persist. The multifocal lesions, however, characteristically disappear without RPE scarring, and may for a time appear in different positions.

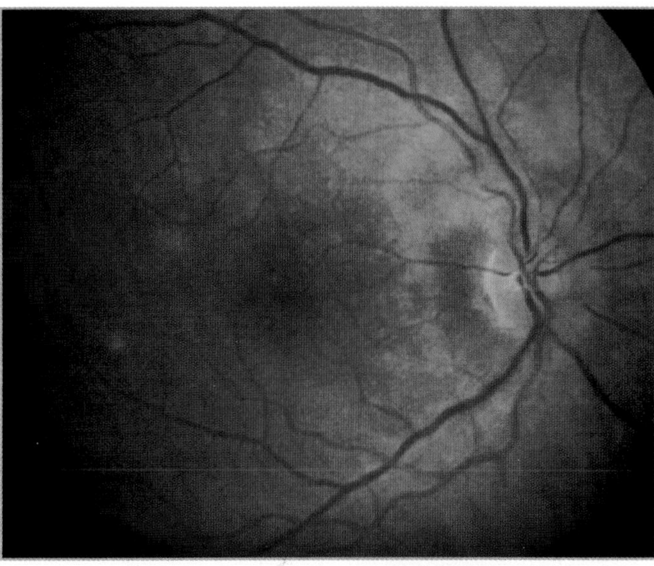

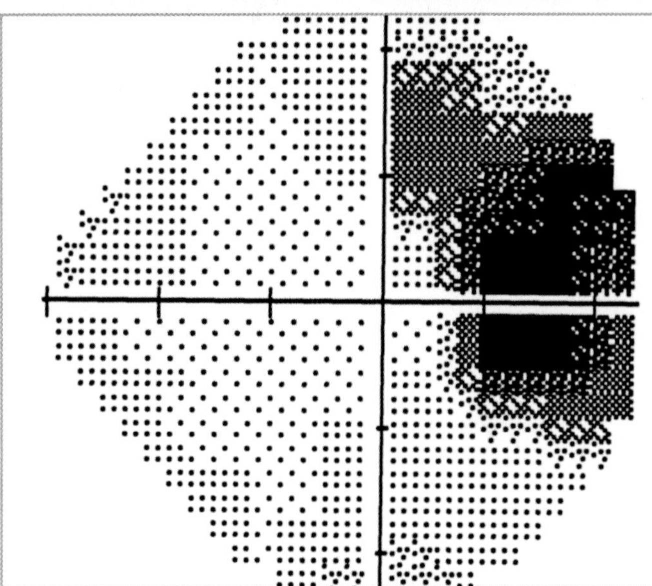

Figure 19.25 Multifocal subtle grayish lesions around the posterior pole in multiple evanescent white dot syndrome. Some peripapillary lesions are confluent. The accompanying (inverted) Humphrey 24/2 field is shown.

Diagnosis

MEWDS has been reported coexistent with acute macular neuroretinopathy (AMN), AIBSE, AZOOR and punctate inner choroidopathy (PIC). Those conditions most likely to be confused include birdshot retinochoroidopathy, which by comparison is less dramatic in onset and bilateral, usually affects older patients, and is associated with more vitreous activity, more vasculitis, disk and macular edema and a more chronic and troublesome course. APMPPE may also sometimes present unilaterally, but the individual lesions are usually more easily seen, larger and distinctly creamy-yellow in color, sometimes associated with retinal edema or focal serous detachment, and a third of patients have a simultaneous systemic upset. Resolution usually leads to profound RPE scarring, in contrast to MEWDS. Retinal pigment epitheliitis may also cause multiple macular lesions but these are usually dark and surrounded by RPE depigmentation. Sarcoidosis may also cause retinal periphlebitis and multiple fundus lesions, but both signs are usually more profound and almost always bilateral.

Fluorescein angiography may show early bright fluorescence and, later, staining of the multifocal lesions and the optic disk. ICG angiography may show more widespread involvement than is seen by ophthalmoscopy and the lesions are hypofluorescent and sustained. A marked effect on the a-wave of the ERG during the acute stage suggests widespread involvement of the RPE. These changes usually return to normal.

Management

Visual loss may be sudden in onset and dramatic in extent, but recovery within a few weeks to 3 months is the rule, with disappearance of the characteristic lesions. However, as for other post-inflammatory maculopathies, a degree of permanent RPE scarring may be seen. Recurrences or sequential involvement of the second eye have been reported and may be more common than had initially been suspected. Some patients go on to develop AZOOR (Fine et al. 2009) and the prognosis must therefore be guarded. A few patients have been treated with systemic steroids and this has been felt to be effective, but most would argue that treatment is unnecessary. A few patients develop subretinal neovascularization despite the apparent absence of disruption of the RPE–Bruch's membrane interface. Anecdotally both intraocular bevacizumab and ranibizumab have been successful in treatment.

OTHER MULTIFOCAL OR ZONAL SYNDROMES

Acute macular neuroretinopathy

First described in four young women in 1975 (Bos and Deutman 1975), AMN typically presents with acute unilateral or bilateral central visual disturbance, usually including scotomas, sometimes following a flu-like illness. The condition is much more common in young women, and therefore the claimed association with oral contraceptive use may not be statistically significant. On examination the macula shows dark-red or brown, wedge-shaped lesions that may radiate in a petalloid fashion around the fovea; the lesions may be mistaken for subretinal blood. They correlate accurately with scotomas on central field testing. The lesions are felt to be in the neurosensory retina with hyper-reflective zones on ocular coherence tomography (OCT) examination showing above the RPE, which seems unaffected. No vitreous cells are seen. Electroretinography has not been abnormal, and fluorescein angiography has not shown significant abnormalities. Resolution may occur over a period of months, but the outcome is guarded and paracentral scotomas may remain (Turbeville et al. 2003). A few cases have been reported after the administration of intravenous adrenergics, and it has been suggested that chorioretinal vasoconstriction may be responsible (Corver et al. 2007). No effective treatment is known.

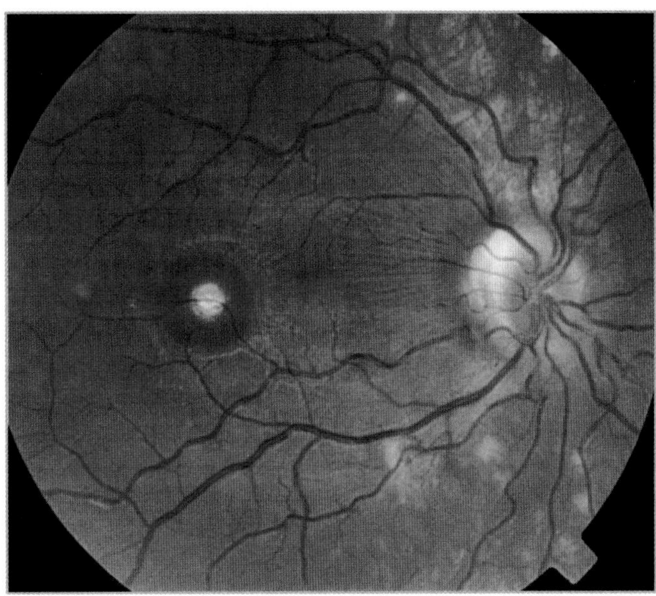

Figure 19.26 The acute phase of multifocal choroiditis with panuveitis in a 12-year-old girl showing multiple small cream lesions, substantial peripapillary swelling with retinal striae and a paramacular subretinal neovascular membrane.

Multifocal choroiditis with panuveitis and PIC

In 1973, Nozik and Dorsch described two patients with fundal signs strongly suggestive of the presumed ocular histoplasmosis syndrome (POHS), but, unlike that disorder, with signs of intraocular inflammation. The fundal lesions are similar to those of POHS. Indeed, the name 'pseudo-POHS' is one of several synonyms for this group of similar disorders, the preferred term being **multifocal choroiditis with panuveitis** (MCP). However, MCP occurs outside areas endemic for histoplasmosis, in patients seronegative for exposure to that fungus.

MCP is a bilateral inflammation, more commonly seen in women, especially those who are myopic. The active lesions if seen (many patients present with scars but inactive inflammation) are creamy, quite well demarcated and usually multiple. Some patients present with papillary or peripapillary swelling (**Fig. 19.26**). In contrast old inactive lesions are clearly defined, pale, punched-out scars, sometimes with dark edges, and sometimes quite large; circumpapillary scarring is characteristic (**Fig. 19.27**). The lesions may be scattered throughout the fundus, especially in nasal retina. Linear streak lesions may be seen near the equator as in POHS (**Fig. 19.28**) and, similar to POHS, subretinal neovascularization is a significant risk; unlike POHS however, a significant amount of intraocular inflammation is seen, most obviously in the vitreous cavity, but often mildly in the AC. The condition can be recurrent or chronic, and macular edema is quite common.

In 1984 Watzke and others described 10 young myopic women with symptomatic clusters of punctate chorioretinal lesions at the macula, sometimes in clusters or linear groups, often with localized exudative detachment, showing no signs of vitritis and with no tendency to peripapillary scarring (**Fig. 19.29**). Subsequently such patients are described as showing particularly frequent and early subretinal neovascular membrane formation (**Fig. 19.30**) (Gerstenblith et al. 2007). Watzke and coworkers (1984) considered this a separate entity and called it **punctate inner choroidopathy** but did not refer to Nozik's paper on MCP.

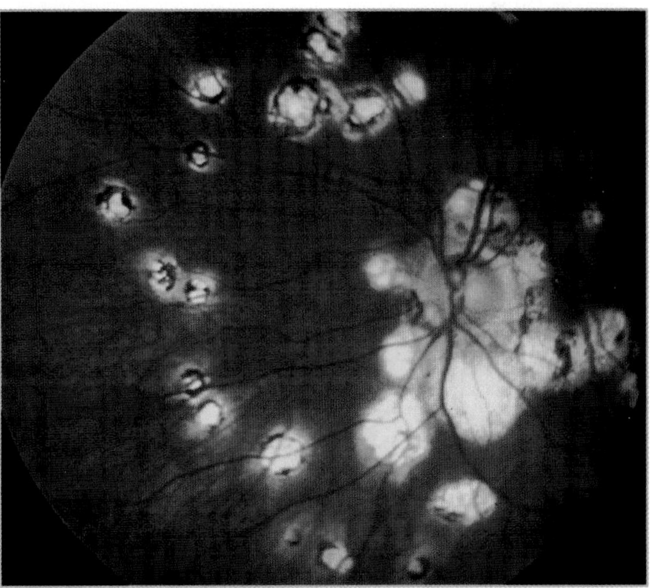

Figure 19.27 Multiple deep chorioretinal scars in quiescent multifocal choroiditis with panuveitis, including substantial peripapillary scarring.

Over subsequent years, some authors remain convinced that MCP and PIC are separate entities, distinguishable from each other and from POHS on clinical examination alone (Kedhar et al. 2007). This author, in the absence of a known etiology for either condition, has never shared that view and regards it as pragmatic to manage these patients as showing variations in a very similar process; others agree (Essex et al. 2010). The number, size, morphology and distribution of lesions

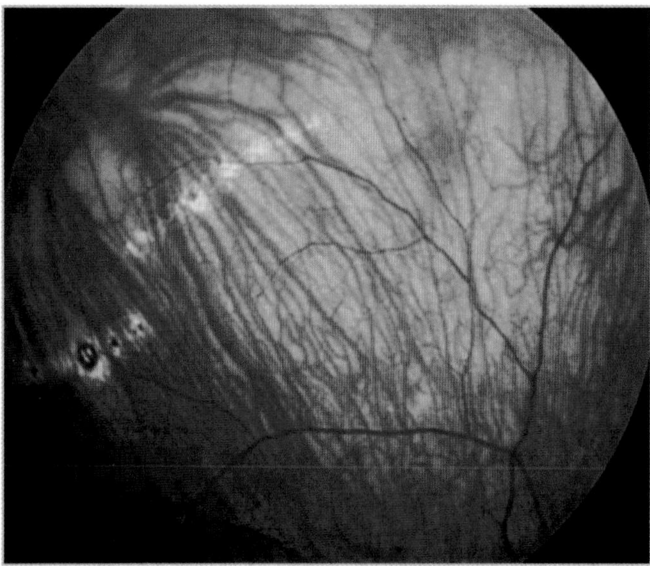

Figure 19.28 Linear grouped scars in the midperiphery in quiescent multifocal choroiditis with panuveitis.

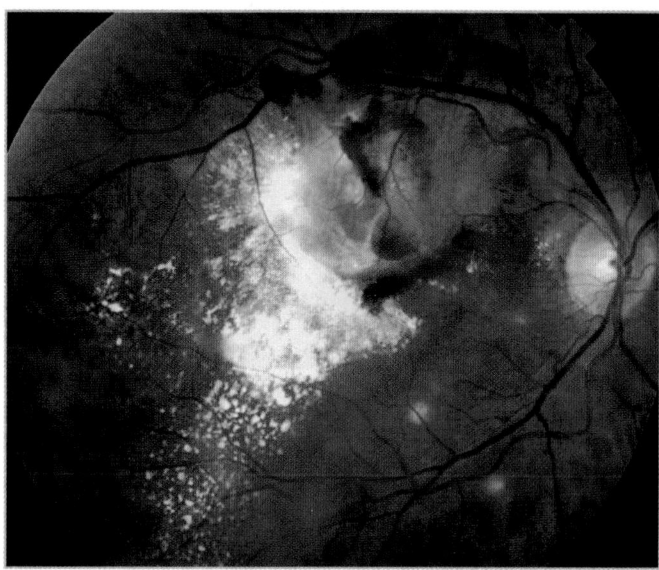

Figure 19.30 Early development of a massive exudative subretinal neovascular membrane in a young woman still exhibiting the early lesions of punctate inner choroidopathy.

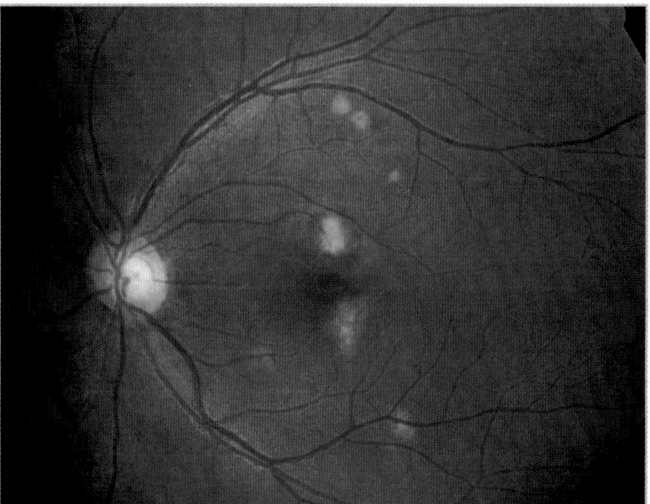

Figure 19.29 The acute phase of punctate inner choroidopathy with multiple grouped lesions at the posterior pole.

may vary, but all go on to form deep scalloped chorioretinal scarring with a high tendency to secondary neovascular membrane formation (**Fig. 19.31**). The age and symptoms at presentation may vary, as may the degree of intraocular inflammation (ranging from undetectable to mild) but the conditions both tend to affect young myopic women. A proportion of patients develop substantial subretinal fibrosis (**Fig. 19.32**). Each patient should be managed on the merits of presenting signs, with aggressive management of neovascularization and progressive or recurrent scarring.

The cause(s) of MCP and PIC is unknown, but anecdotes of underlying sarcoidosis have appeared, and non-caseating sarcoid granulomas have been found on blind conjunctival biopsy from 7 of 10 patients with MCP (Hershey et al. 1994), 4 of whom had supportive evidence of sarcoid in the form of raised angiotensin-converting enzyme or an abnormal chest radiograph. Some patients with sarcoidosis develop very densely packed peripheral multifocal scars and some (Lardenoye et al. 1997) feel that this may be a distinct entity, named **peripheral multifocal chorioretinitis** (**Fig. 19.33**). Evidence of recent infection with Epstein–Barr virus has been identified by others.

Untreated, some patients with MCP develop chronic remitting intraocular inflammation and are at high risk of subretinal neovascularization. The use of systemic steroid treatment has been found helpful in some patients but the responsiveness of subretinal neovascularization to such treatment has been disputed. Before the introduction of photodynamic therapy (PDT) and anti-VEGF (vascular endothelial growth factor) monoclonal antibodies our experience was of clear symptomatic improvement and reduction in membrane size with moderate-dose steroid treatment for several weeks. The introduction of PDT in our experience and that of others (Postlemans et al. 2005) provided a marked improvement in the management of inflammatory subretinal neovascularization, and its rapid demise in favor of anti-VEGF injections may yet prove premature. Both bevacizumab and ranibizumab have been successful in the short-term management but comparative studies for this particular group of patients are needed. Some patients with progressive or recurrent disease clearly require long-term immunosuppression and there is good evidence that this favorably affects the outcome (Michel et al. 2002).

Progressive subretinal fibrosis and uveitis syndrome

In 1984 a syndrome of **progressive subretinal fibrosis and uveitis** was reported (Palestine et al. 1984), a chronic vitritis associated with progressive subretinal lesions (presumed to be fibrosis) which slowly formed a subretinal sheet (**Fig. 19.34**) and, if involving the posterior pole, caused permanent visual loss. Most cases of this rare disease have been in young women and in several patients it has occurred in association with multifocal choroiditis. As subretinal fibrosis may follow several subretinal disorders, it was suggested that the condition may be a non-specific fibrous metaplasia, which may be particularly dramatic after MCP (Gass et al. 1996). More recently the histological examination of an affected eye and the demonstration of autoantibodies against photoreceptor and RPE led to the suggestion that this may be a variant of sympathetic ophthalmia (Wang et al. 2002).

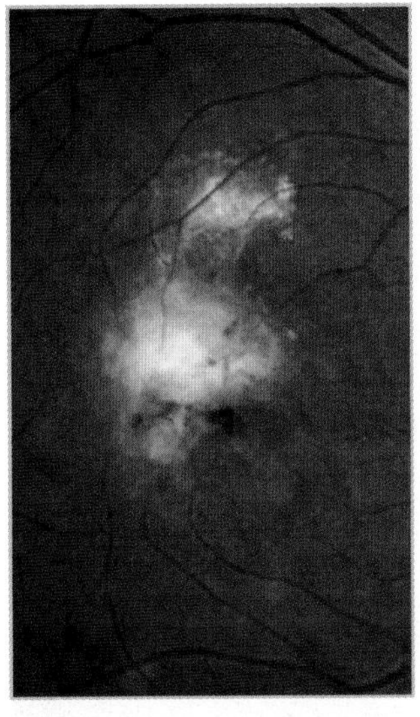
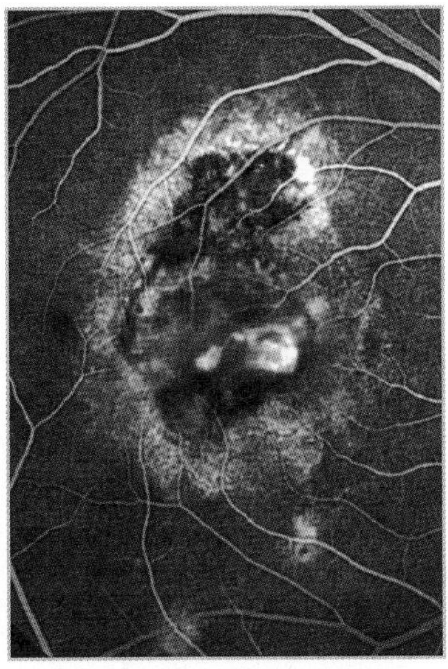
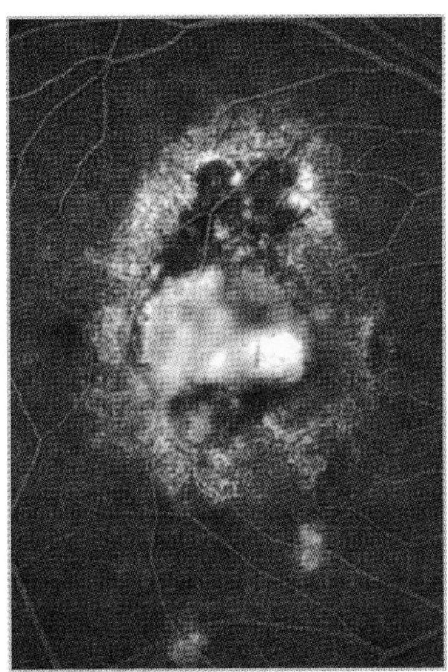

Figure 19.31 An early onset central neovascular membrane with associated subretinal fibrosis in punctate inner choroidopathy.

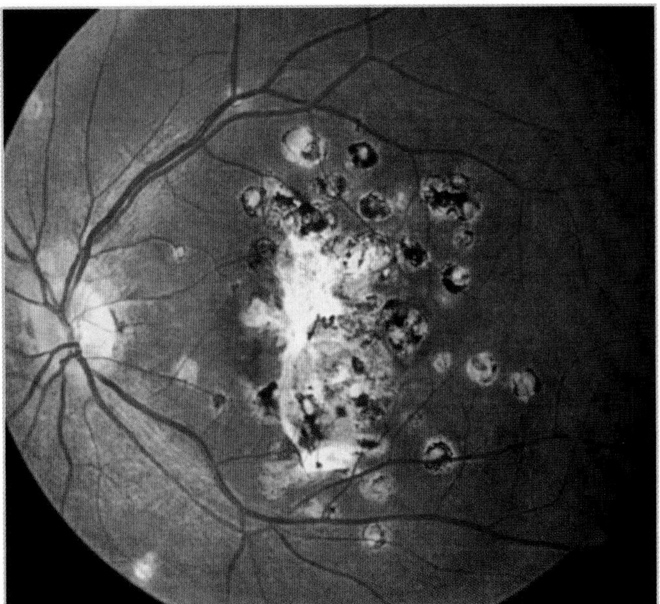

Figure 19.32 A dense cluster of punched-out chorioretinal scars at the posterior pole in quiescent punctate inner choroidopathy associated with substantial subretinal fibrosis.

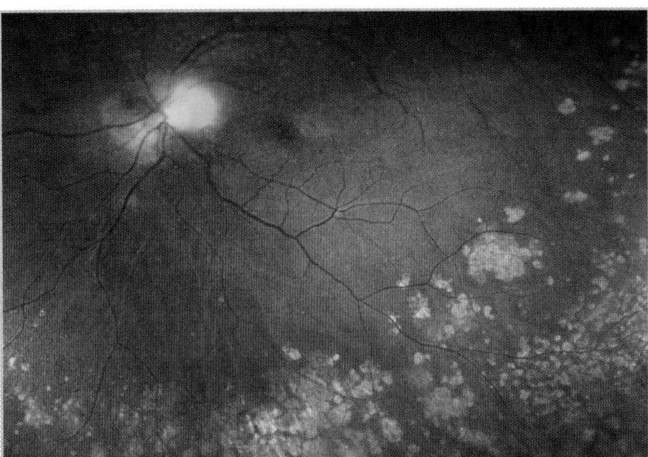

Figure 19.33 Myriad peripheral chorioretinal scars with peripapillary atrophy in peripheral multifocal chorioretinitis.

The syndrome is notorious for its inexorable progression and difficulty in treatment.

Retinal pigment epitheliitis

This entity was first reported in 1972 (Krill and Deutman 1972) and is rare. Presentation is typically in young adults, often after viral infection, with acute central visual loss or distortion, almost always unilaterally. Ophthalmoscopy may be normal at presentation but within a few days reveals groups of tiny dark spots at the posterior pole, each surrounded by a 'halo' of lighter or orange color (**Fig. 19.35**); these lesions, which appear on OCT to be outer retinal, stain on fluorescein angiography. The lesions disappear spontaneously within weeks to leave mild but permanent RPE granularity or clumping (**Fig. 19.36**). Serous retinal detachment may temporarily occur in the acute stage. Spontaneous resolution is the rule within months rather than weeks and treatment is unnecessary; complete visual recovery is common but not guaranteed.

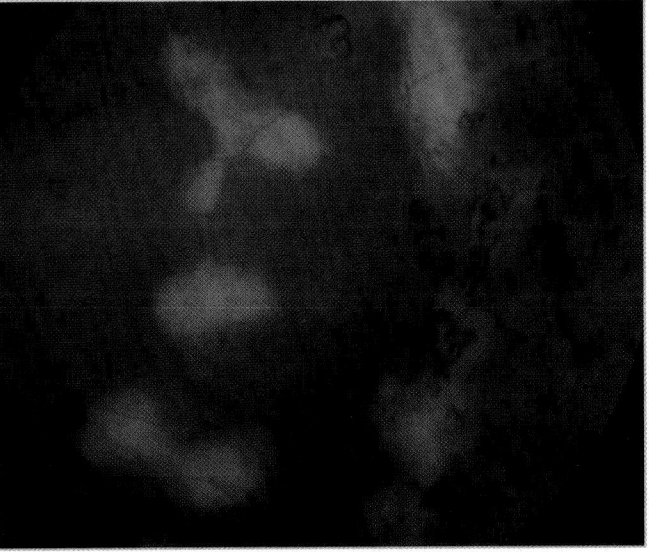

Figure 19.34 Large interconnecting plaques of dense subretinal fibrosis, associated with multifocal choroiditis with panuveitis-like lesions, in the subretinal fibrosis and uveitis syndrome. (Courtesy of Mr I Pearce.)

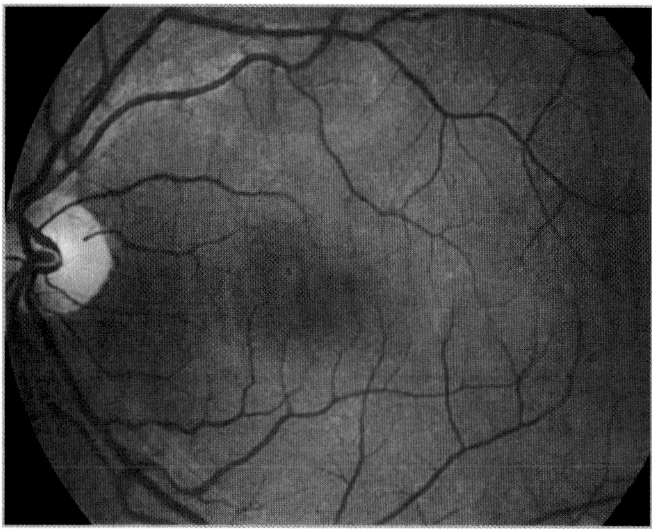

Figure 19.35 Acute retinal pigment epitheliitis. Two tiny adjacent dark parafoveal lesions each have a halo of lighter color.

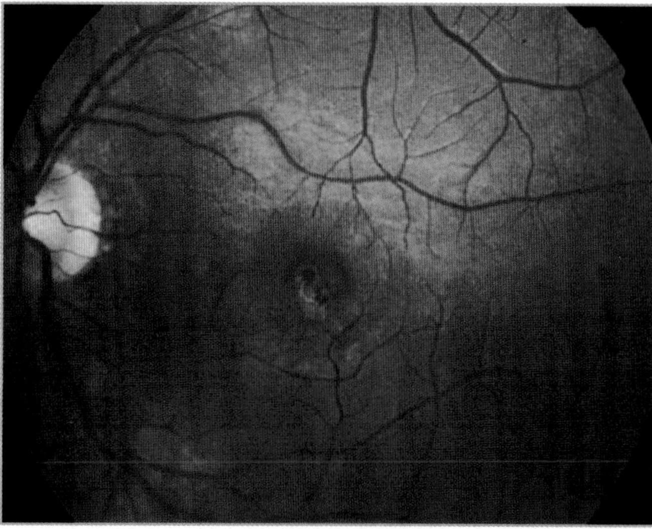

Figure 19.36 Resolved retinal pigment epitheliitis showing pigmented retinal pigment epithelium scars with surrounding depigmentation.

Unilateral acute idiopathic maculopathy

First described in 1991, including nine patients of both sexes with a mean age of 32 years (Yanuzzi et al. 1991), this disorder presents with sudden, almost exclusively unilateral visual loss, usually after a flu-like illness. It has been described several times during pregnancy. There may be some vitreous cells, overlying a central retinal elevation, possibly serous, within which is characteristically a patch of gray or cream thickening (**Fig. 19.37**). Fluorescein angiography may mimic occult choroidal neovascularization. The OCT findings are usually of outer retinal thickening with apparent RPE disruption. The differential diagnosis will include adult-onset vitelliform dystrophy (which is usually bilateral and presents less abruptly) and acquired macular toxoplasmosis (in which the active focus is usually much whiter).

Most cases resolve within weeks to near-normal acuity, others may take months to improve and a minority do not regain good central vision. In most cases, RPE derangement typically remains in the form of a bull's eye lesion, with central hyperpigmentation surrounded by a halo of depigmentation. The role of systemic steroid treatment in this condition has not been clarified. The disorder is presumed to be inflammatory and reports of a clear association with Coxsackievirus-induced hand, foot and mouth disease (Beck et al. 2004) require further study.

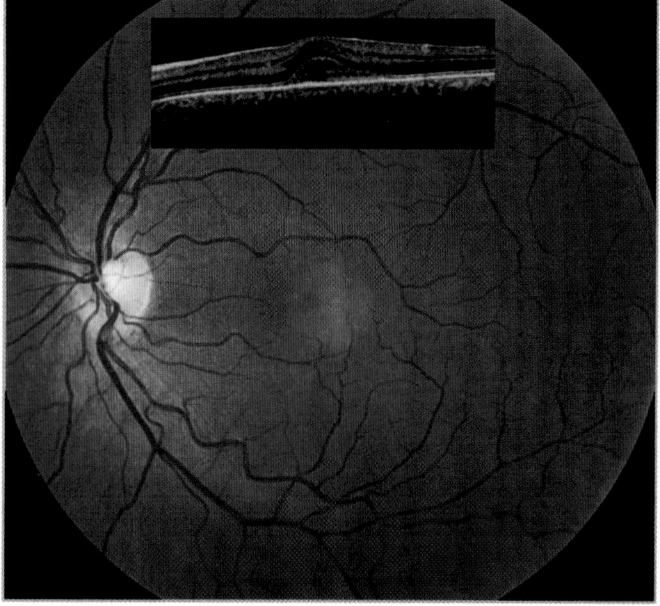

Figure 19.37 Unilateral acute idiopathic maculopathy exhibiting a central raised creamy zone. The ocular coherence tomography findings are superimposed. (Courtesy of Dr M Jumper.)

SUMMARY: ONE OR MANY DISEASES?

The past 40 years have seen the description of a large number of either new or newly recognized syndromes, most of which have acquired a complex descriptive acronym, and this bewildering array has been perceptively described by Jampol and others as an 'alphabet soup.' Of the syndromes described in this chapter, APMPPE, serpiginous choroidopathy and birdshot retinochoroidopathy are, despite some intrinsic variation, distinct conditions.

For the remainder of the conditions described above, although the paradigm for each may be distinctive, there are multiple reports of the simultaneous or sequential occurrence of two types in a single patient, distinct overlapping tendencies in both symptomatology and signs, uniform involvement of the outer retina, and the majority, sometimes the very great majority, occur in young myopic women, often after an apparent viral illness. Logically, therefore, the concept that some of the syndromes may represent different manifestations of an essentially similar process has been aired, with differing conclusions (BenEzra and Forrester 1995, Jampol and Wiredu 1995). Nevertheless there is now a tendency to include MCP, PIC, MEWDS, unilateral acute idiopathic maculopathy, AMN and AIBSE under the umbrella term 'AZOOR-complex diseases.' The concept of a multifocal microgranulomatous inflammation, which differs depending on factors including trigger factors and host immunity to give inflammations varying from the brief and completely evanescent to the chronic, progressive and severe, is interesting and attractive; whether such a theory can explain the many and varied clinical manifestations of these syndromes remains to be seen.

REFERENCES

Akpek EK, Jabs DA, Tessler HH, et al. Successful treatment of serpiginous choroiditis with alkylating agents. *Ophthalmology* 2002;**109**:1506–13.

Beck AP, Jampol LM, Glasser DA, Pollack JS. Is coxsackievirus the cause of unilateral acute idiopathic maculopathy? *Arch Ophthalmol* 2004;**122**;121–3.

BenEzra D, Forrester JV. Fundal white dots: the spectrum of a similar pathological process. *Br J Ophthalmol* 1995;**79**:856–860.

Bos PJ, Deutman AF. Acute macular neuroretinopathy. *Am J Ophthalmol* 1975;**80**:573–584.

Christmas NJ, Oh KT, Oh DM, Folk JC. Long-term follow-up of patients with serpiginous choroiditis. *Retina* 2002;**22**:550–6.

Comu S, Verstraeten T, Rinkoff JS, et al. Neurological manifestations of acute posterior multifocal placoid pigment epitheliopathy. *Stroke* 1996;**27**:996–1001.

Corver HD, Ruys J, Kestelyn-Stevens AM, et al. Two cases of acute macular neuroretinopathy. *Eye* 2007;**21**:1226–9.

Essex RW, Wong J, Fraser-Bell S, et al. Punctate inner choroidopathy: clinical features and outcomes. *Arch Ophthalmol* 2010;**128**:982–7.

Fekrat S, Wilkinson CP, Chang B, et al. Acute annular outer retinopathy: report of four cases. *Am J Ophthalmol* 2000;**130**:636–44.

Fine HF, Spaide RF, Ryan EH, et al. Acute zonal occult outer retinopathy in patients with multiple evanescent white dot syndrome. *Arch Ophthalmol* 2009;**127**:66–70.

Fiore T, Iaccheri B, Androudi S, et al. Acute posterior multifocal placoid pigment epitheliopathy: outcome and visual prognosis. *Retina* 2009;**29**:994–1001.

Fletcher WA, Imes RK, Goodman D, et al. Acute idiopathic blind spot enlargement. *Arch Ophthalmol* 1988;**106**:44–49.

Francis PJ, Marinescu A, Fitzke FW, et al. Acute zonal occult outer retinopathy: towards a set of diagnostic criteria. *Br J Ophthalmol* 2005;**89**:70–3.

Gass JDM. Acute posterior multifocal placoid pigment epitheliopathy. *Arch Ophthalmol* 1968;**80**:177–85.

Gass JDM. Vitiliginous chorioretinitis. *Arch Ophthalmol* 1981;**99**:1778–87.

Gass JDM. Acute zonal occult outer retinopathy. *J Clin Neuroophthalmol* 1993;**13**:79–97.

Gass JDM, Stern C. Acute annular outer retinopathy as a variant of acute zonal occult outer retinopathy. *Am J Ophthalmol* 1995;**119**:330–4.

Gass JDM, Margo CE, Levy MH. Progressive subretinal fibrosis and blindness in patients with multifocal granulomatous chorioretinitis. *Am J Ophthalmol* 1996;**122**:76–85.

Gass JDM, Agarwal A, Scott IU. Acute zonal ocular outer retinopathy: a long-term follow-up study. *Am J Ophthalmol* 2002;**134**:329–39.

Gerstenblith AT, Thorne JE, Sobrin L, et al. Punctate inner choroidopathy: a survey analysis of 77 persons. *Ophthalmology* 2007;**114**:1201–4.

Giuliari GP, Pujari S, Dhaikh M, et al. Microperimetry findings in patients with birdshot chorioretinopathy. *Can J Ophthalmol* 2010;**45**:399–403.

Golchet PR, Jampol LM, Wilson D, et al. Persistent placoid maculopathy: a new clinical entity. *Trans Am Ophthalmol Soc* 2006;**104**:108–20.

Gupta V, Gupta A, Arora S, et al. Presumed tubercular serpiginouslike choroiditis: clinical presentations and management. *Ophthalmology* 2003;**110**:1744–9.

Hershey JM, Pulido JS, Folberg R, et al. Non-caseating conjunctival granulomas in patients with multifocal choroiditis and panuveitis. *Ophthalmology* 1994;**101**:596–601.

Jampol LM, Wiredu A. MEWDS, MFC, PIC, AMN, AIBSE and AZOOR: One disease or many? *Retina* 1995;**15**:373–8.

Jampol LM, Sieving PA, Pugh D, et al. Multiple evanescent white dot syndrome. I. Clinical findings. *Arch Ophthalmol* 1984;**102**:671–4.

Jones BE, Jampol LM, Yanuzzi LA, et al. Relentless placoid chorioretinitis: a new entity or an unusual variant of serpiginous chorioretinitis? *Arch Ophthalmol* 2000;**118**:931–8.

Jones NP. Acute posterior multifocal placoid pigment epitheliopathy. *Br J Ophthalmol* 1995;**79**:384–9.

Kappel PJ, Monnet D, Yu F, et al. Contrast sensitivity among patients with birdshot chorioretinopathy. *Am J Ophthalmol* 2009;**147**:351–6.

Kedhar SR, Thorne JE, Wittenberg S, et al. Multifocal choroiditis with panuveitis and punctate inner choroidopathy: comparison of clinical characteristics at presentation. *Retina* 2007;**27**:1174–9.

Kiss S, Ahmed M, Letko E, Foster CS. Long-term follow-up of patients with birdshot retinochoroidopathy treated with corticosteroid-sparing systemic immunomodulatory therapy. *Ophthalmology* 2005;**112**:1066–71.

Krill AE, Deutman AF. Acute retinal pigment epitheliitis. *Am J Ophthalmol* 1972;**78**:177–85.

Lardenoye CW, Van der Lelij A, de Loos WS, et al. Peripheral multifocal chorioretinitis: a distinct clinical entity? *Ophthalmology* 1997;**104**:1820–6.

Mahajan VB, Stone EM. Patients with an acute zonal occult outer retinopathy-like illness rapidly improve with valacyclovir treatment. *Am J Ophthalmol* 2010;**150**:511–18.

Michel SS, Ekong A, Baltatzis S, et al. Multifocal choroiditis and panuveitis: immunomodulatory therapy. *Ophthalmology* 2002;**109**:378–83.

Monson DM, Smith JR. Acute zonal occult outer retinopathy. *Surv Ophthalmol* 2011;**56**:23–35.

Nozik RA, Dorsch W. A new chorioretinopathy associated with anterior uveitis. *Am J Ophthalmol* 1973;**76**:758–62.

Nussenblatt RB, Mittal KK, Ryan S, et al. Birdshot retinochoroidopathy associated with HLA-A29 antigen and immune responsiveness to retinal S-antigen. *Am J Ophthalmol* 1982;**94**:147–58.

Nussenblatt RB, Whitcup SM, Palestine AG. Uveitis. Fundamentals and clinical practice, 2nd edn. St Louis, MO: *Mosby*, 1996: 364–370.

O'Halloran HS, Berger JR, Lee WB, et al. Acute multifocal placoid pigment epitheliopathy and central nervous system involvement: nine new cases and a review of the literature. *Ophthalmology* 2001;**108**:861–8.

Palestine AG, Nussenblatt RB, Parver LM, et al. Progressive subretinal fibrosis and uveitis. *Br J Ophthalmol* 1984;**68**:667–673.

Pisa D, Ramos M, Garcia P, et al. Fungal infection in patients with serpiginous choroiditis or acute zonal ocular outer retinopathy. *J Clin Microbiol* 2008;**46**:130–5.

Postelmans L, Pasteels B, Coquelet P, et al. Photodynamic therapy for subfoveal classical choroidal neovascularisation related to punctate inner choroidopathy (PIC) or presumed ocular histoplasmosis-like syndrome (POHS-like). *Ocul Immunol Inflamm* 2005;**13**:361–6.

Rothova A, Berendschott TT, Probst K, et al. Birdshot chorioretinopathy: long-term manifestations and visual prognosis. *Ophthalmology* 2004;**111**:954–9.

Ryan SJ, Maumenee AE. Birdshot retinochoroidopathy. *Am J Ophthalmol* 1980;**89**:31–45.

Singh K, deFrank MP, Schults WT, et al. Acute idiopathic blind spot enlargement: a spectrum of disease. *Ophthalmology* 1991;**98**:497–502.

Sobaci G, Bayraktar Z, Bayer A. Interferon alpha-2a treatment for serpiginous choroiditis. *Ocul Immunol Inflamm* 2005;**13**:59–66.

Sobrin L, Huang JJ, Christen W, et al. Daclizumab for treatment of birdshot chorioretinopathy. *Arch Ophthalmol* 2008;**126**:186–91.

Thorne JE, Jabs DA, Kedhar SR, et al. Loss of visual field among patients with birdshot chorioretinopathy. *Am J Ophthalmol* 2008;**145**:23–8.

Trinh L, Bodaghi B, Fardeau C, et al. Clinical features, treatment methods, and evolution of birdshot chorioretinopathy in 5 different families. *Am J Ophthalmol* 2009;**147**:1042–7.

Turbeville SD, Cowan LD, Gass JDM. Acute macular neuroretinopathy: a review of the literature. *Surv Ophthalmol* 2003;**48**:1–11.

Vianna RN, Ozdal PC, Deschenes J, Burnier MN. Combination of azathioprine and corticosteroids in the treatment of serpiginous choroiditis. *Can J Ophthalmol* 2006;**41**:183–9.

Vitale AT, Rodriguez A, Foster CS. Low-dose cyclosporine therapy in the treatment of birdshot retinochoroidopathy. *Ophthalmology* 1994;**101**:822–31.

Volpe NJ, Rizzo JF, Lessell S. Acute idiopathic blind spot enlargement syndrome: a review of 27 new cases. **Arch Ophthalmol** 2001;**119**:59–63.

Wang RC, Zamir E, Dugel PU et al. Progressive subretinal fibrosis and blindness associated with multifocal granulomatous chorioretinitis: a variant of sympathetic ophthalmia. *Ophthalmology* 2002;**109**:1527–31.

Watzke RC, Packer AJ, Folk JC, et al. Punctate inner choroidopathy. *Am J Ophthalmol* 1984:**98**:572–84.

Yannuzzi LA, Jampol LM, Rabb MF, et al. Unilateral acute idiopathic maculopathy. *Arch Ophthalmol* 1991;**109**:1411–16.

Chapter 20 Masquerade syndromes

The European masquerade or masked ball began in the sixteenth century as an elite social event. It was only later that the word was used to imply a deliberate attempt to infiltrate in disguise. The term has been used for decades by physicians to describe a malignancy presenting in a way that mimics a benign condition, usually an inflammation. It may be more appropriate for the term 'masquerade syndrome,' with these sinister undertones, to be limited in ophthalmology to malignant disease presenting as uveitis. However, this would be to ignore the well-recognized but frequently misinterpreted non-malignant mimics of inflammation, which are therefore included here. In addition a variety of drugs, either topical or systemic, are known to induce intraocular inflammation or reaction. and they too appear here because there is no better home for them.

MALIGNANT MASQUERADE SYNDROMES

A number of abnormal ocular signs may be shared between uveitis and intraocular malignancy. White cells in the anterior chamber and sometimes hypopyon are an occasional feature of malignancy, particularly of the leukemias. Pigmented cells from intraocular melanomas may also disperse and be wrongly identified as inflammatory cells. Iris nodules may be neoplastic or inflammatory. Cellular inflammation into the vitreous humor, especially when chronic and resembling intermediate uveitis, can be a presentation of lymphoma, the diagnosis of which is notoriously difficult. Endophytic retinoblastoma may seed into the vitreous humor. Posterior segment masses, unifocal or multifocal, may be primary or secondary tumor, or manifestations of inflammations such as sarcoidosis. This section discusses those malignancies that are capable of such mimicry, and their diagnosis and management. Primary central nervous system (CNS)/ocular lymphoma is the most important of these:

PRIMARY CNS AND OCULAR LYMPHOMA (box 20.1)

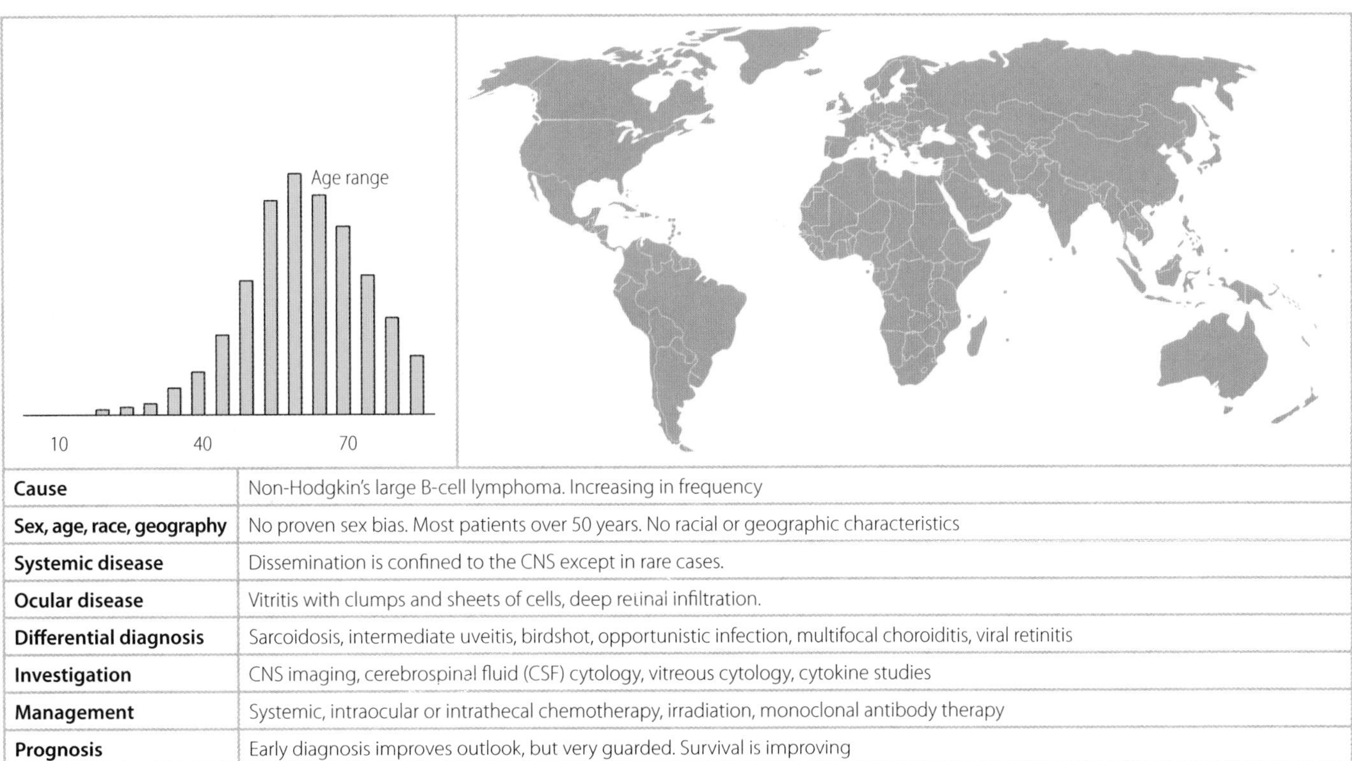

Cause	Non-Hodgkin's large B-cell lymphoma. Increasing in frequency
Sex, age, race, geography	No proven sex bias. Most patients over 50 years. No racial or geographic characteristics
Systemic disease	Dissemination is confined to the CNS except in rare cases.
Ocular disease	Vitritis with clumps and sheets of cells, deep retinal infiltration.
Differential diagnosis	Sarcoidosis, intermediate uveitis, birdshot, opportunistic infection, multifocal choroiditis, viral retinitis
Investigation	CNS imaging, cerebrospinal fluid (CSF) cytology, vitreous cytology, cytokine studies
Management	Systemic, intraocular or intrathecal chemotherapy, irradiation, monoclonal antibody therapy
Prognosis	Early diagnosis improves outlook, but very guarded. Survival is improving

Box 20.1 Primary CNS and ocular lymphoma

Introduction

The lymphomas are a complex group of malignancies affecting the immune system. Together they form some 5% of all adult malignancies. Tumors may be localized (e.g. to skin or CNS) or systemic. The degree of malignancy ranges from a mild, chronic indolent disorder to a rapidly fulminating and fatal disease. The classification of the lymphomas has continuously evolved, with contributions from the presumed cell of origin, the location and the aggressiveness of the tumor. More recently a complex system of cell surface markers has permitted more accurate management decisions and prognostication. The 1993 REAL system (Revised European–American Lymphoma) recognizes the B-cell or T-cell division (the majority being B-cell tumors), but histological appearance and surface immunotypes take a predominant role. Primary CNS/ocular lymphoma (PCNSOL) is almost always a high-grade large-cell non-Hodgkin's lymphoma derived from B cells. It was historically known as reticulum cell sarcoma. Although there is clear evidence that the incidence of this malignancy has increased substantially over the past 30 years, it remains a rare tumor.

Systemic disease

Primary CNSOL originates in the CNS rather than the eye in most patients but will involve the eye in about a quarter of cases. In contrast, those originating in the eye will involve the CNS in up to 80% of cases at some time (Coupland et al. 2009). Although any part of the CNS and meninges can be involved there is a tendency for periventricular infiltration. Presenting symptoms and signs may range from ataxia to personality change, through focal cranial nerve or cord lesions (**Fig. 20.1**).

It is unknown whether the occurrence of CNSOL at two or more sites within the CNS and eye is the result of dissemination from the CNS to the eye (down the optic nerve, intravascular or via CSF), vice versa or the simultaneous or sequential occurrence at several different susceptible sites. Although there is a clear tendency, after the discovery of a single tumor, for the appearance of others within the CNS, the occurrence of tumor outside the CNS and eye is extremely rare.

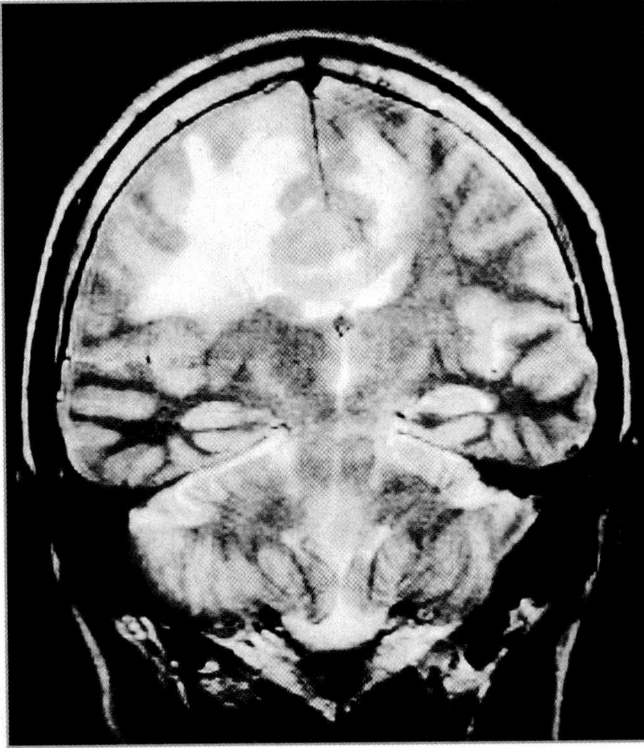

Figure 20.1 A large frontoparietal non-Hodgkin's central nervous system lymphoma with intraocular involvement.

Ocular disease

A few young adults have been described with PCNSOL affecting the eye, but the disease is predominantly one of the over-50s. Unilateral presentations are not uncommon, although eventual bilateral involvement is seen in 80%. Characteristically, patients present with painless visual blurring. There may apparently be a panuveitis, with nondescript anterior segment involvement, although occasionally keratic precipitate (KP) distribution (**Fig. 20.2**) or other manifestations may be peculiar and give rise to suspicion. Sometimes a hypopyon is seen. Vitritis may also be nondescript or exhibit a distribution of cells and opacities into sheets or clumps which again cause suspicion. Opacification may be dense. Subretinal or deep retinal infiltration may be seen (**Fig. 20.3**), manifesting as poorly defined pale patches of varying size and shape, randomly coalescent. Late-phase fluorescein angiography tends to show sustained dark patches (**Fig. 20.4**), probably corresponding to multifocal tumor involvement of the retinal pigment epithelium (RPE)/Bruch's membrane junction. Often eyes initially unsuspected of harboring PCNSOL develop suggestive features over a period of time. However, a high index of suspicion is required if early diagnosis is to be achieved.

Diagnosis

Suspicion of PCNSOL should arise where an older patient presents with a peculiar panuveitis or vitritis, especially where retinal infiltration is observed. The diagnosis is notoriously difficult and the ophthalmologist should be aware that even vigorous and repeated investigation may prove non-diagnostic, only to be followed by the development of overt tumor at a later date. However, diagnostic methods continue to improve. Depending on the clinical manifestations, the differential diagnosis may include sarcoidosis (often the most likely differential in this age group), intermediate uveitis, birdshot retinochoroidopathy, tuberculosis, chronic peripheral toxoplasmosis and, in unusual circumstances, viral retinitis, because lymphoma can mimic necrotizing retinopathy (**Fig. 20.5**).

All suspects should undergo CNS computed tomography (CT) or preferably magnetic resonance imaging (MRI). Newer techniques have improved both sensitivity and specificity for diagnosis: fluoro-D-glucose positron emission tomography (PET) provides 100% sensitivity

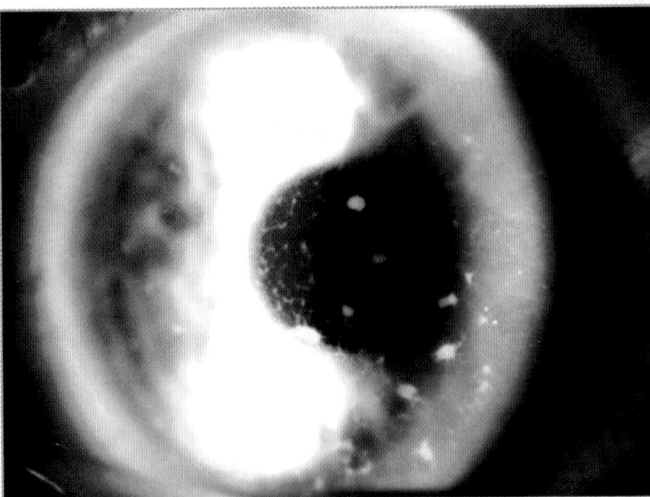

Figure 20.2 Scattered large peculiar-shaped keratic precipitates in a patient with ocular/central nervous system lymphoma. Same patient as Fig. 20.1.

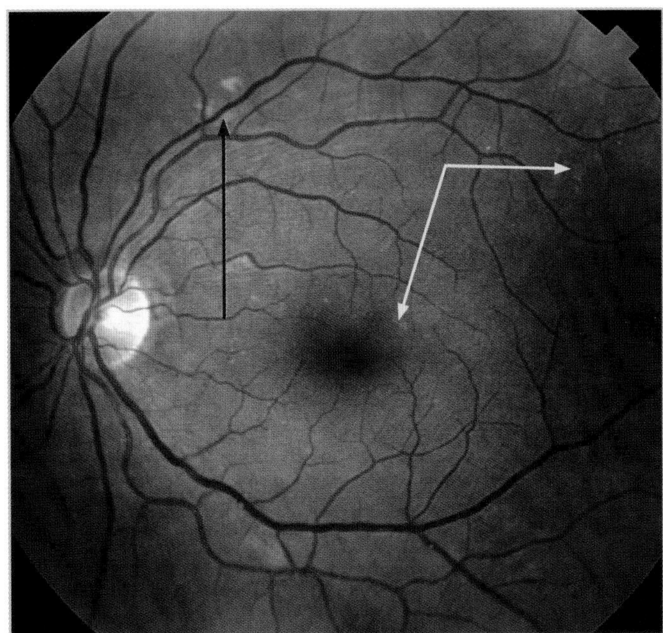

Figure 20.3 The fundus of a patient with vitreous biopsy-confirmed B-cell lymphoma. There is a cluster of fairly well-defined, small, deep retinal lesions under the superior arcade (black arrow), but also very many tiny, less well-defined, retinal lesions scattered throughout the fundus (yellow arrows, examples).

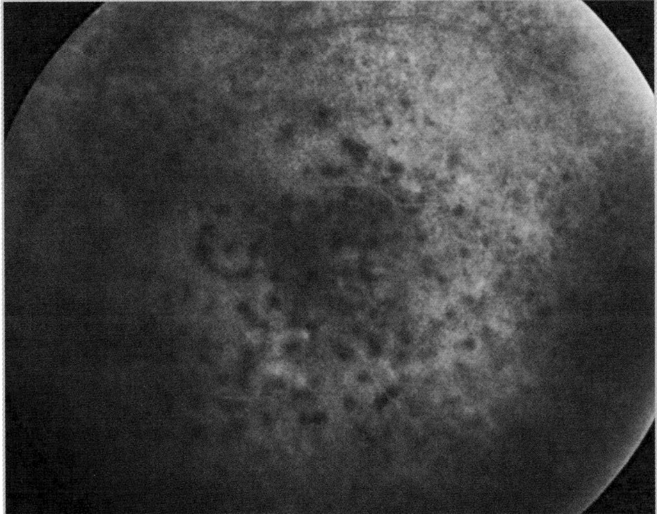

Figure 20.4 Late-phase fluorescein angiography in a patient with retinal lymphoma showing multifocal small dark patches.

for lymphoma (Kawase et al. 2010). In complementary fashion, MRI provides better soft-tissue contrast and high spatial resolution. Software fusional techniques can combine these attributes to enhance tumor imaging (**Fig. 20.6**).

Cytology of CSF should also be performed. If CSF cytology confirms a diagnosis of PCNSOL, intraocular involvement may be presumed to be directly related without the need for intraocular sampling (Sen et al. 2009). If findings are negative (as they may be in over 50%), whether or not mass lesions are detected on neuroradiological imaging, diagnostic vitrectomy is necessary. Cytology of vitreous specimens requires as much sample as possible, and considerable expertise. Total pars plana vitrectomy, rather than

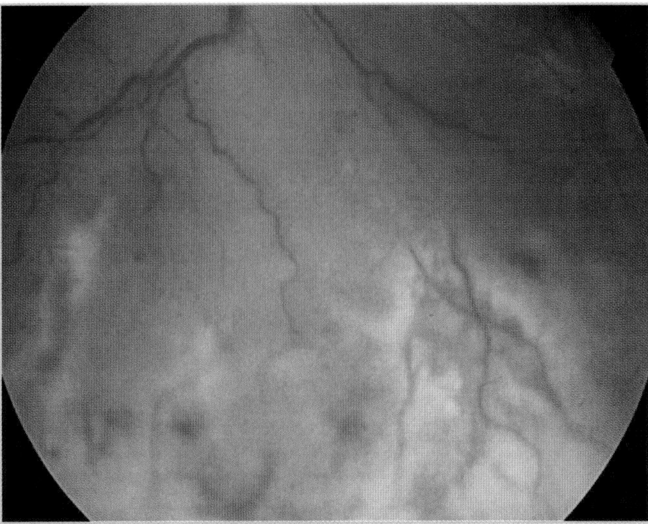

Figure 20.5 Intraocular lymphoma can mimic herpetic necrotizing retinopathy by inducing peripheral or central necrotizing retinal change, with or without retinal vasculitis.

vitreous aspiration, is used because even those eyes with considerable vitreous opacification may produce frustratingly small numbers of cells for the cytologist. It is recommended that a large core vitrectomy (at least 1 ml and preferably 2 ml) be obtained without infusion, by applying extraocular pressure. This can be withdrawn neat from the aspiration line before then infusing and completing the vitrectomy. The remaining diluted sample can be spun down for further cytology and cytokine studies. Cellular fragility is high – care is necessary both when obtaining the specimen (requiring a low vitreous cutting rate) and afterwards: it is recommended that the core sample be placed immediately into cell culture medium and transported warm directly to the cytopathologist. The specimen should be examined as quickly as possible. After spinning down cells for examination, the supernatant can be retained for cytokine and polymerase chain reaction (PCR) studies. Patients who are on treatment with systemic steroids are less likely to produce helpful cytology, and the treatment should be stopped for up to 2 weeks before vitrectomy. A failure to produce diagnostic cells from vitrectomy in a patient with highly suspicious retinal lesions may suggest subretinal aspiration or chorioretinal biopsy. Alternatively a second fluid aspiration may produce abnormal cells.

Primary CNSOL cells are typically large with little cytoplasm, large bean-shaped or lobulated nuclei and prominent nucleoli (**Fig. 20.7**). The great majority are monoclonal B-cell tumors that therefore express CD19, CD20 (**Fig. 20.8**) and CD22. The very rare T-cell types cannot be identified morphologically, but are positive for CD3 or other markers. Flow cytometry can be valuable but requires enough cells, a rare luxury for vitreous samples. Molecular analysis, which requires microdissection, can show rearrangement of the Ig heavy chain (IgH) and this has been found in 100% of a series of 85 patients with PCNSOL (Buggage et al. 2001).

Malignant B cells tend to express high levels of interleukin IL-10, whereas inflammatory lymphocytes tend to express IL-6. The ratio IL-10:IL-6 has therefore been used on aqueous or vitreous humor samples as an aid to diagnosis, a ratio of > 1.0 being supportive. In terms of absolute concentration, an aqueous IL-10 concentration of 50 pg/ml or more has been found to carry an 89% sensitivity and 93% specificity for CNSOL in 51 patients (Cassoux et al. 2007).

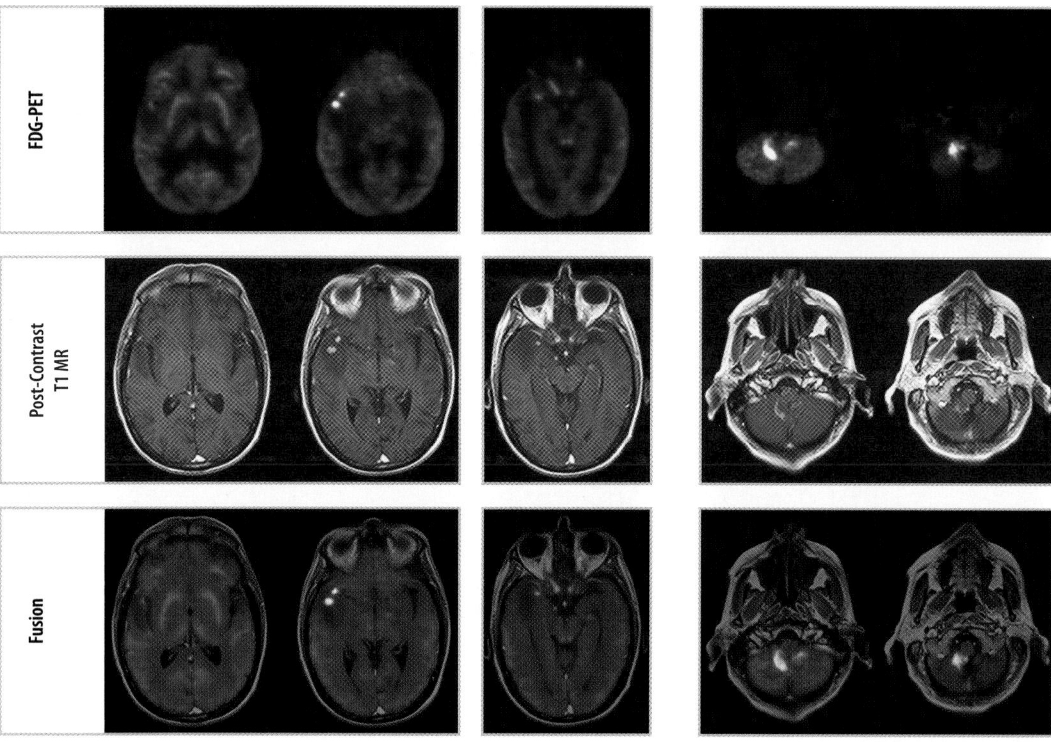

Figure 20.6 Positron emission tomography images (top line) and MR images (middle line) can be fused by software (bottom line) to enhance pickup rate in primary CNS lymphoma. (Courtesy of Dr R Cowan.)

Figure 20.7 A vitreous cytology specimen showing large lymphocytes with large lobulated nuclei typical of B-cell lymphoma. May–Grunwald–Giemsa stain. (Courtesy of Dr L Irion.)

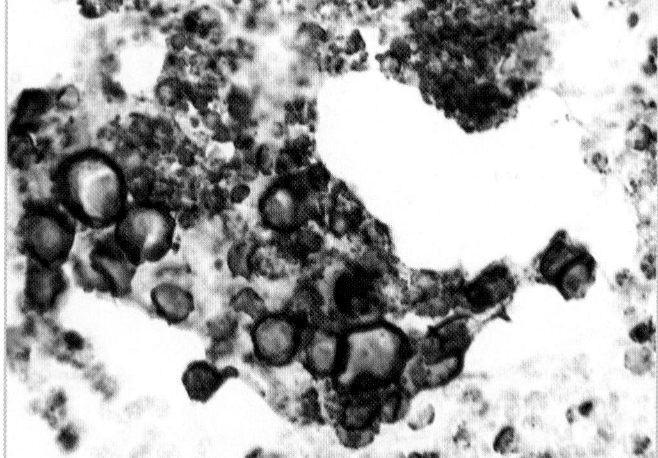

Figure 20.8 Vitreous lymphocytes showing positivity for a CD20 marker, confirming B-cell lineage. (Courtesy of Dr L Irion.)

Where the ophthalmologist remains suspicious of non-Hodgkin's lymphoma (NHL) even after negative investigations, it is legitimate to pursue such suspicions with subsequent repeated investigation, which may ultimately prove positive. Both neurosarcoidosis and demyelinating disease are occasionally part of the differential diagnosis of a patient presenting with intraocular inflammation and focal neurological signs, and in some circumstances the diagnosis can be extremely challenging. Brain or meningeal biopsy is occasionally justified.

Management

The management of PCNSOL is complex and evolving. It is affected by some known difficulties and some imponderables: the blood-brain barrier renders CNS tumors relatively inaccessible to systemic chemotherapy, the eye even less so, so that CNS lymphoma responds less well than systemic lymphoma. Intrathecal chemotherapy may achieve a better response in the CNS but has no ocular therapeutic effect. Intraocular chemotherapy does not reach the CNS. Irradiation is a once-only treatment. Where a lesion is diagnosed in either eye or CNS, should treatment be aimed solely at that area or should all conceivable sites be treated, either 'prophylactically' or on the assumption that preclinical tumors are likely to be elsewhere too? Or should that treatment, especially irradiation, be reserved for a definite lesion, in the knowledge that it cannot be repeated?

Irradiation has been used as primary treatment for PCNSOL with ocular involvement for many years (Pe'er et al. 2009), including the eye fields and the CNS either where tumors were detected or in some cases prophylactically. Most receive about 40 Gy, fractionated into 20–30 doses. This treatment alone has never achieved tumor clearance in 100% of patients, but does so in most, although remission may not be sustained. In an attempt to improve success rates a wide variety of chemotherapy combinations have been used, but increasing experience has concentrated efforts into methotrexate-based regimens. High-dose (8 g/m^2) methotrexate alone achieves poor intraocular concentration (Batchelor et al. 2003) and a correspondingly poor ocular tumor clearance rate. For a time, the combination of intravenous methotrexate 4–8 g/m^2 with irradiation was considered the best available (Kim et al. 2005) but the added value of irradiation to intravenous methotrexate has since been challenged in a large series (Thiel et al. 2010), in which the median progression-free survival was a mere 18 months. Intrathecal methotrexate has been supplemented for CNS involvement. In order to achieve better brain penetration from intravenous therapy, therapeutic blood–brain barrier disruption can be achieved with intra-arterial mannitol followed by intra-arterial methotrexate. Coincidentally this tends to cause macular edema among other side effects. Enhanced chemotherapy including CHOP (cyclophosphamide, hydroxydaunorubicin [doxorubicin], Oncovin [vincristine] prednisolone) and or C5R (cyclophosphamide, vincristine, systemic and intrathecal methotrexate and ara-C, and hydrocortisone) regimens may increase survival rates, at the cost of high morbidity including irradiation-induced cognitive change and chemotherapy-induced leukoencephalopathy. Radiation retinitis and optic neuropathy are also seen, as are mediastinal fibrosis, myelosuppression and opportunistic infection. The treatment-induced mortality rate is as high as 25%. Regimens must be modified for older patients and, where maximal treatment is not possible, the 5-year survival rate remains poor at 17% (Ghesquieres et al. 2010).

The suboptimal ocular responses to the above regimens have led to the use of intravitreal chemotherapy. Methotrexate 400 µg has been shown to be acceptably safe (albeit with some possible side effects including cataract, uveitis and keratopathy) and can be repeated twice-weekly for 4 weeks which is necessary for induction, followed by less frequent injections up to a maximum of 12. This has proved very successful against ocular involvement (Frenkel et al. 2008) and can also be effective to treat recurrence. Concurrent systemic or intrathecal treatment for CNS involvement is necessary. Tumors can occasionally be methotrexate resistant.

In the search for more tolerable treatment, the anti-CD20 monoclonal antibody rituximab has been employed both intrathecally and intravitreally. Intraocular doses of 1 mg appear to be well tolerated and anecdotally useful but further data are awaited. Animal studies on daclizumab and others may introduce further possibilities. Previously the outlook for vision was extremely poor, but there is little doubt that earlier diagnosis can substantially improve this. However, despite improvements in systemic therapy, most patients with PCNSOL do not survive for longer than 2 or 3 years, and overall some 80% will die of their tumor. There is much yet to be done.

Systemic lymphoma with intraocular metastasis

Ocular involvement in patients with systemic (almost invariably non-Hodgkin's) lymphoma is rarer still than PCNSOL. Patients presenting to an ophthalmologist with visual symptoms will have either an established diagnosis or clear symptoms and signs of systemic disease. Such signs depend on the site of primary involvement. Patients do not present with ocular signs in advance of systemic involvement, so all new patients with a suspicion of intraocular lymphoma should undergo a detailed medical history and general examination. In those patients with established NHL who are treated with chemotherapy, the ophthalmologist will also consider opportunistic infection in the differential diagnosis.

Intraocular involvement in NHL is characteristically uveal, in contrast to PCNSOL, which is vitreoretinal. The fundal picture is usually more dramatic in NHL, with solitary or multiple choroidal yellowish lesions (**Fig. 20.9**) which may, if untreated, coalesce to involve most of the posterior segment. Infiltration of the anterior uvea may also occur, sometimes causing secondary glaucoma or other complications. The differential diagnosis may include causes of multifocal choroiditis and other choroidal tumors both primary and secondary.

The management of NHL is constantly under review as survival times and cure rates increase. High-grade tumors are often very radiosensitive and for CNS and ocular involvement in NHL this will usually be the first line of treatment, either alone or with chemotherapy.

Leukemias and the eye

The leukemias are malignant monoclonal proliferations of hemopoietic stem cells. In general the acute leukemias produce immature blast cells whereas the chronic leukemias produce mature leukocytes. Diagnosis and differentiation are by blood and bone marrow cytology. Management varies with subtype, disease staging, patient age and other factors. Both myeloid and lymphoid leukemias may involve the eye, the former somewhat more often. Ocular involvement at

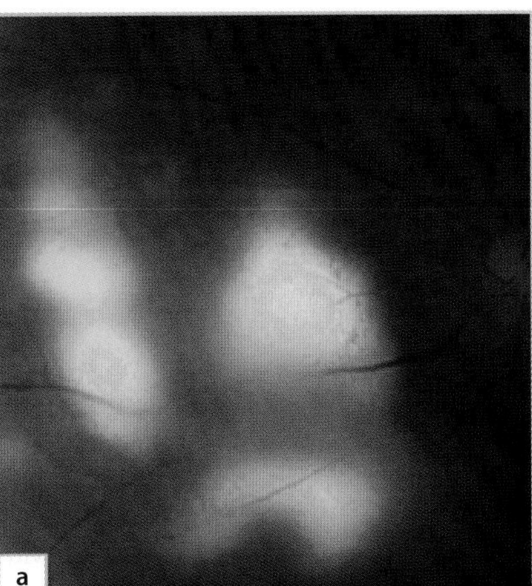

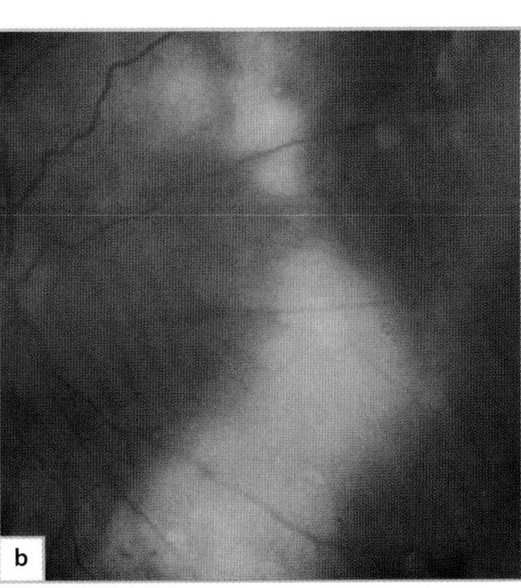

Figure 20.9 Two patients with choroidal involvement in widespread systemic-onset lymphoma, the primary being thoracic (a) and gastrointestinal (b). Large multifocal but coalescing masses are typical.

presentation, including direct retinal involvement by leukemic infiltrate (**Fig. 20.10**), is rare, but also the white centre of Roth's spots, when seen (**Fig. 20.11**), may contain leukemic cells. Rarely choroidal tumor masses (chloromas) may be seen. Serous retinal detachment may also occur, overlying diffuse choroidal involvement expressed as multifocal RPE leakage on fluorescein angiography.

Involvement of the anterior segment is rare, but may mimic acute anterior uveitis, with ciliary injection and a large hypopyon, sometimes streaked with blood (**Fig. 20.12**). The phenomenon is most commonly seen in children with known acute lymphoblastic leukemia. The iris may change color as a result of diffuse leukemic infiltration and. if unilateral or asymmetrical, heterochromia will result. Occasionally iris nodules appear, usually at the pupil margin. Angle infiltration may lead to glaucoma. Both anterior and posterior segment leukemic infiltrate is sensitive to irradiation and, where optic nerve head involvement is present, such treatment becomes urgent. After ocular recurrence, CSF examination is necessary to exclude leukemic infiltration.

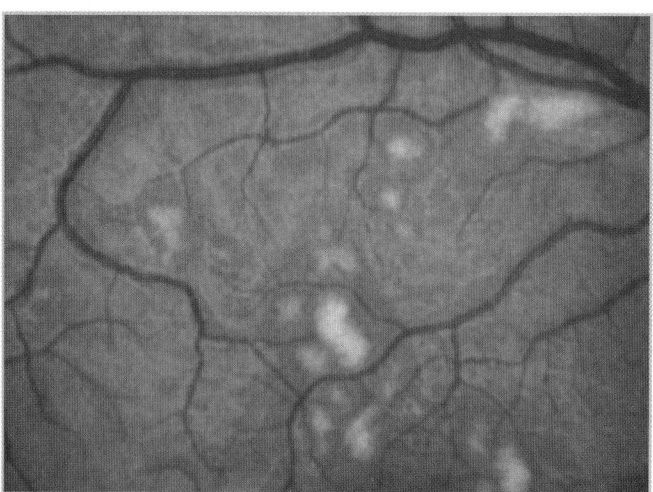

Figure 20.10 Multifocal retinal infiltration by chronic myeloid leukemic cells.

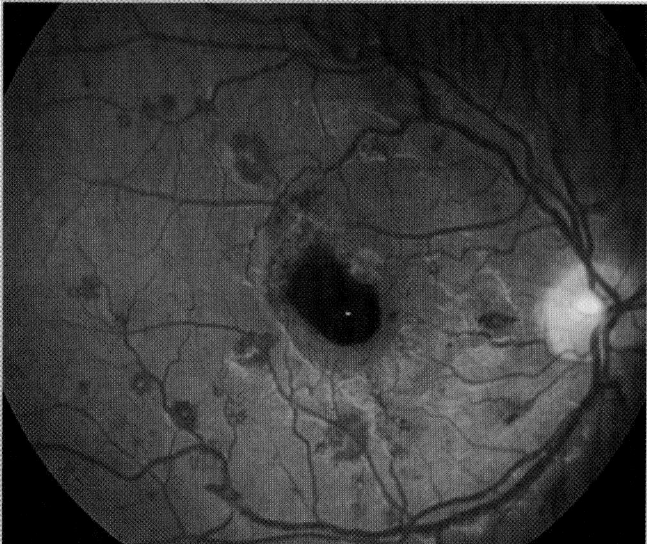

Figure 20.11 Multiple Roth's spots and retinal hemorrhages in a patient with chronic myeloid leukemia. The pale centers to Roth's spots may include embolic clusters of leukemic cells.

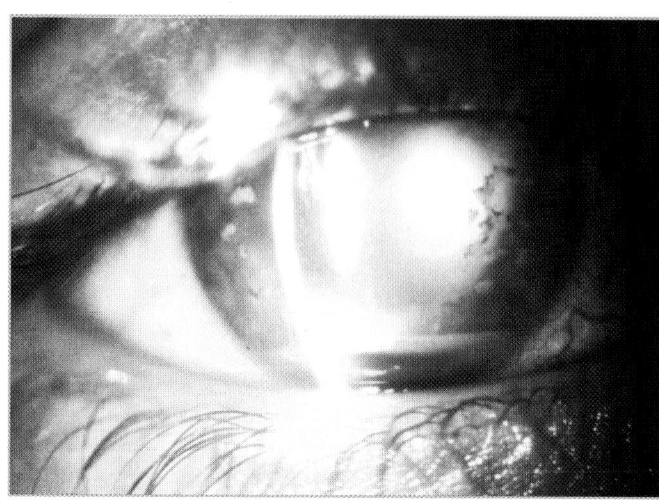

Figure 20.12 Bloody hypopyon in patient with acute lymphoblastic leukemia. (Courtesy of Mr JJ Kanski.)

Primary intraocular tumors

Retinoblastoma

Retinoblastoma is a malignant intraocular neoplasm affecting one child in 20 000, bilaterally in about a third of these. Children may present late with retinoblastoma, with signs of intracranial extension or metastatic disease. Full systemic examination is therefore required when the diagnosis is suspected. The exophytic form of retinoblastoma usually presents a well-defined white mass with prominent vessels. However, it is the endophytic form that most commonly masquerades as ocular inflammation. In addition to a posterior segment white mass (or masses), fluffy white preretinal and vitreous opacities may be seen (**Fig. 20.13a**), with diffuse vitreous cells. Occasionally AC cells or even a pseudohypopyon are seen, but never in isolation. Iris nodules (**Fig. 20.13b**) and heterochromia are rare.

Retinoblastoma is capable of mimicking several forms of intraocular inflammation, and vice versa (Shields and Shields 1992). Toxocariasis is perhaps the most frequent confusion, and many enucleations have been performed on eyes that were feared to contain retinoblastoma but later proved to have toxocariasis. Both may cause a posterior segment white mass, sometimes poorly observed through opacified vitreous humor, and both may cause leukocoria and esotropia in children of similar ages. The characteristics of toxocara uveitis are discussed in Chapter 14. Secondary cataract, although sometimes a feature of toxocariasis, is rare in retinoblastoma. Bilateral ocular toxocariasis is rare. Ultrasonography may be helpful; only retinoblastoma tends to produce the high-intensity echoes caused by calcium deposition. These are also visible on CT. Aqueous humor aspiration allows a comparison of lactate dehydrogenase levels with those of plasma; levels > 1 are seen in retinoblastoma but not in toxocariasis.

Intermediate uveitis in children may show focal peripheral snowbanking and vitreous opacification, and therefore may be confused with an endophytic retinoblastoma that has seeded, in 'snowball' fashion, into the vitreous humor. However, intermediate uveitis is almost always bilateral and the second eye usually shows rather more typical signs of intermediate uveitis. It tends to be diagnosed in older children than in those presenting with retinoblastoma, although there is considerable overlap. Indirect ophthalmoscopy with indentation will often reveal circumferential snowbanking which strengthens the diagnosis of intermediate uveitis.

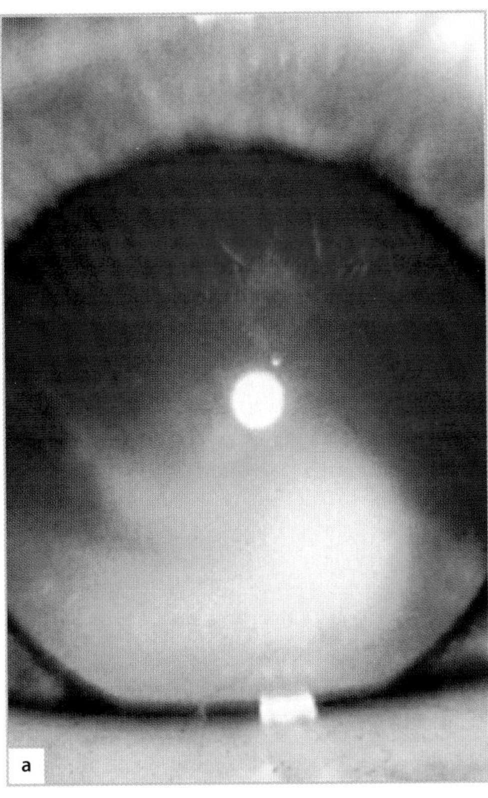

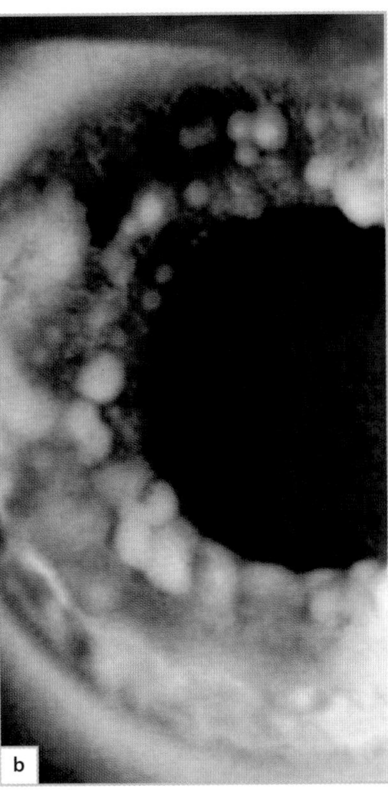

Figure 20.13 Retinoblastoma may masquerade as inflammation, either as an endophytic fluffy vitreous infiltrate (a) or rarely, by multifocal nodular iris infiltration. (b courtesy of Mr JJ Kanski.)

Rarely, other focal posterior segment inflammations may be confused with retinoblastoma. A large, late-presenting focus of toxoplasma retinochoroiditis with substantial vitreous opacification and no visible prior chorioretinal scar may provide a diagnostic challenge, but it is rare in early childhood. Congenital herpes simplex retinitis may cause substantial vitreous involvement and be confused with endophytic retinoblastoma. Concurrent dermatological herpes or encephalitis, and herpes serology will serve to differentiate. In doubtful cases the ocular oncologist should be urgently involved.

Uveal melanoma

Uveal melanoma only rarely masquerades as uveitis. An amelanotic iris tumor may mimic an inflammatory nodule, and diffuse iris melanoma may cause heterochromia. Occasionally, choroidal melanoma that has broken through the retina may seed pigmented cells into vitreous humor, superficially resembling a vitritis. True uveitis accompanying a primary tumor, affecting either anterior chamber or vitreous, is reported, as is scleritis and choroidal effusion. Any level of inflammation up to and including panophthalmitis may occur. The value of B-scan ultrasonography in atypical inflammations with severe media opacification is clear.

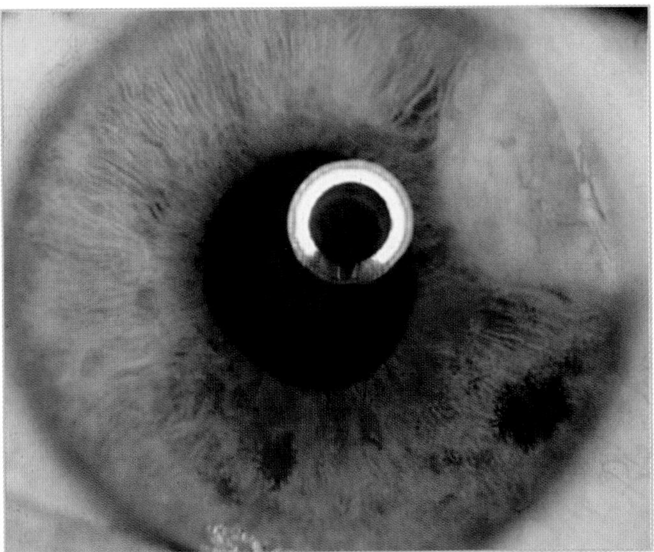

Figure 20.14 Juvenile xanthogranuloma: a vascularized iris mass accompanied by iris heterochromia.

Juvenile xanthogranuloma

This benign histiocytosis occurs usually in those aged <2 years but rarely in adults and comprises multiple orange–brown skin nodules often of the head and neck. The eye is involved in perhaps 1% of patients, the iris being by far the most likely site (Karcioglu and Mullaney 1997). There may be a single mass (**Fig. 20. 14**) or diffuse infiltration, with a tendency to recurrent micro- or macrohyphema and iris xanthochromia. Uveitis can be simulated or, on occasion, provoked. Diagnosis is by skin biopsy. In contrast to skin nodules, iris lesions are unlikely to be self-limiting and are often troublesome, with glaucoma the common end-point. They can respond to subconjunctival steroid injection but on occasion local radiotherapy or chemotherapy has been necessary.

Secondary intraocular tumors

Intraocular metastases, most commonly from lung or breast, usually present as a non-pigmented, elevated choroidal lesion. Overlying RPE mottling is a common feature (**Fig. 20.15**), but when the lesion is rather diffuse, and flat or regressed, inflammatory conditions may enter into the differential diagnosis. Less commonly anterior

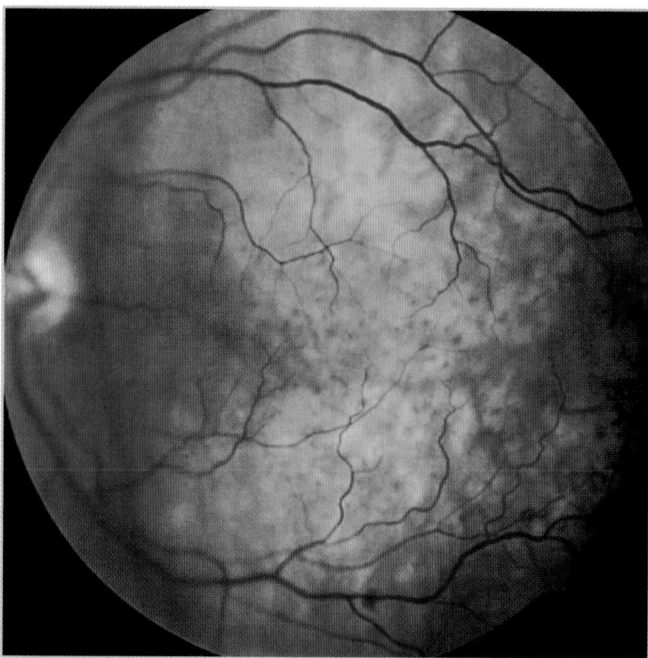

Figure 20.15 Choroidal metastasis from primary breast cancer. Small, flat or irregular metastases may simulate inflammatory foci.

segment metastases may occur and ocular pain and anterior uveitis have been reported in association, as have multiple iris nodules and pseudohypopyon. Ocular involvement in multiple myeloma is rare, but again may masquerade as uveitis. Reactive lymphoid hyperplasia is protean in its involvement of both eye and orbit, but at some stage may resemble anterior uveitis, cyclitis or posterior uveitis. More rarely, cutaneous melanoma may metastasize to the eye and cause free-floating aqueous or vitreous cells, without an intraocular mass lesion. On occasion vitreous involvement has simulated intermediate uveitis.

Paraneoplastic retinopathy

Autoimmune damage to retina or optic nerve secondary to primary cancer elsewhere may be mediated by several antibodies simultaneously, and is rare. Cancer-associated retinopathy is characteristically linked to small-cell lung cancer, and melanoma-associated retinopathy to a primary either cutaneous or intraocular. Visual symptoms may precede identification of the primary tumor. Symptoms usually include asymmetrical gradual blurring, central or paracentral scotomas, nyctalopia (especially associated with melanoma) or shimmering photopsia. Relative afferent pupil defects, variable visual field loss (but, characteristically, ring scotomas) and mild retinal arteriolar narrowing may be the only signs, although vitreous cells are quite common (Keltner et al. 2001) and retinal phlebitis occasional. Progressive visual loss is characteristic. Eventually widespread outer retinal atrophy may appear, accompanied by optic atrophy. Immunosuppression is usually effective (Ferreyra et al. 2009).

NON-MALIGNANT MASQUERADE SYNDROMES

Uveitis has many intraocular manifestations and other conditions can occasionally mislead at least the trainee diagnostician. A proper appraisal of history and full ocular examination almost always serve to differentiate. Nevertheless the expert will forgive the inclusion of a few brief examples of possible confusion.

Abnormalities of the cornea and anterior chamber

Keratic precipitates are very variable in size, number and distribution and sometimes are pigmented. These variations are discussed in Chapter 2. The classic Krukenberg spindle (and associated iris atrophy) of the pigment dispersion syndrome has been confused with active uveitis, especially after mydriasis has released a few pigmented cells into the AC. Very severe pseudoexfoliation can on occasion release material that adheres to corneal endothelium, again mimicking inflammatory precipitates.

Leukocytes, or clumps of these in the AC, are of variable appearance in uveitis. They are distinguishable by light reflection, and their color is distinguishable but their size is not. Other materials may also float in the AC: red or siderotic blood cells are distinguishable by color; ghost cells have an identifiable size and shape; lens material is of variable but generally crystalline shape and size; and most non-inflammatory causes of AC cells are unaccompanied by flare. These conditions are illustrated below.

Abnormalities of the iris and lens

Iris heterochromia is an important feature of some forms of uveitis, but inflammation is by no means the only cause. In particular siderosis and melanosis have caused confusion occasionally. Cicatricial posterior synechiae (PS) are a common feature of previous uveitis but can be distinguished from congenital iridolenticular adhesions because they form from the pupil margin, whereas the latter, being remnants of the fetal pupillary membrane, originate from the collarette (**Fig. 20.16**). Peripheral anterior synechiae (PAS) are a feature of chronic uveitis but anterior embryotoxon (which unlike PAS shows as a regular white line) or forms of the iridocorneal–endothelial syndrome can occasionally be misinterpreted (**Fig. 20.17**). The latter can also mimic previous uveitis by causing irregular corectopia, albeit without PS. Iris nodules can be seen in neurofibromatosis, which should not confuse, and xanthogranuloma, which can, especially when accompanied by AC cells and flare. Broken PS leave pigmented deposits stuck to the anterior lens surface, which are different in appearance from congenital epicapsular stars or siderotic deposits (**Fig. 20.18**).

Abnormalities of the vitreous, retina and choroid

The various causes of intravitreal opacification are usually distinguishable by density, color, size, shape and vitreous quality, the last sometimes being associated with retinal abnormalities. Thus, to the retinal expert, asteroid hyalosis, synchysis scintillans, amyloidosis and vitreous pigment are easily diagnosed; the beginner may need guidance (**Fig. 20.19**). Most dystrophic or degenerative retinal or choroidal diseases are characteristic, but a few can challenge even the experienced, e.g. adult-onset Best's disease, butterfly or Sorsby's dystrophy can mimic inflammatory maculopathies. Coat's disease, especially its atypical forms, can mimic an inflammatory vasculitis; non-inflammatory retinal venous occlusion occasionally exhibits perivenous sheathing.

Four well-known syndromes that mimic uveitis are now described, and finally there will follow a short diatribe on the sometimes enormous difficulty in differentiating between a progressive tapetoretinal degeneration and chronic indolent outer retinitis.

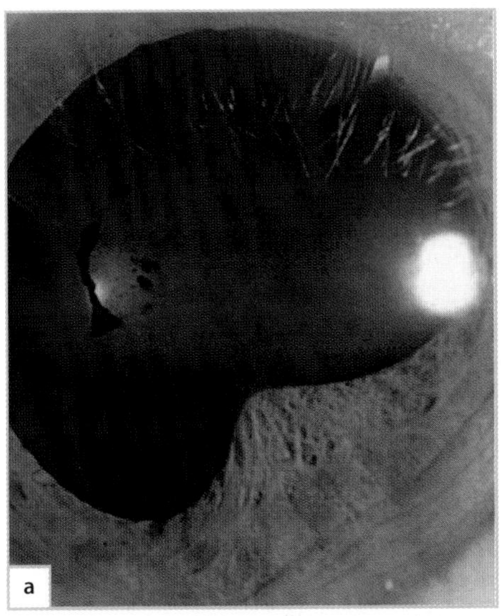

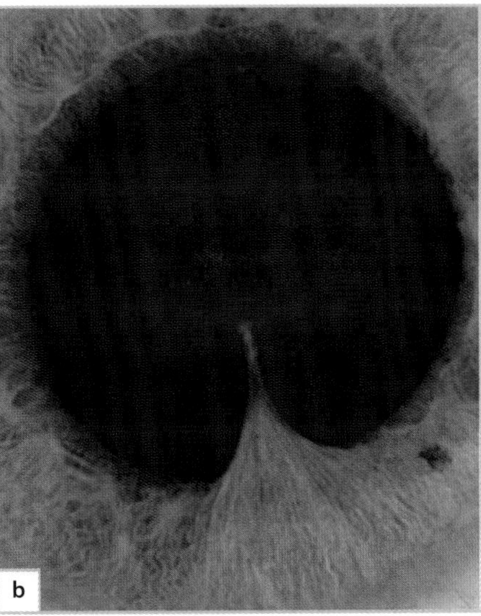

Figure 20.16 Inflammatory posterior synechiae (a) adhere to the lens from the pigmented epithelium of the pupil margin and posterior iris surface, whereas congenital adhesions (b) originate from the collarette and over-reach a normal pupil margin.

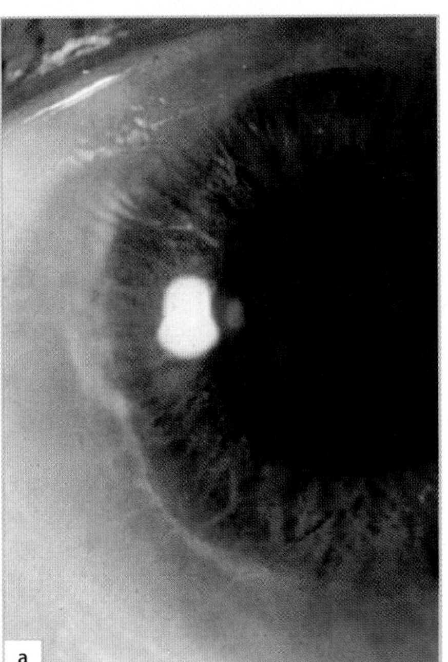

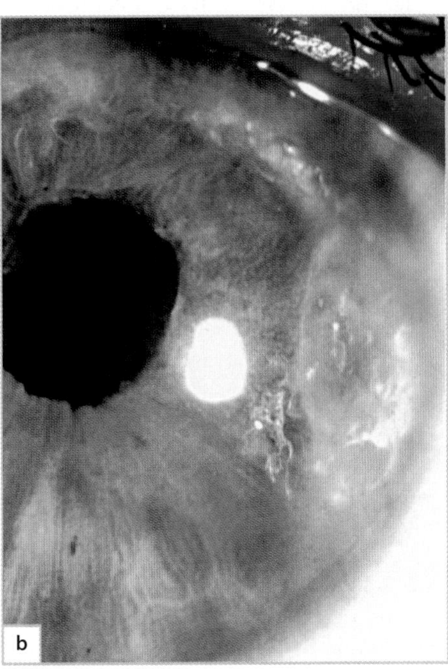

Figure 20.17 Axenfeld's anomaly (a) may resemble inflammatory peripheral anterior synechiae (PAS) but shows a white corneal adhesion and a degree of regularity. True PAS are usually patchy and associated with posterior synechiae and other post-inflammatory scarring.

Retained intraocular foreign body

A small minority of penetrating injuries with tiny, almost invariably ferrous, intraocular foreign bodies are occult because the injury caused negligible symptoms to the patient. Characteristically, at some later stage the presentation will comprise unilateral steroid-resistant uveitis accompanied by siderotic coloration of iris and vitreous. The characteristic yellow iris, orange–brown deposits on the cataractous lens surface and orange vitreous (**Fig. 20.20**) are unmistakable (Ugarte et al. 2009) but unfortunately indicate a late presentation often with permanently damaged retinal function. Diagnosis at an earlier stage, when the condition simply mimics uveitis albeit with some unusual features, requires a high degree of suspicion, a careful search for a healed entry wound and peripheral retinal indentation, and careful imaging to search for the embedded missile. Removal during vitrectomy is the modern approach.

Ocular ischemia

The gradual depletion of the ocular vascular supply, almost always secondary to severe carotid occlusive disease but occasionally secondary to either more local disease or systemic vasculitis, predominantly affects the posterior segment, but may progress to cause anterior segment ischemia. Red eye, anterior chamber cells (occasionally) and flare (usually) may mimic anterior uveitis (Mendrinos et al. 2009). Corneal edema, rubeosis, hypotony or glaucoma may occur, and discomfort and poor vision are frequent. The observation of retinal blossom hemorrhages, retinal vascular tortuosity or microvascular abnormalities assists the diagnosis. Some inexorably progress to painful blindness, whereas others may remain relatively stable for months or years. Panretinal photocoagulation is usually performed and may reverse anterior segment rubeosis and cellular activity. Assessment of the carotid circulation is important, but, although cerebral aspects also require consideration,

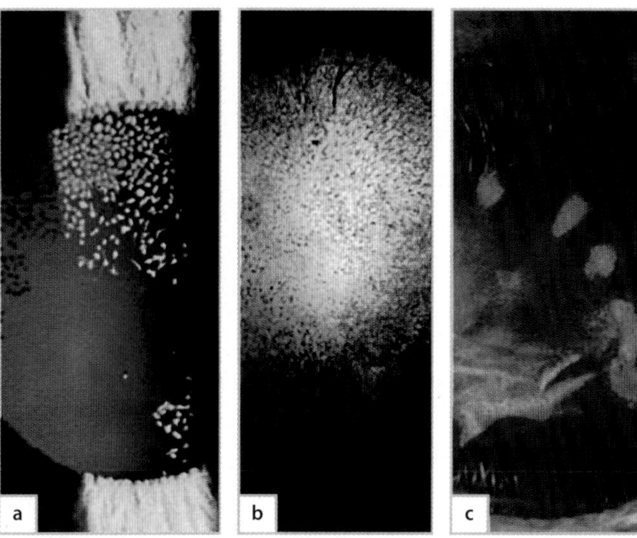

Figure 20.18 Congenital epicapsular stars (a) are often spidery and stellate; post-inflammatory pigmented fibrocytes (b) may resemble them, but are associated with severe posterior synechiae; siderotic deposits (c) may mimic iris pigment deposits but are orange and do not underlie the pupil margin.

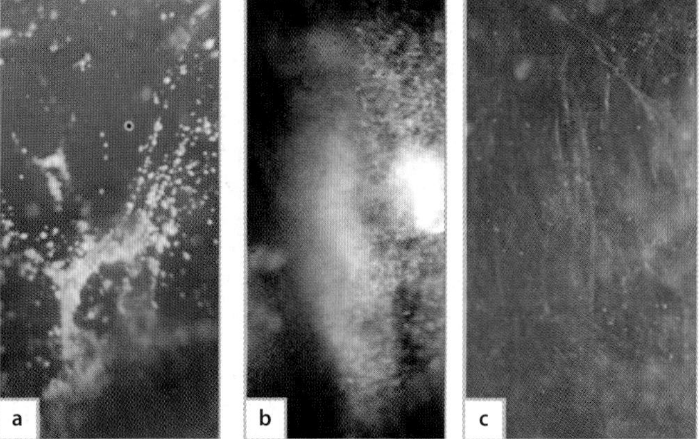

Figure 20.19 Vitreous humor in asteroid hyalosis (a) where the opacities are bright and white; amyloidosis (b) forming a complex filigree pattern (courtesy of Professor D McLeod); and in true inflammatory vitritis (c) in which, although prominence of vitreous architecture may be enhanced, it is the only one of the three showing individual or small clumps of inflammatory cells in the lacunae.

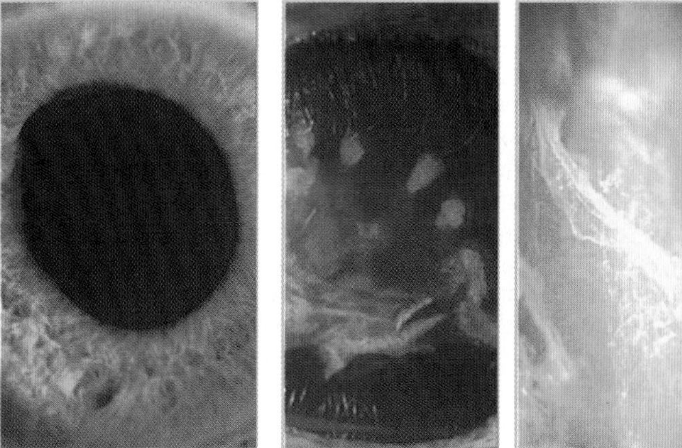

Figure 20.20 A long-retained ferrous intraocular body causes (from left to right) xanthochromia of the iris, siderotic deposits on the lens and orange-colored vitreous infiltration.

the usefulness to the eye of carotid endarterectomy has been disputed and, in those eyes masquerading as uveitis because anterior segment ischemia has already supervened, it is thought unlikely to help.

Retinal detachment and Schwartz syndrome

Rhegmatogenous retinal detachment is sometimes accompanied by a few cells in the anterior chamber, and a low intraocular pressure (IOP) is often encountered. However, Schwartz (1973) described a particular syndrome of rhegmatogenous retinal detachment, raised IOP and apparent uveitis. It has been shown that the condition is more likely to occur in the presence of chronic open peripheral breaks or dialyses. The great majority of affected patients have been young males. Analysis of aqueous humor has shown that the apparent 'cells' are not inflammatory, but are fragments of photoreceptor outer segments of variable size. It is likely that microscopic blockage of trabecular meshwork by these fragments is responsible for the IOP rise, analogous to the effect of swollen erythrocytes in ghost-cell glaucoma. The pseudouveitis does not of course respond to topical corticosteroid treatment. Retinal reattachment surgery with tamponade of all breaks is necessary. Why this syndrome should develop in only a small minority of those with peripheral retinal breaks is unknown.

Ghost cell glaucoma

For reasons unknown, erythrocytes from a persistent vitreous hemorrhage may lose most of their hemoglobin and become tumescent. They are capable of passing into the anterior segment (most commonly in aphakic individuals) where the cells tend to become impacted in the trabecular meshwork, leading to glaucoma. The peculiarly large cells (**Fig. 20.21**) are visible in the AC, mimicking anterior uveitis. However, the size of individual cells and the absence of flare are characteristic. Rarely there may be enough to deposit as a pseudohypopyon. The presence of a posterior segment hemorrhage should serve to distinguish the condition from uveitis. Removal of the reservoir of cells is necessary (El-Asrar and Al-Obeidan 1995).

Chronic indolent outer retinitis or progressive tapetoretinal degeneration? A diagnostic no-man's land

Typical retinitis pigmentosa (RP) is among the most straightforward of ophthalmic diagnoses. However, formes frustes of this group of tapetoretinal dystrophies can mislead. It may be asymmetrical or show atypical RPE damage with less-than-usual or morphologically different bone spicule pigmentation. A few cells, and in some cases a few more, may be seen in the vitreous. Such cases, especially when sporadic, may be referred to a uveitis clinic questioning whether this is truly a dystrophy or an atypical outer retinal inflammation. Electrophysiology studies are usually unable to differentiate.

Despite increasing knowledge of the genetic background for several types of tapetoretinal dystrophy/degeneration, the pathogenesis remains incompletely understood. It has been known for many years that a proportion of such patients exhibit an autoinflammatory response to retinal S-antigen or inter-photoreceptor-binding protein (Tamm et al. 2001). It is not unreasonable to suppose that an element of inflammation is involved in the progressive destruction of the outer retina in such 'inherited' conditions. The description of such possibly inflammatory cases as 'misdiagnoses' (Nagpal and Biswas 2006)

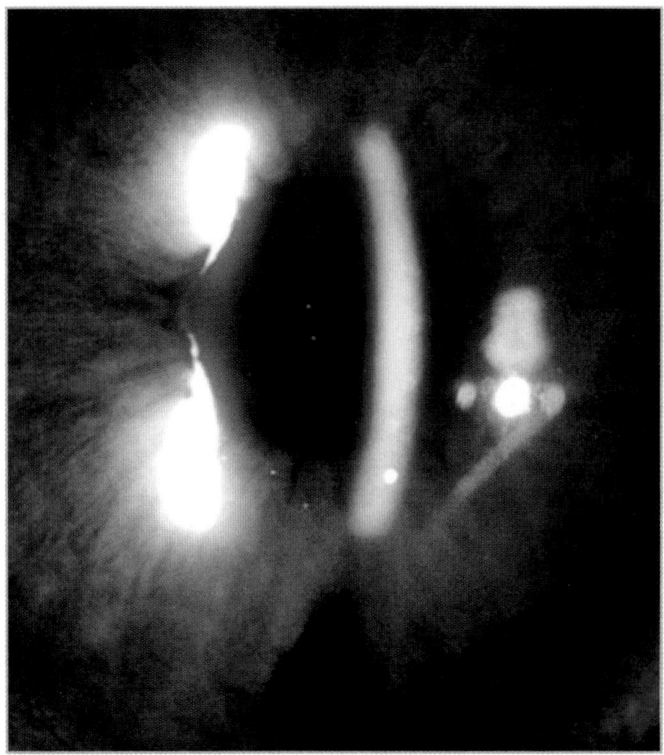

Figure 20.21 Depigmented tumescent erythrocytes ('ghost cells') in the anterior chamber.

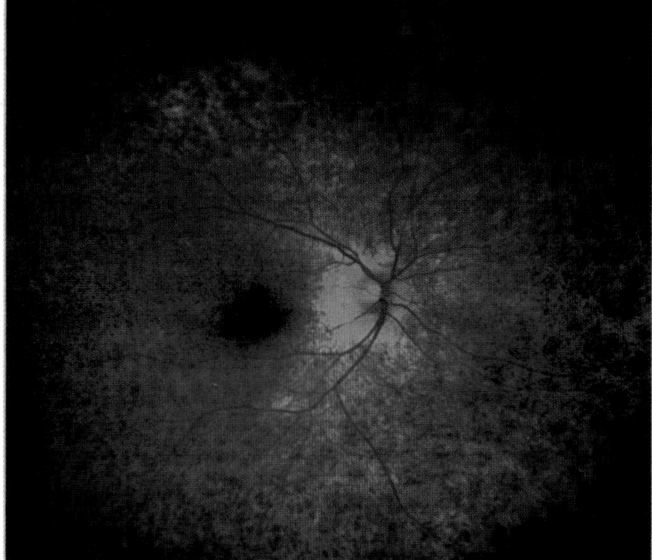

Figure 20.22 Widespread outer retinal disruption with nyctalopia, visual field loss and vitreous cells: dystrophy or inflammation?

may therefore be premature. The association of RP with Fuchs' heterochromic uveitis, which we have also seen, has been well described over the years (Chowers et al. 2000) and is intriguing; there may be a stronger association with Usher's syndrome (Lichtinger et al. 2010).

Pigmented paravenous retinochoroidal atrophy is a rare but well-recognized syndrome with similarities to RP; it is often familial, and investigations have revealed at least one relevant genetic mutation. It manifests as paravenous bone-spicule pigmentation, usually initially asymptomatic, and sometimes progressing to extensive visual field loss. Anecdotes of an association with measles are intriguing. Occasionally signs of intraocular inflammation are described in association (Batioglu et al. 2002). The question of an inflammatory pathogenesis again raises itself.

When confronted, as we are occasionally in a uveitis clinic, with a young adult with severely constricted visual fields, clinical evidence of widespread tapetoretinal damage that may be dystrophic or post-inflammatory or both (**Fig. 20.22**), and some suggestion of mild intraocular inflammation, the question to be answered should perhaps not be 'Is this a dystrophy or an inflammation?' but 'In the presence of these signs should we be offering immunosuppression?' Our answer to that question has pragmatically, usually been 'yes,' taking care to explain to the patient the speculative nature of our diagnosis, the unpredictable benefit of treatment and the virtual impossibility of assessing that benefit. Most patients wish to try.

Drug-induced uveitis

The ocular and visual side effects of drugs are a broad and complex field outside the scope of this text and have been reviewed elsewhere (Santaella and Frauenfelder 2007). This section deals only with drugs reported as causing anterior uveitis and/or vitritis or other intraocular reactions clearly simulating inflammation. Corneal effects, chorioretinal deposition, maculopathy and optic neuropathy are excluded.

Anecdotes of intraocular inflammation after drug or vaccine administration must be interpreted with caution. Ideally such reported reactions should be more than anecdotal: clearly recovering on withdrawal and recurring on re-challenge; dose related; and possibly extrapolated to other drugs within the same chemical group (Moorthy et al. 1998). Anterior uveitis is most commonly seen and, with the exception of rifabutin, severe vitritis or panuveitis is rare. Identification and withdrawal of the offending drug are clearly paramount, with supportive anti-inflammatory medication if indicated. **Table 20.1** summarizes the most common and important reactions, including those with many anecdotes but unproven etiology, e.g. evidence for the association with hepatitis B vaccine is increasing (Fraunfelder et al. 2010), although a few of particular importance are mentioned individually below.

Rifabutin

Rifabutin is used, often together with clarithromycin, in the management and prophylaxis of *Mycobacterium avium* complex disease in immunocompromised individuals. Uveitis occurs in up to 8% of those on 600 mg/day, is often unilateral, may occur either early or late after commencing the drug, and ranges from mild anterior uveitis and vitritis to severely opacified vitreous with fibrinous uveitis and hypopyon. The risk is dose related, 300 mg/day giving much lower risk. However, clarithromycin and other macrolides (Bhagat et al. 2001), and also protease inhibitors, increase serum rifabutin levels, increasing that risk. It has been suggested that, rather analogous to the Jarisch–Herxheimer reaction in syphilis, the uveitis may be caused by an immune reaction to intraocular killed mycobacteria. This, however, does not explain the frequent recurrence of inflammation on re-challenge. Spontaneous improvement follows withdrawal, but severe cases require systemic steroid treatment.

Bisphosphonates

It is ironic that a drug that ophthalmologists may prescribe in the management of steroid-induced bone loss may induce uveitis. Although several in the group have been reported to cause inflammation, intravenous pamidronate is the greatest culprit, risedronate following

Table 20.1 Drugs and vaccines associated with uveitis

Drug		Reported inflammations
Systemic drugs	Rifabutin	Mild-to-severe anterior to panuveitis
	Bisphosphonates	Mild/moderate AU, episcleritis, scleritis
	Sulfonamides	AU
	Cidofovir	AU or mild panuveitis
	Streptokinase	AU
	Oral contraceptives	
Systemic vaccines	Hepatitis B	AU, APMPPE
	Influenza	AU, vitritis
Topical (ocular) drugs	Metipranolol	AU, sometimes granulomatous
	Latanoprost	AU mild
Intraocular drugs	Cidofovir	Mild to very severe fibrinous panuveitis
	Triamcinolone	Moderate-to-severe panuveitis
	Bevacizumab	AU, vitritis occasionally severe
	Ranibizumab	AU, vitritis occasionally severe

APMPPE, Acute posterior multifocal placoid pigment epitheliopathy; AU, anterior uveitis.

closely behind. Non-granulomatous anterior uveitis of variable severity is the usual presentation, sometimes with episcleritis or even scleritis. Withdrawal and topical steroid are usually adequate.

Latanoprost and other prostaglandin analogs

Latanoprost was the first of this new class of glaucoma treatments. The small but significant incidence of mild non-granulomatous uveitis was realized and is now well reported, the drug simply being withdrawn if necessary. A few anecdotes, but no more, of a similar reaction to bimatoprost have appeared. A laser flare cell meter study (Cellini et al. 2004) demonstrated that only latanoprost caused a significant breakdown of the blood–ocular barrier, travoprost and bimatoprost being innocent of this. What exercises the uveitis practitioner in practice is the safety of these drugs for patients with known uveitis, either intermittent or chronic. Although anecdotes of both worsened uveitis and macular edema appear, studies have suggested that there is little to suggest a genuine concern, and that, probably, both latanoprost (Marchomichelakis et al. 2009) and bimatoprost (Fortuna et al. 2008) are safe in patients with secondary glaucoma associated with uveitis. Pragmatically most specialists would avoid these drugs soon after intraocular surgery. These results are reassuring because there are few more challenging glaucoma groups to treat.

REFERENCES

Batchelor TT, Kolak G, Ciordia R, et al. High-dose methotrexate for intraocular lymphoma. *Clin Can Res* 2003;**9**:711–15.

Batioglu F, Atmaca LS, Atilla H, Arslanpence A. Inflammatory pigmented paravenous retinochoroidal atrophy. *Eye* 2002;**16**:81–4.

Bhagat N, Read RW, Rao NA, et al. Rifabutin-associated hypopyon uveitis in human immunodeficiency virus-negative immunocompetent individuals. *Ophthalmology* 2001;**108**:750–2.

Buggage RR, Chan CC, Nussenblatt RB, et al. Ocular manifestations of central nervous system lymphoma. *Curr Opin Oncol* 2001;**13**:137–42.

Cassoux N, Giron A, Bodaghi B, et al. IL-10 measurement in aqueous humour for screening patients with suspicion of primary intraocular lymphoma. *Invest Ophthalmol Vis Sci* 2007;**48**:3253–9.

Cellini M, Caramazza R, Bonsanto D, et al. Prostaglandin analogs and blood-aqueous barrier integrity: a flare cell meter study. *Ophthalmologica* 2004;**218**:312–17.

Chowers I, Zamir E, Banin E, Merin S. Retinitis pigmentosa associated with Fuchs' heterochromic uveitis. *Arch Ophthalmol* 2000;**118**:800–2.

Coupland SE, Chan CC, Smith J. Pathophysiology of retinal lymphoma. *Ocul Immunol Inflamm* 2009;**17**:227–37.

El-Asrar A, Al-Obeidan A. Pars plana vitrectomy in the management of ghost cell glaucoma. *Int Ophthalmol* 1995;**19**:121–4.

Ferreyra HA, Jayasundera T, Khan NW, et al. Management of autoimmune retinopathies with immunosuppression. *Arch Ophthalmol* 2009;**127**:390–97.

Fortuna E, Cervantes-Castaneda RA, Bhat P, et al. Flare-up rates with bimatoprost therapy in uveitic glaucoma. *Am J Ophthalmol* 2008;**146**:876–82.

Frauenfelder FW, Suhler EB, Frauenfelder FT. Hepatitis B vaccine and uveitis: an emerging hypothesis suggested by review of 32 case reports. *Cutan Ocul Toxicol* 2010;**29**:26–9.

Frenkel S, Hendler K, Siegal T, et al. Intravitreal methotrexate for treating vitreoretinal lymphoma: ten years of experience. *Br J Ophthalmol* 2008;**92**:282–88.

Ghesquieres H, Ferlay C, Sebban C, et al. Long-term follow-up of an age-adapted C5R protocol followed by radiotherapy in 99 newly diagnosed primary CNS lymphomas: a prospective multicentre phase II study of the Group d'Etude des Lymphomes de l'Adulte (GELA). *Ann Oncol* 2010;**21**:842–50.

Karcioglu ZA, Mullaney PB. Diagnosis and management of iris juvenile xanthogranuloma. *J Pediatr Ophthalmol Strabismus* 1997;**34**:44–51.

Kawase Y, Yamamoto Y, Kameyama R, et al. Comparison of (11)C-methionine PET and (18)F-FDG PET in patients with primary central nervous system lymphoma. *Mol Imaging Biol* 2010;Epub.

Keltner JL, Thirkill CE, Yip PT. Clinical and immunological characteristics of melanoma-associated retinopathy syndrome: eleven new cases and a review of 51 previously published cases. *J Neuroophthalmol* 2001;**21**:173–87.

Kim SK, Chan CC, Wallace DJ. Management of primary intraocular lymphoma. *Curr Oncol Rep* 2005;**7**:74–9.

Lichtinger A, Chowers I, Amer R. Usher syndrome associated with Fuchs' heterochromic uveitis. *Graefes Arch Clin Exp Ophthalmol* 2010;**248**:1481–5.

Marchomichelakis NN, Kostakou A, Halkaidakis I, et al. Efficacy and safety of latanoprost in eyes with uveitic glaucoma. *Graefes Arch Clin Exp Ophthalmol* 2009;**247**:775–80.

Mendrinos E, Machinis TG, Pournaras CJ. Ocular ischaemic syndrome. *Surv Ophthalmol* 2009;**55**:2–34.

Michelson JB, Grossman KR, Lozier JR, et al. Iridocyclitis masquerade syndrome. *Surv Ophthalmol* 1986;**31**:125–30.

Moorthy RS, Valluri S, Jampol LM. Drug-induced uveitis. *Surv Ophthalmol* 1998;**42**:557–70.

Nagpal A, Biswas J. Pseudouveitis – analysis of cases misdiagnosed as posterior uveitis. *Ocul Immunol Inflamm* 2006;**14**:13–20.

Pe'er J, Hochberg FH, Foster CS. Clinical review: treatment of vitreoretinal lymphoma. *Ocul Immunol Inflamm* 2009;**17**:299–306.

Santaella RM, Frauenfelder FW. Ocular adverse effects associated with systemic medications: recognition and management. *Drugs* 2007;**67**:75–93.

Schwartz A. Chronic open-angle glaucoma secondary to rhegmatogenous retinal detachment. *Am J Ophthalmol* 1973;**75**:205–11.

Sen NS, Bodaghi B, Le Hoang P, Nussenblatt R. Primary intraocular lymphoma: diagnosis and differential diagnosis. *Ocul Immunol Inflamm* 2009;**17**: 133–41.

Shields JA, Shields CL. Differential diagnosis of retinoblastoma. In: *Intraocular Tumours*. Philadelphia, PA: WB Saunders, 1992: 341–62.

Tamm SA, Whitcup SM, Gery I, et al. Immune response to retinal antigens in patients with gyrate atrophy and other hereditary retinal dystrophies. *Ocul Immunol Inflamm* 2001;**9**:75–84.

Thiel E, Korfel A, Martus P, et al. High-dose methotrexate with or without whole brain radiotherapy for primary CNS lymphoma (G-PCNSL-SG-1): a phase 3, randomised, non-inferiority trial. *Lancet Oncol* 2010;**11**:1036–47.

Ugarte M, Nicol DA, Jones NP, et al. Chronic intraocular copper foreign body and candida: a unique combination. *Ocul Immunol Inflamm* 2009;**17**: 356–60.

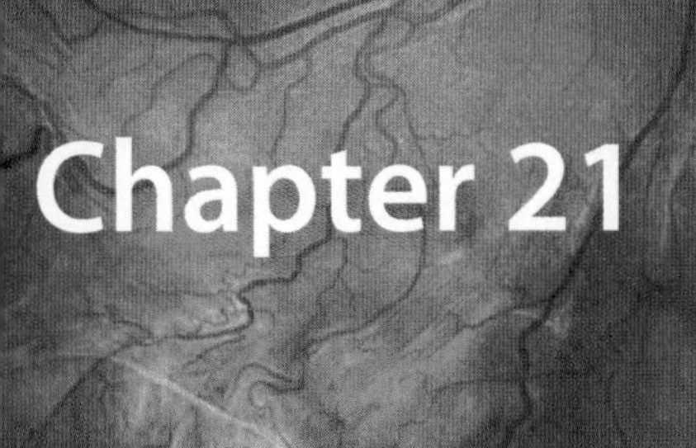

Chapter 21 Cases from the Manchester Uveitis Clinic

Reading the theory of uveitis is one thing. Managing the individual patient is quite another. Although straightforward, self-limiting uveitis lends itself well to management protocols, the peculiar, the complex or the chronic each carry its own challenge. Every patient is different, and the wise ophthalmologist always treats the patient, not the eye. To a firm basis of knowledge about diagnosis, drug safety, surgical risks and prognoses must be added the patient's individual circumstances: the patient is about to undergo a series of important examinations; is pregnant or wishes to be soon; has already lost one eye to trauma; is at risk of redundancy if taking too much time off work; cannot understand the treatment instructions given or is physically or mentally incapable of administering it; fails to attend regular follow-up; cannot afford the treatment; or simply does not trust doctors. Each provides a different dilemma, where the ophthalmologist's wish to pursue best-quality treatment may have to be compromised by pragmatism. Sometimes decision-making on treatment is best understood by hearing of individual cases rather than trying to absorb taught principles. Included here are the abbreviated stories of a few of the 3000 or so patients treated in the Manchester Uveitis Clinic (MUC). They have not been chosen to represent a cross-section of subjects covered in this text and therefore there may be some diagnostic duplication. They have been selected because each is thought to present some interest to the reader. They have been illustrated to challenge the viewer's diagnostic skills, and each has provided the opportunity to pose questions to the reader, followed by our own approach. Doubtless some experts would disagree with some management decisions, but discussion at this level is healthy and the few veterans who may browse this text may have different approaches. Whatever the level of expertise of the reader, it is hoped that these cases will give a flavor of the work done in a specialist uveitis clinic and provide pointers to those who may encounter similar situations in the future.

CASE 1: OCCLUSIVE OR NON-OCCLUSIVE?

With Tim DeKlerk

A 21-year-old woman was referred to the MUC having been diagnosed with bilateral panuveitis and started on treatment with oral prednisolone. Apart from a single episode of arthralgia affecting her right wrist she gave no history of significant medical illness. She had antinuclear antibodies at a titer of 1/160, but her ESR, ACE, chest radiograph, syphilis serology, FBC and ANCA were all normal. She had developed right macular edema, and had already received two orbital floor injections of methylprednisolone, with little effect.

When first assessed in our clinic she was taking 15 mg prednisolone orally, and was using topical dexamethasone 0.1% 2-hourly in her right eye, four times daily in her left. Her visual acuity was R 6/24, L 6/12. Despite this treatment she had mild bilateral anterior uveitis and vitritis with right posterior synechiae. Funduscopy revealed left disk swelling, gross right cystoid macular edema, bilateral widespread patchy periphlebitis, bilateral widespread retinal atrophy and preretinal gliosis. **Fig. 21.1** shows the left fluorescein angiogram. **In the light of the above investigation results, what would your diagnosis be?**

The fluorescein angiogram shows widespread vessel wall staining, disk leak, diffuse retinal leakage, including cystoid macular edema, and patches of retinal staining. She had no clinical or investigational evidence of associated systemic disease. She was diagnosed with primary retinal vasculitis. She was clearly undertreated and the prednisolone dosage was increased to 60 mg/day (1 mg/kg per day). Two weeks later she had gained 5 kg in weight and developed facial swelling. She still had bilateral macular edema. The prednisolone dosage was reduced to 30 mg/day and oral sustained-release acetazolamide 250 mg twice daily was commenced. Three weeks later her macular edema was persistent and she was tolerating acetazolamide poorly. Her retinal vasculitis was clinically improved, and her R VA had improved marginally to 6/18. **What would be your next step in managing her inflammation?**

It was clearly unacceptable for her to continue on this dosage of prednisolone and she needed oral immunosuppression. As was our practice at the time (2002), for patients with severe uveitis, male or female, our first-choice immunosuppressive was ciclosporin and she was provided with information with a view to commencing that drug. However, 1 week later her R VA had dropped to hand movements secondary to a dense intravitreal hemorrhage. The left was now 6/9. She was started on ciclosporin 5 mg/kg per day. Her vitreous hemorrhage cleared gradually but the R macular edema persisted. Intravitreal triamcinolone was injected, her macular edema disappeared and she saw 6/9 in both eyes, with early posterior subcapsular cataract. There was no visible evidence of retinal vascular occlusion. She was maintained on ciclosporin with prednisolone 5 mg/day. Her blood pressure rose to 152/117. **Why, and what would you do?**

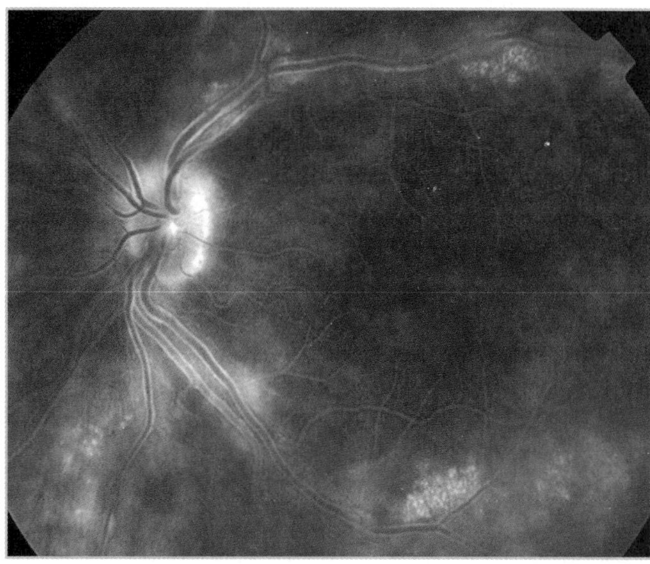

Figure 21.1 Case 1: the left fluorescein angiogram.

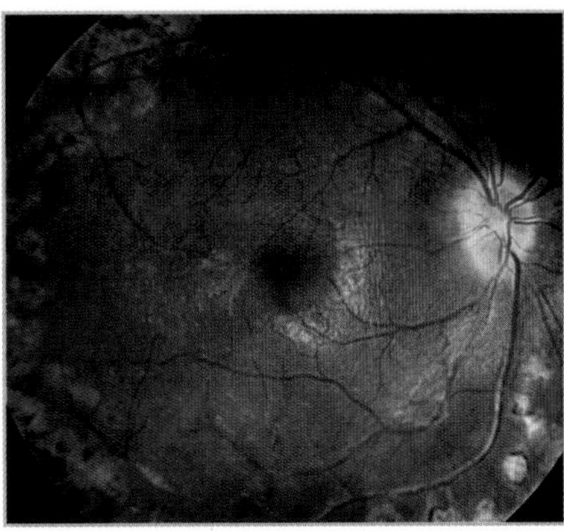
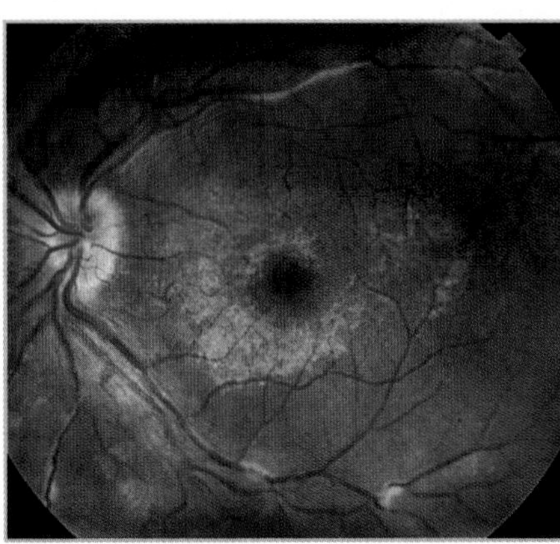

Figure 21.2 Case 1: the fundi after right phakovitrectomy.

Both prednisolone and ciclosporin may cause hypertension. At these dosages the ciclosporin is the culprit. Therefore the dosage was reduced by 25%. This was followed within weeks by a flare-up of her uveitis and vasculitis, requiring an increase in prednisolone. Despite this her inflammation persisted; this regimen was clearly unsatisfactory. **What would your alternative immunosuppressive be in her case?**

In young women, and increasingly in preference over ciclosporin, we use mycophenolate mofetil. This drug was introduced and the ciclosporin dose was tapered, being discontinued after 4 months. At this stage she had a further right vitreous hemorrhage and showed minimal iris rubeosis. There was no fundal view. **What would you do?**

Clearly she had occlusive retinal vasculitis with retinal neovascularization and was at risk of fibroproliferative disease. Her rubeosis made it clear that rapid intervention was necessary. Waiting for spontaneous clearance of vitreous hemorrhage was unsatisfactory. She underwent R phakovitrectomy with panretinal endolaser photocoagulation. Angiography also showed L peripheral vascular shutdown and she also underwent panretinal photocoagulation to this eye. Her R rubeosis regressed and she maintained normal IOP. Her fundal pictures are shown in **Fig. 21.2**.

Mycophenolate was not considered adequately to have adequately controlled her uveitis and so low-dose ciclosporin was reintroduced. We were able to taper her oral steroids to 5 mg/day. Bone densitometry remained normal. The uveitis has remained stable over the following 8 years. During that period she developed bilateral macular epiretinal membrane, and her L cataract was removed. Her recent VA was R 6/9, L 6/7.5 unaided. She was completely well on treatment. **What is her life expectancy?**

She has had retinal vasculitis for 10 years. She may retain intraocular inflammation indefinitely with a potential lifespan of a further 50 years. Clearly the very long-term implications of steroid and immunosuppressive treatment are significant. As a patient with occlusive retinal vasculitis, however, she has a substantially increased risk of coronary artery disease and stroke. In due course stringent precautions should be recommended; serum lipids will continue to be monitored (but statins interfere with ciclosporin synthesis). Low-dose aspirin may at some stage be desirable.

CASE 2: BILATERAL HYPERTENSIVE UVEITIS

With Karl Mercieca

A 47-year-old white woman presented with painful loss of vision in the left eye. There were no previous ophthalmic problems. Her only significant past medical history included a recovered left lower motor neuron facial nerve palsy, 2 months earlier; a cause had not been found and she had been diagnosed with Bell's palsy.

On examination she saw R 6/9, L 6/24. She had bilateral inferior medium-sized white keratic precipitates (KPs), with marked corneal edema in the left eye. There was bilateral anterior uveitis, with cells ++ R and cells +++ with flare L. The IOPs were R 33 mmHg, L 58 mmHg. Gonioscopy showed open angles in all four quadrants on the right with no PAS. Left gonioscopy was not possible owing to corneal edema. Dilated funduscopy of the right eye revealed a circumscribed atrophic chorioretinal scar temporal to the macula, localized intraretinal hemorrhage in the superotemporal midperiphery and three inferior vitreous snowballs. After treatment for raised IOP (including oral acetazolamide), the left cornea cleared enough to permit a view of moderately active vitritis, and multiple round creamy choroidal lesions nasal to the optic disk (**Fig. 21.3**). **What are the causes of hypertensive uveitis? What is the differential diagnosis? What investigations would you order?**

Raised IOP secondary to uveitis is common. Taken alone, the sign may suggest Fuchs' heterochromic uveitis, herpetic anterior uveitis, sarcoidosis, toxoplasmosis, VKH syndrome (but not at presentation) or the Posner–Schlossman syndrome. However, the association with granulomatous KPs narrows this to herpetic uveitis, toxoplasmosis and sarcoidosis. Multifocal choroidal lesions suggest sarcoidosis. Basic blood tests including a FBC, renal function, ESR and CRP were all normal. Syphilis and *Toxoplasma* serology were both negative. She worked in a hospital with exposure to tuberculosis patients, so a Mantoux test and interferon-γ testing were performed, and were negative. Her serum ACE was elevated at 182 IU. The chest radiograph was normal.

The presence of a partially pigmented chorioretinal scar in the right eye raised the possibility of previous *Toxoplasma* infection, but multifocal choroiditis is not in keeping with this diagnosis. A diagnosis of left multifocal choroiditis and bilateral hypertensive uveitis secondary to sarcoidosis was made. The facial palsy was also probably related to the sarcoidosis. **What are the potential mechanisms for raised IOP in uveitis? How would you manage this case in the first instance and in the long term?**

Raised IOP in uveitis may occur by angle closure (directly from PAS, indirectly from PS, or ciliary body or lens swelling leading to pupil block); open-angle mechanisms include trabeculitis or inflammatory exudate and steroid induction. A combination of mechanisms is quite common. Gonioscopy is a key component of the examination. Management should treat both the uveitis and the raised IOP, and aim to prevent complications such as synechiae. Miotics should be avoided owing to the risk of synechiae. Prostaglandin analogs are not routinely avoided, except in cases with macular edema. Systemic acetazolamide is an important and effective short-term agent.

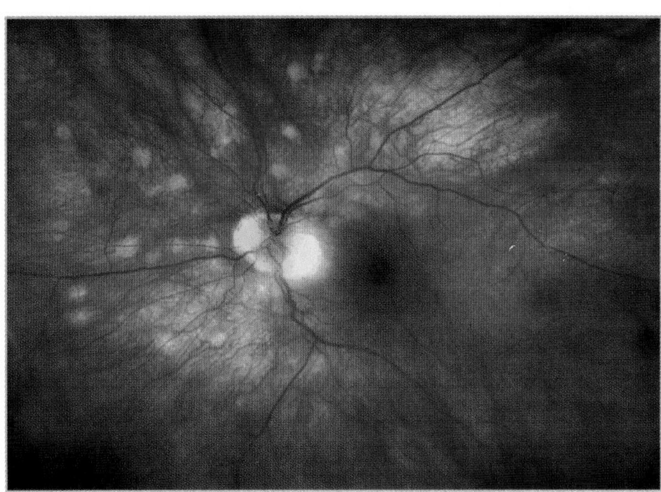

Figure 21.3 Case 2: the left fundus at presentation.

In this case the IOP was controlled in the acute phase with systemic acetazolamide and a topical β blocker/carbonic anhydrase combination. Topical prednisolone acetate 1% 1-hourly and atropine 1% three times daily were also administered. Vision improved to R 6/6, L 6/9. The anterior uveitis settled well on this treatment, with accompanying spontaneous reduction in IOP. At 3 months she required only infrequent topical steroid. Multifocal choroiditis in the absence of macular involvement or occlusive vasculitis does not require systemic medication.

CASE 3: UVEITIS AND BRAIN PATHOLOGY – CRUCIAL TO IDENTIFY A DIAGNOSIS

With Assad Jalil

A 19-year-old man presented with 2-week history of a painful, red left eye with reducing vision. He had a vague recent history of spontaneous weight loss over the previous year, and four years previously had undergone a left inferior oblique recession after a 4th nerve palsy of unknown cause. On examination he was found to have severe non-granulomatous left anterior uveitis with a VA of 3/60 and was treated with hourly topical prednisolone acetate and cycloplegia. The inflammation continued to worsen; 3 days later vitritis and peripheral retinitis were identified and he was referred urgently to the MUC. On presentation he had a L VA of hand movement, severe panuveitis with occlusive retinal vasculitis, and 360° peripheral retinal whitening and necrosis. There was also pale swelling of the optic disk and a localized inferior retinal detachment with two visible breaks in the necrotic area. **What is your differential diagnosis, what investigations would you undertake, and do you think that the previous history may be of relevance?**

A diagnosis of acute retinal necrosis (ARN) was secure owing to the typical clinical appearance, with secondary retinal detachment and optic neuropathy. In this circumstance intraocular fluid sampling is not mandatory. However, where any doubt exists, urgent sampling for PCR should be arranged. Intravenous aciclovir 800 mg three times daily was immediately started for this patient. In view of the retinal detachment being inferior and peripheral in the context of severe intraocular inflammation, surgical intervention was deferred. Systemic examination was normal but he was very thin. Investigations showed a normal ACE and negative serology for syphilis, *Toxoplasma* and HIV. Viral serology showed previous exposure to HSV-2 (IgG) but not to VZV. Chest radiograph and lumbar puncture were normal. However, MRI of the brain (**Fig. 21.4**) showed hyperintense areas in left temporal and parietal lobes and cerebellum of uncertain etiology but reported as indicating old injury or encephalitis. **Do you think this may be connected with his past history or his current retinal necrosis, and if so what etiology does it suggest?**

In most patients with ARN, VZV is the causative agent and a proportion has had shingles within the past year. However, a significant minority has HSV as the cause and, in children and young adults, HSV-2 is the more likely. A previous history of undiagnosed encephalopathy of any degree, in a patient presenting days or even years later with ARN, is highly suggestive of HSV-1 or -2. A previous herpetic encephalitis may well have caused his trochlear palsy. After 3 days of intravenous aciclovir, 40 mg oral prednisolone was added. His retinal detachment showed signs of gradual progression but its edge was still under the inferior arcade. **Do you feel that he should undergo surgery at this stage?**

Wherever possible, surgery should be performed on an uninflamed eye otherwise there is severe risk of exacerbation of inflammation.

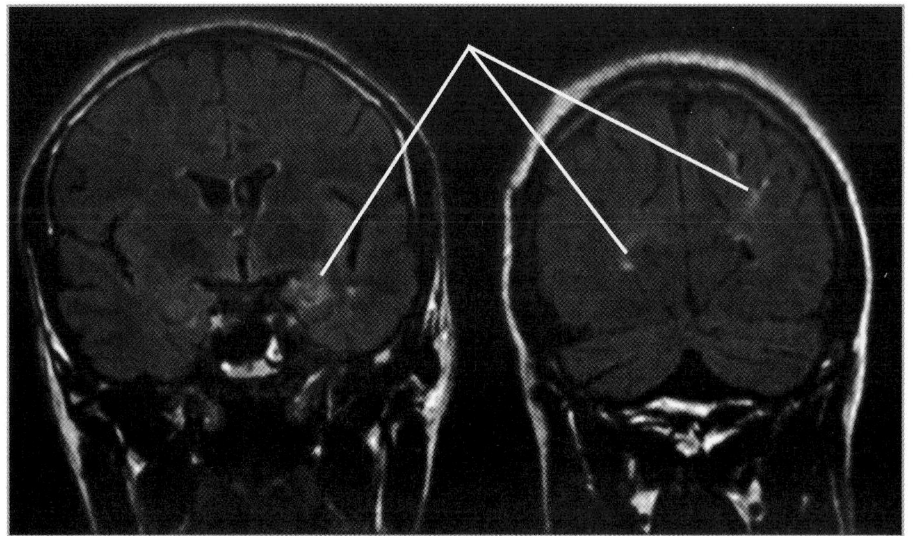

Figure 21.4 Case 4: focal high-intensity signals in left parietal and temporal lobes, and right medial temporal lobe, on presentation.

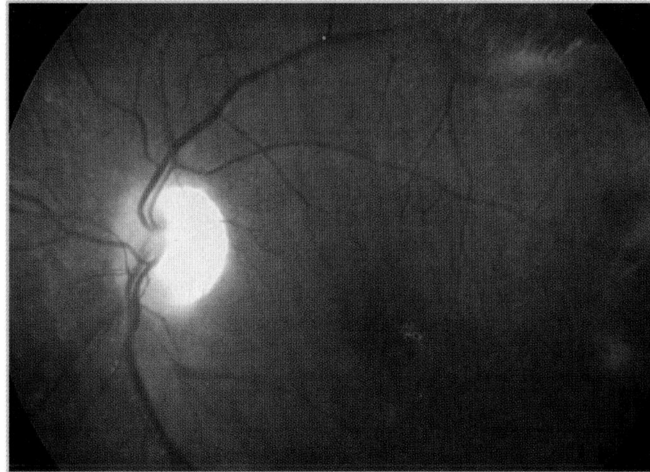

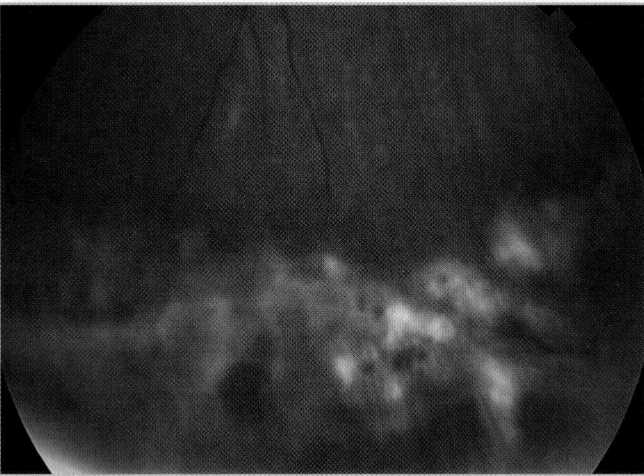

Figure 21.5 Case 3: central and peripheral views after retinal reattachment surgery showing stark optic atrophy and peripheral retinal loss following retinectomy.

The risk of a macula-off detachment may override this in an eye with good visual potential, but in this case the prognosis was quite poor owing to clear associated optic neuropathy. Pragmatically a decision was made to intervene surgically 1 week after the initial diagnosis (after 4 days of oral prednisolone), at which point the macula was still attached. Vitrectomy, retinectomy of peripheral necrotic retina, 360° endolaser and injection of silicone oil 5700 CS was carried out, together with phakoemulsification and intraocular lens implantation. A vitreous sample was submitted for PCR for herpesviruses and was strongly positive for HSV-2 but negative for HSV-1, VZV and CMV. The retina was successfully reattached (**Fig. 21.5**), but he developed optic disk pallor and the VA remained at HM. Optic neuropathy is a common accompaniment to ARN especially when diagnosis is delayed as in this case. This and retinal detachment are the most important causes of central visual loss.

After 10 days of intravenous aciclovir, oral valacicloir 1 g three times daily was given for 10 days after which aciclovir 800 mg four times daily was used, reducing to 400 mg twice daily for a total of 1 year. Oral steroids were tapered and discontinued at 3 months after initial presentation. The right eye remained uninflamed throughout.

The possibility that previous subclinical HSV-2 encephalitis had caused trochlear palsy is considered likely. He underwent extensive investigations including thyroid function tests, Synacthen test, abdominal ultrasonography and HIV serology, all of which proved normal. He went on to develop recurrent hemicranial headache and grand mal epilepsy, both considered postencephalitic by his neurologist.

CASE 4: THE TWO MOST COMMON COMPLICATIONS OF CHRONIC UVEITIS ENCOUNTERED IN UVEITIS CLINICS

With Assad Jalil

A 33-year-old Asian man presented with panuveitis and cystoid macular edema in his left eye. His investigations included a raised ACE level, and high-resolution chest CT led to a diagnosis of sarcoidosis. He was treated with a tapering course of moderate-dose oral steroid, which was then discontinued, leaving him in clinical remission. Four years later he developed a left unilateral flare-up of panuveitis with macular edema, which was treated by orbital floor injection of methylprednisolone 80 mg. The macular edema persisted and he underwent intravitreal triamcinolone injection 2 mg. The edema resolved and his visual acuity returned to 6/6. His IOP rose to 36 mmHg and he was treated with topical latanoprost, timolol and dorzolamide. His IOP remained persistently above 30 mmHg and he underwent left cyclodiode ablation. His IOP returned to normal. Six months later he developed persistent panuveitis and was treated with a tapering dose of prednisolone commencing at 40 mg/day and immunosuppression was started with ciclosporin 150 mg twice daily. He developed systemic hypertension and his ciclosporin dosage was progressively reduced to 50 mg twice daily. Azathioprine was added at 50 mg twice daily. Three months later his uveitis was controlled on these two immunosuppressives and prednisolone 7.5 mg/day. During the preceding months he had developed progressive posterior subcapsular cataract and left VA was now 6/48. He had extensive posterior synechiae. He wished to undergo cataract surgery. **What issues concern you about his forthcoming cataract surgery, and what precautions would you take before, during and after surgery?**

Any patient with chronic uveitis is at risk of flare-up from cataract surgery. There is a clear history of macular edema, which may also recur. Intravitreal steroid injection during surgery is probably unwise owing to his clear previous IOP response. If recurrent macular edema was a particular concern over and above that of increased inflammation (which is not the case here), then preoperative intravitreal anti-VEGF injection could be considered. Division of posterior synechiae and iris hooks will be necessary, which will increase postoperative inflammation. Intensive postoperative topical steroid may induce raised IOP.

As usual in this clinic, a comprehensive information pamphlet was given to the patient, and supplementary discussion ensured that informed consent was obtained. Uveitis was quiescent on systemic immunosuppression for at least 6 months before cataract surgery was performed. To optimize perioperative control of inflammation, oral prednisolone was increased to 25 mg/day for 1 week before surgery and this dose was maintained for 1 week postoperatively before reducing to 15 mg/day for 1 week and then 10 mg/day. Oral immunosuppression was not modified preoperatively because this does not reduce postoperative inflammation in those with inflammation. The initial postoperative visual acuity was 6/9 with pinhole but by week 4 postoperatively it had dropped to 6/24 with OCT evidence of cystoid macular edema (**Fig. 21.6**). **What options were available for treating cystoid macular edema in this patient considering that he**

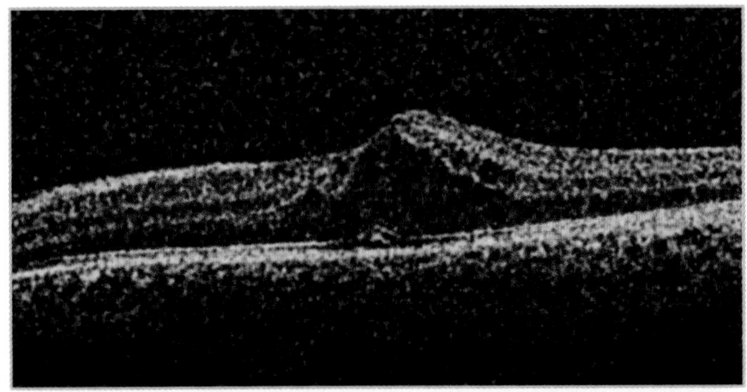

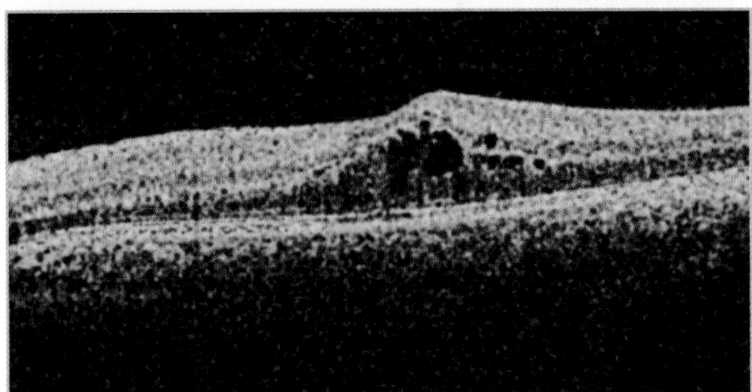

Figure 21.6 Case 4: left macular edema 1 year before cataract surgery (top) and 4 weeks postoperatively (bottom).

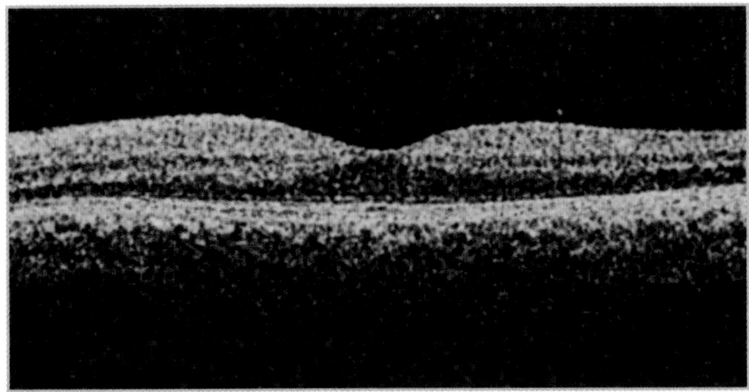

Figure 21.7 Case 4: resolved left macular edema after intravitreal bevacizumab injection.

was already on systemic immunosuppression and had a history of substantially raised IOP after low-dose intravitreal steroid injection?

The options include higher-dose oral steroid, low-dose orbit-floor injection, oral acetazolamide or intravitreal anti-VEGF injection. In fact he was given an orbit-floor injection of methylprednisolone 40 mg together with oral acetazolamide 250 mg twice daily for 2 weeks. In some situations this combination can be very effective to treat inflammatory cystoid macular edema. However, 4 weeks later the cystoid macular edema was persistent with no improvement in vision. He therefore underwent intravitreal injection of bevacizumab 1.25 mg; 2 weeks later the VA had improved to 6/6 with completely resolved cystoid macular edema on OCT. At 3 months after intravitreal bevacizumab injection, VA remained good at 6/6 with no evidence of cystoid macular edema (**Fig. 21.7**) and the patient had returned to baseline treatment of prednisolone 7.5 mg/day, ciclosporin 50 mg twice daily and azathioprine.

This sequence of events during chronic uveitis and cataract surgery is not unusual. It is imperative to control inflammation before surgery is performed, yet postoperative cystoid macular edema is in a sense a failure of control. It is usually straightforward to control but a substantial minority of patients are 'steroid responders' which adds complication. Although not helpful in this case, in inflammatory cystoid macular edema the possibility of oral acetazolamide as adjunctive treatment should always be considered, especially in those with glaucoma where it can 'kill two birds with one stone'.

CASE 5: AN ATYPICAL MACULAR INFLAMMATION

With Robyn Troutbeck

A 33-year-old white man presented with a 2-month history of progressive left paracentral scotomas. He was fit and well with no significant medical history. He had never traveled outside the UK. Visual acuity was R 6/5 and L 6/15. Examination of his anterior segments was normal. He had only a few cells in the L anterior vitreous. His posterior pole is shown in **Fig. 21.8**. **Describe the lesions and make a differential diagnosis.**

There is a combination of active and old lesions. The former seem to be at the level of chorioretinal interface and are contiguous with the old lesions, which appear as pigmented chorioretinal scars. The lesions are irregular, perhaps 'geographic' in shape, rather than roundish 'placoid' lesions. The wider retina cannot be seen in this image but there are similar lesions extending, in decreasing density, to the equator. There is no peripapillary involvement.

The differential diagnosis includes causes of multifocal choroiditis, atypical serpiginous choroiditis, atypical placoid pigment epitheliopathy, and syphilitic and tubercular chorioretinitis. **What investigations would you perform?**

Investigations included fluorescein angiography, FBC, ESR, CRP, U&Es, ACE, LFT, syphilis serology and chest radiograph. All of these results were normal or negative. He had no history of TB and no known contacts, had received BCG immunization as a child, had a clear chest radiograph, and had not traveled to an endemic area or worked with high-risk contacts. On this basis, we considered him very low risk and did not perform further investigations to rule out TB (which if required would include Mantoux and interferon-γ testing).

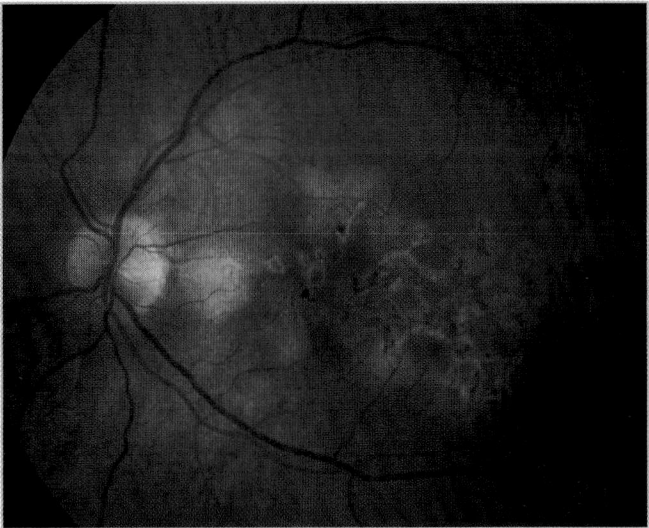

Figure 21.8 Case 5: the left macula at presentation.

Early and late phase fluorescein angiography is shown in **Fig. 21.9**. This reveals the early hypofluorescence and late hyperfluorescence (but no leakage) of active lesions; this pattern is seen in cases of both APMPPE and serpiginous choroidopathy. **What diagnosis would you make?**

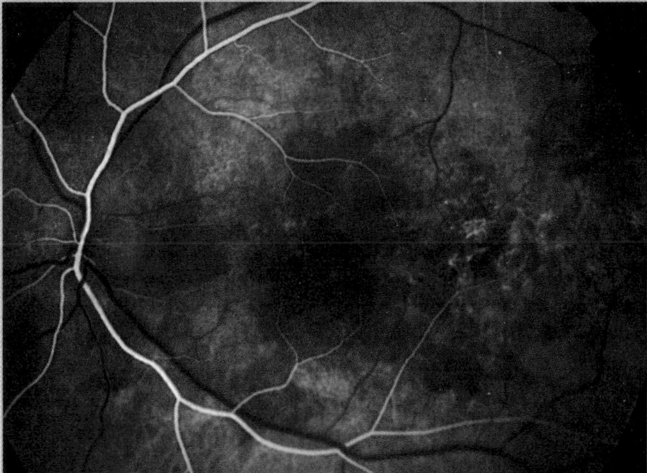

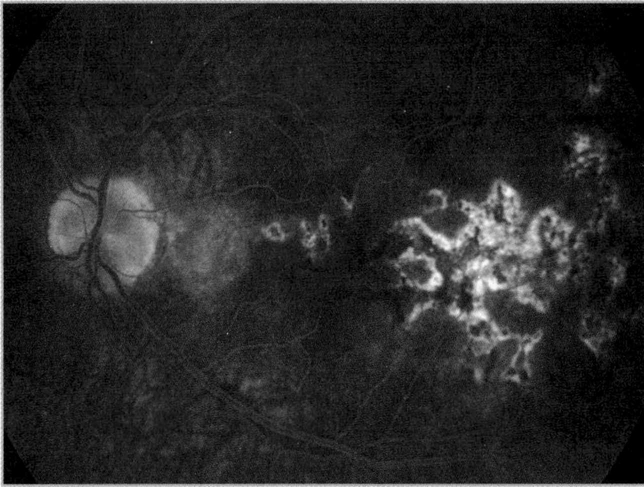

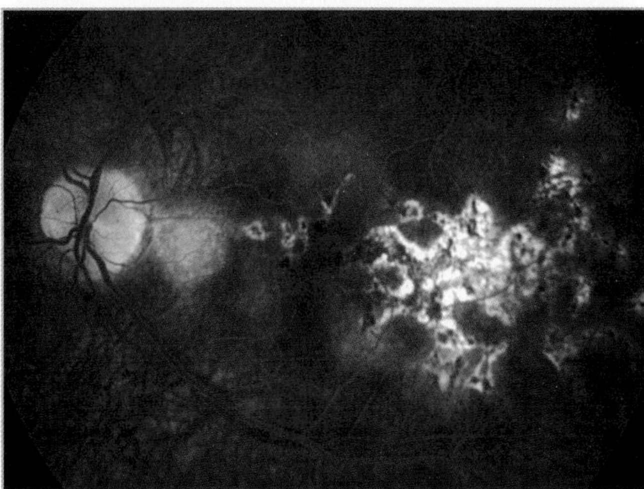

Figure 21.9 Case 5: the FFA sequence in which early dark lesions do not stain until the 4-min (bottom) frame. The middle frame is at 2 min.

On the basis of the widespread foci, peculiar lesion shapes, subacute and progressive behavior incorporating edge reactivations, a diagnosis of ampiginous choroiditis (relentless placoid chorioretinitis) was made. The patient was commenced on moderate-dose prednisolone (60 mg/day) but new foci of inflammation continued to appear. The dose was increased to 100 mg/day (1 mg/kg per day) and after informed consent ciclosporin was also started. No further new foci have appeared, and his vision has remained at L 6/12. The right eye has thus far remained unaffected. The final image shows the change in appearance over 6 months of follow-up, at which time he was using ciclosporin 150 mg twice daily and prednisolone 10 mg/day (**Fig. 21.10**). His blood pressure was 135/95, he had gained 5 kg in weight, his creatinine level was 95 (baseline 70), blood glucose normal, he had normal bone density but had no adverse symptoms on his medication. **How would you manage this over the next 1–2 years?**

Even mild hypertension in an obese patient should be managed with caution. Both oral steroid and ciclosporin contribute to this but, with a creatinine somewhat higher than baseline, it would be appropriate to reduce ciclosporin first by a reasonable increment, probably to 125 mg twice daily. If creatinine were stable at that dosage, it would then be appropriate to reduce prednisolone slowly to 5 mg/day and revisit ciclosporin dosage further. If no further inflammation became apparent (using serial photography) after 1–2 years, it would be reasonable to discontinue treatment (steroid first). If at any stage recurrent disease supervened, we would investigate for TB while reintroducing prednisolone first. Some patients with serpiginous choroiditis and its variants develop recurrent disease after several years of quiescence, so careful observation is necessary.

CASE 6: CLASSIC DIAGNOSIS, DIFFICULT MANAGEMENT

With Tim DeKlerk

A 12-year-old boy attended the emergency eye centre at our hospital with a 3-month history of blurred right vision. He had no significant past medical or ophthalmic history, and pre-school screening had apparently shown symmetrical vision. His VA was R 6/36, L 6/5. He had a right relative afferent pupil defect. There was no anterior uveitis but he had mild vitritis. Dilated funduscopy revealed a large, dense vitreous opacity overlying the right inferotemporal retinal vascular arcade and stretching into the inferior periphery, with tractional retinal folds, as seen in **Fig. 21.11**. **What is the most likely diagnosis and how would you try to confirm it?**

The image shows a broad white band within the vitreous, with tractional attachments to the optic disk and temporal to the macula, with resultant tractional macular dystopia and retinal elevation. The band extends into the periphery. This appearance is classical for ocular toxocariasis. This is a rare diagnosis in the UK, where the great majority of affected children are younger, but the clinical appearance places the diagnosis virtually beyond doubt. However. he was seronegative for *Toxocara* sp. Screening tests were also unremarkable, including seronegativity for *Toxoplasma* sp. (which can rarely cause tractional change). **Would these results make you re-think the diagnosis? How would you manage this situation?**

Serology for *Toxocara* sp. does not have as reliable a sensitivity as that for many other microorganisms; immunity to the antigen is mixed and often fades over time. Therefore, although positive serology is a supportive result in an eye with classic signs, negative serology is merely neutral. There was no need to reconsider the diagnosis. So why did we

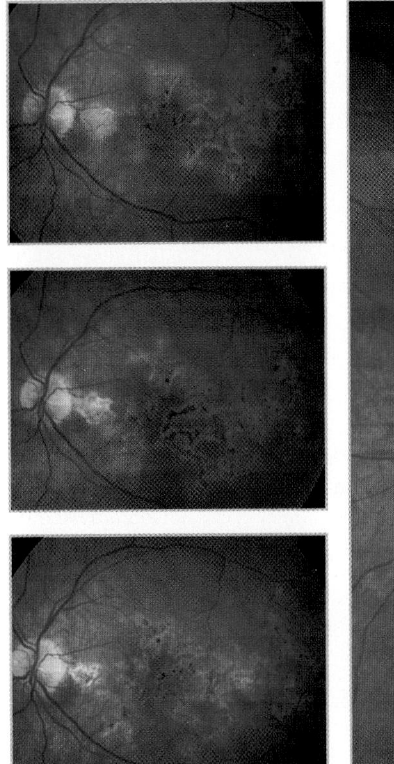

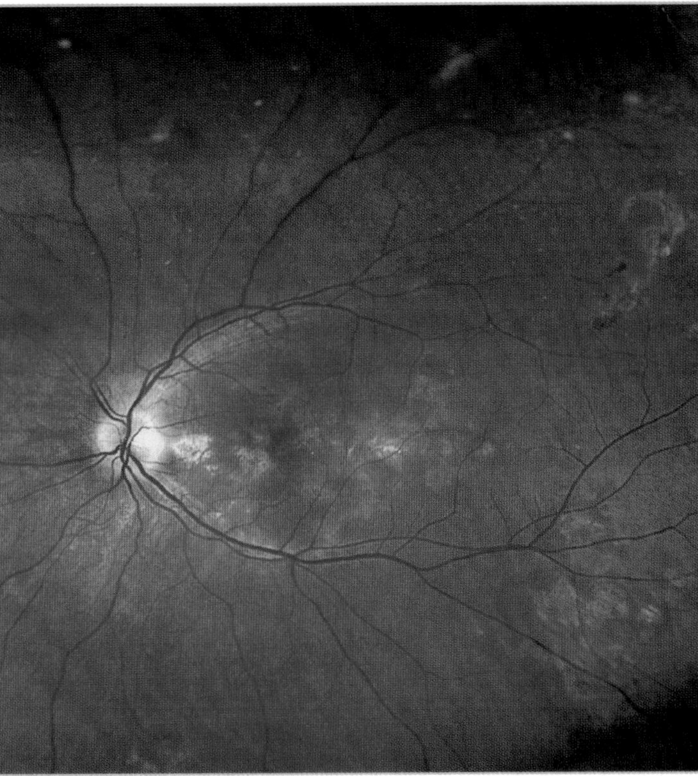

Figure 21.10 Case 5: the sequence of macular photographs show appearance at presentation (top), after 1 month (middle) and after 6 months (bottom). The widefield angiogram also shows the lesions in the temporal midperiphery (the nasal periphery was also patchily involved).

bother to ask for the test? Because seropositivity (had it been present), in a country where it is rare, is essentially a confirmation of diagnosis.

Views differ on the validity of anthelmintic drugs such as thiabendazole, in the management of ocular toxocariasis, especially in children where drug toxicity is an issue. Most uveitis specialists avoid these drugs because they do not counteract the inflammatory or tractional elements of infestation. He was commenced on oral prednisolone 0.5 mg/kg per day. The vitritis settled completely and there was evidence of settling of subretinal fluid. However, as steroids were tapered, his macular dystopia continued to worsen and a decision was made for him to undergo vitrectomy with relief of retinal traction. At surgery the tractional band was deeply embedded within the retina both centrally and peripherally, and it was only possible to divide the band and excise its central part. However, he did very well after surgery with relief of retinal traction and improvement in acuity up to 6/12. His prednisolone was stopped. Soon after this he developed moderate anterior uveitis requiring topical steroids, which have continued long term. Within 6 months he developed further macular traction and visual distortion, with a decline in VA to 6/24. The fundal appearance at this stage is shown in **Fig. 21.12**. **What would you do?**

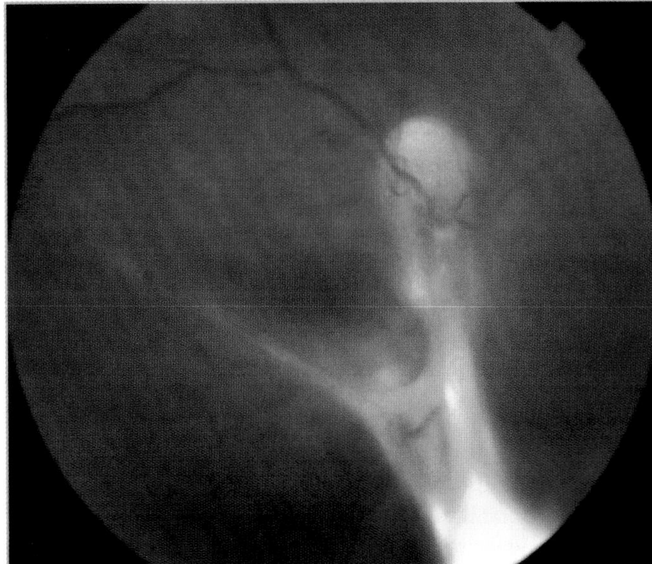

Figure 21.11 Case 6: the left eye at presentation.

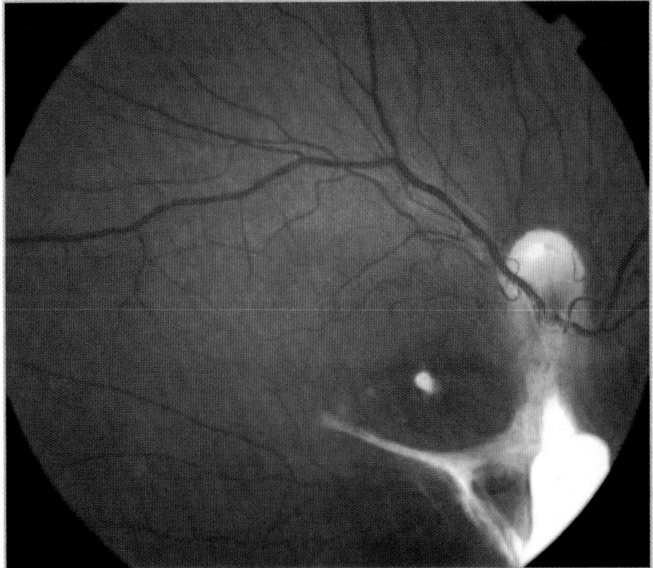

Figure 21.12 Case 6: the is increasing retinal elevation with macular exudate and epiretinal fibrosis.

After careful discussion the vitreoretinal team felt that further surgery to perform macular epiretinal membrane peel and tractional band segmentation would be worthwhile, and he duly underwent this surgery under oral steroid cover. He developed increased postoperative vitritis requiring orbit floor methylprednisolone injection. He was subsequently lost to follow-up and discontinued all treatment. However, on his return 3 years later he had no active inflammation, the macular profile was unchanged and his VA was 6/36, where it has remained.

CASE 7: A CLASSIC DIAGNOSIS WITH TYPICAL COMPLICATIONS

With Robyn Troutbeck

A 54-year-old white man presented to the emergency department in respiratory distress and with gastrointestinal symptoms. He was known to be HIV+ and he was diagnosed with pneumocystis pneumonia and systemic CMV infection. His CD4 count was 50. His CMV infection was treated with oral valganciclovir induction followed by lower-dose maintenance. Once stabilized he described floaters in the right eye, with a scotoma that had increased in size in the previous 4–6 weeks. He was referred to the MUC. On examination, his visual acuity was R 6/12, L 6/6. The left eye showed no abnormality. The right anterior chamber had a moderate cellular reaction and there was mild vitritis. The fundus of the right eye is shown in **Fig. 21.13**. **What is the most likely diagnosis, and how would you manage it?**

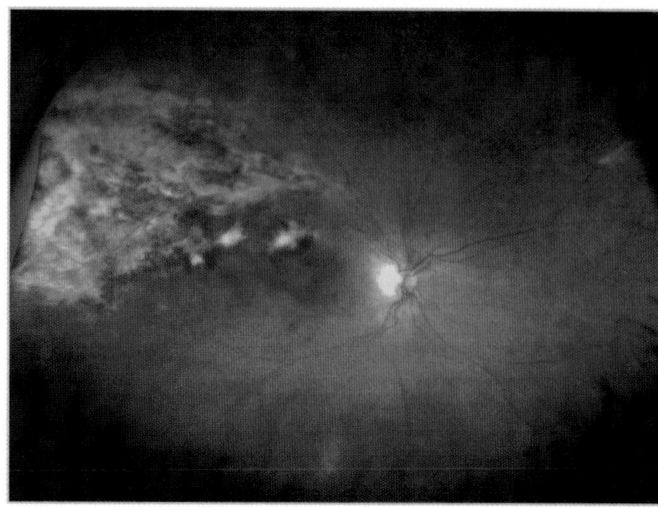

Figure 21.13 Case 7: the right fundus at presentation.

The image shows several areas of retinitis, one particularly substantial that had started in the temporal periphery but is extending into the macula, with hemorrhage along the superior temporal arcade. In the patient's context, the diagnosis must be CMV retinitis. Pneumocystis retinitis looks completely different from this. Other opportunistic infections are very unlikely and it is reasonable to confirm diagnosis by response to treatment, reinvestigating if necessary. The leading edge of his retinitis was close to his macula, so, in addition to reinduction with oral valganciclovir (to which the CMV was proven to be sensitive), we offered intravitreal ganciclovir injection, which he declined. The lesions slowly resolved, leaving him with typical postinflammatory retinal scarring, shown in **Fig. 21.14**, and a VA of 6/9. He was subsequently commenced on HAART and his CD4 count improved. **What are potential complications of CMV retinitis?**

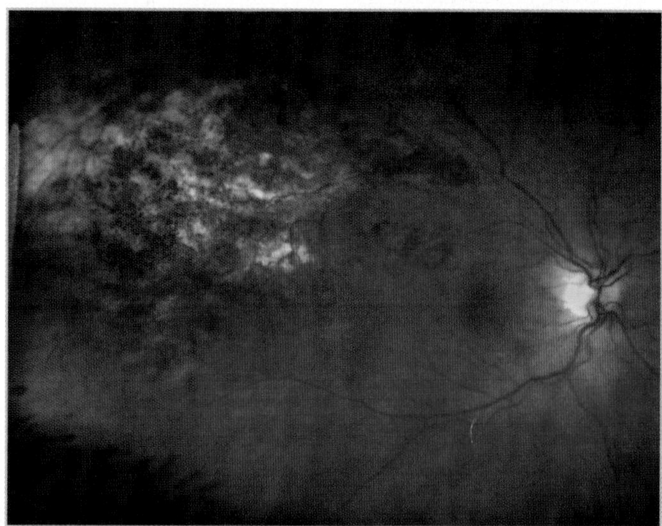

Figure 21.14 Case 7: the right fundus 2 months after reinduction of anti-CMV treatment.

Recurrent disease is a problem in those with AIDS whose HAART cannot raise the CD4 count adequately. Diagnosis of minor edge reactivation can be challenging. Rhegmatogenous retinal detachment is common. Other opportunistic infections may occur if the patient remains immunodeficient. Paradoxically, a recovering immune system may cause inflammation in the form of immune recovery uveitis. Four months after presentation to the uveitis clinic, on routine review, the patient was noted to have a small superior rhegmatogenous retinal detachment secondary to a break in necrotic retina. He underwent vitrectomy with SF_6 gas injection, avoiding silicone oil because the detachment was so localized. The retina remained flat and secure. One month later he developed new significant vitritis in the right eye, with cystoid macular edema and VA of 6/18. There was no sign of active retinitis nor any other fundal lesions. At this stage his CD4 count had risen to 215. **What might be causing this reaction?**

There is a small possibility that the macular edema was induced by vitrectomy, but arising anew 1 month postoperatively, not by the vitritis. In view of the rising CD4 count in the context of previous CMV retinitis this was diagnosed as immune recovery uveitis. An orbital floor depot injection of methylprednisolone 40 mg was given and a review appointment arranged. Unfortunately, he failed to attend this and two other arranged appointments over the next 2 months. He subsequently presented again to the emergency service with sudden right visual deterioration and was found to have a macula-off subtotal rhegmatogenous detachment, with a new break in necrotic retina. He underwent repair with silicone oil injection and currently sees 6/60. The left eye remains normal.

CASE 8: MUCH MORE THAN JUST AN EYE PROBLEM

With Assad Jalil

A 30-year-old white man presented to his general ophthalmologist with subacute visual loss in his left eye. On presentation his VA was R 6/5, L 6/18, and he showed unilateral left anterior uveitis, vitritis and what was described as 'hemorrhagic macular exudation.' He was initially treated with topical steroids and an orbital floor injection of methylprednisolone. Investigations showed normal ACE and chest radiograph, and negative serology for syphilis and herpesviruses. One month later he presented with further profound loss of vision in the same eye. The VA had deteriorated to counting fingers and he had severe panuveitis with liquid hypopyon, together with multifocal retinal infiltrates with associated hemorrhage, as seen in **Fig. 21.15**. He was referred to the MUC. **What diagnosis does this suggest to you, and what questions would you ask?**

Acute panuveitis with hypopyon and hemorrhagic retinitis is very suggestive of Behçet's disease. On closer questioning he gave a history of recurrent mouth ulcers for the previous 5 years, with occasional scrotal ulceration. There was no skin rash, arthropathy or headache. He was diagnosed with Behçet's disease and was initially treated with two pulses of intravenous methylprednisolone 1 g followed by high-dose oral steroid. He was also commenced on ciclosporin 5 mg/kg per day. Subsequently despite treatment he developed non-destructive polyarthropathy. As intraocular inflammation subsided, oral steroids were tapered and discontinued. His anti-inflammatory treatment removed his severe acute retinitis to reveal a scarred macula with central VA not improving beyond count fingers. His systemic symptoms gradually improved and he remained stable for 12 months, but then developed acute panuveitis in his previously uninvolved right eye with VA deteriorating to 6/24. He was treated with intravenous methylprednisolone, and oral prednisolone was recommenced at 80 mg/day. This was successful and the R VA improved to 6/6. Oral prednisolone was gradually tapered over 6 months to 10 mg/day; mild nephrotoxicity, shown by rising creatinine and mild systemic hypertension, was resulting from ciclosporin, which was reduced in dosage. One year later his better, right eye again developed hemorrhagic retinitis with VA dropping to 3/60. **Clearly his immunosuppression is not completely preventing exacerbations. What options are available either immediately or in due course, to treat this severe ocular inflammation?**

As previously the acute phase was managed with intravenous pulsed methylprednisolone and increased oral prednisolone. He was becoming Cushingoid. Combined immunosuppression

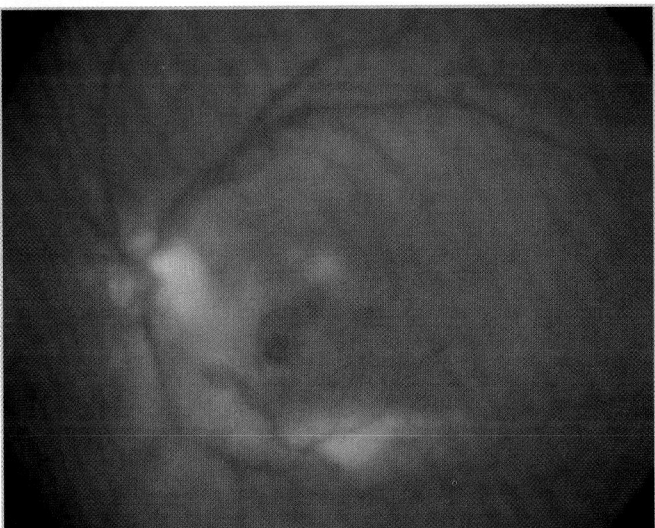

Figure 21.15 Case 8: the left eye showing, through hazy vitreous, macular retinitis with hemorrhage.

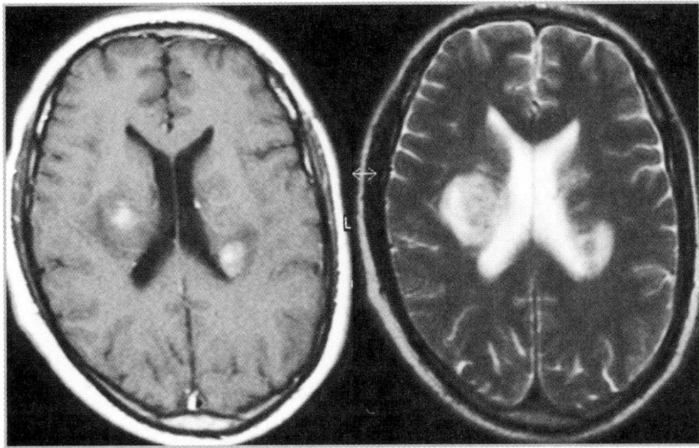

Figure 21.16 Case 8: MRI of the CNS at the time of his acute neurological symptoms.

(adding azathioprine or mycophenolate) was an option. Anti-TNF biologics were at this stage (2002) becoming increasingly used in this disease. After informed consent the patient was commenced on intravenous infliximab at 5 mg/kg, receiving two pulses. The second led to a severe post-infusion reaction, and the inflammatory lesion at the right macula remained recalcitrant; infliximab was therefore discontinued. Mycophenolate mofetil 1 g twice daily was therefore added to the ciclosporin, and was well tolerated. The ocular inflammation in the right eye improved, with VA recovering to 6/9.

Three months later the patient presented with a 2-day history of nausea and vomiting followed by rapid-onset of left hemiparesis and brief loss of consciousness. He underwent CNS imaging (**Fig. 21.16**). **What is the differential diagnosis and how would you manage this?**

The main differential at this point was acute neuro-Behçet's disease, thrombotic stroke (he also had anticardiolipin antibodies), opportunistic infection associated with immunosuppression or ciclosporin neurotoxicity. Ciclosporin has been reported to increase the risk of neurological involvement in Behçet's disease. Blood tests were resolutely normal with no markers of infection and no acute phase response. MRI showed changes typical of Behçet's vasculitis. CSF cytology showed mild pleocytosis only. His immunosuppression was discontinued and he was treated with three pulses of intravenous methylprednisolone 1 g, and intravenous cyclophosphamide was initiated using the Birmingham vasculitis protocol. The neurological signs subsided allowing a complete symptomatic recovery. Mycophenolate immunosuppression was then resumed, together with low-dose prednisolone.

For 8 years subsequently he remained very well on treatment, with no signs of right intraocular inflammation or neurological problems. The left eye continued to have mild-to-moderate flare-ups of inflammation, treated with topical and orbital floor steroids with occasional moderate-dose oral steroid. During this period he presented with subacute bilateral knee pain and MRI demonstrated bilateral osteonecrosis, necessitating cessation of oral steroids but recovering without surgical decompression. Ten years after presentation, the VA was R 6/5, L HM. At routine follow-up he had recently developed increasing paraesthesiae down his left arm and chest, numbness of left hand and left foot drop. Urgent CNS imaging was requested.

CASE 9: A COMMON CONDITION WITH AN UNCOMMON OUTCOME

With Romi Chhabra

A 34-year-old white man presented to the emergency clinic with a 1-day history of photopsiae, blurred vision and ache in his right eye. There was no significant past ocular or medical history. Visual acuity was R 3/60, L 6/6.

On examination the left anterior segment was normal. The right eye showed AC cells 1+ with fine KPs and the IOP was 38 mmHg. Gonioscopy was normal. Dilated funduscopy showed mild posterior vitritis and a parafoveal white infiltrate adjacent to old chorioretinal scars. A few small chorioretinal scars were also noted in his left fundus. **What is your differential diagnosis?**

Active chorioretinal inflammation adjacent to an old chorioretinal scar is the paradigm of ocular toxoplasmosis, which also often causes anterior segment inflammation (granulomatous or otherwise) and this is frequently associated with raised IOP. Serpiginous choroiditis causes edge reactivations adjacent to old scarring, but not with significant vitritis and not with anterior uveitis. Atypical placoid pigment epitheliopathy may present similarly but again without significant vitritis and usually with bilateral macular involvement. Fungal infection or TB might be considered in those at risk.

A provisional diagnosis of ocular toxoplasmosis was made and he was prescribed oral clindamycin 300 mg three times daily, acetazolamide SR 250 mg twice daily, with topical steroid and timolol. He was referred to the MUC and was seen 48 hours later. At this stage the active focus had enlarged significantly and involved the macula. His clindamycin was continued (four times daily) and he was commenced on oral prednisolone 60 mg/day and co-trimoxazole 960 mg twice daily. Antibiotics were continued for 4 weeks and his oral steroid was tapered over 6 weeks, leaving him with a quiet eye, a perifoveal scar and visual acuity of 6/24. He was discharged with information on possible recurrence. He presented again after 5 months with a contiguous recurrence and was treated similarly, leading again to resolution but a worse VA of 6/60. As a result of this fairly early macular recurrence, he was prescribed prophylaxis with co-trimoxazole 480 mg twice weekly. Despite this he developed a third recurrence that was treated similarly and resolved.

There were no further incidents for 4 years, but he then presented again with VA of R HM and a sudden increase in floaters. He had fibrinous anterior uveitis and severe vitritis with a poor fundal view. He was again started on oral prednisolone with co-trimoxazole and clindamycin. Within 1 week his uveitis was substantially improved, revealing large vitreous condensations on the posterior hyaloid, multiple macular scars and several foci of active retinitis adjacent to widespread, contiguous midperipheral scars (**Fig. 21.17**). Despite having had clindamycin previously without problem, on this occasion he developed severe diarrhea; clindamycin was therefore discontinued and a stool sample was negative for *Clostridium difficile*. **What further steps would you take at this stage?**

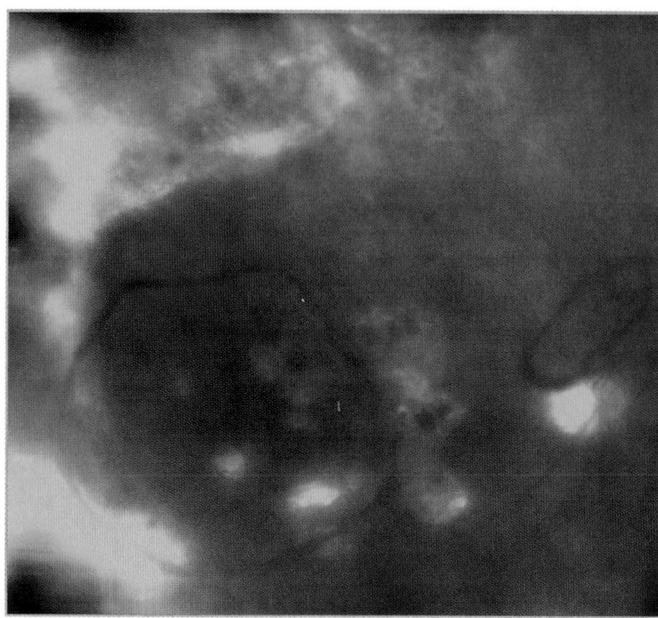

Figure 21.17 Case 9: vitreous opacification, multifocal scars and active retinitis at the most recent presentation.

Statistically, any patient presenting with a first attack of ocular toxoplasmosis has about a 50:50 chance of a recurrence at some stage. Only a few develop frequent recurrences, only a few go on to develop treatment-resistant chronic inflammation and multifocal active lesions are rare. Any of these less common presentations should provoke a search for underlying predisposition (and the astute observer will comment, with some justification, that we could have investigated earlier in his course). At this stage, he was questioned further about his general health. There was no history of significant infections but he admitted to being tired frequently. He agreed to undergo HIV serology and this was combined with hematology and cellular immunity testing.

He was found to be HIV+ with a viral load of 737 863 copies and a CD4 count of 122, and was referred to our genitourinary physician colleagues. He was prescribed high-dose co-trimoxazole and subsequently three-drug HAART. His ocular toxoplasmosis has settled, CD4 count has risen substantially and he has undetectable viral load.

It could be argued that any patient with recurrent ocular toxoplasmosis should undergo HIV serology but in our population this seems an over-reaction. However, in retrospect we feel that his third episode, developing early on co-trimoxazole prophylaxis, should have provoked investigation, in which case his HIV (which was presumably positive at that stage) would have been detected 4 years earlier.

CASE 10: CONFLICTING PRIORITIES

With Romi Chhabra

A 36-year-old woman with Algerian ancestry presented with sore red eyes and mild global headache. Visual acuity was normal and she was fit. One week before presentation she had a mild self-limiting sore throat with pyrexia. She was noted to have mild conjunctival chemosis and anterior chamber inflammation for which topical prednisolone succinate was prescribed. After 5 days the inflammation had resolved completely and drops were discontinued. However, within a week she returned with sore eyes and blurred vision and was found to have substantial bilateral anterior uveitis with posterior synechiae. Funduscopy revealed engorged optic nerve heads, retinal striae and severe macular edema with VA of R 6/24 L 6/12 (**Fig. 21.18**) and she was referred to the MUC. **What is your differential diagnosis?**

This is bilateral, symmetrical, acute-onset uveitis with serous macular elevation. The differential diagnosis includes Vogt–Koyanagi–Harada disease, severe APMPPE, posterior scleritis and lupus choroidopathy. There are no APMPPE-type lesions to be seen and

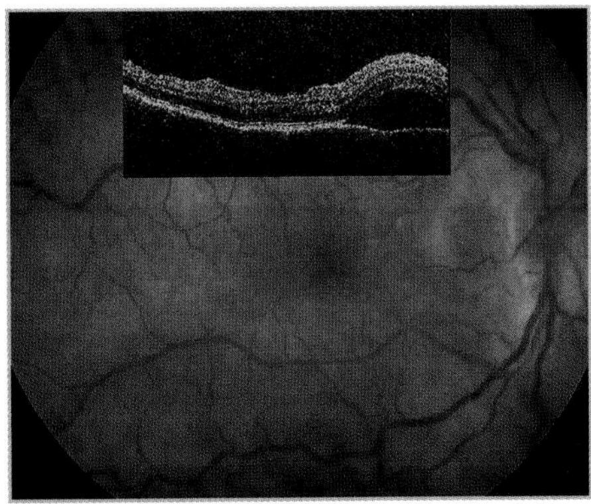
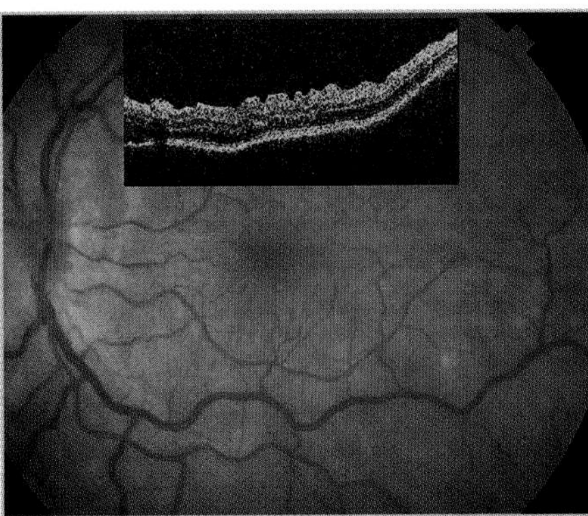

Figure 21.18 Case 10: bilateral pink engorged disks with retinal thickening and subretinal fluid, seen especially on the R OCT. The L OCT demonstrates retinal striae well.

she does not have lupus. The severe loculated serous retinal elevation with congested disks makes the diagnosis of VKH syndrome clear. She was commenced on oral prednisolone 80 mg/day, with calcium supplementation, proton pump inhibitor and semi-intensive topical prednisolone acetate. After 1 week her vision had improved to R 6/12, L 6/6. The AC inflammation was minimal. The serous detachments settled completely and the optic disks showed only mild congestion. She underwent baseline bone densitometry scan which was reported normal. **What treatment plan would you now institute and what potential problems might ensue?**

The VKH syndrome is usually a very chronic process, often beginning with a severe phase but going on to develop chronic uveitis, usually in the anterior segment, and often with secondary glaucoma. Other late disease-related complications include alopecia, poliosis, vitiligo and dysacusia. Long-term oral steroid treatment in a woman carries a high risk of induced bone loss. If potent long-term treatment is considered necessary, oral immunosuppression is usually preferable.

After 2 weeks her IOPs both became raised and she was commenced on a topical β blocker. The IOP did not respond very well but the ACs in both eyes were quiet and topical steroid was reduced, leading to a period of fluctuating anterior segment inflammation with raised IOP. After several weeks her oral prednisolone had been reduced to 10 mg/day. She developed mild tinnitus but audiometry was normal. The behavior of her intraocular inflammation suggested that she should be treated with oral immunosuppression and she was provided with an information pamphlet on mycophenolate mofetil, to consider treatment. At her next review, about 4 months after presentation, she announced that she was 7 weeks' pregnant and not only did not wish to commence oral immunosuppression but wished to come off oral steroid treatment. **How would you advise her at this stage?**

Mycophenolate mofetil carries a 25% risk of fetal malformation and should be avoided in pregnancy. Methotrexate also carries some risk. Both azathioprine and ciclosporin are regularly used during pregnancy, especially in organ transplant recipients, with little risk to the fetus. In some forms of uveitis, high intrinsic estrogen and progesterone levels (both of which are anti-inflammatory) can contribute a little to disease control. It may therefore be possible to reduce oral steroid dosage during pregnancy. Oral prednisolone carries a small but well-identified risk of clefting abnormalities in the child. Women requiring significant doses of oral steroid should be more closely monitored during pregnancy, because of increased risks of hypertension and diabetes.

Following a discussion of risks, at her request oral prednisolone was tapered and stopped over 3 weeks and she was managed throughout her pregnancy on topical medication alone, with fluctuating inflammation and IOP. She presented urgently, 12 days post-term and in early labor, very anxious with blurred vision, at which point her IOP was 40 mmHg in each eye, with mild active anterior uveitis. She was already using topical latanoprost, dorzolamide and timolol in each eye, together with topical steroid. **What would you do?**

It was not appropriate to use oral acetazolamide in this situation. Gt apraclonidine 0.5% three times daily was added and she underwent uneventful labor and delivered a healthy child. At 5 days post partum there was an opportunity for a rather more relaxed review. Vision had remained good at R 6/7.5, L 6/6, IOP was R 19 mmHg, L 24 mmHg on maximal topical treatment but her optic disks had remained healthy with only a 0.1 cup. There was generalized fundal depigmentation with a multitude of small peripheral chorioretinal scars, typical of late VKH syndrome (**Fig. 21.19**). Again oral immunosuppression was recommended but refused as she was breast-feeding.

At 4 months post partum the IOPs were raised at R 28 mmHg, L 30 mmHg with increased cupping. She was commenced on oral acetazolamide and again advised to use oral immunosuppression. She wished to defer the onset of treatment until after a holiday, but returned from this after a further 3 weeks with painful visual loss in the right eye. The R VA was now 6/15 with substantial cupping and grossly raised IOP. She urgently underwent right cyclodiode ablation and is awaiting Baerveldt glaucoma drainage tube surgery. She is finally using mycophenolate immunosuppression. She is aware that conventional contraception is unreliable on mycophenolate and has been advised to use barrier methods. We anticipate better disease control and hope that further visual field loss can be prevented.

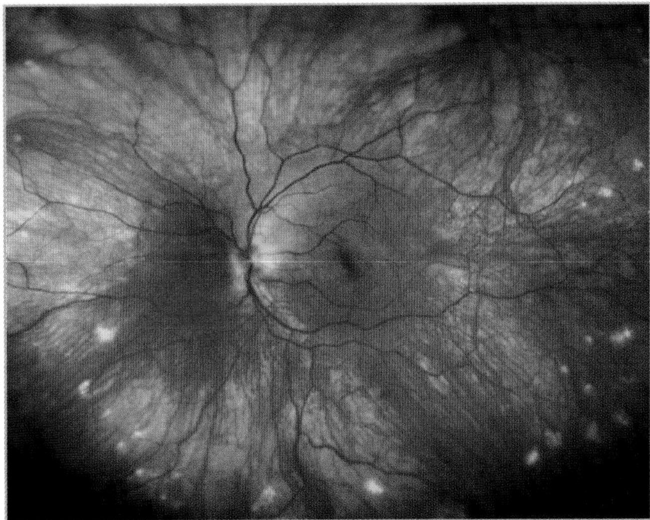

Figure 21.19 Case 10: widespread fundal depigmentation with peripheral punctuate chorioretinal scars.

CASE 11: A PRAGMATIC TREATMENT DECISION

With Robyn Troutbeck

A 23-year-old undergraduate student, recently arrived from India to study in the UK, presented with a 2-day history of dense floaters in his left eye. He had a recent history of dry cough but was otherwise well. He had no history of TB or of known contact with the disease. He had undergone BCG immunization. The VA was R 6/6, L 6/6. He had no anterior segment abnormality and normal IOPs. Dilated funduscopy showed the right fundus to be normal. The left fundus, seen through recent vitreous hemorrhage, demonstrated clear abnormalities. He also underwent fluorescein angiography which identified mild subclinical disease in the right eye. The left fundus and its angiogram are shown in **Fig. 21.20. What is the differential diagnosis, and what investigations would you arrange?**

There is clearly left (unilateral) peripheral retinal ischemia complicated by neovascularization and vitreous hemorrhage. In a patient emanating from an endemic area, TB must always be considered a cause of occlusive retinal vasculitis. Other causes include syphilis (but a complete absence of retinitis is unusual), sarcoidosis (not usually occlusive and not usually asymmetrical), primary retinal vasculitis (probably never unilateral) and non-inflammatory causes. He was not diabetic. His ACE level was normal and syphilis serology was negative. Organ function tests were unremarkable.

He also underwent investigations for TB. His chest radiograph showed old fibrotic changes with an emphysematous bulla in the left upper lobe, suggestive of previous TB but with no sign of activity. His interferon-γ test was positive and his Mantoux test was positive at 14 mm. **Is there enough evidence now to diagnose TB-related occlusive retinal vasculitis, and if so what treatment should he undergo?**

The chest radiograph is virtually pathognomonic of previous TB. Mantoux test positivity is common in those undergoing previous BCG Immunization and is therefore not in itself evidence of exposure to TB unless a substantial reaction is seen. It is unlikely that a 14-mm reaction would be seen solely due to previous BCG immunization. Interferon-γ testing is specific for wild TB and is therefore not confounded by BCG immunization (because BCG, derived from *M. bovis* rather than *M. tuberculosis*, has a different antigenic structure). Interferon-γ testing does not have 100% specificity or sensitivity but a positive result is highly relevant in this patient. There is acceptable evidence that this patient has had primary TB in the past and that the organisms therefore remain at least latent, if not active (interferon-γ testing cannot tell the difference) within the body. Does this mean that it is responsible for the retinal vasculitis? Having excluded other common causes, it seems likely. In the UK, it is recommended that any patient under 35 years with latent TB be treated to prevent the risk of future reactivation. However, this requires only 3 months of two anti-tuberculous drugs. As it is likely that TB is responsible for the retinal vasculitis (which is active) there is a good rationale for full anti-tuberculous chemotherapy in such patients, and this trial of therapy, if arresting deterioration, may effectively prove the etiology. He is therefore undergoing a standard full course of anti-tuberculous chemotherapy, comprising 2 months of rifampicin, isoniazid, pyrizinamide (together prescribed as Rifater) and ethambutol, to be followed by a further 4 months of rifampicin and isoniazid (together prescribed as Rifinah) alone.

He also underwent extensive sectoral peripheral retinal laser treatment to the areas of ischemia (**Fig. 21.21**). This was started promptly and completed as the vitreous hemorrhage cleared.

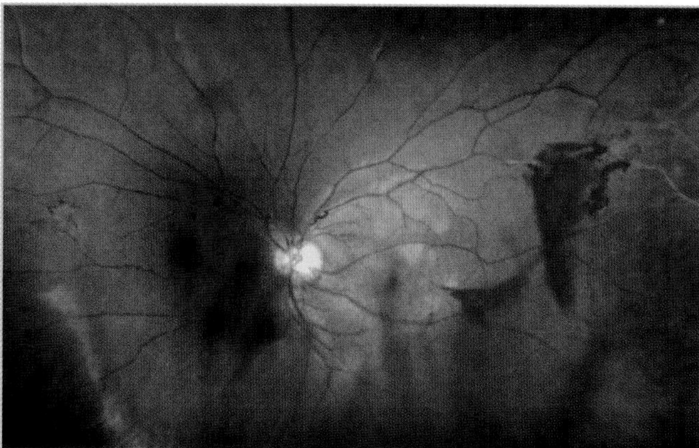

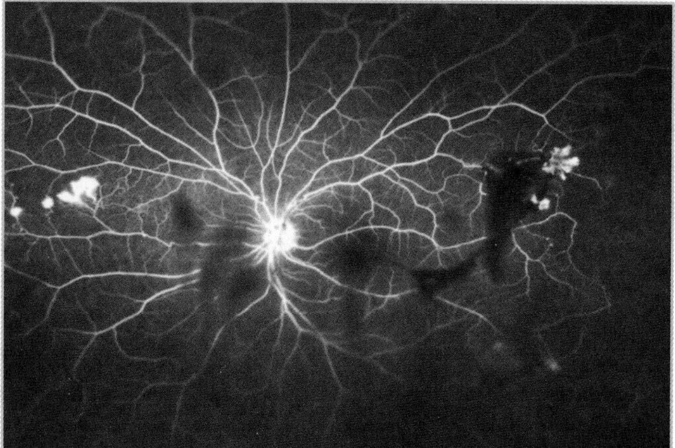

Figure 21.20 Case 11: widefield left fundus photography showing preretinal and vitreous hemorrhage emanating from fronds of retinal new vessels adjacent to ischemic areas.

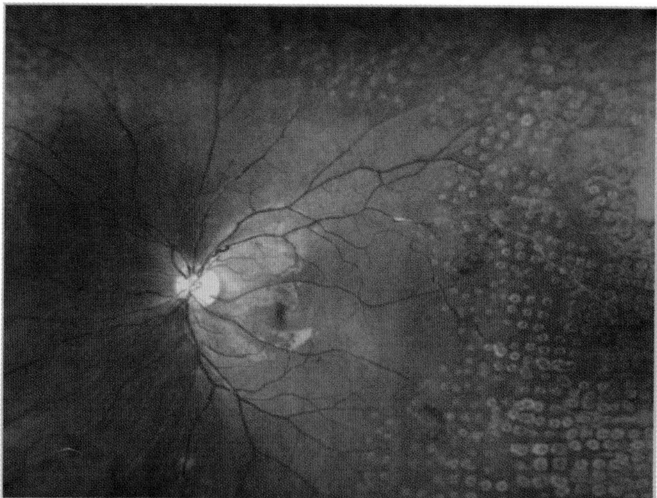

Figure 21.21 Case 11: left fundus after peripheral laser ablation showing regressing retinal new vessels and silver-wiring.

The neovascularization is now regressing, he has developed no further vitreous hemorrhage and he retains good central vision.

CASE 12: A FROSTY FUNDUS

With Karl Mercieca

A 26-year-old man presented with a 1-week history of bilateral, progressive, painless, visual loss. He had no significant past ocular history. He had a history of IgA nephropathy leading to renal failure and transplantation 1 year previously. The donor kidney was CMV positive and consequently the recipient underwent 3 months of prophylactic oral valganciclovir. He was immunosuppressed with tacrolimus 2.5 mg twice daily and prednisolone 20 mg once daily.

Shortly after finishing the post-transplant course of valganciclovir he had developed pyrexia and weight loss, and was diagnosed with systemic CMV infection. Treatment with oral valganciclovir was recommenced but proved ineffective, and intravenous foscarnet was administered, leading to a gradual reduction of the CMV load down to zero. This drug had been discontinued 2 weeks before the onset of his ocular symptoms. He had not undergone funduscopy before presentation.

At presentation his best-corrected VA was R 2/36 and L 2/18. He showed substantial bilateral anterior uveitis with 2+ cells and 2+ flare. IOPs were R 36 mmHg and L 30 mmHg. There was significant vitritis with cells and haze. Funduscopy revealed bilateral extensive frosted branch angiitis associated with peripheral intraretinal hemorrhages and retinal atrophy (**Fig. 21.22**). **What is the differential diagnosis? What investigations would you perform? Would you initiate treatment while waiting for results, and if so what?**

Many forms of retinal vasculitis (particularly phlebitis) cause significant exudation. Florid widespread perivascular exudation, colloquially known as 'frosted branch angiitis,' has a rather narrower differential diagnosis including primary idiopathic, CMV retinitis, other viral retinitis, toxoplasmosis, leukemia, lymphoma and Behçet's disease.

CMV retinitis often presents without systemic symptoms so the diagnosis must always be considered in post-transplantation patients. In this case, a clear history of CMV disease is already apparent. The probable diagnosis in this case is CMV retinitis; we considered it likely that he had developed a chronic indolent CMV retinitis which had been present for several weeks, masked by a partial response to systemic antiviral treatment, which then acutely worsened with extensive perivascular exudate, after withdrawal of the foscarnet. In view of the clinical history intravenous foscarnet 60 mg/kg three times daily was recommenced together with intravenous aciclovir 10 mg/kg three times daily, topical steroid and IOP-lowering agents.

Investigations revealed a moderately raised serum creatinine and herpesvirus serology. The CMV viral load was high at 912 789 copies/ml, log 5.96. He underwent AC tap for PCR testing, and intravitreal ganciclovir 2 mg was injected bilaterally. Despite the above treatment, the fundal picture remained unchanged with extensive exudative perivasculitis. Aqueous PCR testing was negative for VZV and HSV but highly positive for CMV (6140 000 copies/ml, log 6.96). Serological and aqueous fluid analysis using SANGER nucleotide sequencing confirmed ganciclovir resistance secondary to a combination of *UL97* and *L595S* mutations.

Fundus fluorescein angiography demonstrated extensive retinal ischemia, and OCT demonstrated substantial macular subretinal fluid (**Fig. 21.23**). **What treatment options would you consider at this stage? What are the potential side effects of such treatments?**

Ganciclovir either systemically or intravitreally will clearly be ineffective. High-dose foscarnet is nephrotoxic and the patient already has compromised renal function. It can be injected intravitreally but this would need to be frequent and bilateral. Cidofovir can be used intravenously and is also nephrotoxic, but cannot be injected intravitreally because it induces severe intraocular inflammation. In view of the ganciclovir-resistant CMV retinitis and the limited response to lower-dose systemic foscarnet, treatment was modified to higher-dose foscarnet and intravenous cidofovir. A better response was observed and therefore oral prednisolone was increased to 40 mg daily to treat the inflammatory component of the retinitis. VA improved to 6/24 in both eyes over a week, with significant reduction in the perivasculitis. **His creatinine level rose to 290. What would you do?**

The nephrotoxicity of foscarnet and cidofovir assumes particular relevance in patients who have undergone renal transplantation. It can be extremely difficult, for both patient and clinician, to weigh the benefit of vision-saving treatment against the risk of potential loss of a donor kidney. Intravitreal foscarnet could be used, avoiding systemic side effects, but weekly bilateral injections into the foreseeable future would be required, introducing risks including intraocular infection, hemorrhage and retinal tears in eyes that are highly prone to retinal detachment. In due course, as the retinitis settled, cidofovir was discontinued. Two weeks later the VA had improved to 6/9.5 bilaterally. However, new, bilateral, intravitreal, round, white to gray lesions were discovered. **What suspicion might this new finding raise and why?**

Our first thought with this new presentation was the possibility of fungal endophthalmitis relating to his intravenous access and immunosuppression. The patient's indwelling central venous

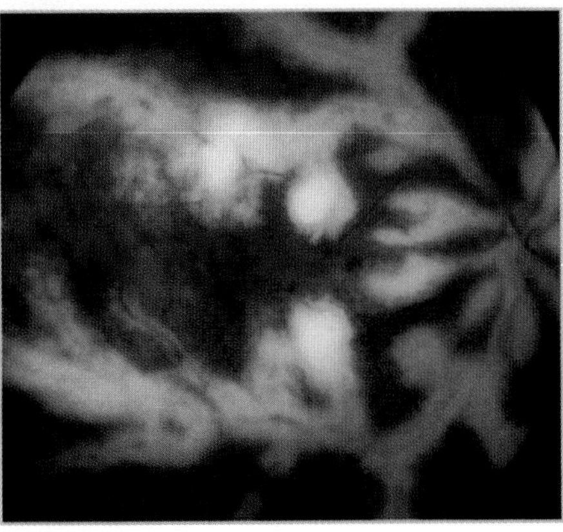

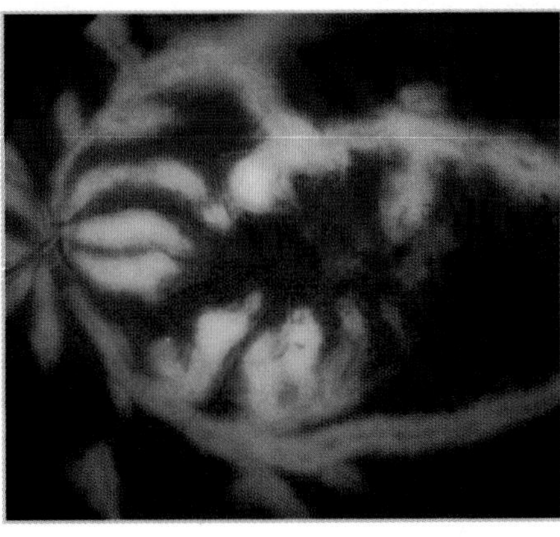

Figure 21.22 Case 12: bilateral florid frosted branch angiitis with massive perivascular exudation.

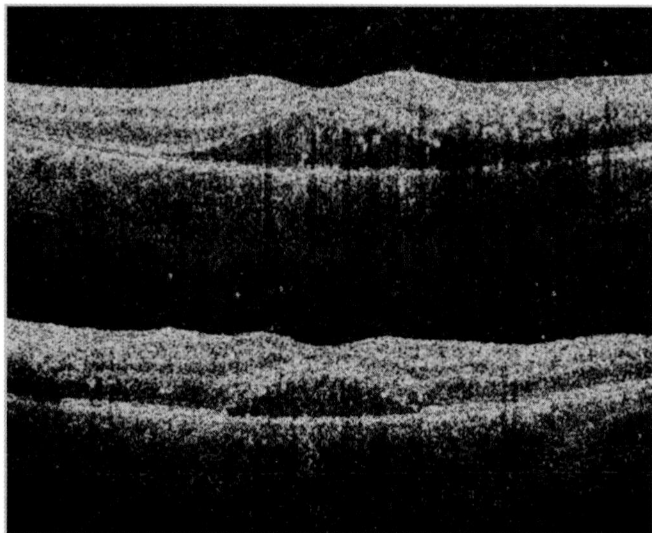

Figure 21.23 Case 12: right (above) and left (below) OCT of maculae.

catheter was a potential source and was removed for culture (which was negative). An AC tap was performed for fungal PCR analysis, which was also negative. The second possibility was that peripheral necrotic retina was fragmenting as a prelude to retinal detachment. However, careful funduscopy did not reveal a suspicion of incipient detachment. In due course, however, he did develop bilateral macula-on retinal detachment requiring vitrectomy, endolaser and silicone oil injection. Six months later his vision was 6/36 in both eyes (6/15 pinhole) (**Fig. 21.24**). On lower-dose foscarnet, renal function has remained poor but sustainable, and dialysis has not been required.

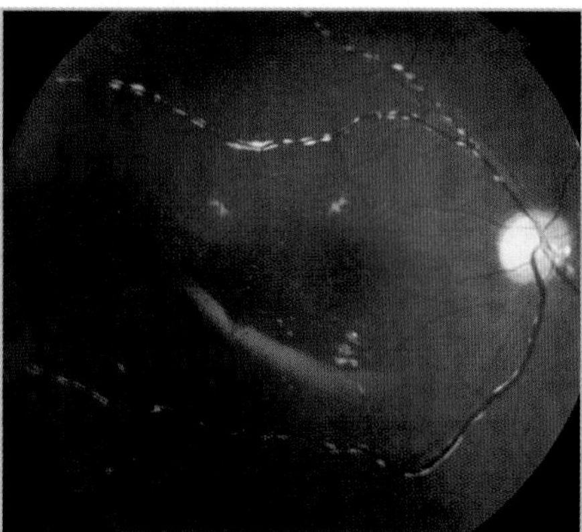

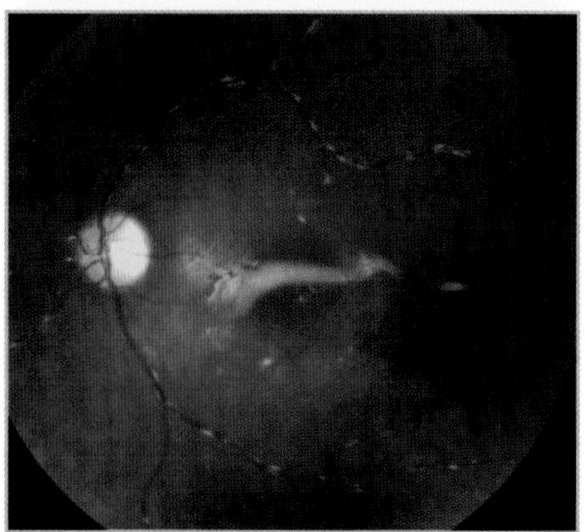

Figure 21.24 Case 12: following vitrectomy and silicone oil injection bilaterally for retinal detachment, the retinas are flat and he has residual perivascular exudate.

CASE 13: OLD DIAGNOSIS, NEW PERSPECTIVES ON IMAGING

With Robyn Troutbeck

A 42-year-old white man presented with decreased vision and floaters in his right eye over a 1-week period. He had previously undergone a kidney transplant after chronic renal failure resulting from recurrent pyelonephritis secondary to vesicoureteric reflux. He was using mycophenolate mofetil 1 g twice daily and prednisolone 10 mg once daily. Four weeks before his ophthalmic presentation he had developed chickenpox, which had resolved on a 7-day course of intravenous high-dose aciclovir. The VZV viral load was initially monitored, with a clear downward trend, and he was discharged from hospital. On presentation to the emergency eye centre his left eye saw 6/6 and showed no abnormality. However, his right eye demonstrated mild anterior uveitis, mild vitritis and gross peripheral fundal lesions as shown in **Fig. 21.25. What is your differential diagnosis, and how would you manage him?**

This is about as straightforward a diagnosis as possible in the context of these very typical signs and a strongly suggestive history. He clearly has ARN caused by VZV. This is the most common virus to cause ARN and is usually the most severe in presentation. A significant minority presenting with VZV ARN have a recent history of shingles (rather than chickenpox) but the latter will do as a clear indicator. Interestingly, he had little inflammation either in AC or vitreous (because he was significantly immunosuppressed). Stretching possibilities to make a differential diagnosis, lymphoma occasionally presents, mimicking ARN, as does toxoplasmosis. Other infections do not. If the diagnosis had not been so clear, he would have undergone an immediate aqueous tap, to be sent for viral PCR for herpesviruses including HSV-1 and -2, VZV and CMV.

He was immediately started on aciclovir intravenously; the dose was carefully calculated in consultation with his nephrologist in view

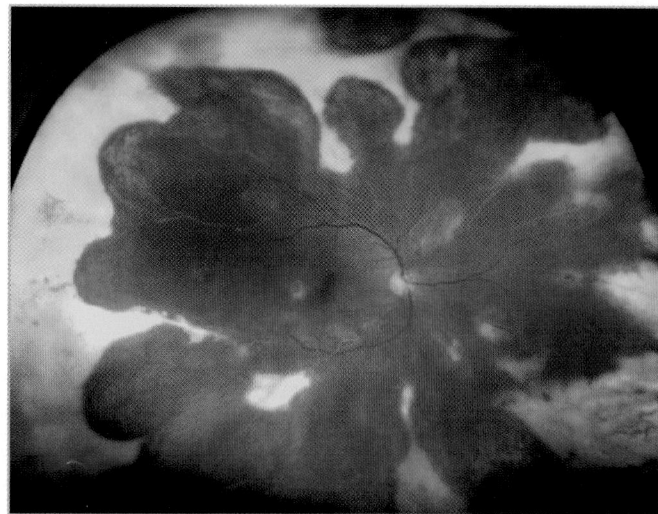

Figure 21.25 Case 13: widefield fundus photography showing almost circumferential, confluent acute retinal necrosis with tongues of extension posteriorly, and occlusive arteriolitis.

of his deranged glomerular filtration rate. As a result of his widespread severe vascular occlusion we elected to give an intravitreal injection of ganciclovir (2 mg in 0.1 ml). For the same reason he was commenced on aspirin 75 mg once daily. The vitritis was mild and so his steroid dosage was unaltered. His intravenous treatment continued for 10 days, during which time his serum viral load again decreased and his retinitis clearly began to settle. He was therefore discharged home on adjusted full-dose oral valaciclovir (**Fig. 21.26**). **Would you do anything else?**

In a patient presenting with ARN and no clear predisposing factors, we would always check for innate or acquired immune deficiency. However, in this case iatrogenic immunosuppression was clearly present (and would be required in future). The evidence for the efficacy of a laser barrage to prevent subsequent rhegmatogenous detachment is mixed and, although we are normally proactive in this way, in this case the extent and complexity of retinal involvement made effective barrage too difficult to consider. Antiviral was reduced to a maintenance dose of aciclovir 400 mg twice daily after 3 months

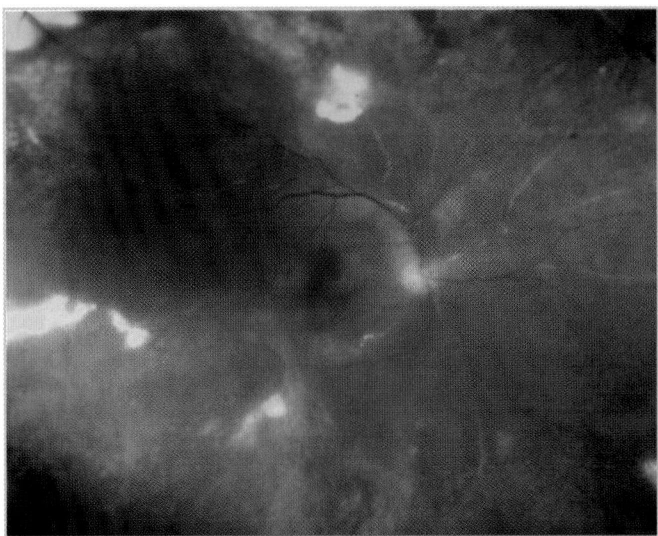

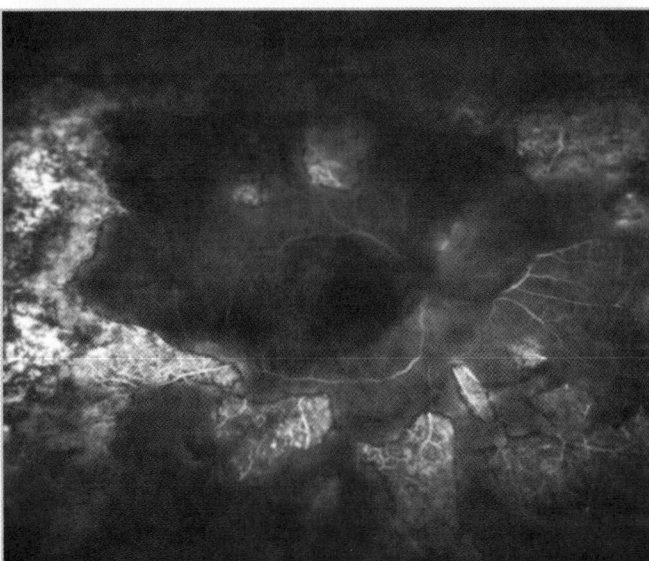

Figure 21.26 Case 13: the fundus 4 weeks after commencing treatment shows resolving retinitis leaving atrophy with residual exudate, and central vitreous condensation. After a further 2 months an FFA shows the extent of vascular shutdown and peripheral ischemia.

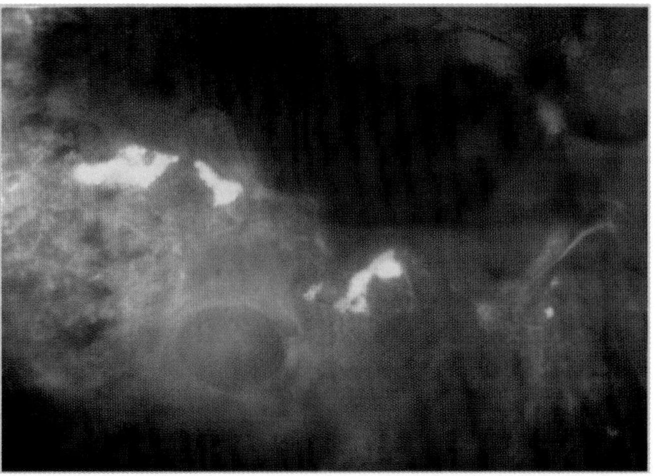

Figure 21.27 Case 13: inferior retinal detachment with a large break.

(at which time he had an undetectable serum viral load). It is our normal practice to continue maintenance treatment for 12 months. The other eye remains unaffected. Nine months after presentation, at routine review he retains 6/12 acuity (despite central vitreous condensation), but was found to have inferior retinal detachment with a large break (**Fig. 21.27**) and will undergo vitrectomy with silicone oil injection.

CASE 14: WHEN THE EYE DOESN'T FIT THE PATIENT

With Romi Chhabra

A 68-year-old farmer's wife lived all of her life in the mountains of Albania but for the first time left her country to visit her son in the UK. She presented with a 2-month history of a left upper visual field defect, floaters and photopsia, with intermittent frontal headache. She was otherwise fit and well. There was no history of exposure to TB and she had received BCG immunization as a child.

At presentation her VA was R 6/7.5, L 6/60. The right eye was normal on examination. There was no anterior segment inflammation in the left eye but it showed mild vitritis, subtle macular edema and, inferiorly, dense vitreous opacification overlying a pale peripheral retinal elevation (**Fig. 21.28**). **What is your differential diagnosis?**

Inferior vitreous opacification with underlying density is strongly suggestive of intermediate uveitis, but this is only very rarely unilateral and does not present in this age group. This presentation is entirely compatible with toxocariasis, but this disease is virtually unheard of in this age group. Fungal infection might be considered but there were no underlying risk factors. Peripheral nodular telangiectasis might be a possibility. Other neoplasia should be considered, as might longstanding organized vitreous hemorrhage overlying a retinal detachment.

Clinically, despite her age, toxocariasis was thought most likely on the basis of clinical appearance. Toxocara serology was arranged, together with ACE and basic bloods. In the meantime it was considered appropriate to commence prednisolone 30 mg/day.

Two weeks later vision had improved to 6/24 and toxocara serology was strongly positive. The inferior vitreous had cleared substantially to reveal a peripheral granuloma with surrounding gliosis and a band of vitreoretinal adhesion with its apex towards the optic disk (**Fig. 21.29**). **Now that the diagnosis of ocular toxocariasis seems secure, how would you treat it?**

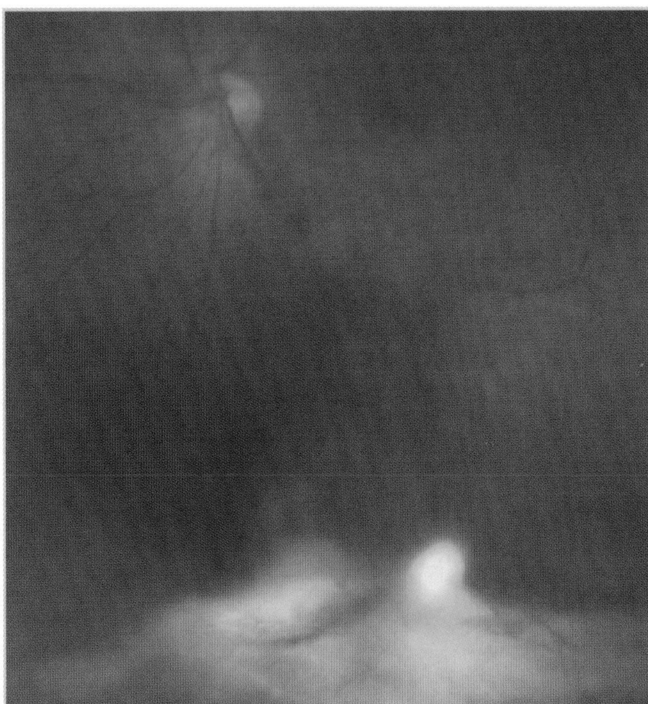

Figure 21.28 Case 14: on presentation, an inferior pale elevation with dense overlying vitritis.

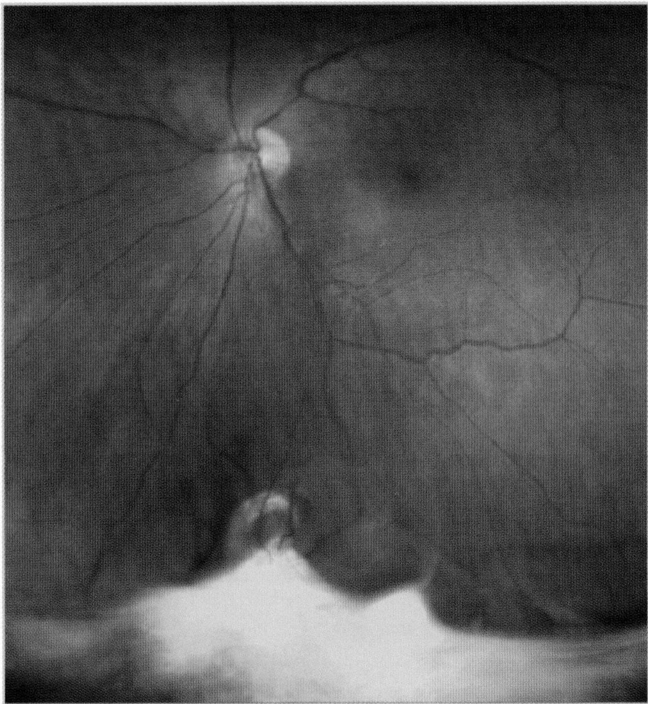

Figure 21.29 Case 14: oral steroid treatment has cleared vitreous substantially, to reveal a typical peripheral toxocara granuloma.

There is no good evidence that systemic anthelmintic treatment is effective for ocular toxocariasis. Initial treatment with systemic steroid is clearly reducing inflammation. There is no evidence of retinal traction sufficient to justify surgery. Both surgery and cryotherapy have led to worsened inflammation. It was decided to administer a tapering regimen of oral steroid during her remaining weeks in the UK.

At her final visit 8 weeks after presentation, using prednisolone 7.5 mg/day vision had improved to 6/12 with resolution of macular edema and negligible central vitritis. Instructions on a further slow treatment taper were given and she returned home to Albania with a recommendation that she be reviewed if possible by an ophthalmologist within 3 months. Had she remained in the UK our preference would be for her to be re-started on oral steroid with a slow subsequent taper and to remain on low-dose treatment if necessary. Retinal traction of vitreal traction bands may necessitate future surgery.

Had this patient been a 10-year-old child, the clinical appearance would have immediately suggested toxocariasis. However, to our knowledge no patient of this age has been described with ocular toxocariasis. This woman lived in a rural environment with several unwormed dogs at her farm. Such environments raise the risk of adult-onset toxocariasis.

CASE 15: CONFLICTING INTERESTS FOR MOTHER AND BABY

With Laura Steeples

A healthy 25-year-old woman presented during week 35 of her first pregnancy with acute painless loss of vision in her left eye. Her past medical, ocular and obstetric histories were unremarkable.

The visual acuity was R 6/6, L 1/60. Granulomatous KPs, AC cells + and vitritis ++ were noted in the left eye. Funduscopy revealed a single white elevated focus of inflammation with poorly defined margins on the inferotemporal vascular arcade (**Fig. 21.30**). There was associated vasculitis with sheathing and attenuation, particularly affecting the superior and inferior temporal arcades. The macular OCT demonstrated substantial subretinal fluid. The right eye was unaffected. **What is the differential diagnosis? Would you arrange any investigations? While awaiting the results of these, is immediate treatment necessary?**

A single focus of acute retinitis with panuveitis may have several causes, but toxoplasmosis is the most common, with or without associated chorioretinal scarring. The differential diagnosis includes TB, syphilis, Behçet's disease, atypical viral retinitis, bartonellosis and fungal endophthalmitis. Most of these are associated with systemic disease or clear underlying predisposition. A working diagnosis of primary ocular toxoplasmosis was made (because the focus of inflammation was typical for this condition, but no clinical evidence of an old chorioretinal scar could be found in either eye). The proximity of this lesion to essential structures, and the primary and secondary inflammatory effects mandate immediate steroid treatment, covered by anti-toxoplasma antibiotic. Nevertheless, serology was arranged because true negative toxoplasma serology requires further investigation. **This woman was in the third trimester of pregnancy. Which treatment for toxoplasmosis is safe at this stage?**

Toxoplasmosis during pregnancy must be managed with care. In addition to the potential direct risk to the fetus of primary toxoplasmosis, some antibiotics can be harmful. In practice the risk at week 35 is very small, but in this case oral spiramycin 1 g three times daily and prednisolone 40 mg/day, together with topical steroids and mydriasis, were prescribed. Toxoplasma serology was IgM negative but IgG positive. **How do you interpret this result?**

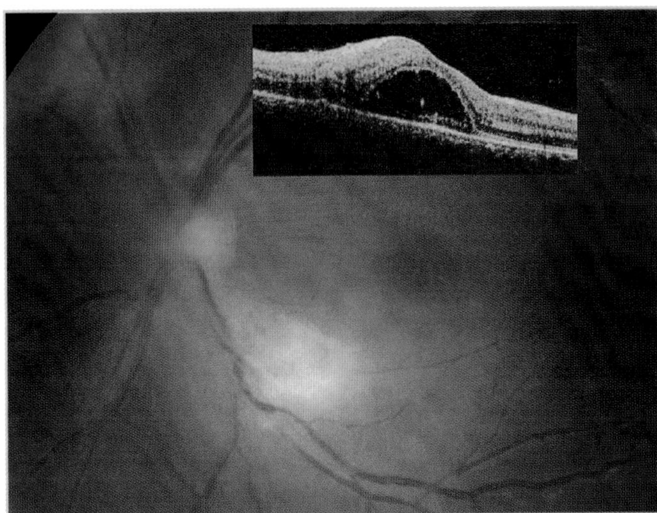

Figure 21.30 Case 15: a focus of inner retinal inflammation is associated with substantial subretinal fluid under the macula as shown on OCT.

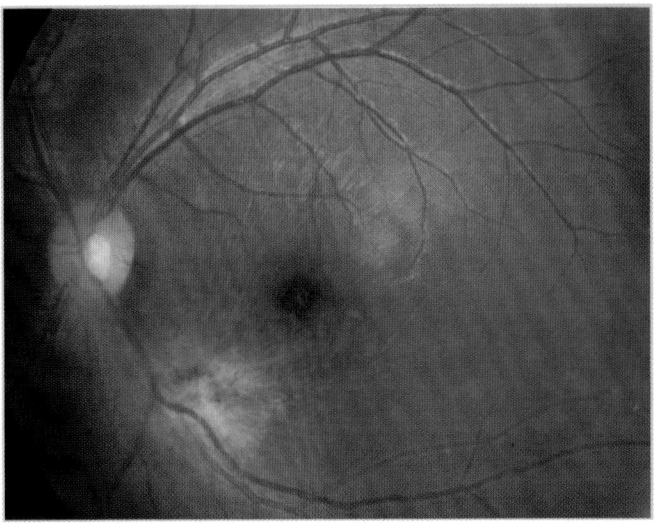

Figure 21.31 Case 15: the resolved focus of inflammation showing slight epiretinal fibrosis.

Positive IgG serology (at any titer) proves previous exposure to *Toxoplasma* sp. Negative IgM serology may indicate that this is indeed recurrent toxoplasmosis rather than primary disease, or that the sample was too early; if necessary it can be repeated, and IgM positivity will confirm primary disease. In this instance no change in management would result so no further testing was performed. Occasionally a small chorioretinal scar of previous toxoplasmosis can be covered by a new focus, rendering it invisible. If in doubt, intraocular fluid sampling for toxoplasma PCR can prove infection.

After 2 weeks the left vision improved to 6/24 and inflammation was settling. A healthy baby was delivered at 39 weeks' gestation, with no evidence of congenital infection. Spiramycin was stopped after delivery and prednisolone was tapered over 4 weeks. The retinal lesion changed to a chorioretinal pigmented scar, and all vasculitis and macular edema settled leaving VA of 6/9 (**Fig. 21.31**). **If this patient had presented at week 15 of pregnancy with primary toxoplasmosis, what management decisions would have been necessary?**

Management choices depend upon, first, whether the infection is primary (where there is a risk of fetal malformation or TORCH syndrome) or recurrent (where the risk is very small to negligible unless the mother is immunodeficient), gestational stage (because major problems may affect the fetus earlier in pregnancy), maternal co-morbidities, and the site of ocular pathology and its risk to vision. Systemic treatment should be strongly considered in primary infection (or reactivated disease in immunocompromised mothers) because the fetus may also be infected. Sight-threatening lesions require treatment. The obstetrician should become involved early, during the first trimester. Surveillance including regular ultrasonography is important; therapeutic abortion may be considered.

All treatments carry a risk of fetal toxicity, particularly in the first trimester. Patients must be informed of these risks. Treatment requires multidisciplinary decisions on the risks and benefits to maternal and fetal health. Intravitreal clindamycin injection is an alternative strategy with potential to limit systemic effects and fetal toxicity. Lastly, it may be appropriate to observe, without treatment, non-sight threatening recurrences in pregnancy.

CASE 16: THE EYE WAS TYPICAL, BUT NOTHING ELSE WAS

With Laura Steeples

A 34-year-old healthy white man presented with a 2-day history of acute painless loss of vision in the left eye. He had no significant past medical or ophthalmic history. He had not traveled abroad recently. The visual acuity was R 6/6 and L HM. The right eye was entirely normal. He had severe left panuveitis with cells +++ in the anterior chamber (no fibrin, no hypopyon), severe vitritis and florid occlusive vasculitis with severe perivenous exudate, involving the inferior retina and the left macula (**Fig. 21.32**). **What is your differential diagnosis? What specific questions would you ask?**

The fundus image shows, through severe viritis (clearly of acute onset), occlusive retinal vasculitis with substantial perivascular exudate and hemorrhage, together with some patches of retinitis. There is a clear differential diagnosis: rapid-onset unilateral inflammation with occlusive retinal vasculitis is very suggestive of Behçet's disease and therefore we enquired into other potential symptoms; he had no history of oral ulceration, no genital ulceration, no skin rash, no arthropathy, no bowel problems, no chest problems, no headache or neurological symptoms, and no thrombotic episodes. He therefore offered no other evidence of Behçet's disease.

Viral retinitis with vasculitis was considered. CMV infection was very unlikely in a healthy immunocompetent patient and the disease behavior was much more aggressive than typical CMV retinitis. However, hematology with viral serology and immune function was checked, all being normal. Both HSV and VZV could conceivably (but very unusually) cause such a picture. Although unlikely, he nevertheless immediately underwent an AC tap, which showed no evidence of herpesviruses on PCR. Syphilis was considered; serology was negative. Rarely, florid perivenous exudation occurs in sarcoidosis (although more commonly bilaterally and never this acutely) but his ACE level and chest radiograph were normal. Aggressive TB-related Eales' disease may also cause such florid perivenous exudate, but not with an acute history in the absence of vitreous hemorrhage. His risk of TB

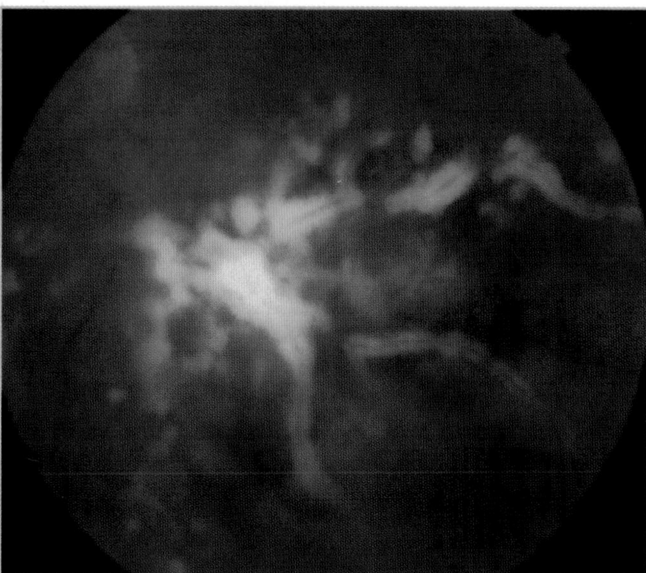

Figure 21.32 Case 16: the left fundus at presentation.

Figure 21.33 Case 16: the fundus 1 week after reintroducing high-dose oral steroid shows resolving multifocal retinitis and optic atrophy.

was carefully considered; he had no personal or contact history, had undergone BCG immunization and did not work in a risk occupation. He had not traveled to an endemic area. It was thought highly unlikely that TB was the cause and he required immediate anti-inflammatory treatment so that TB testing was not feasible. A working diagnosis of ocular Behçet's disease was made, on the basis of a typical ocular presentation. **What treatment would you initiate and how urgently?**

High-dose oral corticosteroids or intravenous methylprednisolone forms the mainstay of treatment of all acute-onset, non-infective, sight-threatening uveitis. In this instance oral prednisolone 80 mg/day (1.25 mg/kg per day) was initiated immediately alongside valaciclovir 1 g three times daily (to cover for herpetic infection while awaiting the result of aqueous PCR; this was shortly discontinued). Intensive topical steroid and mydriatic agent were used to treat the anterior uveitis. The panuveitis gradually improved and the steroids were tapered to 30 mg/day over several weeks. Unfortunately it was clear from the outset that he had sustained irreversible ischemic macular damage and he retained only hand movement vision in the upper hemifield. While on prednisolone 30 mg/day he developed a severe recurrence of posterior inflammation incorporating multifocal retinitis in both hemifields, with vasculitis (**Fig. 21.33**), and higher-dose steroid was resumed. **What would you do at this stage of his management?**

He clearly cannot manage on oral steroid alone. Despite early central visual loss the remaining left vision needs protection, first because it is navigationally useful and second because there is a high likelihood of right eye involvement at some stage. He was commenced on immunosuppression with ciclosporin 5 mg/kg per day. This drug was poorly tolerated and he developed intractable and persistent tremor with peripheral paraesthesiae and malaise. Dose reduction was attempted but he developed two further episodes of acute flare-up of left panuveitis. Further immunosuppression with mycophenolate mofetil was commenced at 1 g twice daily and subsequently 1.5 g twice daily after discontinuing ciclosporin. He developed a further flare-up while reducing prednisolone below 45 mg/day. He was now Cushingoid but bone densitometry was normal. He had glycosuria. **What would you do? What is the risk to the other eye?**

The majority of cases are eventually bilateral, although there may be a delay of a decade or more before involvement of the other eye. Long-term steroids are inadequate to prevent recurrence or progression. In this man's case, despite combined immunosuppression the disease remained active and the risk to the second eye is a significant concern to the medical team and the patient. One option was to be pragmatic and explain that the left eye was effectively lost and that treatment should be tailed off. However, he remained adamant in support of aggressive treatment despite at all times being fully appraised of the potential for steroid-induced problems including permanent diabetes. He underwent a glucose tolerance test, which was clearly abnormal and was started on hypoglycemic treatment. Anti-TNF biologic agents are not routinely funded in the UK for ocular inflammation. Cyclophosphamide may be used and can induce disease remission, but he wished to have another child. An appeal for special funding was made and granted for three infusions of infliximab. He underwent Mantoux and interferon-γ testing for TB (despite the difficulty in interpretation forced by the confounding factor of his current oral steroid and immunosuppressive treatment). His Mantoux was completely negative, as was his interferon-γ test. He was considered to be a true negative (which is important to establish before using anti-TNF treatment). He underwent the first at 5 mg/kg and after 2 days developed severe intractable headache, malaise and dysphoria. Nevertheless he agreed to a second infusion at 2 weeks, which caused a similar but less severe reaction. Currently he continues to reduce prednisolone dosage and is using 20 mg/day; he continues full-dose mycophenolate and awaits his next infusion. To date his right eye has remained uninvolved: VA R 6/5, L HM.

CASE 17: PRIMUM NON NOCERE (HIPPOCRATES): IS THE TREATMENT WORSE THAN THE DISEASE?

With Romi Chhabra

A 64-year-old white man presented to his local hospital with a 10-day history of cobwebs in the right vision. This eye had always been slightly the weaker of the two. He was noted to have mild panuveitis in both eyes. Funduscopy revealed scattered, subtle, creamy, oval retinal lesions (**Fig. 21.34**), and a diagnosis of birdshot retinochoroidopathy was suggested. He proved to be HLA-A29 positive and underwent fluorescein angiography. He was commenced on oral prednisolone 20 mg/day. He was referred to the MUC for further management. **Do you agree with the diagnosis? What parameters would you use to initiate and monitor treatment?**

At his first visit (using prednisolone 20 mg/day) he saw R 6/12 and L 6/7.5. Although his anterior chamber was quiet, there was moderate vitritis. He had subtle active retinitis. OCT showed bilateral macular edema. This clinical appearance, together with his HLA-A29 positivity, is entirely in keeping with the diagnosis of birdshot retinochoroidopathy. We excluded sarcoidosis by finding a normal ACE and chest radiograph.

Birdshot retinochoroidopathy is a condition with widely variable severity but is usually an inexorable low-grade inflammation with accumulating macular damage. A few patients do not need treatment. However, chronic macular edema (sometimes diffuse rather than cystoid) necessitates adequate treatment. The starting dose of prednisolone was not adequate. It was increased to 50 mg/day for 2 weeks, then 40 mg/day for a further 2 weeks (he was 80 kg). It was clear at 4 weeks that he had an inadequate response to oral steroids alone. **What would you do?**

Most patients with birdshot need oral immunosuppression to prevent deterioration. Raising the steroid dosage to 1 mg/kg per day may well be helpful in the short term but would only delay the start of immunosuppression. Our first-choice agent in normotensive men with birdshot is ciclosporin, which was started at 150 mg twice daily (about 4 mg/kg per day). **What potential for side effects would you mention to patients starting treatment?**

Our patients are provided with comprehensive information on the potential for side effects (which are not often severe and rarely abruptly so) with instructions to persist with treatment if mild, but to stop if severe. We review after 2 weeks of treatment. Within a few hours of taking his first tablet, he developed severe problems including nausea, shivers, numbness and weakness in arms and legs, and cramps. He discontinued treatment after 2 days. After further discussion and a delay to permit symptoms to subside, azathioprine 50 mg twice daily was started. He developed no adverse symptoms but his lymphocyte count fell from 1.85 to 0.74 in 4 weeks, and was 0.55 at 6 weeks. Thiopurine *S*-methyltransferase (TPMT) assay demonstrated a slightly low secretion. **What would you do?**

Lymphopenia is an intrinsic part of azathioprine action, up to a point. Opinions on tolerable lymphopenia differ among doctors, and physicians dealing with multisystem inflammation tend to be less tolerant. Infection rates in these patients are higher and prophylactic co-trimoxazole is frequently prescribed if the count falls to 0.6 or below. The risk is far lower for fit ophthalmological patients. At this stage his azathioprine appeared to have contributed significantly because VA had improved to R 6/9, L 6/6, with OCT confirming a dry L macula but persistent mild residual R edema. Azathioprine was reduced to 50 mg once daily and an orbital floor injection of methylprednisolone 80 mg was administered. Four weeks later the R macula was dry with normal VA. Oral steroids continued to taper but at 15 mg/day he developed increased floaters and his VA was R 6/18, L 6/7.5 with reactivated vitritis and OCT scans as shown in **Fig. 21.35. What would you do?**

He did not appear to be able safely to tolerate normal-dose azathioprine and could clearly not tolerate ciclosporin. He demonstrated ongoing sight-threatening inflammation despite an unacceptable dose of oral steroid. We discontinued azathioprine, provided him with information on mycophenolate mofetil and injected R intravitreal triamcinolone. It is necessary to allow azathioprine to 'wash out,' preferably for 4 weeks, before commencing mycophenolate. His R IOP rose to 44 mmHg and this was treated topically. He underwent bone densitometry which showed osteopenia. Bone risk was assessed; he was advised (again) to stop smoking and weight-bearing exercise was encouraged. Mycophenolate mofetil was commenced at 500 mg twice daily and, as this was well tolerated at 2 weeks, it was increased to the standard dosage of 1 g twice daily. After 3 months his prednisolone dosage was 10 mg/day, he had residual bilateral macular edema and the R IOP was back up to 34 mmHg on maximal topical medication. He was commenced on acetazolamide sustained release 250 mg twice daily (with the intention of both lowering IOP and hopefully contributing to macular edema reduction). Three weeks later, he reported intense right-sided loin pain and mild

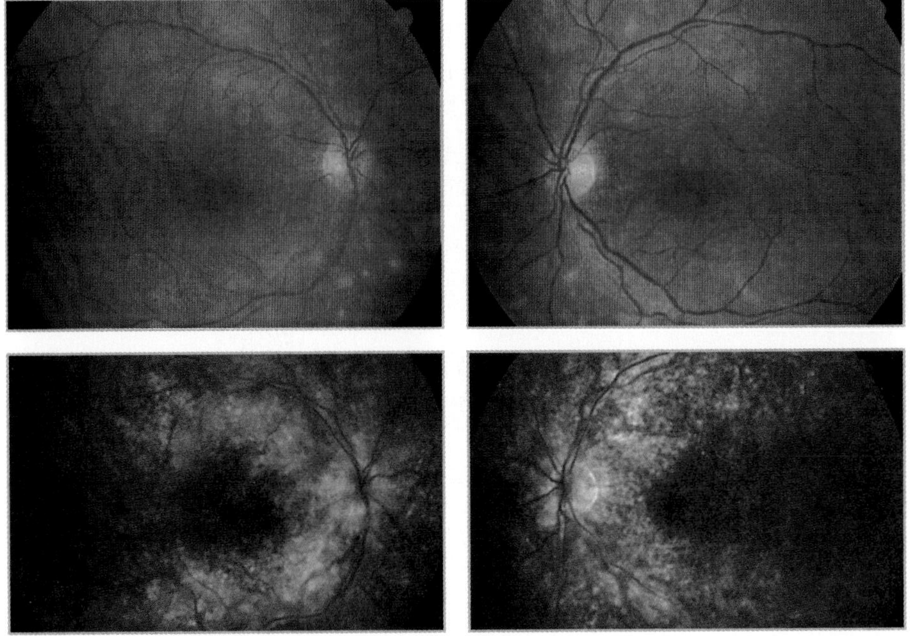

Figure 21.34 Case 17: the fundi at presentation.

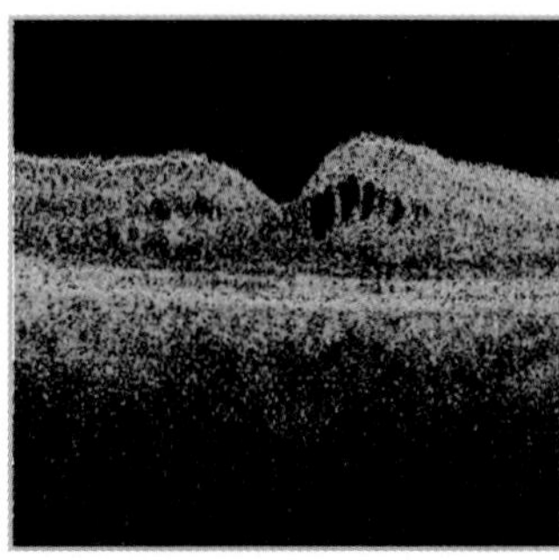
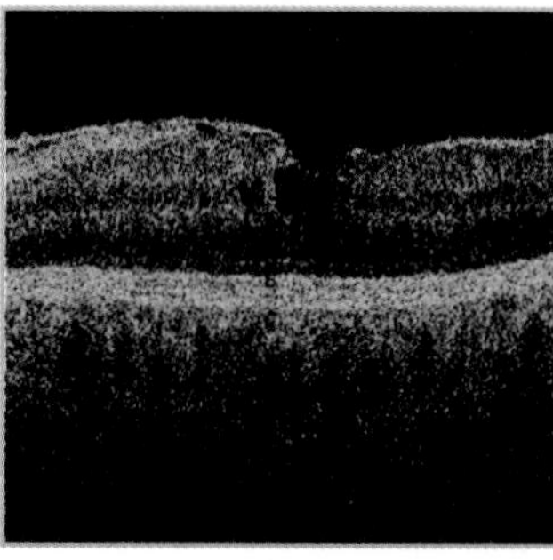

Figure 21.35 Case 17: recurrent bilateral macular edema following a taper of oral steroid treatment.

hematuria, and was hospitalized by the general surgeons and found to have renal calculi. He was prescribed an antispasmodic and, after a further episode of renal colic, passed stones and became symptom free. **Is this iatrogenic?**

Acetazolamide is well known to cause renal calculi after chronic use, but such a rapid response must be rare. His other drugs do not cause stones. As a precaution it was necessary to stop his acetazolamide. His lymphocyte count dropped further to 0.4 and he developed mild thrombocytopenia at 133. His oral steroids were reduced to 10 mg/day and his mycophenolate to 500 mg twice daily. He was started on co-trimoxazole prophylaxis 960 mg three times weekly. Fortunately his IOP improved and his maculae were dry. Currently he has acceptable visual acuity but mild vitritis. We continue to monitor him closely.

CASE 18: UNILATERAL PANUVEITIS IN A YOUNG ASIAN MAN

With Karl Mercieca

An 18-year-old healthy male Asian student presented with a 2-day history of left ocular pain and blurred vision. There was no previous ophthalmic history and, particularly, no eye trauma. There was no relevant past medical history and he denied the use of recreational drugs. He was apyrexial.

Visual acuity was R 6/5 and L CF. The right eye was entirely normal on examination. The left eye had panuveitis including very severe fibrinous anterior uveitis with hypopyon, extensive posterior synechiae, severe vitritis and a poor fundal view. The IOP was 15 mmHg in both eyes. **What is your differential diagnosis? What tests would you carry out? How would you treat this in the first instance?**

Our differential diagnosis included infective endophthalmitis, syphilis, TB, toxoplasmosis, toxocariasis, HSV and VZV infection. Investigation results included a normal chest radiograph, normal ACE, negative serology for syphilis, toxoplasmosis, toxocariasis and HLA-B27 positivity. His ESR was not raised. Blood cultures found no evidence of bacteremia or fungemia. Oral prednisolone 1 mg/kg per day and aciclovir 800 mg five times daily were commenced, in addition to intensive topical steroids and mydriatic. He underwent an urgent diagnostic vitrectomy. Intraoperative findings included dense vitreous haze and an opaque vitreous base with snowbanking and peripheral vascular sheathing. Intravitreal cefuroxime and vancomycin were injected. Microbiological samples were negative on microscopy and culture, and herpesvirus PCRs were negative. His aciclovir was discontinued. A working diagnosis was made, of very severe HLA-B27-associated uveitis, mimicking endophthalmitis. **What are the potential complications of his management so far?**

Acute side effects of high-dose systemic steroid include increased appetite and weight gain, mood swings and psychosis, fluid retention, osteonecrosis, and myopathy or pancreatitis. However, he tolerated treatment well. The risks of pars plana vitrectomy include lens touch, cataract formation, infection and iatrogenic retinal tears/detachment. In this case, there was inadvertent lens touch during surgery. He therefore underwent lensectomy during the procedure; there was no possibility of IOL implantation during acute inflammation and he was left aphakic. Postoperatively the IOP was low (3–7 mmHg) for a prolonged period, and improvement in inflammation was slow. On attempting tapering of prednisolone the uveitis flared up very substantially on three occasions, with a drop in IOP to 0–3 mmHg, necessitating enhanced steroid treatment. He refused intravitreal steroid injection. In the months after presentation he developed low back pain with stiffness and was diagnosed by a rheumatologist with ankylosing spondylitis. The corrected VA 2 months postoperatively was 6/6 but he was using semi-intensive topical medication and could not tolerate a contact lens. **What other treatment options would you consider?**

He clearly required oral immunosuppression. Methotrexate was chosen, rising to 20 mg weekly, with folic acid 5 mg weekly. This lowed a prednisolone taper initially down to below 10 mg/day but a further severe flare-up necessitated high-dose steroid again. His bone densitometry was normal. Nine months after starting methotrexate he developed problematic nausea, and the option of alternative immunosuppression was considered. At this stage he was using prednisolone 5 mg/day. After discussion with the rheumatologists his methotrexate was reduced to 5 mg weekly and mycophenolate mofetil 500 mg twice daily was started. However, he could not tolerate this owing to increased nausea and bowel upset, so azathioprine 50 mg twice daily was used. He tolerated this well and methotrexate was stopped. His eye remained uninflamed and over several months his prednisolone was gingerly tapered and discontinued. However, within 4 weeks he again presented with painful panuveitis and hypopyon. After urgent steroid treatment his azathioprine dose was increased to 150 mg daily. Owing to recurrent inflammation on conventional immunosuppression, adalimumab injection 40 mg every 2 weeks was instituted. Five years after presentation the uveitis is quiescent using azathioprine 50 mg twice daily, adalimumab 40 mg every 2 weeks and topical prednisolone acetate twice daily. The right eye remains unaffected. The left remains aphakic with best-corrected VA of 6/7.5 (but he chooses not to wear a contact lens), moderate intraocular flare and an IOP <10 mmHg but not falling. His macula is dry. His back is pain free.

CASE 19: SUSPICIONS CORRECT …

A 28-year-old man, born and raised in Kashmir but recently arrived in the UK, presented with a 3-month history of painless blurred vision in the right eye. He was fit and well with no previous medical history of significance. His VA was R6/18, L6/6. He had normal anterior segments, no cells in aqueous or vitreous, but an abnormal right fundus showing multiple, patchy, irregularly shaped chorioretinal scars in the posterior pole, with no sign of active inflammation. The left fundus was normal. He was referred to MUC for a further opinion, and was seen 2 months later. At this time, although VA was unchanged, his fundi were as shown in **Fig. 21.36. How would you investigate this?**

It is now clear that he has a bilateral atypical placoid-like chorioretinitis, with active contiguous extensions of inflammation on the left side. It is clearly progressive. This is 'ampiginous choroidopathy.' He had spent most of his life in a TB-endemic area. Although he had no personal history of the disease, two family members had been treated for this before he arrived in the UK. He had received no prophylaxis and had not undergone BCG immunization. TB testing was therefore arranged, which showed a highly positive Mantoux test at 18 mm with central ulceration, and a positive interferon-γ test. His chest radiograph was normal. He was seronegative for syphilis.

A working diagnosis of TB-related chorioretinitis was made. He was commenced on the UK-standard anti-tuberculous chemotherapy course including 2 months of Rifater (combined isoniazid, rifampicin and pyrazinamide) with ethambutol and pyridoxine, followed by 4 months of Rifinah 300 (combined isoniazid and rifampicin). He tolerated treatment well, with no abnormality of liver function and no neurological side effects. His intraocular inflammation became quiescent. At the latest review he saw R 6/9, L 6/9, and was inflammation-free and well (**Fig. 21.37**).

TB may or may not have been the cause of this atypical placoid-like chorioretinitis but, where placoid disease is atypical in appearance or progressive, investigating for, and treating, TB, if located, is essential.

CASE 20: TO TREAT OR NOT TO TREAT?

With Romi Chhabra

A 50-year-old white woman was referred to her local ophthalmologist after presenting to her optometrist with right metamorphopsia of 4 weeks' duration. She saw R 6/12, L 6/6. On examination there were no cells in aqueous or vitreous. The L eye was normal. Her R retina showed multiple, apparently longstanding chorioretinal scars, both macular and peripapillary. She was also felt to have an active extrafoveal lesion, shown in **Fig. 21.38**, and was referred to the MUC. **What is your differential diagnosis?**

These smallish, atrophic scars, specifically with some peripapillary involvement, are indicative of PIC or POHS. She was a nurse but not exposed occupationally to TB. She had traveled previously to the West Indies and had worked in Afghanistan. She underwent histoplasma serology which was negative. The angiogram shows a small choroidal neovascular membrane inferior to the fovea, which looked partly fibrosed. Her symptoms were improving spontaneously without treatment and her VA had risen to 6/7.5. **What would you do?**

The choice is: observe; give oral steroid; use PDT; or inject intravitreal anti-VEGF. We chose to observe. One month later she re-presented with sudden deterioration of vision to 6/36 and her retinal appearance is shown in **Fig. 21.39. What would you do now?**

Her angiogram clearly showed a large, predominantly classic, choroidal neovascular membrane with significant leak, and

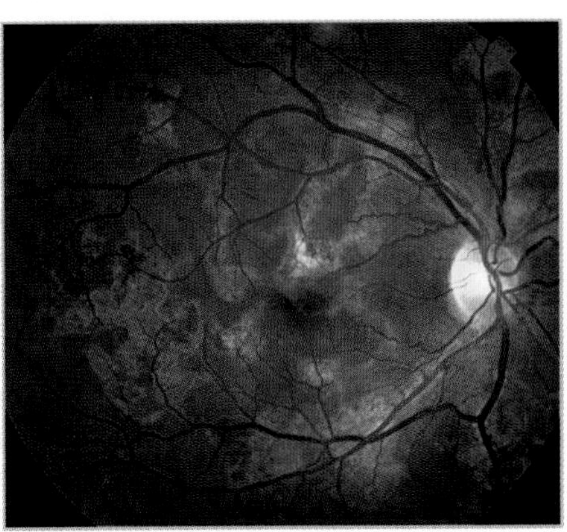
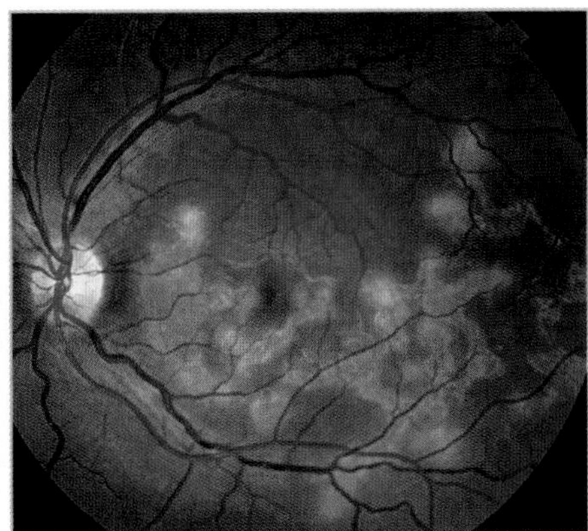

Figure 21.36 Case 19: the fundi at his second visit.

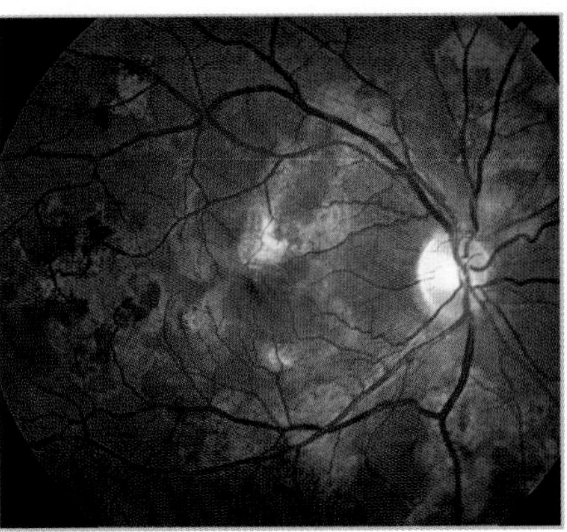
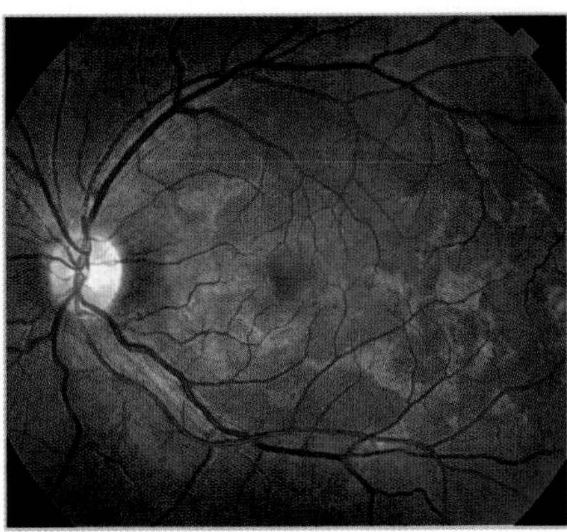

Figure 21.37 Case 19: the fundi after treatment.

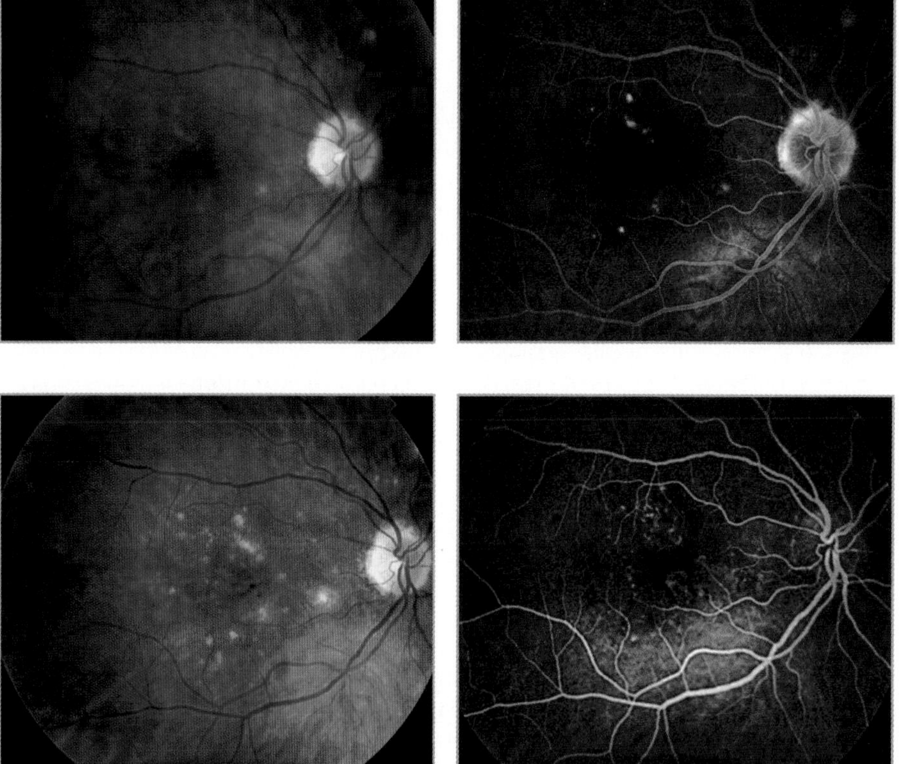

Figure 21.38 Case 20: the right fundus at presentation.

Figure 21.39 Case 20: the right fundus 1 month later.

a further probable membrane above. She therefore underwent intravitreal bevacizumab injection; within 1 month her vision had improved to 6/7.5 and an OCT scan confirmed a dry macula. However, 1 month after that an OCT showed recurrent shallow subretinal fluid. She underwent a second injection of bevacizumab. Four weeks later, although there was minor subretinal fibrosis, her VA improved to 6/6 and she was symptom free. She remains under regular review.

Index

Note: Page numbers in **bold** or *italic* refer to tables or figures, respectively.

U

V